Acid–Base Disorders and Their Treatment

Acid–Base Disorders and Their Treatment

Edited by

F. John Gennari
University of Vermont College of Medicine
Burlington, Vermont, U.S.A.

Horacio J. Adrogué
Baylor College of Medicine
Houston, Texas, U.S.A.

John H. Galla
University of Cincinnati College of Medicine
Cincinnati, Ohio, U.S.A.

Nicolaos E. Madias
Caritas St. Elizabeth's Medical Center
Tufts University School of Medicine
Boston, Massachusetts, U.S.A

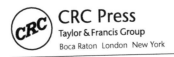
CRC Press
Taylor & Francis Group
Boca Raton London New York

CRC Press is an imprint of the
Taylor & Francis Group, an **informa** business
A TAYLOR & FRANCIS BOOK

CRC Press
Taylor & Francis Group
6000 Broken Sound Parkway NW, Suite 300
Boca Raton, FL 33487-2742

First issued in paperback 2019

© 2005 by Taylor & Francis Group, LLC
CRC Press is an imprint of Taylor & Francis Group, an Informa business

No claim to original U.S. Government works

ISBN-13: 978-0-8247-5915-5 (hbk)
ISBN-13: 978-0-367-39234-5 (pbk)

Library of Congress Cataloging-in-Publication Data

Catalog record is available from the Library of Congress

Visit the Taylor & Francis Web site at
http://www.taylorandfrancis.com

and the CRC Press Web site at
http://www.crcpress.com

Foreword

In the middle of the last century, acid–base and electrolyte metabolism was perceived by medical students and physicians as a muddled and hopelessly complex field with few important clinical implications. Though names of notable early researchers such as Darrow, Singer, Hastings, Gamble, Peters, Davenport, Henderson, and Hasselbalch were recognized by many, their observations were not easily translated into a transparent form of physiology, pathophysiology, and clinical action. The elegant studies of many investigators, especially William B. Schwartz (our intellectual mentor), Donald W. Seldin, and Arnold S. Relman in the decades thereafter, dramatically enhanced the fundamental understanding of acid–base processes in humans and changed how the information was used in emergency departments, intensive care units, and ordinary hospital rooms. By the late 1970s and early 1980s, the focus on hydrogen ion concentration and the use of the Henderson equation ($H^+ = 24 \times P_aCO_2/HCO_3^-$) made caring for most patients with acid–base disorders more or less routine. With major discoveries such as "confidence bands" delineating the normal whole body responses to a primary change in $PaCO_2$ or plasma bicarbonate concentration, the role of chloride, potassium, and volume in the development and correction of metabolic alkalosis, and the delineation of the various forms of metabolic acidosis, the acid–base mystery slowly evolved into the straightforward application of acid–base pathophysiology.

In the early 1980s, together with two of the editors of *Acid–Base Disorders* (Nicolaos E. Madias and F. John Gennari), we were the proud co-authors of *Acid–Base,* the first book devoted exclusively to the integration of basic acid–base physiology and explicit clinical applications. But the world of biological sciences has exploded again, and an extraordinary amount of information has accrued since, particularly at the cellular and molecular level. Acid–base retains its critical clinical importance because of two fundamental facts. First, characterization of the specific type of acid-base disorder can lead to appropriate therapy directly improving a patient's outcome, and second, careful and rigorous analysis of a complex acid-base disorder can provide critical clues to detect underlying diseases.

The current cadre of editors, Horacio J. Adrogué, F. John Gennari, Nicolaos E. Madias, and John H. Galla, has created a rich, comprehensive book with the aid of some 26 authors from around the USA, Canada, and Europe. *Acid–Base Disorders* will be the basis for further research and clinical applications and the new encyclopedia of acid-base.

Jordan J. Cohen, M.D.
President, Association of American Medical Colleges

John T. Harrington, M.D.
Professor of Medicine
Dean Emeritus, Tufts University School of Medicine

Jerome P. Kassirer, M.D.
Distinguished Professor, Tufts University School of Medicine
Editor-in-Chief Emeritus, *New England Journal of Medicine*

Preface

Over twenty years ago, two of us (Nicolaos E. Madias and F. John Gennari) were fortunate to contribute to writing a unique book, entitled *Acid–Base*. That book combined a comprehensive review of acid–base physiology and pathophysiology with straightforward clinical applications of the principles derived from this knowledge. Over the ensuing years, our knowledge of acid–base physiology and pathophysiology has changed dramatically, and it became clear that it was time for a new look at this subject. Hence the origin of *Acid–Base Disorders*.

As we looked at the breadth of this new body of knowledge, we saw that the task was larger than the four of us. To that end, we have recruited a select group of acid–base experts as contributors to the new book. Although now a multi-authored work, we have written many of the chapters ourselves, and have carefully edited the remaining chapters to avoid unnecessary redundancy and ensure a consistency of style throughout the book.

Our goal is to present the normal physiology of acid–base homeostasis as we know it in the early 21st century, and to review current information about the pathophysiology of acid–base disorders from both a molecular and an integrative perspective. Most important, *Acid–Base Disorders* continues the tradition of *Acid–Base* by bringing these new experimental observations to the bedside and providing straightforward guidelines for diagnosing and managing disturbances of acid–base homeostasis. A key feature of this new book is to link molecular and cellular information about epithelial transport in the kidney to observations in intact animals and humans in an effort to explain unanswered questions about acid–base physiology and pathophysiology.

The book is divided into seven sections. Section I encompasses normal chemistry and physiology. This section reviews the current state of our knowledge of acid–base chemistry, and includes a discussion of the Stewart approach to analyzing acid–base chemistry in terms of the independent and dependent variables. It reviews recent advances in the molecular biology of renal acid–base transporters, as well as animal and human studies of acid balance, and ends with a novel hypothesis concerning diet and acid–base balance (Chapter 8). Section II is devoted to a comprehensive view of metabolic acidosis, with separate chapters on all the major forms. The controversy concerning whether acid is retained in chronic kidney disease is discussed in Chapter 14. Section III covers metabolic alkalosis, and comes to grips with the roles of chloride, potassium, and extracellular fluid volume in the pathophysiology of this disorder. Section IV reviews our current knowledge of respiratory and mixed acid–base disorders, including the recently described "pseudorespiratory alkalosis" that occurs in patients with profound depression of cardiac function. Section V covers the unique nature of acid-balance and acid–base disorders in patients with end-stage renal disease receiving renal replacement therapy. Section VI is devoted to acid–base disorders in infants and children, and Section VII reviews the measurement techniques for diagnosing acid–base disorders, but its main focus is on providing clinical tools for diagnosis, and to demonstrate the use of these tools in diagnosing and managing patients with acid–base disorders using cases culled from our combined experience.

Our goal has been to produce a complete review of this broad topic, directed both to experts in the field, and also to the many clinicians who must deal with acid–base disorders in their daily practice. Our readers will judge whether our goal was accomplished.

F. John Gennari
Horacio J. Adrogué
John H. Galla
Nicolaos E. Madias

Contents

29. Illustrative Cases *817*
F. John Gennari, John H. Galla, Horacio J. Adrogué, and
Nicolaos E. Madias

Contributors

Horacio J. Adrogué Baylor College of Medicine, VA Medical Center, Houston, Texas, U.S.A.

Robert J. Alpern Yale University School of Medicine, New Haven, Connecticut, U.S.A.

Daniel Batlle Division of Nephrology, Northwestern University Feinberg School of Medicine, Chicago, Illinois, U.S.A.

Michel Baum University of Texas Southwestern Medical Center, Dallas, Texas, U.S.A.

Alan N. Charney NYU School of Medicine, Nephrology Section, VA Medical Center, New York, New York, U.S.A.

Mark Donowitz Hopkins Center for Epithelial Disorders, Johns Hopkins University School of Medicine, Baltimore, Maryland, U.S.A.

Michael Emmett Baylor University Medical Center, Dallas, Texas, U.S.A.

Lynda A. Frassetto Department of Medicine, University of California San Francisco, San Francisco, California, U.S.A.

John H. Galla Department of Medicine, University of Cincinnati College of Medicine, Cincinnati, Ohio, U.S.A.

F. John Gennari Department of Medicine, University of Vermont College of Medicine, Burlington, Vermont, U.S.A.

Mitchell L. Halperin Division of Nephrology, St. Michael's Hospital, University of Toronto, Toronto, Canada

L. Lee Hamm Section of Nephrology and Hypertension, Department of Medicine, Tulane University Health Sciences Center, New Orleans, Louisiana, U.S.A.

Virginia L. Hood University of Vermont College of Medicine, Burlington, Vermont, U.S.A.

Henry N. Hulter Genentech, Inc., South San Francisco, California, U.S.A.

Shahrokh Javaheri Department of Veterans Affairs Medical Center, University of Cincinnati College of Medicine, Cincinnati, Ohio, and Sleepcare Diagnostics, Mason, Ohio, U.S.A.

Reto Krapf Department of Medicine, Kantonsspital Bruderholz, Basel, Switzerland

Melvin Laski Departments of Internal Medicine and Physiology, Texas Tech University Health Sciences Center, Lubbock, Texas, U.S.A.

Robert G. Luke Department of Medicine, University of Cincinnati College of Medicine, Cincinnati, Ohio, U.S.A.

Nicolaos E. Madias Department of Medicine, Caritas St. Elizabeth's Medical Center, Tufts University School of Medicine, Boston, Massachusetts, U.S.A.

Renée L. Merriam Department of Medicine, University of California San Francisco, San Francisco, California, U.S.A.

Orson W. Moe University of Texas Southwestern Medical Center, Dallas, Texas, U.S.A.

K. M. L. S. T. Moorthi Division of Nephrology, Northwestern University Feinberg School of Medicine, Chicago, Illinois, U.S.A.

R. Curtis Morris, Jr. Department of Medicine, University of California San Francisco, San Francisco, California, U.S.A.

Man S. Oh Department of Medicine, State University of New York, Health Science Center at Brooklyn, Brooklyn, New York, U.S.A.

Asghar Rastegar   Department of Nephrology, Yale University School of Medicine, New Haven, Connecticut, U.S.A.

George J. Schwartz   Departments of Pediatrics and Medicine, University of Rochester School of Medicine, Rochester, New York, U.S.A.

Anthony Sebastian   Department of Medicine, University of California San Francisco, San Francisco, California, U.S.A.

Deborah E. Sellmeyer   Department of Medicine, University of California San Francisco, San Francisco, California, U.S.A.

Manoocher Soleimani   Division of Nephrology and Hypertension, University of Cincinnati College of Medicine, Cincinnati, Ohio, U.S.A.

Donald E. Wesson   Departments of Internal Medicine and Physiology, Texas Tech University Health Sciences Center, Lubbock, Texas, U.S.A.

Acid–Base Chemistry and Buffering

F. John Gennari

University of Vermont College of Medicine, Burlington, Vermont, U.S.A.

John H. Galla

Department of Medicine, University of Cincinnati College of Medicine, Cincinnati, Ohio, U.S.A.

INTRODUCTION

Acid–base biochemistry encompasses the physical chemistry of the constituents of biological solutions that influence the dissociation of, and therefore the concentration of, hydrogen ions (H^+) in those solutions. In the biological solutions that comprise the body fluids, these constituents include electrolytes that are essentially completely dissociated at the solute strength that exists in the body fluids, termed "strong ions" (1,2), a wide variety of weak acids and, most importantly, the volatile weak acid H_2CO_3 (carbonic acid). Central to an understanding of acid–base homeostasis is knowledge of the chemistry of weak acids and, in particular, carbonic acid. In this chapter, we review the physical chemistry that underlies acid–base homeostasis, incorporating the concepts of Brønsted and Lowry, who defined acids as H^+ donors and bases as H^+ acceptors (3,4). The additional role of strong ions, which are regulated independently of the dictates of acid–base homeostasis but influence $[H^+]$ is discussed at the end of this chapter.

Van Slyke (5) revolutionized our ability to approach and deal with the acid–base status of biological solutions, using the concepts of Brønsted and Lowry to focus on $[H^+]$ through evaluation of a single weak acid, H_2CO_3 (carbonic acid). Stewart (1,2) added the constraints of electroneutrality to the assessment of $[H^+]$ and separated the quantities that can be manipulated external to the solution, i.e., the concentrations of strong ions, buffer content, and PCO_2, from the quantities that are dependent on the nature of the solution, i.e., $[H^+]$ and $[HCO_3^-]$. Although Stewart's analysis provides a more complete description of all the events influencing $[H^+]$ in biological solutions, it is cumbersome to use in clinical medicine. Both approaches describe the state of the biological solution at the moment of analysis and are not mutually exclusive, neither provides any insight into regulatory processes. The mystery of how acid–base homeostasis is sensed and regulated remains unsolved and is discussed in later chapters in this book.

Central Role of H$^+$: The Brønsted/Lowry Formulation

A wide array of molecules contains hydrogen atoms that may dissociate in solution, yielding H^+. Once dissociated, these same molecules become sites for potential recombination with H^+. This cycle of dissociation and recombination led to the following definitions by Brønsted and Lowry (3,4). An acid is any molecular species that can function as a proton donor (i.e., that can dissociate an H^+). A base is a proton acceptor (i.e., a compound that can bind to and remove H^+ from solution). The anion remaining when an acid (HA) gives up H^+ is termed the conjugate base (A^-) of that acid, because it becomes a potential proton acceptor. These concepts are illustrated by the following formula:

$$\begin{array}{cc} Acid & Base \end{array}$$
$$HA \leftrightarrow A^- + H^+ \tag{1}$$

This simple formula provides the basis for measurement of acidity, that is, the amount of free H^+ released from HA at equilibrium in any given setting, and avoids the confusion that arose with other approaches to describing the acid–base status of the body fluids such as defining cations as bases and anions as acids (6,7). The relative ease with which a given molecule in a given milieu dissociates H^+ under equilibrium conditions is a measure of acid strength. In the mixture of weak acids that comprise biological fluids, the concentration of H^+ ($[H^+]$) is vanishingly small in comparison to HA and A^-, and its measurement requires the use of the pH electrode. The technique for measuring $[H^+]$ in biological solutions, and its nomenclature, is described below.

Units of Measurement: [H$^+$] and pH

The degree of acidity of a solution is a measure of the activity of H^+ in that solution. Because H^+ activity in chemical solutions can range so widely and because small changes have such a large impact on enzyme reactions, Sørensen (8) developed the pH unit to describe acidity and set the standards for its measurement. He defined pH as the negative logarithm of hydrogen ion concentration, $[H^+]$:

$$pH = -\log_{10}[H^+] \tag{2}$$

Because pH is a logarithm, it has no units. $[H^+]$ in this equation is expressed in mol or equivalents per liter.

Sørensen measured pH using an electrode that generates a voltage proportional to the difference in H^+ activity, α_{H^+}, rather than $[H^+]$, between a test solution and a standard solution. Unfortunately, his standard was based on a value for α_{H^+} corrected for ionic interaction that did not precisely reflect activity. A later correction was introduced, but in fact a precise definition of α_{H^+} is not possible with electrode technology (9). Thus, while pH is a highly accurate and reproducible measure of "acidity," it is not an exact measure of either α_{H^+} or $[H^+]$. These two entities are related as follows:

$$\alpha_{H^+} = \gamma_{H^+}[H^+] \tag{3}$$

In this equation, γ_{H^+} is the activity coefficient for H^+. The value for γ_{H^+} is directly related to the temperature and inversely related to the ionic strength of the solution (9). In biological solutions of interest to physiologists and clinicians, γ_{H^+} is close to 1.0 and varies only very slightly because temperature and ionic strength are both closely regulated. As a result (and because there is no completely precise measure of either), $[H^+]$ and α_{H^+} are used interchangeably in human acid–base analyses. Unless otherwise noted, $[H^+]$ will be used throughout this book instead of α_{H^+} when this measure rather than pH is used to denote acidity. Because of the very low concentrations found in biological fluids, $[H^+]$ is expressed in nanoequivalents per liter (nEq/L), rather than in equivalents or milliequivalents. To convert the measured pH to $[H^+]$ in nEq/L, the following formula is used:

$$[H^+] = 10^{(9-pH)} \tag{4}$$

The use of pH units to assess acidity is well established among chemists because it allows the wide range of $[H^+]$ encountered to be designated by a manageable numerical scale (pH 0–14). The range encountered in living biological systems is considerably narrower, however, and some acid–base experts have advocated using $[H^+]$ rather than pH to evaluate clinical acid–base problems (2,10). The relationship between pH and $[H^+]$ over the range of values of interest is shown in Fig. 1 and Table 1. This conversion has two main virtues. The first is to make manipulation of the Henderson–Hasselbalch equation (see later) simpler by removing logarithms, and the second is to call attention to the impact of changes in acidity on mass balance in any quantitative analysis (1). The two modes of assessing acidity are used interchangeably in this book.

Hydrogen Ion Activity in Water: Law of Mass Action

In his discussion of the milieu intérieur or "inner environment" of the body fluids, Claude Bernard (12) stated, "Water is the first indispensable

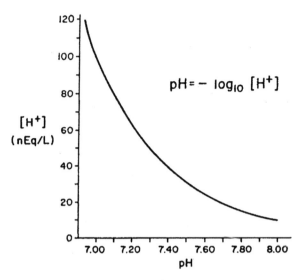

Figure 1   Relationship between pH and [H⁺] (in nEq/L) over a range of pH values of interest. *Source*: From Ref. 11.

condition of every vital manifestation . . . ." The properties of this remarkable molecule are therefore worthy of consideration. Because of its structure, water behaves as a dipole with a weak positive charge in the region of the hydrogen atoms and a weak negative charge in the region of the oxygen atom. This property of water causes substances whose atoms are kept together primarily by electrostatic bonds to dissociate into their

Table 1   Relationship Between H^+ and pH

H^+ (nEq/L) $= 10^{(9-\mathrm{pH})}$	
pH	H^+ (nEq/L)
7.80	16
7.70	20
7.60	25
7.50	32
7.40	40
7.30	50
7.20	63
7.10	80
7.00	100
6.90	126
6.80	159

component ions when they dissolve in it. In addition, this property of water causes it to dissociate slightly into H^+ and OH^-. Although this dissociation is minute, it can be measured with the pH electrode. Water dissociation follows the law of mass action. According to this principle, the cycle of dissociation and recombination is a continuous and reversible process:

$$HOH \leftrightarrow H^+ + OH^- \tag{5}$$

The H^+ in Eq. (5) actually combines with an undissociated HOH to produce a hydronium ion, H_3O^+, but by convention the symbol H^+ is used to designate hydrogen ions in solution (9). At any given moment, a particular molecule is either dissociated or recombined. The fraction of all such molecules in one or the other state is stable at equilibrium because the more molecules dissociate [movement to the right-hand side of Eq. (5)], the stronger the drive for recombination (movement to the left-hand side), and vice versa. At equilibrium, conditions are defined as follows:

$$[H^+] \times [OH^-]/[HOH] = K'_{HOH} \tag{6}$$

This equation states that at equilibrium the ratio of the concentration products of the opposing reactions is a predictable value (K'_{HOH}). K'_{HOH} is not a constant, but varies with temperature. Because the high concentration of undissociated water ($[HOH] = 55.5\,M$) varies negligibly in dilute solutions, the equation simplifies to

$$[H^+] \times [OH^-] = K'_{HOH} = 10^{-14} \tag{7}$$

The prime symbol indicates that concentrations rather than activities are used, and the concentration of HOH is included in the value of K. At $25°C$, K' is 10^{-14}. In pure water, $[H^+] = [OH^-]$ and therefore $[H^+]$ is equal to the square root of 10^{-14} or 10^{-7}. Thus, pH = 7.0, defined as neutrality. In body fluids, the pH optimum is 7.40 at $37°C$, defined by functionality rather than equivalence of $[H^+]$ and $[OH^-]$. The ability of water to dissolve ionic compounds reflects the development of electrostatic linkages between water molecules and the cations and anions of the solute. For example, when NaCl is placed in water, Cl^- bonds weakly with the positive pole and Na^+ bonds weakly with the negative pole of the water molecule.

The Concept of Acid Strength

The dissociation of acids in solution follows the same law of mass action described earlier for water, and at equilibrium the following formula applies:

$$[H^+] \times [A^-]/[HA] = K'_A \tag{8}$$

In this equation, $[A^-]$ is the concentration of the dissociated anion of the acid in question, and $[HA]$ is the concentration of the undissociated acid. Each acid has a unique value for K_A'. Because concentrations rather than activities are used to calculate K_A', the value for K_A' varies with temperature, ionic strength, and to a small degree with pH as well (see later under carbonic acid). In all subsequent equations, K' is used to denote K_A' for ease of notation. Rearranging Eq. (8), we can highlight the determinants of $[H^+]$ in a solution containing HA:

$$[H^+] = K' \times [HA]/[A^-] \qquad (9)$$

This equation, developed by Henderson (13) in 1907 and named for him, indicates that $[H^+]$ is determined by the equilibrium dissociation constant of HA multiplied by the ratio of the concentrations of the undissociated acid and its conjugate base. When expressed in pH units, this equation (Hasselbalch's modification (14), now termed the Henderson–Hasselbalch equation) takes the form

$$pH = pK' + \log_{10}([A^-]/[HA]) \qquad (10)$$

In this equation, $pK' = -\log K'$. The dissociation constant (K' or pK') of a given acid at standard conditions is a measure of its strength because it connotes the ease with which H^+ is released from the undissociated acid. The tenacity of H^+ binding varies greatly among acid–base pairs. Strong acids, such as hydrochloric and sulfuric acid, dissociate freely when placed in solution because their conjugate bases have virtually no affinity for H^+. For strong acids, the equilibrium concentration of the undissociated acid ($[HA]$) is negligible and $[H^+]$ is high. As a result, K' is high and pK' is low. Most organic acids dissociate only partially and are less strong. For example, acetic acid only dissociates about 1% at equilibrium in solution at 25°C (i.e., 99% exists in the form CH_3OOH and only 1% exists as CH_3OO^-). These acids have a much lower K' and higher pK'.

BUFFERING

When a weak acid is placed in solution, it dissociates only partially and both the undissociated acid and its conjugate base are present. Such solutions have the ability to resist a change in acidity following the addition of another acid or base. This property is termed buffering and the acid–conjugate base pairs are termed buffers. In essence, buffered solutions act like bases with regard to added acids and like acids with respect to added bases. When a strong acid is added to a solution containing a buffer, some of the added H^+ combines with the base form of the buffer (increasing the acid form) rather than remaining free in solution. Thus, the increase in $[H^+]$ (or decrease in pH) is less than would have occurred in the absence of the buffer. Similarly, addition of a strong base to a buffered solution limits the decrease in [H$^+$] (or increase in pH) that would otherwise occur.

Buffering can be illustrated by considering the change in [H$^+$] that occurs when 10 mmol of HCl is added to 1 L of water. This strong acid is virtually completely dissociated, changing [H$^+$] in the solution from 100 nEq/L (pH = 7.00, pure water) to 10,000,000 nEq/L (pH = 2.00). The same amount of HCl added to a solution containing 30 mmol of the buffer sodium phosphate at the same starting pH (7.00), however, has a much smaller effect on [H$^+$], as demonstrated by the following calculation. The K' of the $H_2PO_4^-/HPO_4^{2-}$ buffer pair is 160 nEq/L (p$K' = 6.8$), and thus the initial ratio of its two components at a pH of 7.00 ([H$^+$] = 100 nEq/L) is

$$[H^+] = 160 \times ([H_2PO_4^-]/[HPO_4^{2-}]) \tag{11}$$

Transposing:

$$[H_2PO_4^-]/[HPO_4^{2-}] = [H^+]/160 = 100/160 = 5/8 \tag{12}$$

Thus, of the total phosphate concentration (30 mM), 5/13 (11.5 mM) is $H_2PO_4^-$ and 8/13 (18.5 mM) is HPO_4^{2-}. When the 10 mmol of HCl is added to this solution, virtually all the free H$^+$ binds immediately to the conjugate base, HPO_4^{2-} forming its conjugate acid, $H_2PO_4^-$. As a result, [$H_2PO_4^-$] increases from 11.5 to 21.5 mM, and the concentration of HPO_4^{2-} decreases from 18.5 to 8.5 mM. At this new equilibrium,

$$[H^+] = 160 \times 21.5/8.5 = 405 \text{ nEq/L (pH} = 6.39) \tag{13}$$

Thus, adding 10 mmol/L of HCl to this buffered solution increases [H$^+$] by only 305 nEq/L, as compared to the increase of 9,999,900 nEq/L in water. With continued addition of either a strong acid or base to a solution, the corresponding weak acid or base eventually becomes saturated. In the example above, this happens when all available base (HPO_4^{2-}) combines with the added H$^+$ to form the acid, $H_2PO_4^-$. When this occurs, all further added H$^+$ will remain in solution, rapidly lowering the pH until $H_2PO_4^-$ becomes a proton acceptor (pH < 3.0). This behavior leads to the typical sigmoid titration curves in Fig. 2.

Quantitation of Buffer Effect on Acidity

Figure 2 depicts the titration curves of three buffers: acetic acid/acetate, uric acid/monourate, and monobasic phosphate/dibasic phosphate. The midpoint of each of the curves denotes the setting in which the concentrations of the acid and its conjugate base are equal. From Eqs. (9) and (10), one can see that when these concentrations are equal, [H$^+$] = K' or pH = pK'. As illustrated in Fig. 2, the buffering ability or capacity is also the greatest when pH = pK'.

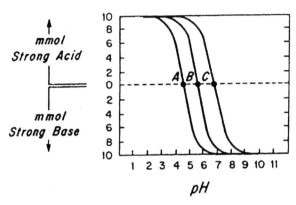

Figure 2 Titration curves of three buffer systems (**A**) Acetic acid/acetate, (**B**) Uric acid/monourate, (**C**) Monobasic/dibasic phosphate). In each case, 1 L of a 20 mM solution is titrated with strong acid and strong base. The midpoint of each titration curve corresponds to the pK' of the system (4.6, 5.6, and 6.8, respectively). *Source*: From Ref. 11.

The capacity of a specific buffer to resist a change in pH is defined as its buffer value (β), the first derivative of the titration curve:

$$\beta = d(\text{acid or base})/d\text{pH} \tag{14}$$

Buffer value is conventionally expressed as mol/L or mmol/L of strong acid or base added per unit change in pH. Given the curves in Figure 2, it is apparent that β varies with pH and reaches a maximum when pH $= pK'$. This unit of measure has been named the slyke, in honor of Donald D. Van Slyke (15), a pioneer in the study of acids and bases in biological fluids. In a seminal paper, he deduced that β is a function of the concentration of the weak acid in a solution (C), the K' (or pK') of the buffer, and the prevailing $[H^+]$ (16). He also showed that for any weak acid, the maximal value for β (i.e., when $[H^+] = K'$ or pH $= pK'$) is 0.575. Thus, if one added HCl to the 30 mM phosphate solution discussed earlier at a starting pH of 6.8 (the pK' for $H_2PO_4^-/HPO_4^{2-}$), 0.575 × 30 or 17.25 mmol of HCl would be required to lower pH by 1 unit, to 5.8.

Complex Solutions Containing Multiple Buffers

The buffer value of a solution containing more than one buffer is equal to the additive effects of all buffers in the solution. In solutions containing multiple buffers with pK' values that are reasonably close to one another, or one that contains a complex buffer with multiple dissociation constants (e.g., hemoglobin), the titration curve may approach linearity over the range of pH values of interest. In this setting, β can be approximated by a single value (see later). Blood, extracellular and intracellular fluids are examples of such complex solutions. In the extracellular compartment, the principal buffers are carbonic acid, phosphate, and proteins. Hemoglobin, although located within red cells, is considered by convention as one of the proteins contributing to extracellular buffering. The intracellular compartment is more complex (see Chapter 2), comprised of multiple subcompartments containing different proteins, and both inorganic and organic phosphates. Carbonic acid is also an important intracellular buffer.

Isohydric Principle

Although most biological solutions contain a variety of simple and complex buffers, such solutions have only a single value for $[H^+]$ at any given time if they are well mixed and homogeneous. It follows from Eq. (9) above that

$$[H^+] = K_1'[HA_1]/[A_1] = K_2'[HA_2]/[A_2] = K_3'[HA_3]/[A_3] = K_n'[HA_n]/[A_n]$$

$$(15)$$

In such a complex solution, the equilibrium value for $[H^+]$ is determined by the composite effect of the concentrations of the buffer pairs and their respective dissociation constants. The beauty of this formulation is that one can quickly and easily determine the value for $[H^+]$ in a given solution from a knowledge of the K' and concentrations of just one acid and its conjugate base in the system. Thus, regardless of the complexity of the solution evaluated, the Brønsted/Lowry approach provides a powerful means for analysis of its acid–base status by focusing on a single buffer. The buffer system most commonly used for this analysis in biological fluids is carbonic acid/bicarbonate. It should be emphasized, however, that any buffer pair would serve the purpose. The features of carbonic acid that make it such a powerful buffer are discussed below.

Carbonic Acid/Bicarbonate Buffer System

Carbon dioxide is the end product of oxidative metabolism and is therefore ubiquitous in biological systems. In addition, it freely equilibrates between the intracellular and extracellular compartments. Carbon dioxide is highly soluble in water and behaves as a weak acid in solution because a small fraction of dissolved CO_2 interacts with water forming HCO_3^- and H^+, and these ions rapidly combine to form carbonic acid (H_2CO_3). Central to acid–base physiology is an understanding of the relationships among CO_2, H_2CO_3, and HCO_3^-.

CO₂ Solubility

The concentration of CO_2 in solution is directly proportional to the partial pressure of CO_2 in the gas phase in equilibrium with the solution, a relationship known as Henry's law:

$$[CO_{2\ dis}] = \alpha PCO_2 \tag{16}$$

In this equation, $[CO_{2\ dis}]$ is expressed in mmol/L and PCO_2 in mmHg. The proportionality constant α is the solubility coefficient for CO_2. The value of α decreases with increasing temperature (i.e., the hotter the solution, the less CO_2 dissolved for any given PCO_2) and with increasing ionic strength (i.e., the more concentrated the solution, the less CO_2 dissolved for any given PCO_2). In plasma at 37°C, $\alpha = 0.0308$ mmol/L/mmHg (17–19). Thus, for either arterial or venous blood:

$$[CO_{2\ dis}] = 0.0308 \times PCO_2 \tag{17}$$

At a normal PCO_2 in arterial blood (40 mmHg), $[CO_{2\ dis}] = 1.2$ mmol/L.

Hydration of Dissolved CO_2

As mentioned above, a small fraction of dissolved CO_2 combines with water forming the weak acid, H_2CO_3:

$$CO_{2\ dis} + H_2O \leftrightarrow H_2CO_3 \tag{18}$$

This relationship indicates the end products of this reversible reaction, but not a key intermediate step. This step is the reaction of $CO_{2\ dis}$ with OH^-, yielding HCO_3^-. It is catalyzed by carbonic anhydrase in most cells in the body assuring equilibration within a few milliseconds (20–22):

$$\overset{carbonic\ anhydrase}{H^+ + OH^- + CO_{2\ dis} \leftrightarrow HCO_3^- + H^+ \leftrightarrow H_2CO_3} \tag{19}$$

Although the catalytic effects of carbonic anhydrase are critical for human biology, it is noteworthy that even in the absence of this enzyme, equilibrium is probably reached in less than 1 min (21–23). Equilibrium relationships can be evaluated for any part of this reaction. The equilibrium conditions for the end products tell us about the relationship between $CO_{2\ dis}$ and H_2CO_3:

$$K' = [H_2CO_3]/[CO_{2\ dis}] \tag{20}$$

At 37°C, $K' = 0.0029$, indicating that each molecule of H_2CO_3 is in equilibrium with approximately 340 molecules of dissolved CO_2 (23,24). Because $[H_2CO_3]$ is difficult to measure directly and its concentration is so small compared to dissolved CO_2, the two species are incorporated in the variable, $[CO_{2 \text{ dis}}]$. As shown in Eq. (17), the latter variable is simple to calculate from the measured PCO_2.

Equilibrium Relationships for Bicarbonate/Carbonic Acid

Carbonic acid is a weak acid, and therefore at equilibrium

$$K' = [H^+] \times [HCO_3^-]/[H_2CO_3] \tag{21}$$

The value for K' in this equation is 0.27 mmol/L ($pK' = 3.57$) at 37°C (22–24). Because H_2CO_3 is difficult to measure and is directly related to $[CO_{2 \text{ dis}}]$ ($[H_2CO_3] = 0.0029 \times [CO_{2 \text{ dis}}]$, see above), a more convenient way to measure and assess the equilibrium conditions is to substitute $[CO_{2 \text{ dis}}]$ for $[H_2CO_3]$ in Eq. (21), as follows:

$$K_a' = [H^+] \times [HCO_3^-]/[CO_{2 \text{ dis}}] \tag{22}$$

In this equation, K_a' signifies the *apparent* dissociation constant for the HCO_3^-/H_2CO_3 system, "apparent" because the denominator is no longer an acid, but a species directly proportional to an acid. If one substitutes αPCO_2 for $[CO_{2 \text{ dis}}]$ in this Eq. (27), one obtains a practical tool for assessing acid–base status. In the Henderson format [see Eq. (9)], the new relationship is

$$[H^+] = K_a' \times \alpha PCO_2/[HCO_3^-] \tag{23}$$

Recast in terms of pH, this becomes the Henderson–Hasselbalch equation:

$$PH = pK_a' + \log_{10}[HCO_3^-]/\alpha PCO_2 \tag{24}$$

The numerical value for pK_a' (or K_a') varies with temperature, ionic strength and pH (19). The effect of pH is minimal, varying the value for pK_a' from only 6.11 at pH 7.00 to 6.09 at pH 7.60 at a temperature of 37°C (Table 2). In a similar fashion, over a range of temperatures compatible with life, the effect on pK_a' is small. Thus, by convention, the value of pK_a' is taken as 6.10 (the value at 7.40 and 37°C, at the ionic strength of normal plasma). The corresponding value for K_a' is 794 nmol/L.

In clinical practice, the working form of the Henderson equation (23) is

$$[H^+] = 23.8 \times PCO_2/[HCO_3^-] \tag{25}$$

In this equation, K_a' (794 nM) and α (0.03) have been combined, yielding 23.8. For ease of computation in clinical practice, this number is rounded to 24 or, in some instances, to 25 (26,27).

Table 2   Effects of Temperature and pH on the Apparent Dissociation Constant of
the Carbonic Acid–Bicarbonate System (pK_a') in Human Serum

Temperature (°C)	Serum pH			
	7.00	7.20	7.40	7.60
25	6.173	6.139	6.129	6.116
30	6.148	6.139	6.129	6.116
35	6.124	6.117	6.108	6.097
36	6.119	6.112	6.104	6.093
37	6.114	6.108	6.099	6.089
38	6.109	6.103	6.095	6.085
39	6.104	6.099	6.090	6.081
40	6.099	6.094	6.086	6.077

Source: From Ref. 25.

Is the pK_a' OK?

As indicated above, pK_a' is not a constant but is affected by temperature and
ionic strength, and to a minor degree by pH. This uncertainty is one of the
arguments for evaluating the effects of strong ions on the relationship (28).
Measurements of pK_a' in acutely ill patients have been reported to yield
values more divergent from 6.10 than can be accounted for by known effects
on this variable (29,30). These observations have led some investigators to
conclude that nonequilibrium conditions may prevail in the acute care
setting, invalidating the Henderson–Hasselbalch relationship (29–31). Evaluation of these observations, however, indicates that measurement errors
rather than nonequilibrium conditions can account for the results (32). This
conclusion is buttressed by two careful studies in acutely ill patients, in
which no such divergence can be found (33,34). In addition, nonequilibrium
conditions are virtually impossible given that the time to reach equilibrium
is measured in seconds even in the absence of carbonic anhydrase (21–23).
Using a pK_a' value of 6.10 (or a K_a' of 794 nM) is more than sufficiently
precise for evaluating acid–base status in clinical practice and, with the
minor corrections shown in Table 2, for research studies as well.

Role of the $CO_2/H_2CO_3/HCO_3^-$ Buffer System in the
Regulation of Acidity

The volatile nature of H_2CO_3 makes it a powerful buffer, even though its
dissociation constant ($pK_a' = 6.1$) is far from pH values compatible with life.
Because of its volatility, H_2CO_3 does not accumulate when a strong acid is
added and combines with HCO_3^-. As a result, the reduction in pH that
would otherwise occur is minimized. This effect is illustrated in Fig. 3, in

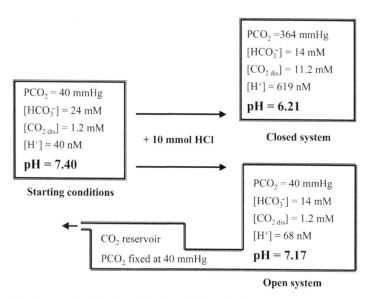

Figure 3 Change in pH induced by the addition of acid to a solution containing the carbonic acid/bicarbonate buffer pair (starting conditions), in a closed system (*above*) and in an open system (*below*). In the closed system, the total quantity of buffer (acid plus base components) remains constant. In the open system, PCO_2 (and thus [dissolved CO_2]) is maintained at a fixed level by continuous equilibration of the liquid phase with a gas reservoir at a constant PCO_2 of 40 mmHg.

which a solution containing HCO_3^- at a concentration of 24 mEq/L is equilibrated with a PCO_2 of 40 mmHg at 37°C. In this solution, $[CO_{2\ dis}] = 1.2$ mM $(0.0308 \times PCO_2)$ and pH is 7.40 $([H^+] = 40$ nEq/L). If 10 mmol of HCl is added to a liter of this solution, the 10 mEq of H^+ dissociated from this strong acid will immediately combine with HCO_3^-, forming H_2CO_3 and reducing $[HCO_3^-]$ from 24 to 14 mEq/L. This reaction will increase $[H_2CO_3]$ and therefore $[CO_{2\ dis}]$ from 1.2 to 11.2 mM. Given the relationship between H_2CO_3 and CO_2 [see Eq. (17)], however, such an increase could only occur if the partial pressure of CO_2 rose to 364 mmHg! If the solution was in a sealed chamber and such a high PCO_2 could be sustained, the pH in the system would fall to 6.21, a value obviously incompatible with life. If, however, the same solution is equilibrated continuously with a reservoir set at a PCO_2 of 40 mmHg, then the newly formed CO_2 will escape from the system, $[CO_{2\ dis}]$ would remain at 1.2 mM, and pH would drop only to 7.17. In humans, the PCO_2 reservoir, of course, is not fixed at 40 mmHg, but is variable and regulated in its own right (see Chapter 3). As a result, $[CO_{2\ dis}]$ and therefore $[H_2CO_3]$ actually decrease (as a result of hyperventilation) when a strong acid is added to the body fluids, minimizing the fall in pH even further. The ubiquitous, abundant, and variable amounts of CO_2 and

HCO$_3^-$ make this buffer pair unique and central to the maintenance of a stable pH in our body fluids.

Nonbicarbonate Buffers

Although many organic and inorganic constituents in the body fluids function as buffers, proteins (particularly hemoglobin) are quantitatively the most important, after the CO$_2$/HCO$_3^-$ buffer pair.

Proteins

Proteins are complex buffers, containing a number of dissociable groups and, as a result, their titration curves approach a straight-line function over the range of pH values of interest to physiologists (Fig. 4). Thus, buffer capacity (β, see earlier discussion) can be considered to be constant at a single value (17,35–37). Most of the buffer capacity of proteins resides in the imidazole group of histidine (Fig. 5). The pK' of this moiety ranges between 5.0 and 8.0 in various proteins, because of variations in the effect of local electrostatic forces due to differences in protein structure (38). A lesser contribution is provided by the dissociable N-terminal α-amino groups, which have operational pK' values of 7.4–7.9. Other dissociable groups play no significant role in buffering because their pK' values are well beyond the physiological range of pH (Table 3).

The behavior of the dissociable groups on a protein in relation to changes in pH defines the net charge of that protein for any given pH.

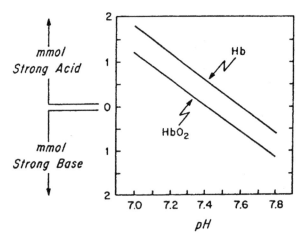

Figure 4   Idealized titration curves of 1 mM oxyhemoglobin (HbO$_2$) and 1 mM reduced hemoglobin (Hb). *Source:* From Ref. 11.

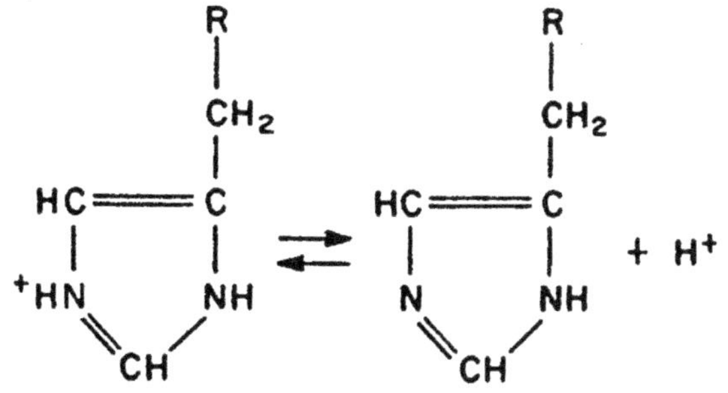

Figure 5 Reversible dissociation of the imidazole group of histidine. *Source*: From Ref. 11.

Titration with acid reduces the net negative charge, as anionic groups bind to H^+, and alkali titration conversely increases net negative charge as anions are created by the release of H^+. The pH at which there is no net charge is termed the isoelectric point and is unique for each protein. If the isoelectric point is at a pH lower (more acid) than the physiological level, then the protein exists in vivo as a polyanion. If the isoelectric point is more alkaline, then the protein is a polycation in vivo. The dominant proteins in plasma exist as polyanions, contributing to the anion gap (see Chapter 28) (36–38).

Extracellular Nonbicarbonate Buffers

Plasma Proteins

The buffer value (β) of the composite mixture of plasma proteins is approximately 0.1 mmol/g/pH (17,36,37). From this value and normal protein concentration (70 g/L), one can calculate that their contribution to buffer-

Table 3 Intrinsic pK' Values for Dissociable Groups of Various Body Proteins

Dissociable groups (amino acid)	pK'
α-carboxyl	3.6–3.8
β-carboxyl (aspartic acid)	~4.0
γ-carboxyl (glutamic acid)	~4.0
Imidazole (histidine)	6.4–7.0
α-amino	7.4–7.9
Sulfhydryl (cysteine)	~9.0
ε-amino (lysine)	9.8–10.6
Phenolic (tyrosine)	8.5–10.9
Guanidino (arginine)	11.9–13.3

Source: From Ref. 39.

ing is 7 slykes, a low value compared to the 55 slykes contributed by the CO_2/HCO_3^- buffer system. In whole blood (55% plasma), β for plasma proteins is only $\sim 1/6$ that of hemoglobin (see later). With rare exception, plasma proteins have isoelectric points well below the pH of the body fluids and thus exist as polyanions. At a normal pH, the net negative charge of these proteins (primarily albumin) is $\sim 12\,mEq/L$ (36,37). Albumin is the major buffer protein in plasma, containing 16 histidine residues per molecule (36,37). Globulins contribute little if at all to buffering (38).

Hemoglobin

Although it resides within red cells, hemoglobin is regarded as an extracellular buffer because historically extracellular buffering was studied by titrating whole blood (40). Hemoglobin is the preeminent nonbicarbonate buffer in the extracellular compartment defined in this manner, due both to its high concentration and high buffer value. Hemoglobin is a unique protein in that its isoelectric point is shifted to a more alkaline pH (from 6.65 to 6.80) when it releases O_2 (Fig. 4). This rightward shift indicates that some dissociable groups have increased affinity for H^+, that is, they behave as weaker acids when the molecule releases O_2 (35,41). This change in H^+ affinity, termed the Bohr effect, is an adaptation that allows the molecule to facilitate the movement of CO_2 from tissues to the lungs with a smaller change in pH than would otherwise occur. In addition, the buffer value of reduced hemoglobin is slightly greater than oxygenated hemoglobin. The titration curves of both reduced and oxygenated hemoglobin approach a straight line over the range of pH values of interest. The buffer value of either form of hemoglobin is approximately 3 slykes (15,41). Expressed per gram of hemoglobin, β is $0.18\,mmol/g/pH$ unit. At a normal concentration in whole blood of $150\,g/L$, hemoglobin contribute 27 slykes to buffer capacity (15). Its buffering power can be attributed almost exclusively to the nine histidine residues in each of its four peptide chains. An additional small contribution is made by the four terminal α-amino groups on the molecule (15).

Inorganic Phosphate

Inorganic phosphate compounds are present in the extracellular fluid and have three dissociable hydrogen ions. Phosphoric acid (H_3PO_4) is a relatively strong acid ($pK' = 2.0$) and, as such, does not exist in the body. Monobasic phosphate ($H_2PO_4^-$) has a pK' value of 6.8 and as a result is a very effective buffer (with its conjugate base, dibasic phosphate, HPO_4^{2-}). At a pH of 7.4, 80% of phosphate is present as the base, HPO_4^{2-}, and 20% as the acid, $H_2PO_4^-$. Nonetheless, phosphate contributes only a small amount to overall buffering in the extracellular fluid because of its low concentration. Phosphates are present in the urine in much higher concentration, and this buffer pair contributes importantly to buffering excreted acid (see Chapter 6). The third species, tribasic phosphate (PO_4^{3-}) is the conjugate base for HPO_4^{2-} ($pK' = 12.4$), and also does not exist in the body fluids.

Intracellular Nonbicarbonate Buffers

The buffer characteristics and regulation of intracellular $[H^+]$ are discussed in Chapter 2. Below is a description of contribution of cell proteins and organic phosphates to cell buffering.

Proteins

A wide variety of proteins in cells contain histidine residues and thus contribute to intracellular buffering. One can calculate from the histidine content of striated muscle homogenates, for example, that at least 57% of the aggregate buffer value of nonbicarbonate buffers in this tissue is accounted for by proteins and by the low-molecular-weight peptides carnosine and anserine.

Organic Phosphates

Organic phosphates are a heterogeneous group of compounds composed principally of 2,3-diphosphoglycerate (2,3-DPG), glucose-1-phosphate, and various nucleotide phosphates such as adenosine mono-, di-, and triphosphate (AMP, ADP, and ATP, respectively). The phosphate moiety in each of these compounds functions as a buffer, in a similar fashion as described above for the inorganic phosphates in the extracellular fluid (see earlier). The H^+ affinity of the base component, however, varies to some degree because of local electrostatic influences and, as a result, pK' values range from 6.0 to 9.0 (42,43). Organic phosphates are abundant in cells and are important contributors to their buffering capacity.

THE ROLE OF STRONG IONS

Stewart (1,2) has advanced a more comprehensive analysis of acid–base biochemistry by adding the constraints of electroneutrality to the assessment of $[H^+]$. His analysis adds evaluation of the strong ions in solution to the chemistry discussed earlier in this chapter. Most biological solutions contain an array of electrolytes that for all practical purposes dissociate completely, including Na^+, K^+, Ca^{2+}, Cl^-, and SO_4^{2-}, which are termed strong ions. A few important organic anions of sufficiently strong acids (e.g., lactate) have pK' values sufficiently lower than the pH of the body fluids and also behave as strong ions. As with $[H^+]$, the activities of these strong ions vary with temperature and concentration. With the exception of Na^+ and Cl^-, the concentrations of all other strong ions are low.

A second and important feature of Stewart's (1,2) approach is that he differentiates the quantities that are independent variables in biological fluids (strong ions, PCO_2, and total concentration of weak acids) from the quantities that are determined by the nature of the solution, i.e., $[H^+]$ and $[HCO_3^-]$. This approach emphasizes the fact that $[H^+]$ and $[HCO_3^-]$ are dependent variables, a concept not apparent from evaluation of the Henderson or Henderson–Hasselbalch equation.

To begin an analysis of a given solution in terms using Stewart's approach, consider the addition of only Na^+ and Cl^- to water. First, electroneutrality must be satisfied:

$$([Na^+] + [H^+]) - ([Cl^-] + [OH^-]) = 0 \qquad (26)$$

Solved simultaneously with the equation for the dissociation of water [Eq. (6)], which always must be satisfied, yields

$$[H^+]^2 + ([Na^+] - [Cl^-]) \times [H^+] - K'_{HOH} = 0 \qquad (27)$$

Rearranged in quadratic form and solved for $[H^+]$, Eq. (27) yields the following expression:

$$[H^+] = \sqrt{K'_{HOH} + ([Na^+] - [Cl^-])^2/4} - ([Na^+]-[Cl^-])/2 \qquad (28)$$

In this equation, $[H^+]$ is a dependent variable and a function of the difference between the charges of the strong electrolytes and K'_{HOH}, both *independent* variables. Note that in this example $[Na^+]=[Cl^-]$, because only salt was added.

If a mixture of unequal amounts of HCl and NaOH are added instead of NaCl, the resulting difference between $[Na^+]$ and $[Cl^-]$, termed the strong ion difference (SID), would become the dominant determinant of $[H^+]$ because SID is orders of magnitude greater than K'_{HOH}. For substances that behave as strong ions, SID equals the sum of all the strong cations minus the sum of all the strong anions in the solution, and is the single most important determinant of $[H^+]$ or $[OH^-]$ in solution, regardless of how these concentrations have been brought about. The essential feature of SID is the difference in charge and *not* the ion species. For example, if Ca^{2+} and SO_4^{2-} are added to the solution of NaCl, SID is expressed as

$$([Na^+] + [Ca^{2+}]) - ([Cl^-] + [SO_4^{2-}]) = SID \qquad (29)$$

In solutions with a positive SID such as in various body fluids, $[H^+]$ is small and $[OH^-]$ predominates. For example, Eq. (26) can be rearranged to solve for $[OH^-]$:

$$([Na^+] - [Cl^-]) + [H^+] = [OH^-] \qquad (30)$$

Because Eq. (6) must always be satisfied, if $[Na^+]=140\,mEq/L$ and $[Cl^-]=100\,mEq/L$, $SID=40\,mEq/L$. Under these conditions, $[OH^-]=$ $\sim 40\,mEq/L$ and $[H^+]$ is $1 \times 10^{-9}\,mEq/L$ [calculated from Eq. (6)].

Whether the SID is positive or negative, electroneutrality must be preserved; in Eq. (30), the difference between $[H^+]$ and $[OH^-]$ is equal to SID. Substituting SID for $([Na^+] - [Cl^-])$ in Eq. (28) yields

$$[H^+] = \sqrt{K'_{HOH} + ([SID]/2)^2} - [SID]/2 \qquad (31)$$

Table 4 illustrates the effect of SID depending on the initial pH and SID of the solution. In this illustration, 2 mEq of HCl is added to a liter of solution at three different initial SID values. Although the added H^+ and Cl^- are completely dissociated, equal changes in strong ions (Cl^- in this instance) evoke markedly different changes in $[H^+]$ depending on the initial or ambient $[H^+]$ of the solution.

In a strongly alkaline solution (pH $\sim$ 12), addition of 2 mEq HCl has a trivial effect on $[H^+]$ whereas, in a strongly acidic solution (pH $\sim$ 1.5), $[H^+]$ increases mole for mole. The reason is that, in alkaline solutions, H^+ reacts with OH^- to form H_2O while the added Cl^- remains as an anion. In the acidic solution, H^+ does not react with OH^- because virtually none is present and each mEq of H^+ added remains a proton while Cl^- remains as an anion. The effect of 2 mEq HCl at initial pH 10.5 is intermediate as it passes through the neutral point for water (pH 7.00). The effect of this titration on pH is much more difficult to visualize. In contrast to the change in $[H^+]$, the effect of the 2 mEq of HCl on pH is most dramatic at the neutral point for water and is numerically similar at both high and low initial pH's. This difference, of course, is because pH is a logarithmic function that obscures the effect of HCl on $[H^+]$.

Thus far, this analysis has dealt with solutions that do not contain the CO_2/HCO_3^- buffer pair. In such solutions, $[HCO_3^-]$ and $[CO_3^{2-}]$ as well as $[OH^-]$ are considered as dependent variables and analysis is more complex, although the same principles hold. Such solutions are discussed below.

Quantitative Analysis of All Plasma Constituents

Stewart's analysis focuses on the dependent nature of $[H^+]$ and $[HCO_3^-]$, a fact not emphasized in the Brønsted/Lowry approach. He considers the

Table 4 The Effect of a 2 mEq/L Change in SID,[a] Induced by the Addition of HCl, on pH and $[H^+]$ in a Solution at Three Different Initial SID Values

SID (mEq/L)			pH			$[H^+]$ (Eq/L)		
Initial	Final	Δ	Initial	Final	Δ	Initial	Final	Δ
41	39	−2	11.97	11.95	−0.02	1.07×10^{-12}	1.13×10^{-12}	$+5.5 \times 10^{-14}$
1	−1	−2	10.36	3.00	−7.36	4.40×10^{-11}	1.0×10^{-3}	$+1.0 \times 10^{-3}$
−39	−41	−2	1.41	1.39	−0.02	3.90×10^{-2}	4.1×10^{-3}	$+2.0 \times 10^{-3}$

[a]SID, strong ion difference (see text for definition).

concentrations of strong ions, buffers, and PCO_2, all of which are regulated separately by organ transport, metabolism, or the central nervous system, as the independent variables for acid–base base evaluation of plasma. Buffers (with the exception of the CO_2/HCO_3^- buffer pair) are the second variable considered here and include the total concentration of plasma buffers, C. The plasma buffers are nearly all proteins (primarily albumin), the concentration of which is reasonably stable. Thus the total amount, $[C]$, described by the conservation of mass is

$$[HA] + [A^-] = [C] \tag{32}$$

The third variable, PCO_2, determines the concentration of HCO_3^- and CO_3^{2-}.

In the final analysis, there are six unknowns ($[H^+]$, $[OH^-]$, $[HA]$, $[A^-]$, $[HCO_3^-]$, and $[CO_3^{2-}]$), and therefore six equations that must be satisfied to solve for $[H^+]$. These are: (1) water dissociation [Eq. (6)], (2) electroneutrality, for which the SID is included ($[SID] + [H^+] - [HCO_3^-] - [A^-] - [CO_3^{2-}] - [OH^-] = 0$), (3) the total weak acid dissociation equilibrium [Eq. (8)], (4) the conservation of mass for the total weak acid [Eq. (32)], (5) HCO_3^-/CO_2 equilibrium [Eq. (23)], and (6) CO_3^{2-}/HCO_3^- equilibrium ($K_3' = [H^+] \times [CO_3^{2-}]/[HCO_3^-]$). When solved simultaneously, they yield a fourth-order equation:

$$[H^+]^4 + ([SID] + K_A') \times [H^+]^3 + (K_A' \times ([SID] - [C]) - K_{HOH}'$$
$$- K_A' \times PCO_2) \times [H^+]^2 - (K_A' \times (K_{HOH}' + K_A' \times PCO_2)$$
$$- K_3' \times K_A' \times PCO_2) \times [H^+] - K_A' \times K_3' \times K_A' \times PCO_2 = 0 \tag{33}$$

Rearranging this formula to solve for $[H^+]$, and using the values from normal plasma, this expression yields a value of 40 nEq/L.

CONCLUSION

The value of the Stewart analysis is that it impels one to consider all the factors that influence pH. Several independent mechanisms regulate strong ion metabolism and alter their total body contents. However, because the plasma concentration of total solute and, therefore, of total strong cations in biological systems is governed closely by the regulation of water balance, changes in concentrations are small. In addition, changes in strong anion concentration are reflected by changes in serum $[HCO_3^-]$ whether effected by increases in other strong anions such as lactate or by reciprocal transport of chloride, e.g., by the gut in the setting of diarrhea. Thus, viewed from a clinical perspective, changes in SID, while undeniably a powerful influence on pH, are reflected by changes in serum $[HCO_3^-]$ and need not be calculated by the painstaking method proposed by Stewart. This approach also requires additional laboratory testing for each analysis. Notwithstanding the nearly ubiquitous availability of computers and calculators, the use of which Stewart champions, the classical approach of Van Slyke to consider only the three variables of the Henderson equation [Eq (25)], by virtue of the isohydric principle, provides a faster, simpler, and equally accurate determination of the ambient plasma pH. In the final analysis, the Van Slyke approach provides all the information needed for acid–base assessment and is a far superior tool for clinical application.

REFERENCES

1. Stewart PA. Modern quantitative acid–base chemistry. Can J Physiol Pharmacol 1983; 61:1444–1461.
2. Stewart PA. Independent and dependent variables of acid–base control. Respir Physiol 1978; 33:9–26.
3. Brønsted JN. Einige bemerkungen über den begriff der säuren und basen. Rec Trav Chim Pays-Bas 1923; 42:718–728.
4. Lowry TM. The uniqueness of hydrogen. J Soc Chem Indust 1923; 42:43–47.
5. Van Slyke DD, Cullen GE. Studies on acidosis. I. The bicarbonate concentration of the blood plasma; its significance and its determination as a measure of acidosis. J Biol Chem 1917; 30:289–346.
6. Gamble JL, Ross GS, Tisdall FF. The metabolism of fixed base during fasting. J Biol Chem 1923; 57:633–695.
7. Christensen HN. Anions versus cations?. Am J Med 1957; 23:163–165.
8. Sørensen SPL. Enzymstudien. II. Mitteilung. Über die messung und die bedeutung der wasserstoffionenkonzentration beienzymatischen prozessen. Biochem Z 1909; 21:131–200.
9. Bates RC. Determination of pH. Theory and Practice. New York: Wiley and Sons, 1964.
10. Hills AG. pH and the Henderson–Hasselbalch equation. Am J Med 1973; 55:131–133.
11. Madias NE, Cohen JJ. Acid–base chemistry and buffering. In: Cohen JJ, Kassirer JP, eds. Acid–Base. Boston: Little Brown, 1982:3–24.
12. Bernard C. An Introduction to the Study of Experimental Medicine. New York: Henry Schuman, Inc., 1949.
13. Henderson LJ. The theory of neutrality regulation in the animal organism. Am J Physiol 1908; 21:427–448.
14. Hasselbalch KA. Die berechnung der wasserstoffzahl des blutes uas der freien und gebundedn kohlensäure desselben, und die sauerstoffbindung des blutes alk funktion der wasserstoffzahl. Biochem Z 1917; 78:112–144.
15. Woodbury DM. Regulation of pH. In: Ruch TC, Patton HD, eds. Physiology and Biophysics. Philadelphia: Saunders, 1965:899–930.
16. Van Slyke DD. On the measurement of buffer values and on the relationship of buffer value to the dissociation constant of the buffer and the concentration and reaction of the buffer solution. J Biol Chem 1922; 52:525–571.

17. Van Slyke DD, Hastings AB, Hiller A, Sendroy J. Studies of gas and electrolyte equilibria. XIV. The amounts of alkali bound by serum albumin and globulin. J Biol Chem 1928; 79:769–780.

18. Austin WH, Lacombe E, Rand PW, Chatterjee M. Solubility of carbon dioxide in serum from 15 to 38 C. J Appl Physiol 1963; 18:301–304.

19. Severinghaus JW, Stupfel M, Bradley AF. Accuracy of blood pH and PCO$_2$ determinations. J Appl Physiol 1956; 9:189–196.

20. Maren TH. Carbonic anhydrase: chemistry, physiology, and inhibition. Physiol Rev 1967; 47:595–781.

21. Garg LC, Maren TH. The rates of hydration of carbon dioxide and dehydration of carbonic acid at 37 degrees. Biochim Biophys Acta 1972; 261:70–76.

22. Geers C, Gros G. Carbon dioxide transport and carbonic anhydrase in blood and muscle. Physiol Rev 2000; 80:681–715.

23. Gibbons BH, Edsall JT. Rate of hydration of carbon dioxide and dehydration of carbonic acid at 25 degrees. J Biol Chem 1963; 238:3502–3507.

24. Malnic G, Giebisch G. Symposium on acid–base homeostasis. Mechanism of renal hydrogenion secretion. Kidney Int 1972; 1:280–296.

25. Severinghaus JW, Stupfel M, Bradley AF. Variations of serum carbonic acid pK with pH and temperature. J Appl Physiol 1956; 9:197–200.

26. Valtin H, Gennari FJ. Acid–Base Disorders. Boston: Little Brown, 1987.

27. Kassirer JP, Bleich HL. Rapid estimation of plasma carbon dioxide tension from ph and total carbon dioxide content. N Engl J Med 1965; 272:1067–1068.

28. Constable PD. A simplified strong ion model for acid–base equilibria: application to horse plasma. J Appl Physiol 1997; 83:297–311.

29. Trenchard D, Noble MI, Guz A. Serum carbonic acid pK 1 abnormalities in patients with acid–base disturbances. Clin Sci 1967; 32:189–200.

30. Natelson S, Nobel D. Effect of the variation of pK of the Henderson–Hasselbalch equation on values obtained for total CO$_2$ calculated from pCO$_2$ and pH values. Clin Chem 1977; 23:767–769.

31. Hood I, Campbell EJ. Is pK' ok? N Engl J Med 1982; 306:864–866.

32. Gennari FJ. Is pK' ok? New Engl J Med 1982; 307:683.

33. Austin WH, Ferrante V, Anderson C. Evaluation of whole blood pK in the acutely ill patient. J Lab Clin Med 1968; 72:129–135.

34. DeRaedt M, Vandenbergh E, Van de Woestijne KP. Direct and indirect determination of partial pressure of CO$_2$ in the arterial blood of patients with respiratory insufficiency. Clin Sci 1968; 35:347–352.

35. Van Slyke DD, Hastings AB, Hiller A, Sendroy J. Studies of gas and electrolyte equilibria in blood. XVII. The effect of oxygenation and reduction on the carbon dioxide absorption curve and the pK of whole blood. J Biol Chem 1933; 102:505–519.

36. Figge J, Rossing TH, Fencl V. The role of serum proteins in acid–base equilibria. J Lab Clin Med 1991; 117:453–467.

37. Figge J, Mydosh T, Fencl V. Serum proteins and acid–base equilibria: a follow-up. J Lab Clin Med 1992; 120:713–719.

38. Bos OJ, Labro JF, Fischer MJ, Wilting J, Janssen LH. The molecular mechanism of the neutral-to-base transition of human serum albumin. Acid/base

titration and proton nuclear magnetic resonance studies on a large peptic and a large tryptic fragment of albumin. J Biol Chem 1989; 264:953–959.

39. Edsall JT, Wyman J. Biophysical Chemistry. New York: Academic Press, 1966.
40. Singer RB, Hastings AB. Improved clinical method for estimation of disturbances of acid–base balance in human blood. Medicine 1948; 27:223–242.
41. Rossi-Bernardi L, Roughton FJW. The specific influence of carbon dioxide and carbamate compounds on the buffer power and Bohr effects in human haemoglobin solutions. J Physiol 1967; 189:1–29.
42. German B, Wyman J. The titration curves of oxygenated and reduced hemoglobin. J Biol Chem 1937; 117:533–550.
43. Phillips R, Eisenberg P, George P, Rutman RJ. Thermodynamic data for the secondary phosphate ionizations of adenosine, guanosine, inosine, cytidine, and uridine nucleotides and triphosphate. J Biol Chem 1965; 240:4393–4397.

2

Intracellular Acid–Base Homeostasis

F. John Gennari

University of Vermont College of Medicine, Burlington, Vermont, U.S.A.

INTRODUCTION

Maintenance of a stable intracellular pH is central to cell metabolic processes and therefore for life itself. Regulation of intracellular $[H^+]$ involves active transport processes, modulation of production and utilization of organic acids, and chemical buffering. Characterization of these regulatory processes is extremely difficult because of the complex nature of the intracellular environment and remains a work in progress. Historically, most attempts at assessment of intracellular $[H^+]$ have been based on the assumption that the interior of the cell is a uniform solution. In fact, the interior milieu is extremely heterogeneous, containing vesicles, mitochondria, and multiple other structures that are known to create microenvironments in the cell with varying pH values (Fig. 1). In addition, cells differ widely in their metabolic and transport characteristics and therefore have differences in the nature of their acid–base homeostasis. Despite these shortcomings, extensive information has been acquired about cell pH and its regulation. This chapter reviews this information, covering both pH measurements and the nature of the transporters that regulate intracellular $[H^+]$ at the cell membrane and within its interior microenvironments.

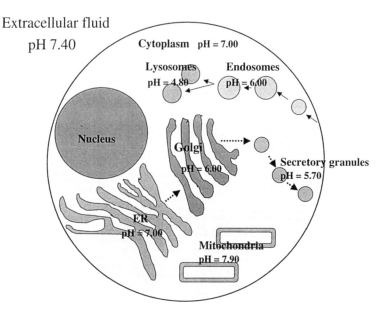

Figure 1 Schematic diagram of a generic mammalian cell, showing only the nucleus, cell membrane and the organelles discussed in this chapter. As shown in the figure, there is an inward pathway (endosomes to lysosomes) and an outward pathway (endoplasmic reticulum to secretory granules), both of which demonstrate progressive acidification. The interior of the mitochondria is highly alkaline. The pH values shown for each organelle and for the cytoplasm are approximations.

ASSESSMENT OF INTRACELLULAR pH

Historical Measurements

Our initial knowledge about cell pH came primarily from two techniques—microelectrode impalement of cells and the use of the weak acid dimethylox-azolidinedione (DMO), whose concentration in cells is pH dependent. Both approaches have major limitations, discussed below, the most important being the assumption that the interior of the cell is a uniform solution. Nonetheless, results obtained from these two techniques have provided the foundation for investigation into the regulation of cell pH. Both techniques demonstrated that cell $[H^+]$ is much lower than it should be if electrochemical forces were the only determinants of its distribution.

Microelectrode Impalement

Specially designed pH-sensitive and reference microelectrodes, with tip sizes $<1\ \mu m$, are used to assess cell pH (1,2). To measure pH, a double impalement is required (pH and reference electrode). Obviously, such a technique has a high probability of cell injury, and problems with electrode seal also

Table 1 Microelectrode Cell pH Measurements[a]

	Cell	ECF	Reference
Mammalian muscle			
Rat	6.88	7.41	4
	6.91	7.40	5
	5.99	7.41	1
Mouse	7.07	7.40	6
Nonmammalian muscle			
Barnacle	7.31	7.50	7
Crab	6.91	7.80	4
Axon			
Snail	7.44	7.80	2

[a]Representative studies.

affect the accuracy of measurement (3). These limitations were partially overcome by electrode design, and by limiting measurements to relatively large cells such as the squid axon. Table 1 summarizes measurements made in muscle and nerve cells in a variety of species. With a few notable exceptions, these measurements demonstrated intracellular pH values at or near 7.00. In four studies, pH was measured in mammalian muscle cells, and in three out of four of these studies, the pH value obtained is remarkably similar to measurements made with a less invasive technique, evaluating the pH-dependent distribution of DMO (see below and Table 2).

Table 2 Cell pH Determined by the Distribution of DMO[a]

	Cell	ECF	Reference
Human total body	6.94	7.37	8
	6.77	7.40	9
	6.88	7.43	10
Muscle			
Human	6.87	7.40	9
	6.90	7.36	11
Dog	7.04	7.37	12
	6.93	7.30	13
Rat	6.92	7.49	14
	6.75	7.34	15
Rabbit	6.79	7.36	16
Brain			
Dog	7.05	7.36	17
Rat	7.07	7.40	18

[a]Representative studies.

Dimethyloxazolidinedione

Dimethyloxazolidinedione is a weak acid (pK' = 6.13) that diffuses across cell membranes in its undissociated form, but not when the H^+ is dissociated (3,19). Thus, when DMO is added to the extracellular compartment, the amount of DMO that enters and remains in cells at equilibrium is directly related to the transmembrane pH gradient, with concentration falling as cell pH falls. A limitation in the use of DMO to assess cell pH is the indirect nature of the measurement. For example, errors in assessing the volumes of the intra- and extracellular compartments in which the DMO is distributed will affect the estimate of cell pH. Distribution could also be affected by protein binding, or to differential binding to intracellular organelles of differing pH. Finally, one cannot know with certainty whether DMO is toxic to the cell, or that it alters cell metabolism in some way that may affect pH. The limitations and utility of DMO for measuring cell pH have been reviewed in detail (19,20). Despite these limitations, estimates of cell pH using DMO have been remarkably consistent (Table 2), yielding values of 6.8–7.1.

Newer Techniques

New techniques for assessing cell pH have largely replaced the use of DMO and microelectrodes. These techniques have addressed the mechanisms maintaining the relative alkalinity of the intracellular milieu, as well as pH differences among different cell types and within the various microenvironments of the cell. Most widely used is the pH-dependent fluorescent probe 2,7-bis(carboxyethyl)-5,6-carboxyfluorescein (BCECF) (21). This probe is an ester that does not fluoresce until the ester linkage is cleaved. The lipidophilic ester crosses the cell membrane and is cleaved by intracellular esterases, leaving the native pH-dependent fluorescent compound trapped within the cell. Other trapped pH-dependent fluorescent dyes used for cell pH measurements include acridine orange and the esterified agent, seminaphthorhodafluor-1 (SNARF-1) (22). All these probes have a relatively uniform cytoplasmic distribution, and thus give data similar to that obtained using DMO. Their major advantage is that they provide information about changes in pH in seconds. Techniques to characterize pH in subcellular compartments have used physically targeted substances to localize, for example, in lysosomes, golgi, or mitochondria (22–25). In addition, spectral imaging microscopy has been coupled with fluorescent dyes to localize activity to specific subcellular sites (22,25). The results obtained with these newer techniques are discussed later in the chapter.

NONEQUILIBRIUM DISTRIBUTION OF H^+

Given the normal potential difference across most cell membranes (cell interior 90 mV negative as compared to the exterior), intracellular pH would be 5.8–6.0 if H^+ was distributed passively across the cell membrane (20).

The measurements shown in Tables 1 and 2 thus not only established values for cell pH, but also demonstrated that $[H^+]$ is notably lower than expected if its transcellular distribution were determined solely by electrical and chemical forces. The only exception to this finding appears to be the red blood cell, in which cell $[H^+]$ is consistent with electrochemical equilibrium (19). In all other cells, regardless of the buffer properties of the intracellular compartment, energy (i.e., O_2 consumption) is continually required to either remove H^+ from the cell or to add OH^- in order to maintain the relative alkalinity of the intracellular environment. This selective ion movement is accomplished by active (or secondary active) transport of H^+ and HCO_3^-, often linked to the transport of other ions (most notably Na^+, K^+, and Cl^-).

REGULATION OF CELL pH

To maintain cell pH stable at a higher level than its equilibrium value, active and regulated H^+ extrusion must be an ongoing process, and the rate of extrusion of H^+ must equal its rate of entry (26). Because HCO_3^- can also cross the cell membrane (see below), the rate of HCO_3^- entry must also equal the rate of HCO_3^- exit. Cell buffers can minimize the change in pH induced by the addition of H^+ or the loss of alkali, but these buffers will not restore pH to its baseline level. In the face of H^+ entry, in fact, H^+ extrusion (or alkali entry) must be sufficient to back-titrate cell buffers in order to restore pH to its resting level.

Because, as in any biological solution, $[H^+]$ and $[OH^-]$ in cells are determined by the strong ion difference (in addition to carbonic and organic acid concentrations) (27), one could consider regulation of cell pH from the perspective of the strong ion transport processes that establish the intracellular concentrations of these ions, rather than looking primarily at H^+ and HCO_3^- movement. As an example, Na^+- and K^+ -linked Cl^- movement across cell membranes modulate intracellular $[Na^+]$ and $[Cl^-]$ in a fashion to promote intracellular alkalinity. Attempting to determine which strong ions are key in the regulation of cell pH is a huge undertaking, however, as they all are likely to participate. In addition, such an approach adds unnecessary complexity. In this chapter (as in most reviews on the subject), the focus is on H^+ and HCO_3^- entry and exit from the cell or organelle.

H^+ Entry into Cells

As shown in Fig. 2, H^+ has ready access to cells, through its relationship with the volatile weak acid, H_2CO_3, as well as through its linkage to a variety of weak organic acids (e.g., lactic acid) (20,28). Carbon dioxide readily traverses the cell membrane, reacting reversibly with water to form H_2CO_3, a fraction of which dissociates to H^+ and HCO_3^-. As H^+ dissociates from H_2CO_3, the electrochemical forces at play drive it to remain in the cell and drive the associated HCO_3^- to leave the cell, decreasing cell pH (26). In

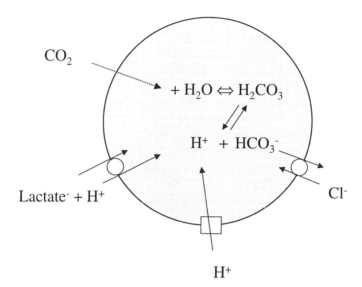

Figure 2 Pathways for H^+ entry and HCO_3^- exit from cells. Carbon dioxide (CO_2) diffuses readily across the membrane and adds H^+ to the cell by combining with water to form the weak acid, H_2CO_3. H^+ also can enter the cell on an organic anion cotransporter (*circle*), or via an H^+ channel (*rectangle*). HCO_3^- exits the cell in exchange for Cl^- entry on one of the AE family of exchange transporters (*circle*), with both ions moving down their electrochemical gradient.

addition to these modes of H^+ entry, H^+ channels are present in the cell membrane (Fig. 2) (29), although their role in modulating H^+ entry is unclear. These channels may in fact be an elegant way to promote H^+ exit from nerve and muscle cells during depolarization (26).

The ability of H^+ to enter cells has been used to study the transporters that respond to this entry. Isolated cells can be acidified acutely by a variety of techniques, including increasing bath PCO_2 or using NH_4Cl (20,30). These agents induce a rapid fall in intracellular pH, followed by rapid recovery (Fig. 3). The role of various membrane transport proteins in the recovery process can then be assessed by adding specific inhibitors or removing key ions from the bath (see below).

Alkali Exit from Cells

A variety of transporters have been identified, many of which have been cloned (see Chapter 5), that carry HCO_3^- across the cell membrane. In mammalian cells, most of these normally operate in mode of HCO_3^- exit from cells and thus will reduce intracellular pH if not counterbalanced by H^+ extrusion. Membrane transporters that facilitate alkali loss include the Na^+-independent Cl^-/HCO_3^- exchanger, the Na^+–HCO_3^- cotransporter,

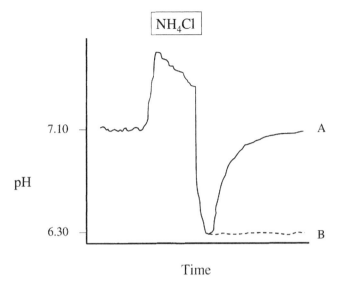

Figure 3 Schematic representation of the change in intracellular pH induced in an isolated cell by NH₄Cl addition to and then removal from the bath. Addition of NH₄Cl rapidly alkalinizes the cell due to NH₃ entry and recombination with intracellular H^+. Following this alkalinization, NH_4^+ slowly enters, causing a gradual fall in pH. With removal of NH₄Cl from the bath, NH₃ rapidly diffuses out of the cell, releasing H^+ from NH_4^+ and markedly acidifying the cell. This drop in pH is followed by rapid recovery to baseline pH due to active H^+ extrusion (line A). When the bath solution contains no CO_2 or HCO_3^-, inhibition of cell membrane Na^+/H^+, or removal of Na^+ from the bath blocks this recovery (line B), indicating a key role for this transporter in cell pH recovery. Time across the entire abscissa is less than 10 min. *Source*: Abstracted from many experimental observations (see Ref. 31).

the K^+–HCO_3^- cotransporter, and the Cl^-/organic anion exchangers. The energetics and characteristics of these transporters are reviewed in Chapter 5, and in Ref. 26. Most are only present in certain cell types (e.g., epithelial cells). Only the Cl^-/HCO_3^- exchanger will be discussed further here.

The AE family of electroneutral Na^+-independent Cl^-/HCO_3^- exchangers are widely extant, and in mammalian cells virtually always operate to extrude HCO_3^- from cells, exchanging this anion for Cl^- on a one-to-one basis (Fig. 2) (26,32). The best characterized of these is the so-called band-3 protein (AE1) which is abundant in red blood cell membranes (33). The direction of exchange is dependent on the Cl^- and HCO_3^- transcellular electrochemical gradients, and can be reversed by manipulating extracellular and/or intracellular ion concentrations (26). Because intracellular Cl^- is lower and HCO_3^- is higher than at electrochemical equilibrium in most mammalian cells, the transporter normally brings Cl^- into the cell in exchange for HCO_3^- exit (Fig. 2). Related Na^+-independent Cl^-/HCO_3^-

exchangers, AE2 and AE3, are present on many epithelial cells, and in smooth and cardiac muscle (26). These isoforms also normally operate to cause a loss of alkali from cells. In some experimental models, the Cl^-/HCO_3^- exchanger appears to be activated by an increase in intracellular pH and to be inactivated by low cell pH, thus serving to regulate cell pH homeostatically in states of alkalemia (34). This property appears to occur primarily in cells of renal origin.

Regulatory Control of Cell pH

Cells contain a variety of membrane transporters that are candidates for regulatory H^+ extrusion. A few are active transporters (e.g., the H^+-ATPase) but most are dependent on the activity of cell membrane Na^+/K^+ ATPase to develop the necessary chemical and electrical gradients for linked H^+ extrusion or alkali entry. The principal regulatory transporters are diagrammed in Fig. 4. Of these, the Na^+/H^+ exchanger is predominant. Virtually all vertebrate cells rely primarily on this exchanger to mediate regulatory H^+ extrusion (31,32). As discussed below, notable differences

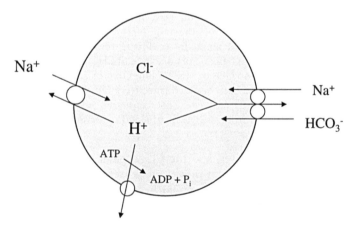

Figure 4 Examples of membrane transport proteins involved in removing acid from, or adding alkali to, mammalian cells. The Na^+/H^+ exchanger, shown on the left, plays a central role in regulating cell pH in most cells. This exchanger depends on the electrochemical gradients favoring Na^+ entry set up by the Na^+/K^+ ATPase (not shown). Using the same gradient for Na^+ entry, the Na^+-dependent Cl^-/HCO_3^- exchanger, shown on the right, moves HCO_3^- into cells as well as removing H^+. This transporter is present in muscle cells, fibroblasts, neurons and glomerular mesangial cells, and accounts for a varying portion of pH regulation in these cells. The H^+-ATPase shown at the bottom is present only on a subset of cells (mainly epithelial cells), but when present appears to participate in regulation of cell pH.

exist among cell types in the presence and participation of other membrane H^+ or HCO_3^- transporters in maintaining a low intracellular $[H^+]$.

Na^+/H^+ Exchanger

Several isoforms of the Na^+/H^+ exchanger have been cloned and characterized (see Chapter 5 and Ref. 35). The first of these transporters cloned, NHE1 (termed the "housekeeper" transporter), is ubiquitous, located on the cell membranes of both nonepithelial and epithelial cells (26,32). NHE1 uses the Na^+ electrochemical gradient generated by the Na^+/K^+ ATPase to extrude H^+ across the cell membrane in electroneutral exchange for Na^+ entry. Recovery of cell pH after acid loading is markedly attenuated after inhibition of this exchanger in a wide variety of cells (see example in Fig. 3) (31,32,36–38). In addition to its importance in restoring cell pH in the face of an acute acid load, NHE1 is central to steady-state pH regulation. Inhibition of this transporter uniformly results in a sustained fall in intracellular pH (38,39). Cell membrane Na^+/H^+ exchange activity is pH dependent for several isoforms of the NHE family; the transporter is activated by a fall in intracellular pH, and is largely inactivated at alkaline pH levels in the cell (35–37,40,41). In addition to intracellular pH, the transporter is affected by the pH in the fluid surrounding the cell; an increase in bath pH increases its activity and a decrease inhibits it (42,43).

Six isoforms of NHE family have been identified (NHE1-6) (35). Of these, NHE2 and 3 are confined to the apical membranes of intestinal and kidney epithelial cells. Both are activated by a decrease in intracellular pH and are key transporters for H^+ secretion into the gut and urine. NHE4 is confined to the basolateral membrane of stomach and renal epithelial cells and is also found in brain. This transporter appears to have no pH dependence. NHE5 is also found in brain tissue, and NHE6 appears to be a mitochondrial transporter (44).

H^+-ATPase

The vacuolar H^+-ATPase is an electrogenic active transporter present in a subset of specialized cells in the body, including renal tubule and corneal epithelial cells, neutrophils, macrophages, and osteoclasts (Fig. 4) (26). In all these cells, H^+-ATPase on the cell membrane can be shown to play a role in restoring intracellular pH in response to acute acidification when Na^+/H^+ exchange is inhibited (36,45–47). Under normal conditions, cell membrane H^+-ATPase, a relatively slow transporter, most likely works in concert with an Na^+/H^+ exchanger (most commonly NHE1) to control cell pH. A decrease in cell pH induced by increasing PCO_2 increases the insertion of vacuolar H^+-ATPase into the apical membranes of renal tubular epithelial cells, presumably increasing their capacity for H^+ secretion (41,48,49). Exposure of renal cells to extracellular metabolic acidosis or alkalosis, however, has shown conflicting results; one study shows a decrease in activity with metabolic acidosis (41), while another shows an increase in activity (50). In neither of these studies was intracellular pH monitored. Vacuolar H^+-ATPases are key transporters for producing local areas of increased $[H^+]$ within cells, rather than maintaining the low overall cytoplasmic $[H^+]$ (see later) (51).

H^+/K^+-ATPase

Certain epithelial cells (stomach, kidney, and colon) contain an H^+/K^+-ATPase on their limiting membranes that secretes H^+ in exchange for entry of K^+ (52). This transporter could function as a regulatory H^+ extrusion mechanism in these cells. Recovery of cell pH after acid loading in intercalated cells of rabbit cortical collecting ducts appears to have a K^+-dependent component that is blocked by inhibition of gastric-type H^+/K^+-ATPase (53). As with the H^+-ATPase, this effect can only be demonstrated after inactivation of the Na^+/H^+ exchanger. In other studies, expression or activity of either the gastric or colonic isoforms of this transporter was not upregulated by the induction of metabolic acidosis, but was by respiratory acidosis (54–56). The colonic H^+/K^+-ATPase in the kidney is upregulated in states of K^+ depletion (52,55), reflecting its primary role in K^+ homeostasis. Whether the gastric isoform contributes to the maintenance of cell pH is unclear, but it is unlikely to play an important role.

Na^+-Dependent Cl^-/HCO_3^- Exchanger

An Na^+-dependent Cl^-/HCO_3^- transporter is present on the cell membrane of cultured fibroblasts, glomerular mesangial cells and neurons, carrying Na^+ and HCO_3^- into cells in exchange for H^+ and Cl^- exit (Fig. 4) (57–60). The precise exchange is unclear, as one cannot differentiate the above exchange from one that involves 2 HCO_3^- or a $CO3^{2-}$ in rather than an H^+ out (26). Regardless of the ions carried, however, the net effect is to reduce intracellular $[H^+]$. Thus, the Na^+-dependent Cl^-/HCO_3^- transporter could play a role in maintaining cell $[H^+]$ below its equilibrium value. The activity of this transporter is enhanced by a reduction in intracellular pH, and the transporter becomes inactive above a threshold pH of around 7.40 (42). Transport activity is highly dependent on the presence of Na^+ in the extracellular compartment, and also appears to be related to the $[HCO_3^-]$ in the extracellular compartment (26,57,61). In glomerular mesangial cells, the Na^+-dependent Cl^-/HCO_3^- exchanger participates along with the Na^+/H^+ exchanger in maintaining a low cell $[H^+]$ (59). In an HCO_3^--free bathing medium, pH recovery from an acid load is mediated entirely by the Na^+/H^+ exchanger. With the addition of HCO_3^- to the bath, approximately 50% of pH recovery is mediated by the Na^+-dependent Cl^-/HCO_3^- exchanger. In mammalian neurons, this exchanger appears to be the major acid-extrusion mechanism (57). Whether it plays a role in other cell types in mammals remains to be determined.

Lactate$^-$/H$^+$ Cotransporter

The lactate/H$^+$ cotransporter, present on the cell membrane of striated skeletal muscle cells, serves to carry H$^+$ and lactate ions out of these cells during times of high production rate, ameliorating cell acidity (62). In resting striated muscle cells, Na$^+$/H$^+$ is the predominant transporter controlling intracellular pH, but a membrane HCO$_3^-$ transporter is also involved (6,63). With intense exercise, cell pH falls and H$^+$ secretion by the lactate$^-$/H$^+$ cotransporter is greater than by Na$^+$/H$^+$ exchange (64).

Other Potential Regulatory Transporters

The present discussion has reviewed the most likely candidates for regulating cell pH in mammalian cells. Many other acid–base transporters are present on various cells, which may also contribute to the regulatory control on intracellular [H$^+$]. These include the NBC class of Na$^+$–HCO$_3^-$ cotransporters, which may operate during cell alkalemia (26). In addition, cell membrane K$^+$–Cl$^-$ and K$^+$–alkali transporters are present in some cells. For a more complete review of the regulatory control of intracellular pH, see Ref. 26.

CELL BUFFER PROPERTIES

Cells provide a major component of body buffers. In response to an acid load, approximately 50% of the buffer response that minimizes changes in extracellular fluid (ECF) pH is accounted for by uptake and buffering of the added acid by cells (see Chapters 1 and 6) (65,66). If ECF [HCO$_3^-$] is already reduced prior to an acid challenge, an even greater percentage is accounted for by cells (66). This "buffer" response includes both chemical buffering (primarily titration of intracellular phosphates and proteins) and metabolic events (e.g., changes in organic acid production). In intact animals and humans, a reduction in ECF pH inhibits the production of both lactic and β-hydroxybutyric acids and an increase stimulates their production (67). The buffer response also includes changes in the activity of H$^+$ and HCO$_3^-$ transport proteins (see above), which may enhance the "buffer capacity" of cells, but diminish the cellular contribution to buffering the ECF.

Cell buffer capacity (β, see Chapter 1) has been assessed using a variety of techniques. The simplest and earliest method used was homogenization of tissue (usually muscle) followed by titration of the homogenates with acid or base (or CO$_2$) (68,69). These techniques yielded buffer values (β) of 50–65 slykes, but their relevance to living cells is questionable. Whether all the buffer substances exposed during homogenization are available to H$^+$ in living cells is unknown, for example, and any metabolic component or change in H$^+$ transport in or out of the cell is eliminated. A second approach was to use DMO to assess intracellular pH in intact tissue (most commonly muscle) after titration with acid or base (or CO$_2$) (70–72). This technique includes chemical and metabolic events, as well as changes in H^+ transport across the membrane, but suffers the problem of the weak acid or base's effect on cellular processes. Studies in muscle tissue have yielded widely varying results and these variations remain unexplained. The combined results of these early studies showed that muscle cells have a high capacity to buffer-added acid, but little attention should be paid to the actual values obtained.

The buffer properties of isolated or cultured cells have also been examined, using the fluorescent dye, BCECF (see earlier), to assess the change in cell pH induced by acid or alkali (NH_3) loading after inhibition of membrane H^+ transport and removal of CO_2/HCO_3^- (42,60,73). The results uniformly show a dependence of β on resting cell pH, with increasing values for β as pH falls. Thus, the CO_2/HCO_3^--independent component of cell buffering increases as cell pH falls, an effect probably related to the pK' values of most nonbicarbonate intracellular buffers. While not strictly comparable, the buffer values obtained in these cells are lower than those reported by earlier techniques, ranging from $\sim$10 to 30 slykes, depending on initial cell pH (42,60,73).

EFFECT OF CHANGES IN ECF pH ON CELL pH

Given the ready access of CO_2, H^+, and HCO_3^- to cells, it is not surprising that changes in ECF acid–base status are reflected by the intracellular milieu. Indeed, this access is part of the buffer response to changes in ECF acid–base status (see above). A reduction in ECF pH caused either by respiratory or metabolic acidosis produces a predictable steady-state decrease in intracellular pH (20,72,74,75). Although cell buffering determines the degree to which cell pH changes in response to a change in ECF pH, it does not play a role in maintaining the new steady state. The new steady state is due to a resetting of the balance between H^+ entry and exit from the cell (26). In metabolic acidosis, this resetting most likely reflects inhibition of H^+ exit via the Na^+/H^+ exchanger due to the increase in ECF $[H^+]$, and inhibition of HCO_3^- entry via the Na^+-dependent Cl^-/HCO_3^- exchanger due to the reduction in ECF $[HCO_3^-]$. In respiratory acidosis, intracellular pH falls rapidly, followed by a partial recovery (75). The degree to which cell pH recovers is dependent on ECF $[H^+]$ (76). When ECF H^+ is low in respiratory or metabolic alkalosis, cell H^+ falls as well, an effect in the steady state explained by forces affecting the activity of membrane acid–base transporters (26).

CELL PCO_2 AND $[HCO_3^-]$

Direct measurement of intracellular PCO_2 is not technically feasible but, given the high permeability of cell membranes to CO_2 (77,78), it is generally assumed that PCO_2 within cells is essentially equal to ECF PCO_2. This assumption is not precisely correct, of course, because cell metabolism provides the source for virtually all the CO_2 in the body and therefore a small diffusion gradient must exist between cells and the extracellular space. Measurements of PCO_2 in the proximal tubule of the rat kidney provide experimental support both for the rapid diffusion of CO_2 across cell membranes and the presence of small standing gradients in areas of very high CO_2 production, such as the very early segment (78). Additional evidence is the rapid change in intracellular pH that occurs in response to increasing the PCO_2 in the bath solution surrounding isolated cells (72,75).

Knowledge of the value for intracellular PCO_2 as well as cell pH allows for calculation of $[HCO_3^-]$. At a cell pH of 7.00 and a PCO_2 of 40 mmHg, for example, calculated $[HCO_3^-]$ is 9.5 mEq/L at 37°C, assuming pK' and solubility coefficient for CO_2 are similar in cells and the ECF. Intracellular $[HCO_3^-]$ can also be measured independently. Two techniques have been used. The first is simply to measure the total CO_2 concentration of minced or homogenized tissue (79,80). The second technique is to use a HCO_3^--sensitive ion-exchange electrode (74,81). Despite the technical problems and shortcomings of both approaches, these techniques have yielded remarkably similar values, 10–13 mEq/L, for $[HCO_3^-]$ in mammalian muscle cells (74,79–81). This value also fits well with calculated $[HCO_3^-]$ (see above). Microelectrode measurements have also shown that cell $[HCO_3^-]$ is responsive to ECF acid–base status, increasing in metabolic alkalosis and decreasing in metabolic acidosis (74).

pH IN INTRACELLULAR ORGANELLES

Most cells in the body contain many organelles with widely differing pH values, and these differences are maintained by H^+ transporters on their limiting membranes (Fig. 1). Some have very acid environments (lysosomes, golgi) and one has a notably alkaline environment (the mitochondrion). Maintenance of differing pH values in these organelles is critical for normal cell function. New insights have been gained about organelle pH and its regulation using targeted fluorescent dyes and molecular biology techniques (25). These studies have shown that endocytic vesicles become progressively more acid as they progress to lysosomes, and that the pH becomes progressively more acid from the endoplasmic reticulum to the trans-golgi network (25).

Mitochondria

Measurements of pH in isolated mitochondria and within living cells have consistently shown very alkaline values (82–85). In HeLa cells and rat cardiomyocytes, mitochondrial matrix pH values are 7.98 and 7.91, respectively (85). Replacement of bath glucose with lactate and pyruvate reversibly reduces pH, presumably promoting H^+ entry via an organic anion cotransporter, and addition of a proton ionophore rapidly reduces mitochondrial pH to 7.0 (85). The high pH in mitochondria is a key feature of the mechanism that links cell respiration to the generation of high-energy phosphate bonds. In 1965, Mitchell and Moyle (82) postulated that phosphorylation of adenosine diphosphate (ADP) is driven by the influx of H^+ across the mitochondrial membrane down its electrochemical gradient. This key insight has been borne out by subsequent experiments (86). As shown in Fig. 5, the final stages of oxidative phosphorylation are carried out by specialized proteins, the so-called respiratory chain, embedded in the inner mitochondrial membrane. These proteins accept H^+ from NADH and deliver them the intermembranous space, increasing both pH and the negative

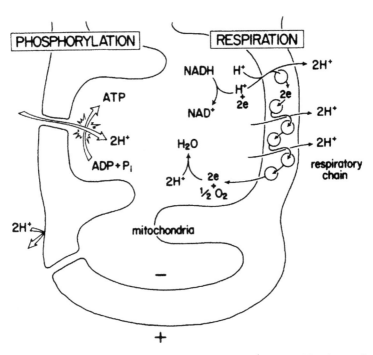

Figure 5   Schematic diagram of the linkage between H^+ removal by the respiratory chain and oxidative phosphorylation in mitochondria. The interior of the mitochondrion is highly alkaline (pH—7.9–8.0) and negatively charged due to the extrusion of H^+ by the proteins in the respiratory chain that are embedded in the inner membrane (right-hand side). The electrochemical gradient generated by this extrusion creates a strong driving force for H^+ reentry into the interior of the mitochondrion, but the inner membrane is impermeant to H^+ except through specific transport pores. One of these pores, shown on the left side of the diagram, is the F_1F_0 H^+-ATP synthase. H^+ passage through this pore activates the ATP synthase, which then phosphorylates ADP to form a new ATP molecule. *Source*: From Ref. 87.

electrical potential within the mitochondrial matrix. This extrusion of H^+ across the inner membrane creates a huge electrochemical gradient for H^+ reentry, and reentry is largely limited to a pathway involving an F_0F_1 H^+-ATP synthase in this membrane (88). Passage of H^+ through the F_0F_1 H^+-ATP synthase activates it to phosphorylate ADP to produce new ATP (89). The F_0F_1 H^+-ATP synthase normally acts to phosphorylate ADP, but it can be reversed to function as an ATPase by reversing the direction of H^+ movement (86). In addition to the F_0F_1 H^+-ATP synthase, the inner membranes of mitochondria appear to have a full panoply of H^+ transporters, including an Na^+/H^+ and K^+/H^+ exchanger as well as a Cl^-/HCO_3^- exchanger (44,88). These transporters presumably operate to modulate and help maintain the H^+ gradient needed for phosphorylation. This gradient is essential for cell life; its collapse is a feature of programmed cell death. The outer membrane of the mitochondrion is freely permeable to H^+.

Acidic Organelles

The acidic organelles of the cell can be characterized as forming a vacuolar system, with an inward and outward pathway (Fig. 1). The inward pathway begins at the plasma membrane with early endosomes, progressing to late endosomes and then to lysosomes, and the outward pathway begins with the endoplasmic reticulum, progressing to the golgi complex, and then the secretory granules. Both pathways demonstrate progressive intraorganelle acidification along their course (25,90). These organelles are all acidified by a common mechanism, an inwardly directed vacuolar H^+-ATPase (Fig. 6). The vacuolar H^+-ATPase is an electrogenic pump that moves H^+ from the cytoplasm into the organelle at a steady rate, independent of pH. Because it is electrogenic, the pump can also produce a transmembrane electrical gradient (interior positive), but this does not develop because of inward Cl^- and outward K^+ and H^+ movement (Fig. 6) (25). Because the H^+-ATPase does not change its rate of transport in response to changes in pH, another regulatory mechanism must be responsible for the maintenance of stable intraorganelle acidity. Although some studies suggested that the pH in organelles was regulated by changes in Cl^- conductance (51,85), it is currently thought to be regulated primarily by the rate of H^+ leak, presumably through an as yet undefined H^+ channel (25,91). One also cannot exclude the possibility that changes in K^+ and Cl^- conductances contribute to the regulation in some organelles. The characteristics of some members of the inward and outward pathways are described below.

Endosomes and Lysosomes

The lysosome was first shown to be acidic in 1893, by Metchnikoff, who fed litmus paper to protozoans and observed a red color change in the vacuoles (90). Measurements in intact cells indicate that the pH of

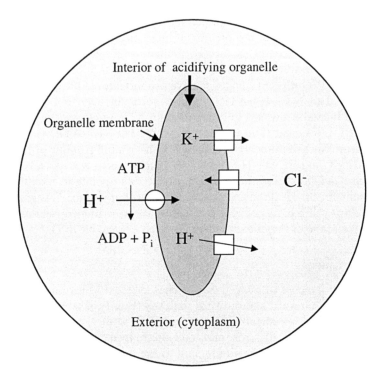

Figure 6 Schematic diagram of the acidification process in an intracellular organelle. Hydrogen ions are pumped at a steady rate into all acidified organelles by a vacuolar H^+-ATPase. This electrogenic H^+ pump also makes the interior of the organelle positively charged, which provides the driving force for the movement of H^+ and K^+ out of the organelle and/or Cl^- entry, via specific ion channels (*squares*). The final steady-state pH of the interior of the organelle appears to be determined primarily by the rate of H^+ exit.

lysosomes is 4.6–5.0, the most acidic environment in living cells (90). The low pH in the lysosome is generated by the vacuolar H^+-ATPase, and is presumably maintained by a low rate of H^+ exit. Endosomes are acidified by the same H^+-ATPase, but are less acidic than lysosomes; pH values measured in early endosomes average 5.5–6.0, and in endosomes recycling to the plasma membrane, 6.2 (90,92).

Endoplasmic Reticulum and Golgi

Using a targeted fluoroprobe, the pH of the endoplasmic reticulum of cultured HeLa cells was found to be 7.1, virtually identical to the cytoplasm (93). This organelle was found to be highly permeable to H^+, and to have a buffer value identical to the cytoplasm. No evidence of a vacuolar H^+-ATPase could be found in this organelle. By contrast, the pH of the golgi was 6.56 in these cells, and was unaffected by maneuvers to acidify the organelle, suggesting much tighter regulation of pH (93). Other investigators using similar techniques have shown the pH in the golgi complex to be notably more acid than the cytoplasm (23,24,85,94). Inhibition of the vacuolar H^+-ATPase rapidly alkalinizes this compartment, indicating the key role of this ATPase in maintaining the acid pH within this microenvironment of the cell (23,85). Acidification of the golgi by the H^+-ATPase is dependent on the presence of Cl^-, which presumably enters the complex as a counterion, but maintenance of a stable pH could still be dependent primarily on the rate of H^+ efflux. The pH in the *trans*-golgi, the terminal portion of the complex (forming the secretory vesicles) falls to approximately 6.0 (24,94).

Secretory Vesicles

Measurement of pH in a variety of secretory vesicles, including chromaffin granules, platelet dense granules, neurosecretory granules from the pituitary, and cholinergic secretory granules have uniformly demonstrated a low pH coupled with the presence of a membrane H^+-ATPase (90). Chromaffin granules from bovine adrenal gland have an internal pH of approximately 5.7.

SUMMARY

Living cells are complex machines with a highly regulated pH. Historical measurements demonstrated conclusively that, with rare exception, H^+ is not distributed passively across cell membranes. Regulation of cell pH begins at the cell membrane where H^+ entry and HCO_3^- loss is countered by a variety of acid–base transporters. Of these, the most universal appears to be the Na^+/H^+ exchanger, which uses gradients developed by the membrane Na^+/K^+ ATPase to move H^+ out of cells. In addition, cells have a high capacity to buffer H^+ that enters the cells and can alter organic acid production, minimizing changes in ECF pH brought on by acid–base perturbations. The cell regulates $[H^+]$ at varying levels within its organelles, maintaining mitochondria highly alkaline to create the driving force of high-energy phosphorylation, and maintaining vacuoles and the golgi more acid than the cytoplasm to facilitate protein synthesis and catabolism.

REFERENCES

1. Carter NW, Rector FC Jr, Campion DS, Seldin DW. Measurement of intracellular pH of skeletal muscle with pH-sensitive glass microelectrodes. J Clin Invest 1967; 46:920–933.
2. Thomas RC. Intracellular pH of snail neurones measured with a new pH-sensitive glass mirco-electrode. J Physiol 1974; 238:159–180.

3. Boron WF, Roos A. Comparison of microelectrode, DMO, and methylamine methods for measuring intracellular pH. Am J Physiol 1976; 231:799–809.
4. Paillard M, Sraer JD, Leviel F, Claret M. Direct measurement of intracellular pH in crab and rat muscle. J Physiol (Paris) 1971; 63:148A.
5. Lavallee M. Intracellular pH of rat atrial muscle fibers measured by glass micropipette electrodes. Circ Res 1964; 15:185–193.
6. Aickin CC, Thomas RC. Micro-electrode measurement of the intracellular pH and buffering power of mouse soleus muscle fibres. J Physiol 1977; 267: 791–810.
7. Boron WF. Intracellular pH transients in giant barnacle muscle fibers. Am J Physiol 1977; 233:C61–C73.
8. Manfredi F. Calculation of total body intracellular pH in normal human subjects from the distribution of 5,5-dimethyl-2,4-oxazolidinedione (DMO). J Lab Clin Med 1963; 61:1005–1014.
9. Grantham JJ, Schloerb PR. Measurments of intracellular hydrogen ion concentration in patients. Surg Forum 1964; 15:81–82.
10. Lambie AT, Anderton JL, Cowie J, Simpson JD, Tothill P, Robson JS. Intracellular hydrogen ion concentration in renal acidosis. Clin Sci 1965; 28:237–249.
11. Bittar EE, Watt MF, Pateras VR, Parrish AE. The pH of muscle in Laennec's cirrhosis and uremia. Clin Sci 1962; 23:265–276.
12. Waddell WJ, Butler TC. Calculation of intracellular pH from the distribution of 5,5-dimethyl-2,4-oxazolidinedione (DMO). Application to skeletal muscle of dog. J Clin Invest 1959; 38:720–729.
13. Brown EB, Goott B. Intracellular hydrogen ion changes and potassium movement. Am J Physiol 1963; 204:765–770.
14. Irvine RO, Dow J. Intracellular pH and electrolyte content of voluntary muscle in renal acidosis. Clin Sci 1966; 31:317–324.
15. Butler TC, Kuroiwa Y, Waddell WJ, Poole DT. Effects of 5,5-dimethyl-2,4-oxazolidinedione (DMO) on acid–base and electrolyte equilibria. J Pharmacol Exp Ther 1966; 152:62–66.
16. Poole-Wilson PA, Cameron IR. Intracellular pH and K^+ of cardiac and skeletal muscle in acidosis and alkalosis. Am J Physiol 1975; 229:1305–1310.
17. Arieff AI, Kerian A, Massry SG, DeLima J. Intracellular pH of brain: alterations in acute respiratory acidosis and alkalosis. Am J Physiol 1976; 230:804–812.
18. Roos A. Intracellular pH and buffering power of rat brain. Am J Physiol 1971; 221:176–181.
19. Waddell WJ, Bates RG. Intracellular pH. Physiol Rev 1969; 49:285–329.
20. Roos A, Boron WF. Intracellular pH. Physiol Rev 1981; 61:296–434.
21. Alpern RJ. Cell mechanisms of proximal tubule acidification. Physiol Rev 1990; 70:79–114.
22. Gillies RJ, Lynch RM. Frontiers in the measurement of cell and tissue pH. Novartis Found Symp 2001; 240:7–19; discussion 19–22, 152–153.
23. Kim JH, Lingwood CA, Williams DB, Furuya W, Manolson MF, Grinstein S. Dynamic measurement of the pH of the golgi complex in living cells using retrograde transport of the verotoxin receptor. J Cell Biol 1996; 134:1387–1399.

24. Seksek O, Biwersi J, Verkman AS. Direct measurement of *trans*-golgi pH in living cells and regulation by second messengers. J Biol Chem 1995; 270: 4967–4970.

25. Demaurex N. pH homeostasis of cellular organelles. News Physiol Sci 2002; 17:1–5.

26. Bevensee MO, Alper SA, Aronson PS, Boron WF. Control of intracellular pH. In: Seldin DW, Giebisch G, eds. The Kidney: Physiology and Pathophysiology. Vol. 1. Philadelphia: Lippincott Williams & Wilkins, 2000:391–442.

27. Stewart PA. Independent and dependent variables of acid-base control. Respir Physiol 1978; 33:9–26.

28. Mason MJ, Mainwood GW, Thoden JS. The influence of extracellular buffer concentration and propionate on lactate efflux from frog muscle. Pflugers Arch 1986; 406:472–479.

29. DeCoursey TE, Cherny VV. Voltage-activated hydrogen ion currents. J Membr Biol 1994; 141:203–223.

30. Boron WF, De Weer P. Intracellular pH transients in squid giant axons caused by CO_2, NH_3, and metabolic inhibitors. J Gen Physiol 1976; 67:91–112.

31. Aickin CC. Intracellular pH regulation by vertebrate muscle. Annu Rev Physiol 1986; 48:349–361.

32. Hoffmann EK, Simonsen LO. Membrane mechanisms in volume and pH regulation in vertebrate cells. Physiol Rev 1989; 69:315–382.

33. Jennings ML. Structure and function of the red blood cell anion transport protein. Annu Rev Biophys Biophys Chem 1989; 18:397–430.

34. Olsnes S, Tonnessen TI, Sandvig K. pH-regulated anion antiport in nucleated mammalian cells. J Cell Biol 1986; 102:967–971.

35. Counillon L, Pouyssegur J. The members of the Na^+/H^+ exchanger gene family: their structure, function, expression, and regulation. In: Seldin DW, Giebisch G, eds. The Kidney. Physiology and Pathophysiology. Vol. 1. Philadelphia: Lippincott Williams and Wilkins, 2000:223–234.

36. Ravesloot JH, Eisen T, Baron R, Boron WF. Role of Na–H exchangers and vacuolar H^+ pumps in intracellular pH regulation in neonatal rat osteoclasts. J Gen Physiol 1995; 105:177–208.

37. Boyarsky G, Ganz MB, Cragoe EJ Jr, Boron WF. Intracellular-pH dependence of Na–H exchange and acid loading in quiescent and arginine vasopressin-activated mesangial cells. Proc Natl Acad Sci USA 1990; 87:5921–5924.

38. Moolenaar WH, Tertoolen LG, de Laat SW. The regulation of cytoplasmic pH in human fibroblasts. J Biol Chem 1984; 259:7563–7569.

39. Moolenaar WH, Tsien RY, van der Saag PT, de Laat SW. Na^+/H^+ exchange and cytoplasmic pH in the action of growth factors in human fibroblasts. Nature 1983; 304:645–648.

40. Aronson PS, Nee J, Suhm MA. Modifier role of internal H^+ in activating the $Na^+–H^+$ exchanger in renal microvillus membrane vesicles. Nature 1982; 299:161–163.

41. Soleimani M, Bookstein C, Singh G, Rao MC, Chang EB, Bastani B. Differential regulation of Na^+/H^+ exchange and H(+)-ATPase by pH and HCO_3^- in kidney proximal tubules. J Membr Biol 1995; 144:209–216.

42. Boron WF, McCormick WC, Roos A. pH regulation in barnacle muscle fibers: dependence on intracellular extracellular pH. Am J Physiol 1979; 237: C185–C193.

43. Gennari FJ, Helmle-Kolb C, Murer H. Influence of extracellular pH and perfusion rate on Na^+/H^+ exchange in cultured opossum kidney cells. Pflugers Arch 1992; 420:153–158.

44. Numata M, Petrecca K, Lake N, Orlowski J. Identification of a mitochondrial Na^+/H^+ exchanger. J Biol Chem 1998; 273:6951–6959.

45. Swallow CJ, Grinstein S, Rotstein OD. A vacuolar type H(+)-ATPase regulates cytoplasmic pH in murine macrophages. J Biol Chem 1990; 265:7645–7654.

46. Wagner CA, Giebisch G, Lang F, Geibel JP. Angiotensin II stimulates vesicular H^+-ATPase in rat proximal tubular cells. Proc Natl Acad Sci USA 1998; 95:9665–9668.

47. Selvaggio AM, Schwartz JH, Bengele HH, Gordon FD, Alexander EA. Mechanisms of H^+ secretion by inner medullary collecting duct cells. Am J Physiol 1988; 254:F391–F400.

48. Gluck S, Cannon C, Al-Awqati Q. Exocytosis regulates urinary acidification in turtle bladder by rapid insertion of H^+ pumps into the luminal membrane. Proc Natl Acad Sci USA 1982; 79:4327–4331.

49. Schwartz GJ, Al-Awqati Q. Carbon dioxide causes exocytosis of vesicles containing H^+ pumps in isolated perfused proximal and collecting tubules. J Clin Invest 1985; 75:1638–1644.

50. Chambrey R, Paillard M, Podevin RA. Enzymatic and functional evidence for adaptation of the vacuolar H(+)-ATPase in proximal tubule apical membranes from rats with chronic metabolic acidosis. J Biol Chem 1994; 269:3243–3250.

51. Rudnick G. ATP-driven H^+ pumping into intracellular organelles. Annu Rev Physiol 1986; 48:403–413.

52. Silver RB, Soleimani M. H^+–K^+-ATPases: regulation and role in pathophysiological states. Am J Physiol 1999; 276:F799–F811.

53. Silver RB, Frindt G. Functional identification of H–K-ATPase in intercalated cells of cortical collecting tubule. Am J Physiol 1993; 264:F259–F266.

54. Eiam-ong S, Laski ME, Kurtzman NA, Sabatini S. Effect of respiratory acidosis and respiratory alkalosis on renal transport enzymes. Am J Physiol 1994; 267:F390–F399.

55. DuBose TD Jr, Codina J, Burges A, Pressley TA. Regulation of H(+)–K(+)-ATPase expression in kidney. Am J Physiol 1995; 269:F500–F507.

56. Fejes-Toth G, Rusvai E, Longo KA, Naray-Fejes-Toth A. Expression of colonic H–K-ATPase mRNA in cortical collecting duct: regulation by acid/base balance. Am J Physiol 1995; 269:F551–F557.

57. Schwiening CJ, Boron WF. Regulation of intracellular pH in pyramidal neurones from the rat hippocampus by Na(+)-dependent Cl(−)-HCO_3^- exchange. J Physiol 1994; 475:59–67.

58. L'Allemain G, Paris S, Pouyssegur J. Role of a Na^+-dependent Cl^-/HCO_3^- exchange in regulation of intracellular pH in fibroblasts. J Biol Chem 1985; 260:4877–4883.

59. Boyarsky G, Ganz MB, Sterzel RB, Boron WF. pH regulation in single glomerular mesangial cells II. Na^+-dependent and -independent $Cl(-)$-HCO_3^- exchangers. Am J Physiol 1988; 255:C857–C869.

60. Boyarsky G, Ganz MB, Sterzel RB, Boron WF. pH regulation in single glomerular mesangial cells I. Acid extrusion in absence and presence of HCO_3. Am J Physiol 1988; 255:C844–C856.

61. Boron WF, Knakal RC. $Na(+)$-dependent Cl–HCO_3 exchange in the squid axon. Dependence on extracellular pH. J Gen Physiol 1992; 99:817–837.

62. Juel C. Muscle pH regulation: role of training. Acta Physiol Scand 1998; 162:359–366.

63. Putnam RW, Roos A, Wilding TJ. Properties of the intracellular pH-regulating systems of frog skeletal muscle. J Physiol 1986; 381:205–219.

64. Juel C. Intracellular pH recovery and lactate efflux in mouse soleus muscles stimulated in vitro: the involvement of sodium/proton exchange and a lactate carrier. Acta Physiol Scand 1988; 132:363–371.

65. Swan RC, Pitts RF. Neutralization of infused acid by nephrectomized dogs. J Clin Invest 1955; 34:205–212.

66. Adrogue HJ, Brensilver J, Cohen JJ, Madias NE. Influence of steady-state alterations in acid–base equilibrium on the fate of administered bicarbonate in the dog. J Clin Invest 1983; 71:867–883.

67. Hood VL, Tannen RL. Protection of acid–base balance by pH regulation of acid production. N Engl J Med 1998; 339:819–826.

68. Larsen LA, Burnell JM. Muscle buffer values. Am J Physiol 1978; 234: F432–F436.

69. Heisler N, Piiper J. The buffer value of rat diaphragm muscle tissue determined by PCO_2 equilibration of homogenates. Respir Physiol 1971; 12:169–178.

70. Heisler N, Piiper J. Determination of intracellular buffering properties in rat diaphragm muscle. Am J Physiol 1972; 222:747–753.

71. Adler S. The simultaneous determination of muscle cell pH using a weak acid and weak base. J Clin Invest 1972; 51:256–265.

72. Adler S, Roy A, Relman AS. Intracellular acid–base regulation I. The response of muscle cells to changes in CO_2 tension or extracellular bicarbonate concentration. J Clin Invest 1965; 44:8–20.

73. Grinstein S, Cohen S, Rothstein A. Cytoplasmic pH regulation in thymic lymphocytes by an amiloride-sensitive Na^+/H^+ antiport. J Gen Physiol 1984; 83:341–369.

74. Khuri RN, Agulian SK, Bogharian KK. Intracellular bicarbonate of skeletal muscle under different metabolic states. Am J Physiol 1976; 230:228–232.

75. Aickin CC, Thomas RC. Micro-electrode measurement of the internal pH of crab muscle fibres. J Physiol 1975; 252:803–815.

76. Adler S, Roy A, Relman AS. Intracellular acid–base regulation II. The interaction between CO_2 tension and extracellular bicarbonate in the determination of muscle cell pH. J Clin Invest 1965; 44:21–30.

77. Wang KW, Deen WM. Chemical kinetic and diffusional limitations on bicarbonate reabsorption by the proximal tubule. Biophys J 1980; 31:161–182.

78. Maddox DA, Atherton LJ, Deen WM, Gennari FJ. Proximal HCO_3^- reabsorption and the determinants of tubular and capillary PCO_2 in the rat. Am J Physiol 1984; 247:F73–F81.
79. Wallace WM, Hastings AB. The distribution of the bicarbonate ion in mammalian muscle. J Biol Chem 1942; 144:637–649.
80. Danielson IS, Hastings AB. A method for determining tissue carbon dioxide. J Biol Chem 1939; 130:349–356.
81. Khuri RN, Bogharian KK, Agulian SK. Intracellular bicarbonate in single skeletal muscle fibers. Pflugers Arch 1974; 349:285–294.
82. Mitchell P, Moyle J. Stoichiometry of proton translocation through the respiratory chain and adenosine triphosphatase systems of rat liver mitochondria. Nature 1965; 208:147–151.
83. Chance B, Mela L. Intramitochondrial pH changes in cation accumulation. Proc Natl Acad Sci USA 1966; 55:1243–1251.
84. Addanki S, Cahill FD, Sotos JF. Intramitochondrial pH and intra-extramitochondrial pH gradient of beef heart mitochondria in various functional states. Nature 1967; 214:400–402.
85. Llopis J, McCaffery JM, Miyawaki A, Farquhar MG, Tsien RY. Measurement of cytosolic, mitochondrial, and golgi pH in single living cells with green fluorescent proteins. Proc Natl Acad Sci USA 1998; 95:6803–6808.
86. Hatefi Y. The mitochondrial electron transport and oxidative phosphorylation system. Annu Rev Biochem 1985; 54:1015–1069.
87. Gennari FJ, Cohen JJ. Intracellular acid–base physiology. In: Cohen JJ, Kassirer JP, eds. Acid–Base. Boston: Little Brown, 1982:25–40.
88. Matsuyama S, Reed JC. Mitochondria-dependent apoptosis and cellular pH regulation. Cell Death Differ 2000; 7:1155–1165.
89. Konforti B. Picture story. How proton pumps make ATP. Nat Struct Biol 1999; 6:1090.
90. Mellman I, Fuchs R, Helenius A. Acidification of the endocytic and exocytic pathways. Annu Rev Biochem 1986; 55:663–700.
91. Wu MM, Llopis J, Adams S, et al. Organelle pH studies using targeted avidin and fluorescein-biotin. Chem Biol 2000; 7:197–209.
92. Gagescu R, Demaurex N, Parton RG, Hunziker W, Huber LA, Gruenberg J. The recycling endosome of Madin–Darby canine kidney cells is a mildly acidic compartment rich in raft components. Mol Biol Cell 2000; 11:2775–2791.
93. Kim JH, Johannes L, Goud B, et al. Noninvasive measurement of the pH of the endoplasmic reticulum at rest and during calcium release. Proc Natl Acad Sci USA 1998; 95:2997–3002.
94. Demaurex N, Furuya W, D'Souza S, Bonifacino JS, Grinstein S. Mechanism of acidification of the *trans*-golgi network (TGN). In situ measurements of pH using retrieval of TGN38 and furin from the cell surface. J Biol Chem 1998; 273:2044–2051.

3

Determinants of Carbon Dioxide Tension

Shahrokh Javaheri

Department of Veterans Affairs Medical Center, University of Cincinnati College of Medicine, Cincinnati, Ohio and Sleepcare Diagnostics, Mason, Ohio, U.S.A.

INTRODUCTION

The major function of the respiratory system is to maintain normal arterial blood partial pressures of the two vital respiratory gases, O_2 and CO_2, and a normal pH. This important regulatory function is automatically controlled, and is referred to as the homeostatic (chemostatic or metabolic) function. Homeostatic regulation is achieved by adjustment of ventilation to the metabolic (O_2 consumption/CO_2 production) and acid–base needs of the organism (1). The respiratory system is also utilized for behavioral (nonhomeostatic) functions such as phonation and swallowing. The act of breathing, therefore, is complex and needs to be governed precisely by a set of hierarchically arranged control systems. The focus of this chapter is chemical control of breathing and regulation of PCO_2.

In humans, arterial PCO_2 ($PaCO_2$) is tightly controlled in wakefulness and sleep. $PaCO_2$ remains constant throughout life, in contrast to the progressive decline in arterial PO_2 (PaO_2) that occurs with aging. Thus, any sustained deviation in $PaCO_2$ indicates a major disturbance in its homeostasis.

WHY IS $PaCO_2$ 40 mmHg IN MAN?

Values for $PaCO_2$ differ considerably among various species. In sea animals with gill ventilation, for example, water is the respiratory vehicle. Because of the low solubility of O_2 in water, a large amount of gill ventilation is required to extract sufficient O_2 to meet metabolic demands. Because CO_2 is $\sim$30 times more soluble in water than O_2, the large volume of ventilation results in CO_2 washout and a very low PCO_2, 1–4 mmHg (2). With an equal exchange of O_2 and CO_2 (respiratory quotient equal to one), PO_2 in water drops by about 30 mmHg as it flows over the gills, whereas PCO_2 rises by $\sim$1 mmHg.

With land invasion and air breathing, high-level ventilation was no more necessary to provide adequate O_2 delivery. Land invasion, therefore, set the stage for ventilation to decrease. This change had the advantage of decreasing the metabolic cost of breathing and providing considerable ventilatory reserve. At the same time, PCO_2 had to rise with two consequent problems. First, PCO_2 is a key determinant of acid–base status and secondly, with air breathing, a reciprocal relation (almost 1 for 1) between PO_2 and PCO_2 was established. As a result, hypoxemia limited the reduction in ventilation that could occur.

Given these considerations, the PCO_2, PO_2, and pH values that evolved in humans are the result of a complex interaction between optimization and prioritization of respiratory functions to fulfill a number of important physiological demands (3). Issues such as efficiency of breathing at rest and exercise, acid–base status, and optimal PO_2 for interaction with hemoglobin in arterial blood contributed to the evolution of "normal" arterial PCO_2, PO_2, and pH values in terrestrial organisms. Maintaining proper acid–base balance is of utmost biological importance, because changes in pH alter the charged state of enzymes and impair their function. At a $PaCO_2$ of 40 mmHg, intracellular pH at 37°C is $\sim$6.8. At this temperature, the pH of pure water is also 6.8, by definition at neutrality. This intracellular pH appears to serve biologically important functions well (see Chapters 1 and 2) (2–8). Thus, an arterial PCO_2 of 40 mmHg was an excellent evolutionary choice to set intracellular pH close to neutrality at 37°C. Given other biochemical determinants of $[H^+]$ in blood and $PaCO_2$ of 40 mmHg, arterial blood pH had to be 7.40 at 37°C.

THE IMIDAZOLE α-STAT HYPOTHESIS

The pH of water is inversely related to temperature. In pure water at all temperatures, of course, $[H^+]$ and $[OH^-]$ are equal and therefore by definition, water always has a neutral pH. Blood and intracellular fluid pH also change with temperature. The intracellular pH of various ectotherms at their normothermic temperatures is equal to the pH value of water at that temperature. In other words, intracellular pH remains virtually neutral as temperature changes. Blood pH is alkaline relative to intracellular pH, but in vivo changes in blood pH parallel changes in intracellular pH as temperature changes such that relative alkalinity (blood pH vs. intracellular pH) remains constant. A similar change in human blood pH is observed in vitro as temperature changes. This adaptation is a reflection of the fact that pH is an important determinant for enzymatic functions in living cells (2–11).

Based on observations in animals with different core temperatures and the behavior of imidazole moiety of histidine, Reeves (4,12) advanced the α-stat hypothesis. At 37°C, intracellular pH is close to the pK of the imidazole group of histidine, and changes in the pK of imidazole parallel changes in pH, as the latter changes with temperature (7). The α-stat hypothesis states that the charge state or fractional dissociation (the ratio of protonated to total protein) of the imidazole group of histidine remains constant as pH changes with temperature (2–8). Histidine is present at the active site of key enzymes, and the charge state of these enzymes is critical for their function (5,6,9–13). Central to the regulation of ventilation, a protein conforming to the α-stat hypothesis appears to be involved in central chemosensitivity (7,9,14). In fresh water turtles, ventilation was not related to cerebrospinal fluid pH changes, induced by changing water temperature, but was a function of α-imidazole (15).

Another important benefit of maintaining intracellular pH close to neutral is that most water-soluble biosynthetic intermediates have pK values that render them fully ionized at neutrality (10). A cell pH near neutrality retains these ionized molecules inside the boundaries of cell membranes without energy expenditure.

QUANTITATIVE COMPONENTS OF VENTILATION

Minute Volume

Minute volume (also referred to as minute ventilation) is the product of respiratory rate (RR, or breathing rate) and tidal volume (VT):

$$\dot{V}I \text{ or } \dot{V}E = RR \times VT \tag{1}$$

In this equation, $\dot{V}I$ and $\dot{V}E$ stand for minute volume measured during inspiration or expiration, respectively. Tidal volume is usually measured during expiration. Therefore, the minute volume usually measured is VE. If inspiratory tidal volume is being recorded, the minute volume measured is $\dot{V}I$. Normally $\dot{V}I$ is somewhat greater than $\dot{V}E$, because O_2 consumption ($\dot{V}O_2$) is greater than CO_2 production ($\dot{V}CO_2$).

Some of the volume of each breath is distributed to areas where gas exchange does not occur (Fig. 1). This area is called the anatomical dead space and includes the nose, mouth, trachea, and bronchi up to and including terminal bronchioles. The more distal airways take part in gas exchange and are referred to as respiratory airways (Fig. 1). In various cardiopulmonary disorders (e.g., pulmonary embolism) some alveoli are ventilated but not perfused, and these unperfused alveoli act as extra dead space. The new dead space along with anatomical dead space is collectively referred to as physiological dead space.

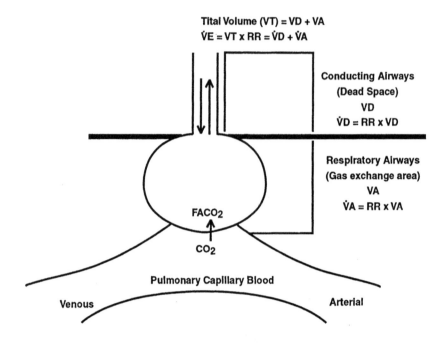

Tital Volume (VT) = VD + VA
$\dot{V}E = VT \times RR = \dot{V}D + \dot{V}A$

Conducting Airways
(Dead Space)
VD
$\dot{V}D = RR \times VD$

Respiratory Airways
(Gas exchange area)
VA
$\dot{V}A = RR \times VA$

$FAco_2$

CO_2

Pulmonary Capillary Blood

Venous

Arterial

$\dot{V}co_2$ = Venous CO_2 Content - Arterial CO_2 Content

Figure 1 A simplified two-compartment model of the lung and airways. The anatomical dead space (upper part of diagram) includes the conducting airways where gas exchange does not occur. The alveolar space (lower part of diagram) contains the respiratory airways, adjacent to the pulmonary capillary bed, where gas exchange occurs. When dead space (VD) and alveolar volumes (VA) are multiplied by respiratory rate (RR), dead space ventilation (VD) and alveolar ventilation (VA) are obtained. The sum of dead space and alveolar volume is equal to the tidal volume. The sum of dead space and alveolar ventilation is equal to minute ventilation (VE).

In a simplified model, the volume of each breath consists of two components, the dead space (VD) volume and the alveolar volume (VA):

$$VT = VD + VA \tag{2}$$

Multiplying both sides of the equation by respiratory rate:

$$RR \times VT = VD \times RR + VA \times RR \text{ or} \tag{3}$$

$$\dot{V}E = \dot{V}D + \dot{V}A \tag{4}$$

As indicated by Eq. (4), minute volume ($\dot{V}E$) consists of two "separate" ventilation volumes, dead space ($\dot{V}D$) and alveolar ventilation ($\dot{V}A$). The gas composition of $\dot{V}E$ is the sum of the gas compositions of $\dot{V}D$ and

$\dot{V}A$. For a given minute volume, the higher the dead space ventilation, the lower the alveolar ventilation and the higher the $PaCO_2$.

Alveolar Ventilation

PCO_2 is determined by the balance between CO_2 production ($\dot{V}CO_2$) and excretion under steady-state conditions (16). Excretion of CO_2 is determined by its pulmonary clearance, alveolar ventilation ($\dot{V}A$):

$$PACO_2 = PaCO_2 = K \times \dot{V}CO_2 / \dot{V}A \tag{5}$$

In Eq. (5), $\dot{V}CO_2$ is CO_2 production in mL/min, $\dot{V}A$ is CO_2 clearance in mL/min, $PACO_2$ is alveolar carbon dioxide tension, which is assumed to be equal to $PaCO_2$ in mmHg, and K is a number, which relates the different units in this equation. Equation (5) is called the alveolar ventilation equation.

Clearance of a substance is the amount of the substance removed from plasma per unit time, divided by the average plasma concentration. Equation (5) is a clearance equation. The relationship between $\dot{V}A$ and $PaCO_2$ (assumed to be equal to $PACO_2$) is depicted in Fig. 2. In the context of clearance,

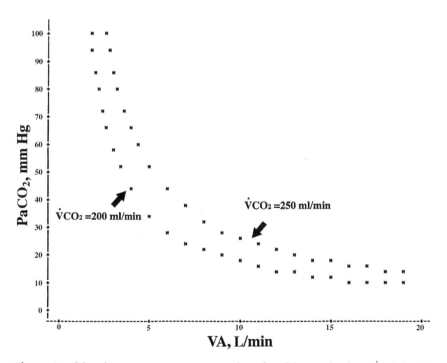

Figure 2 CO_2 clearance curves at two values for CO_2 production ($\dot{V}CO_2$), 200 and 250 mL/min. For a given level of CO_2 production, $PaCO_2$ increases as alveolar ventilation ($\dot{V}A$) falls.

alveolar ventilation is the virtual volume that removes all the CO_2 produced by the body per unit time in the steady state.

The same principle that relates serum creatinine to creatinine clearance also operates to relate $PaCO_2$ to alveolar ventilation. In this regard, the following applies:

$$\text{Creatinine production} = U_{creatinine} \times V \tag{6}$$

Because urine volume (V) is analogous to exhaled volume ($\dot{V}E$) and urine creatinine concentration ($U_{creatinine}$) is analogous to CO_2 concentration in the mixed exhaled air ($FECO_2$), CO_2 production ($\dot{V}CO_2$) is related to CO_2 excretion in the steady state as follows:

$$\dot{V}CO_2 = \dot{V}E \times FECO_2 \tag{7}$$

As noted earlier, minute ventilation ($\dot{V}E$) includes both alveolar ventilation and dead space ventilation. Because venous CO_2 is cleared only by alveolar ventilation:

$$\dot{V}CO_2 = FECO_2 \times \dot{V}E = FACO_2 \times \dot{V}A \tag{8}$$

In Eq. (8), $FACO_2$ is the fractional concentration of CO_2 in alveolar air (also analogous to serum creatinine) and can be converted to $PACO_2$, partial pressure of CO_2 in alveolar air:

$$PACO_2 = FACO_2 \times (\text{Barometric pressure} - 47\,\text{mmHg}) \tag{9}$$

In this equation, 47 mmHg is the water vapor pressure at 37°C. Normally, we assume that partial pressure of PCO_2 in the alveolar air is equal to $PaCO_2$. Therefore, $FACO_2$, $PACO_2$, and $PaCO_2$ are all analogous to serum creatinine.

The alveolar ventilation equation [Eq. (5)] shows that when metabolism is stable (constant CO_2 production), $PACO_2$ is inversely proportional to $\dot{V}A$. Thus, if $\dot{V}A$ decreases by 50%, $PACO_2$ and $PaCO_2$ will double. The alveolar ventilation equation can be applied to a single lung unit or to a homogeneous normal lung if one assumes that $PACO_2$ is equal to $PaCO_2$ (17). In the presence of ventilation–perfusion mismatch, however, this assumption is invalid, because $PaCO_2$ and $PACO_2$ diverge. Therefore, alveolar ventilation cannot be accurately assessed. Despite this problem, the equation is commonly used to calculate $\dot{V}A$ in the presence of ventilation–perfusion mismatch. Under such circumstances, it is assumed that some lung units with homogenous gas exchange are present and the equation represents ventilation of these lung units. In the presence of hypercapnia, the calculated $\dot{V}A$ will be low, but the latter does not mean that the total air movement into and out of all lung units is necessarily low. In such settings, hypercapnia should not be equated with hypoventilation (discussed later).

When $PaCO_2$ is within the normal range, large changes in alveolar ventilation are required before appreciable changes in $PaCO_2$ are observed (Fig. 2). In contrast, when $PaCO_2$ is elevated, small changes in alveolar ventilation result in major changes in $PaCO_2$. This has important consequences with regard to oxygenation, because of the reciprocal relation between alveolar PO_2 and PCO_2. Administration of small doses of respiratory depressants, for example, may result in a major rise in $PaCO_2$ and a major drop in PaO_2 in hypercapnic states such as severe asthma and chronic obstructive pulmonary disease. When ventilation decreases during sleep, $PaCO_2$ normally rises by 4–6 mmHg. In a hypercapnic subject, however, the same decrement in ventilation increases $PaCO_2$ to a much greater extent, causing clinically significant oxygen desaturation.

PATHOPHYSIOLOGY OF ALTERATIONS IN $PaCO_2$

$PaCO_2$ is determined by the balance between CO_2 production and alveolar ventilation. $PaCO_2$ will increase when either CO_2 production increases or alveolar ventilation decreases or a combination of the two, and will decrease when either CO_2 production decreases or alveolar ventilation increases. During wakefulness at sea level, normal $PaCO_2$ is 40 mmHg. When $PaCO_2$ is <36 mmHg, hypocapnia is diagnosed, and when $PaCO_2$ is >44 mmHg hypercapnia is diagnosed. The term hypoventilation is not synonymous with hypercapnia. Although hypoventilation results in hypercapnia (see earlier), it is not the only cause. In many disorders causing hypercapnia, minute ventilation and therefore air movement into and out of lung may be normal or increased. In fact, hypercapnia frequently occurs in the absence of hypoventilation in disorders such as chronic obstructive pulmonary disease. Hyperventilation and tachypnea are also often used synonymously. However, hyperventilation is defined as an increase in alveolar ventilation and tachypnea simply means rapid breathing.

Steady-state changes in CO_2 production reflect changes in metabolic rate (Table 1). Examples of increased CO_2 production include exercise, increased body weight, hyperthermia, hyperthyroidism, and carbohydrate utilization. Under normal conditions, an increase or decrease in CO_2 production does not change $PaCO_2$ because alveolar ventilation changes appropriately. For example, CO_2 production increases several folds during exercise, but $PaCO_2$ does not rise because alveolar ventilation increases in direct proportion to the increase in production [see Eq. (5)]. The mechanisms coupling CO_2 production to alveolar ventilation are complex and are not discussed further in this chapter.

If alveolar ventilation is kept constant and CO_2 production changes, $PaCO_2$ has to change proportionately [see Fig. 2 and Eq. (5)]. For example, under conditions of fixed mechanical ventilation, if CO_2 production

Table 1 Factors Altering CO_2 Production

Increased	Decreased
Exercise	Sleep, inactivity
Increased work of breathing	Decreased work of breathing; respiratory muscles rest; use of mechanical ventilation, paralyzing or sedating agents
Weight gain	Weight loss
Hyperthermia	Hypothermia
Hyperthyroidism	Hypothyroidism
Carbohydrate utilization	Fat utilization

increases, due to excessive utilization of carbohydrates, fever, use of respiratory muscles when fighting the ventilator, $PaCO_2$ will increase. Sedating agents are used to decrease excessive work of breathing and metabolic rate in order to lower CO_2 production. Maneuvers to decrease CO_2 production help to lower $PaCO_2$ and reciprocally increase PaO_2. Such maneuvers are particularly helpful when gas exchange is severely impaired. Under these conditions, high positive end-expiratory pressure, high fractional concentration of O_2 in inhaled air, or excessive ventilation may be necessary to provide acceptable levels of PaO_2 and $PaCO_2$. Lowering CO_2 production allows for decreasing the amount of inhaled O_2 to avoid O_2 toxicity, or lowering the tidal volume to avoid damage to the lung due to intermittent stretch. In the absence of fixed ventilation, alterations in $PaCO_2$ are invariably caused by alterations in alveolar ventilation rather than CO_2 production. The disorders causing hyper- and hypocapnia are discussed elsewhere (Chapters 20 and 21), but the major control mechanisms relating ventilation to $PaCO_2$ are reviewed here.

NORMAL CONTROL OF BREATHING

Overview

The respiratory apparatus controlling breathing has three components: sensors, controllers, and effectors (Fig. 3) (1). The controllers are the respiratory centers, which are the sites of respiratory rhythmogenesis, the most basic function underlying automatic breathing. The centers receive inputs from sensors located at various sites (Fig. 3). The sensors perceive changes in PCO_2, PO_2, [H^+] and lung inflation and send information (in the form of increased or decreased activity) to the controllers. After processing this information, the controllers alter the level of activity via efferent pathways (cranial, spinal, and phrenic nerves) to multiple effectors to modify their level of function (Figs. 3 and 4).

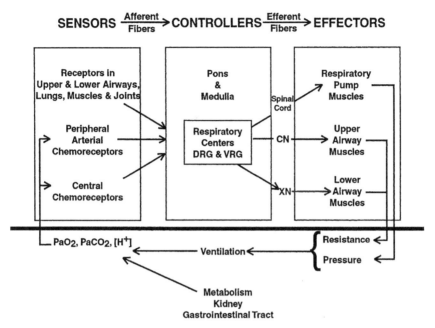

Figure 3 A simplified diagram of respiratory control system with its three major components. DRG = Dorsal respiratory group; VRG = Ventral respiratory group; CN = Cranial nerves; XN = 10th Cranial nerve.

The effectors are the thoracic inspiratory pump muscles, the muscles of the upper and lower airways, and expiratory abdominal muscles. The main inspiratory pump muscle is the diaphragm. The major respiratory muscles of the upper airways are the so-called upper airway dilators that regulate cross-sectional area and resistance. The activity of thoracic pump muscles provides the force behind inspiration (pressure, P), and the activity of muscles of the upper and lower airways determine airway resistance (R). Flow of air into the lung is determined according to

$$\text{Airflow} = P/R \tag{10}$$

Inspiration is an active process. Contraction of the inspiratory muscles (primarily the diaphragm) causes airflow into the lung by decreasing intrathoracic pressure. The rate of airflow, however, is determined by force of contraction reflected as Δ pressure, and the resistance of the respiratory system [Eq. (10)]. Normally, expiration is passive. During inspiration, the lung progressively increases in volume (and in its recoil) and when the diaphragm begins to relax at the end of inspiration, the unopposed inward recoil (created by inspiration) increases intrathoracic pressure and results in airflow

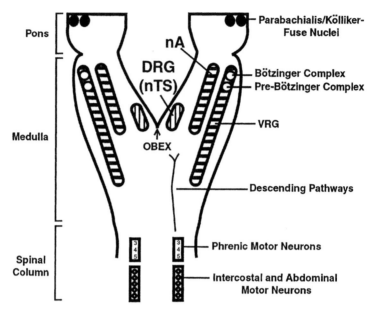

Figure 4   A cross-section of brainstem and spinal cord showing respiratory centers and some of the descending pathways. VRG, ventral respiratory group; DRG, dorsal respiratory group; NA, nucleus ambiguus.

out of the lung. During active expiration, contraction of the internal intercostal and abdominal muscles further facilitates airflow out of the lungs.

Pontomedullary Respiratory Centers

Breathing ceases in the absence of efferent output from the central nervous system. Respiratory rhythm persists after removal of the brain above the brainstem, but ceases after transection of the brainstem at the medullary-spinal level (18). Thus, rhythmogenesis is localized to the brainstem. The brainstem contains multiple neural aggregates located bilaterally (Fig. 4), whose activities have an oscillation linked to respiratory output (e.g., phrenic nerve motor activity) (19–23).

The pontine respiratory group (PRG) consists of two pairs of rostral pontine nuclei, the parabrachialis medialis and Kolliker–Fuse nuclear complex (NPBM-KF), corresponding to the pneumotaxic center. The function of these nuclei is to facilitate an earlier cut-off of inspiration, similar to that of vagal afferent pathway originating in the lung. Lesions of PRG in man cause apneustic breathing.

The medullary centers consist of two separate groups of nuclei, the dorsal (DRG) and ventral (VRG) respiratory groups (Fig. 4). The DRG is located in the dorsomedial part of the medulla, corresponding to the ventrolateral nucleus of the tractus solitarius (nTS in Fig. 4) and contains mainly inspiratory-related neurons. They receive afferent information from the peripheral arterial chemoreceptors, via the glossopharyngeal nerves, and from intrathoracic receptors, via the vagus nerves. The axonal projections of DRG exhibit discharge patterns similar to those of the phrenic or inspiratory intercostal activities. These projections cross the midline of medulla and terminate in the cervical and thoracic anterior spinal motor neurons of the phrenic and intercostal nerves.

The VRG is more diffuse than the DRG, consisting of many neural aggregates extending from the rostral to the caudal medulla. The VRG consists of the Bötzinger complex, pre-Bötzinger complex, nucleus ambiguus (NA), nucleus paraambigualis (NPA), and nucleus retroambigualis (NRA) (Fig. 4). The pre-Bötzinger complex is probably the site of respiratory rhythm generation (22). The VRG contains neurons that are active both during inspiration and expiration, projecting to inspiratory and expiratory motor neurons.

Destruction of respiratory centers may result in respiratory failure. However, because these centers are bilateral, a pathological process, such as an infarct, would have to be bilateral or otherwise very extensive, in order to cause complete cessation of respiration.

Efferent Pathways

The inspiratory and expiratory pump muscles and the muscles of the upper airway all receive rhythmic activity from the respiratory centers via descending neural pathways (Figs. 3 and 4). The pump muscles provide the pressure and the airway muscles determine the resistance. Pressure and resistance are the two determinants of airflow through airways [Eq. (10)].

The diaphragm, intercostal and abdominal muscles are activated by spinal α-motor neurons (Fig. 4). Phrenic motor neurons lie in the third, fourth, and fifth cervical segments and motor neurons of intercostal and abdominal muscles extend from thoracic to upper lumbar spinal cord. Because the diaphragm is the main inspiratory muscle (see below), cervical pathology involving third, fourth, and fifth segments results in hypoventilation and respiratory failure.

Cranial nerves innervate muscles of the upper and lower airways. The neural mechanisms controlling upper airway muscles are of critical importance in upper airway occlusion and obstructive sleep apnea–hypopnea. The vagus nerves control the tone of the smooth muscles of the intrathoracic airways. Increases in vagal activity to these muscles decrease airway cross-sectional area, resulting in airway constriction and bronchospasm. In severe asthma and exacerbation of chronic obstructive pulmonary disease, increased airway resistance could contribute to hypercapnia by increasing work of breathing.

Peripheral Arterial Chemoreceptors (PCR) and PO_2 Homeostasis

The peripheral arterial chemoreceptors include the carotid and aortic bodies, which show chemosensitivity to changes in blood PO_2, PCO_2, and $[H^+]$. The carotid bodies are located in the tissue between the internal and external carotid arteries and the aortic bodies are located at the arch of aorta (Fig. 5). The carotid bodies should not be mistaken for the carotid sinuses, which are located in the wall of the internal carotid arteries and are baroreceptors sensing changes in blood pressure.

The carotid bodies are the predominant arterial chemoreceptors, stimulating ventilation in response to decreased PaO_2 (hypoxemia) (Fig. 5). In the absence of carotid bodies, hypoxemia causes ventilatory depression (23,24). There are two cell types in the carotid bodies, type I and II cells. Type I cells (the glomus cells) are the cells involved in chemotransduction (25) via transmission to the sensory endings of the carotid sinus nerve, a branch of the glossopharyngeal nerve. The afferent information from the carotid body goes to the nucleus tractus solitarius in the medulla (Fig. 4).

The feedback loop involving the carotid bodies is illustrated in Fig. 6. Hypoxemia stimulates the carotid bodies causing an increase in afferent impulses to the brainstem respiratory centers (nTS). Increased activity from the respiratory centers to the upper airway muscles decreases airway

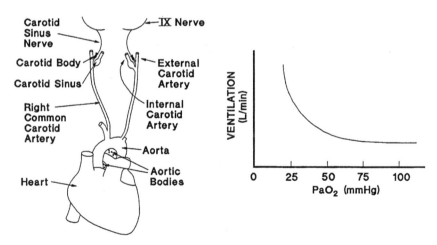

Figure 5 Diagram showing locations of peripheral arterial chemoreceptors and the related ventilatory response to hypoxemia mediated primarily by carotid bodies. Note the hyperbolic nature of ventilatory response, and that arterial PO_2 must decrease considerably before appreciable changes in ventilation are noted.

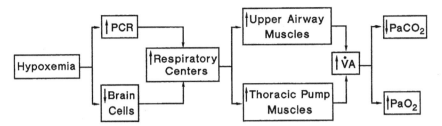

Figure 6 The feedback loop involving carotid bodies (PCR) in the response to hypoxemia. Hypoxemia results in both an increase in the force of breathing and a decrease in airway resistance, increasing airflow into the lung. Increased ventilation increases the clearance of CO_2 and therefore $PaCO_2$ decreases as PaO_2 increases.

resistance, and to the thoracic pump muscles increases the force of breathing. Alveolar ventilation thus increases [see Eq. (10)], delivering more O_2 and removing more CO_2. As a result, PaO_2 increases (and $PaCO_2$ decreases), removing the initial stimulus of hypoxemia.

The importance of the carotid and aortic bodies in O_2 homeostasis is demonstrated by travel to high altitude. Despite a progressive drop in atmospheric PO_2, compensatory hyperventilation allows for maintenance of adequate PO_2 for survival (26). In various cardiopulmonary disorders the ventilation–perfusion mismatch results in impairment of gas exchange across alveolar-capillary membrane (17,27,28). If no ventilatory compensation occurred, severe hypoxemia and hypercapnia would ensue. These adverse events are minimized by the actions of the peripheral chemoreceptors.

As shown in Fig. 5, PaO_2 falls to 55–60 mmHg before the receptors are stimulated to increase ventilation. Thus, hyperventilation cannot be ascribed to hypoxemia unless $PaO_2 \leq 55$–60 mmHg. As PaO_2 decreases further, ventilation progressively increases. These characteristics are due to the hyperbolic nature of the changes in the rate of discharge of afferent nerve fibers from the carotid body, and are reflected in the hyperbolic changes in ventilation when PO_2 decreases. The carotid bodies sense PaO_2, not hemoglobin saturation or the O_2 content of the arterial blood. Thus, anemia and carbon monoxide inhalation are not associated with compensatory hyperventilation.

The ventilatory response to hypoxemia is quite variable, but the scatter diminishes within family members, suggesting that genetic factors may play an important role (29–31). Individuals with diminished O_2-chemosensitivity could be prone to develop hypercapnia in the face of ventilatory stress, such as asthma or chronic obstructive pulmonary disease (32–36).

Although the carotid bodies show chemosensitivity to changes in $PaCO_2$ and $[H^+]$ in addition to changes in PaO_2, their most important function is O_2 chemosensitivity. In metabolic acidosis, for example, the ventilatory response to an increase in arterial $[H^+]$ is preserved in animals with peripheral chemodenervation (37–40). This is not to say that the peripheral arterial chemoreceptors are H^+-insensitive; indeed they may be involved in initiating hyperventilation in metabolic acidosis (see later).

A low $PaCO_2$ can be seen in a variety of cardiopulmonary disorders in the absence of sufficient hypoxemia to stimulate the carotid bodies, and is due to stimulation of pulmonary airway and parenchymal receptors by pathological processes in the lung (Fig. 3) (41,42). This information is transferred from intrapulmonary receptors via vagus nerves to the nucleus tractus solitarius (Fig. 3), resulting in an increase in respiratory rate and ventilation.

Central Chemoreceptors and PCO_2 Homeostasis

The central chemoreceptors are located in the brain within the medulla (43–45), but are different from the respiratory centers discussed above. Evidence for their existence stems from the observation that infusion of acidic solution into cerebral ventricles stimulates ventilation (45–47). This response is maintained in animals with peripheral arterial chemodenervation (37–40). The central chemoreceptors are exquisitely sensitive to changes in $[H^+]$; small changes induced either by acid infusion or changes in PCO_2 elicit a brisk ventilatory response (46,47).

This information is signaled to respiratory centers (Fig. 2) and causes changes in alveolar ventilation and $PaCO_2$ that mitigate the changes in $[H^+]$ induced initially by the acid–base perturbation. This feedback loop is similar to that described earlier for peripheral chemoreceptors when PO_2 changes. However, the ventilatory response of central chemoreceptors to changes in $[H^+]$ is linear (Fig. 7).

Early studies (43,44) identified superficial areas on the ventrolateral aspect of the medulla, designated M, S, and L for the scientists who discovered them (Fig. 7). Areas M and L are chemosensitive and presumably their outputs converge into area S which is not chemosensitive. Deeper chemoreceptors are present as well (48–50).

The stimulus to the central chemoreceptors is the $[H^+]$ in their environment, although PCO_2 may have an independent effect (51–53).

The central chemoreceptors are separated from the blood by the blood–brain barrier, which is formed anatomically by the tight junctions between the endothelial cells of the cerebral capillaries (54). Because the blood–brain barrier resists ionic diffusion, it takes several minutes for changes in plasma $[H^+]$ to be reflected in cerebral fluids (55,56). As noted earlier, it is therefore conceivable that the initial hyperventilatory response to metabolic acidosis, particularly if the process is mild, is mediated via carotid bodies.

Changes in brain extracellular fluid $[H^+]$ are smaller than corresponding changes in plasma $[H^+]$ in both metabolic acidosis and alkalosis (55,56). This difference occurs because the blood–brain barrier can transport various

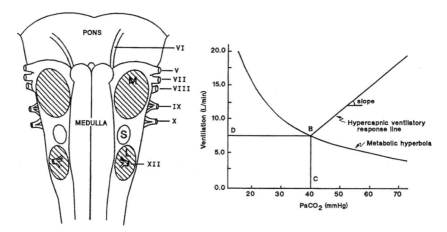

Figure 7 Location of the central chemoreceptors (labeled M, S, and L) and the related ventilatory response to CO_2. Note that resting $PaCO_2$ is at the point where the line defining ventilatory response and the curve defining the CO_2 hyperbola meet. Also note that ventilatory response to CO_2 is linear and any increment in PCO_2 elicits a response.

ions into and out of extracellular fluid, thereby regulating ionic composition of the brain extracellular fluid (57–59).

In contrast to somewhat slow changes in cerebral fluid [H^+] during metabolic acid–base changes in plasma, brain extra- and intracellular fluid [H^+] increases rapidly with acute increases in $PaCO_2$ (55,60). This rapid increase in [H^+] occurs because CO_2 diffuses quickly across the blood–brain barrier. In brain fluids, CO_2 is hydrated to form carbonic acid, which is dissociated to H^+ and HCO_3^-. The excess [H^+] stimulates the central chemoreceptors. The opposite occurs with hypocapnia.

The sensitivity or gain of the central chemoreceptors to changes in PCO_2 exceeds that of the peripheral chemoreceptors. Overall, most of the steady-state ventilatory response to changes in [H^+] (metabolic or respiratory) is mediated by the central chemoreceptors. As noted earlier, in response to severe metabolic acidosis, hyperventilation occurs equally before and after denervation of the peripheral chemoreceptors (37–40).

Carbon dioxide chemosensitivity varies considerably among normal individuals. There are the so-called low and high responders. In low responders the rise in ventilation as PCO_2 increases is smaller than in high responders. Diminished CO_2 chemosensitivity may predispose an individual to CO_2 retention in the face of asthma and chronic obstructive pulmonary disease (31–35) when gas exchange abnormalities occur. In contrast, high responders may be predisposed to instabilities in breathing. For example, patients with heart failure and increased CO_2 chemosensitivity may be predisposed to develop central apnea during sleep (Cheyne–Stokes respiration) (61).

OVERVIEW OF MECHANISMS CAUSING CHANGES IN $PaCO_2$

Hypercapnia

Hypercapnia occurs when the rate of alveolar ventilation is insufficient for elimination of CO_2. Four pathogenetic mechanisms can cause hypercapnia (Table 2): (1) ventilation–perfusion inequality (V/Q mismatch), (2) hypoventilation (decreased $\dot{V}E$), (3) a pattern of breathing characterized by shallow breaths (low tidal volume), and (4) increased CO_2 production. In three of these, V/Q mismatch, shallow breathing, or increased CO_2 production, "compensatory" increases in ventilation may occur that can ameliorate or eliminate the hypercapnia. For example, the increase in CO_2 production that accompanies exercise is coupled with a parallel increase in $\dot{V}A$, such that $PaCO_2$ remains constant.

Clinical causes of hypercapnia can be divided into three categories: (1) pathophysiological processes affecting chemoreflex system, (2) disorders of neuromuscular system, and (3) disorders of ventilatory apparatus (airways, lung parenchyma, and chest wall). Hypoventilations due to metabolic alkalosis or administration of respiratory depressants are examples of reversible processes affecting the chemoreflex system. Severe asthma, severe acute respiratory distress syndrome, and kyphoscoliosis are, respectively, examples of disorders of airways, lung parenchyma and chest wall causing hypercapnia. Table 3 shows some of the processes mediating hypercapnia in part based on factors controlling respiration shown in Fig. 3. For further details of disorders causing hypercapnia, see Chapter 20.

Hypocapnia

Hyperventilation occurs when alveolar ventilation exceeds the amount necessary for elimination of CO_2. Alveolar hyperventilation is caused by an abnormally excessive ventilatory drive, persisting despite the resultant

Table 2 Pathogenic Mechanisms of Hypercapnia

1.	V/Q mismatch (most common)	Various CP disorders
2.	Hypoventilation	Respiratory depression
3.	Shallow breathing	Various CP disorders
4.	Increased CO_2 production	Unlikely cause of hypercapnia

In 1, 3, and 4, "compensatory" mechanisms may occur that can prevent development of hypercapnia.
V/Q, ventilation/perfusion; CP, cardiopulmonary.

Table 3 Some Disorders and Their Mechanisms Mediating Hypercapnia

Sites	Stimuli/factors	Conditions
I. Controllers (DRG/VRG)	Necrosis, inflammation	Brainstem infract (usually bilateral), encephalitis
II. Descending pathways, spinal cord, nerves, neuromuscular junction	Inflammation, injury, autoimmune drugs	ALS, GBS, C_{3-5} trauma, MG, procainamide toxicity
III. Effectors		
Muscles	Inflammation, energetics	Muscular dystrophy, diaphragmatic fatigue
Chest wall	Congenital/genetic	Kyphoscoliosis, obesity, and OSAHS
Airways	Bronchospasm	Severe asthma, COPD
Lungs	V/Q mismatch	Severe asthma or COPD, severe pulmonary edema, severe ARDS
IV. PCR	a. Hyperoxia	COPD with hypercapnia
	b. Alkalemia	Metabolic alkalemia
	c. Decreased hypoxic chemosensitivity	COPD, asthma
V. CCR	a. Alkalemia	Metabolic alkalemia
	b. Drugs	Opiates, benzodiazepines
	c. Decreased CO_2 chemosensitivity	Primary alveolar hypo-ventilation syndrome COPD, asthma, OSAHS

DRG, dorsal respiratory groups; VRG, ventral respiratory group; ALS, amyotrophic lateral sclerosis; MG, myasthenia gravis; GBS, Gillian Barre syndrome; V/Q, ventilation/perfusion; PCR, peripherial arterial chemoreceptors; CCR, central chemoreceptors; CNS, central nervous system; CSF, cerebrospinal fluid; ARDS, acute respiratory distress syndrome; COPD, chronic obstructive pulmonary disease; OSAHS, obstructive sleep apnea–hypopnea syndrome.

fall in PCO_2, which should decrease ventilation by the feedback loop discussed earlier in this chapter.

The excessive ventilatory drive is mediated by disorders affecting either the metabolic or behavioral control system. Engagement of the automatic metabolic pathway in hyperventilation occurs via stimulation of peripheral arterial or central chemoreceptors or pulmonary airway or parenchymal receptors (Fig. 3). Psychogenic hyperventilation is an example of a behavioral (cortical) mechanism of hyperventilation. Using Fig. 3 as a model, some of the causes of hyperventilation are depicted in Table 4. For further details of the disorders causing hypocapnia, see Chapter 21.

Table 4 Some Disorders and Their Mechanisms Mediating Hypocapnia

Sensors	Stimuli/factors	Conditions
I. PCR	a. Hypoxemia	High-altitude cardiopulmonary disorders[a]
	b. Acidemia	Metabolic acidemia
	c. Drugs	Almitrine, doxapram
II. CCR	a. Hormones & drugs, progesterone, salicylate	Pregnancy; liver disease, salicylate poisoning
	b. Acidemia	Metabolic acidemia
	c. CSF lactacidosis	Central neurogenic hyperventilation, intracranial hemorrhage, CNS malignancy
III. Cortical	Anxiety	Psychogenic hyperventilation
IV. Pulmonary receptors (J or irritant)	Inflammatory mediators, increased interstitial pressure	Cardiopulmonary disorders

[a]Cardiopulmonary disorders such as pulmonary congestion/edema, pulmonary embolism, pneumonias, interstitial lung disorders, and mild asthma.
PCR, peripheral arterial chemoreceptors; CCR, central chemoreceptors; CSF, cerebro spinal fluid; CNS, central nervous system.

CHANGES IN PaCO$_2$ IN METABOLIC ACID–BASE DISTURBANCES

Metabolic Alkalosis

Metabolic alkalosis increases PaCO$_2$ in a predictable fashion (62,63). The fall in [H$^+$] in the blood and brain caused by metabolic alkalosis decreases the activity of the peripheral and central chemoreceptors (Fig. 8). As a result, medullary respiratory output to inspiratory muscles decreases and minute and alveolar ventilation decrease, increasing alveolar and arterial PCO$_2$. The rise in PaCO$_2$ increases [H$^+$], which mitigates the initial drop in [H$^+$] due to metabolic alkalosis (see Chapter 16).

Metabolic alkalosis causing hypercapnia is an example of hypoventilation (Table 2). The decreased minute and alveolar ventilation is brought about primarily by a reduction in tidal volume (Table 5) (62). Assuming a constant dead space, a fall in tidal volume decreases alveolar ventilation. As an example, with dead space of 150 mL and tidal volume of 450 mL, VD/VT ratio is 1/3 and alveolar volume of each breath is 300 mL (Fig. 1). With respiratory rate of 15/min, alveolar ventilation is 4.5 L/min. If tidal volume is decreased to 300 mL per breath (about 30% reduction from

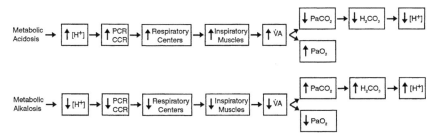

Figure 8 Diagram of the negative feedback loop involving the carotid bodies (PCR) and central chemoreceptors (CCR) in mediating hyper- or hypoventilation as [H⁺] changes in metabolic acid–base disorders.

baseline), then VD/VT ratio is 1/2 and alveolar volume of this breath is 150 mL. With the same respiratory rate of 15/min, alveolar ventilation becomes 2.25 L/min, doubling arterial PCO_2. In order to decrease alveolar ventilation by the same amount with only a reduction in respiratory rate, the respiratory rate would have to fall from 15 to 7.5 breaths/min (50% reduction). Therefore, decreasing tidal volume is a very efficient way to decrease alveolar ventilation.

Metabolic Acidosis

Metabolic acidosis decreases $PaCO_2$ in a predictable fashion (62,64) (see Chapter 9). The rise in [H⁺] caused by metabolic acidosis is reflected in the environment of the peripheral and central chemoreceptors, which collectively increase afferent activity to respiratory centers. This, in turn, causes augmented output to the respiratory muscles (Fig. 8), causing a rise in alveolar ventilation and a fall in $PaCO_2$. The fall in PCO_2 reduces extra- and intracellular [H⁺] mitigating the initial rise due to metabolic acidosis.

In response to metabolic acidosis, $PaCO_2$ is decreased primarily by increasing tidal volume. As discussed earlier, this is a more efficient way to achieve a given change in alveolar ventilation than is an increase in respiratory rate (Table 6). For example, to increase alveolar ventilation from 4.5 to 6.7 L/min, the respiratory rate has to increase from 15 to 22.5 if tidal volume remains constant (Table 6). However, the same increment in alveolar ventilation can be achieved by increasing tidal volume form 450 to 600 mL without changing respiratory rate.

Because small increases in tidal volume can decrease $PaCO_2$ considerably, it is often difficult to notice the compensatory hyperventilation at the bedside, unless metabolic acidosis is so severe to make the increase in the depth of breathing visually apparent (Kussmaul's sign). The difficulty in appreciating an increase in the depth of breathing contrasts with the easily recognizable tachypnea observed in various diseases such as pneumonia,

Table 5 Ventilation Under Baseline, Acidotic, and Alkalotic Conditions in Six Normal Subjects

	[H$^+$] (nmol/l)	PaCO$_2$ (mmHg)	[HCO$_3^-$] (mmol/L)	PaO$_2$ (mmHg)	V̇E (L/min)	RR (/min)	VT (ml)	V̇A (L/min)	VD (ml)	VD/VT (%)	V̇CO$_2$ (ml/min)
Baseline	38±1	38±1	24±0.4	94±4	6±0.2	12±2	522±72	4.4±0.3	90±10	18±3	177±18
Metabolic alkalosis	31*±1	44*±1	34*±2	85*±4	5*±0.1	13±2	422*±55	3.2*±0.2	101±6	29*±3	156±14
Metabolic acidosis	46*±1	32*±1	17*±0.2	109*±4	7*±0.1	12±2	624*±92	—	—	—	—

Values are means ± 1SE. There were 14 episodes of metabolic alkalosis and seven episodes of metabolic acidosis.
V̇E = exhaled volume; RR = respiratory rate; V̇CO$_2$ = carbon dioxide production; VT = tidal volume; V̇A = alveolar ventilation; VD = dead space.
*Significant vs. baseline. *Source*: Modified from Ref. 62.

Table 6 Theoretical Examples Showing Differences in Respiratory Rate vs. Tidal Volume to Achieve the Same Alveolar Ventilation

	VT (mL)	RR (/min)	$\dot{V}E$ (mL/min)	VD (mL)	$\dot{V}A$ (mL/min)	$\dot{V}D$ (mL/min)
Baseline	450	15	6750	150	4500	2250
Increased RR	450	22.5	10125	150	6750	3375
Increased VT	600	15	9000	150	6750	2250

A higher minute ventilation is necessary to achieve the same alveolar ventilation with tachypnea than by increasing tidal volume. In this example, dead space was kept constant, though with an increase in tidal volume and lung stretch, the anatomical dead space also increases slightly. VT = tidal volume; RR, respiratory rate; VD = dead space; $\dot{V}A$ = alveolar ventilation; $\dot{V}E$ = minute ventilation; $\dot{V}D$ = dead space ventilation.

pulmonary embolism, congestive heart failure, or interstitial lung diseases. As is discussed below, the rise in respiratory rate in these disorders is almost always due to stimulation of pulmonary airway and parenchymal receptors brought about by the pathological process in the lung (Fig. 3).

CHANGES IN PaCO$_2$ IN CARDIOPULMONARY DISORDERS

Decreased PaCO$_2$

Hypocapnia occurs in a variety of cardiopulmonary disorders, including pulmonary edema, asthma, interstitial lung diseases, and pulmonary embolism. Assuming that these disorders do not alter or minimally affect CO_2 production, the fall in PaCO$_2$ is primarily due to an increase in alveolar ventilation [Eq. (5)]. The increase in alveolar ventilation in these disorders is due to an increase in respiratory rate. Increasing alveolar ventilation primarily by a change in rate (Table 6), tachypnea, is easily recognizable at the bedside and is characteristic of a pathological process in the lung. Typically, the pattern of breathing is rapid and shallow.

In all these disorders, ventilation and perfusion are increasingly mismatched. In lung units with a low ventilation/perfusion ratio, the amount of ventilation is inadequate for the corresponding blood flow, resulting in inadequate O_2 delivery and insufficient CO_2 removal. Consequently, regional alveolar PO$_2$ (and therefore regional capillary PO$_2$) is reduced, and regional alveolar PCO$_2$ (and therefore regional capillary PCO$_2$) is increased. Without an increase in ventilation, hypoxemia and hypercapnia will develop (17,27,28). However, alveolar ventilation typically increases by a variety of signaling and effector mechanisms (discussed earlier). When PCO$_2$ increases because of the V/Q mismatch, ventilation is stimulated primarily by central chemoreceptors. The ventilatory response to CO_2 is linear and any small increment in PCO$_2$ will increase ventilation. This feedback mechanism is an attempt to maintain PCO$_2$ close to normal and should not cause hypocapnia. However, when PaO_2 decreases, ventilation is stimulated by peripheral chemoreceptors. As noted earlier, hypoxemia must be relatively severe before noticeable chemostimulation occurs, but this feedback mechanism can result in hypocapnia. Alveolar ventilation may also increase due to an increase in respiratory rate. Tachypnea is caused by stimulation of intrapulmonary receptors by the pathological process in the lung. Depending, collectively, on the severity of V/Q mismatch, CO_2 production and the three compensatory mechanisms to increase alveolar ventilation, $PaCO_2$ may be normal or decreased, or rarely increased.

Although patients with V/Q mismatch commonly have normal or a low $PaCO_2$, hypoxemia is invariably present. PaO_2 decreases because the O_2 content of the blood leaving areas with high V/Q ratios is not sufficiently increased to compensate for the low O_2 content of the blood emanating from low V/Q areas. Therefore, the characteristic arterial blood gas findings in these disorders are hypoxemia with either normal $PaCO_2$ or chronic hypocapnia (chronic respiratory alkalosis).

In the presence of hypocapnia, the severity of gas exchange abnormalities is commonly underestimated. As noted earlier, when PCO_2 decreases (or increases), the PO_2 should rise (or decrease) almost equally. A PaO_2 of 75 mmHg thus signifies a considerably greater abnormality in gas exchange across the alveolar capillary membrane if $PaCO_2$ is 20 rather than 40 mmHg.

Increased PaCO$_2$

Hypercapnia is observed in the course of a variety of cardiopulmonary disorders as the severity of the pathological process intensifies. In chronic obstructive pulmonary disease and asthma, hypercapnia is observed when forced expiratory volume in 1 sec (a surrogate of severity of the disorder) has decreased to values approaching 1 L/sec, about 20–30% of predicted (Fig. 9) (65–79). Milder obstructive defects are not associated with hypercapnia unless additional factors contribute. For example, a eucapnic individual with moderate chronic obstructive pulmonary disease may develop hypercapnia if pneumonia or congestive heart failure develops, increasing ventilation–perfusion mismatch.

The mechanisms of hypercapnia in severe asthma and chronic obstructive pulmonary disease are multifactorial and relate to a complex interaction of severity of ventilation perfusion mismatch, work of breathing and CO_2 production, pattern of breathing, and O_2–CO_2 chemosensitivity. The role of diminished O_2–CO_2 chemosensitivity in predisposing an individual with chronic obstructive pulmonary disease (34–36) or asthma (32,33) to hypercapnia has already been discussed (see earlier). Increased work of breathing due to elevated airway resistance and mechanical impediment results in excessive CO_2 production and contributes to hypercapnia [Eq. (6)].

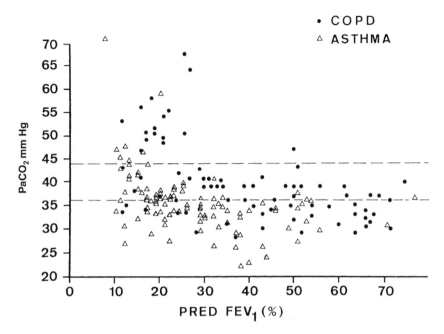

Figure 9 Diagram showing that in both chronic obstructive pulmonary disease and asthma, CO_2 retention occurs mostly when mechanical impairment, as measured by forced expiratory volume in one second (FEV_1), is severe. PRED = Predicted.*Source*: Modified from Refs. 65, 66.

The two major reasons for hypercapnia, however, are probably ventilation–perfusion mismatch impairing CO_2 clearance (26–28) and shallow tidal volume (71,72). When hypercapnic and eucapnic subjects are matched for severity of mechanical impairment and CO_2 production, the breathing pattern appears to be the main factor determining $PaCO_2$ (72). Both groups had similar minute ventilation, metabolic rate (CO_2 production), and absolute volume of dead space (Table 7). Hypercapnic subjects, however, breathed faster and shallower than eucapnic subjects and the lower tidal volume resulted in lower alveolar ventilation (Table 7). Recall that for any given minute ventilation and dead space, a reduction in tidal volume due to shallower breathing causes an increase in VD/VT, resulting in "wasted" breathing, that is, a decrease in alveolar ventilation. Thus, for any minute ventilation, dead space volume and CO_2 production rate, low tidal volume causes CO_2 retention, as the proportion of alveolar ventilation decreases.

Although not well studied, shallow breathing may also contribute to hypercapnia in severe pulmonary edema, acute respiratory distress syndrome, and during exacerbation of chronic obstructive pulmonary

Table 7   Chronic Hypercapnia in Chronic Obstructive Pulmonary Disease

$PaCO_2$ (mmHg)	RR (min)	VT (mL)	$\dot{V}E$ (L/min)	VD (mL)	$\dot{V}D$ (L/min)	$\dot{V}A$ (L/min)	$\dot{V}CO_2$ (mL/min)
40	16	463	7.6	179	3.0	4.7	212
50*	22*	355*	7.8	181	4.0*	3.8*	222

In the face of similar minute ventilation ($\dot{V}E$), dead space volume (VD), and CO_2 production ($\dot{V}CO_2$), hypercapnia occurred. This was due to shallow breathing resulting in decreased alveolar ventilation. Note that in each group, the sum of alveolar and dead space ventilation is equal to minute ventilation. *Source*: Values have been rounded from Ref. 72.
* $P < 0.05$.

disease. As these disorders are appropriately treated with antibiotics, bronchodilators and diuretics, the depth of breathing increases, the VD/VT ratio and wasted ventilation decrease while alveolar ventilation increases. Treatment also improves ventilation–perfusion mismatch, facilitating effective gas exchange.

Stable patients with interstitial lung diseases rarely develop hypercapnia, despite hypoxemia (66). In 60 subjects mostly diagnosed by lung biopsy, only two had a $PaCO_2$ > 44 mmHg (66). Hypercapnia in interstitial lung disease is rare for a variety of reasons. The main reason is that the decrease in tidal volume is counterbalanced by an increase in respiratory rate, so that adequate minute and alveolar ventilation are maintained. In addition, CO_2 production does not increase as mechanical impairment worsens (66).

HYPERCAPNIA IN NEUROMUSCULAR DISORDERS

Neuromuscular disorders comprise a major category of diseases causing hypercapnia (73). These disorders may involve the brainstem respiratory centers, the motor neurons located in the anterior horns of the spinal cord or their axons, the neuromuscular junctions or the muscle cells themselves (Fig. 3). The common final pathway in diseases causing hypercapnia, however, is diaphragmatic weakness or paralysis.

If respiratory centers are damaged by medullary infarction, hypoventilation may ensue. Because respiratory centers are widespread and bilateral (see earlier), the infarct must be extensive. Neuromuscular disorders involving the spinal cord (e.g., multiple sclerosis, amyotrophic lateral sclerosis), nerves (C_3–C_5 trauma causing phrenic nerve injury and diaphragmatic paralysis) or neuromuscular junction (Guillain Barre syndrome) are common causes of hypercapnia (Fig. 5).

Patients with neuromuscular disorders involving the diaphragm may present with orthopnea because diaphragmatic dysfunction is worse in the supine position. Therefore, they may be misdiagnosed as having congestive heart failure (74). An important physical finding is paradoxical thoracoabdominal excursions, which should alert the clinician that diaphragmatic weakness is present (74). Subjects with neuromuscular disorders may first manifest hypercapnia only during sleep, or when another pathological process such as pneumonia stresses the respiratory system.

If hypercapnia is due solely to hypoventilation, hypoxemia should be proportional to hypercapnia and alveolar–arterial PO_2 difference should remain normal. If hypoxemia is greater than predicted by the rise in $PaCO_2$, the presence of a parenchymal process such as aspiration pneumonia or pulmonary embolism should be suspected. Subjects with neuromuscular disorders are prone to develop aspiration pneumonia (due to involvement of pharyngeal muscles) or pulmonary embolism (due to sedentary status).

OBESITY–HYPOVENTILATION SYNDROME

The obesity–hypoventilation syndrome is characterized by obesity and hypercapnia. Subjects with the syndrome commonly have excessive daytime sleepiness, high hematocrit and, in more advanced cases, cardiovascular complications such as right heart failure. Although the disorder is called obesity–hypoventilation syndrome, no systematic studies measuring minute and alveolar ventilation have been reported.

Most subjects with obesity–hypoventilation syndrome have obstructive sleep apnea–hypopnea syndrome. Characteristically, repetitive episodes of complete (obstructive apnea) or incomplete upper airway occlusion (obstructive hypopnea) occur during sleep and are terminated by arousal (75). On awakening, upper airway patency is restored and normal ventilation resumes until sleep recurs. Occlusive episodes are due to relaxation of dilator muscles of the upper airway during sleep, occurring in an individual with an anatomically small upper airway, most commonly due to obesity. Obesity is the most important risk factor for of obstructive sleep apnea–hypopnea syndrome. Episodes of apnea and hypopnea may be repeated hundreds of times during sleep in the form of periodic breathing. As a result, hypoxemia and hypercapnia develop, which eventually can cause cardiovascular complications such as hypertension, heart failure, and stroke. Daytime sleepiness is due to repetitive arousals and poor sleep quality.

A minority of patients with obstructive sleep apnea–hypopnea syndrome have daytime hypercapnia. Daytime hypercapnia in this disorder is probably multifactorial in pathogenesis (Fig. 10) (75). While asleep, hypercapnia occurs when ventilation ceases or decreases. The magnitude and duration of this nocturnal hypercapnia depends on the number and duration of these episodes. Upon termination by arousal, hyperpnea occurs correcting the blood gas abnormalities. The magnitude of hyperpnea required to excrete

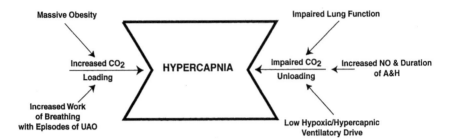

Figure 10   Mechanisms mediating CO_2 retention in obstructive sleep apnea–hypopnea syndrome. There is an imbalance between CO_2 loading and unloading processes during sleep. Eventually, nocturnal hypercapnia leads to diurnal hypercapnia. *Source*: Modified from Ref. 75.

the accumulated CO_2 (and replenish O_2) depends on the ability to increase ventilation, intrinsic chemosensitivity, and normal gas exchange. Mechanical impediments, due to chronic obstructive pulmonary disease or severe obesity (restrictive defect), may decrease the ability to respond appropriately to hypercapnia and hypoxemia and thereby limit CO_2 excretion (the "cannot breathe" mechanism). A subject with diminished hypoxic and hypercapnic chemosensitivity may not unload the accumulated CO_2 (and replenish O_2) during the intervals between apneic periods when hyperpnea should occur (the "won't breathe" mechanism). In parenchymal lung disorders with V/Q mismatch, CO_2 unloading is further impaired during hyperpnea. Excessive CO_2 production due to massive obesity also increases the CO_2 load and may contribute to hypercapnia (Fig. 10) (75).

With sustained impairment in CO_2 unloading during sleep, nocturnal CO_2 retention leads eventually to daytime CO_2 retention, perhaps due to a resetting in central chemosensitivity (76). A resetting of peripheral chemo-receptors may also occur as demonstrated in other disorders with chronic hypoxemia (77). Familial variations in chemosensitivity do not appear to be contributing to the likelihood of sustained hypercapnia in the obesity–hypoventilation syndrome (78).

A subset of patients with obesity but without evidence of obstructive sleep apnea–hypopnea may also develop hypercapnia. The mechanisms of hypercapnia in these patients remain unclear, but probably include high CO_2 production, reduced chest wall compliance, V/Q mismatch and decreased respiratory muscle strength. Subjects with obesity and hypercap-nia should always undergo testing to determine if obstructive sleep apnea–hypopnea is present, because this problem can be treated effectively with mechanical ventilatory devices such as nasal continuous positive airway pressure or bilevel ventilation. In some of these patients, hypercapnia may improve or be reversed and morbidity decreased (79–82).

SUMMARY

The major function of the lungs is to regulate the partial pressures of both O_2 and CO_2 in the arterial blood in the face of varying metabolic and environmental conditions. From an acid–base perspective, this regulation acts to maintain intracellular pH close to neutrality, resulting in an arterial blood pH of 7.40. Arterial PCO_2 is regulated by a complex hierarchical system of peripheral and central nervous system sensors that respond to changes in pH and signal appropriate changes in alveolar ventilation. This regulation requires an intact neuromuscular signal-effector pathway, as well as an appropriate match between ventilation and perfusion of the lungs. Hypocapnia and hypercapnia can be the result of a normal adaptive response to superimposed acid–base disorders, or disruption of normal regulation by pulmonary, cardiopulmonary, neurologic, or neuromuscular disorders.

REFERENCES

1. Javaheri S, Anderson DK. Control of ventilation during wakefulness. In: Sperekalis N, Banks RO, eds. Essentials of Basic Science: Physiology. 2nd ed. Boston: Little Brown, 1996:387–396.
2. Rahn H, Baumgardner FW. Temperature and acid–base regulation in fish. Respir Physiol 1972; 14:171–182.
3. Rahn H. Why are pH of 7.4 and PCO_2 of 40 normal values for man?. Bull Eur Physiopath Respir 1976; 12:5–13.
4. Reeves HR, Howell BJ. Hydrogen ion regulation, temperature, and evolution. The 1975 J. Burns Aberson Lecture. Am Rev Respir Dis 1975; 112:165–172.
5. Rahn H. Body temperature and acid–base regulation. Pneumonologie 1974; 151:87–94.
6. Reeves RB. An imidazole alphastat hypothesis for vertebrate acid–base regulations: tissue carbon dioxide content and body temperature in bullfrogs. Respir Physiol 1972; 14:219–236.
7. Nattie EE. The alphastat hypothesis in respiratory control and acid–base balance. J Appl Physiol 1990; 69:1201–1207.
8. Hitzig BM, Perng WC, Burt T, Okunieff P, Johnson DC. ^{1}H-NMR measurement of fractional dissociation of imidazole in intact animals. Am J Physiol 1994; 266:R1008–R1015.
9. Somero GN. Protons, osmolytes, and fitness of internal milieu for protein function. Am J Physiol 1986; R251:R197–R213.
10. Davis BD. On the importance of being ionized. Arch Biochem Biophys 1958; 78:497–509.
11. Busa WB, Nuccitelli R. Metabolic regulation via intracellular pH. Am J Physiol 1984; 246:R409–R438.
12. Reeves RB. Temperature-induced changes in blood acid-base status: PH and PCO_2 in a binary buffer. J Appl Physiol 1976; 40:762–767.
13. Somero GN, White FN. Enzymatic consequences under alphastat regulation. In: Rahn H, Prakash O, eds. Acid–Base Regulation and Body Temperature. Hingham, MA: Nijhoff, 1985:55–80.

14. Burton RF. The role of imidazole ionization in the control of breathing. Comp Biochem Physiol 1986; 83:333–336.
15. Hitzig BM. Temperature-induced changes in turtle CSF pH and central control of ventilation. Respir Physiol 1982; 49:205–222.
16. Goldring RM, Heinemann HO, Turino GM. Regulation of alveolar ventilation in respiratory failure. Am J Med Sci 1975; 269:161–170.
17. West JB. Assessing pulmonary gas exchange. N Engl J Med 1987; 316: 1336–1338.
18. Lumsden T. Observation on the respiratory centres in the cat. J Physiol 1923; 57:153–160.
19. Euler CV. Brain stem mechanisms for generation and control of breathing pattern. In: Cherniack NS, Widdicombe JG, eds. Harbook of Physiology. The Respiratory System. Vol. II. New York: Oxford University Press, 1986.
20. Rekling JC, Feldman JL. Prebötzinger complex and pacemaker neurons: hypothesized site and kernel for respiratory rhythm generation. Ann Rev Physiol 1998; 60:385–405.
21. Ramirez JM, Richter DW. The neuronal mechanisms of respiratory rhythm generation. Curr Opin Neurobiol 1996; 6:817–825.
22. Funk GD, Feldman JL. Generation of respiratory rhythm and pattern in mammals: insights from development studies. Neurobiology 1995; 5:778–785.
23. Duffin J, Ezure K, Lipski J. Breathing rhythm generation: focus on the rostral ventrolateral medulla. NIPS 1995; 10:133–139.
24. Javaheri S, Teppema LJ. Ventral medullary extracellular fluid pH and PCO_2 during hypoxemia in anesthetized spontaneously breathing cats. J Appl Physiol 1987; 63:1567–1571.
25. Gonzales C, Dinger BG, Fidone SJ. Mechanisms of carotid body chemoreception. In: Dempsy JA, Pack AI, eds. Regulation of Breathing. 2nd ed. New York: Marcel Dekker, Inc., 1995; 291–448.
26. Winslow RM, Samaja M, West JB. Red cell function at extreme altitude on Mount Everest. J Appl Physiol 1984; 56:109–116.
27. West JB. Causes of carbon dioxide retention in lung disease. N Engl J Med 1971; 284:1232–1236.
28. Hughes JMB. Hypercapnia and gas exchange. Bull Eur Physiopath Respir 1979; 15:129–133.
29. Weil JV. Pulmonary hypertension and cor pulmonale in hypoventilating patients. In: Weir EK, Reeves TJ, eds. Pulmonary Hypertension. New York: Futura Publishing Company, Inc., 1984:321–339.
30. Scoggin CH, Doekel RD, Kryger MH, Zwillich W, Weil JV. Familial aspects of decreased hypoxic drive in endurance athletes. J Appl Physiol 1978; 44: 464–468.
31. Collins DD, Scoggin CH, Zwillich CW, Weil JV. Hereditary aspects of decreased hypoxic drive. J Clin Invest 1976; 62:105–110.
32. Rebuck AS, Read J. Patterns of ventilatory response to CO_2 during recovery from severe asthma. Clin Sci 1971; 41:13–21.
33. Hudgel DW, Weil JV. Asthma associated with decreased hypoxic ventilatory drive. A family study. Ann Intern Med 1974; 80:622–625.

34. Mountain R, Zwillich CW, Weil J. Hypoventilation in obstructive disease; the role of familial factors. N Engl J Med 1978; 298:521–525.
35. Fleetham JA, Arnup ME, Anthonisen NR. Familial aspects of ventilatory control in patients with chronic obstructive pulmonary disease. Am Rev Respir Dis 1984; 129:3–7.
36. Kawakami Y, Irie T, Shida A, Yoshikawa T. Familial factors affecting arterial blood gas values and respiratory chemosensitivity in chronic obstructive pulmonary disease. Am Rev Respir Dis 1982; 125:420–425.
37. Javaheri S, Herrera L, Kazemi H. Ventilatory drive in acute metabolic acidosis. J Appl Physiol 1979; 46:913–918.
38. Nattie EE. Ventilation during acute HCl infusion in intact and chemodenervated conscious rabbits. Respir Physiol 1983; 54:97–107.
39. Steinbrook RA, Javaheri S, Gabel RA, Donovan JC, Leith DE, Fencl V. Respiration of chemodenervated goats in acute metabolic acidosis. Respir Physiol 1984; 56:51–60.
40. Kaehny WD, Jackson JT. Respiratory response to HCl acidosis in dogs after carotid body denervation. J Appl Physiol Environ Exercise Physiol; 46: 1138–1142.
41. Paintal AS. The nature and effects of sensory inputs into the respiratory centers. Fed Proc 1977; 36:2428–2432.
42. Paintal AS. Vagal sensory receptors and their reflex effects. Physiol Rev 1973; 53:159–227.
43. Loeschcke HH. Respiratory chemosensitivity in the medulla oblongata. Acta Neurobiol Exp 1973; 33:97–112.
44. Schläfke ME, Pokorski M, See WR, Prill RK, Loeschcke HH. Chemosensitive neurons on the ventral medullary surface. Bull Physiopath Respir 1975; 11: 277–284.
45. Leusen IR. Chemosensitivity of the respiratory center. Influence of CO_2 in the cerebral ventricles on respiration. Am J Physiol 1954; 1976:39–44.
46. Pappenheimer JR, Fencle V, Heisey SR, Held D. Role of cerebral fluids in control of respiration as studied in unanesthetized goats. Am J Physiol 1965; 208:436–450.
47. Fencl V, Miller TB, Pappenheimer JR. Studies on the respiratory response to disturbances of acid–base balance, with deductions concerning the ionic composition of cerebral interstitial fluid. Am J Physiol 1966; 210:459–472.
48. Nattie EE, Li A. Central chemoreception in the region of the ventral respiratory group in the rat. J Appl Physiol 1996; 81:1987–1995.
49. Coates EL, Li A, Nattie EE. Widespread sites of brain stem ventilatory chemoreceptors. J Appl Physiol 1993; 75:5–14.
50. Nattie E. CO_2 brainstem chemoreceptors and breathing. Prog Neurobiol 1999; 59:299–331.
51. Teppema LJ, Barts PW, Folgering HT, Evers JA. Effects of respiratory and (isocapnic) metabolic arterial acid–base cats. Respir Physiol 1983; 53:379–395.
52. Eldrigde FL, Kiley JP, Millhorn DE. Respiratory responses to medullary hydrogen ion changes in cats: different effects of respiratory and metabolic acidosis. J Physiol (London); 358:285–297.

53. Shams H. Differential effects of CO_2 and H^+ as central stimuli of respiration in the cat. J Appl Physiol 1985; 58:357–364.
54. Sauders NR, Habgood MD, Dziegielewska. Barrier mechanisms in the brain, I. Adult brain. Clin Exp Pharmacol Physiol 1999; 26:11–19.
55. Javaheri S, Clendening A, Papadakis N, Brody JS. Changes in brain surface pH during acute isocapnic metabolic acidosis and alkalosis. J Appl Physiol 1981; 51:276–281.
56. Javaheri S, de Hemptinne A, Vanheel B, Leusen I. Changes in brain ECF pH during metabolic acidosis and alkalosis: a microelectrode study. J Appl Physiol 1983; 55:1849–1853.
57. Javaheri S, Wagner KR. Bumetanide decreases canine cerebrospinal fluid production. J Clin Invest 1993; 92:2257–2261.
58. Javaheri S, Weyne J, Demeester G, Leusen I. Effects of SITS, an anion transport blocker, on CSF ionic composition in metabolic alkalosis. J Appl Physiol Respir Environ Exercise Physiol 1984; 57:92–97.
59. Javaheri S, Weyne J. Effects of "DIDS", an anion transport blocker, on CSF $[HCO_3]$ in respiratory acidosis. Respir Physiol 1984; 57:365–376.
60. Rapoport SI. Cortical pH and the blood brain barrier. J Physiol London 1964; 170:238–249.
61. Javaheri S. A mechanism of central sleep apnea in patients with heart failure. N Engl J Med 1999; 341:949–954.
62. Javaheri S, Shore NS, Rose B, Kazemi H. Compensatory hypoventilation in metabolic alkalosis. Chest 1982; 81:296–301.
63. Javaheri S, Kazemi H. Metabolic alkalosis causes compensatory hypoventilation in man. Am Rev Respir Dis 1987; 136:1011–1016.
64. Alberts MS, Dell RB, Winters RW. Quantitative displacement of acid–base equilibrium in metabolic acidosis. Ann Intern Med 1967; 66:312–322.
65. McFadden ER Jr, Lyons HA. Arterial-blood gas tension in asthma. N Engl J Med 1968; 278:1027–1032.
66. Javaheri S, Sicilian L. Lung function, breathing pattern, and gas exchange in interstitial lung disease. Thorax 1992; 47:93–97.
67. Burrows B, Sakesena FB, Diener CF. Carbon dioxide tension and ventilatory mechanics in chronic obstructive pulmonary disease. Ann Intern Med 1966; 65:685–700.
68. Javaheri S. $PaCO_2$ in emphysema. (By invitation) Pflugers Arch 1987; 408:S29.
69. Kelsen SG. Control of breathing. Montenegro HD, ed. Chronic Obstructive Pulmonary Disease. New York: Curchill Livingstone, 1984:65–116.
70. Howell JBL. Ventilatory control in chronic airways obstruction. Bull Physiopathologie Respir 1973; 9:661–671.
71. Sorli J, Grassino A, Lorange G, et al. Control of breathing in patients with chronic obstructive lung disease. Clin Sci Mole Med 1978; 54:295–304.
72. Javaheri S, Blum J, Kazemi H. Pattern of breathing and CO_2 retention in chronic obstructive lung disease. Am J Med 1981; 71:228–234.
73. Fanburg BL, Sicilian L. Respiratory Dysfunction in Neuromuscular Disease. Clinics in Chest Medicine, No. 4. Vol. 15. Philadelphia: W.B. Saunders, 1994.
74. Javaheri S, Logemann TN, Corser BC, Guerra LF, Means E. Diaphragmatic paralysis. Am J Med 1989; 86:623–624.

75. Javaheri S, Colangelo G, Lacey W, Gartside PS. Chronic hypercapnia in obstructive sleep apnea–hypopnea syndrome. Sleep 1994; 17:416–423.

76. Schaefer KE, Hastings BJ, Carey CR, Nichols G Jr. Respiratory acclimatization to carbon dioxide. J Appl Physiol 1963; 18:1071–1078.

77. Edelman NH, Lahiri S, Braudo L, Cherniack NS, Fishman AP. The blunted ventilatory response to hypoxia in cyanotic congenital heart disease. N Engl J Med 1970; 282:405–411.

78. Javaheri S, Colangelo G, Corser B, Zahedpour MR. Familial respiratory chemosensitivity does not predict hypercapnia of patients with sleep apnea–hypopnea syndrome. Am Rev Respir Dis 1992; 145:837–840.

79. Sullivan CE, Berthon-Jones M, Issa FG. Remission of severe obesity–hypoventilation syndrome after short-term treatment during sleep with nasal continuous positive airway pressure. Am Rev Respir Dis 1983; 128:177–181.

80. Berthon-Jones M, Sullivan CE. Time course of change in ventilatory response to CO_2 with long-term CPAP therapy for obstructive sleep apnea. Am Rev Respir Dis 1987; 135:144–147.

81. Mason JF, Celli BR, Riesco JA, Hernandez M, Sanclez de Cos J, Disdier C. The obesity hypoventilation syndrome can be treated with noninvasive mechanical ventilation. Chest 2001; 119:1102–1107.

82. Berg G, Delaive K, Manfreda J, Walld R, Kryger MH. The use of health-care resources in obesity–hypoventilation syndrome. Chest 2001; 120:377–383.

4

Renal Regulation of Hydrogen Ion Balance

L. Lee Hamm

Section of Nephrology and Hypertension, Department of Medicine, Tulane University Health Sciences Center, New Orleans, Louisiana, U.S.A.

INTRODUCTION AND OVERVIEW

The kidneys are responsible for day-to-day acid–base homeostasis, with the lungs regulating $PaCO_2$ on a minute-to-minute basis. This renal regulation is accomplished by recapturing filtered HCO_3^- and excretion of "nonvolatile" or "fixed" acids. The terms "nonvolatile" or "fixed" acids refer to all dietary or endogenously produced acid except CO_2, the "volatile" acid excreted by the lungs. Each day, a large amount of HCO_3^- is filtered (some 4300 mEq/day at a glomerular filtration rate (GFR) of 120 mL/min), and loss of even a fraction of this HCO_3^- would represent a major loss of body alkali stores. Acid excretion is much smaller in magnitude, some 50–100 mEq/day, but is equally vital for acid–base homeostasis and is carefully regulated to maintain acid–base balance. This chapter addresses the transport processes along the renal tubules that reabsorb HCO_3^- and excrete acid. The results of these two processes are summarized in Fig. 1. As discussed in what follows, both processes are accomplished primarily by H^+ secretion by tubule epithelial cells, and much of the chapter is devoted to the nature and regulation of these H^+ transport events. The references are selective with emphasis on more recent papers, which will refer the reader to older papers.

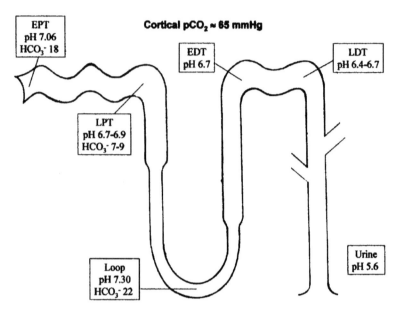

Figure 1   Model of lumen pH and HCO_3^- profile along the nephron. pH and $[HCO_3^-]$ are shown in the following sequential nephron segments: early superficial proximal tubule (EPT), late superficial proximal tubule (LPT), bend of Henle's loop (loop), early superficial distal tubule (EDT), and late superficial distal tubule (LDT). The PCO_2 in the renal cortex has been determined to be ~65 mmHg (266). See text for additional details. *Source*: Derived from Ref. 16, 17, and 267.

CARBONIC ANHYDRASE

The enzyme, carbonic anhydrase (CA), is an important component of acid–base transport because it catalyzes the reversible reaction (1):

$$CO_2 + OH^- \leftrightarrow HCO_3^-$$

In aqueous physiologic solutions:

$$CO_2 + H_2O \leftrightarrow H_2CO_3 \leftrightarrow HCO_3^- + H^+$$

In the absence of CA, this reaction reaches equilibrium in <1 min, but CA accelerates the rate by several orders of magnitude (see Chapter 1). The uncatalyzed rate is slow enough that at high rates of epithelial H^+ secretion, H^+ accumulates above the equilibrium in the tubule lumen. This accumulation lowers pH and slows subsequent H^+ secretion. The converse is true with HCO_3^- secretion or transport (i.e., the rate of back-flux will increase). Thus CA facilitates acid–base transport all along the nephron.

Two functionally important isoforms of CA are present in the kidney, type II (cytoplasmic) and type IV (membrane-bound) (1). Type II is present in most cells along the nephron involved in acid–base transport. Membrane-bound type IV is less widespread but where present is also key for H^+ transport (2). Carbonic anhydrase IV is present both on the apical and the basolateral membranes of epithelial cells in the S1 and S2 segments of the proximal tubule, facilitating H^+ secretion and probably HCO_3^- efflux from the cell. Carbonic anhydrase IV is also present on the apical and basolateral membranes of the epithelium lining the thick ascending limb (TAL) (2). Some cells of the distal tubule and collecting duct also have CA IV on their luminal membrane (3–5). However, most segments of the collecting duct and the final portion of the proximal tubule, the S3 segment, do not have luminal CA IV (2,6). The nephron segments with no luminal CA absorb HCO_3^- at slower rates (due to the accumulation of H^+), and luminal pH is lower. The exact importance of the lower luminal pH in these segments is unknown, although it clearly augments NH_4^+ trapping (see in what follows). Both CA II and CA IV increase with metabolic acidosis, presumably facilitating increased rates of acid–base transport (7,8).

Two additional isoforms of CA are present in the kidney, CA XII and CA XIV (9,10). Carbonic anhydrase XII is present in the basolateral membranes of the TAL, the distal tubule, and principal cells of the collecting duct (9) and is also present in the proximal tubule and collecting tubules of some species (11). Carbonic anhydrase XIV appears to be present in the proximal tubule and thin descending limb (10).

BICARBONATE REABSORPTION

Proximal Tubule

The proximal tubule reabsorbs about 75% of the filtered HCO_3^- and is composed of at least three specific segments (S1, S2, and S3). Acid–base transport in these segments differ both quantitatively and qualitatively to some extent (12), but most of the mechanisms and regulation of acid–base transport are similar. The general features include apical H^+ secretion, basolateral Na^+-coupled HCO_3^- exit from the cell, and facilitation by both membrane bound and cellular CA (Fig. 2). Secreted H^+ reacts with luminal HCO_3^- to form CO_2 and H_2O, both of which readily cross all membranes of the proximal tubular epithelium. For each H^+ secreted, this reaction removes a HCO_3^- from the tubular lumen. To complete the process of HCO_3^- reabsorption, cellular HCO_3^- derived from $CO_2 + H_2O$ is extruded out the basolateral membrane. Both the apically secreted H^+ and the basolaterally secreted HCO_3^- derive from CO_2 and H_2O. The reversible hydration and dehydration reaction, $HCO_3^- + H^+ \leftrightarrow CO_2 + H_2O$, is catalyzed (accelerated) by CA II in the cytoplasm, as well as by apical and basolateral

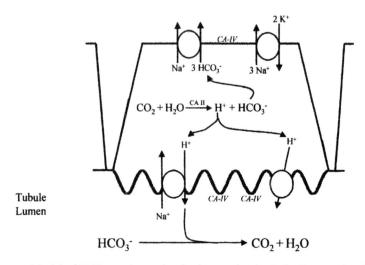

Figure 2   Model of HCO_3^- reabsorption in the proximal tubule. See text for details. *Source*: Adapted from Ref. 267.

membrane-bound CA IV. In the absence or inhibition of CA, HCO_3^- reabsorption is marked inhibited.

Apical H^+ secretion occurs both via an apical Na^+/H^+ exchanger and a H^+-ATPase. However, because of the thermodynamics of Na^+/H^+ exchange (13) and the relatively high permeability of the proximal tubule to H^+ and HCO_3^- (14,15), the proximal tubule is only able to lower the luminal pH to ~6.7 and the luminal $[HCO_3^-]$ to ~7–8 mEq/L (16,17). Therefore, the proximal tubule can be considered a "high capacity, low gradient" system for H^+/HCO_3^- transport, in contrast to the distal nephron discussed in what follows.

Na^+/H^+ Exchanger

More than three decades ago, classic studies established that HCO_3^- reabsorption in the proximal tubule results from H^+ secretion rather than HCO_3^- reabsorption (18). This conclusion derived from pH measurements of an acid disequilibrium pH using microelectrodes in the proximal tubule lumen during CA inhibition. Equally important, most HCO_3^- reabsorption was later found to be Na^+ dependent and electroneutral. Subsequently, it was established that the mechanism of H^+ secretion involves a Na^+/H^+ exchanger that exchanges one luminal Na^+ for one cellular H^+ (19,20). This exchanger is responsible for approximately two-thirds of HCO_3^- reabsorption and is also the major mode of Na^+ reabsorption in the proximal tubule. The driving force is the large $[Na^+]$ gradient between the lumen and cell (~140 and 10–15 mEq/L, respectively), maintained by the basolateral Na^+/K^+-ATPase. Owing to the near-equivalent reabsorption of Na^+ and water in the proximal tubule, the luminal Na^+ concentration remains $\sim$140 mEq/L along its entire length. This exchange process is inhibited by amiloride and its analogs (21) and transports other ions such as lithium and NH_4^+ (22). It is stimulated by intracellular acidosis via both kinetic and allosteric mechanisms (23). The Na^+/H^+ exchanger on the apical membrane is predominantly Na^+/H^+ exchanger 3 (NHE3), a member of the ubiquitous family of Na^+/H^+ exchangers that function in nonepithelial cells to regulate intracellular pH and volume (see Chapter 5). Other as yet unidentified NHE isoforms (24) may contribute to H^+ secretion, but immunohistochemical studies and studies of NHE3 knockout animals are most consistent with a predominant role for NHE3 (24–26).

H^+-ATPase

Approximately one-third of HCO_3^- reabsorption in the proximal tubule lumen occurs via H^+ secretion by an apical membrane, multisubunit vacuolar type H^+-ATPase (see Chapter 5) (27). This pump is electrogenic and shares most subunits with the distal nephron H^+-ATPase, discussed in detail in what follows. This pump likely accounts for virtually all of the residual H^+ secretion in the proximal tubule when Na^+/H^+ exchange is blocked by inhibitors, Na^+ removal, or genetic knockout (25). The vacuolar H^+-ATPases are blocked by N,N'-dicyclohexylcarbodiimide and more specifically by bafilomycin A1 (28).

Other Apical Transporters

The apical membrane of the proximal tubule also contains several Cl^-/anion exchangers (anions include such bases as OH^-, formate, oxalate), but these appear to function for NaCl rather than HCO_3^- reabsorption (29). Cl^-/base exchange, in parallel with Na^+/H^+ exchange (Na^+ and Cl^- moving into the cell, and H^+ and base moving into the lumen), has no net effect on acid–base transport but results in NaCl absorption. Citrate and other organic anions are reabsorbed in the proximal tubule by Na^+-coupled mechanisms. This reabsorption prevents the loss of excess "potential base" into the urine. "Potential base" represents organic anions that could be metabolized to HCO_3^- (see later under "Organic Anions").

Basolateral HCO_3^- Extrusion

Efflux of HCO_3^- out of the basolateral cell membrane into the blood is as important as apical H^+ secretion for transepithelial HCO_3^- reabsorption. Extrusion of cellular HCO_3^-, derived from CO_2 and H_2O in the presence of CA II, into the interstitium and capillary blood completes the process of net HCO_3^- reabsorption (Fig. 2). Basolateral HCO_3^- extrusion is mediated by an electrogenic Na^+/HCO_3^--coupled transporter [sodium bicarbonate cotransporter (NBC)] that transports one Na^+ with the equivalent of three HCO_3^- ions (30,31). Whether this transporter always functions in a 3:1

$HCO_3^-:Na^+$ mode, in a $1HCO_3^-:1CO_3^{-2}:1Na^+$ mode (32), or sometimes in a 2:1 mode is not clear (33,34). The driving force for cotransport is the transmembrane voltage (cell negative). The NBC isoform in the proximal tubule is NBC1 (35), with the possible exception of the late proximal where a different isoform may be present (36). The NBC transporters are sensitive to inhibition by DIDS and other disulfonic stilbenes (see Chapter 5).

Other HCO_3^- or base transporters (in particular, a Na^+-coupled Cl^-/HCO_3^- exchanger) are present in the basolateral membrane but probably do not contribute to transepithelial acid–base transport (37). A basolateral Na^+/H^+ exchanger, NHE1, is also present but probably functions to regulate cell volume and pH (38).

Organic Anions

Changes in organic anion reabsorption in the proximal tubule could theoretically contribute to regulation of net acid–base homeostasis, as these anions generate HCO_3^- when they are reabsorbed and metabolized to CO_2 and H_2O. In the rat, for example, renal excretion of urinary citrate and other organic anions contributes substantially to the removal of excess alkali during recovery from metabolic alkalosis (39). Citrate is the most abundant organic anion found in urine (40), but changes in citrate excretion (or other organic anions) do not affect acid–base balance notably in humans. Citrate excretion does change as expected in acid–base disturbances, but the magnitude is small (only ~5–10 mEq/day) (41).

General Ionic Permeability

The proximal tubule is a so-called "leaky epithelium" with high permeabilities to many ions and to water, as well as to H^+, HCO_3^-, and CO_2 (14,15,42). The high CO_2 permeability allows for near-instantaneous equilibration of CO_2 in each of the adjacent structures of the kidney (e.g., tubule lumen, cell, and interstitium). The high paracellular HCO_3^- permeability limits reabsorption in late proximal tubule (where luminal $[HCO_3^-]$ is low compared with the peritubular interstitium) (43).

Regulation of Proximal Tubule H⁺ Secretion

Regulation of H^+ secretion in the proximal tubule normally functions to maintain acid–base homeostasis. However, during disease states, some of the regulatory features actually cause changes in acid–base transport that can potentially cause or perpetuate acid–base disorders. For instance, metabolic alkalosis with severe vomiting is accompanied by increased proximal tubule HCO_3^- reabsorption (i.e., H^+ secretion), induced by a variety of factors, including an increase in angiotensin II and in filtered HCO_3^-, a decrease in HCO_3^- backleak across the paracellular pathway, and K^+ depletion—each a component of the regulatory aspects discussed in what follows (44).

Acidemia

Proximal tubule H^+ secretion increases when systemic pH falls secondary to a number of mechanisms. In response to metabolic acidosis, an acute increase in Na^+/H^+ exchange occurs secondary to kinetic effects (increased cell $[H^+]$) and an allosteric stimulation of the exchanger (23). Over a more prolonged period, both apical Na^+/H^+ exchange and basolateral Na^+–HCO_3^- cotransport increase in activity (45). This increase is associated with an increase in NHE3 protein in the apical membrane but not an increase in NHE3 mRNA; the increase in protein results from both increased translation and probably more importantly from increased exocytic insertion from subapical membrane vesicles (46–48). Hormonal responses perhaps also play a critical role, with increased renal endothelin-1 (ET-1) (49,50) and cortisol from the adrenal (51) stimulating transport (see later). Cortisol increases both NHE3 protein and exocytic insertion of vesicles. The increase in basolateral membrane Na^+–HCO_3^- cotransport with metabolic acidosis may be secondary to post-translational modifications of NBC1, as protein levels do not change (52). Despite stimulation of both H^+ secretion and HCO_3^- extrusion, proximal tubule HCO_3^- reabsorption is sharply limited by the reduction in filtered HCO_3^- that occurs in metabolic acidosis.

In respiratory acidosis, peritubular and cell pH decrease, but filtered HCO_3^- is increased, allowing for an increase in reabsorption to occur. The cellular response to respiratory acidosis is similar to chronic metabolic acidosis. Both apical Na^+/H^+ exchange and basolateral Na^+–HCO_3^- cotransport are increased (53). Increases in PCO_2 also increase the exocytic insertion of vesicles containing H^+-ATPase (54). Hydrogen ion secretion appears to be stimulated directly by an increase in basolateral PCO_2, independent of pH, suggesting the presence of a "CO_2 sensor" in the basolateral membrane of the proximal tubule (55,56).

Potassium Depletion

Potassium depletion induces many of the same changes in acid–base transport as metabolic acidosis (57), despite the usual clinical accompaniment of metabolic alkalosis. In fact, the acid–base transport changes with K^+ depletion likely contribute to sustaining the metabolic alkalosis (see Chapter 18). The acid–base transport changes are likely due to intracellular acidosis secondary to cell hyperpolarization (58,59).

Extracellular Fluid Volume and Luminal Flow Rate

Changes in extracellular fluid (ECF) volume and luminal flow both influence proximal tubule HCO_3^- reabsorption. Increasing luminal flow increases reabsorption both by maintaining luminal $[HCO_3^-]$ high and by a more direct effect of flow rate on Na^+/H^+ exchange and H^+-ATPase. Increases in luminal pH increase H^+ secretion as might be expected from kinetic effects on the apical Na^+/H^+ exchanger (lower luminal [H^+]). Proximal tubule HCO_3^- reabsorption increases with increasing luminal [HCO_3^-], likely due to both the pH effect and the improved [HCO_3^-] gradient across the epithelium (60–65). By these effects, volume expansion increases proximal HCO_3^- reabsorption to the extent that GFR, filtered HCO_3^-, and luminal flow increase. An important consequence of increasing proximal tubule HCO_3^- reabsorption with increasing delivery is to limit delivery of HCO_3^- to the distal nephron. In addition to these immediate effects, chronic adaptations in Na^+/H^+ exchange and $Na^+–HCO_3^-$ cotransport occur in the same direction as GFR (66). Extracellular fluid volume contraction, in which GFR and filtered HCO_3^- may be decreased, is often also accompanied by increased proximal tubule HCO_3^- reabsorptive capacity as well, as is seen in metabolic alkalosis. This may be secondary to increased angiotensin II or catecholamines causing increased Na^+/H^+ exchange (67) but is also aided by decreased paracellular HCO_3^- permeability (68).

Hormones

Glucocorticoids: Cortisol levels increase with metabolic acidosis, and this increase appears to be necessary for the increase in Na^+/H^+ exchange in metabolic acidosis (69). Glucocorticoids increase Na^+/H^+ exchange by multiple mechanisms, including an increased insertion of NHE3 protein into the apical membrane (51). Glucocorticoids also increase NBC1 mRNA levels and activity in the proximal tubule (70).

Endothelin-1: Endothelin-1, working through the endothelin B (ETB) receptor in proximal tubules, may also be a critical factor in the response to acidosis (50,71). Endothelin-1 in very low concentrations increases proximal tubule HCO_3^- reabsorption (72). Both apical Na^+/H^+ exchange and basolateral $Na^+–HCO_3^-$ cotransport increase (50,73). A decrease in intracellular pH increases ET-1 synthesis in the kidney, specifically by microvascular endothelial cells and proximal tubule cells (71,74,75). The mechanism whereby acidosis stimulates ET-1 synthesis appears to involve sequential activation of Pyk2 (a nonreceptor tyrosine kinase), c-Src (another nonreceptor tyrosine kinase), followed by ERK activation, c-fos/c-jun (immediate early genes) activating the AP-1 promoter site of the ET-1 gene (71,76–78). The ETB activation leads to a phosphorylation of NHE3 and its insertion in the apical membrane (48–50,71,79). A calcium sensitive pathway also plays a role (80). Similar signaling pathways have been implicated in the stimulation of basolateral $Na^+–HCO_3^-$ cotransport (81,82).

Angiotensin II: Angiotensin II at low concentrations increases HCO_3^- reabsorption by co-ordinated increases in apical H^+ secretion and basolateral HCO_3^- transport (83). Endogenously produced angiotensin II may stimulate luminal receptors to augment HCO_3^- reabsorption in the proximal tubule (84). Angiotensin II increases NHE3 activity and exocytic insertion of NHE3-containing vesicles into the brush border (85) and directly stimulates basolateral Na^+–HCO_3^- transport (86,87). The cellular mechanisms implicated in these responses include decreased cAMP, activation of protein kinase C, and activation of tyrosine kinase (src)/MAPK pathways (88–90). These effects are likely important in the response to volume depletion and metabolic alkalosis.

Other Hormones: A variety of other hormones have also been shown to regulate proximal tubule acid–base transport. However, their importance has not been clearly delineated. Parathyroid hormone (PTH) decreases proximal HCO_3^- reabsorption via an increase in cAMP activity (91,92). The increase in cAMP activates PKA, which then phosphorylates and inhibits NHE3 (93). Parathyroid hormone also inhibits basolateral Na^+–HCO_3^- cotransport (94). On a more chronic basis, cAMP (as well as hormones that stimulate cAMP) may actually increase Na^+/H^+ exchange (95). Catecholamines stimulate HCO_3^- reabsorption (96) by binding to α-2 receptors that activate NHE3 by interacting with Na^+/H^+ exchange regulatory factor (NHERF) (97). The NHERF is a protein cofactor important for cAMP-mediated regulation of NHE3 activity (98,99). The NHERF (as well as the related NHERF2) links ezrin, NHE3, and PKA to the actin cytoskeleton (98,99). The NHERF may also regulate basolateral Na^+–HCO_3^- cotransport (100). Insulin (101), dopamine (102,103), adenosine (104), and cholinergic agents (105) also modulate proximal HCO_3^- transport, but the physiologic significance of these effects is unclear.

Loop of Henle

The loop of Henle reabsorbs much of the HCO_3^- that remains in the nephron after the proximal tubule (106,107). Reabsorption in the loop has been estimated from measurements of HCO_3^- delivery from the end of the accessible superficial proximal tubule and to the beginning of the distal tubule (106,108,109). Between these two sites, several nephron segments exist— the S3 segment of the proximal tubule, the thin descending and ascending limbs, as well as the medullary and cortical TAL. Between 15% and 20% of the filtered HCO_3^- is reabsorbed in these segments, but only the S3 segment and the TALs have the capacity for active transport. The S3 segment can reabsorb HCO_3^- via both Na^+/H^+ exchange and H^+-ATPase (110), but the extent of reabsorption is probably low because of the low $[HCO_3^-]$ in this segment. Thus, the TAL is likely responsible for most of the HCO_3^- reabsorption between the end of the accessible proximal tubule and the early distal tubule.

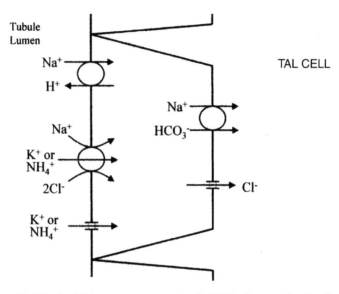

Figure 3 Model of acid–base transporters in the TAL. See text for details. *Source*: Adapted from Ref. 214.

The major H^+-secretory mechanism in the TAL is the Na^+/H^+ exchanger (Fig. 3). Apical membrane NHE3 is abundantly present (111) as is NHE2 (112). Some features of Na^+/H^+ exchange in the TAL (e.g., relative pH independence) differ from that in other epithelia (113,114). The H^+-ATPase is also present (106,115). At the basolateral membrane, a Na^+–HCO_3^- cotransporter is present and may mediate HCO_3^- transport into the peritubular interstitium (116). The isoform in the TAL is the electroneutral NBC2 (also known as NBCn1) (117,118). Basolateral Cl^-/HCO_3^- exchangers and K^+–HCO_3^- cotransporters are also present and may be important mediators of transepithelial HCO_3^- transport (119–121). The role of each of these transporters is not clear, but some may serve to regulate cell pH and volume during transepithelial transport of NaCl, HCO_3^-, and NH_4^+. Basolateral Na^+/H^+ exchangers, NHE1 and probably NHE4, are also present and appear to regulate apical Na^+/H^+ exchange (see in what follows) (122,123).

Regulation of HCO_3^- Transport in the TAL

Delivery Dependence

Reabsorption of HCO_3^- in the TAL is concentration—as well as delivery—dependent, so that reabsorption increases as delivery increases (106,124). Concentration dependence is physiologically important because [HCO_3]

rises to above $20\,mEq/L$ in the descending loop of Henle as H_2O is reabsorbed (125). Reabsorption of HCO_3^- in the TAL is sensitive to CA inhibition and to high concentrations of amiloride and its analogs (106,124). Loop diuretics stimulate HCO_3^- reabsorption, possibly via decreases in cell Na^+ concentration (109).

Acid–Base Responsiveness

HCO_3^- reabsorption in the loop of Henle responds to perturbations in systemic acid–base balance (108,126). Na^+/H^+ exchange and basolateral Na^+–HCO_3^- cotransport increase in response to acidosis (118,127). There are similar adaptations in NH_4^+ transport as well (see later). Bicarbonate transport, however, does not appear to change in the TAL in response to either metabolic alkalosis or respiratory acid–base disturbances (109,128), despite changes in NHE3 activity in metabolic alkalosis (129). The lack of effect in these disorders may relate to countervailing influences of changes in delivery to this part of the nephron.

Sodium Intake and Hormonal Effects

Changes in dietary Na^+ intake and a variety of hormones affect HCO_3^- transport in the loop of Henle. An increase in dietary Na^+ intake increases loop segment and more specifically TAL HCO_3^- reabsorption (108,126). This effect occurs without a measurable change in NHE3 (129). The effect of dietary Na^+ intake could be secondary to inhibition of aldosterone secretion. Aldosterone appears to inhibit TAL HCO_3^- reabsorption by a nongenomic mechanism (130), although glucocorticoid replacement restores loop HCO_3^- reabsorption after adrenalectomy (131). Angiotensin II, nerve growth factor, prostaglandin E_2, PTH, and glucagon all can affect TAL HCO_3^- transport. These hormones influence TAL HCO_3^- transport via diverse signaling pathways (such as extracellular signal-regulated kinase ERK, cytochrome P-450, and phosphatidylinositol 3-kinase) in addition to the cAMP pathway (132–136). In contrast to its effects in the proximal tubule, angiotensin II inhibits TAL HCO_3^- reabsorption (134). The physiologic significance of many of these hormonal effects is not clear, in part because of the large amount of HCO_3^- reabsorption in the proximal nephron and the downstream regulation of urine acidification in the collecting duct. A novel mechanism of regulation of TAL HCO_3^- transport appears to be a regulation of apical Na^+/H^+ exchange by basolateral Na^+/H^+ exchange (122,137). The mechanism of this interaction between exchangers is not clear.

Osmolality

HCO_3^- transport in the TAL is also sensitive to hyper- and hypo-osmolality (135,138–140). Hypertonicity inhibits and hypotonicity stimulates HCO_3^- reabsorption. This action occurs via a tyrosine kinase-dependent pathway

(139). The effect of hypotonicity may be pertinent to the stimulation of urinary acidification with loop diuretics. Antidiuretic hormone (ADH), which promotes medullary hypertonicity, also reduces TAL HCO_3^- reabsorption (141,142).

Distal Nephron

The nephron segments beyond the TAL (distal nephron) are responsible for reabsorption of the remaining filtered HCO_3^- ($\sim$5–10% of filtered load), generation of additional titratable acid, and NH_4^+ "trapping" for excretion into the final urine (see later section Ammonium Excretion). All these functions are accomplished, in large part, by apical H^+ secretion. The distal nephron is composed of several distinct segments, some of which have multiple cell types. These segments include the distal convoluted tubule, the connecting segment, the cortical collecting duct, the medullary collecting duct (outer and inner stripe portions), and the inner medullary collecting duct (IMCD)(with initial and terminal portions). Despite this anatomic and functional heterogeneity, many features of H^+ secretion by the segments of the distal nephron are shared.

The general model for H^+ secretion in the distal nephron is depicted in Fig. 4. This model most closely approximates the type A or α intercalated cells in the cortical collecting duct (CCD), but similar mechanisms exist in other distal nephron acid-secreting cells. Type A intercalated cells are

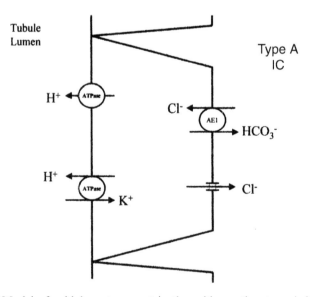

Figure 4   Model of acid–base transport in the acid-secreting type A intercalated cells of the CCD. See text for details. *Source*: Adapted from Ref. 214.

acid-secreting cells in the collecting duct interspersed among the more numerous principal cells, whose predominant function is Na^+, K^+, and H_2O transport. In type A intercalated cells, H^+ is secreted across the apical membrane predominantly via a vacuolar-type H^+-ATPase. A second H^+ transporter, the H^+/K^+-ATPase, discussed in what follows, secretes H^+ in some distal nephron segments during states of K^+ deficiency. On the basolateral membrane of type A intercalated cells, a Cl^-/HCO_3^- exchanger mediates HCO_3^- extrusion into the peritubular interstitium. Intercalated cells in the distal nephron (and other acid-secreting cells in the papillary collecting duct) all have abundant cytoplasmic CA II. As discussed earlier, a minority of cells along the distal nephron also has functional luminal CA. In addition to the model shown in Fig. 4, the distal convoluted tubule and connecting segments contain an apical Na^+/H^+ exchanger (probably NHE2) (111,143,144). Although this general model of H^+ secretion pertains to many cells along the distal nephron, there are differences among the various segments and between experimental species.

Bicarbonate Secretion

Bicarbonate secretion occurs in the superficial distal tubule and cortical-collecting duct of rats, rabbits, and mice (145–147). Bicarbonate secretion is electroneutral, Na^+ independent, and coupled to Cl^- reabsorption and occurs in type B or β intercalated cells (Fig. 5). Basolateral H^+-ATPase

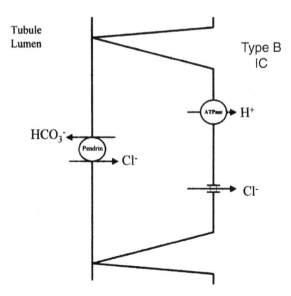

Figure 5 Model of HCO_3^--secreting type B intercalated cells of the CCD. See text for details. *Source*: Adapted from Ref. 214.

probably provides the active component of this process, with apical HCO_3^- transport occurring via an apical Cl^-/HCO_3^- exchanger. Bicarbonate secretion is stimulated by metabolic alkalosis, mineralocorticoids, and isoproterenol (148–150), inhibited by acid loads (150,151), and enhanced in recovery from metabolic alkalosis (152,153).

Distinct Features of Distal Tubule Nephron Segments

Superficial Distal Tubule

In the early portion of the superficial distal tubule (predominantly distal convoluted tubule), no intercalated cells are present, but the epithelial cells secrete H^+ via both a Na^+/H^+ exchanger (likely NHE2) and H^+-ATPase (111,143). The connecting tubule (more distal aspect of the superficial distal tubule) has intercalated cells, and in these cells, an apical membrane H^+-ATPase accounts for most of the H^+ secretion (154). The superficial distal tubule (as well as connecting segment specifically) also secretes HCO_3^- with alkali loading (see later) (147,155,156).

Cortical Collecting Duct

The CCD has both type A and type B intercalated cells and thus can either reabsorb or secrete HCO_3^- [157]. Type B intercalated cells predominate in the initial CCD, and type A intercalated cells predominate in the more distal CCD in rabbit, whereas in rat, there is less distinction. With acid loading, tubules reabsorb HCO_3^-, whereas with alkali loading, HCO_3^- secretion predominates (145). Under normal conditions, simultaneous secretion and reabsorption of HCO_3^- probably occur (see later section on regulation).

In addition to type A and type B intercalated cells, intermediate cell types have been identified that may function to regulate the amount and direction of HCO_3^- transport (158). These cells contain both apical and basolateral Cl^-/HCO_3^- exchangers (159). In some studies, interconversion of IC cell types (between A and B or intermediate types) in the CCD has been demonstrated (160–162).

Outer Medullary Collecting Duct

The outer medullary collecting duct has two distinct segments: the outer and the inner stripes. The outer stripe has both principal cells and type A intercalated cells; the transepithelial voltage is lumen negative due to Na^+ reabsorption by the principal cells (163). In contrast, the inner stripe has no Na^+ transport and, as in the outer stripe, only type A intercalated cells, and therefore, has a lumen positive voltage (163). In the rabbit, all cells in the inner stripe, particularly the inner most aspect, are a single cell type that secretes acid but with variation in transport rates (164,165). The inner stripe, in contrast to most segments of the distal tubule, has luminal CA, facilitating a high rate of HCO_3^- reabsorption (4).

Inner Medullary Collecting Duct

The IMCD has three segments, but few functional differences are found with regard to H^+ secretion. The outermost part has distinct intercalated cells, at least in several species, whereas the inner part has none. Nonetheless, it secretes H^+ very effectively (166). Cellular localization of key acid–base transport proteins is not well defined in the IMCD.

H^+-ATPase in the Distal Nephron

H^+ secretion along the distal nephron is accomplished primarily by an apical membrane H^+-ATPase (27,167,168). The H^+-ATPase in the distal nephron is a multisubunit "vacuolar-type" ATPase (see Chapter 5) (27,167). This H^+-ATPase is the same as that found in many intracellular organelles such as lysosomes and clathrin-coated vesicles, although some subunits may vary. The distal nephron H^+-ATPase also shares most subunits with the one in the proximal tubule. In the proximal tubule, however, the H^+-ATPase has a distinct 56 K subunit (B2 subunit or "brain isoform") that differs from that in the distal nephron (B1 or "kidney isoform") (169). Other subunits also differ (170). The H^+-ATPase is electrogenic and therefore influenced by membrane voltage. In the distal nephron, the current from the H^+-ATPase is shunted via the paracellular pathway (Cl^- enters the lumen via a paracellular pathway), rather than via a parallel apical anion channel as in intracellular organelles, although there may be an exception in the superficial distal tubule (171).

Regulation of H^+-ATPase activity in the distal nephron occurs predominantly via insertion (and retrieval) of the pump in the apical membrane via fusion of subapical vesicles (27,167). Insertion of the H^+-ATPase occurs in response to intracellular acidification or increased PCO_2, possibility acting via an increase in intracellular calcium (172,173). Regulatory proteins of H^+-ATPase have been identified in the cytosol, but their role remains uncertain (174,175). Transcriptional and translational regulation appears to be a less-important mechanism of regulation (158). Basolateral H^+-ATPase mediates HCO_3^- secretion from type B intercalated cells (157).

H^+/K^+-ATPase

Collecting duct intercalated cells contain a second apical membrane H^+-secreting protein, the H^+/K^+-ATPase. This transporter also plays an important role in distal nephron H^+ secretion particularly in the setting of K^+ depletion (176–178). The H^+/K^+-ATPase secretes H^+ in a coupled exchange for K^+ entry and is therefore electroneutral and not influenced by membrane voltage. There are at least two isoforms of H^+/K^+-ATPase, gastric and colonic, present in the kidney (see Chapter 5). An additional type may also be present in the distal tubule. These pumps are K^+-dependent ATPases of the E1, E2 class (P-type ATPase). Both known pumps contain a unique α subunit ($\alpha 1$ for gastric and $\alpha 2$ for the colonic isoform) and a β subunit (a unique isoform for the gastric or the β subunit of Na–K-ATPase for the colonic pump) (176–181). Animals lacking either the gastric or colonic H^+/K^+-ATPase have normal acid–base status (182,183). Thus either these ATPases do not play an important role in overall renal H^+ secretion or their inactivation is compensated for by an increase in the activity of other H^+ transporters. The colonic isoform may also substitute Na^+ for H^+ in the kidney and function as Na^+/K^+-ATPase (184) or substitute NH_4^+ for K^+ and secrete NH_4^+ (185,186).

Potassium depletion upregulates H^+/K^+-ATPase activity and mRNA for the colonic isoform, particularly in the medullary collecting duct (143,187–190). There is also an adaptation of H^+/K^+-ATPase in the CCD during K^+ depletion that may involve gastric H^+/K^+-ATPase (191). Metabolic acidosis also stimulates H^+/K^+-ATPase activity (187). The H^+/K^+-ATPase may play a role in HCO_3^- secretion, but this has not been completely characterized; H^+/K^+-ATPase in the type B intercalated cell is located at the apical membrane (148,192,193). The H^+/K^+-ATPase transporter may also play a role in Na^+ reabsorption in the collecting duct, through substitution of Na^+ for K^+ (creating a functional Na^+/H^+ exchanger) (184,194).

The exact isoforms of H^+/K^+-ATPase that mediate H^+ and K^+ transport in the collecting duct remain controversial. In large part, this controversy derives from differences between studies in different cell systems and the responses to various inhibitors. For instance, colonic H^+/K^+-ATPase is sensitive to high concentrations of ouabain but not to SCH28080; however, in the distal tubule, some studies have identified acid secretion sensitive to SCH28080 simultaneous with upregulation of colonic H^+/K^+-ATPase and downregulation of gastric H^+/K^+-ATPase (177). At least three distinct H^+/K^+-ATPases have been identified in studies of enzyme activities (177). However, the identity of a third isoform (in addition to gastric and colonic) has not been established in mammals.

Basolateral Cl^-/HCO_3^- Exchange

Basolateral HCO_3^- transport in H^+-secreting cells of the distal nephron occurs predominantly via a truncated form of the exchange transporter AE1 (anion exchanger 1), also known as Band 3 protein, the red cell exchanger involved in CO_2 transport (195,196). The kidney form of AE1 has an alternate start site from erythroid AE1 and lacks the C-terminal portion that binds to the cytoskeleton in red cells (197,198). Anion exchanger 1 (both renal and red cell forms) exchanges one Cl^- for one HCO_3^- in an electroneutral fashion. The interstitium-to-cell Cl^- concentration gradient provides the driving force, at least in part, for HCO_3^- extrusion from the cell. Anion exchanger 1 is present in the basolateral membrane of type A intercalated cells and probably all distal tubule acid-secreting cells, including those in the IMCD (199).

Apical Cl⁻/HCO₃⁻ Exchange

The Cl^-/HCO_3^- exchanger in the apical membrane of type B intercalated cells is now postulated to be pendrin, the gene product responsible for Pendred's Syndrome—an autosomal recessive deafness and goiter (200–202). In addition to an appropriate cellular localization, pendrin expression and distribution appears to be regulated as expected for a HCO_3^- secretory process (202–204). One study has suggested that a novel anion exchanger AE4 accounts for apical Cl^-/HCO_3^- exchange, at least in the rabbit (205,206). Interestingly, the apical Cl^-/HCO_3^- exchanger in vivo is DIDS insensitive, an unusual feature of a HCO_3^- transporter.

Other Transporters

Several other acid–base transporters are present in the distal nephron, which can potentially contribute to transepithelial H^+ or HCO_3^- flux. A basolateral Na^+/H^+ exchanger (NHE1) is present in virtually all cells along the distal nephron (207). Na^+/H^+ exchanger 1 regulates intracellular pH and volume but does not appear to function in transepithelial acid–base transport. Basolateral Cl^- channels in the collecting duct recycle Cl^- that enters the cell via the basolateral Cl^-/HCO_3^- exchanger (208). In this manner, these Cl^- channels could regulate transepithelial acid–base transport. The Cl^- channels ClC-5 and ClC-3 have been found in type A and type B intercalated cells, respectively, but their functions there are unknown (209,210). Cystic fibrosis transmembrane regulator (CFTR) (the cystic fibrosis Cl^- channel) is also found in the collecting duct, but its function is unknown (211). An electroneutral Na^+–HCO_3^- cotransporter, NBC-3, has been localized to the apical membrane of type A intercalated cells in the outer medullary collecting duct and to the basolateral membrane of type B intercalated cells (212,213). It probably has only a minor role, if any, in transepithelial acid–base transport (34).

Regulation of Distal Nephron H⁺ and HCO₃⁻ Secretion

Acid–Base Balance and pH: With the exception of metabolic alkalosis, the distal nephron responds as expected to systemic acid–base changes. In metabolic alkalosis, the high serum [HCO_3^-] is sustained in part by maladaptive changes in distal nephron H^+ secretion caused by hormones and other stimuli (see in what follows and chapters 16–18).

Acidosis stimulates distal nephron H^+ secretion in several segments (reviewed in Refs. 157, 214). Lowering basolateral pH by either lowering peritubular HCO_3^- or raising PCO_2 increases collecting duct luminal H^+ secretion and HCO_3^- reabsorption (215,216). A fall in peritubular [HCO_3^-] will kinetically stimulate basolateral Cl^-/HCO_3^- exchange, but most of the acute effects result from decreases in intracellular pH that promote insertion of H^+-ATPase into the apical membrane (172). This process is calcium and microtubule/microfilament dependent (216–218). Luminal pH also affects

H^+ secretion. Decreasing luminal pH thermodynamically inhibits the H^+-ATPase by increasing the gradient against which it secretes H^+. However, all distal nephron segments have low ionic and solute permeability (i.e., all are tight epithelia), and therefore, relatively high H^+ gradients can be sustained.

Chloride concentration gradients can influence transepithelial HCO_3^- transport through effects on apical Cl^-/HCO_3^- exchanger in type B cells and the basolateral Cl^-/HCO_3^- exchanger in type A cells (219). For instance, a low luminal Cl^- concentration inhibits HCO_3^- secretion (151,220).

Additional mechanisms come into play when abnormalities in acid–base equilibrium are sustained. For instance, with chronic acid loading the HCO_3^--secreting type B cells undergo both morphologic and functional changes (160,221,222). Some data suggest interconversion between type B and type A intercalated cells (160). Immunocytochemical studies have shown changes in the distributions of intercalated cells with acid or alkali loads (158). In addition, polarity reversal of transporters (Cl^-/HCO_3^- exchange) has been observed both in cultured cells and, more recently, in freshly isolated CCD tubules, an effect mediated in part by the extracellular protein hensin (161,221,223,224).

Transcriptional regulation of H^+-ATPase has not been considered a major mechanism of the response to acidosis (158), but there is some evidence of response in at least the 31 kDa subunit of H^+-ATPase in acidosis (225). For AE1, an increase in the mRNA and protein levels occurs with acidosis (226,227). The mechanism(s) by which systemic acidosis (or alkalosis) signals the distal nephron segments to respond are not certain, although endothelin has recently been proposed to play a role (74). Renal cortical acid content may also be altered even when systemic pH is normal (228).

In segments that both reabsorb and secrete HCO_3^-, changes in HCO_3^- secretion appear to predominant over changes in HCO_3^- reabsorption in mediating changes in net HCO_3^- transport (150,151,229). Regulation of HCO_3^- secretion is paralleled by changes in expression and localization of pendrin (203,204).

Sodium Delivery, Voltage, and Mineralocorticoids: Sodium delivery, along with its accompanying anions, and mineralocorticoid status have major effects on distal nephron H^+ secretion. These factors are probably responsible for the effects of ECF volume on H^+ and HCO_3^- transport in the distal nephron (157,214,230,231). In epithelial cells transporting Na^+ (e.g., principal cells), most of these effects are probably mediated by changes in transepithelial voltage. A larger transepithelial voltage gradient (lumen negative) stimulates H^+ secretion, because the H^+ ATPase is an electrogenic pump. Increasing Na^+ delivery, poorly transported accompanying anion (e.g., anions other than Cl^-), and mineralocorticoids will increase the lumen-negative transepithelial voltage (232,233). Changes in luminal Cl^- and in the transepithelial Cl^- gradient will influence HCO_3^- reabsorption and secretion by effects on the apical and basolateral Cl^-/HCO_3^- transporters (220). In addition to voltage effects, mineralocorticoids directly stimulate H^+-ATPase (231). At the same time, mineralocorticoids also stimulate HCO_3^- secretion by type B cells, although this may be secondary to the associated metabolic alkalosis (150).

Potassium: Potassium depletion is well known to increase acid excretion; this results not only from increased NH_4^+ production and H^+ secretion in the proximal tubule, but also from increased distal nephron H^+ secretion (234,235). A major component of the effect of K^+ depletion is stimulation of distal nephron H^+/K^+-ATPase activity (177,236–238). Increased H^+/K^+-ATPase activity increases K^+ reabsorption and thereby H^+ secretion. The mRNA of the colonic isoform of H/K-ATPase increases with K^+ depletion, but functional H^+/K^+-ATPase activity is sensitive to SCH28080, to which the colonic isoform is insensitive (177,190,239,240). This finding and other conflicting results suggest that neither the colonic nor the gastric isoform of H^+/K^+-ATPase is stimulated by hypokalemia, and that perhaps a third and unique isoform is (177,241).

Endothelin: Endothelin-1 is released from microvascular endothelial cells in response to acidosis and may be an important regulator of H^+ secretion (242). Renal interstitial levels of ET-1 are increased in acidotic rats and this hormone stimulates superficial distal tubule H^+ secretion via the ETB receptor (74,242). Endothelin may increase H^+ secretion by stimulation of apical Na^+/H^+ exchange (154). Endothelin may also decrease HCO_3^- secretion, an effect that increases net HCO_3^- reabsorption (242).

Other Hormones: Other hormones, including vasopressin, isoproterenol, VIP, angiotensin II, PTH, PGE_2, PGI_2, and glucagon, have been shown to modulate distal nephron H^+ and HCO_3^- transport, but the physiologic significance of these effects has not been established (157,214).

Overview of Renal H^+ Secretion and Titratable Acid Excretion

Over 90% of H^+ secretion by the kidney is directed at recapturing filtered HCO_3^- and this process is accomplished by specialized transport proteins on the apical membrane of epithelial cells. H^+ secretion also reduces pH in the tubules, titrating nonbicarbonate buffer substances, such as phosphate and creatinine. As a result, the same process that removes HCO_3^- from the tubule fluid allows for H^+ to be excreted as titratable acid. The primary contributor to this form of acid excretion is phosphate, which is converted from HPO_4^{2-} to $H_2PO_4^-$ by secreted H^+ (see Chapter 6). In addition, H^+ secretion in the collecting ducts is a key factor contributing to NH_4^+ excretion, as discussed in what follows.

AMMONIUM EXCRETION

Renal excretion of ammonium (NH_4^+) normally accounts for approximately two-thirds of net acid excretion and can adaptively increase more than any other component of net acid excretion. Ammonium is a weak acid ($NH_4^+ \leftrightarrow NH_3 + H^+$) with a pK_a of ~9.0. As a result, it is not an effective buffer because over 99% of this weak base exists as NH_4^+ at the pH of the body fluids. The mechanism by which NH_4^+ excretion in the urine represents acid excretion is complex and, as discussed in what follows, depends on the metabolism of glutamine.

NH_4^+ Production and Excretion

Ammonium is produced by proximal tubule epithelial cells predominantly by the deamidation of glutamine, a process that yields two NH_4^+ molecules (Fig. 6) (157,243,244). The first deamidation produces glutamate and one NH_4^+. When ammoniagenesis is stimulated, glutamate is deamidated as well, yielding a second NH_4^+ and α-ketoglutarate. Excretion of this newly formed NH_4^+ allows for subsequent metabolism of these deamidation products to produce new HCO_3^- (Fig. 6). If the newly formed NH_4^+ were not excreted

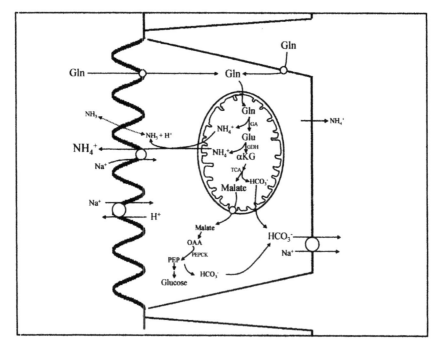

Figure 6   Major pathway of ammoniagenesis in the proximal tubule. *Source*: Adapted from Ref. 249.

by the kidney, it would return to the liver and be used either to resynthesize glutamine or combine with HCO_3^- to form urea, and neither process would generate new HCO_3^- (see Chapter 6). Thus, excretion of NH_4^+ is an essential step for subsequent metabolic processes within the body to generate new HCO_3^-. Many of the steps of NH_4^+ production and secretion into the urine are regulated by acid–base balance and by other factors.

Regulation of Ammoniagenesis

Production of NH_4 in the kidney (renal ammoniagenesis) is regulated by the effects of acid–base equilibrium on the activity of key deamidation enzymes and also by the effects on enzymes that metabolizes the carbon skeleton of glutamine (243,244). Deamidation is mediated primarily by the activities of mitochondrial glutaminase 1 (also called phosphate-dependent glutaminase) and glutamate dehydrogenase in the proximal tubule epithelial cells. Glutaminase is present in other nephron segments in small amounts but in these locations is not regulated by acid–base balance. Glutaminase-mediated deamidation of glutamine yields glutamate, and glutamate dehydrogenase deamidates glutamate to form α-ketoglutarate. Glutaminase I and glutamate dehydrogenase are upregulated by acid loading, predominantly by an increase in mRNA stability of these enzymes (245–248). Coupled with Krebs cycle enzymes, deamidated glutamine is metabolized to malate, which is then transported to the cytoplasm and converted to oxaloacetate and finally to phosphoenolpyruvate by the enzyme phosphoenolpyruvate carboxykinase (PEPCK). The PEPCK is also regulated by acid–base homeostasis. Phosphoenolpyruvate is primarily metabolized to CO_2 and H_2O but can also be used as a substrate for gluconeogenesis. In either case, a new HCO_3^- is produced. Glutamine is metabolized by other pathways to yield NH_4^+, but these pathways appear to be less important (243,244).

Ammonium production is increased by both acute and chronic acidosis (243). This increase appears to be mediated by acidosis-induced activation of glutaminase I, glutamate dehydrogenase, and PEPCK (243,244,249). Chronic hypokalemia also stimulates ammoniagenesis, probably via a decrease in intracellular pH. Hyperkalemia reduces both ammoniagenesis and transport into the collecting duct (250). A variety of hormones, including angiotensin II, have been found to increase ammoniagenesis. Angiotensin II not only increases ammoniagenesis, but also transport of NH_4^+ from the proximal tubule cell into the lumen (see in what follows) (251). Insulin, PTH, dopamine, and α-adrenergic agonists also increase ammoniagenesis, but the physiologic significance of these effects is unclear (243,252). Prostaglandins inhibit ammoniagenesis (253).

NH_4^+ Transport

Proximal Tubule: NH_4^+ produced in the proximal tubule is secreted preferentially into the tubule lumen, but a substantial portion of NH_4^+

ultimately exits the kidney via the renal veins (40,243,244). Secretion of total ammonia occurs both by NH_3 diffusion across the apical membrane and NH_4^+ transport on the apical Na^+/H^+ exchanger (NH_4^+ substituting for H^+) (22,254). NH_3 diffusion is facilitated by the lower luminal NH_3 concentration that results from the fall in pH in the tubule lumen created by H^+ secretion. Therefore, both NH_3 diffusion and NH_4^+ transport are accelerated by increased Na^+/H^+ exchange. Increased secretion into the proximal tubule also results from increasing luminal flow rate and from increased angiotensin II levels (251). Greater than 20% of ammonium produced in the proximal tubule is released across the basolateral membrane and reaches the renal venous blood (244,255). Although essentially all of the NH_4^+ that reaches the urine is produced in the proximal tubule, the pathway to the final urine is not simply down the tubule lumen.

Loop of Henle: In the loop segment, NH_3 diffuses out and NH_4^+ is transported out of the tubule, so that only about 50% of the ammonia delivered out of the proximal tubule reaches the early distal tubule (256,257). In the loop of Henle, recycling and countercurrent concentration occur and this process is critical for NH_4^+ excretion in the urine. Total ammonia concentration in the renal interstitium increases from the outer medullary region to the deep papilla (Fig. 7). NH_3 diffuses into the tubule in the descending limb and diffuses out of the tubule in the ascending limb, but the driving force for this medullary concentration of total ammonia is the secondary active reabsorption of NH_4^+ in the TAL (257,258). Ammonium is reabsorbed in the TAL by substitution for K^+ on the $Na^+–K^+–2Cl^-$ cotransporter, by the apical membrane K^+ channel, and by other pathways (259–261). Some NH_4^+ uptake may also be driven by the lumen positive voltage in the TAL. NH_4^+ transport in the TAL is decreased by increasing K^+ concentration (262). Another unique characteristic of the TAL is an apical membrane that has extremely low permeability to NH_3 (263).

Collecting Tubules: Ammonia secretion into the collecting tubules occurs in large part by diffusion of NH_3 across the epithelial cells. The NH_3 and NH_4^+ reabsorbed by the loop of Henle accumulate in the renal medulla and papilla, and the fraction that is NH_3 diffuses into the collecting tubules where it is converted back to NH_4^+ by combining with H^+ secreted into the lumen by collecting duct epithelial cells (see the earlier section). Acidification of the collecting duct urine by H^+ secretion is critical for reducing the NH_3 concentration in the collecting duct urine, thereby facilitating NH_3 diffusion into the tubule. As a result of this ammonia "trapping," urinary NH_4^+ excretion is inversely related to urinary pH. In addition to transepithelial NH_3 diffusion, NH_4^+ may be transported on H^+/K^+ ATPase or into collecting duct cells by substituting for K^+ on the basolateral Na^+/K^+-ATPase (264,265).

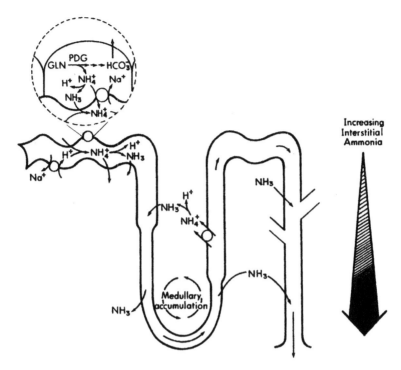

Figure 7 Overall scheme of ammonia transport along the nephron. *Source*: Adapted from Ref. 214.

Overview of NH_4^+ Excretion

Ammonium excretion is a flexible and carefully regulated resource for regenerating body alkali stores. It is regulated through control of NH_4^+ production in the renal cortex, by control of transport into the proximal tubule, and by control of H^+ secretion into the collecting duct. Countercurrent concentration in the loop of Henle is also a key determinant of NH_4^+ excretion. Disruption of any of these processes results in impaired renal NH_4^+ excretion. Given this complexity, it is not surprising that the earliest defect that occurs with renal injury is impaired NH_4^+ excretion (see Chapter 14).

REFERENCES

1. Schwartz GJ. Physiology and molecular biology of renal carbonic anhydrase. J Nephrol 2002; 15(suppl 5):S61–S74.
2. Brown D, Zhu XL, Sly WS. Localization of membrane-associated carbonic anhydrase type IV in kidney epithelial cells. Proc Natl Acad Sci USA 1990; 87(19):7457–7461.

3. Dobyan DC, Magill LS, Friedman PA, Hebert SC, Bulger RE. Carbonic anhydrase histochemistry in rabbit and mouse kidneys. Anat Rec 1982; 204(3):185–197.

4. Star RA, Burg MB, Knepper MA. Luminal disequilibrium pH and ammonia transport in outer medullary collecting duct [corrected and issued with original paging in Am J Physiol 1987 Aug; 253(2 Pt 2)]. Am J Physiol 1987; 252(6 Pt 2): F1148–F1157.

5. Wall SM, Flessner MF, Knepper MA. Distribution of luminal carbonic anhydrase activity along rat inner medullary collecting duct. Am J Physiol 1991; 260(5 Pt 2):F738–F748.

6. Kurtz I, Star R, Balaban RS, Garvin JL, Knepper MA. Spontaneous luminal disequilibrium pH in S3 proximal tubules. Role in ammonia and bicarbonate transport. J Clin Invest 1986; 78(4):989–996.

7. Brion LP, Zavilowitz BJ, Suarez C, Schwartz GJ. Metabolic acidosis stimulates carbonic anhydrase activity in rabbit proximal tubule and medullary collecting duct. Am J Physiol 1994; 266(2 Pt 2):F185–F195.

8. Tsuruoka S, Kittelberger AM, Schwartz GJ. Carbonic anhydrase II and IV mRNA in rabbit nephron segments: stimulation during metabolic acidosis. Am J Physiol 1998; 274(2 Pt 2):F259–F267.

9. Parkkila S, Parkkila AK, Saarnio J, et al. Expression of the membrane-associated carbonic anhydrase isozyme XII in the human kidney and renal tumors. J Histochem Cytochem 2000; 48(12):1601–1608.

10. Mori K, Ogawa Y, Ebihara K, et al. Isolation and characterization of CA XIV, a novel membrane-bound carbonic anhydrase from mouse kidney. J Biol Chem 1999; 274(22):15701–15705.

11. Schwartz GJ, Kittelberger AM, Watkins RH, O'Reilly MA. Carbonic anhydrase XII mRNA encodes a hydratase that is differentially expressed along the rabbit nephron. Am J Physiol Renal Physiol 2003; 284(2):F399–F410.

12. Sheu JN, Quigley R, Baum M. Heterogeneity of chloride/base exchange in rabbit superficial and juxtamedullary proximal convoluted tubules. Am J Physiol 1995; 268(5 Pt 2):F847–F853.

13. Aronson PS. Kinetic properties of the plasma membrane Na^+–H^+ exchanger. Annu Rev Physiol 1985; 47:545–560.

14. Hamm LL, Pucacco LR, Kokko JP, Jacobson HR. Hydrogen ion permeability of the rabbit proximal convoluted tubule. Am J Physiol 1984; 246(1 Pt 2): F3–F11.

15. Preisig PA, Alpern RJ. Contributions of cellular leak pathways to net $NaHCO_3$ and NaCl absorption. J Clin Invest 1989; 83(6):1859–1867.

16. DuBose TD Jr, Pucacco LR, Lucci MS, Carter NW. Micropuncture determination of pH, PCO_2, and total CO_2 concentration in accessible structures of the rat renal cortex. J Clin Invest 1979; 64(2):476–482.

17. Buerkert J, Martin D, Trigg D. Segmental analysis of the renal tubule in buffer production and net acid formation. Am J Physiol 1983; 244(4):F442–F454.

18. Rector FC Jr, Carter NW, Seldin DW. The mechanism of bicarbonate reabsorption in the proximal and distal tubules of the kidney. J Clin Invest 1965; 44:278–290.

19. Murer H, Hopfer U, Kinne R. Sodium/proton antiport in brush-border-membrane vesicles isolated from rat small intestine and kidney. Biochem J 1976; 154(3):597–604.

20. Kinsella JL, Aronson PS. Properties of the Na^+-H^+ exchanger in renal microvillus membrane vesicles. Am J Physiol 1980; 238(6):F461–F469.

21. Kinsella JL, Aronson PS. Amiloride inhibition of the Na^+-H^+ exchanger in renal microvillus membrane vesicles. Am J Physiol 1981; 241(4):F374–F379.

22. Kinsella JL, Aronson PS. Interaction of $NH4^+$ and Li^+ with the renal microvillus membrane Na^+-H^+ exchanger. Am J Physiol 1981; 241(5):C220–C226.

23. Aronson PS, Nee J, Suhm MA. Modifier role of internal H^+ in activating the Na^+-H^+ exchanger in renal microvillus membrane vesicles. Nature 1982; 299(5879):161–163.

24. Choi JY, Shah M, Lee MG, et al. Novel amiloride-sensitive sodium-dependent proton secretion in the mouse proximal convoluted tubule. J Clin Invest 2000; 105(8):1141–1146.

25. Wang T, Yang CL, Abbiati T, et al. Mechanism of proximal tubule bicarbonate absorption in NHE3 null mice. Am J Physiol 1999; 277(2 Pt 2):F298–F302.

26. Ledoussal C, Lorenz JN, Nieman ML, Soleimani M, Schultheis PJ, Shull GE. Renal salt wasting in mice lacking NHE3 Na^+/H^+ exchanger but not in mice lacking NHE2. Am J Physiol Renal Physiol 2001; 281(4):F718–F727.

27. Nakhoul NL, Hamm LL. Vacuolar H(+)-ATPase in the kidney. J Nephrol 2002; 15(suppl 5):S22–S31.

28. Bank N, Aynedjian HS, Mutz BF. Evidence for a DCCD-sensitive component of proximal bicarbonate reabsorption. Am J Physiol 1985; 249(5 Pt 2):F636–F644.

29. Aronson PS, Giebisch G. Mechanisms of chloride transport in the proximal tubule. Am J Physiol 1997; 273(2 Pt 2):F179–F192.

30. Alpern RJ. Mechanism of basolateral membrane H^+/OH^-/HCO_3^- transport in the rat proximal convoluted tubule. A sodium-coupled electrogenic process. J Gen Physiol 1985; 86(5):613–636.

31. Akiba T, Alpern RJ, Eveloff J, Calamina J, Warnock DG. Electrogenic sodium/bicarbonate cotransport in rabbit renal cortical basolateral membrane vesicles. J Clin Invest 1986; 78(6):1472–1478.

32. Soleimani M, Aronson PS. Ionic mechanism of Na^+-HCO_3^- cotransport in rabbit renal basolateral membrane vesicles. J Biol Chem 1989; 264(31): 18302–18308.

33. Gross E, Hawkins K, Abuladze N, et al. The stoichiometry of the electrogenic sodium bicarbonate cotransporter NBC1 is cell-type dependent. J Physiol 2001; 531(Pt 3):597–603.

34. Gross E, Kurtz I. Structural determinants and significance of regulation of electrogenic Na(+)–HCO(3)(–) cotransporter stoichiometry. Am J Physiol Renal Physiol 2002; 283(5):F876–F887.

35. Burnham CE, Amlal H, Wang Z, Shull GE, Soleimani M. Cloning and functional expression of a human kidney Na^+:HCO_3^- cotransporter. J Biol Chem 1997; 272(31):19111–19114.

36. Maunsbach AB, Vorum H, Kwon TH, et al. Immunoelectron microscopic localization of the electrogenic Na/HCO(3) cotransporter in rat and ambystoma kidney. J Am Soc Nephrol 2000; 11(12):2179–2189.

37. Alpern RJ, Chambers M. Basolateral membrane Cl/HCO_3 exchange in the rat proximal convoluted tubule. Na-dependent and -independent modes. J Gen Physiol 1987; 89(4):581–598.

38. Biemesderfer D, Reilly RF, Exner M, Igarashi P, Aronson PS. Immunocytochemical characterization of Na(+)–H+ exchanger isoform NHE-1 in rabbit kidney. Am J Physiol 1992; 263(5 Pt 2):F833–F840.

39. Cheema-Dhadli S, Lin SH, Halperin ML. Mechanisms used to dispose of progressively increasing alkali load in rats. Am J Physiol Renal Physiol 2002; 282(6):F1049–F1055.

40. Hamm LL, Simon EE. Roles and mechanisms of urinary buffer excretion. Am J Physiol 1987; 253(4 Pt 2):F595–F605.

41. Hamm LL, Hering-Smith KS. Pathophysiology of hypocitraturic nephrolithiasis. Endocrinol Metab Clin North Am 2002; 31(4):885–893, viii.

42. Schwartz GJ, Weinstein AM, Steele RE, Stephenson JL, Burg MB. Carbon dioxide permeability of rabbit proximal convoluted tubules. Am J Physiol 1981; 240(3):F231–F244.

43. Alpern RJ, Cogan MG, Rector FC Jr. Effect of luminal bicarbonate concentration on proximal acidification in the rat. Am J Physiol 1982; 243(1):F53–F59.

44. Maddox DA, Gennari FJ. Load dependence of proximal tubular bicarbonate reabsorption in chronic metabolic alkalosis in the rat. J Clin Invest 1986; 77(3):709–716.

45. Soleimani M, Bizal GL, McKinney TD, Hattabaugh YJ. Effect of in vitro metabolic acidosis on luminal Na^+/H^+ exchange and basolateral $Na^+:HCO_3^-$ cotransport in rabbit kidney proximal tubules. J Clin Invest 1992; 90(1): 211–218.

46. Wu MS, Biemesderfer D, Giebisch G, Aronson PS. Role of NHE3 in mediating renal brush border $Na^+–H^+$ exchange. Adaptation to metabolic acidosis. J Biol Chem 1996; 271(51):32749–32752.

47. Ambuhl PM, Amemiya M, Danczkay M, et al. Chronic metabolic acidosis increases NHE3 protein abundance in rat kidney. Am J Physiol 1996; 271(4 Pt 2):F917–F925.

48. Yang X, Amemiya M, Peng Y, Moe OW, Preisig PA, Alpern RJ. Acid incubation causes exocytic insertion of NHE3 in OKP cells. Am J Physiol—Cell Physiol 2000; 279(2):C410–C419.

49. Peng Y, Amemiya M, Yang X, et al. ET(B) receptor activation causes exocytic insertion of NHE3 in OKP cells. Am J Physiol—Renal Fluid Electrol Physiol 2001; 280(1):F34–F42.

50. Laghmani K, Preisig PA, Moe OW, Yanagisawa M, Alpern RJ. Endothelin-1/endothelin-B receptor-mediated increases in NHE3 activity in chronic metabolic acidosis. J Clin Invest 2001; 107(12):1563–1569.

51. Ambuhl PM, Yang X, Peng Y, Preisig PA, Moe OW, Alpern RJ. Glucocorticoids enhance acid activation of the Na^+/H^+ exchanger 3 (NHE3). J Clin Invest 1999; 103(3):429–435.

52. Amlal H, Chen Q, Greeley T, Pavelic L, Soleimani M. Coordinated down-regulation of NBC-1 and NHE-3 in sodium and bicarbonate loading. Kidney Int 2001; 60(5):1824–1836.
53. Ruiz OS, Arruda JA, Talor Z. Na–HCO_3 cotransport and Na–H antiporter in chronic respiratory acidosis and alkalosis. Am J Physiol 1989; 256(3 Pt 2): F414–F420.
54. Schwartz GJ, Al Awqati Q. Carbon dioxide causes exocytosis of vesicles containing H^+ pumps in isolated perfused proximal and collecting tubules. J Clin Invest 1985; 75(5):1638–1644.
55. Nakhoul NL, Chen LK, Boron WF. Effect of basolateral CO_2/HCO_3^- on intracellular pH regulation in the rabbit S3 proximal tubule. J Gen Physiol 1993; 102(6):1171–1205.
56. Chen LK, Boron WF. Acid extrusion in S3 segment of rabbit proximal tubule. II. Effect of basolateral CO_2/HCO_3^-. Am J Physiol 1995; 268(2 Pt 2):F193–F203.
57. Soleimani M, Bergman JA, Hosford MA, McKinney TD. Potassium depletion increases luminal Na^+/H^+ exchange and basolateral $Na^+:CO_3^-:HCO_3^-$ cotransport in rat renal cortex. J Clin Invest 1990; 86(4):1076–1083.
58. Amemiya M, Tabei K, Kusano E, Asano Y, Alpern RJ. Incubation of OKP cells in low-K^+ media increases NHE3 activity after early decrease in intracellular pH. Am J Physiol 1999; 276(3 Pt 1):C711–C716.
59. Adam WR, Koretsky AP, Weiner MW. 31P-NMR in vivo measurement of renal intracellular pH: effects of acidosis and K^+ depletion in rats. Am J Physiol 1986; 251(5 Pt 2):F904–F910.
60. Alpern RJ, Cogan MG, Rector FC Jr. Flow dependence of proximal tubular bicarbonate absorption. Am J Physiol 1983; 245(4):F478–F484.
61. Preisig PA. Luminal flow rate regulates proximal tubule H–HCO_3 transporters. Am J Physiol 1992; 262(1 Pt 2):F47–F54.
62. Gennari FJ, Helmle-Kolb C, Murer H. Influence of extracellular pH and perfusion rate on Na^+/H^+ exchange in cultured opossum kidney cells. Pflugers Arch 1992; 420(2):153–158.
63. Maddox DA, Fortin SM, Tartini A, Barnes WD, Gennari FJ. Effect of acute changes in glomerular filtration rate on Na^+/H^+ exchange in rat renal cortex. J Clin Invest 1992; 89(4):1296–1303.
64. Maddox DA, Barnes WD, Gennari FJ. Effect of acute increases in filtered HCO_3^- on renal hydrogen transporters: II. H(+)-ATPase. Kidney Int 1997; 52(2):446–453.
65. Maddox DA, Gennari FJ. The early proximal tubule: a high-capacity delivery-responsive reabsorptive site. Am J Physiol 1987; 252(4 Pt 2):F573–F584.
66. Preisig PA, Alpern RJ. Increased Na/H antiporter and Na/$3HCO_3$ symporter activities in chronic hyperfiltration. A model of cell hypertrophy. J Gen Physiol 1991; 97(2):195–217.
67. Moe OW, Tejedor A, Levi M, Seldin DW, Preisig PA, Alpern RJ. Dietary NaCl modulates Na(+)–H^+ antiporter activity in renal cortical apical membrane vesicles. Am J Physiol 1991; 260(1 Pt 2):F130–F137.
68. Alpern RJ, Cogan MG, Rector FC Jr. Effects of extracellular fluid volume and plasma bicarbonate concentration on proximal acidification in the rat. J Clin Invest 1983; 71(3):736–746.

69. Kinsella J, Cujdik T, Sacktor B. Na^+-H^+ exchange activity in renal brush border membrane vesicles in response to metabolic acidosis: the role of glucocorticoids. Proc Natl Acad Sci USA 1984; 81(2):630–634.

70. Ali R, Amlal H, Burnham CE, Soleimani M. Glucocorticoids enhance the expression of the basolateral $Na^+{:}HCO_3^-$ cotransporter in renal proximal tubules. Kidney Int 2000; 57(3):1063–1071.

71. Laghmani K, Preisig PA, Alpern RJ. The role of endothelin in proximal tubule proton secretion and the adaptation to a chronic metabolic acidosis. J Nephrol 2002; 15(suppl 5):S75–S87.

72. Garcia NH, Garvin JL. Endothelin's biphasic effect on fluid absorption in the proximal straight tubule and its inhibitory cascade. J Clin Invest 1994; 93(6):2572–2577.

73. Eiam-Ong S, Hilden SA, King AJ, Johns CA, Madias NE. Endothelin-1 stimulates the Na^+/H^+ and Na^+/HCO_3^- transporters in rabbit renal cortex. Kidney Int 1992; 42(1):18–24.

74. Wesson DE. Endogenous endothelins mediate increased distal tubule acidification induced by dietary acid in rats. J Clin Invest 1997; 99(9):2203–2211.

75. Wesson DE, Simoni J, Green DF. Reduced extracellular pH increases endothelin-1 secretion by human renal microvascular endothelial cells. J Clin Invest 1998; 101(3):578–583.

76. Chu TS, Tsuganezawa H, Peng Y, Cano A, Yanagisawa M, Alpern RJ. Role of tyrosine kinase pathways in ETB receptor activation of NHE3. Am J Physiol 1996; 271(3 Pt 1):C763–C771.

77. Yamaji Y, Tsuganezawa H, Moe OW, Alpern RJ. Intracellular acidosis activates c-Src. Am J Physiol 1997; 272(3 Pt 1):C886–C893.

78. Tsuganezawa H, Sato S, Yamaji Y, Preisig PA, Moe OW, Alpern RJ. Role of c-SRC and ERK in acid-induced activation of NHE3. Kidney Int 2002; 62(1):41–50.

79. Peng Y, Moe OW, Chu T, Preisig PA, Yanagisawa M, Alpern RJ. ETB receptor activation leads to activation and phosphorylation of NHE3. Am J Physiol 1999; 276(4 Pt 1):C938–C945.

80. Chu TS, Peng Y, Cano A, Yanagisawa M, Alpern RJ. Endothelin(B) receptor activates NHE-3 by a Ca^{2+}-dependent pathway in OKP cells. J Clin Invest 1996; 97(6):1454–1462.

81. Ruiz OS, Robey RB, Qiu YY, et al. Regulation of the renal Na–HCO(3) cotransporter. XI. Signal transduction underlying CO(2) stimulation. Am J Physiol 1999; 277(4 Pt 2):F580–F586.

82. Espiritu DJ, Bernardo AA, Robey RB, Arruda JA. A central role for Pyk2-Src interaction in coupling diverse stimuli to increased epithelial NBC activity. Am J Physiol Renal Physiol 2002; 283(4):F663–F670.

83. Geibel J, Giebisch G, Boron WF. Angiotensin II stimulates both $Na(+)-H^+$ exchange and Na^+/HCO_3^- cotransport in the rabbit proximal tubule. Proc Natl Acad Sci USA 1990; 87(20):7917–7920.

84. Baum M, Quigley R, Quan A. Effect of luminal angiotensin II on rabbit proximal convoluted tubule bicarbonate absorption. Am J Physiol 1997; 273(4 Pt 2): F595–F600.

85. Bloch RD, Zikos D, Fisher KA, et al. Activation of proximal tubular Na(+)–H$^+$ exchange by angiotensin II. Am J Physiol 1992; 263(1 Pt 2):F135–F143.

86. Eiam-Ong S, Hilden SA, Johns CA, Madias NE. Stimulation of basolateral Na(+)-HCO$_3^-$ cotransporter by angiotensin II in rabbit renal cortex. Am J Physiol 1993; 265(2 Pt 2):F195–F203.

87. Ruiz OS, Qiu YY, Wang LJ, Arruda JA. Regulation of the renal Na–HCO$_3$ cotransporter: IV. Mechanisms of the stimulatory effect of angiotensin II. J Am Soc Nephrol 1995; 6(4):1202–1208.

88. Liu FY, Cogan MG. Role of protein kinase C in proximal bicarbonate absorption and angiotensin signaling. Am J Physiol 1990; 258(4 Pt 2):F927–F933.

89. Tsuganezawa H, Preisig PA, Alpern RJ. Dominant negative c-Src inhibits angiotensin II induced activation of NHE3 in OKP cells. Kidney Int 1998; 54(2):394–398.

90. Robey RB, Ruiz OS, Espiritu DJ, et al. Angiotensin II stimulation of renal epithelial cell Na/HCO$_3$ cotransport activity: a central role for Src family kinase/classic MAPK pathway coupling. J Membr Biol 2002; 187(2):135–145.

91. McKinney TD, Myers P. PTH inhibition of bicarbonate transport by proximal convoluted tubules. Am J Physiol 1980; 239(2):F127–F134.

92. Puschett JB, Zurbach P, Sylk D. Acute effects of parathyroid hormone on proximal bicarbonate transport in the dog. Kidney Int 1976; 9(6):501–510.

93. Moe OW, Amemiya M, Yamaji Y. Activation of protein kinase A acutely inhibits and phosphorylates Na/H exchanger NHE-3. J Clin Invest 1995; 96(5):2187–2194.

94. Ruiz OS, Qiu YY, Wang LJ, Arruda JA. Regulation of the renal Na–HCO$_3$ cotransporter: V. Mechanism of the inhibitory effect of parathyroid hormone. Kidney Int 1996; 49(2):396–402.

95. Cano A, Preisig P, Alpern RJ. Cyclic adenosine monophosphate acutely inhibits and chronically stimulates Na/H antiporter in OKP cells. J Clin Invest 1993; 92(4):1632–1638.

96. Nord EP, Howard MJ, Hafezi A, Moradeshagi P, Vaystub S, Insel PA. Alpha 2 adrenergic agonists stimulate Na$^+$–H$^+$ antiport activity in the rabbit renal proximal tubule. J Clin Invest 1987; 80(6):1755–1762.

97. Hall RA, Premont RT, Chow CW, et al. The beta2-adrenergic receptor interacts with the Na$^+$/H$^+$-exchanger regulatory factor to control Na$^+$/H$^+$ exchange. Nature 1998; 392(6676):626–630.

98. Shenolikar S, Weinman EJ. NHERF: targeting and trafficking membrane proteins. [Review] [66 refs]. Am J Physiol—Renal Fluid Electrol Physiol 2001; 280(3):F389–F395.

99. Weinman EJ. New functions for the NHERF family of proteins. [letter; comment.]. J Clin Invest 2001; 108(2):185–186.

100. Bernardo AA, Kear FT, Santos AV, et al. Basolateral Na(+)/HCO(3)(-) cotransport activity is regulated by the dissociable Na(+)/H(+) exchanger regulatory factor. J Clin Invest 1999; 104(2):195–201.

101. Klisic J, Hu MC, Nief V, et al. Insulin activates Na(+)/H(+) exchanger 3: biphasic response and glucocorticoid dependence. Am J Physiol Renal Physiol 2002; 283(3):F532–F539.

102. Felder CC, Campbell T, Albrecht F, Jose PA. Dopamine inhibits Na(+)–H$^+$ exchanger activity in renal BBMV by stimulation of adenylate cyclase. Am J Physiol 1990; 259(2 Pt 2):F297–F303.

103. Hu MC, Fan L, Crowder LA, Karim-Jimenez Z, Murer H, Moe OW. Dopamine acutely stimulates Na$^+$/H$^+$ exchanger (NHE3) endocytosis via clathrin-coated vesicles: dependence on protein kinase A-mediated NHE3 phosphorylation. J Biol Chem 2001; 276(29):26906–26915.

104. Di Sole F, Cerull R, Casavola V, Moe OW, Burckhardt G, Helmle-Kolb C. Molecular aspects of acute inhibition of Na(+)–H(+) exchanger NHE3 by A(2)-adenosine receptor agonists. J Physiol 2002; 541(Pt 2):529–543.

105. Robey RB, Ruiz OS, Baniqued J, et al. SFKs, Ras, and the classic MAPK pathway couple muscarinic receptor activation to increased Na–HCO(3) cotransport activity in renal epithelial cells. Am J Physiol Renal Physiol 2001; 280(5):F844–F850.

106. Capasso G, Unwin R, Agulian S, Giebisch G. Bicarbonate transport along the loop of Henle. I. Microperfusion studies of load and inhibitor sensitivity. J Clin Invest 1991; 88(2):430–437.

107. Good DW. The thick ascending limb as a site of renal bicarbonate reabsorption. Semin Nephrol 1993; 13(2):225–235.

108. Capasso G, Unwin R, Ciani F, et al. Bicarbonate transport along the loop of Henle. II. Effects of acid–base, dietary, and neurohumoral determinants. J Clin Invest 1994; 94(2):830–838.

109. Capasso G, Unwin R, Rizzo M, Pica A, Giebisch G. Bicarbonate transport along the loop of Henle: molecular mechanisms and regulation. J Nephrol 2002; 15(suppl 5):S88–S96.

110. Kurtz I. Apical Na$^+$/H$^+$ antiporter and glycolysis-dependent H$^+$-ATPase regulate intracellular pH in the rabbit S3 proximal tubule. J Clin Invest 1987; 80(4):928–935.

111. Wang T, Hropot M, Aronson PS, Giebisch G. Role of NHE isoforms in mediating bicarbonate reabsorption along the nephron. Am J Physiol—Renal Fluid Electrol Physiol 2001; 281(6):F1117–F1122.

112. Sun AM, Liu Y, Dworkin LD, Tse CM, Donowitz M, Yip KP. Na$^+$/H$^+$ exchanger isoform 2 (NHE2) is expressed in the apical membrane of the medullary thick ascending limb. J Membr Biol 1997; 160(1):85–90.

113. Watts BA III, Good DW. Apical membrane Na$^+$/H$^+$ exchange in rat medullary thick ascending limb. pH-dependence and inhibition by hyperosmolality. J Biol Chem 1994; 269(32):20250–20255.

114. Good DW, Watts BA III. Functional roles of apical membrane Na$^+$/H$^+$ exchange in rat medullary thick ascending limb. Am J Physiol 1996; 270(4 Pt 2): F691–F699.

115. Brown D, Hirsch S, Gluck S. Localization of a proton-pumping ATPase in rat kidney. J Clin Invest 1988; 82(6):2114–2126.

116. Krapf R. Basolateral membrane H/OH/HCO$_3$ transport in the rat cortical thick ascending limb. Evidence for an electrogenic Na/HCO$_3$ cotransporter in parallel with a Na/H antiporter. J Clin Invest 1988; 82(1):234–241.

117. Vorum H, Kwon TH, Fulton C, et al. Immunolocalization of electroneutral Na–HCO(3)(–) cotransporter in rat kidney. Am J Physiol Renal Physiol 2000; 279(5):F901–F909.
118. Kwon TH, Fulton C, Wang W, et al. Chronic metabolic acidosis upregulates rat kidney Na–HCO cotransporters NBCn1 and NBC3 but not NBC1. Am J Physiol—Renal Fluid Electrol Physiol/Renal Physiol 2002; 282(2):F341–F351.
119. Blanchard A, Leviel F, Bichara M, Podevin RA, Paillard M. Interactions of external and internal K^+ with $K(+)$–HCO_3^- cotransporter of rat medullary thick ascending limb. Am J Physiol 1996; 271(1 Pt 1):C218–C225.
120. Leviel F, Eladari D, Blanchard A, Poumarat JS, Paillard M, Podevin RA. Pathways for HCO_3^- exit across the basolateral membrane in rat thick limbs. Am J Physiol 1999; 276(6 Pt 2):F847–F856.
121. Bourgeois S, Masse S, Paillard M, Houillier P. Basolateral membrane Cl(–)-, Na(+)-, and K(+)-coupled base transport mechanisms in rat MTALH. Am J Physiol Renal Physiol 2002; 282(4):F655–F668.
122. Good DW, George T, Watts BA III. Basolateral membrane Na^+/H^+ exchange enhances HCO_3^- absorption in rat medullary thick ascending limb: evidence for functional coupling between basolateral and apical membrane Na^+/H^+ exchangers. Proc Natl Acad Sci USA 1995; 92(26):12525–12529.
123. Chambrey R, St John PL, Eladari D, et al. Localization and functional characterization of Na^+/H^+ exchanger isoform NHE4 in rat thick ascending limbs. Am J Physiol—Renal Fluid Electrol Physiol 2001; 281(4):F707–F717.
124. Good DW. Sodium-dependent bicarbonate absorption by cortical thick ascending limb of rat kidney. Am J Physiol 1985; 248(6 Pt 2):F821–F829.
125. DuBose TD Jr, Lucci MS, Hogg RJ, Pucacco LR, Kokko JP, Carter NW. Comparison of acidification parameters in superficial and deep nephrons of the rat. Am J Physiol 1983; 244(5):F497–F503.
126. Good DW. Adaptation of HCO_3^- and NH_4^+ transport in rat MTAL: effects of chronic metabolic acidosis and Na^+ intake. Am J Physiol 1990; 258(5 Pt 2): F1345–F1353.
127. Laghmani K, Borensztein P, Ambuhl P, et al. Chronic metabolic acidosis enhances NHE-3 protein abundance and transport activity in the rat thick ascending limb by increasing NHE-3 mRNA. J Clin Invest 1997; 99(1):24–30.
128. Unwin R, Stidwell R, Taylor S, Capasso G. The effects of respiratory alkalosis and acidosis on net bicarbonate flux along the rat loop of Henle in vivo. Am J Physiol 1997; 273(5 Pt 2):F698–F705.
129. Laghmani K, Chambrey R, Froissart M, Bichara M, Paillard M, Borensztein P. Adaptation of NHE-3 in the rat thick ascending limb: effects of high sodium intake and metabolic alkalosis. Am J Physiol 1999; 276(1 Pt 2): F18–F26.
130. Good DW, George T, Watts BA III. Aldosterone inhibits HCO absorption via a nongenomic pathway in medullary thick ascending limb. Am J Physiol Renal Physiol 2002; 283(4):F699–F706.
131. Unwin R, Capasso G, Giebisch G. Bicarbonate transport along the loop of Henle effects of adrenal steroids. Am J Physiol 1995; 268(2 Pt 2):F234–F239.

132. Good DW. Nerve growth factor regulates HCO$_3^-$ absorption in thick ascending limb: modifying effects of vasopressin. Am J Physiol 1998; 274(4 Pt 1): C931–C939.

133. Watts BA III, Di Mari JF, Davis RJ, Good DW. Hypertonicity activates MAP kinases and inhibits HCO$_3^-$ absorption via distinct pathways in thick ascending limb. Am J Physiol 1998; 275(4 Pt 2):F478–F486.

134. Good DW, George T, Wang DH. Angiotensin II inhibits HCO$_3^-$ absorption via a cytochrome P-450-dependent pathway in MTAL. Am J Physiol 1999; 276(5 Pt 2):F726–F736.

135. Good DW, Di Mari JF, Watts BA III. Hyposmolality stimulates Na(+)/H(+) exchange and HCO(3)(-) absorption in thick ascending limb via PI 3-kinase. Am J Physiol Cell Physiol 2000; 279(5):C1443–C1454.

136. Watts BA III, Good DW. ERK mediates inhibition of Na(+)/H(+) exchange and HCO(3)(-) absorption by nerve growth factor in MTAL. Am J Physiol Renal Physiol 2002; 282(6):F1056–F1063.

137. Watts BA III, George T, Good DW. Nerve growth factor inhibits HCO$_3^-$ absorption in renal thick ascending limb through inhibition of basolateral membrane Na$^+$/H$^+$ exchange. J Biol Chem 1999; 274(12):7841–7847.

138. Good DW. Effects of osmolality on bicarbonate absorption by medullary thick ascending limb of the rat. J Clin Invest 1992; 89(1):184–190.

139. Good DW. Hyperosmolality inhibits bicarbonate absorption in rat medullary thick ascending limb via a protein-tyrosine kinase-dependent pathway. J Biol Chem 1995; 270(17):9883–9889.

140. Watts BA III, Good DW. Hyposmolality stimulates apical membrane Na(+)/H(+) exchange and HCO(3)(-) absorption in renal thick ascending limb. J Clin Invest 1999; 104(11):1593–1602.

141. Good DW. Inhibition of bicarbonate absorption by peptide hormones and cyclic adenosine monophosphate in rat medullary thick ascending limb. J Clin Invest 1990; 85(4):1006–1013.

142. Bichara M, Mercier O, Houillier P, Paillard M, Leviel F. Effects of antidiuretic hormone on urinary acidification and on tubular handling of bicarbonate in the rat. J Clin Invest 1987; 80(3):621–630.

143. Wang T, Malnic G, Giebisch G, Chan YL. Renal bicarbonate reabsorption in the rat. IV. Bicarbonate transport mechanisms in the early and late distal tubule. J Clin Invest 1993; 91(6):2776–2784.

144. Chambrey R, Warnock DG, Podevin RA, et al. Immunolocalization of the Na$^+$/H$^+$ exchanger isoform NHE2 in rat kidney. Am J Physiol 1998; 275 (3 Pt 2):F379–F386.

145. McKinney TD, Burg MB. Bicarbonate transport by rabbit cortical collecting tubules. Effect of acid and alkali loads in vivo on transport in vitro. J Clin Invest 1977; 60(3):766–768.

146. Knepper MA, Good DW, Burg MB. Ammonia and bicarbonate transport by rat cortical collecting ducts perfused in vitro. Am J Physiol 1985; 249(6 Pt 2): F870–F877.

147. Levine DZ, Iacovitti M, Nash L, Vandorpe D. Secretion of bicarbonate by rat distal tubules in vivo. Modulation by overnight fasting. J Clin Invest 1988; 81(6):1873–1878.

148. Gifford JD, Rome L, Galla JH. H(+)–K(+)-ATPase activity in rat collecting duct segments. Am J Physiol 1992; 262(4 Pt 2):F692–F695.
149. Hayashi M, Yamaji Y, Iyori M, Kitajima W, Saruta T. Effect of isoproterenol on intracellular pH of the intercalated cells in the rabbit cortical collecting ducts. J Clin Invest 1991; 87(4):1153–1157.
150. Garcia-Austt J, Good DW, Burg MB, Knepper MA. Deoxycorticosterone-stimulated bicarbonate secretion in rabbit cortical collecting ducts: effects of luminal chloride removal and in vivo acid loading. Am J Physiol 1985; 249(2 Pt 2):F205–F212.
151. Hamm LL, Hering-Smith KS, Vehaskari VM. Control of bicarbonate transport in collecting tubules from normal and remnant kidneys. Am J Physiol 1989; 256(4 Pt 2):F680–F687.
152. Wesson DE, Dolson GM. Enhanced HCO3 secretion by distal tubule contributes to NaCl-induced correction of chronic alkalosis. Am J Physiol 1993; 264(5 Pt 2):F899–F906.
153. Galla JH, Gifford JD, Luke RG, Rome L. Adaptations to chloride-depletion alkalosis. Am J Physiol 1991; 261(4 Pt 2):R771–R781.
154. Wesson DE. Na/H exchange and H–K ATPase increase distal tubule acidification in chronic alkalosis. Kidney Int 1998; 53(4):945–951.
155. Wesson DE. Dietary HCO3 reduces distal tubule acidification by increasing cellular HCO3 secretion. Am J Physiol 1996; 271(1 Pt 2):F132–F142.
156. Tsuruoka S, Schwartz GJ. Mechanisms of HCO(–)(3) secretion in the rabbit connecting segment. Am J Physiol 1999; 277(4 Pt 2):F567–F574.
157. Alpern RJ. Renal acidification mechanisms. In: Brenner B, ed. The Kidney. Philadelphia: W. B. Saunders Company, 2000:455–519.
158. Bastani B, Purcell H, Hemken P, Trigg D, Gluck S. Expression and distribution of renal vacuolar proton-translocating adenosine triphosphatase in response to chronic acid and alkali loads in the rat. J Clin Invest 1991; 88(1):126–136.
159. Emmons C, Kurtz I. Functional characterization of three intercalated cell subtypes in the rabbit outer cortical collecting duct. J Clin Invest 1994; 93(1): 417–423.
160. Schwartz GJ, Barasch J, Al Awqati Q. Plasticity of functional epithelial polarity. Nature 1985; 318(6044):368–371.
161. Schwartz GJ, Tsuruoka S, Vijayakumar S, Petrovic S, Mian A, Al Awqati Q. Acid incubation reverses the polarity of intercalated cell transporters, an effect mediated by hensin. J Clin Invest 2002; 109(1):89–99.
162. Al Awqati Q, Vijayakumar S, Takito J, Hikita C, Yan L, Wiederholt T. Phenotypic plasticity and terminal differentiation of the intercalated cell: the hensin pathway. Exp Nephrol 2000; 8(2):66–71.
163. Hamm LL, Hering-Smith KS. Acid–base transport in the collecting duct. Semin Nephrol 1993; 13(2):246–255.
164. Ridderstrale Y, Kashgarian M, Koeppen B, et al. Morphological heterogeneity of the rabbit collecting duct. Kidney Int 1988; 34(5):655–670.
165. Weiner ID, Wingo CS, Hamm LL. Regulation of intracellular pH in two cell populations of inner stripe of rabbit outer medullary collecting duct. Am J Physiol 1993; 265(3 Pt 2):F406–F415.

166. Madsen KM, Clapp WL, Verlander JW. Structure and function of the inner medullary collecting duct. Kidney Int 1988; 34(4):441–454.

167. Brown D, Breton S. Structure, function, and cellular distribution of the vacuolar H+ATPase (H+V-ATPase/proton pump). In: Seldin DW, Giebisch G, eds. The Kidney: Physiology and Pathophysiology. Philadelphia: Lippincott Williams & Wilkins, 2000:171–191.

168. Gluck S, Nelson R. The role of the V-ATPase in renal epithelial H^+ transport. J Exp Biol 1992; 172:205–218.

169. Nelson RD, Guo XL, Masood K, Brown D, Kalkbrenner M, Gluck S. Selectively amplified expression of an isoform of the vacuolar H(+)-ATPase 56-kilodalton subunit in renal intercalated cells. Proc Natl Acad Sci USA 1992; 89(8):3541–3545.

170. Hemken P, Guo XL, Wang ZQ, Zhang K, Gluck S. Immunologic evidence that vacuolar H^+ ATPases with heterogeneous forms of Mr = 31,000 subunit have different membrane distributions in mammalian kidney. J Biol Chem 1992; 267(14):9948–9957.

171. Fernandez R, Bosqueiro JR, Cassola AC, Malnic G. Role of Cl^- in electrogenic H^+ secretion by cortical distal tubule. J Membr Biol 1997; 157(2):193–201.

172. Gluck S, Cannon C, Al Awqati Q. Exocytosis regulates urinary acidification in turtle bladder by rapid insertion of H^+ pumps into the luminal membrane. Proc Natl Acad Sci USA 1982; 79(14):4327–4331.

173. Schwartz GJ, Al Awqati Q. Regulation of transepithelial H^+ transport by exocytosis and endocytosis. [Review] [28 refs]. Annu Rev Physiol 1986; 48:153–161.

174. Zhang K, Wang ZQ, Gluck S. Identification and partial purification of a cytosolic activator of vacuolar H(+)-ATPases from mammalian kidney. J Biol Chem 1992; 267(14):9701–9705.

175. Zhang K, Wang ZQ, Gluck S. A cytosolic inhibitor of vacuolar H(+)-ATPases from mammalian kidney. J Biol Chem 1992; 267(21):14539–14542.

176. Wingo CS, Smolka AJ. Function and structure of H–K-ATPase in the kidney. Am J Physiol 1995; 269(1 Pt 2):F1–F16.

177. Doucet A, Horisberger J. Renal Ion-translocating ATPases: the P-type family. In: Seldin D, Giebisch G, eds. The Kidney: Physiology and Pathophysiology. Philadelphia: Lippincott Williams & Wilkins, 2000:140–170.

178. Caviston TL, Campbell WG, Wingo CS, Cain BD. Molecular identification of the renal H^+,K^+-ATPases. Semin Nephrol 1999; 19(5):431–437.

179. Kraut JA, Hiura J, Shin JM, Smolka A, Sachs G, Scott D. The Na(+)-K(+)-ATPase beta 1 subunit is associated with the HK alpha 2 protein in the rat kidney. Kidney Int 1998; 53(4):958–962.

180. Codina J, Delmas-Mata JT, DuBose TD Jr. The alpha-subunit of the colonic H^+,K^+-ATPase assembles with beta1-Na^+,K^+-ATPase in kidney and distal colon. J Biol Chem 1998; 273(14):7894–7899.

181. Sangan P, Kolla SS, Rajendran VM, Kashgarian M, Binder HJ. Colonic H–K-ATPase beta-subunit: identification in apical membranes and regulation by dietary K depletion. Am J Physiol 1999; 276(2 Pt 1):C350–C360.

182. Spicer Z, Miller ML, Andringa A, et al. Stomachs of mice lacking the gastric H,K-ATPase alpha-subunit have achlorhydria, abnormal parietal cells, and ciliated metaplasia. J Biol Chem 2000; 275(28):21555–21565.

183. Meneton P, Schultheis PJ, Greeb J, et al. Increased sensitivity to K$^+$ deprivation in colonic H,K-ATPase-deficient mice. J Clin Invest 1998; 101(3):536–542.

184. Cougnon M, Bouyer P, Planelles G, Jaisser F. Does the colonic H,K-ATPase also act as an Na,K-ATPase?. Proc Natl Acad Sci USA 1998; 95(11):6516–6520.

185. Cougnon M, Bouyer P, Jaisser F, Edelman A, Planelles G. Ammonium transport by the colonic H(+)–K(+)-ATPase expressed in Xenopus oocytes. Am J Physiol 1999; 277(2 Pt 1):C280–C287.

186. Codina J, Pressley TA, DuBose TD Jr. The colonic H$^+$,K$^+$-ATPase functions as a Na$^+$-dependent K$^+$(NH4$^+$)-ATPase in apical membranes from rat distal colon. J Biol Chem 1999; 274(28):19693–19698.

187. Silver RB, Mennitt PA, Satlin LM. Stimulation of apical H–K-ATPase in intercalated cells of cortical collecting duct with chronic metabolic acidosis. Am J Physiol 1996; 270(3 Pt 2):F539–F547.

188. Ahn KY, Park KY, Kim KK, Kone BC. Chronic hypokalemia enhances expression of the H(+)–K(+)-ATPase alpha 2-subunit gene in renal medulla. Am J Physiol 1996; 271(2 Pt 2):F314–F321.

189. Marsy S, Elalouf JM, Doucet A. Quantitative RT–PCR analysis of mRNAs encoding a colonic putative H,K-ATPase alpha subunit along the rat nephron: effect of K$^+$ depletion. Pflugers Arch 1996; 432(3):494–500.

190. Nakamura S, Wang Z, Galla JH, Soleimani M. K$^+$ depletion increases HCO$_3^-$ reabsorption in OMCD by activation of colonic H(+)–K(+)-ATPase. Am J Physiol 1998; 274(4 Pt 2):F687–F692.

191. Ahn KY, Turner PB, Madsen KM, Kone BC. Effects of chronic hypokalemia on renal expression of the "gastric" H(+)–K(+)-ATPase alpha-subunit gene. Am J Physiol 1996; 270(4 Pt 2):F557–F566.

192. Weiner ID, Milton AE. H(+)–K(+)-ATPase in rabbit cortical collecting duct B-type intercalated cell. Am J Physiol 1996; 270(3 Pt 2):F518–F530.

193. Silver RB, Frindt G. Functional identification of H–K-ATPase in intercalated cells of cortical collecting tubule. Am J Physiol 1993; 264(2 Pt 2):F259–F266.

194. Zhou X, Wingo CS. H–K-ATPase enhancement of Rb efflux by cortical collecting duct. Am J Physiol 1992; 263(1 Pt 2):F43–F48.

195. Schuster VL, Bonsib SM, Jennings ML. Two types of collecting duct mitochondria-rich (intercalated) cells: lectin and band 3 cytochemistry. Am J Physiol 1986; 251(3 Pt 1):C347–C355.

196. Drenckhahn D, Schluter K, Allen DP, Bennett V. Colocalization of band 3 with ankyrin and spectrin at the basal membrane of intercalated cells in the rat kidney. Science 1985; 230(4731):1287–1289.

197. Kudrycki KE, Shull GE. Primary structure of the rat kidney band 3 anion exchange protein deduced from a cDNA. J Biol Chem 1989; 264(14):8185–8192.

198. Brosius FC III, Alper SL, Garcia AM, Lodish HF. The major kidney band 3 gene transcript predicts an amino-terminal truncated band 3 polypeptide. J Biol Chem 1989; 264(14):7784–7787.

199. Obrador G, Yuan H, Shih TM, et al. Characterization of anion exchangers in an inner medullary collecting duct cell line. J Am Soc Nephrol 1998; 9(5):746–754.

200. Soleimani M, Greeley T, Petrovic S, et al. Pendrin: an apical Cl$^-$/ OH$^-$/HCO$_3^-$ exchanger in the kidney cortex. Am J Physiol Renal Physiol 2001; 280(2):F356–F364.

201. Royaux IE, Wall SM, Karniski LP, et al. Pendrin, encoded by the Pendred syndrome gene, resides in the apical region of renal intercalated cells and mediates bicarbonate secretion. Proc Natl Acad Sci USA 2001; 98(7):4221–4226.

202. Kim YH, Kwon TH, Frische S, et al. Immunocytochemical localization of pendrin in intercalated cell subtypes in rat and mouse kidney. Am J Physiol Renal Physiol 2002; 283(4):F744–F754.

203. Wagner CA, Finberg KE, Stehberger PA, et al. Regulation of the expression of the Cl^-/anion exchanger pendrin in mouse kidney by acid–base status. Kidney Int 2002; 62(6):2109–2117.

204. Petrovic S, Wang Z, Ma L, Soleimani M. Regulation of the apical Cl^-/HCO_3^- exchanger pendrin in rat cortical collecting duct in metabolic acidosis. Am J Physiol Renal Physiol 2003; 284(1):F103–F112.

205. Tsuganezawa H, Kobayashi K, Iyori M, et al. A new member of the $HCO_3(-)$ transporter superfamily is an apical anion exchanger of beta-intercalated cells in the kidney. J Biol Chem 2001; 276(11):8180–8189.

206. Ko SB, Luo X, Hager H, et al. AE4 is a DIDS-sensitive $Cl(-)$/$HCO(-)(3)$ exchanger in the basolateral membrane of the renal CCD and the SMG duct. Am J Physiol Cell Physiol 2002; 283(4):C1206–C1218.

207. Weiner ID, Hamm LL. Regulation of intracellular pH in the rabbit cortical collecting tubule. J Clin Invest 1990; 85(1):274–281.

208. Koeppen BM. Conductive properties of the rabbit outer medullary collecting duct: inner stripe. Am J Physiol 1985; 248(4 Pt 2):F500–F506.

209. Gunther W, Luchow A, Cluzeaud F, Vandewalle A, Jentsch TJ. ClC-5, the chloride channel mutated in Dent's disease, colocalizes with the proton pump in endocytotically active kidney cells. Proc Natl Acad Sci USA 1998; 95(14):8075–8080.

210. Obermuller N, Gretz N, Kriz W, Reilly RF, Witzgall R. The swelling-activated chloride channel ClC-2, the chloride channel ClC-3, and ClC-5, a chloride channel mutated in kidney stone disease, are expressed in distinct subpopulations of renal epithelial cells. J Clin Invest 1998; 101(3):635–642.

211. Todd-Turla KM, Rusvai E, Naray-Fejes-Toth A, Fejes-Toth G. CFTR expression in cortical collecting duct cells. Am J Physiol 1996; 270(1 Pt 2): F237–F244.

212. Kwon TH, Pushkin A, Abuladze N, Nielsen S, Kurtz I. Immunoelectron microscopic localization of NBC3 sodium-bicarbonate cotransporter in rat kidney. Am J Physiol—Renal Fluid Electrol Physiol/Renal Physiol 2000; 278(2):F327–F336.

213. Pushkin A, Abuladze N, Lee I, Newman D, Hwang J, Kurtz I. Cloning, tissue distribution, genomic organization, and functional characterization of NBC3, a new member of the sodium bicarbonate cotransporter family. J Biol Chem 1999; 274(23):16569–16575.

214. Hamm LL, Alpern RJ. Cellular mechanisms of renal tubular acidification. Seldin DW, Giebisch G, eds. The Kidney: Physiology and Pathophysiology. Philadelphia: Lippincott Williams & Wilkinns, 2000.

215. Breyer MD, Kokko JP, Jacobson HR. Regulation of net bicarbonate transport in rabbit cortical collecting tubule by peritubular pH, carbon dioxide tension, and bicarbonate concentration. J Clin Invest 1986; 77(5):1650–1660.

216. McKinney TD, Davidson KK. Effects of respiratory acidosis on HCO_3^- transport by rabbit collecting tubules. Am J Physiol 1988; 255(4 Pt 2):F656–F665.

217. Banerjee A, Li G, Alexander EA, Schwartz JH. Role of SNAP-23 in trafficking of H^+-ATPase in cultured inner medullary collecting duct cells. Am J Physiol—Cell Physiol 2001; 280(4):C775–C781.

218. Banerjee A, Shih T, Alexander EA, Schwartz JH. SNARE proteins regulate H(+)-ATPase redistribution to the apical membrane in rat renal inner medullary collecting duct cells. J Biol Chem 1999; 274(37):26518–26522.

219. Laski ME, Warnock DG, Rector FC Jr. Effects of chloride gradients on total CO_2 flux in the rabbit cortical collecting tubule. Am J Physiol 1983; 244(2):F112–F121.

220. Star RA, Burg MB, Knepper MA. Bicarbonate secretion and chloride absorption by rabbit cortical collecting ducts. Role of chloride/bicarbonate exchange. J Clin Invest 1985; 76(3):1123–1130.

221. Satlin LM, Schwartz GJ. Cellular remodeling of $HCO_3(-)$-secreting cells in rabbit renal collecting duct in response to an acidic environment. J Cell Biol 1989; 109(3):1279–1288.

222. Madsen KM, Verlander JW, Kim J, Tisher CC. Morphological adaptation of the collecting duct to acid–base disturbances. Kidney Int Suppl 1991; 33:S57–S63.

223. Yasoshima K, Satlin LM, Schwartz GJ. Adaptation of rabbit cortical collecting duct to in vitro acid incubation. Am J Physiol 1992; 263(4 Pt 2):F749–F756.

224. Al Awqati Q. Terminal differentiation of intercalated cells: the role of hensin. Annu Rev Physiol 2003; 65:567–583.

225. Fejes-Toth G, Naray-Fejes-Toth A. Effect of acid/base balance on H-ATPase 31 kD subunit mRNA levels in collecting duct cells. Kidney Int 1995; 48(5):1420–1426.

226. Silva Junior JC, Perrone RD, Johns CA, Madias NE. Rat kidney band 3 mRNA modulation in chronic respiratory acidosis. Am J Physiol 1991; 260(2 Pt 2):F204–F209.

227. Sabolic I, Brown D, Gluck SL, Alper SL. Regulation of AE1 anion exchanger and H(+)-ATPase in rat cortex by acute metabolic acidosis and alkalosis. Kidney Int 1997; 51(1):125–137.

228. Wesson DE. Dietary acid increases blood and renal cortical acid content in rats. Am J Physiol 1998; 274(1 Pt 2):F97–F103.

229. Wesson DE. Reduced bicarbonate secretion mediates increased distal tubule acidification induced by dietary acid. Am J Physiol 1996; 271(3 Pt 2):F670–F678.

230. Schwartz WB. JRRA. Acidification of the urine and increased ammonium excretion without change in acid–base equilibrium: sodium reabsorption as a stimulus to the acidifying process. J Clin Invest 1955; 34:673–680.

231. Stone DK, Seldin DW, Kokko JP, Jacobson HR. Mineralocorticoid modulation of rabbit medullary collecting duct acidification. A sodium-independent effect. J. Clin Invest 1983; 72(1):77–83.

232. Laski ME, Kurtzman NA. Characterization of acidification in the cortical and medullary collecting tubule of the rabbit. J Clin Invest 1983; 72(6):2050–2059.

233. Tam SC, Goldstein MB, Stinebaugh BJ, Chen CB, Gougoux A, Halperin ML. Studies on the regulation of hydrogen ion secretion in the collecting duct in

vivo: evaluation of factors that influence the urine minus blood PCO_2 difference. Kidney Int 1981; 20(5):636–642.

234. Capasso G, Jaeger P, Giebisch G, Guckian V, Malnic G. Renal bicarbonate reabsorption in the rat. II. Distal tubule load dependence and effect of hypokalemia. J Clin Invest 1987; 80(2):409–414.

235. Hays SR, Seldin DW, Kokko JP, Jacobson HR. Effect of K depletion on HCO_3 transport across rabbit collecting duct segments. Kidney Int 1986; 29:368A.

236. Doucet A, Marsy S. Characterization of K-ATPase activity in distal nephron: stimulation by potassium depletion. Am J Physiol 1987; 253(3 Pt 2):F418–F423.

237. Buffin-Meyer B, Younes-Ibrahim M, Barlet-Bas C, Cheval L, Marsy S, Doucet A. K depletion modifies the properties of Sch-28080-sensitive K-ATPase in rat collecting duct. Am J Physiol 1997; 272(1 Pt 2):F124–F131.

238. Wingo CS. Active proton secretion and potassium absorption in the rabbit outer medullary collecting duct. Functional evidence for proton-potassium-activated adenosine triphosphatase. J Clin Invest 1989; 84(1):361–365.

239. Nakamura S, Amlal H, Galla JH, Soleimani M. Colonic H^+-K^+-ATPase is induced and mediates increased HCO_3^- reabsorption in inner medullary collecting duct in potassium depletion. Kidney Int 1998; 54(4):1233–1239.

240. Kraut JA, Hiura J, Besancon M, Smolka A, Sachs G, Scott D. Effect of hypokalemia on the abundance of HK alpha 1 and HK alpha 2 protein in the rat kidney. Am J Physiol 1997; 272(6 Pt 2):F744–F750.

241. Petrovic S, Spicer Z, Greeley T, Shull GE, Soleimani M. Novel schering and ouabain-insensitive potassium-dependent proton secretion in the mouse cortical collecting duct. Am J Physiology—Renal Fluid Electrol Physiol 2002; 282(1):F133–F143.

242. Wesson DE, Dolson GM. Endothelin-1 increases rat distal tubule acidification in vivo. Am J Physiol 1997; 273(4 Pt 2):F586–F594.

243. Nagami GT. Renal ammonia production and excretion. In: Seldin D, Giebisch G, eds. The Kidney: Physiology and Pathophysiology. Philadelphia: Lippincott Williams & Wilkins, 2000:1996–2013.

244. Tannen RL. Renal ammonia production and excretion. In: Windhager EE, ed. Handbook of Physiology: Renal Physiology. New York: Oxford University Press, 1992:1017–1059.

245. Laterza OF, Curthoys NP. Effect of acidosis on the properties of the glutaminase mRNA pH-response element binding protein. J Am Soc Nephrol 2000; 11(9):1583–1588.

246. Laterza OF, Hansen WR, Taylor L, Curthoys NP. Identification of an mRNA-binding protein and the specific elements that may mediate the pH-responsive induction of renal glutaminase mRNA. J Biol Chem 1997; 272(36):22481–22488.

247. Wright PA, Packer RK, Garcia-Perez A, Knepper MA. Time course of renal glutamate dehydrogenase induction during NH_4Cl loading in rats. Am J Physiol 1992; 262(6 Pt 2):F999–1006.

248. Kaiser S, Hwang JJ, Smith H, Banner C, Welbourne TC, Curthoys NP. Effect of altered acid–base balance and of various agonists on levels of renal glutamate dehydrogenase mRNA. Am J Physiol 1992; 262(3 Pt 2):F507–F512.

249. Curthoys NP, Gstraunthaler G. Mechanism of increased renal gene expression during metabolic acidosis. Am J Physiol Renal Physiol 2001; 281(3):F381–F390.
250. DuBose TD Jr, Good DW. Chronic hyperkalemia impairs ammonium transport and accumulation in the inner medulla of the rat. J Clin Invest 1992; 90(4):1443–1449.
251. Nagami GT. Effect of luminal angiotensin II on ammonia production and secretion by mouse proximal tubules. Am J Physiol 1995; 269(1 Pt 2):F86–F92.
252. Schoolwerth AC. Regulation of renal ammoniagenesis in metabolic acidosis. Kidney Int 1991; 40(5):961–973.
253. Jones ER, Beck TR, Kapoor S, Shay R, Narins RG. Prostaglandins inhibit renal ammoniagenesis in the rat. J Clin Invest 1984; 74(3):992–1002.
254. Nagami GT. Luminal secretion of ammonia in the mouse proximal tubule perfused in vitro. J Clin Invest 1988; 81(1):159–164.
255. Good DW, DuBose TD Jr. Ammonia transport by early and late proximal convoluted tubule of the rat. J Clin Invest 1987; 79(3):684–691.
256. Buerkert J, Martin D, Trigg D. Ammonium handling by superficial and juxtamedullary nephrons in the rat. Evidence for an ammonia shunt between the loop of Henle and the collecting duct. J Clin Invest 1982; 70(1):1–12.
257. Knepper MA, Packer R, Good DW. Ammonium transport in the kidney. Physiol Rev 1989; 69(1):179–249.
258. DuBose TD Jr, Good DW, Hamm LL, Wall SM. Ammonium transport in the kidney: new physiological concepts and their clinical implications. J Am Soc Nephrol 1991; 1(11):1193–1203.
259. Good DW. Active absorption of NH_4^+ by rat medullary thick ascending limb: inhibition by potassium. Am J Physiol 1988; 255(1 Pt 2):F78–F87.
260. Kikeri D, Sun A, Zeidel ML, Hebert SC. Cellular NH_4^+/K^+ transport pathways in mouse medullary thick limb of Henle. Regulation by intracellular pH. J Gen Physiol 1992; 99(3):435–461.
261. Attmane-Elakeb A, Amlal H, Bichara M. Ammonium carriers in medullary thick ascending limb. Am J Physiol Renal Physiol 2001; 280(1):F1–F9.
262. Good DW. Effects of potassium on ammonia transport by medullary thick ascending limb of the rat. J Clin Invest 1987; 80(5):1358–1365.
263. Kikeri D, Sun A, Zeidel ML, Hebert SC. Cell membranes impermeable to NH_3. Nature 1989; 339(6224):478–480.
264. Wall SM, Davis BS, Hassell KA, Mehta P, Park SJ. In rat tIMCD, NH_4^+ uptake by Na^+–K^+-ATPase is critical to net acid secretion during chronic hypokalemia. Am J Physiol 1999; 277(6 Pt 2):F866–F874.
265. Wall SM, Fischer MP, Kim GH, Nguyen BM, Hassell KA. In rat inner medullary collecting duct, NH uptake by the Na,K-ATPase is increased during hypokalemia. Am J Physiol—Renal Fluid Electrol Physiol 2002; 282(1):F91–F102.
266. DuBose TD Jr, Caflisch CR, Bidani A. Role of metabolic CO_2 production in the generation of elevated renal cortical PCO_2. Am J Physiol 1984; 246(5 Pt 2): F592–F599.
267. Hamm LL. Renal acidification mechanisms. In: Brenner B, ed. The Kidney. Philadelphia: W.B. Saunders, 2003:497–534.

$$5$$

Molecular Biology of Renal Acid–Base Transporters

Orson W. Moe and Michel Baum

University of Texas Southwestern Medical Center, Dallas, Texas, U.S.A.

Robert J. Alpern

Yale University School of Medicine, New Haven, Connecticut, U.S.A.

INTRODUCTION

The study and understanding of the renal regulation of acid–base balance has undergone remarkable progress over the last five decades. Starting from clearance studies at the level of the whole organism, the function of individual nephron segments has been defined with in vivo and in vitro microperfusion. The delineation of transport and regulatory mechanisms was further refined with the application of isolated membrane vesicles and model epithelial in cell culture. Recombinant DNA techniques allowed us to secure the identity for individual transporters and regulatory proteins. Two strategies have been used for the cloning of acid–base transporters. For proteins obtained in high abundance (e.g., the Cl^-/HCO_3^- exchanger and H^+-ATPase), classical protein chemistry has been used to purify the proteins of interest. For others, approaches such as functional complementation in mammalian cells for the Na^+/H^+ exchanger or in *Xenopus* oocytes for the Na^+–HCO_3^- cotransporter. In this chapter, the current knowledge of the molecular definition of renal acid–base transporters is summarized, with emphasis on its implications for our understanding of the physiology of acid–base balance.

ACID–BASE TRANSPORTERS IN RENAL EPITHELIA: OVERVIEW

Acidification mechanisms along the nephron are reviewed in Chapter 4. In this chapter, the proteins that translocate H^+/OH^- equivalents across a membrane are discussed. As an introduction, we will review the organization of an acid–base transporting epithelial cell. A polarized epithelial cell (Fig. 1) alters acid–base balance between its two diametric sides by splitting a neutral precursor (carbonic acid or glutamine) into an acid and a base and extruding the two components across opposite membranes. Regardless of whether a renal cell excretes acid or base into the urine, acid and base transporters are simultaneously requisite.

Base transporters. In mammals, the base equivalent transported is primarily HCO_3^-, although there is also functional evidence of Cl^-/OH^- exchange activity (1,2). Because it is difficult to distinguish Cl^-/OH^- exchange from Cl^--H^+ cotransport, we will not analyze OH^- as a primary substrate for practical purposes. Carbon dioxide was present in the planet's atmosphere and $NaHCO_3$ was abundant in the Archean sea when cellular life blossomed some 3.5 billion years ago (3,4), and as a result HCO_3^- has been a biologic substrate even in the most primitive organisms alive today such as cyanobacteria (5,6). In mammals, HCO_3^- is the main buffer for H^+ in the extracellular fluid and the principal substrate for epithelial cell base transporters. Base transporters in renal epithelia primarily extrude HCO_3^- out of the cell, deriving electrochemical energy either from coupling to the low cell $[Cl^-]$ in an electroneutral fashion (Cl^-/HCO_3^- exchange) or to the negative cell interior voltage in an electrogenic fashion ($Na^+-HCO_3^-$ cotransport).

Acid transporters. A preponderance of mammalian renal acid–base transport is devoted to luminal H^+ secretion. Most of secreted H^+ reacts with filtered HCO_3^-, removing this anion from the filtrate and returning a base equivalent to the body fluids (see Chapter 4). The HCO_3^- filtered into Bowman's space under normal circumstances far exceeds any base excess that a human will ever face. Bicarbonate in the urinary lumen is reclaimed by titration with secreted H^+ regardless of systemic acid–base status. To achieve net acid excretion, the amount of secreted H^+ must exceed the amount of HCO_3^- recaptured. The excess H^+ combines with NH_3 and/or inorganic phosphate, allowing for its excretion at a pH >4.5. The electrochemical energy for H^+ extrusion is derived from either direct coupling to ATP hydrolysis (H^+-ATPase, H^+/K^+-ATPase) or to the low cell $[Na^+]$ (Na^+/H^+ exchanger) (Fig. 1C).

H^+-ATPase

Background. The simplest mode of uphill H^+ extrusion from an epithelial cell is via direct coupling to ATP hydrolysis. Ion-translocating ATPases are classified into F-type, V-type and P-type, based on organellar locale

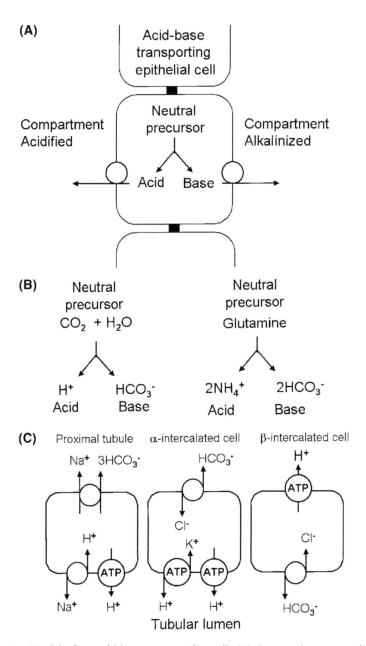

Figure 1 Model of an acid-base transporting cell. (**A**) A neutral precursor is split into its conjugate acid and base, which are then extruded on opposite membranes. (**B**) Two examples of neutral precursors and their cognate acid/base components in renal epithelia. (**C**) Representative acid–base transporting cells in the proximal and distal nephron depicting the H^+-ATPase, the H^+/K^+-ATPase, the Na^+/H^+ exchanger, the Na^+–HCO_3^- cotransporter, and the Cl^-/HCO_3^- exchanger.

and biochemical and molecular characteristics. This section focuses on the V-type H^+-ATPase that acidifies urine. V-type H^+-ATPases are pervasive in eukaryotes and serve many functions. They are intracellular pumps participating in ligand release, receptor-mediated endocytosis, intracellular vesicular trafficking, degradation of macromolecules in lysosomes, and membrane potential-driven transport of small molecules into vesicles for exocytosis (7–9). On the plasma membrane, V-type H^+-ATPases contribute to cell pH defense, generate potential for voltage-driven K^+ transport in insect epithelia, acidify extracellular microenvironment for bone matrix dissolution by osteoclasts, and acidify urine in renal epithelia (10–13).

Distribution and function in mammalian kidney. In the mammalian kidney, H^+-ATPase activity (14) and antigen (15) is present in the apical membrane of the proximal tubule, the apical membrane of the thick ascending limb, the distal convoluted and connecting tubules, and in a distinct subset of cells in the collecting duct, termed intercalated cells. In the proximal tubule, H^+-ATPase activity is expressed intensely and is responsible for about one-third of apical membrane H^+ extrusion (16). It is expressed moderately on the apical membrane of the thick ascending limb, the distal convoluted tubule, and connecting tubule. In the collecting duct, H^+-ATPase is expressed intensely in intercalated cells (ICs), a subset of morphologically distinct cells rich in mitochondria and carbonic anhydrase. In the cortical collecting duct, there are two types of ICs, H^+-secreting A (or α) -IC and HCO_3^--secreting B (or β)-IC, consistent with the ability of this segment to either secrete H^+ or HCO_3^-. In medullary collecting duct, only α-IC are present. In both types of IC, H^+ extrusion from one cell membrane is coupled to HCO_3^- extrusion (via Cl^-/HCO_3^- anion exchanger, see later) from the opposite cell membrane. The H^+-ATPase is present on the apical membrane of α-IC (17) and in the basolateral membrane of β-IC. About 40% of ICs are hybrids where H^+-ATPase is found in both the apical and basolateral membrane and diffusely in the cytoplasm (15,17,18). The significance of these hybrid cells is not clear but may account for the functional category of the β-IC which can extrude base from both apical and basolateral membranes (19,20). All ICs are endowed with striking arrays of intracellular tubulovesicular profiles fusing with clathrin-coated vesicles (17,18). These vesicular structures have 10 nm particles on their surface called studs that are associated with the H^+-ATPase (15). In contrast to all epithelial cells, the ICs exhibit little or no Na^+–K^+-ATPase (21) and have low Na^+ and K^+ conductance (22), rendering them dedicated acid–base transporting cells.

Molecular structure and function. V-type H^+-ATPase is an ancient protein with homologues present in archaebacteria (23). Although a high-resolution structure is not yet available, electron micrographic data supporting a stalk and globular head model with additional peripheral stalks (24), similar to the F-ATPase (25). The current model for the structure of

Table 1 H$^+$-ATPase Subunits

Structure/function	Subunits (Mr/kDa)	Properties and putative function	
V_0			
260 kDa integral complex H$^+$ translocation	a 100–115	H$^+$ transport (?), bafilomycin binding, α-IC specific isoform	
	c 14–17		Highly hydrophobic proteolipids
	c′ 17		
	c″ 19–20	DCCD binding	H$^+$ pore
	d 38–39		
V_1			
570 kDa peripheral complex ATP hydrolysis	A 70–73	A: catalytic site; NEM binding	Nucleotide binding
	B 55–60	B1: renal-specific isoform	
	C 40–44		
	D 34–36	High α-helical content	Critical for function and assembly of V_1
	E 31–33	Potential central stalk	
	F 10–14		
	G 14–15		
	H 50–57	Required for activity but not assembly	

V-ATPase consists of two structural and functional domains: V_0 and V_1 (Table 1 and Fig. 2).

The V_0 domain is a 270 kDa integral complex situated beneath the plasma membrane. The *a* subunit has an N-terminal hydrophilic (cytoplasmic) and C-terminal hydrophobic (transmembrane) domain (26). Although not an integral part of the H$^+$-pore (27), the *a* subunit is postulated to create a water-filled space to permit H$^+$ to enter the pore (28). This may explain the ability of cytoplasmic pH to gate H$^+$ movement even though the H$^+$ pore is deeply embedded in the lipid bilayer (27). The *a* subunit is also the binding

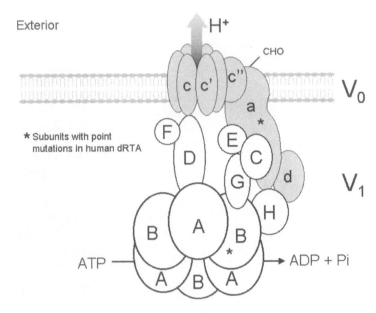

Figure 2   Putative model of the V-type H^+-ATPase. Subunits for the V_0 domain (*grey*): a, b, c, c′, c″; and the V_1 domain (*white*): A, B, C, D, E, F, G, H. CHO: glycosylation. ATP: adenosine trisphosphate. *Subunits where human mutations have been described in association with renal tubular acidosis.

site for the specific V-type H^+-ATPase inhibitor bafilomycin (29). The *c* subunits (*c*, *c′*, *c″*) are extremely lipophilic transmembrane proteolipids and are homologous to their counterparts in the F0 domain of the F-ATPase, which has been shown to form annular structures believed to be the actual pore that allows H^+ to traverse the lipid bilayer (30). The six copies of the *c* and *c′* subunits of V-ATPase form a star-shaped hexameric ring in plasma membranes (31) and probably constitute the H^+-pore. Covalent binding of a single *c* subunit of the V-ATPase by dicyclohexylcarbodiimde (DCCD) is sufficient to block H^+ permeation (32). Subunit *d* is cytoplasmic but has no known function to date.

The V_1 domain is a 570 kDa peripheral complex composed of subunits A to H (Table 1 and Fig. 2). The multimeric A and B subunits both participate in nucleotide binding (33) but the catalytic site resides in the A subunit (34). Critical cysteine residues in the A subunit accounts for their sensitivity to sulfhydryl agents and regulation of H^+-ATPase by intramolecular disulfide bridges (35). The function of the noncatalytic ATP binding sites on the B subunit is unclear as mutation of these sites leads to modest loss of activity. However, ATP binding by the B subunit appears to be necessary to achieve maximal activity (36). A B1 isoform specific to the kidney and placenta has been described (37). Subunits C through H are all

Table 2 Mechanisms of Regulation of V-type H^+-ATPase

---

1. Disulphide oxidation
2. Subunit dissociation
3. H^+ translocation/ATPase uncoupling
4. Activator proteins[a]
5. Trafficking[a]
6. Epithelial switching: Hensin-mediated pathway[a]

---

[a]Operational in renal epithelial cells.

necessary for H^+-ATPase assembly and activity, except that deletion of subunit H does not appear to disrupt function in yeast (38). Subunits C, G, and H are potential candidates for the peripheral stalk protruding into the cytoplasm.

Regulation of H^+-ATPase in the kidney. Changes in acid–base status regulate H^+-ATPase activity. This regulation is clearly evident in the distal nephron, but there is suggestion of regulation in the proximal tubule as well (39). The collecting tubule can either secrete H^+ or HCO_3^- depending on the acid–base status of the organism (40). This change in transport is paralleled by alterations in abundance of H^+-ATPase of α- and β-ICs (41,42).

Table 2 lists the mechanisms for regulation of V-type H^+-ATPase activity. When two cysteines (bovine C254 and C532) in the A subunit are oxidized by a disulfide bridge in vitro, the pump is reversibly inactivated (35). The evidence for this mode of regulation in vivo is largely circumstantial. A substantial fraction of H^+-ATPase in clathrin-coated vesicles isolated from native mammalian tissue is indeed oxidized (43), suggesting that the balance of reduction and oxidation serves to regulate H^+-ATPase (44,45). Consistent with this postulate, cysteine mutants in *Neurospora* are resistant to the nitrate-induced inactivation of H^+-ATPase (44). Currently, there is no information as to whether this mechanism operates in the mammalian kidney, although glutathione-SH depletion (oxidized state) has been implied to cause a distal acidification defect (46). In yeast, glucose starvation or switching to alternative carbon source rapidly inactivates the V-type H^+-ATPase by dissociating the complex into individual V_0 and V_1 subunits (47). This effect is reversible upon glucose repletion. A similar mechanism is utilized in insects where H^+-ATPase energizes K^+/H^+ antiport (48). Although free V_0 and V_1 subunits have been described in mammalian cells (49,50), it is uncertain whether this dissociation is a physiologically regulated process in mammalian kidney. A third mechanism proposed is the tightness of coupling between ATP hydrolysis and H^+ translocation. One can dissociate the ATP hydrolytic activity from the H^+ translocation activity by either gentle proteolysis or azide (51,52). This has been proposed as a mechanism to disengage uncontrolled H^+ extrusion during states of high ATP concentrations. Similar findings have been reported in plant cells

(53). Accessory regulatory proteins have also been proposed to regulate V-ATPase activity. Two heat-stable activating proteins have been purified; a 35 kDa protein from kidney that stimulates V-ATPase only when in pH is low (54) and a 6 kDa membrane-bound activator from brain (55). An inhibitory 6 kDa peptide has been isolated from kidney that acts at high ambient pH (56). The mechanism of action of these cofactors is unknown but they may modify oxidation, dissociation or uncoupling of the V_1V_0 subunits as described above.

In response to changes in systemic acid–base balance, the relative abundance of α- and β-ICs changes dramatically (41,42), raising the fundamental question is whether these terminally differentiated cells can phenotypically interconvert (57). Interconversion of α-/β-ICs occurs in cultured cells. When immortalized α-ICs are seeded at high density, they are converted into β-IC phenotypes with full reversal of polarity of H^+-ATPase and Cl^-/HCO_3^- exchange (58). This conversion is mediated by secretion of the extracellular matrix protein hensin into the basolateral membrane (59). Hensin by itself in a highly polymerized multimeric form (60) appears to be sufficient to induce phenotypic changes including columnarization, development of microvilli, and reversal of polarity (60,61). It is tempting to postulate that Hensin may operate to convert β-ICs to α-ICs in the collecting during acid loading, but there is no evidence to support interconversion.

Important differences exist between the in vitro model and the kidney. While immortalized β-ICs express the Cl^-/HCO_3^- anion exchanger AE1 on the apical membrane (62), the β-ICs in kidney expresses a novel AE4 isoform on its apical membrane (63). An alternative explanation of the immunohistochemical data suggesting interconversion (41,42) is changes in protein trafficking. There is a large intracellular pool of H^+-ATPase (13,15–17) and significant recycling of this pool into the apical membrane (64,65). Lowering of basolateral pH can induce apical insertion of H^+-ATPase in α-ICs (57), thereby intensifying the staining of α-ICs. Likewise, because β-ICs also express some apical H^+-ATPase (16–18,41), and evidence exists for transcytotic pathways for the ICs (66), it is conceivable that acidosis can cause shuttling of more H^+-ATPase from the basolateral to apical membrane in β-IC.

Whole organism phenotype of H^+-ATPase abnormalities. Defects in H^+-ATPase can cause disturbances in acid–base balance. Absence of staining for H^+-ATPase has been described in patients with Sjogren's syndrome, an acquired disorder of distal renal tubular acidosis, suggesting possible autoimmune destruction of the protein (67). Although there are autoantibodies from patient sera that label intercalated cells, no evidence has been found to date of a circulating antibody against the H^+-ATPase (68). Patients with systemic lupus and transplant allografts, who have the hyperkalemic variety of distal renal tubular acidosis, appear to have intact expression of H^+-ATPase in the collecting duct (69). While the gene for the c proteolipid subunit of the H^+-pore is haplosufficient, homozygous disruption of this gene leads to embryonic death (70). Mutations in an osteoclast-specific a subunit of the V-ATPase in the mouse impairs H^+-ATPase-mediated bone resorption, leading to osteosclerosis (71). Natural mutations in the human homologue leads to autosomal dominant osteopetrosis (72,73). As expected for an osteoclast-specific subunit, no renal lesion has been described in these animals or humans.

In several human kindreds with autosomal recessive distal renal tubular acidosis (dRTA) and sensorineural deafness, a variety of mutations (frame-shift, nonsense, and nonconservative missense) have been found in the B1 subunit of the V-type ATPase (Table 3) (74). In the autosomal recessive variant without hearing loss, homozygous mutations were found in a novel renal α-intercalated cell-specific isoform of the 116 kDa a subunit (Table 3) (75). The H^+-ATPases in the proximal tubule and thick ascending limb are presumably normal. This finding implies that a singular defect in H^+-secretion in the α-intercalated cell is sufficient to cause systemic acidosis. Regardless of whether acquired or congenital, disruption of subunits of the V-type H^+-ATPase in the kidney results in a distal renal tubular acidosis, underscoring the importance of this protein in renal acid excretion.

H^+/K^+-ATPase

Background. The H^+/K^+-ATPase is a P-type ATPase that is also involved in urinary acidification. The prototypic P-type ATPase is the Na^+–K^+-ATPase, the principal powerhouse of renal epithelial transport that is indirectly responsible for energizing H^+ secretion by the mammalian Na^+/H^+ exchanger. Other members include the sarcoplasmic and endoplasmic reticulum Ca^{2+}-ATPase (SERCA), the plasma membrane Ca^{2+}-ATPase (PMCA), and the gastric and colonic H^+–K^+-ATPases (gH^+/K^+-ATPase and cH^+/K^+-ATPase) (76–78). The Na^+–K^+-ATPase, and the gastric and colonic H^+–K^+-ATPases have been categorized as X^+/K^+-ATPases based on their functional and sequence similarities. In this chapter, we will discuss the two H^+/K^+-ATPases that secrete H^+ into the urine—the gastric (g) and colonic (c) isoforms.

Distribution and function in mammalian kidney. Transport energized by H^+–K^+-ATPase is ancient in vertebrate nephrons. Both functional and immunologic evidence for apical H^+ secretion via an H^+/K^+-ATPase are present in both proximal and distal nephrons of the elasmobranch dogfish (79,80). The functional presence of H^+–K^+-ATPase in the cortical and medullary collecting duct of the mammalian kidney has been demonstrated by three separate approaches, electroneutral K^+-dependent SCH-28080-sensitive H^+ secretion, bicarbonate absorption and cell pHi regulation (81–85). Isoform distribution along the nephron is based on pharmacologic and immunohistochemical data. Difficulties abound in both fronts.

Table 3   Human Mutations Resulting in Congenital Renal Tubular Acidosis (RTA)

	Gene/chromosome	Inheritance	Phenotype
Epithelial transporter			
H^+-ATPase 55 kDa B_1 subunit	*ATP6B1*/2p13	Autosomal, recessive	Distal RTA with sensorineural deafness
H^+-ATPase 55 kDa B_1 subunit	*ATP6N1*/7q33–34	Autosomal, recessive	Distal RTA with preserved hearing
Cl^-/HCO_3^- exchanger, anion exchanger AE1	*SLC4A1*/17q21–22	Autosomal, dominant	Distal RTA
		Autosomal, recessive	Distal RTA
		Autosomal, dominant, or recessive	Distal RTA associated with southeast Asian ovalocytosis
		Autosomal, dominant	Distal RTA associated with hereditary spherocytosis
Na^+–HCO_3^- cotransporter NBC	*SCL4A4*/4p21	Autosomal, recessive	Proximal RTA with ocular abnormalities
Proteins other than transporters			
Carbonic anhydrase CAII	*CA2*		
Hepatic nuclear factor HNF			

The three related P-type ATPases (Na^+/K^+-ATPase, gH^+/K^+-ATPase, and cH^+/K^+-ATPase) exhibit distinct yet overlapping inhibitor profiles. That fact H^+/K^+-ATPase can accept Na^+ as substrate (86–89), a property akin to the mixed cation selectivity described for the Na^+/K^+-ATPase (90), further confounds the functional-molecular correlation. There are at least four functional categories proposed for X^+/K^+-ATPases based on differential sensitivities to ouabain and SCH28080 (91). There is also simultaneous expression of g and c H^+/K^+-ATPase in some nephron segments. At present, it is very difficult to correlate these activities to specific molecular isoforms. It is best to keep the functional and antigenic data separate. The g H^+/K^+-ATPase protein is expressed in the intercalated cells in the collecting duct (92,93) but g H^+/K^+-ATPase transcript is more widespread in the collecting duct with weaker hybridizations in proximal straight tubule, thick ascending limb, and distal convoluted tubule (94,95). Differences between mRNA and protein may be due to differential sensitivity of the methods. Gastric H^+/K^+-ATPase protein colocalizes with H^+-ATPase in the apical membrane of α-IC and basolateral membrane of β-IC (96,97). Contrary data showing absence of g H^+/K^+-ATPase in the kidney also exist (98).

Colonic H^+/K^+-ATPase mRNA is present in the thick ascending limb, distal convoluted tubule, and connecting tubule, and is highly expressed throughout the collecting duct (99–101). Unlike g H^+/K^+-ATPase, the immunolocalization of c H^+/K^+-ATPase in the mammalian nephron is controversial. Theoretically, apical H^+/K^+-ATPase on the α-IC can secrete H^+ with apical K^+ recycling or absorb K^+ with basolateral K^+ exit. Basolateral H^+/K^+-ATPase on the β-IC can participate in base excretion with basolateral K^+ recycling. Some functional data suggest apical H^+/K^+-ATPase in β-ICs (102). Theoretically, apical H^+/K^+-ATPase in conjunction with Cl^-/HCO_3^- exchange and H_2CO_3 recycling can function as an apical KCl cotransporter.

Molecular structure and function. The definition of isoforms within the H^+/K^+-ATPases has been controversial. As one peruses the sequence of all P-type ATPases, there is higher homology within the same transporter across divergent species than across different P-type ATPases (103). Within the X^+/K^+-ATPases, approximately 66% homology exists among the α-subunits of Na^+/K^+-ATPase (NaKα1,2,3), g H^+/K^+-ATPase (HKα1), and c H^+/K^+-ATPases (HKα2) (104,105). Cross-species comparisons of given α-subunits of Na^+/K^+-ATPase and g H^+/K^+-ATPase are more than 95% homologous. The cDNAs for α-subunits of the c H^+/K^+-ATPases from rat, human, *Bufo marinus*, rabbit, and guinea pig shares only about 85% homology (HKα2–6) (99,106), however, which is only marginally higher than what is conventionally qualified to be separate genes (103). Multiple transcripts within species have been attributed to alternative splicing of the same primary transcript (106,107). At present, it is unresolved whether there are multiple genes for the α-subunit of c and g H^+/K^+-ATPases. Four β subunits have been identified for the X^+/K^+-type of P-ATPases with approximately 35% cross homology: NaKβ1, NaKβ2, NaKβ3 (or HKcβ), and HKβ. Although the data are incomplete, the presence and role of specific β subunits in the kidney has been implied based on transcript expression, coprecipitation and coassembly with α subunits in native tissue or heterologous systems. HKβ is present in the kidney (108,109).

In the family of ion-translocating ATPases, there is a distinct difference between the P- vs. the F- and V-type ATPases. The F- and V-type ATPases are multimeric proteins where the ATPase domain is segregated from the ion-translocating domain and uses rotational energy for ion-translocation, while the P-ATPases are monomers or dimers that harbor both ATPase and ion-transport function in a single molecule and uses alterations in membrane helix interactions to transport ions (110,111). Little is known about the structure of the c H^+/K^+-ATPase. Based on its primary sequence resemblance to the g H^+/K^+-ATPase which has more structure data, and to more distant relatives, the sarcoplasmic reticulum Ca^{2+}-ATPase and the *Neurospora* monomeric H^+-ATPase (which both have substantial crystallographic characterization), one can speculate on a tentative model of the c H^+/K^+-ATPase (Fig. 3) (111). The α-subunit is predicted to span the membrane 10 times (112). The first six transmembrane domains are believed to form a core structure akin to the rectangular central array seen in two-dimensional crystals of other P-type ATPases, with the ATP binding signature (DKTGTLT) and phosphorylation site in the large cytoplasmic loop between M4 and M5 (113,114). M9/10 transmembrane segments are likely in proximity with M5/6 (111). Both biochemical and yeast-two-hybrid data suggest that the β-subunit associates stably with the α-subunit M8 helix (115,116). The β-subunit consists of a single transmembrane polypeptide in a type II orientation that is heavily glycosylated on the exoplasmic surface (Fig. 3). Although there are monomeric (α only) forms of P-type ATPases, expression of intact H^+/K^+-ATPase β-subunit is essential for pump function (117,118) and for stability of the α-subunit (119). The enzyme undergoes a cycle of phosphorylation and dephosphorylation coupled to the electroneutral exchange of H^+ extrusion and K^+ influx. Interestingly,

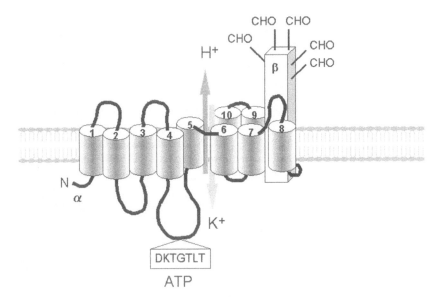

Figure 3 Putative model of the P-type H^+/K^+-ATPase. The 10-membrane spanning α subunit is shown as cylinders and the highly glycosylated (CHO) β subunit is shown as a rectangular prism. DKTGTLT is the signature adenosine trisphosphate-binding site.

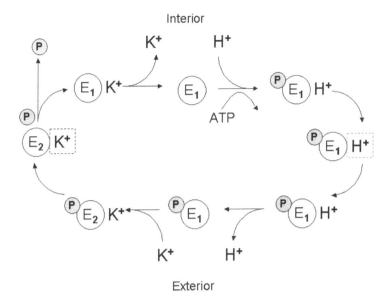

Figure 4 The E1/E2 cycle of ATP hydrolysis and ion translocation for P-type ATPases. The inward-facing E1 state binds an H^+ and gets phosphorylated. With the H^+ in a occluded state (dotted square), the protein changes conformation sending the bound H^+ to an outward-facing locale. Release of H^+ to the extracellular side is tightly coupled to binding of K^+, which switches the enzyme to an E2 state. With K^+ in the occluded site, the protein once again changes conformation to face the interior of the cell. With hydrolysis of the phosphodiester bond of ATP, the enzyme changes from the E2 back to the E1 state and now is positioned to start a new cycle.

modeling of these conformational changes was conceptualized prior to the availability of cDNA for any of the P-ATPases (120,121). This scheme is summarized in Fig. 4.

Regulation of H^+/K^+-ATPase in the kidney. In the stomach, g H^+/K^+-ATPase is regulated by secretagogue-dependent endocytosis and exocytosis (122). Data at this level of precision have not been reported in the kidney. If renal H^+/K^+-ATPase serves to excrete H^+ and conserve K^+, it should be upregulated in acidosis and K^+ depletion. Chronic K depletion in rats leads to a robust increase in HK $\alpha2$ mRNA in the collecting duct with no change in cortex (100,101,123). These findings are compatible with increased ouabain-sensitive K^+, HCO_3^- and NH_4^+ flux (124,125) in the collecting duct and increased enzyme activities with chronic K^+ depletion (126,127). In contrast to c H^+/K^+-ATPase, g H^+/K^+-ATPase is not regulated in the kidney in response to K^+ depletion (100). However, discrepancies exist as increases in SCH-28080-sensitive flux (presumed to be g H^+/K^+-ATPase) has been described (128). Increased H^+/K^+-ATPase activity occurs in both chronic hypercapnia (129,130) and chronic metabolic acidosis (84,131).

This increased activity has not been correlated with increases in c H^+/K^+-ATPase or g H^+/K^+-ATPase transcript abundance (100). To date, we still lack concordance between transport, pharmacologic, and molecular data. Possible explanations include translational or trafficking changes, yet unidentified isoforms, or alterations in inhibitor pharmacokinetics with regulation.

Whole organism phenotype of H^+/K^+-ATPase abnormalities. Changes in H^+/K^+-ATPase enzymatic activity have been reported in dissected tubules in numerous animal models with distal acidification defects (132,133). The functional significance of these changes in ATPase activities remains uncertain. High soil vanadium levels has been implied as a potential cause of an endemic form of distal renal tubular acidosis and achlorhydria in northeastern Thailand (134), but a pathogenetic link remains to be proven. No spontaneous mutations of c H^+/K^+-ATPase have been described in animals or humans.

The phenotype of c H^+/K^+-ATPase $-/-$ mice is primarily confined to the inability of the gastrointestinal tract to conserve K^+ on a K^+-restricted diet (135). Although the difference was small, there was also a trend for the c H^+/K^+-ATPase $-/-$ animals to waste more K^+ in the urine despite hypokalemia. Plasma pH and $[HCO_3^-]$ were normal under both baseline and low K^+ conditions. A tyrosine-based internalization motif in the β-subunit has been shown to mediate g H^+/K^+-ATPase endocytosis (136) and mutant β-subunits leads to gastric acid hypersecretion in transgenic animals (137). The animals expressing the mutant β-subunit in the kidney also exhibit reduced fractional K^+ excretion suggesting similar endocytotic regulation in the kidney (138).

Na$^+$/H$^+$ Exchanger

Background. In addition to coupling to ATP hydrolysis, uphill H^+ extrusion from cells is also achieved by coupling to the downhill influx of Na^+. Energetically, the inward 10-fold Na^+ electrochemical gradient can support up to one pH unit acidification of the urinary lumen by 1:1 Na^+/H^+ exchange. Whereas this pH gradient is inadequate for the collecting duct, it is quite sufficient for the pH gradients in the proximal tubule and thick ascending limb. The energy is derived from ATP expended by the basolateral Na^+–K^+-ATPase, which lowers cell $[Na^+]$. Na^+/H^+ exchangers are present in and vital to all cells from microorganisms (139) to plants (140) and animals. Amongst all living organisms, only one prokaryotic naturally devoid of any Na^+/H^+ exchange genes is known to date (141). Na^+/H^+ exchange is not universally utilized for Na^+-driven H^+ extrusion (pH-gradient-driven Na^+ transport in prokaryotes and yeast) (142) and is not always electroneutral ($Na^+/2H^+$ in prokaryotes, $2Na^+/H^+$ in crustaceans) (142,143). In mammals, Na^+/H^+ exchange is encoded by the NHE gene

family. NHE1 was cloned using functional reconstitution by genetic complementation in Na^+/H^+ exchange null cells (144) and the other members were
cloned subsequently by homologous hybridization. Eight members with distinct pharmacokinetics and tissue and subcellular distribution have been
identified (145–147). No splice variants have been described. Primary
sequence analysis of all isoforms yields a similar predicted topology with
a transmembrane N-terminal of approximately 400 amino acids and a dili-
gent C-terminal cytoplasmic region domain of varying number and primary
sequence of amino acids (Fig. 5).

Distribution and function in mammalian kidney. The tissue distribution
and intrarenal localization of the NHE isoforms are summarized in Table 4.
An exhaustive discussion of each isoform is beyond the scope of this
chapter. From the standpoint of urinary acidification, we will focus mainly
on NHE3. NHE3 is localized in the apical membrane of the proximal tubule

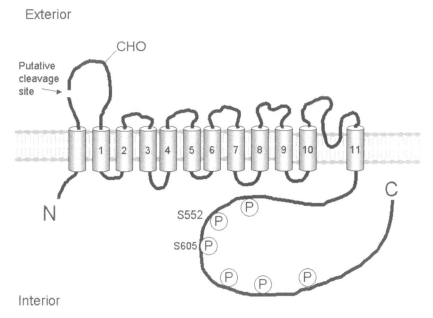

Figure 5 Putative model of the Na/H exchanger (NHE). The holoprotein contains
10–12 transmembrane spans at the N-terminal half (~400 aa) of the protein, which
mediates Na^+ and H^+ transport. The transmembrane domain also a putative cleaved
signal peptide, glycosylation site in the first extracellular loop, the putative H^+-
sensing region and the amiloride-analogues binding site. The C-terminal half
(~400 aa) of the protein contains multiple phosphorylation sites (P) with phosphoserines 552 and 605 (rat NHE3) having proven regulatory significance. Not shown
are also multiple binding regions to regulatory cofactors. An alternative model
proposes an extracellular location of the extremely C-terminal tail.

Table 4   Na$^+$/H$^+$ Exchanger (NHE) Gene Family

Isoform	Tissue distribution	Intrarenal localization
NHE1	Ubiquitous	Along the entire nephron; basolateral
NHE2	Epithelial	Distal convoluted tubule; apical membrane
NHE3	Epithelial	Proximal tubule and thick ascending limb, apical membrane
NHE4	Epithelial	Thick ascending limb basolateral membrane
NHE5	Neuronal	Unknown[a]
NHE6	General	Intracellular organelle[a]
NHE7	General	Intracellular organelle[a]

[a]Not specifically examined in the kidney.

of most species studied (148,149) except the pig (150), and on the apical membrane of the thick ascending limb (149). NHE3 mediates a substantial part of NaHCO$_3$ and NaCl absorption in the proximal tubule via coupling with parallel Cl$^-$/base$^-$ exchange (16,151). In the thick ascending limb, NHE3 mediates primarily NaHCO$_3$ absorption (152).

NHE1 is widely distributed in the nephron on the basolateral membrane (153) and is likely responsible for cell pH and volume regulation. The role of NHE2 in the kidney is unknown. It is expressed in the apical membrane of the thick ascending limb, distal convoluted tubule and connecting tubule (154). There is no pharmacokinetic evidence of NHE2 function in native cortical brush border vesicles (155) and NHE2 $-/-$ animals have NHE activity in the proximal tubule indistinguishable from wild type (156). NHE2$-/-$NHE3$-/-$ animals are identical to NHE3 $-/-$ animals (156). NHE4 is present on the basolateral membrane of the thick ascending limb (157), and it may mediate basolateral NH$_4^+$ exit from the thick limb into the interstitium (158). NHE5 transcript is extremely low in abundance in renal tissue and no data are available on tissue distribution. NHE6 and 7 are ubiquitous intracellular NHEs. NHE8 is expressed in the proximal tubule but there is no functional characterization at this isoform thus far (147).

Molecular structure and function. Whereas the prokaryotic NHEs (NhaA and NhaB) have different predicted topology (142), the Na$^+$/H$^+$ exchangers in yeast are remarkably similar to the mammalian NHEs (159). The conventional cartoon for the mammalian Na$^+$/H$^+$ exchanger is shown in Fig. 5, although no definitive structural information is available. Although imprecise, the linear array of beer cans is often drawn for convenience. The exact number of membrane-spanning domains is still undetermined although a model with 11 transmembrane spans and a P-loop (a structure well known in ion channels) between transmembrane spans 10 and 11 has been proposed (160) (Fig. 5). The predicted secondary structure for all NHEs are very similar and functionally NHEs have similar turnover rates (161). From data derived from NHE1, inaccessibility of putative external loops near the C-terminal end suggest folding into an aqueous pore in this region (161,162).

The N-terminal transmembrane half of NHE1 is believed to mediate Na^+/H^+ exchange (160,163). The ability for NHE1 to transport without the first 150 amino acids in a heterologous system is compatible with an N-terminal signal peptide (161). In addition to transport, the N-terminal half of the protein likely mediates acute regulation of NHE3 by hypertonicity (164,165), in contrast to NHE1 (166). Based on extrapolation from NHE1, the pH-sensing region of NHE3 is thought to reside somewhere in the transmembrane region (167). pH sensing endows transport with typical cooperative H^+ kinetics (168), with its set point modulated by interaction with the regulatory cytoplasmic domain (169,170). The H^+-dependence of *Escherichia coli* Na^+/H^+ exchanger isoform NhaA is opposite to mammalian NHE in that it is activated by alkaline pH (142). NhaA is the only definitive proof of a built-in sensor to date because NhaA exhibits identical pH dependence when reconstituted in proteoliposomes in purified form (171). Histidine 226 at the junction of a transmembrane domain and cytoplasmic loop has been identified to be a pH sensor for NhaA (172). The identity of the pH sensor in mammalian NHEs has not been defined.

The putative cytoplasmic C-terminal domain of NHE has more diversity in primary sequence between isoforms, and functions to coordinate incoming signals and exert regulatory control over the transporting transmembrane domain. The C-terminus harbors numerous phosphorylation sites as well as binding domains for regulatory factors (163,173,174). An alternative model for an extracellular location of the extreme C-terminus has been proposed (175).

Regulation of NHE3 function in the kidney. NHE3 is one of the most extensively studied renal epithelial acid–base transporters. There is a vast body of literature regarding the acute and chronic regulation of NHE3 in renal epithelia involving myriad mechanisms at multiple levels. A number of hormones acutely regulate NHE3 activity in intact tubules, membrane vesicles, and cultured cells (α-adrenergic agonists, angiotensin, endothelin, and insulin stimulate NHE3; dopamine, parathyroid hormone, adenosine inhibit NHE3) (173). Regulation of NHE3 can proceed via either changes in intrinsic transport or changes in amount of plasma membrane NHE3 protein. There is clear evidence that NHE3 activity can be altered acutely without changing its surface protein abundance in whole animals (176), in cultured cells (177–181), and in a series of membrane vesicles studies where there is no possibility of trafficking (182).

Changes in NHE3 activity are associated with modification of NHE3 phosphorylation (166,176,178,180,181,183–187). The functional significance of phosphoserine 552 and 605 (rat NHE3 numbering) in mediating protein kinase A (PKA) inhibition has been shown in transfected fibroblasts (184,185). The neighboring peptides flanking these two sites are highly conserved in NHE3 from all species (181). Dopamine-mediated stimulation of NHE3 endocytosis (see below) appears to be absolutely dependent on phosphorylation of serines in the equivalent positions of 552 and 605 by PKA. The NHE regulatory factor (NHERF) family of proteins are docking proteins that contain PDZ (postsynaptic density, disc large, ZO-1) protein–protein interaction domains. The current model proposed is that the NHE3/NHERF/ezrin complex tethers NHE3 to the cytoskeleton as well as acts as an A kinase anchoring protein (AKAP) to shuttle the PKA holoenzyme to NHE3 (Fig. 6A). Phosphorylation of NHE3 by PKA occurs without changes in the phosphorylation of NHERF or NHERF/NHE3 association (187–190). The NHERF-1 isoform is expressed primarily in the proximal tubule while NHERF-2 is expressed in the glomerulus, the vasculature, and the principal cells in the collecting duct (191). Activation of PKA does not universally lead to inhibition of NHE3. Sequestering of NHERF by the β-adrenergic receptor/ligand complex, for example, may be a physiologic mechanism to spare NHE3 from PKA activation (192).

Phosphorylation-independent mechanisms also exist as changes in NHE3 activity can be dissociated from changes in NHE3 phosphorylation (184,193). Despite the association with NHE3 phosphorylation, the mechanism by which NHE3 activity is inhibited is still elusive. In transfected fibroblasts, an intact actin cytoskeleton is required for surface NHE3 to be active (177). Inhibition of one of multiple steps upstream to actin polymerization (RhoA, Rho-associated kinase, or myosin light chain phosphorylation) all lead to reduction of surface NHE3 activity without changing surface protein expression (194). Changes in interaction between NHE3 and the actin cytoskeleton may be a mechanism to alter activity of surface NHE3 molecules. More can be learned about acute regulation of NHE3 from studies performed in its cousin, NHE1. ATP depletion inhibits NHE1 activity (195), and this effect is due, at least in part, to depletion of cellular phosphatidylinositol-4,5-bisphosphate (PIP_2). Phosphatidylinositol-4,5-bisphosphate directly binds to the cytoplasmic domain of NHE1 and activates NHE1 (196). Although no published data are yet available, NHE3 has consensus motifs for PIP_2 binding and ATP depletion is associated with inhibition of NHE3 (197). Direct modulation of ion channel activity by PIP_2 has been described for inward rectifiers (198). Another model has been proposed that portrays NHE3 in two forms; a 9.6S form present in the microvillus which is functionally active, and a 21S multimeric complex with megalin in the intermicrovillar microdomain of the apical membrane which is relatively inactive (199,200). According to this model, alteration of NHE3 activity in the apical membrane is achieved by shuttling NHE3 between these two states. To summarize a wealth of data, cell surface

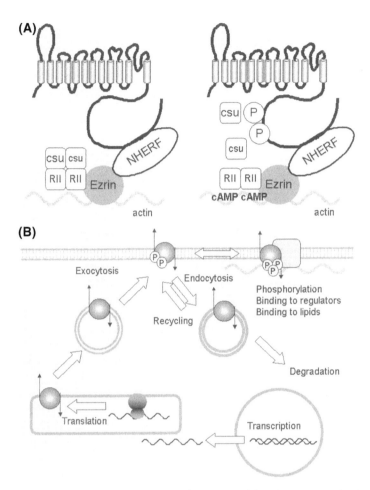

Figure 6 Regulation of NHE3. (**A**) Model proposed for the NHERF/ezrin complex as an anchor to bring the protein kinase A (PKA) holoenzyme to the actin filament as well as to the vicinity of NHE3 so that PKA can phosphorylate NHE3 in response to cAMP. NHERF, Na^+/H^+ exchanger regulatory protein; CSU, catalytic subunit of PKA; RII, regulatory subunit of PKA; cAMP, cyclic adenosine monophosphate. (**B**) Levels of regulation of NHE3: (1) Regulation of NHE3 activity on the plasma without changes in NHE3 protein amount can potentially be achieved by changes in interaction with the actin cytoskeleton, megalin, or PIP_2. In addition NHE3 phosphorylation per se can potentially alter NHE3 activity. (2) Exocytosis and endocytosis. (3) Translation. (4) Transcription.

NHE3 activity can potentially be modified by interaction with the actin cytoskeleton, megalin, lipids, or by modulation of NHE3 phosphorylation per se (Fig. 6B). PTH (176,178,201) and dopamine (180,181) both decrease the intrinsic activity of surface NH3 acutely, and then with sustained exposure, decrease the abundance of NH3 in the apical cell membrane. In intact kidneys, PTH-induced endocytosis of NHE3 is dependent on microtubules (180). In cultured epithelial cells, NHE3 endocytosis most likely proceeds via a nonadaptin-related but dynamin-dependent pathway, such as the caveolae pathway (181). Phosphorylation of NHE3 by PKA appears to be necessary for NHE3 to associated with the adaptor protein complex (181). In addition to PTH and dopamine, changes in surface NHE3 protein abundance mediate the changes in NHE3 activity in response to endothelin-1 (202), acidosis (203), and pressure natriuresis (204). Both endothelin and acid incubation stimulate exocytosis of NHE3, an effect that is dependent on an intact actin cytoskeleton (202,203). In transfected fibroblasts, there is a large intracellular pool of NHE3, which contains functional NHE3 units and are constantly recycled back to the plasma membrane in a phosphatidylinositol-3-kinase-dependent fashion and requires the last 142 amino acids of the NHE3 C-terminal tail (205–208). In contrast to epithelial cells, baseline endocytosis of NHE3 in fibroblasts appears to proceed via clathrin-coated vesicles (209).

While acute regulation of NHE3 alters intrinsic activity and membrane trafficking, the mechanisms responsible for chronic regulation are less clear. Chronic regulation of NHE3 is effected at different levels. A number of chronic conditions stimulate proximal tubule transport capacity and NHE3 activity (metabolic acidosis, respiratory acidosis, hyperfiltration, K^+ deficiency, hyperosmolarity, glucocorticoid, thyroid hormone). More comprehensive reviews are available (210,211). Increased NHE3 protein expression occurs in chronic acidosis (155,212–214) K^+ depletion (215), hyperosmolarity (216), glucocorticoid excess (217), and thyroid hormone excess (170). In chronic acidosis, NHE3 protein is increased in the proximal tubule, thick ascending limb, and in cultured cells, but an increase in NHE3 transcript can only be detected in the latter two settings (212,213). Given these findings, acidosis either produces a change in transcript that is undetectable by present techniques or increases NHE3 protein directly without changing its mRNA abundance.

Physiologic concentrations of glucocorticoids synergizes activation of NHE3 by acidosis at the level of the transcript, total cellular protein and apical insertion (214). Glucocorticoids may serve a permissive role for NHE3 adaptation to other stimuli. Both glucocorticoids and thyroid hormone increase NHE3 expression by activating NHE3 transcription (170,217). Glucocorticoids and dopamine may have translational or posttranslational effects on NHE3 expression (214). Our present understanding of the complex regulation of NHE3 is summarized in Fig. 6 B.

Whole organism phenotypes of abnormal NHE function. No human mutations of NHE have been described to date. One human study specifically excluded any linkage between the NHE1 locus and polygenic primary hypertension (218). Rodents with a spontaneous mutation in NHE1 have slow-wave epilepsy (219). A similar but not identical neurologic syndrome occurs in mice with targeted NHE1 disruption (220). Although cell pH regulation is impaired in the parotid gland (221), no renal abnormality has been described in either of these rodent strains. As mentioned earlier, NHE2-deficient mice have no identified renal phenotype (222), but NHE3-deficient mice exhibit numerous ion transport defects (223–226). Fluid and HCO_3^- absorption in the proximal tubule are both decreased in NHE3 $-/-$ mice by the magnitude predicted from pharmacologic inhibition of NHE3. They are hypotensive and have metabolic acidosis. NHE3 $+/-$ mice seem to exhibit an intermediate phenotype (224). The absence of NHE3-mediated HCO_3^- transport in the proximal tubule is not compensated by appearance of other NHE isoforms or by H^+–K^+-ATPase activity, or by an increase in H^+-ATPase activity (225). A yet undefined Na^+-dependent acidification mechanism seems to exist (155). The increased distal delivery is compensated primarily by increased thick limb absorption in NHE3 $+/-$ mice and also by drastic lowering of GFR (via tubuloglomerular feedback) in NHE3 $-/-$ mice (224). In addition, the Na^+-dependent phosphate cotransporter is upregulated in the proximal tubule and the epithelial Na^+ channel and Cl^-/HCO_3^- exchanger are upregulated in the distal tubule (226). Due to multiple compensatory mechanisms, incomplete activating or inactivating mutations of NHE3 may not be detectable even if present in humans.

Cl^-/HCO_3^- Exchanger

Background. Luminal H^+ secretion in renal epithelia requires commensurate basolateral base exit. In addition, certain specialized cells secrete base into the tubular lumen and thus are instrumental for rectifying systemic base excess. Finally, direct absorption of base equivalents may occur. In mammalian renal epithelia, this transfer of base occurs primarily via a transporter that directly couples HCO_3^- to Cl^- in an electroneutral fashion. With the exception of the highly unusual high cell $[Cl^-]$ in promyelocytic leukemic cells (227), Cl^-/HCO_3^- exchangers function exclusively as base extruders. This family of proteins is referred to as the anion exchangers (AEs). Anion exchangers perform multiple functions in mammalian cells. In erythrocytes, an AE constitutes 50% of the membrane protein and is primarily responsible for two functions (228): it enables vertebrates to carry CO_2 as HCO_3^- in both the plasma and intraerythrocyte space, and it maintains the integrity of the red cell membrane by anchoring the protein skeleton to the lipid bilayer. Anion exchangers also participate in cell pH homeostasis (229), inward cell Cl^- transport (230), and cell volume regulation (231). In this chapter, we will focus on the role of AEs in transepithelial Cl^- and HCO_3^- movement. The prototype AE1, also known as band 3, was purified from erythrocytes and AE2 and AE3 were cloned by homology to AE1 (232). The latest member, AE4, is actually closer in sequence to the Na^+, HCO_3^- cotransporter (NBC) family (see below) but has been shown to mediate Cl^-/HCO_3^- exchange (63). Although there are only four genes, alternative transcript splicing has produced more than 10 AE proteins to date (232).

Distribution and function in mammalian kidney. Functional evidence for stilbene-sensitive Cl^--dependent HCO_3^- extrusion is well established in α- and β-ICs in the collecting duct (233–235). All four AEs are expressed in the kidney. The distribution is summarized in Table 5. AE1 is expressed in the basolateral membrane of the α-IC in the cortical collecting duct and in the basolateral membrane of the outer medullary collecting duct cells with very little or no staining in the inner medulla (18,236–239). Intracellular staining is also observed (239). Although AE1 transcript and protein are detected in cultured β-ICs (62), there is no expression in intact native renal tissues (18,236–239) or freshly sorted β-ICs (240). AE2 is present in the basolateral membrane of medullary and cortical thick ascending limb, and the macula densa. In the collecting duct, AE2 expression is basolateral and increases in intensity axially towards the medullary tip (241–243). There are no published data on AE3 staining in the kidney but AE3 transcript is abundant. AE4 was originally assigned to the NBC family as it is only about 30% homologous to AEs 1–3. However, AE4 is expressed on the apical membrane of some but not all β-ICs in the cortical collecting duct (63). AE4 induces Na^+-independent DIDS-sensitive Cl^-/HCO_3^- exchange (63). Anion exchangers 1–3 most likely provide the pathway for basolateral base exit, whereas AE4 most likely mediates luminal HCO_3^- secretion. The axial heterogeneity in distribution suggests that AE2 is more suited for base exit in deeper portions of the collecting duct. A major distinction between AE1 and AE2 is that AE2 is activated by cell alkalinization while the pH response of AE1 is relatively flat (244–247). It is conceivable that a higher rate of basolateral base transport in response to apical H^+ pumping is required to enable the apical H^+-ATPase to pump against a high luminal $[H^+]$ in the deeper portions of the collecting duct.

Table 5 Anion Exchanger (AE; Cl^-/HCO_3^- Exchanger) Gene Family

Isoform	Intrarenal localization
AE1	Basolateral membrane CCD (α-IC only), OMCD
AE2	Basolateral membrane mTAL > cTAL, macula densa, IMCD > OMCD
AE3	No published data
AE4	Apical membrane β-IC

m or cTAL, medullary or cortical ascending limb; CCD, cortical collecting duct; OMCD, outer medullary collecting duct; IMCD, inner medullary collecting duct; IC, intercalated cell.

Protein structure and function. The transmembrane topology of AE1 was postulated even before the cloning of the gene. The detailed elaboration of AE structure is beyond the scope of this chapter but is presented in several excellent reviews (248–251). Although knowledge of AE1 structure is still evolving and high-resolution models are not yet available, one current model is presented in Fig. 7. The ∼910 amino acid protein can be partitioned into an N-terminal cytoplasmic regulatory and protein-binding domain (∼360 aa) and a 14-span transmembrane (∼550 aa) glycosylated domain that performs obligatory anion exchange function with both termini facing the cytoplasmic side. Renal AE1 lacks the extreme N-terminal (65 residues, human; 79 residues, rodent) of the red cell AE1, which harbors the ankyrin-binding site due to an alternative promoter within intron 3 (252–254). Direct biochemical evidence confirms the lack of ankyrin binding by renal AE1 (254). While the paradigm of the first eight transmembrane spans (Fig. 7) is supported by topology, the remaining 200 or so residues in the C-terminus are still open to debate (250,251). Residues in the loop between transmembrane region 9 and 10 can be accessed from either the exterior or interior suggesting that this extracellular loop, in conjunction with the P-loop transmembrane span 12, is associated with the translocation pore with flexibility in accessibility secondary to conformational changes during anion transport (255–257). Band 3 is predominantly a dimer in the

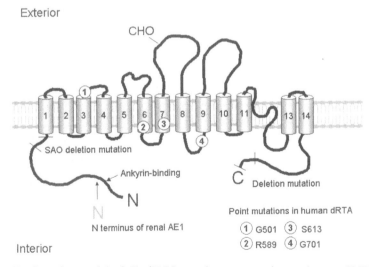

Figure 7 Putative model of Cl^-/HCO_3^- exchanger or anion exchanger (AE). The protein is approximately 900 amino acids with an N-terminal regulatory and anchoring domain and a C-terminal transporting domain. CHO, glycosylation site. The renal AE1 has a different N terminus (grey). Locations of several mutations are shown.

membrane (258,259). Electron microscopic images of two-dimensional crystals show a depression at the dimeric center in a canyon buried within the bilayer (260–262). Two arms protrude upwards from the ends of the dimer, and these may form the anion selectivity and permeability barrier.

The functions of cloned AEs have been studied extensively. AE1 forms a ternary complex with Cl^- and stilbene, with Cl^- and stilbene on distinct and interactive sites (263,264). There is limited information on HCO_3^-–protein interaction. The pH sensitivity of AE1 is relatively flat whereas AE2 is activated by cell alkalinization (244–247). The transmembrane domain of AE2 confers steep activity-pH curves, and is postulated to contain a modifier site in the cytoplasmic domain between aa 99 and 510 that shifts the pH_{2max} of the curve (265). Substitution of a conserved critical glutamic acid residue in the transmembrane domain abolishes pH sensitivity, as well as other functions of the A2 exchanger (266). NH_4^+ per se appears to activate AE2 independent of changes in cytosolic or organellar pH, an effect postulated to be a mechanism of stimulation of apical H^+ secretion in states of high NH_4^+ production (247). Similar notions of NH_4^+ stimulation have been hypothesized for ATP-coupled H^+ secretion in the collecting duct (267,268).

Regulation of AEs in the kidney. The relative number of α- and β-ICs changes in response to acid–base status (269). As discussed earlier, interconversion of α- and β-ICs occurs in cultured cells (62), but definitive evidence is still absent in native kidney. AE1 transcript and protein are both upregulated in α-ICs in chronic metabolic and respiratory acidosis (42,268,269) and decreased in metabolic alkalosis (42,268). These changes are in accord with transport data in α-ICs (270). In contrast to AE1, AE2 mRNA is decreased by acid loading or incubation in acid pH and increased by alkaline loading, and increased in cultured collecting duct cells by incubation in alkaline pH (271). The role of this paradoxical regulation of AE2 is unclear. An unusual feature in this study is expression of AE2 in principal cells as well as in α- and β-ICs (271).

Whole organism phenotype from defects in AE. AE1 mutations produce a myriad of defects in red cell plasma membrane integrity, surface antigen expression, and cellular metabolism (272,273). AE1 mutations in the kidney have been extensively studied (Table 3). Naturally occurring congenital homozygous absence of AE1 occurs in cattle (274) and targeted disruption of AE1 has been carried out in mice (275). Both AE1-null species suffer high perinatal mortality. The stunted growth in survivors has been attributed to metabolic acidosis, but it is difficult to distinguish the effect of acidosis from the severe hemolytic anemia. On a bovine (alkaline) diet, AE1-deficient cattle have a blood pH of 7.3, plasma $[HCO_3^-]$ of 19 mmol/L, and a normal anion gap (274). Although urinary net acid excretion was not reported, the urinary pH remained high at 7.5 despite systemic acidosis, a finding compatible with distal renal tubular acidosis (274). Numerous mutations in AE1 have been reported in humans. Several fascinating enigmas are outstanding. What is the basis for autosomal dominance? How is it that some mutant AE1 proteins seem to function normally when heterologously expressed? How can loss-of-function AE1 mutations that are debilitating in erythrocytes give rise to normal renal phenotypes? Conversely, how is it that patients with AE1 mutations and distal renal tubular acidosis have normal erythrocyte ion transport and membrane integrity? All these issues will permeate the discussion below.

An autosomal dominant form of congenital distal renal tubular acidosis is described in patients of primarily European descent. Heterozygous mutations in AE1 segregate with the distal renal tubular acidosis phenotype in several unrelated kindreds. The most common mutation is in arginine 589 (R589H, R589C, R589S) (276–279) predicted to be at the inner face of the sixth transmembrane span (Fig. 7). This mutant AE1 is associated with reduced erythrocyte SO_4^{2-} (a surrogate of AE1 activity) transport (276,278). In *Xenopus* oocytes, mutant AE1 activity is either normal (276) or partially impaired (278). The lack of relation of the kindreds and the singular de novo R589 mutation in one family (277) suggest mutagenic susceptibility in R589. Interestingly, one member of a kindred with R589H had normal plasma $[HCO_3^-]$ (278). Two other less common mutations have been identified: S613F with paradoxically increased erythrocyte SO_4^{2-} transport (276) and an 11 amino acid deletion at the C-terminus with no functional data (277).

The mechanism for the autosomal dominance is unknown. None of the three mechanisms for autosomal dominance (dominant negative mutant, haploinsufficiency, and the two-hit model) seems to be evident from the current data. When coexpressed with wild-type AE1, $AE1^{R589H}$ did not exert a dominant negative effect (278). It is possible that the dominant negative effect of mutant AE1 is specific to the cellular context of mammalian α-intercalated cells such as apical mistargeting of AE1 (which will not be manifest in oocytes). The lack of a suitable mammalian expression system has impeded further delineation of the defect (280).

An autosomal recessive form of distal RTA without erythrocyte abnormalities has also been described (281). Two siblings from a Thai kindred were homozygous triple mutants for M31T, K56E, and G701D. Both parents were phenotypically normal, and they and an unaffected sibling were found to be heterozygotes. While M31T and K56E appear to be benign polymorphisms, G501D is sufficient to inactivate kidney and erythrocyte AE1 when expressed in *Xenopus* oocytes. The defect in this kindred seems to be an inability of $AE1^{G501D}$ to be targeted to the plasma membrane. Coexpression with the red cell chaperone protein glycophorin A completely rescues the phenotype. This is the first experimental explanation of the differential phenotype in erythrocyte and α-intercalated cells with an identical underlying AE1 mutation.

Southeast Asian ovalocytosis (SAO) results from heterozygosity of an AE1 mutation (deletion of residues 400–408 in *cis* with K56E Memphis I polymorphism) and its gene frequency is enriched in areas with endemic malaria (282) because red cell rigidity is protective against cerebral malaria in children (283). The nonexistence of homozygotes suggests embryonic lethality (284). The SAO AE1 protein has been studied extensively and is laden with severe defects including protein misfolding, self-tetramerization, abnormal glycosylation, and inability to transport or bind inhibitors (285,286). Its dominant negative effect in the red cell appears well founded. It is truly astonishing why acidification by the α-intercalated cell is not completely disrupted in these patients. There must be a drastic difference in the biology of the C-terminal end of the cytoplasmic domain in terms of protein processing in the α-intercalated cell compared to the erythrocyte.

The SAO mutation does affect renal acidification as some patients with SAO and distal renal tubular acidosis have been described (287–289). Thus far, all the patients in the 11 kindreds with unequivocally documented phenotype and genotype are compound heterozygotes with one SAO allele and one other mutation (two missense: G701D, A858D; and one single amino acid deletion: ΔV850) (288,289). With the exception of two patients with A858D who showed true autosomal dominance, no other patients with G701D or ΔV850 have distal RTA unless the mutation is accompanied by the SAO allele (288,289). In other words, in an SAO background, G701D and ΔV850 exhibit pseudodominant inheritance. This can be due to haplosufficiency of the single SAO AE1 alone. Alternatively, the SAO AE1 protein may be permissive for AE1^{G701D} and AE1$^{\Delta V850}$ to exert a dominant negative effect. Again, apical mistargeting in the α-IC is postulated to occur (289). The finding of distal RTA in conjunction with a normal urine-blood PCO_2 (U-B PCO_2) in one patient is compatible with apical mistargeting of AE1 (287). Unfortunately, the genotyping of this patient was restricted only to the SAO mutation (287); compound heterozygosity was not examined. There is an alternative interpretation for the normal U-B PCO_2. First, U-B PCO_2 data are not widely available in patients with distal RTA and AE1 mutations, and many may have normal values. Theoretically, a basolateral slow AE1 in the α-intercalated cells can sustain enough H^+ flux to mount a CO_2 gradient but not enough to maintain a normal plasma $[HCO_3^-]$. In addition, even if AE1 is impaired, intact AE2 deep in the medulla can increase the U-B PCO_2 without AE1. Until immunohistochemical data are available in these patients, apical mistargeting of AE1 remains an intriguing theory.

Hereditary spherocytosis (HS) is an autosomal dominant disorder resulting from a myriad of AE1 mutations primarily affecting red cell membrane integrity (290). Patients with HS rarely have renal acidification defects despite grossly abnormal or absent AE1 in erythrocytes (290). This apparent paradox suggests major differences between erythrocyte and renal processing of AE1 protein and presence of modifiers. Isolated cases of RTA have been reported in HS patients but no genotypic information is available (291). In one report, two HS patients with normal plasma [HCO_3^-] had incomplete RTA (291). The mutation in AE1 was a known one for HS with premature truncation after only three transmembrane domains (291); no other mutations were looked for. It is possible that the HS mutations are like SAO mutations where distal RTA is only apparent with compound heterozygosity.

Na^+–HCO_3^- Cotransporter

Background. A second mode of moving HCO_3^- uphill across the plasma membrane is to couple it to the favorable electrochemical driving force for Na^+. Functionally, Na^+-coupled HCO_3^- cotransport comes in several stoichiometries (292–294). It can also occur as Na^+-coupled Cl^-/HCO_3^- exchange (295). K^+–HCO_3^- cotransport activity has also been described (296). The first cDNA of an Na^+–HCO_3^- cotransporter (NBC) was cloned by functional expression by simultaneously measuring positive current and acidification that is Na^+-dependent, HCO_3^--dependent, and stilbene-sensitive. Numerous cDNAs were subsequently obtained by homology (297).

At present, the nomenclature of Na^+-coupled HCO_3^- transporters is diverging from rather than converging towards a state of unity. A review of all the Na^+–HCO_3^- cotransporter cDNAs is beyond the scope of this chapter. Table 6 is an attempt at a summary and classification. Considerable primary sequence homology exists between the NBC and AE families of HCO_3^- transporters (297). The dual classification of AE4 as NBC5 is one example. Both families have multiple members and an extended number of isoforms due to different transcription start sites and exon splicing. If one adds the Na^+-driven Cl^-/HCO_3^- exchangers (NDAE) (298,299) and the K^+–HCO_3^- cotransporters to these two superfamilies, the number of mammalian gene products devoted to transporting HCO_3^- is quite impressive.

Distribution and function in mammalian kidney. In the kidney, Na^+-coupled HCO_3^- cotransport is found in intact tubules (292,300) and in basolateral membrane vesicles from renal cortex (301–303). NBC-1 is localized to the basolateral membranes of S1 and S2 segments of the proximal convoluted tubule (304). This localization for NBC-1 correlates well with functional studies of basolateral base exit in the proximal tubule (292,300–303). Two other NBC isoforms have been identified in the kidney. Electroneutral NBC-3 is found on the apical membrane of the connecting tubule, and in the cortical, outer and initial inner medullary collecting ducts (305,306). In intercalated cells, NBC-3 is found in subapical vesicles and tubulocisternal structures as well as in the cell membranes (306). NBC-3 is

Table 6 NBC Family of Na-Coupled Bicarbonate Transporters[a]

Subgroup	Function	Synonyms (Reference, year)	Source	
NBC-1	Electrogenic Na^+-$3HCO_3^-$	aNBC, NBC-1B (Romero, 1997)	Ambystoma kidney	Short N-terminus
		hkNBC, kNBC-1, NBC-1A (Burnham, 1997)	Human kidney	
		rNBC (Romero 1998, Burnham, 1998)	Rat kidney	
	Electrogenic Na^+-$3HCO_3^-$, long N-terminus	pNBC, pNBC-1 (Abuladze, 1998)	Human pancreas	Long N-terminus
		rpNBC (Thevenod, 1999)	Rat pancreas	
		hhNBC (Choi, 1999)	Human heart	
	Electrogenic Na^+-$3HCO_3^-$	rb1NBC (Bevensee, 2000)	Rat brain	
		rb2NBC (Bevensee, 2000)	Rat brain	C-terminal deletion
NBC-2	Unknown	NBC-2 (Ishibashi, 1998)	Human retina	
NBC-3	Electroneutral Na^+-HCO_3^-	mNBC3, NBCn1-D (Pushkin, 1999, Choi, 2000)	Human muscle	
		NBC3 (Amlal, 1999)	Human cell line	
		NBCn1-A to C (Choi, 2000)	Rat aortic smooth muscle	
NBC-4	Unknown	NBC4a and b (Pushkin, 2000)	Human database	

[a]Not shown are clones that code for Na^+-driven Cl^-/HCO_3^- exchangers and AE4, which has been classified by some as NBC5.

expressed on the apical membrane of the α-IC and basolateral membrane of β-IC (306). In the α-IC, NBC-3 exhibits almost perfect colocalization with H^+-ATPase (305). The role of an electroneutral Na^+–HCO_3^- cotransporter in these locales is uncertain at present. With a 1:1 stoichiometry, it is unclear how a 5–10-fold lumen-to-cell Na^+ gradient can drive apical HCO_3^- uptake against a potential pH gradient of two units. NBCn-1, an isoform of the NBC-3" class (see Table 6), has been localized to the basolateral membrane of the thick ascending limb in the outer medulla and to α-ICs of the collecting duct and is likely responsible for base exit in these acid-secreting cells (307).

Molecular structure and function. Figure 8 is a cartoon of a 10 membrane-spanning protein based on hydropathy prediction. The approximately 1000 amino acid protein has both termini in the cytoplasmic face. The 5'-end of the reading frame is spliced differently, giving rise to two different N-termini (297). The renal and pancreatic isoforms have a unique span of 41 and 85 amino acids at the N-termini, respectively. The differential stoichiometry

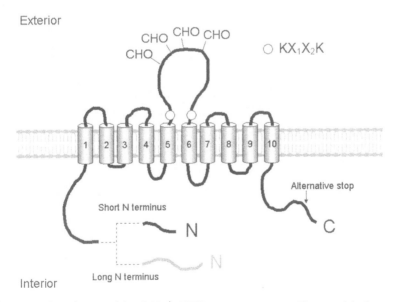

Figure 8 Putative model of Na^+–HCO_3^- cotransporter. The model shown is derived primarily hydropathy plots of NBC1 ($\sim$1000 amino acids). The renal and pancreatic isoforms are 5'-splice variants with divergent N-terminus [renal (*grey*): $\sim$80 aa, long-N-terminus; pancreatic (*black*): $\sim$40 aa, short-N-terminus]. Consensus stilbene binding sites KX_1X_2K (K, lysine, X_1, methionine or leucine, X_2, isoleucine, valine, or tyrosine). CHO, putative glycosylation sites. One isoform (rb1NBC) has an alternative 3'-splice site with an earlier stop codon. Numerous putative kinase sites based solely on consensus motifs have not been experimentally verified.

of the renal (short) and pancreatic (long) isoforms resides not in the divergent N-terminus sequence but rather in the cellular context (308,309). One of the brain isoforms (rb2NBC) has the same start site as the long NBC-1, but has a more proximal stop codon. The functional significance of this truncation is unknown.

NBC-1 function has been studied in *Xenopus* oocytes and in mammalian HEK cells (297). The characteristics of the cloned protein resemble that of the native protein. NBC-1 is Na^+-dependent (K_{Na} ~30 mM), HCO_3^--dependent, DIDS-sensitive, electrogenic, voltage-dependent, and has a stoichiometry of $1Na^+:3HCO_3^-$. Functional evidence in native renal basolateral membranes suggests that the transported species are $Na^+/HCO_3^-/CO_3^{2-}$, which is equivalent to $1Na^+:3HCO_3$ (309). The NBC clones do not support Li^+ or SO_4^{2-} as substrates (310,311), while the native protein appears to do so (302,303,312).

Regulation of NBC in the kidney. Changes in $Na^+-HCO_3^-$ cotransport occur in response to chronic acid–base disturbances in basolateral membrane vesicles (313), intact renal tubules (314), and suspended cortical tubules (315). However, no changes in NBC-1 transcript levels appear to occur with similar chronic acid or alkali loads. One cell culture study, in which inner medullary cells were subjected to a near-lethal acid load, provided evidence that the increase in $Na^+-HCO_3^-$ cotransport activity may be due to isoform switching between NBC-1 and NBC-3 (316). In contrast to metabolic acidosis, stimulation of $Na^+-HCO_3^-$ cotransport activity induced by K^+ depletion (317) is accompanied by increase in NBC-1 transcript in the proximal tubule (318). In addition to proximal tubule adaptation, K^+ depletion induces NBC-1 transcript in the thick ascending limb and inner medullary collecting duct (318). Increased NBC-1 expression is also reported in glucocorticoid excess (319). Due to the multiple isoforms of NBCs in the kidney, we are far from understanding the role of each in either physiologic or pathophysiologic states.

Whole organism phenotype of NBC abnormalities. Several familial forms of proximal tubular acidosis have been reported in humans with features suggestive of NBC dysfunction in whom acidosis occurs without features of the Fanconi syndrome. An autosomal dominant (based on transmission via successive generations) form of isolated proximal renal tubular acidosis was described in Costa Rica years ago, but still does not have published genotypic data (320). An autosomal recessive form associated with mental retardation and multiple ocular abnormalities has been described from Scandinavia, Japan, and Israel (321–323), and the lesion has been mapped to NBC-1 (324). Two (R298S, R510H) of the three (R298S, S427L, R510H) homozygous missense mutations with approximately 50% NBC transport activity when expressed in mammalian cells (324). A nonsense (Q29X) mutation has also been described (325). The same mutation (S427L) was found in Israel and Japan suggesting that the alleles are identical-by-state rather than identical-by-descent, implying a vulnerable mutagenic hot spot.

Because of the defect in NBC1, base exit should be impaired and resting cell pH in the proximal tubule should be higher in order to drive basolateral HCO_3^- extrusion. Two direct physiologic consequences of cellular alkalinization are suppression of ammoniagenesis and paradoxical hypercitraturia in the presence of systemic acidosis. Halperin and associates predicted the lesion of isolated proximal RTA to be proximal tubule cell alkalinization secondary to impaired basolateral HCO_3^- exit based solely on physiologic data prior to the emergence of the molecular tools (326).

OTHER ACID–BASE TRANSPORTERS

Not all acid–base transporters are directly coupled to H^+ or HCO_3^-. Excretion of inorganic anions such as phosphate at a lower valence than in blood is equivalent to H^+ excretion. In addition to the titratable anions in Table 7, NH_3 is a major H^+ acceptor in urine. Excretion of all these H^+-titratable entities in the urine will affect external acid–base balance. Most organic

Table 7 Titrable Anions in the Urine

Anion[a]	pK^a	Metabolized to base equivalent	Approximate range of daily excretion in a normal 70 kg human (mmol/day)
Acetate	4.75	Yes	0.1–3.7
Aceto-acetate	3.8	Yes	<0.1
β-OH-butyrate	4.7	Yes	<0.1
Citrate	5.6/4.3/2.9	Yes	**5–17**
Fumarate	3.0	Yes	0.05–0.3
Lactate	0.3–0.4	Yes	3.1
Proprionate	4.9	Yes	<0.1
Succinate	5.6/4.2	Yes	0.3–1.2
Creatinate	4.9	No	**12**
Formate	3.8	No	0.04–0.73
Glycolic	3.8	No	1–2.2
Oxalate	4.2/1.2	No	0.1–0.5
Phosphate	12.3/6.8/2.1	No	**20–30**
Urate	5.6	No	**4–6**

Anions of substantial quantity are in bold. Cl^- and SO_4^{2-} are excluded because they: (1) are not metabolizable, (2) have pKs too low to accept H^+ in urine. A major H^+ acceptor that is not an anion is NH_3.
[a]Multiple pKs refer to neutral–monovalent–bivalent–trivalent transition.
Source: Values compiled from Refs. 327, 328, 329, 330.

anions are base equivalents, and excreton of these anions in the urine as Na^+ or K^+ salt is equivalent to base loss (Table 7, see also Chapter 6) (328). A number of transporters in the proximal tubule secrete or reabsorb organic anions and are thus capable of altering the concentration of base equivalents in the urine (331). In addition, inorganic anion transporters such as the Na^+–SO_4^{2-} cotransporter can alter the luminal impermeable anions and luminal negativity and hence modulate distal acidification (332). A discussion of all these transporters is beyond the scope of this chapter. The most abundant organic anion is citrate and the most abundant inorganic anion is phosphate (Table 7). We will limit our discussion to the two transporters associated with these ions—the Na^+-coupled dicarboxylate (NaDC) and the Na^+-coupled inorganic phosphate (NaPi) transporter.

Na-citrate cotransporter. Citrate excretion is highly regulated by acid–base status (333). Regulation of citrate excretion occurs at multiple levels (333) including mitochondrial aconitase (334), cytoplasmic citrate lyase (335), and at the apical membrane Na^+-coupled citrate cotransporter (336,337). Analogous to the NBCs, the family of Na-citrate cotransporters have been classified in many ways. Table 8 summarizes the three groups of cDNAs termed NaDC-1, 2, and 3. NaDC-1 (synonyms: hNaDC-1, rNaDC-1, SDCT-1, Ri-19) (338–341) is expressed in the apical membrane of the proximal tubule (337,340). NaDC-1 corresponds to the low affinity dicarboxylate transport of proximal tubule brush border. NaDC-2 is primarily an intestinal isoform (342). NaDC-3 (synonym SDCT-2) is the high-affinity transporter expressed in the kidney (343). It functionally resembles the basolateral transporter that takes up dicarboxylates from the plasma into the proximal tubule (344–346).

A fall in luminal pH instantly stimulates proximal tubule citrate uptake (347) via activation of apical Na^+-citrate cotransport (346,348). The cloned transporter NaDC-1 exhibits similar properties in heterologous systems (349,350). The prevailing consensus is that the pH effect is via titration of citrate^{3-} to the preferred NaDC-1 substrate citrate^{2-} (346,347,351), although kinetic data supporting either H^+ cotransport or allosteric regulation by H^+ also exists (352). Both chronic acid feeding and K^+ depletion

Table 8 Na-Coupled Citrate and Inorganic Phosphate Transporters

Isoform	Function	Distribution
NaDC-1	Low affinity	Proximal tubule apical membrane. Also in intestine, liver lung and adrenals
NaDC-2	Low affinity	Intestine
NaDC-3	High affinity	Strongly expressed in kidney. Intrarenal distribution unknown. Also in brain, placenta and liver

lead to intracellular acidosis, hypocitraturia and increased proximal tubule apical membrane Na^+-citrate cotransport, whereas alkali feeding has no effect on Na^+-citrate cotransport despite hypercitraturia (336,353). Increases in NaDC-1 mRNA occur rapidly in response to acid loading with changes detectable in 3 hr, peaking in 24 hr and plateauing thereafter (337). New NaDC protein appearance is more gradual with peak increase occurring after 7 days. This profile of change in NaDC protein does not correspond to NaDC-1 mRNA appearance and suggests a more complex underlying mechanism of regulation (337). Both the acute and chronic stimulation of NaDC-1 by acid contributes to preservation of base in acidosis.

Na-phosphate cotransporter. Phosphate is an integral component of many biologic molecules including phosphoproteins, nucleic acids, and phospholipids. Whether dietary phosphate constitutes an acid or base load depends on the valence of the phosphate entering and leaving the body. As a result, phosphate balance is intimately intertwined with H^+ homeostasis. In the kidney, phosphate is reabsorbed solely by the proximal tubule via an apical membrane Na^+-coupled cotransport system. The gene family of Na^+-coupled inorganic phosphate transporters (NaPi) is shown in Table 9. NaPi-I has virtually no sequence similarity with the other members of this family (354). Antisense oligonucleotides to NaPi-II almost completely eliminate Na-PO_4 transport from kidney polyA$^+$ RNA (355). NaPi-I is most likely a protein with Cl^-/anion channel activity that activates endogenous Na-PO_4 contransporter activity when expressed, rather than being a phosphate transporter itself (356). NaPi-II is responsible for transepithelial phosphate transport with IIa being the renal-limited and IIb more likely the ubiquitous gastrointestinal isoform (357). NaPi-III consists of two homologous members, originally described as a cell surface receptor for certain viruses (357), and these two members are likely responsible for general phosphate uptake by all cells (357). NaPi-IIIs are ubiquitous, about 20% similar to NaPi-II, and are highly expressed the in the kidney. The role of

Table 9 Na-Coupled Inorganic Phosphate Transporters

Isoform	Function	Distribution
Type I	Likely an anion channel	Multiple tissues including kidney proximal tubule
Type IIa	Transepithelial phosphate transport	Exclusively apical membrane renal proximal tubule
Type IIb	Transepithelial phosphate transport	More general expression. Apical membrane of gastrointestinal tract. Not in kidney
Type III	Cellular phosphate transport (?)	Ubiquitous

Table 10 Proximal Tubule Cellular Adaption to Chronic Acidosis[a]

Effectors	Mechanism
Membrane transporters	
NHE3	Increased mRNA and protein, increased trafficking to apical membrane
NaPi-IIa	Increased protein
NaDC-1	Increased mRNA and protein
Cytosolic/mitochondrial enzymes	
PEPCK	Increased mRNA and protein, increased transcription
PDG	Increased mRNA and protein, increased mRNA T2 via crystallin binding
Aconitase	Increased protein
ATP citrate lyase	Increased protein
Autocrine hormone	
Endothelin	Increased mRNA and protein, activation of ET-1 promoter

[a]Not a complete list. Only a selected number of effectors are shown.
PEPCK, phosphoenolpyruvate carboxykinase; PDG, phosphate-dependent glutaminase; ET-1, endothelin 1.

NaPi-III in renal phosphate and acid–base homeostasis is unknown. We will focus on NaPi-IIa and discuss its relevance to acid–base balance. Acidosis (or an acidic pH) inhibits proximal tubule phosphate absorption and brush border Na-phosphate cotransport activity (357). NaPi-IIa is regulated at three levels by an acidic milieu: (1) direct gating of the protein by pH, (2) titration of phosphate from its dibasic to monobasic form, and (3) alteration of NaPi-IIa protein expression.

The pH-responsive region of NaPi-IIa is in the third extracellular loop, harboring the highly basic triad of arginine–glutamine–lysine (358). The mechanism of sensing is yet to be defined. Direct regulation of NaPi-IIa by acid pH occurs and a theoretical model has been proposed in which H^+ both interacts with the empty carrier, altering the kinetics of its *cis–trans* (inner membrane-facing to outer membrane-facing) transition, and also competes with Na^+ for the Na^+-binding site, increasing the apparent K_{Na} (359). A second mode of inhibition of NaPi-IIa activity by H^+ is simply via H^+ titration of HPO_4^{2-}, the preferred substrate of NaPi-IIa, to $H_2PO_4^-$, which is poorly accepted by the transporter (360–362). In chronic metabolic acidosis, NaPi-IIa protein expression is decreased in both the apical membrane and renal cortex (363). The mechanism by which chronic acid feeding decreases NaPi-IIa expression is unknown.

The physiologic effect of these regulatory mechanisms is to increase urinary buffer capacity. NaPi-II is expressed primarily in the convoluted portion of the proximal tubule (364). When luminal HCO_3^- falls in metabolic acidosis, the instantaneous inhibition of NaPi-II serves to preserve buffering capacity in the early proximal tubule. In chronic acidosis, increased phosphate excretion likely contributes to increased net acid excretion.

In addition to NHE3, Napi-IIa, and NaDC-1, there are other processes that are regulated by acid in the proximal tubule. A short list is provided in Table 10.

CONCLUDING REMARKS

This chapter highlights the impact of molecular reagents and model systems on our understanding of acid–base homeostasis by the kidney. The summary is far from complete, as this field is evolving rapidly. Acid–base physiology is embarking on a phase in which there will be a tremendous outpouring of detailed data about the function of individual molecules in multiple model systems including epithelial and nonepithelial cells, in eukaryotes and prokaryotes, and genetically manipulated animals. The challenge of the acid–base physiologist will be to assimilate the molecular data, and to test their significance and relevance for organ and intact animal physiology.

REFERENCES

1. Baum M. Evidence that parallel Na^+–H^+ and $Cl(^-)$–HCO_3^- (OH^-) antiporters transport NaCl in the proximal tubule. Am J Physiol 1987; 252: F338–F345.
2. Kurtz I, Nagami G, Yanagawa N, Li L, Emmons C, Lee I. Mechanism of apical and basolateral Na(+)-independent Cl^-/base exchange in the rabbit superficial proximal straight tubule. J Clin Invest 1994; 94:173–183.
3. Kempe S, Degens ET. An early soda water ocean? Chem Geol 1985; 53: 95–104.
4. Ohno S. The reason for as well as the consequence of the Cambrian explosion in animal evolution. J Mol Evol 1997; 44:S23–S27.
5. Chen Y, Cann MJ, Litvin TN, Iourgenko V, Sinclair ML, Levin LR, Buck J. Soluble adenylyl cyclase as an evolutionarily conserved bicarbonate sensor. Science 2000; 289:625–628.
6. Smith KS, Ferry JG. Prokaryotic carbonic anhydrases. FEMS Microbio Rev 2000; 24:335–366.
7. Stevens TH, Forgac M. Structure, function and regulation of the vacuolar (H+)-ATPase. Annu Rev Cell Dev Biol 1997; 13:779–808.
8. Clague MJ, Urbe S, Aniento F, Gruenberg. Vacuolar ATPase activity is required for endosomal carrier vesicle formation. J Biol Chem 1994; 269: 21–24.
9. Futai M, Oka T, Sun-Wada G, Moriyama Y, Kanazawa H, Wada Y. Luminal acidification of diverse organelles by V-ATPase in animal cells. J Exp Biol 2000; 203:107–116.

10. Swallow CJ, Grinstein S, Sudsbury RA, Rotstein OD. Relative roles of Na^+/H^+ exchange and vacuolar-type H^+ ATPases in regulating cytoplasmic pH and function in murine peritoneal macrophages. J Cell Physiol 1993; 157:453–460.

11. Wieczorek H, Putzenlechner M, Zeiske W, Klein U. A vacuolar-type protein pump energizes K/H antiport in an animal plasma membrane. J Biol Chem 1991; 266:15,340–15,347.

12. Blair HC, Teitelbaum SL, Ghiselli R, Gluck S. Osteoclastic bone resorption by a polarized vacuolar protein pump. Science 1989; 245:855–857.

13. Gluck SL, Underhill DM, Iyori M, Holliday LS, Kostrominova TY, Lee BS. Physiology and biochemistry of the kidney vacuolar H^+-ATPase. Annu Rev Physiol 1996; 158:427–445.

14. Kinne-Safran E, Beauwens R, Kinne R. An ATP-driven proton pump in brush border membranes from rat renal cortex. J Memb Biol 1982; 64:67–76.

15. Brown D, Hirsch S, Gluck S. Localization of a proton pumping ATPase in rat kidney. J Clin Invest 1988; 82:2114–2126.

16. Preisig PA, Ives HE, Cragoe EJ Jr, Alpern RJ, Rector FC Jr. Role of the Na^+/H^+ antiporter in rat proximal tubule bicarbonate absorption. J Clin Invest 1987; 80:970–978.

17. Brown D, Hirsch S, Gluck S. An H^+-ATPase in opposite membranes domains in a kidney epithelial cell subpopulations. Nature 1988; 331:622–624.

18. Alper SL, Natale J, Gluck S, Lodish HF, Brown D. Subtypes of intercalated cells in rat kidney collecting duct defined by antibodies against erythroid band 3 and renal vacuolar H^+-ATPase. Proc Natl Acad Sci USA 1989; 86:5429–5433.

19. Weiner ID, Hamm LL. Regulation of intracellular pH in the rabbit cortical collecting tubule. J Clin Invest 1990; 85:274–281.

20. Emmons C, Kurtz I. Functional characterization of three intercalated cell subtypes in the rabbit collecting duct. J Clin Invest 1994; 93:417–423.

21. Kashgarian M, Biemesderfer D, Caplan M, Forbush B. Monoclonal antibody to Na–K-ATPase: immunolocalization along nephron segments. Kidney Int 1985; 28:899–913.

22. Koeppen BM. Electrophysiologic identification of principal and intercalated cells in the rabbit outer medullary collecting duct. Pflügers Arch 1987; 409:138–141.

23. Südhof TC, Fried VA, Stone DK, Johnston PA, Xie XS. Human endomembrane H^+ pump strongly resembles the ATP-synthase of archaebacteria. Proc Natl Acad Sci USA 1989; 86:6067–6071.

24. Boekema EJ, Ubbink-Kok T, Lolkema JS, Brisson A, Konings WN. Visualization of a peripheral stalk in V-type ATPase: evidence for the stator structure essential to rotational catalysis. Proc Natl Acad Sci USA 1997; 94: 14, 291–14,293.

25. Wilkens S, Capaldi RA. ATP synthase's second stalk comes into focus. Nature 1998; 393:29.

26. Perin MS, Fried VA, Stone DK, Xie XS, Sudhof TC. Structure of the 116-kDa polypeptide of the clathrin-coated vesicle/synaptic vesicle proton pump. J Biol Chem 1991; 266:3877–3881.

27. Leng XH, Manolson MF, Forgac M. Function of the COOH-terminal domain of Vph1p in activity and assembly of the yeast V-ATPase. J Biol Chem 1998; 273:6717–6723.
28. Vik SB, Antonio BJ. A mechanism of proton translocation by F1F0 ATP synthases suggested by double mutants of the a subunit. J Biol Chem 1994; 269:30,364–30,369.
29. Zhang J, Feng Y, Forgac M. Proton conduction and bafilomycin binding by the V0 domain of the coated vesicle V-ATPase. J Biol Chem 1994; 269:23,518–23,523.
30. Birkenhager R, Hoppert M, Deckers-Hebestreit G, Mayer F, Altendorf K. The F0 complex of the *Escherichia coli* ATP synthase. Investigation by electron spectroscopic imaging and immunoelectron microscopy. Eur J Biochem 1995; 230:58–67.
31. Holzenburg A, Jones PC, Franklin T, Pali T, Heimburg T, Marsh D, Findlay JB, Finbow ME. Evidence for a common structure for a class of membrane channels. Eur J Biochem 1993; 213:21–30.
32. Fillingame RH. Coupling H$^+$ transport and ATP synthesis in F1F0-ATP synthases: glimpses of interacting parts in a dynamic molecular machine. J Exp Biol 1997; 200:217–224.
33. Zhang J, Vasilyeva E, Feng Y, Forgac M. Inhibition and labeling of the coated vesicle V-ATPase by 2-azido-[32P]ATP. J Biol Chem 1995; 270:15,494–15,500.
34. Liu J, Kane PM. Mutational analysis of the catalytic subunit of the yeast vacuolar proton-translocating ATPase. Biochemistry 1996; 35:10,938–10,948.
35. Feng Y, Forgac M. Inhibition of vacuolar H(+)-ATPase by disulfide bond formation between cysteine 254 and cysteine 532 in subunit A. J Biol Chem 1994; 269:13,224–13,230.
36. Liu Q, Kane PM, Newman PR, Forgac M. Site-directed mutagenesis of the yeast V-ATPase B subunit (Vma2p). J Biol Chem 1996; 271:2018–2022.
37. Nelson RD, Guo XL, Masood K, Brown D, Kalkbrenner M, Gluck S. Selectively amplified expression of an isoform of the vacuolar H(+)-ATPase 56-kilodalton subunit in renal intercalated cells. Proc Natl Acad Sci USA 1992; 89:3541–3545.
38. Ho MN, Hirata R, Umemoto N, Ohya Y, Takatsuki A, Stevens TH, Anraku Y. VMA13 encodes a 54-kDa vacuolar H(+)-ATPase subunit required for activity but not assembly of the enzyme complex in Saccharomyces cerevisiae. J Biol Chem 1993; 268:18,286–18,292.
39. Chambrey R, Paillard M, Podevin RA. Enzymatic and functional evidence for adaptation of the vacuolar H(+)-ATPase in proximal tubule apical membranes from rats with chronic metabolic acidosis. J Biol Chem 1994; 269:3243–3250.
40. Tsuruoka S, Schwartz GJ. Adaptation of rabbit cortical collecting duct HCO$_3^-$ transport to metabolic acidosis in vitro. J Clin Invest 1996; 97:1076–1084.
41. Bastani B, Purcell H, Hemken P, Trigg D, Gluck S. Expression and distribution of renal vacuolar proton-translocating ATPase in response to chronic acid and alkali loads in the rat. J Clin Invest 1991; 88:126–136.

42. Sabolic I, Brown D, Gluck SL, Alper SL. Regulation of AE1 anion exchanger and H^+-ATPase in rat cortex by acute metabolic acidosis and alkalosis. Kidney Int 1997; 51:125–137.

43. Feng Y, Forgac M. A novel mechanism for regulation of vacuolar acidification. J Biol Chem 1992; 267:19,769–19,772.

44. Dschida WJ, Bowman BJ. The vacuolar ATPase: sulfite stabilization and the mechanism of nitrate inactivation. J Biol Chem 1995; 270:1557–1563.

45. Oluwatosin YE, Kane PM. Mutations in the CYS4 gene provide evidence for regulation of the yeast vacuolar H+-ATPase by oxidation and reduction in vivo. J Biol Chem 1997; 272:28,149–28,157.

46. Torres AM, Ochoa JE, Elias MM. Role of lipid peroxidation on renal dysfunction associated with glutathione depletion: effects of vitamin E. Toxicology 1991; 70:163–172.

47. Kane PM. Regulation of V-ATPases by reversible disassembly. FEBS Lett 2000; 469:137–141.

48. Sumner JP, Dow JA, Earley FG, Klein U, Jager D, Wieczorek H. Regulation of plasma membrane V-ATPase activity by dissociation of peripheral subunits. J Biol Chem 1995; 270:5649–5653.

49. Zhang J, Myers M, Forgac M. Characterization of the Vo domain of the coated vesicle H^+-ATPase. J Biol Chem 1992; 267:9773–9778.

50. Myers M, Forgac M. Assembly of the peripheral domain of the bovine vascuolar H-ATPase. J Cell Physiol 1993; 156:35–42.

51. Vasilyeva E, Forgac M. Interaction of the clathrin-coated vesicle V-ATPase with ADP and sodium azide. J Biol Chem 1998; 273:23,823–23,829.

52. Forgac M. Structure, function and regulation of the vacuolar (H^+)-ATPases. FEBS Lett 1998; 440:258–326.

53. Muller ML, Irkens-Kiesecker U, Kramer D, Taiz L. Purification and reconstitution of the vacuolar H^+-ATPases from lemon fruits and epicotyls. J Biol Chem 1997; 272:12,762–12,770.

54. Zhang K, Wang ZQ, Gluck S. Identification and partial purification of a cytosolic activator of vacuolar H^+-ATPase from mammalian kidney. J Biol Chem 1992; 267:9701–9705.

55. Xie XS, Crider BP, Stone DK. Isolation of a protein activator of the clathrin-coated vesicle proton pump. J Biol Chem 1993; 268:25,063–25,067.

56. Zhang K, Wang ZQ, Gluck S. A cytosolic inhibitor of vacuolar H^+-ATPase from mammalian kidney. J Biol Chem 1992; 267:14,539–14,542.

57. Schwartz GJ, Barasch J, Al-Awqati Q. Plasticity of functional epithelial polarity. Nature 1985; 318:368–371.

58. van Adelsberg J, Edwards JC, Takito J, Kiss B, Al-Awqati Q. An induced extracellular matrix protein reverses the polarity of band 3 in intercalated cells. Cell 1994; 76:1053–1061.

59. Takito J, Hikita C, Al-Awqati Q. Hensin, a new collecting duct protein involved in the in vitro plasticity of intercalated cell polarity. J Clin Invest 1996; 98:2324–2331.

60. Hikita C, Takito J, Vijayakumar S, Al-Awqati Q. Only multimeric hensin located in the extracellular matrix can induce apical endocytosis and reverse the polarity of intercalated cells. J Biol Chem 1999; 274:17,671–17,676.

61. Vijayakumar S, Takito J, Hikita C, Al-Awqati Q. Hensin remodels the apical cytoskeleton and induces columnarization of intercalated epithelial cells: processes that resemble terminal differentiation. J Cell Biol 1999; 144:1057–1067.

62. van Adelsberg J, Edwards JC, Al-Alwati Q. The apical Cl/HCO₃ exchanger of beta-intercalated cells. J Biol Chem 1993; 268:11,283–11,289.

63. Tsuganezawa H, Kobayashi K, Iyori M, Araki T, Koizumi A, Watanabe SI, Kaneko A, Fukao T, Monkawa T, Yoshida T, Kim DK, Kanai Y, Endou H, Hayashi M, Saruta T. A new member of the HCO_3^- transporter superfamily is an apical anion exchanger of beta-intercalated cells in the kidney. J Biol Chem 2001; 267:8180–8189.

64. Brown D. Membrane recycling and epithelial cell function. Am J Physiol 1989; 256:F1–F12.

65. Brown D, Sabolic I. Endosomal pathways for water channel and proton pump recylcing in kidney epithelial cells. J Cell Sci 1993; 17(suppl):49–59.

66. Brown D, Breton S. H^+-V-ATPase-dependent luminal acidification in the kidney collecting duct and the epididymis/vas deferens: vesicle recycling and transcytotic pathways. J Exp Biol 2000; 203:137–145.

67. Cohen EP, Bastani B, Cohen MR, Kolner S, Hemken P, Gluck SL. Absence of H(+)-ATPase in cortical collecting tubules of a patient with Sjogren's syndrome and distal renal tubular acidosis. J Am Soc Nephrol 1992; 3:264–271.

68. Konoshi K, Hayashi M, Saruta T. Renal tubular acidosis with antibody directed to renal collecting duct cells. N Eng J Med 1994; 331:1494–1593.

69. Bastani B, Underhill D, Chu N, Nelson RD, Haragsim L, Gluck S. Preservation of intercalated cell H(+)-ATPase in two patients with lupus nephritis and hyperkalemic distal renal tubular acidosis. J Am Soc Nephrol 1997; 7: 1109–1117.

70. Inoue H, Noumi T, Nagata M, Murakami H, Kanazawa H. Targeted disruption of the gene encoding the proteolipid subunit of mouse vacuolar H(+)-ATPase leads to early embryonic lethality. Biochim Biophys Acta 1999; 1413:130–138.

71. Li YP, Chen W, Liang Y, Li E, Stashenko P. Atp6i-deficient mice exhibit severe osteopetrosis due to loss of osteoclast-mediated extracellular acidification. Nat Genet 1999; 23:447–451.

72. Kornak U, Schulz A, Friedrich W, Uhlhaas S, Kremens B, Voit T, Hasan C, Bode U, Jentsch TJ, Kubisch C. Mutations in the a3 subunit of the vacuolar H(+)-ATPase cause infantile malignant osteopetrosis. Hum Mol Genet 2000; 9:2059–2063.

73. Frattini A, Orchard PJ, Sobacchi C, Giliani S, Abinun M, Mattsson JP, Keeling DJ, Andersson AK, Wallbrandt P, Zecca L, Notarangelo LD, Vezzoni P, Villa A. Defects in TCIRG1 subunit of the vacuolar proton pump are responsible for a subset of human autosomal recessive osteopetrosis. Nat Genet 2000; 25:343–346.

74. Karet FE, Finberg KE, Nelson RD, Nayir A, Mocan H, Sanjad SA, Rodriguez-Soriano J, Santos F, Cremers CW, Di Pietro A, Hoffbrand BI, Winiarski J, Bakkaloglu A, Ozen S, Dusunsel R, Goodyer P, Hulton SA, Wu DK, Skvorak AB, Morton CC, Cunningham MJ, Jha V, Lifton RP.

Mutations in the gene encoding B1 subunit of H^+-ATPase cause renal tubular acidosis with sensorineural deafness. Nat Genet 1999; 21:84–90.

75. Smith AN, Skaug J, Choate KA, Nayir A, Bakkaloglu A, Ozen S, Hulton SA, Sanjad SA, Al-Sabban EA, Lifton RP, Scherer SW, Karet FE. Mutations in ATP6N1B, encoding a new kidney vacuolar proton pump 116-kD subunit, cause recessive distal renal tubular acidosis with preserved hearing. Nat Genet 2000; 26:71–75.

76. Misquitta CM, Mack DP, Grover AK. Sarco/endoplasmic reticulum Ca^{2+} (SERCA)-pumps: link to heart beats and calcium waves. Cell Calcium 1999; 25:277–290.

77. Carafoli E, Garcia-Martin E, Guerini D. The plasma membrane calcium pump: recent developments and future perspectives. Experientia 1996; 52:1091–1100.

78. Caplan MJ. Gastric H^+/K^+-ATPase: targeting signals in the regulation of physiologic function. Curr Opin Cell Biol 1998; 10:468–473.

79. Hentschel H, Mahler S, Herter P, Elger M. Renal tubule of dogfish, Scyliorhinus caniculus: a comprehensive study of structure with emphasis on intramembrane particles and immunoreactivity for $H(+)$–$K(+)$-adenosine triphosphatase. Anat Rec 1993; 235:511–532.

80. Swenson ER, Fine AD, Maren TH, Reale E, Lacy ER, Smolka AJ. Physiological and immunocytochemical evidence for a putative H–K-ATPase in elasmobranch renal acid secretion. Am J Physiol 1994; 267:F639–F645.

81. Wingo CS. Active protein secretion and potassium absorption in the rabbit outer medullary collecting duct: functional evidence for proton, potassium activated adenosine triphosphatase. J Clin Invest 1989; 84:361–365.

82. Wingo CS, Armitage FE. Rubidium absorption and proton secretion by rabbit outer medullary collecting duct via H^+/K^+-ATPase. Am J Physiol 1992; 263:F849–F857.

83. Silver RB, Frindt G. Functional identification of H^+/K^+-ATPase in intercalated cells of cortical collecting tubule. Am J Physiol 1993; 264:F259–F266.

84. Wall SM, Truong AV, DuBose TD. H^+/K^+-ATPase mediates net acid secretion in rat terminal inner medullary collecting duct. Am J Physiol 1996; 271:F1037–F1044.

85. Weiner ID, Milton AE. H^+/K^+-ATPase in rabbit cortical collecting duct B-type intercalated cell. Am J Physiol 1996; 270:F450–F458.

86. Polvani C, Sachs G, Blostein R. Sodium ions as substitutes for protons in the gastric H,K-ATPase. J Biol Chem 1989; 264:17,854–17,859.

87. Rabon EC, Bassilian S, Sachs G, Karlish SJ. Conformational transitions of the H,K-ATPase studied with sodium ions as surrogates for protons. J Biol Chem 1990; 265:19,594–19,599.

88. Grishin AV, Caplan MJ. ATP1AL1, a member of the non-gastric H,K-ATPase family, functions as a sodium pump. J Biol Chem 1998; 273:27,772–27,778.

89. Cougnon M, Bouyer P, Planelles G, Jaisser F. Does the colonic H,K-ATPase also act as an Na,K-ATPase? Proc Natl Acad Sci USA 1998; 95:6516–6520.

90. Polvani C, Blostein R. Protons as substitutes for sodium and potassium in the sodium pump reaction. J Biol Chem 1988; 263:16,757–16,763.
91. Silver RN, Soleimani M. H–K-ATPases: regulation and role in pathophysiologic states. Am J Physiol 1999; 276:F799–F811.
92. Wingo CS, Madsen KM, Smolka A, Tisher CC. H–K-ATPase immunoreactivity in cortical and outer medullary collecting duct. Kidney Int 1990; 38:985–990.
93. Bastani B. Colocalization of H-ATPase and K–K-ATPase immunoreactivity in the rat kidney. J Am Soc Nephrol 1995; 5:1476–1482.
94. Ahn KY, Kone BC. Expression and cellular localization of mRNA encoding the "gastric" isoform of H(+)–K(+)-ATPase alpha-subunit in rat kidney. Am J Physiol 1995; 268:F99–F109.
95. Kraut JA, Starr F, Sachs G, Reuben M. Expression of gastric and colonic H(+)–K(+)-ATPase in the rat kidney. Am J Physiol 1995; 268:F581–F587.
96. Reinhardt J, Grishin AV, Oberleithner H, Caplan MJ. Differential localization of human nongastric H(+)–K(+)-ATPase ATP1AL1 in polarized renal epithelial cells. Am J Physiol 2000; 279:F417–F425.
97. Cheval L, Elalouf JM, Doucet A. Re-evaluation of the expression of the gastric H,K-ATPase alpha subunit along the rat nephron. Pflugers Arch 1997; 433:539–541.
98. Silver RB, Frindt G, Mennitt P, Satlin L. Characterization and regulation of H–K-ATPase in intercalated cells of rabbit cortical collecting duct. J Exp Zool 1997; 279:443–455.
99. Crowson MS, Shull GE. Isolation and characterization of a cDNA encoding the putative distal colon H–K-ATPase. J Biol Chem 1992; 2267:13,740–13,748.
100. DuBose TD Jr, Codina J, Burges A, Pressley TA. Regulation of H^+/K^+-ATPase expression in kidney. Am J Physiol 1995; 269:F500–F507.
101. Ahn KY, Park KY, Kim KK, Kone BC. Chronic hypokalemia enhances expression of the H(+)–K(+)-ATPase alpha 2-subunit gene in renal medulla. Am J Physiol 1996; 271:F314–F321.
102. Weiner ID, Milton AE. H–K-ATPase in rabbit cortical collecting duct B-type intercalated. Am J Physiol 1996; 270:F518–F530.
103. Palmgren MG, Axelsen KB. Evolution of the P-type ATPases. Biochem Biophys Acta 1998; 1365:37–45.
104. Caviston TL, Campbell G, Wingo CS, Cain BD. Molecular identification of the renal H^+/K^+-ATPase's. Semin Nephrol 1999; 19:431–437.
105. Jaisser F, Beggah AT. The nongastric H^+/K^+-ATPase's: molecular and functional properties. Am J Physiol 1999; 276:F812–F824.
106. Campbell WG, Weiner ID, Wingo CS, Cain BD. H–K-ATPase in the RCCT-28A rabbit cortical collecting duct cell line. Am J Physiol 1999; 276:F237–F245.
107. Kone BC, Higham SC. A novel N-terminal splice variant of the rat $H^+–K^+$-ATPase alpha2 subunit: cloning, functional expression, and renal adaptive response to chronic hypokalemia. J Biol Chem 1998; 273:2543–2552.

108. Campbell-Thompson ML, Verlander JW, Curran KA, Campbell WG, Cain BD, Wingo CS, McGuigan JE. In situ hybridization of H–K-ATPase beta-subunit mRNA in rat and rabbit kidney. Am J Physiol 1995; 269:F345–F354.

109. Callaghan JM, Tan SS, Khan MA, Curran KA, Campbell WG, Smolka AJ, Toh BH, Gleeson PA, Wingo CS, Cain BD. Renal expression of the gene encoding the gastric H(+)–K(+)-ATPase beta-subunit. Am J Physiol 1995; 268:F363–F374.

110. Sachs G. Symposium on ion motive ATPase. Acta Physiol Scand 1998; 643(supp):5–6.

111. Munson K, Lanbrecht N, Shin JM, Sachs G. Analysis of the membrane domain of the gastric H/K ATPase. J Exp Biol 2000; 203:161–170.

112. Bamberg K, Sachs G. Topological analysis of $H^+,K(+)$-ATPase using in vitro translation. J Biol Chem 1994; 269:16,909–16,919.

113. Auer M, Scarborough GA, Kuhlbrandt W. Three-dimensional map of the plasma membrane H^+-ATPase in the open conformation. Nature 1998; 392:840–843.

114. Zhang P, Toyoshima C, Yonekura K, Green NM, Stokes DL. Structure of the calcium pump from sarcoplasmic reticulum at 8-A resolution. Nature 1998; 392:835–839.

115. Shin JM, Sachs G. Identification of a region of the H,K-ATPase alpha subunit associated with the beta subunit. J Biol Chem 1994; 269:8642–8646.

116. Melle-Milovanovic D, Milovanovic M, Nagpal S, Sachs G, Shin JM. Regions of association between the alpha and the beta subunit of the gastric H,K-ATPase. J Biol Chem 1998; 273:11,075–11,081.

117. Chow DC, Browning CM, Forte JG. Gastric H–K-ATPase activity is inhibited by reduction of disulphide bonds in the beat-subunit. Am J Physiol 1992; 263:C39–C46.

118. Caplan M, Gottardi CJ. Molecular requirements for cell surface expression of multi-subunit ion-transporting ATPases. J Biol Chem 1993; 268:24,921–24,931.

119. Beggah AT, Beguin P, Bamberg K, Sachs G, Geering K. Beta subunit assembly is essential for the correct packing and the stable membrane insertion of the H,K-ATPase alpha-subunit. J Biol Chem 1999; 274:8217–8223.

120. Forte JG, Ganser AL, Tanisawa AS. The K+-stimulated ATPase system of microsomal membrane from gastric oxyntic cells. Ann NY Acad Sci 1974; 242:255–267.

121. Sachs G, Chang HH, Rabon E, Schackman R, Lewin M, Saccomani G. A non-electrogenic H^+ pump in plasma membrane of hog stomach. J Biol Chem 1976; 251:7690–7698.

122. Hersey SJ, Sachs G. Gastric acid secretion. Physiol Rev 1995; 75:155–189.

123. Sangan P, Rajendran VM, Mann AS, Kashgarian M, Binder HJ. Regulation of colonic H^+/K^+-ATPase in large intestine and kidney by dietary Na depletion and dietary K depletion. Am J Physiol 1997; 272:C685–C696.

124. Nakamura S, Amlal H, Galla JH, Soleimani M. Colonic H^+–K^+-ATPase is induced and mediates increased HCO_3^- reabsorption in inner medullary collecting duct in potassium depletion. Kidney Int 1998; 54:1233–1239.

125. Nakamura S, Amlal H, Galla JH, Soleimani M. NH_4^+ secretion in inner medullary collecting duct in potassium deprivation: role of colonic H^+–K^+-ATPase. Kidney Int 1999; 56:2160–2167.

126. Doucet A, Marsy S. Characterization of K-ATPase activity in distal nephron: stimulation by K^+ depletion. Am J Physiol 1987; 253:F418–F423.

127. Garg LC, Narang N. Ouabain-insensitive K-adenosine triphosphatase in distal nephron segments of the rabbit. J Clin Invest 1988; 81:1204–1208.

128. DuBose TD Jr, Gitomer J, Codina J. H^+/K^+-ATPase. Curr Opin Nephrol Hypertens 1999; 8:597–602.

129. Eiam-Ong S, Laski ME, Kurtzman NA, Sabatini S. Effects of respiratory acidosis and respiratory alkalosis on renal transport enzymes. Am J Physiol 1994; 267:F390–F399.

130. Zhou X, Wingo CS. Stimulation of total CO_2 flux by 10% CO_2 in rabbit CCD: role of an apical SCH-28080 and Ba-sensitive mechanism. Am J Physiol 1994; 267:F114–F120.

131. Silver RB, Frindt G, Mennitt P, Satlin L. Stimulation of apical H^+/K^+-ATPase in intercalated cells of cortical collecting duct with chronic metabolic acidosis. Am J Physiol 1996; 270:F539–F547.

132. Dafnis E, Spohn M, Lonis B, Kurtzman NA, Sabatini S. Vanadate causes hypokalemic distal renal tubular acidosis. Am J Physiol 1992; 262:F449–F453.

133. Eiam-Ong S, Dafnis E, Spohn M, Kurtzman NA, Sabatini S. H–K-ATPase in distal renal tubular acidosis: urinary tract obstruction, lithium, and amiloride. Am J Physiol 1993; 265:F875–F880.

134. Tosukhowong P, Tungsanga K, Eiam-Ong S, Sitprija V. Environmental distal renal tubular acidosis in Thailand: an enigma. Am J Kidney Dis 1999; 33:1180–1186.

135. Meneton P, Schultheis PJ, Greeb J, Nieman ML, Liu LH, Clarke LL, Duffy JJ, Doetschman T, Lorenz JN, Shull GE. Increased sensitivity to K^+ deprivation in colonic H,K-ATPase-deficient mice. J Clin Invest 1998; 101:536–542.

136. Gottardi CJ, Caplan MJ. An ion-transporting ATPase encodes multiple apical localization signals. J Cell Biol 1993; 121:283–293.

137. Courtois-Coutry N, Roush D, Rajendran V, McCarthy JB, Geibel J, Kashgarian M, Caplan MJ. A tyrosine-based signal targets H/K-ATPase to a regulated compartment and is required for the cessation of gastric acid secretion. Cell 1997; 90:501–510.

138. Wang T, Courtois-Coutry N, Giebisch G, Caplan MJ. A tyrosine-based signal regulates HKATPase-mediated potassium absorption in the kidney. Am J Physiol 1998; 275:F818–826.

139. Padan E, Sculdiner S. Na/H antiporters, molecular devices that couple the Na^+ and H^+ circulation in cells. J Bioenerg Biomembr 1993; 25:647–669.

140. Serrano R. Salt tolerance in plants and microorganisms: toxicity targets and defense responses. Int Rev Cytol 1996; 165:1–52.

141. Speelmans G, poolman B, Abee T, Konings WN. Energy transduction in the thermophilic anerobic bacterium *Colstridium fervifus* is exclusively coupled to Na ions. Proc Natl Acad Sci USA 1993; 90:7975–7979.

142. Padan E, Sculdiner S. Molecular physiology of the Na/H antiporter in *Escherichia coli.* J Exp Biol 1994; 196:443–456.

143. Ahearn GA, Franco P, Clay LP. Electrogenic 2 $Na^+/1\ H^+$ exchange in crustaceans. J Membr Biol 1990; 116:215–226.

144. Sardet C, Counillion L, Franchi A, Pouyssegur. Molecular cloning, primary structure and expression of the human growth factor-activatable Na/H antiporter. Cell 1989; 56:271–280.

145. Orlowski J, Grinstein S. Na^+/H^+ exchangers of mammalian cells. J Biol Chem 1997; 272:22,373–22,376.

146. Numata M, Orlowski J. Molecular cloning and characterization of a novel $(Na^+,K^+)/H+$ exchanger localized to the *trans*-golgi network. J Biol Chem 2001; 276:17,387–17,394.

147. Goyal S, Vanden Heuvel G, Aronson PS. Renal expression of novel Na^+/H^+ exchanger isoform NHE8. Am J Physiol Renal Physiol 2003; 284:F467–F473.

148. Biemesderfer D, Pizzonia J, Abu-Alfa A, Exner M, Reilly R, Igarashi P, Aronson PS. NHE-3: a Na/H exchanger isoform of renal brush border. Am J Physiol 1993; 265:F736–F742.

149. Amemiya M, Loffing J, Lötscher M, Kaissling B, Alpern RJ, Moe OW. Expression of NHE-3 in the apical membrane of rat renal proximal tubule and thick ascending limb. Kidney Int 1995; 48:1206–1215.

150. Shugrue CA, Obermuller N, Bachmann S, Slayman CW, Reilly RF. Molecular cloning of NHE3 from LLC-PK1 cells and localization in pig kidney. J Am Soc Nephrol 1999; 10:1649–1657.

151. Priesig PA, Rector FC Jr. Role of Na/H antiport in rat proximal tubule NaCl absorption. Am J Physiol 1988; 255:F461–F467.

152. Good DW. Sodium-dependent bicarbonate absorption by the cortical thick ascending limb. Am J Physiol 1988; 247:F821–F829.

153. Biemesderfer D, Reilly RF, Exner M, Igarashi P, Aronson PS. Immunocytochemical characterization of $Na(+)-H^+$ exchanger isoform NHE-1 in rabbit kidney. Am J Physiol 1992; 263:F833–F840.

154. Sun AM, Liu Y, Dworkin LD, Tse CM, Donowitz M, Yip KP. Na^+/H^+ exchanger isoform 2 (NHE2) is expressed in the apical membrane of the medullary thick ascending limb. J Membr Biol 1997; 160:85–90.

155. Wu MS, Biemesderfer D, Giebisch G, Aronson PS. Role of NHE3 in mediating renal brush border $Na^+–H^+$ exchange. Adaptation to metabolic acidosis. J Biol Chem 1996; 271:32,749–32,752.

156. Choi JY, Shah M, Lee MG, Schultheis PJ, Shull GE, Muallem S, Baum M. Novel amiloride-sensitive sodium-dependent proton secretion in the mouse proximal convoluted tubule. J Clin Invest 2000; 105:1141–1146.

157. Pizzonia JH, Biemesderfer D, Abu-Alfa AK, Wu MS, Exner M, Isenring P, Igarashi P, Aronson PS. Immunochemical characterization of Na^+/H^+ exchanger isoform NHE4. Am J Physiol 1998; 275:F510–F517.

158. Houillier P, Bourgeois S, Paillard M. Basolateral NH_4 efflux from the rat medullary thick ascending limb cell: a role for the NHE4 Na/H exchanger isoform [abstr]. J Am Soc Nephrol 2000; 11:5A.

159. Wells KM, Rao R. The yeast Na/H exchange Nhx1 is an N-linked glycoprotein. J Biol Chem 2001; 276:3401–3407.

160. Zizak M, Cavet ME, Bayle D, Tse CM, Hallen S, Sachs G, Donowitz M. Na(+)/H(+) exchanger NHE3 has 11 membrane spanning domains and a cleaved signal peptide: topology analysis using in vitro transcription/translation. Biochemistry 2000; 39:8102–8112.

161. Shrode LD, Gan BS, D'Souza SJ, Orlowski J, Grinstein S. Topological analysis of NHE1, the ubiquitous Na^+/H^+ exchanger using chymotryptic cleavage. Am J Physiol 1998; 275:C431–C439.

162. Wakabayashi S, Pang T, Su X, Shigekawa M. A novel topology model of the human Na(+)/H(+) exchanger isoform 1. J Biol Chem Mar 2000; 275: 7942–7949.

163. Wakabayashi S, Shigekawa M, Pouyssegur J. Molecular physiology of vertebrate Na^+/H^+ exchangers. Physiol Rev 1997; 77:51–74.

164. Nath S K, Hang CY, Levine SA, Yun CHC, Montrose MH, Donowitz M, Tse C-M. Hyperosmolarity inhibits the Na/H exchanger isoforms NHE2 and NHE3: an effect opposite to NHE1. Am J Physiol 1996; 270:G431–G441.

165. Wiederkehr MR, Zhao H, Moe OW. Acute regulation of Na/H exchanger NHE-3 by protein kinase C: role of NHE-3 phosphorylation. Am J Physiol 1999; 276:C1205–C1217.

166. Bianchi L, Kapus A, Lukas G, Wasan S, Wakabayashi S, Pouyssegur J, Yu FH, Orlowski J, Grinstein S. Responsiveness of mutants of NHE1 isoform of Na/H antiport to osmotic stress. Am J Physiol 1995; 269:C998–C1007.

167. Wakabayashi S, Fafournoux P, Sardet C, Pouyssegur J. The Na^+/H^+ antiporter cytoplasmic domain mediates growth factor signals and controls "H(+)-sensing." Proc Natl Acad Sci USA 1992; 89:2424–2428.

168. Aronson PS, Nee J, Suhm MA. Modifier role of internal H^+ in activating the Na+-H+ exchanger in renal microvillus membrane vesicles. Nature 1982; 299:161–163.

169. Wakabayashi S, Ikeda T, Iwamoto T, Pouyssegur J, Shigekawa M. Calmodulin-binding autoinhibitory domain controls "pH-sensing" in the Na+/H+ exchanger NHE1 through sequence-specific interaction. Biochemistry 1997; 36:12,854–12,861.

170. Cano A, Baum M, Moe OW. Thyroid hormone stimulates the renal Na/H exchanger NHE-3 by transcriptional activation. Am J Physiol 1999; 276:C102–C108.

171. Taglicht D, Padan E, Schuldiner S. Overproduction and purification of a functional Na+/H+ antiporter coded by nhaA (ant) from *Escherichia coli.* J Biol Chem 1991; 266:11,289–11,294.

172. Gerchman Y, Olami Y, Rimon A, Taglicht D, Schuldiner S, Padan E. Histidine-226 is part of the pH sensor of NhaA, a Na+/H+ antiporter in *Escherichia coli.* Proc Natl Acad Sci USA 1993; 90:1212–1216.

173. Moe OW. Na–H exchange in renal epithelia. Mechanisms of acute regulation by protein kinases. Curr Opin Nephrol Hypertens 1997; 6:440–446.

174. Moe OW. Acute regulation of proximal tubule Na/H exchanger NHE-3: role of NHE-3 phosphorylation, trafficking and regulatory cofactors. J Am Soc Nephrol 1999; 10:2412–2425.

175. Biemesderfer D, DeGray B, Aronson PS. Membrane topology of NHE3. Epitopes within the carboxyl-terminal hydrophilic domain are exoplasmic. J Biol Chem 1998; 273:12,391–12,396.

176. Fan L, Wiederkehr MR, Collazo R, Huang H, Crowder, LA, Moe OW. Dual mechanism of acute regulation of Na/H exchanger NHE-3 by parathyroid hormone in rat kidney. J Biol Chem 1999; 274:11,289–11,295.

177. Kurashima K, D'Souza S, Szaszi K, Ramjeesingh R, Orlowski J, Grinstein S. The apical Na(+)/H(+) exchanger isoform NHE3 is regulated by the actin cytoskeleton. J Biol Chem 1999; 274:29,843–29,849.

178. Collazo R, Fan L, Zhao H, Wiederkehr M, Moe OW. Acute regulation of Na/H exchanger NHE3 by parathyroid hormone via NHE3 phosphorylation and dynamin-dependent endocytosis. J Biol Chem 2000; 276:31,601–31,608.

179. Szaszi K, Kurashima K, Kapus A, Paulsen A, Kaibuchi K, Grinstein S, Orlowski J. RhoA and rho kinase regulate the epithelial Na+/H+ exchanger NHE3. Role of myosin light chain phosphorylation. J Biol Chem 2000; 275:28,599–28,606.

180. Wiederkehr MR, Di Sole F, Fan L, Hu MC, Collazo R, Murer H, Helmle-Kolb C, Moe OW. Characterization of acute regulation of Na/H exchanger NHE-3 by dopamine in opossum kidney cells. Kidney Int 2001; 59:197–209.

181. Hu MC, Fan L, Quiñones H, Crowder LA, Karim-Jimenez Z, Murer H, Moe OW. Dopamine stimulates dynamin-dependent endocytosis of NHE3 via PKA-mediated phosphorylation of NHE3. J Biol Chem 2001; 276:26906–26915.

182. Weinman EJ, Shenolika S, Kahn AM. cAMP-associated inhibition of Na/H exchanger in rabbit kidney. Am J Physiol 1987; 352:F19–F25.

183. Moe OW, Amemiya M, Yamaji Y. Activation of protein kinase A acutely phosphorylates and inhibits Na/H exchanger NHE-3. J Clin Invest 1995; 96:2187–2194.

184. Kurashima K, Yu FH, Cabado AG, Szabo EZ, Grinstein S, Orlowski J. Identification of sites required for down-regulation of Na+/H+ exchanger NHE3 activity by cAMP-dependent protein kinase. phosphorylation-dependent and -independent mechanisms. J Biol Chem 1997; 272:28,672–28,679.

185. Zhao H, Wiederkehr MR, Collazo R, Fan L, Crowder LA, Moe OW. Acute regulation of Na/H exchanger NHE-3 by protein kinase A (PKA): role of protein kinase A and NHE-3 phosphoserines 552 and 605. J Biol Chem 1999; 274:3978–3987.

186. Peng Y, Moe OW, Chu TS, Preisig PA, Yanagisawa M, Alpern RJ. ET_B receptor activation leads to phosphorylation of NHE-3. Am J Physiol 1999; 276:C938–C945.

187. Zizak M, Lamprecht G, Steplock D, Tariq N, Shenolikar S, Donowitz M, Yun CH, Weinman EJ. cAMP-induced phosphorylation inhibition of Na(+)/H(+) exchanger 3 (NHE3) are dependent on the presence but not the phosphorylation of NHE regulatory factor . J Biol Chem 1999; 274:24,753–24,558.

188. Weinman EJ, Steplock D, Donowitz M, Shenolikar S. NHERF associations with sodium–hydrogen exchanger isoform 3 (NHE3) and ezrin are essential

for cAMP-mediated phosphorylation and inhibition of NHE3. Biochemistry 2000; 39:6123–6129.

189. Yun CH, Oh S, Zizak M, Steplock D, Tsao S, Tse CM, Weinman EJ, Donowitz M. cAMP-mediated inhibition of the epithelial brush border Na^+/H^+ exchanger, NHE3, requires an associated regulatory protein. Proc Natl Acad Sci USA 1997; 94:3010–3015.

190. Lamprecht G, Weinman EJ, Yun CHC. The role of NHERF and E3KARP in the cAMP mediated inhibition of NHE-3. J Biol Chem 1998; 273:29,972–29,978.

191. Wade JB, Welling PA, Donowitz M, Shenolikar S, Weinman EJ. Differential renal distribution of NHERF isoforms and their colocalization with NHE3, ezrin, and ROMK. Am J Physiol 2001; 280:C192–C198.

192. Hall RA, Premont RT, Chow CW, Blitzer JT, Pitcher J, Claing A, Stoffel RH, Barak LS, Shenolikar S, Weinman EJ, Grinstein S, Lefkowitz RJ. The b2-adrenergic receptor interacts with the Na/H exchanger regulatory factor to control Na/H exchange. Nature 1998; 392:626–630.

193. Yip JW, Ko WH, Viberti G, Huganir RL, Donowitz M, Tse CM. Regulation of the epithelial brush border Na^+/H^+ exchanger isoform 3 stably expressed in fibroblasts by fibroblast growth factor and phorbol esters is not through changes in phosphorylation of the exchanger. J Biol Chem 1997; 272: 18,473–18,480.

194. Szaszi K, Grinstein S, Orlowski J, Kapus A. Regulation of the epithelial Na(+)/H(+) exchanger isoform by the cytoskeleton. Cell Physiol Biochem 2000; 10:265–272.

195. Demaurex N, Romanek RR, Orlowski J, Grinstein S. ATP dependence of Na^+/H^+ exchange. Nucleotide specificity and assessment of the role of phospholipids. J Gen Physiol 1997; 109:117–128.

196. Aharonovitz O, Zaun HC, Balla T, York JD, Orlowski J, Grinstein S. Intra-cellular pH regulation by Na(+)/H(+) exchange requires phosphatidylinositol 4,5-bisphosphate. J Cell Biol 2000; 150:213–224.

197. Cabado AG, Yu FH, Kapus A, Lukacs G, Grinstein S, Orlowski J. Distinct structural domains confer cAMP sensitivity and ATP dependence to the Na^+/H^+ exchanger NHE3 isoform. J Biol Chem 1996; 271:3509–3590.

198. Huang CL, Feng S, Hilgemann DW. Direct activation of inward rectifier potassium channels by PIP2 and its stabilization by $G\beta$. Nature 1998; 391:803–806.

199. Biemesderfer D, Nagy T, DeGray B, Aronson PS. Specific association of megalin and the Na^+/H^+ exchanger isoform NHE3 in the proximal tubule. J Biol Chem 1999; 274:17,518–17,524.

200. Biemesderfer D, DeGray B, Aronson PS. Active (9.6S) and inactive (21S) oligomers of NHE3 in distinct microdomains of the renal brush border. J Biol Chem. 2001; 276:10161–10167.

201. Hensley CB, Bradley ME, Mircheff AK. Parathyroid hormone-induced translocation of Na/H antiporters in rat proximal tubules. Am J Physiol 1989; 257:C637–C642.

202. Peng Y, Amemiya M, Yang X, Fan L, Moe OW, Yin H, Preisig PA, Yanagisawa M, Alpern RJ. ET(B) receptor activation causes exocytic insertion of NHE3 in OKP cells. Am J Physiol 2001; 280:F34–F42.

203. Yang X, Amemiya M, Peng Y, Moe, OW, Priesig PA, Alpern RJ. Acid incubation causes exocytotic insertion of NHE3 into the apical membrane of OK cells. Am J Physiol 2000; 279:C410–C419.

204. Zhang Y, Mircheff AK, Hensley CB, Makyar CE, Warnock DG, Chambrey R, Yip KP, Marsh DJ, Holstein-Rathlou NH, McDonough AA. Rapid redistribution and inhibition of renal sodium transporters during acute pressure natriuresis. Am J Physiol 1996; 270:F1004–F1014.

205. D'Souza S, Garcia-Cabado A, Yu F, Teter K, Lukacs G, Skorecki K, Moore HP, Orlowski J, Grinstein S. The epithelial sodium–hydrogen antiporter Na+/H+ exchanger 3 accumulates and is functional in recycling endosomes. J Biol Chem 1998; 273:2035–2043.

206. Kurashima K, Szabo EZ, Lukacs G, Orlowski J, Grinstein S. Endosomal recycling of the Na^+/H^+ exchanger NHE3 isoform is regulated by the phosphatidylinositol 3-kinase pathway. J Biol Chem 1998; 273:20,828–20,836.

207. Akhter S, Cavet ME, Tse CM, Donowitz M. C-terminal domains of Na(+)/H(+) exchanger isoform 3 are involved in the basal and serum-stimulated membrane trafficking of the exchanger. Biochemistry 2000; 39:1990–2000.

208. Janecki AJ, Janecki M, Akhter S, Donowitz M. Basic fibroblast growth factor stimulates surface expression and activity of Na^+/H^+ exchanger NHE3 via mechanism involving phosphatidylinositol 3-kinase. J Biol Chem 2000; 275:8133–8142.

209. Chow CW, Woodside M, Demaurex N, Yu FH, Plant P, Rotin D, Grinstein S, Orlowski J. Proline-rich motifs of the Na+/H+ exchanger 2 isoform. Binding of Src homology domain 3 and role in apical targeting in epithelia. J Biol Chem 1999; 74:10,481–10,488.

210. Alpern RJ, Moe OW, Preisig PA. Chronic regulation of the proximal tubular Na/H antiporter: from HCO_3 to SRC. Kidney Int 1995; 48:1386–1396.

211. Paillard M. Na^+/H^+ exchanger subtypes in the renal tubule: function and regulation in physiology and disease. Exp Nephrol 1997; 5:277–284.

212. Ambühl PM, Amemiya M, Danczkay M, Lotscher M, Kaissling B, Moe OW, Preisig PA, Alpern RJ. Chronic metabolic acidosis increases NHE3 protein abundance in rat kidney. Am J Physiol 1996; 271:F917–F925.

213. Laghmani K, Borensztein P, Ambühl P, Froissart M, Bichara M, Moe OW, Alpern RJ, Paillard M. Chronic metabolic acidosis enhances NHE-3 protein abundance and transport activity in the rat thick ascending limb by increasing NHE-3 mRNA. J Clin Invest 1997; 99:24–30.

214. Ambühl PM, Yang X, Peng Y, Preisig PA, Moe OW, Alpern RJ. Glucocorticoids enhance acid activation of the Na+/H+ exchanger 3 (NHE3). J Clin Invest 1999; 103:429–435.

215. Amemiya M, Tabei K, Kusano E, Asano Y, Alpern RJ. Incubation of OKP cells in low-K+ media increases NHE3 activity after early decrease in intracellular pH. Am J Physiol 1999; 276:C711–C716.

216. Ambühl P, Amemiya M, Preisig PA, Moe OW, Alpern RJ. Chronic hyperosmolality increases NHE3 activity in OKP cells. J Clin Invest 1998; 101:170–177.
217. Baum M, Amemiya M, Dwarakanath V, Alpern RJ, Moe OW. Glucocorticoids regulate NHE-3 transcription in OKP cells. Am J Physiol 1996; 270: F164–F169.
218. Lifton RP, Hunt SC, Williams RR, Pouyssegur J, Lalouel JM. Exclusion of the Na^+/H^+ antiporter as a candidate gene in human essential hypertension. Hypertension 1991; 17:8–14.
219. Cox GA, Lutz CM, Yang CL, Biemesderfer D, Bronson RT, Fu A, Aronson PS, Noebels JL, Frankel WN. Sodium/hydrogen exchanger gene defect in slow-wave epilepsy mutant mice. Cell 1997; 91:139–148.
220. Bell SM, Schreiner CM, Schultheis PJ, Miller ML, Evans RL, Vorhees CV, Shull GE, Scott WJ. Targeted disruption of the murine Nhe1 locus induces ataxia, growth retardation, and seizures. Am J Physiol 1999; 276:C788–C795.
221. Evans RL, Bell SM, Schultheis PJ, Shull GE, Melvin JE. Targeted disruption of the Nhe1 gene prevents muscarinic agonist-induced up-regulation of Na(+)/H(+) exchange in mouse parotid acinar cells. J Biol Chem 1999; 274:29,025–29,030.
222. Schultheis PJ, Clarke LL, Meneton P, Harline M, Boivin GP, Stemmermann G, Duffy JJ, Doetschman T, Miller ML, Shull GE. Targeted disruption of the murine Na^+/H^+ exchanger isoform 2 gene causes reduced viability of gastric parietal cells and loss of net acid secretion. J Clin Invest 1998; 101:1243–1253.
223. Schultheis PJ, Clarke LL, Meneton P, Miller ML, Soleimani M, Gawenis LR, Riddle TM, Duffy JJ, Doetschman T, Wang T, Giebisch G, Aronson PS, Lorenz JN, Shull GE. Renal and intestinal absorptive defects in mice lacking the NHE3 Na^+/H^+ exchanger. Nat Genet 1998; 19:282–285.
224. Lorenz JN, Schultheis PJ, Traynor T, Shull GE, Schnermann J. Micropuncture analysis of single-nephron function in NHE3-deficient mice. Am J Physiol 1999; 277:F447–F453.
225. Wang T, Yang CL, Abbiati T, Schultheis PJ, Shull GE, Giebisch G, Aronson PS. Mechanism of proximal tubule bicarbonate absorption in NHE3 null mice. Am J Physiol 1999; 277:F298–F302.
226. Brooks HL, Sorensen AM, Terris J, Schultheis PJ, Lorenz JN, Shull GE, Knepper MA. Profiling of renal tubule Na^+ transporter abundances in NHE3 and NCC null mice using targeted proteomics. J Physiol 2001; 530:359–366.
227. Restrepo D, Kozody DJ, Spinelli LJ, Knauf PA. pH homeostasis in promyelocytic leukemic HL60 cells. J Gen Physiol 1988 1988; 92:489–507.
228. Jennings ML. Structure and function of the red blood cell anion transport system. Annu Rev Biophys Biochem Chem 1989; 18:397–430.
229. Ganz MB, Boyarsky G, Sterzel RB, Boron WF. Arginine vasopressin enhances pHi regulation in the presence of HCO3– by stimulating three acid-base transport systems. Nature 1989; 337:648–651.
230. Vaughn-Jones RD. Anion exchange in sheep Purkinje fibres. J Physiol 1986; 379:377–406.

231. Sun A, Hebert SC. Rapid hypertonic cell volume regulation in the perfused inner medullary collecting duct. Kidney Int 1989; 36(5):831–842.
232. Kopito RR. Molecular biology of the anion exchanger gene family. Int Rev Cytol 1990; 123:177–199.
233. Stone DK, Seldin DW, Kokko JP, Jacobson HR. Anion dependence of rabbit medullary collecting duct acidification. J Clin Invest 1983; 71:1505–1508.
234. Schwartz GJ, Satlin LM, Bergmann JE. Fluorescent characterization of collecting duct cells: a second H+-secreting type. Am J Physiol 1988; 255:F1003–F1014.
235. Star RA, Burg MB, Knepper MA. Bicarbonate secretion and chloride absorption by rabbit cortical collecting ducts. Role of chloride/bicarbonate exchange. J Clin Invest 1985; 76:1123–1130.
236. Drenckhahn D, Schluter K, Allen DP, Bennett V. Colocalization of band 3 with ankyrin and spectrin at the basal membrane of intercalated cells in the rat kidney. Science 1985; 230:1287–1289.
237. Schuster VL, Bonsib SM, Jennings ML. Two types of collecting duct mitochondrial-rich cells: lectin and band 3 cytochemistry. Am J Physiol 1986; 251:C347–C355.
238. Wagner S, Vogel R, Lietzke R, Koob R, Drenckkahn D. Immunochemical characterization of a band-3 like anion exchanger in collecting duct of human kidney. Am J Physiol 1987; 253:F213–F221.
239. Verlander JW, Madsen KM, Low PS, Allen DP, Tisher CC. Immunocytochemical localization of band 3 protein in the rat collecting duct. Am J Physiol 1988; 255:F115–F125.
240. Fejes-Toth G, Chen WR, Rusvai E, Moser T, Naray-Nejes-Toth A. Differential expression of AE1 in renal HCO_3^B-secreting and reabsorbing intercalated cells. J Biol Chem 1994; 269:26,717–26,721.
241. Brosius FC III, Nguyen K, Stuart-Tilley AK, Haller C, Briggs JP, Alper SL. Regional and segmental localization of AE2 anion exchanger mRNA and protein in rat kidney. Am J Physiol 1995; 269:F461–F468.
242. Alper SL, Stuart-Tilley AK, Biemesderfer D, Shmukler BE, Brown D. Immunolocalization of AE2 anion exchanger in rat kidney. Am J Physiol 1997; 273:F601–F614.
243. Stuart-Tilley AK, Shmukler BE, Brown D, Alper SL. Immunolocalization and tissue-specific splicing of AE2 anion exchanger in mouse kidney. J Am Soc Nephrol 1998; 9:946–959.
244. Lee BS, Gunn RB, Kopito RR. Functional differences among nonerythroid anion exchangers expressed in a transfected human cell line. J Biol Chem 1991; 266:11,448–11,454.
245. Jiang L, Stuart-Tilley A, Parkash J, Alper SL. pHi serum regulate AE2-mediated $Cl^-/HCO3^-$ exchange in CHOP cells of defined transient transfection status. Am J Physiol 1994; 267:C845–C856.
246. Humphreys BD, Chernova MN, Jiang L, Zhang Y, Alper SL. NH4Cl activates AE2 anion exchanger in *Xenopus* oocytes at acidic pHi. Am J Physiol 1997; 272:C1232–C1240.

247. Humphreys BD, Jiang L, Chernova MN, Alper SL. Hypertonic activation of AE2 anion exchanger in *Xenopus* oocytes via NHE-mediated intracellular alkalinization. Am J Physiol 1995; 268:C201–C209.

248. Wang DN. Band 3 protein: structure, flexibility, and function. FEBS Lett 1994; 346:26–31.

249. Hamasaki N, Okubo K. Band 3 protein: physiology, function and structure. Mol Cell Biol 1996; 42:1025–1039.

250. Tanner MJA. The structure and function of Band 3(AE1): recent developments. Mol Membr Biol 1997; 14:155–165.

251. Casey JR, Reithmeier RAF. Anion exchangers in the red cell and beyond. Biochem Cell Biol 1998; 76:709–713.

252. Kollert-Jons A, Wagner S, Hubner S, Appelhans H, Drenckhahn D. Anion exchanger 1 in human kidney and oncocytoma differs from erythroid AE1 in its NH2 terminus. Am J Physiol 1993; 265:F813–F821.

253. Schofield AE, Martin PG, Spillett D, Tanner MJ. The structure of the human red blood cell anion exchanger (EPB3, AE1, band 3) gene. Blood 1994; 84:2000–2012.

254. Ding Y, Kobayashi S, Kopito R. Mapping of ankyrin binding determinants on the erythroid anion exchanger, AE1. J Biol Chem 1996; 271:22,494–22,498.

255. Jennings ML, Smith JS. Anion–proton cotransport through the human red blood cell band 3 protein. Role of glutamate 681. J Biol Chem 1992; 267:13,964–13,971.

256. Tang XB, Fujinaga J, Kopito R, Casey JR. Topology of the region surrounding Glu681 of human AE1 protein, the erythrocyte anion exchanger. J Biol Chem 1998; 273:22,545–22,553.

257. Popov M, Li J, Reithmeier RA. Transmembrane folding of the human erythrocyte anion exchanger (AE1, Band 3) determined scanning and insertional Bglycosylation mutagenesis. Biochem J 1999; 339:269–279.

258. Blackman SM, Piston DW, Beth AH. Oligomeric state of human erythrocyte band 3 measured by fluorescence resonance energy homotransfer. Biophys J 1998; 75:1117–1130.

259. Zolotarev AS, Shmukler BE, Alper SL. AE2 anion exchanger polypeptide is a homooligomer in pig gastric membranes: a chemical cross-linking study. Biochemistry 1999; 38:8521–8531.

260. Dolder M, Walz T, Hefti A, Engel A. Human erythrocyte band 3. Solubilization and reconstitution into two-dimensional crystals. J Mol Biol 1993; 231:119–132.

261. Wang DN, Sarabia VE, Reithmeier RA, Kuhlbrandt W. Three-dimensional map of the dimeric membrane domain of the human erythrocyte anion exchanger, Band 3. EMBO J 1994; 13:3230–3235.

262. Wang DN, Kuhlbrandt W, Sarabia VE, Reithmeier RA. Two-dimensional structure of the membrane domain of human band 3, the anion transport protein of the erythrocyte membrane. EMBO J 1993; 12:2233–2339.

263. Salhany JM, Sloan RL, Cordes KA, Schopfer LM. Kinetic evidence for ternary complex formation and allosteric interactions in chloride and stilbene-disulfonate binding to band 3. Biochemistry 1994; 33:11,909–11,916.

264. Salhany JM. Allosteric effects in stilbene disulphonate binding to band 3 protein (AE1). Mol Cell Biol 1996; 42:1065–1096.

265. Zhang Y, Chernova MN, Stuart-Tilley AK, Jiang L, Alper SL. The cytoplasmic and transmembrane domains of AE2 both contribute to regulation of anion exchange by pH. J Biol Chem 1996; 271:5741–5749.

266. Sekler I, Lo RS, Kopito RR. A conserved glutamate is responsible for ion selectivity and pH dependence of the mammalian anion exchangers AE1 and AE2. J Biol Chem 1995; 270:28,751–28,758.

267. Wall SM. NH_4^+ augments net acid secretion by a ouabain-sensitive mechanism in isolated perfused inner medullary collecting ducts. Am J Physiol 1996; 270:F432–F439.

268. Huber S, Asan E, Jons T, Kerscher C, Puschel B, Drenckhahn D. Expression of rat kidney anion exchanger 1 in type A intercalated cells in metabolic acidosis and alkalosis. Am J Physiol 1999; 277:F841–F849.

269. Da Silva JC Jr, Perrone RD, Johns CA, Madias NE. Rat kidney band 3 mRNA modulation in chronic respiratory acidosis. Am J Physiol 1991; 260:F204–F209.

270. Schuster V. Function and regulation of collecting duct intercalated cells. Annu Rev Physiol 1993; 55:267–288.

271. Fejes-Toth G, Rusvai E, Cleaveland ES, Naray-Fejes-Toth A. Regulation of AE2 mRNA expression in the cortical collecting duct by acid/base balance. Am J Physiol 1998; 274:F596–F601.

272. Hanspal M, Palek J. Biogenesis and normal and abnormal red cell membrane skeletons. Semin Hematol 1992; 29:305–325.

273. Delauney. Genetic disorders of red cell membranes. FEBS Lett 1995; 369:34–37.

274. Inaba M, Yawata A, Koshino I, Sato K, Takeuchi M, Takakuwa Y, Manno S, Yawata Y, Kanzaki A, Sakai J, Ban A, Ono K, Maede Y. Defective anion transport and marked spherocytosis with membrane instability caused by hereditary total deficiency of red cell band 3 in cattle due to a nonsense mutation. J Clin Invest 1996; 97:1804–1817.

275. Peters LL, Shivdasani RA, Liu SC, Hanspal M, John KM, Gonzalez JM, Brugnara C, Gwynn B, Mohandas N, Alper SL, Orkin SH, Lux SE. Anion exchanger 1 (band 3) is required to prevent erythrocyte membrane surface loss but not to form the membrane skeleton. Cell 1996; 86:917–927.

276. Bruce LJ, Cope DL, Jones GK, Schofield AE, Burley M, Povey S, Unwin RJ, Wrong O, Tanner MJ. Familial distal renal tubular acidosis is associated with mutations in the red cell anion exchanger (Band 3, AE1) gene. J Clin Invest 1997; 100:1693–1707.

277. Karet FE, Gainza FJ, Gyory AZ, Unwin RJ, Wrong O, Tanner MJ, Nayir A, Alpay H, Santos F, Hulton SA, Bakkaloglu A, Ozen S, Cunningham MJ, di Pietro A, Walker WG, Lifton RP. Mutations in the chloride-bicarbonate exchanger gene AE1 cause autosomal dominant but not autosomal recessive distal renal tubular acidosis. Proc Natl Acad Sci USA 1998; 95:6337–6342.

278. Jarolim P, Shayakul C, Prabakaran D, Jiang L, Stuart-Tilley A, Rubin HL, Simova S, Zavadil J, Herrin JT, Brouillette J, Somers MJ, Seemanova E, Brugnara C, Guay-Woodford LM, Alper SL. Autosomal dominant distal renal tubular acidosis is associated in three families with heterozygosity for

the R589H mutation in the AE1 (band 3) Cl^-/HCO_3^- exchanger. J Biol Chem 1998; 273:6380–6388.

279. Weber S, Soergel M, Jeck N, Konrad M. Atypical distal renal tubular acidosis confirmed by mutation analysis. Pediatr Nephrol 2000; 15:201–204.

280. DuBose TD. Autosomal dominant distal renal tubular acidosis and the AE1 gene. Am J Kidney Dis 1999; 33:1190–1197.

281. Tanphaichitr VS, Sumboonnanonda A, Ideguchi H, Shayakul C, Brugnara C, Takao M, Veerakul G, Alper SL. Novel AE1 mutations in recessive distal renal tubular acidosis. Loss-of-function is rescued by glycophorin A. J Clin Invest 1998; 102:2173–2179.

282. Bruce LJ, Tanner MJ. Structure-function relationships of band 3 variants. Cell Mol Biol 1996; 42:953–973.

283. Genton B, Al-Yaman F, Mgone CS, Alexander N, Paniu MM, Alpers MP, Mokela D. Ovalocytosis and cerebral malaria. Nature 1995; 378:564–565.

284. Liu SC, Jarolim P, Rubin HL, Palek J, Amato D, Hassan K, Zaik M, Sapak P. The homozygous state for the band 3 protein mutation in Southeast Asian ovalocytosis may be lethal. Blood 1994; 84:3590–3591.

285. Sarabia VE, Casey JR, Reithmeier RA. Molecular characterization of the band 3 protein from Southeast Asian ovalocytes. J Biol Chem 1993; 268:10,676–10,680.

286. Liu SC, Palek J, Yi SJ, Nichols PE, Derick LH, Chiou SS, Amato D, Corbett JD, Cho MR, Golan DE. Molecular basis of altered red blood cell membrane properties in Southeast Asian ovalocytosis: role of the mutant band 3 protein in band 3 oligomerization and retention by the membrane skeleton. Blood 1995; 86:349–358.

287. Kaitwatcharachai C, Vasuvattakul S, Yenchitsomanus PT, Thuwajit P, Malasit P, Chuawatana D, Mingkum S, Halperin ML, Wilairat P, Nimmannit S. Distal renal tubular acidosis and high urine carbon dioxide tension in a patient with southeast Asian ovalocytosis. Am J Kidney Dis 1999; 33:1147–1152.

288. Vasuvattakul S, Yenchitsomanus PT, Vachuanichsanong P, Thuwajit P, Kaitwatcharachai C, Laosombat V, Malasit P, Wilairat P, Nimmannit S. Autosomal recessive distal renal tubular acidosis associated with Southeast Asian ovalocytosis. Kidney Int 1999; 56:1674–1682.

289. Bruce LJ, Wrong O, Toye AM, Young MT, Ogle G, Ismail Z, Sinha AK, McMaster P, Hwaihwanje I, Nash GB, Hart S, Lavu E, Palmer R, Othman A, Unwin RJ, Tanner MJ. Band 3 mutations, renal tubular acidosis and south-east Asian ovalocytosis in Malaysia and Papua New Guinea: loss of up to 95% band 3 transport in red cells. Biochem J 2000; 15:41–51.

290. Hassoun H, Palek J. Hereditary spherocytosis: a review of the clinical and molecular aspects of the disease. Blood Rev 1996; 10:129–147.

291. Rysava R, Tesar V, Jirsa M, Brabec V, Jarolim P. Incomplete distal renal tubular acidosis coinherited with a mutation in the band 3 (AE1) gene. Nephrol Dial Transplant 1997; 12:1869–1867.

292. Boron WF, Boulpaep EL. Intracellular pH regulation in the renal proximal tubule of the salamander. Basolateral HCO_3^- transport. J Gen Physiol 1983; 81:53–94.

293. Deitmer JW, Schlue WR. The regulation of intracellular pH by identified glial cells and neurones in the central nervous system of the leech. J Physiol 1987; 388:261–283.

294. Dart C, Vaughan-Jones RD. Na(+)–HCO3–symport in the sheep cardiac Purkinje fibre. J Physiol 1992; 451:365–385.

295. Russell JM, Boron WF. Role of chloride transport in regulation of intracellular pH. Nature 1976; 264:73–74.

296. Hogan EM, Cohen MA, Boron WF. K(+)- and HCO3(−)-dependent acid-base transport in squid giant axons. J Gen Physiol 1995; 106:821–862.

297. Romero MF, Boron WF. Electrogenic Na^+/HCO_3^- cotransporters: cloning and physiology. Annu Rev Physiol 1999; 61:699–723.

298. Romero MF, Henry D, Nelson S, Harte PJ, Dillon AK, Sciortino. Cloning and characterization of a Na^+-driven anion exchanger (NDAE1): a new transporter. J Biol Chem 2000; 275:24,552–24,559.

299. Wang CZ, Yano H, Nagashima K, Seino S. The Na^+-driven Cl^-/HCO_3^- exchanger. Cloning, tissue distribution, and functional characterization. J Biol Chem 2000; 275:35,486–35,490.

300. Alpern RJ. Mechanism of basolateral membrane $H^+/OH^-/HCO_3^-$ transport in the rat proximal convoluted tubule. A sodium-coupled electrogenic process. J Gen Physiol 1985; 86:613–636.

301. Akiba T, Alpern RJ, Eveloff J, Calamina J, Warnock DG. Electrogenic sodium/bicarbonate cotransport in rabbit renal cortical basolateral membrane vesicles. J Clin Invest 1986; 78:1472–1478.

302. Soleimani M, Grassi SM, Aronson PS. Stoichiometry of $Na^+–HCO_3^-$ cotransport in basolateral membrane vesicles isolated from rabbit renal cortex. J Clin Invest 1987; 79:1276–1280.

303. Soleimani M, Aronson PS. Ionic mechanism of $Na^+–HCO_3^-$ cotransport in rabbit renal basolateral membrane vesicles. J Biol Chem 1989; 264: 18,302–18,308.

304. Schmitt BM, Biemesderfer D, Romero MF, Boulpaep EL, Boron WF. Immunolocalization of the electrogenic $Na^+–HCO_3^-$ cotransporter in mammalian and amphibian kidney. Am J Physiol 1999; 276:F27–F38.

305. Pushkin A, Yip KP, Clark I, Abuladze N, Kwon TH, Tsuruoka S, Schwartz GJ, Nielsen S, Kurtz I. NBC3 expression in rabbit collecting duct: colocalization with vacuolar H^+-ATPase. Am J Physiol 1999; 277:F974–F981.

306. Kwon TH, Pushkin A, Abuladze N, Nielsen S, Kurtz I. Immunoelectron microscopic localization of NBC3 sodium-bicarbonate cotransporter in rat kidney. Am J Physiol 2000; 278:F327–F336.

307. Vorum H, Kwon TH, Fulton C, Simonsen B, Choi I, Boron W, Maunsbach AB, Nielsen S, Aalkjaer C. Immunolocalization of electroneutral Na–HCO(3)(−) cotransporter in rat kidney. Am J Physiol 2000; 279:F901–F909.

308. Gross EZ, Abuladze N, Pushkin A, Kurtz I, Cotton CU. The stoichiometry of the sodium bicarbonate cotransporter is mouse pancreatic cells is $2HCO_3^-:1Na^+$ [abstr]. J Am Soc Nephrol 2000; 11:4A.

309. Gross EZ, Abuladze N, Pushkin A, Hopfer U, Kurtz I. The $HCO_3^-:Na^+$ stoichiometry of pNBC1is organ specfic [abstr]. J Am Soc Nephrol 2000; 11:5A.

310. Sciortino CM, Romero MF. Cation and voltage dependence of rat kidney electrogenic Na^+-HCO_3^- cotransporter, rkNBC, expressed in oocytes. Am J Physiol 1999; 277:F611–F623.

311. Grichtchenko II, Romero MF, Boron WF. Extracellular HCO (3) (−) dependence of electrogenic Na/HCO(3) cotransporters cloned from salamander and rat kidney. J Gen Physiol 2000; 115:533–546.

312. Soleimani M, Lesoine GA, Bergman JA, Aronson PS. Cation specificity and modes of the Na^+:CO_3^{2-}:HCO_3^- cotransport in renal basolateral membrane vesicles. J Biol Chem 1991; 266:8706–8710.

313. Akiba T, Rocco VK, Warnock DG. Parallel adaptation of the rabbit renal cortical sodium/proton antiporter and sodium/bicarbonate cotransporter in metabolic acidosis and alkalosis. J Clin Invest 1987; 80:308–315.

314. Preisig PA, Alpern RJ. Chronic metabolic acidosis causes an adaptation in the apical membrane Na/H antiporter and basolateral membrane $Na(HCO_3)_3$ symporter in the rat proximal convoluted tubule. J Clin Invest 1988; 82:1445–1453.

315. Soleimani M, Bizal GL, McKinney TD, Hattabaugh YJ. Effect of in vitro metabolic acidosis on luminal Na^+/H^+ exchange and basolateral Na^+:HCO_3^- cotransport in rabbit kidney proximal tubules. J Clin Invest 1992; 90:211–218.

316. Amlal H, Wang Z, Soleimani M. Functional upregulation of H+-ATPase by lethal acid stress in cultured inner medullary collecting duct cells. Am J Physiol 1997; 273:C1194–C1205.

317. Soleimani M, Bergman JA, Hosford MA, McKinney TD. Potassium depletion increases luminal Na^+/H^+ exchange and basolateral Na^+:CO_3^{2-}:HCO_3^- cotransport in rat renal cortex. J Clin Invest 1990; 86:1076–1083.

318. Amlal H, Habo K, Soleimani M. Potassium deprivation upregulates expression of renal basolateral Na(+)–HCO(3)(−) cotransporter (NBC-1). Am J Physiol 2000; 279:F532–F543.

319. Ali R, Amlal H, Burnham CE, Soleimani M. Glucocorticoids enhance the expression of the basolateral Na+:HCO3− cotransporter in renal proximal tubules. Kidney Int 2000; 57:1063–1071.

320. Brenes LG, Brenes JM, Hernandez MM. Familial proximal tubular acidosis: a distinct disease entity. Am J Med 1977; 63:244–252.

321. Winsnes RW, Monn E, Stokke O, Feyling T. Congenital persistent proximal type renal tubular acidosis in two brothers. Acta Pediatr Scand 1979; 68: 861–868.

322. Braverman DE, Snyder WE. A case report and review of band keratopathy. Metab Pediatr Syst Ophthalmol 1987; 10:39–41.

323. Igarashi T, Ishii T, Watanabe K, Hayakawa H, Horio K, Sone Y, Ohga K. Persistent isolated proximal renal tubular acidosis—a systemic disease with a distinct clinical entity. Pediatr Nephrol 1994; 8:70–71.

324. Igarashi T, Inatomi J, Sekine T, Cha SH, Kanai Y, Kunimi M, Tsukamoto K, Satoh H, Shimadzu M, Tozawa F, Mori T, Shiobara M, Seki G, Endou H. Mutations in SLC4A4 cause permanent isolated proximal renal tubular acidosis with ocular abnormalities. Nat Genet 1999; 23:264–266.

325. Igarashi T, Inatomi J, Sekine T, Takeshima Y, Yoshikaa N, Endou H. A nonsense mutation in the Na/HCO_3 cotransporter gene (SLC4a4) in a patient with permanent isolated proximal renal tubular acidosis and bilateral glaucoma [abstr]. J Am Soc Nephrol 2000; 11:106A.

326. Halperin ML, Kamel KS, Ethier JH, Magner PO. What is the underlying defect in patients with isolated, proximal renal tubular acidosis? Am J Nephrol 1989; 9:265–268.

327. Thompson JA, Miles BS, Fennessey PV. Urinary values quantified by age groups in a healthy pediatric population. Clin Chem 1977; 23:1734–1738.

328. Hamm LL, Simon EE. Roles and mechanisms of urinary buffer excretion. Am J Physiol 1987; 22:F595–F605.

329. Urine, volume, and physio chemical data. In: Lenter C, ed. Geigy Scientific Tables. Bassel, Switzerland: Ciba-Geigy, 1981:53–95.

330. Lide DR, ed. CRC Handbook of Chemistry and Physics. Boca Raton, Ann Arbor: CRC Press, 1991.

331. Van Aubel RA, Masereeuw R, Russel FG. Molecular pharmacology of renal organic anion transporters. Am J Physiol 2000; 279:F216–F232.

332. Markovich D. Physiological roles and regulation of mammalian sulfate transporters. Physiol Rev 2001; 81:1499–1533.

333. Simpson DP. Citrate excretion: a window to renal metabolism. Am J Physiol 1983; 244:F223–F234.

334. Melnick JZ, Preisig PA, Moe OW, Srere P, Alpern RJ. Renal cortical mitochondrial aconitase is regulated in hypo- and hypercitraturia. Kidney Int 1998; 54:160–165.

335. Melnick JZ, Srere PA, Elshourbagy NA, Moe OW, Preisig PA, Alpern RJ. Adenosine triphosphate citrate lyase mediates hypocitraturia in rats. J Clin Invest 1996; 98:2381–2387.

336. Jenkins AD, Dousa TP, Smith LH. Transport of citrate across brush border membrane: effect of dietary acid and alkali loading. Am J Physiol 1985; 249:F590–F595.

337. Aruga S, Wehrli S, Kaissling B, Moe OW, Preisig PA, Pajor AM, Alpern RJ. Chronic metabolic acidosis increases NaDC-1 mRNA and protein abundance in rat kidney. Kidney Int 2000; 58:206–215.

338. Pajor AM. Sequence and functional characterization of a renal sodium/dicarboxylate cotransporter. J Biol Chem 1995; 270:5779–5785.

339. Pajor AM. Molecular cloning and functional expression of a sodium-dicarboxylate cotransporter from human kidney. Am J Physiol 1996; 270:F642–F658.

340. Sekine T, Cha SH, Hosoyamada M, Kanai Y, Watanabe N, Furuta Y, Fukuda K, Igarashi T, Endou H. Cloning, functional characterization, and localization of a rat renal Na^+-dicarboxylate transporter. Am J Physiol 1998; 275:F298–F305.

341. Chen XZ, Shayakul C, Berger UV, Tian W, Hediger MA. Characterization of a rat Na^+-dicarboxylate cotransporter. J Biol Chem 1998; 273:20, 972–20,981.

342. Bai L, Pajor AM. Expression cloning of NaDC-2, an intestinal Na(+)- or Li(+)-dependent dicarboxylate transporter. Am J Physiol 1997; 273:G267–G274.

343. Kekuda R, Wang H, Huang W, Pajor AM, Leibach FH, Devoe LD, Prasad PD, Ganapathy V. Primary structure and functional characteristics of a mammalian sodium-coupled high affinity dicarboxylate transporter. J Biol Chem 1999; 274:3422–3429.

344. Jorgensen KE, Kragh-Hansen U, Roigaard-Petersen H, Iqbal Sheikh M. Citrate uptake by basolateral and luminal membrane vesicles from rabbit kidney cortex. Am J Physiol 1983; 244:F686–F695.

345. Burckhardt G. Sodium-dependent dicarboxylate transport in rat renal basolateral membrane vesicles. Pflugers Arch 1984; 401:254–261.

346. Wright SH, Wunz TM. Succinate and citrate transport in renal basolateral and brush-border membranes. Am J Physiol 1987; 253:F432–F439.

347. Brennan S, Hering-Smith K, Hamm LL. Effect of pH on citrate reabsorption in the proximal tubule. Am J Physiol 1988; 255:F301–F306.

348. Barac-Nieto M. Effects of pH, calcium, and succinate on sodium citrate cotransport in renal microvilli. Am J Physiol 1984; 247:F282–F290.

349. Pajor AM, Sun N. Functional differences between rabbit and human Na(+) -dicarboxylate cotransporters, NaDC-1 and hNaDC-1. Am J Physiol 1996; 271:F1093–F1099.

350. Pajor AM, Valmonte HG. Expression of the renal Na^+/dicarboxylate cotransporter, NaDC-1, in COS-7 cells. Pflugers Arch 1996; 431:645–651.

351. Pajor AM. Sodium-coupled transporters for Krebs cycle intermediates. Annu Rev Physiol 1999; 61:663–683.

352. Grassl SM, Heinz E, Kinne R. Effect of K and H on sodium/citrate cotransport in renal brush border vesicles. Biochem Biophy Acta 1983; 736:178–188.

353. Levi M, McDonald LA, Preisig PA, Alpern RJ. Chronic K depletion stimulates rat renal brush-border membrane Na-citrate cotransporter. Am J Physiol 1991; 261:F767–F773.

354. Werner A, Moore ML, Mantei N, Biber J, Semenza G, Murer H. Cloning and expression of cDNA for a Na/Pi cotransport system of kidney cortex. Proc Natl Acad Sci USA 1991; 88:9608–9612.

355. Miyamoto K, Tatsumi S, Sonoda T, Yamamoto H, Minami H, Taketani Y, Takeda E. Cloning and functional expression of a Na-dependent phosphate transporter from human kidney. Biochem J 1995; 305:81–85.

356. Broer S, Schuster A, Wagner CA, Broer A, Forster I, Biber J, Murer H, Werner A, Lang F, Busch AE. Chloride conductance and Pi transport are separate functions induced by the expression of NaPi-1 in *Xenopus* oocytes. J Membr Biol 1998; 164:71–77.

357. Murer H, Hernando N, Forster I, Biber J. Proximal tubular phosphate reabsorption: molecular mechanism. Physiol Rev 2000; 80:1373–1409.

358. De la Horra C, Hernando N, Lambert G, Forster I, Biber J, Murer H. Molecular determinants of pH sensitivity of the type IIa Na-Pi cotransporter. J Biol Chem 2000; 275:6284–6287.

359. Forster IC, Biber J, Murer H. Proton-sensitive transitions of renal type II Na-coupled phosphate cotransporter kinetics. Biophys J 2000; 79:215–230.

360. Cheng L, Sacktor B. Sodium gradient-dependent phosphate transport in renal brush border membrane vesicles. J Biol Chem 1981; 256:1556–1564.

361. Bindels RJM, van den Broek LAM, van Os CH. Effect of pH on the kinetics of Na-dependent phosphate transport in rat renal brush border membranes. Biochem Biophys Acta 1987; 897:83–92.
362. Forster I, Hernando N, Biber J, Murer H. The voltage dependence of a cloned mammalian renal type II Na+/Pi cotransporter (NaPi-2). J Gen Physiol 1998; 112:1–18.
363. Ambhhl PM, Zajicek HK, Wang H, Puttaparthi K, Levi M. Regulation of renal phosphate transport by acute and chronic metabolic acidosis in the rat. Kidney Int 1998; 53:1288–1298.
364. Custer M, Lotscher M, Biber J, Murer H, Kaissling B. Expression of Na-P(i) cotransport in rat kidney: localization by RT-PCR and immunohistochemistry. Am J Physiol 1994; 266:F767–F774.

6

Regulation of Acid–Base Balance: Overview

F. John Gennari

University of Vermont College of Medicine, Burlington, Vermont, U.S.A.

INTRODUCTION

The pH of the extracellular fluid is maintained within narrow limits by a complex and incompletely understood control system. Arterial blood pH is stabilized between 7.39 and 7.41 indirectly through control of bicarbonate concentration ($[HCO_3^-]$) and carbon dioxide tension ($PaCO_2$). The prevailing $PaCO_2$ is itself in turn regulated by a tightly linked feedback system to pH through control of ventilation (see Chapter 3). The present chapter focuses on the regulation and maintenance of $[HCO_3^-]$, where the control systems are less well defined.

Bicarbonate ions are consumed and generated continuously by metabolic processes and buffer reactions, and these events are reflected by changes in serum $[HCO_3^-]$ (Fig. 1). Regardless of whether consumption or generation prevails, serum $[HCO_3^-]$ is maintained at a constant level over time by homeostatic adjustments in H^+ secretion along the renal tubules. Secretion of H^+ by the epithelial cells lining the renal tubules accomplishes both the reabsorption of filtered HCO_3^- and the generation of new HCO_3^- (see Chapters 4 and 5). A wide variety of factors have been shown to influence these renal transporters, but our understanding of the signals and effectors in the kidney that lead to the renal maintenance of normal acid–base

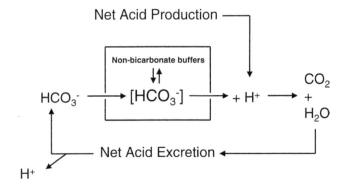

Steady state: Net acid excretion = Net acid production

Figure 1   Normal H^+ balance. Endogenous acid production produces new H^+, which acutely consumes HCO_3^- (and other buffers, see Fig. 2). In the steady state, net acid production is balanced by net acid excretion, leading to the excretion of an equivalent amount of H^+ (as NH_4^+ and titratable acid) and resulting in regeneration of body buffers, thereby stabilizing extracellular fluid $[HCO_3^-]$ (shown in the central box).

equilibrium remains incomplete (1). In the ensuing discussion, those factors likely to play a role in normal $[H^+]$ homeostasis are emphasized.

BODY BUFFERS

All organic and inorganic acids with a $pK < 5.0$ produced by metabolic activity or added to the body fluids are essentially completely dissociated at the pH of the body fluids. The free H^+ produced is bound immediately by a wide variety of buffers in the intracellular and extracellular compartments, minimizing changes in body pH (Fig. 2). Approximately 40–50% of newly formed or added H^+ is buffered by HCO_3^- in the extracellular compartment, and the remainder is buffered by intracellular HCO_3^- and by nonbicarbonate buffers (2,3). Bicarbonate is consumed in buffering H^+ by the following reaction:

$$H^+ + HCO_3^- \rightarrow H_2CO_3 \rightarrow H_2O + CO_2 \qquad (1)$$

The CO_2 produced by this reaction is rapidly excreted by the lungs together with the vastly greater quantity produced by cell metabolism. The major nonbicarbonate buffer in the blood is hemoglobin, which contributes about 10% of the whole body buffering (3). Other extracellular buffers, plasma proteins, and extracellular inorganic phosphates, contribute less than 1% (3). Intracellular proteins, organic and inorganic phosphates,

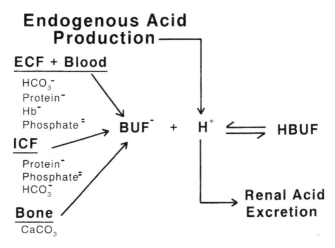

Figure 2 Sources of buffers for reaction with H^+ added to the body fluids. *Source*: From Ref. 1.

and the small amount of HCO_3^- that resides in cells buffer the remainder. All nonbicarbonate buffers (e.g., hemoglobin, phosphate) bind reversibly with H^+ in a pH-dependent manner, effectively removing this ion from solution, and are restored to their original state when back-titrated by H^+ removal (equivalent to HCO_3^- addition, see below). Balance is achieved when the H^+ produced is equivalent to the new HCO_3^- added (or H^+ removed), a process that restores pH and alkali stores to their baseline levels (Fig. 1).

Bicarbonate "Space of Distribution"

The amount of HCO_3^- needed to titrate body buffers back to their pretreatment level can be assessed by measuring the increase in serum $[HCO_3^-]$ that occurs after administering an intravenous HCO_3^- load. The increase in this setting reflects not only the addition of HCO_3^- to the body but also the consumption of administered HCO_3^- by titration of nonbicarbonate buffers, both within cells and in the extracellular fluid (ECF) compartment. The resultant change (Δ) in $[HCO_3^-]$ is traditionally expressed as a "space of distribution" in L:

$$HCO_3^- \text{ space (L)} = (\text{mEq alkali given})/\Delta[HCO_3^-] \qquad (2)$$

When ECF $[HCO_3^-]$ is in the normal range prior to HCO_3^- administration, the HCO_3^- space is approximately twice as large as the ECF compartment, reflecting the fact that approximately half combines with intracellular buffers. The volume of this space, however, varies as a function of

ECF [HCO_3^-] and the time after challenge (2). At a normal initial ECF [HCO_3^-], the space of distribution is twice the ECF volume when assessed at 30 min, but it rises to three times the ECF volume after 90 min (2). This increase reflects further consumption of administered HCO_3^- by H^+ released from newly recruited buffers and newly produced organic acids (see later).

The space also increases when ECF [HCO_3^-] is low, rising to over 80% of body weight when [HCO_3^-] is 5 mEq/L prior to alkali administration. The increase is unrelated to pH and depends solely on the initial ECF [HCO_3^-], as it is due to the greater titration of nonbicarbonate buffers by added alkali when [HCO_3^-] is low (2). The relationship between the space of distribution and initial ECF [HCO_3^-] 30 min after alkali administration is:

$$HCO_3^- \text{ space (\% of body weight)} = (244/\text{serum }[HCO_3^-]) + 36 \qquad (3)$$

These observations in dogs, on which the above equation is based, are supported by measurements in patients with severe metabolic acidosis (4), and provide practical guidelines for acute treatment of metabolic acidosis. They are of course based on the assumption that no further acid or alkali is being produced by body metabolic processes, and thus serve only as "ballpark" estimates for the amount of alkali needed (see Chapters 15 and 29—illustrative cases).

In addition to the buffer reactions described above, which are virtually instantaneous, calcium and sodium carbonates and phosphates contained in bone contribute to the buffer response to added H^+ or alkali (2,5–7). This component of buffering is difficult to quantitate, and it appears to change both qualitatively and quantitatively with the duration of the acid challenge to the body. The initial buffer response of bone is to release Na^+ (and presumably HCO_3^-) from a transcellular pool on its surface (5,6,8). With sustained reductions in HCO_3^-, calcium is released from bone (6,9). Initially calcium release is a physicochemical event, but continued acidosis stimulates osteoclast activity and inhibits osteoblast activity, facilitating calcium carbonate and phosphate release (10,11). This response is independent of parathyroid hormone (12,13). Strikingly, none of these bone buffer events occur when pH is reduced by hypercapnia; thus, a reduction in [HCO_3^-] appears to be the key change initiating the response (10,14). The extent to which calcium salts in bone continue to be released when acidosis is present for months or years rather than days to weeks is uncertain and an ongoing area of debate (see Chapters 8 and 14).

Metabolic Regulation of Acid Production

Organic acid production and consumption are important modulators of the minute-to-minute balance between H^+ and HCO_3^- in the body fluids. Lactic acid, for example, is produced in cells by a variety of metabolic processes, including incomplete oxidation of glucose. Because the pK' of lactic acid is 3.0, it dissociates essentially completely to a lactate anion and H^+:

$$\text{Metabolism} \leftrightarrow \text{Buffering}$$

$$HCO_3^- + CO_2 + H_2O \leftarrow \text{Lactate}^- + H^+ + HCO_3^- \rightarrow CO_2 + H_2O + \text{Lactate}^-$$

As indicated by the two arrows in this equation, buffering of newly formed lactic acid (rightward direction) consumes HCO_3^-, replacing it with a lactate ion, and lactic acid metabolism (leftward direction) generates HCO_3^- and removes lactate from the body fluids. The equilibrium in this reaction is regulated by metabolic events and serum [lactate$^-$] is maintained at ~ 1 mEq/L. When lactic acid production is increased, however, systemic pH becomes a modulating factor. An alkaline pH promotes production and an acid pH suppresses it (see Chapter 11) (15). Regulation of organic acid production by pH extends to other organic acids as well, including β-hydroxybutyric acid, in states of increased production (e.g., fasting, exercise) (15). The response is rapid, occurring within minutes and is rapidly terminated when the superimposed acid–base disorder is corrected. With the exception of these special settings, pH regulation of organic acid production does not appear to be an important factor in acid-base homeostasis and it does not play any role in day-to-day acid balance.

ACID BALANCE

Day-to-day maintenance of body alkali stores involves both the consumption and generation of HCO_3^-. These processes can be assessed either in terms of H^+ or HCO_3^- because the generation and consumption of these two ions are mirror images of each other. Each new H^+ added to the body fluids is immediately buffered, a process that leads to the consumption of a HCO_3^- (see Figs. 1 and 2). To maintain balance, H^+ must be removed from the body fluids, causing regeneration of the lost HCO_3^-. Traditionally, the process has been analyzed in terms of H^+, and the analysis termed acid balance. This approach reflects the fact that the usual challenge to acid–base equilibrium is H^+ addition and the renal generation of new HCO_3^- is accomplished by H^+ excretion. Unlike the strong ions, H^+ is not ingested as acid per se, but rather is generated by metabolic events.

Sources of Acid

The single major source of acid in a normal Western diet is sulfuric acid, generated by oxidative metabolism of the sulfur-containing amino acids in animal proteins (Table 1) (16). Oxidation of these amino acids produces H^+, which is immediately buffered, and sulfate ions, which are rapidly excreted in the urine. In individuals eating meat, this process accounts for

Table 1   Sources of Endogenous Acid and Alkali Production by Metabolic Events

Metabolic events	Acids produced	Alkali produced
Oxidation		
Sulfur-containing amino acids	H_2SO_4	
Glucose (incomplete)	Lactic/pyruvic acids	
Triglycerides	Acetoacetic/β-OH butyric acids	
Nucleoproteins	Uric acid	
Organic cations	HCl	
Organic anions		HCO_3^-
Hydrolysis		
Phospholipids, phosphoproteins	H_3PO_4	
Dibasic phosphoester salts		HCO_3^-

approximately 50% of acid production. The remainder comes from a variety of metabolic events. These include the hydrolysis of phosphoproteins and phospholipids, yielding H^+ and phosphate anions, and the production of organic acids from neutral precursors (17). Loss of organic anions in the stool and urine also reflect addition of H^+ to the body fluids, as these anions (if retained) generate HCO_3^- when oxidized to CO_2 and water.

Production of H^+ is offset by its removal through other metabolic events. The major source for H^+ removal, and therefore generation of new HCO_3^-, is oxidative metabolism of dietary organic anions (Table 1). Diets rich in vegetables contain large amounts of organic anions and can result in net alkali rather than acid production (16). Dibasic phosphoesters are a second potential alkali source, as they combine with H^+ when hydrolyzed.

Measurement of Acid Production and Excretion

Assessment of acid (or alkali) production from dietary precursors is an arduous and difficult undertaking, involving diet, stool, and urine analyses. The components of acid production are assessed as follows:

$$\text{Net acid production} = (U_{[\text{sulfate}]} V + U_{[\text{organic anion}]} V)$$
$$- (\text{diet} - \text{stool}[\text{organic anion}]) \times V) \quad (5)$$

In this equation, urinary sulfate excretion ($U_{[\text{sulfate}]}V$) is a measure of H^+ produced by the metabolism of sulfur-containing amino acids. The other components are captured in the net gain or loss of organic cations and anions (diet–stool [organic anion]) $\times V$) and ($U_{[\text{organic anion}]}V$). The contribution of metabolism of phosphate-containing amino acids to acid production is covered in this calculation by "titrating" diet minus stool phosphate to a pH of 7.4, that is, by using a valence of 1.8. This valence correction adjusts organic anion absorption for acid production or consumption by phosphoesters (17,18).

The difference between diet and stool [organic anion] is assessed by burning the diet and stool to ash and measuring the resultant *inorganic* cation and anion concentrations (cations $= Na^+$, K^+, Ca^{2+}, Mg^{2+}; anions $= Cl^-$ and $1.8 \times P$). The difference (cations − anions) is equal to the net organic anions (or cations) present in the diet and stool (17,18). Urinary organic anion excretion is measured by precipitating the phosphate in the urine with calcium hydroxide, converting all organic anions to acids by titrating the urine to a pH of 2.7 with HCl, and then back-titrating the urine to its original pH with NaOH (17,18).

To assess acid balance (i.e., acid production − acid excretion), one must also measure acid excretion, given by the formula:

$$\text{Net acid excretion} = NH_4^+ \text{ excretion} + \text{titratable acid excretion}$$
$$- HCO_3^- \text{ excretion} \qquad (6)$$

The components of this equation are discussed later. Using these measurements in a series of classic balance experiments, humans ingesting diets causing widely varying endogenous acid production were found to maintain acid balance by varying net acid excretion to match production (17).

This technique has been simplified to eliminate diet and stool analysis, based on the assumption that the difference between urinary noncombustible cations and anions is equal to net dietary organic anion absorption plus any endogenous alkali addition (19). Using this approach in normal human subjects, acid excretion was again found to balance production (20). These careful measurements have been substantiated by observations that variations in dietary endogenous acid production from 30 to 130 mEq/day have only a trivial effect on serum $[HCO_3^-]$ in normal humans (21). Thus, renal homeostatic mechanisms allow for wide variations in dietary intake without concerns about acid balance.

Although the measurements described above support the view that acid balance is readily achieved without regard for or concern about dietary intake in normal individuals, measurements in patients with chronic renal insufficiency have raised questions about the accuracy of the technique (20,22,23). These observations are discussed in detail in Chapter 14, but in brief they uniformly demonstrate a small but consistently positive acid balance, a result that seems difficult to square with the clinical course of chronic renal insufficiency. Of all these measurements described above, two have been targeted as possible sources of error. The first is titratable acid. This measurement takes its name from the technique—titration of the urine to a pH of 7.40 with added alkali. Virtually all of measured titratable acid is due to conversion of dibasic to monobasic phosphate between the pH of blood and urine, and physical titration is actually not necessary. Titratable acid excretion can be calculated from measured urinary phosphate excretion and pH, using the appropriate pK' value for the buffer pair $HPO_4^{2-}/H_2PO_4^-$ (24). This calculated value is essentially equivalent to the amount measured by actual titration of the urine. The controversy resides in whether this measurement (or calculation) systematically overestimates H^+ excretion because it fails to account for organic cations in the urine (20,22,23). The second measurement is urinary organic anion excretion. Because it is impossible to identify and quantitate all organic acids in the urine, the nonspecific titration procedure described above is used. This technique could easily under- or overestimate the actual organic anion loss in the urine (20,22,23). It has been argued that errors in these two measurements and perhaps other errors may fortuitously cancel each other out in subjects with normal renal function, but not in individuals with renal insufficiency. The issue remains unresolved (see Chapter 14) (25).

Nondietary Influences on Acid Balance

Strenuous exercise and catabolic states including sepsis, major trauma, and starvation all increase endogenous acid production. Starvation causes a major increase in β-hydroxybutyric acid production as body fat stores replace carbohydrates as a source of energy (26). Although acid excretion increases in response to increased production in these settings, mild to moderate metabolic acidosis is a characteristic feature (27). The acidosis seen in these settings is multifactorial in origin. Factors such as a limitation in sodium delivery to the distal nephron or in NH_4^+ production and excretion due to volume contraction (see later) undoubtedly contribute, in addition to the high rate of acid production. Diabetic ketoacidosis and lactic acidosis are associated with much larger increases in acid production, due to runaway organic acid production, and can cause more severe acidosis (see Chapters 10 and 11).

The Role of the Liver in Acid Balance

Catabolism of amino acids produces HCO_3^- and NH_4^+, providing the substrate for urea synthesis (Fig. 3). To the extent that these substances are brief intermediates in a tightly linked urea synthetic pathway, protein catabolism will not change net alkali balance, save for its component sulfur and phosphate containing amino acids (see earlier). The production of these intermediates and subsequent urea synthesis, however, are not completely linked reactions, a finding that has led some to conclude that the liver is

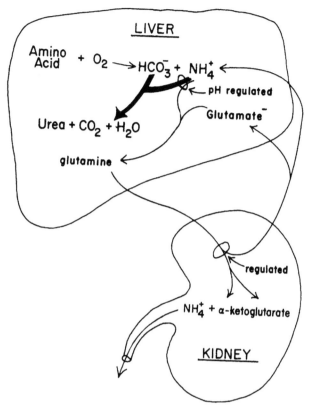

Figure 3 Role of the liver in modulating urea synthesis in response to perturbations in acid-base homeostasis. An acid pH in the liver diverts NH_4^+ from urea production to glutamine synthesis, providing additional glutamine for delivery to the kidney where it is deaminated in response to a stimulus for renal NH_4^+ excretion. *Source:* From Ref. 1.

the key regulator of body alkali stores (28,29). In fact, a small fraction of the NH_4^+ produced in the liver by amino acid breakdown is diverted to gluta-mine synthesis (Fig. 3). This reaction does not consume the companion HCO_3^- and therefore adds to body alkali stores. Acidemia, moreover, pro-motes diversion of NH_4^+ to glutamine synthesis and alkalemia suppresses this reaction (29–31). Because of the large amount of protein catabolized each day, producing as much as 700 mmol of NH_4^+ and HCO_3^-, small changes in the rate of glutamine synthesis driven by changes in pH could have a major impact on acid–base equilibrium. Diversion of NH_4^+ away from urea and towards glutamine synthesis, however, is limited by gluta-mine accumulation (31). Unless the newly synthesized glutamine is deami-nated in the kidney, it returns to the liver and is deaminated there again promoting urea synthesis and consumption of HCO_3^- (31). The ultimate control of net glutamine synthesis thus resides in the renal regulation of glutamine deamination. Hepatic stimulation of glutamine synthesis by acidemia serves a facilitating role, increasing glutamine production when its deamination by the kidney is stimulated. When alkalosis develops, hepatic glutamine synthesis is suppressed preventing its accumulation when renal deamination is inhibited.

RENAL HCO_3^- REABSORPTION AND ACID EXCRETION

The key locus for determining steady-state serum $[HCO_3^-]$ is the kidney. To maintain body alkali stores, the kidney has the dual task of recapturing filtered HCO_3^- and generating the new HCO_3^- needed both to back-titrate nonbicarbonate buffers and to replace HCO_3^- lost in buffering endogenously produced acids. The renal processes responsible for these tasks are discussed in detail in Chapters 4 and 5. Here, the task itself is summarized briefly, and attention focused on its regulation. Both HCO_3^- removal and generation of new HCO_3^- are accomplished by the secretion of H^+ into the tubule lumen by epithelial cells, primarily via two apical membrane transporters, the Na^+/H^+ exchanger and the H^+-ATPase (1). When H^+ is secreted, new HCO_3^- is formed in the cell and secreted across the opposite (basolateral) membrane into the peritubular capillaries by means of specific anion transporters (see Chapters 4 and 5).

Bicarbonate Reabsorption

Throughout the nephron, >98% of secreted H^+ reacts with HCO_3^- in the tubule fluid (Table 2), yielding carbonic acid, which is rapidly dehydrated

Table 2 Percentage of Total H^+ Secretion Utilized for HCO_3^- Reabsorption at Varying Levels of Steady-State Serum $[HCO_3^-]$[a]

Serum $[HCO_3^-]$ (mEq/L)	Filtered HCO_3^-	Titratable acid (mEq/day)	NH_4^+	Total H^+	%[b]
30	5100	30	30	5160	98.8
25	4250	30	30	4310	98.6
20	3400	30	50	3480	97.7
15	2550	35	60	2640	96.6
10	1700	40	80	1820	93.4

[a]Assumes all filtered HCO_3^- reabsorbed, GFR of 170 L/day. NH_4^+ and titratable acid excretion are assumed to increase when serum $[HCO_3^-]$ is low.
[b]Percentage of total H^+ secretion utilized for HCO_3^- reabsorption.

to CO_2. The CO_2 formed by this reaction diffuses back across the tubular epithelium and is excreted by the lungs. As a result, H^+ secretion removes HCO_3^- from the tubular fluid. Secretion of H^+ also generates new HCO_3^- in the cell, which in turn is secreted across the basolateral membrane. Thus, reaction of secreted H^+ with filtered HCO_3^- is equivalent to HCO_3^- reabsorption.

Reabsorption of HCO_3^- is an avid process; over 90% of filtered HCO_3^- is recaptured before the early distal tubule under a wide variety of conditions, and little is ever excreted in the urine (1). Most is reabsorbed in the proximal tubule and over 50% is recaptured within the first mm in this segment (32). Avid reabsorption is essential for recapturing the HCO_3^- lost into the glomerular filtrate, but it does not generate new alkali. The latter task is accomplished when secreted H^+ reacts not with filtered HCO_3^- but with other filtered buffers (primarily phosphate), or when NH_4^+ is secreted in place of H^+, and the resultant products are excreted in the urine (see later). These events are facilitated by the removal of HCO_3^- from the glomerular filtrate in the earliest portions of the nephron, reducing the $[HCO_3^-]$ and pH in the tubular fluid.

Titratable Acid Excretion

Titratable acid excretion is defined as the combination of secreted H^+ with filtered buffers in the tubular fluid that are destined for excretion. The amount of secreted H^+ that can combine with a particular buffer depends on the pK' of the buffer, the fall in pH between the blood and final urine, and the quantity excreted. Because of its favorable pK' (6.8 for $HPO_4^{2-}/H_2PO_4^-$) and the quantity excreted, phosphate accounts for virtually all titratable acid excretion under normal circumstances (24,33). At the pH of the blood, 80% of phosphate exists as the dibasic form (HPO_4^{2-}) and 20% is monobasic ($H_2PO_4^-$). At a urine pH of 5.8, by contrast, only 10% exists as the dibasic form and, at a urine pH of 4.8, only 1% is dibasic. Thus, a reduction in the pH of the tubule fluid between the glomerulus and the final urine from 7.4 to 4.8 is accompanied by the combination of 0.79 mEq of H^+ with each mmol of phosphate excreted. Given the usual rate of phosphate excretion (40–60 mmol/day), 30–40 mEq/day of H^+ excretion can be accomplished by converting dibasic phosphate to monobasic phosphate. Most other filtered buffers (e.g., organic anions and creatinine) have much lower pK' values and are excreted in lesser amounts. For example, approximately 12–16 mmol of creatinine are excreted in the urine each day but, given its pK' (4.97), only ~1 mEq of H^+ combines with it at a pH of 5.8, and only 6–8 mEq combines with it when the urine is maximally acid. Organic anions have even lower pK' values and account for less than 1 mEq of titratable acid excretion under normal conditions.

Ammonium Excretion

By contrast with titratable acid, excretion of NH_4^+ is a more flexible mechanism for the generation of new HCO_3^- because excretion of this cation is not dependent on filtration. Ammonium ions are produced in the renal cortex by deamination of organic amines (almost exclusively glutamine). Glutamine uptake into proximal tubular epithelial cells, its deamination to produce NH_4^+ and secretion of NH_4^+ into the tubular fluid are all regulated by acid–base status (34). Ammonium ions are excreted in the urine as a result of a complex process involving secretion, reabsorption, countercurrent concentration, diffusion (as NH_3) and then recombination with H^+ by a process known as diffusion trapping (34) (see Chapters 4 and 5).

Acidification of the urine by H^+ secretion in the medullary collecting duct is essential for NH_4^+ excretion, preventing back-diffusion of NH_3. Generation of new alkali from excretion of NH_4^+, however, is not the direct result of H^+ secretion in the terminal portions of the nephron because this process simply reunites NH_3 with the H^+ that was secreted with it in the proximal tubule (34,35). Excretion of NH_4^+ produces new HCO_3^- because α-ketoglutaric acid, the endproduct of the deamination of glutamine, produces HCO_3^- when metabolized to CO_2 and H_2O (or to any other neutral substance) (35). Ammonium production and excretion varies widely and is regulated by the same processes that regulate H^+ secretion itself (see below). Variations in NH_4^+ excretion account for over 90% of the day-to-day variations in net acid excretion, varying from negligible amounts when excess alkali must be excreted to over 400 mmol/day in severe metabolic acidosis (33).

FACTORS INFLUENCING HCO_3^- REABSORPTION AND ACID EXCRETION

Many factors have been shown to have a regulatory influence on renal H^+ secretion (see Tables 3 and 4). The specific cellular effects of these factors and their mechanisms of action are discussed in Chapter 4. In this chapter,

Table 3 Nonhormonal Factors Influencing Renal H^+ Secretion

Factor	Effect
pH	H^+ secretion inversely related
PCO_2	H^+ secretion directly related
HCO_3^- delivery	H^+ secretion directly related
Distal Na^+ delivery	H^+ secretion directly related
K^+ depletion	H^+ and NH_4^+ secretion stimulated
Cl^- depletion	Indirectly stimulates H^+ secretion

Table 4 Hormonal Influences on H^+ Secretion[a]

Hormone	Effect
May affect serum [HCO_3^-]	
Aldosterone	Stimulates H^+ secretion in CD
Parathyroid hormone (acute)	Inhibits Na^+/H^+ exchanger
Parathyroid hormone (chronic)	Increases H^+ secretion indirectly
Calcitriol	Increases H^+ secretion indirectly
No effect on serum [HCO_3^-]	
Angiotensin (low level)	Stimulates Na^+/H^+ exchanger
Angiotensin (high level)	Inhibits Na^+/H^+ exchanger
α-Adrenergic activity	Stimulates Na^+/H^+ exchanger
Glucocorticoids	Stimulate Na^+/H^+ exchanger
Thyroid hormone	Stimulates Na^+/H^+ exchanger
Dopamine	Inhibits Na^+/H^+ exchanger
Nitric oxide	Stimulates H^+ secretion in epithelia
Endothelin	Stimulates H^+ secretion in epithelia

[a]Based on experimental evidence in intact animals, isolated tubules or cultured epithelial cells.

we review the overall impact of these influences on HCO_3^- reabsorption and acid excretion.

Systemic pH

Given the narrow range of arterial pH values seen in normal humans and experimental animals, a logical scheme for acid balance would be one in which the kidney sensed changes in pH and responded directly with appropriate changes in H^+ and NH_4^+ secretion. In fact, changes in pH uniformly do affect secretion of both these cations in the expected fashion in isolated perfused tubule segments, cultured renal epithelial cells, and in membrane vesicles. In all these experimental settings, alkalemia inhibits H^+ secretion and acidemia stimulates it (36–39). Acidemia has also been shown to increase glutamine uptake, facilitating NH_4^+ production, but this entry step is not rate limiting (40–42). Acidemia stimulates NH_4^+ production and secretion, and alkalemia inhibits these events (34). Despite this evidence that pH influences both the secretion of H^+ and the production and secretion of NH_4^+, it is difficult to show a clear linkage between changes in pH and changes in HCO_3^- reabsorption and acid excretion in intact animals and human subjects (43). In fact, no connection between pH and renal acid excretion is discernable in the day-to-day variations in acid excretion that occur in response dietary-induced variations in endogenous acid production (21). One explanation for this dissociation is that a wide variety of factors, all seemingly unrelated to acid balance, influence renal HCO_3^- reabsorption and acid excretion (see later). Systemic pH may affect renal H^+ secretion indirectly through its effect on $PaCO_2$. Ventilatory rate, and therefore $PaCO_2$, is exquisitely sensitive to changes in arterial pH (see Chapter 3), and PCO_2 influences H^+ secretion by the kidney (see below).

Systemic PCO_2

Changes in arterial PCO_2 affect renal HCO_3^- reabsorption and acid excretion and produce significant changes in steady-state serum $[HCO_3^-]$ in intact animals and humans. These effects are best illustrated by the response of the kidney to sustained hypercapnia or hypocapnia (44,45). The renal response does not occur immediately, but takes 48–72 hr to develop fully. During adaptation, net acid excretion increases transiently in respiratory acidosis and falls transiently in respiratory alkalosis, producing a change in body alkali stores and in serum $[HCO_3^-]$. In the new steady state, serum $[HCO_3^-]$ increases by ~ 3 mEq/L for each 10 mmHg increase in $PaCO_2$, and falls to a similar degree when $PaCO_2$ is reduced (44–46). Changes in PCO_2 influence H^+ secretion (and therefore HCO_3^- reabsorption) in the expected fashion in both the proximal and distal nephron (47,48). The effect appears to be specific for peritubular PCO_2 and is independent of both pH and $[HCO_3^-]$ (47).

In a series of inventive balance studies in intact animals, changes in PCO_2 have also been shown to influence renal H^+ secretion in a fashion that is independent of pH and $[HCO_3^-]$ (49–51). In dogs with metabolic acidosis, a superimposed sustained reduction in $PaCO_2$ paradoxically reduces renal acid excretion and HCO_3^- reabsorption, lowering serum $[HCO_3^-]$ and exacerbating the acidemia (Fig. 4) (49). In a related study, prevention of the usual adaptive hyperventilation in dogs with metabolic acidosis resulted in a higher steady-state serum $[HCO_3^-]$ for any given acid load (50). Moreover, when PCO_2 was then allowed to fall as part of the normal response to the metabolic acidosis, $[HCO_3^-]$ fell as well, so that pH was unaffected by the "adaptive" hyperventilation. In animals with metabolic alkalosis, manipulation of $PaCO_2$ also caused parallel changes in serum $[HCO_3^-]$, hypercapnia worsening the increase in serum $[HCO_3^-]$ and hypocapnia ameliorating it (51). Although changes in $PaCO_2$ in intact animals have many effects (e.g., changes in renal hemodynamics, hormone levels), it seems likely, given the evidence from isolated cells and tubules, that these effects are mediated primarily by the influence of PCO_2 on renal H^+ secretion.

In addition to these experimental manipulations, minor variations in $PaCO_2$ within the normal range influence steady-state serum $[HCO_3^-]$ (52,53). In normal human subjects, serum $[HCO_3^-]$ correlates directly with variations in $PaCO_2$ (Fig. 5).

Acid–Base Disorders

Acid–base disorders are characterized by sustained alterations in serum pH. Nonetheless, elucidation of specific effects of these changes in pH on renal

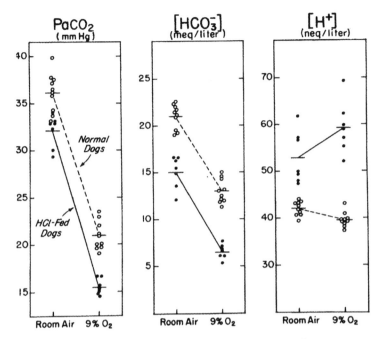

Figure 4 Changes in PCO_2 ($PaCO_2$), plasma [HCO_3^-] and [H^+] produced by sustained hypocapnia (induced by exposure to an environment containing 9% oxygen) in normal dogs (*dashed lines*) and in dogs with chronic metabolic acidosis induced by HCl feeding (*solid lines*). Note that in both groups of animals, plasma [HCO_3^-] fell to the same degree, an effect which minimized the fall in [H^+] in the normal dogs, but which paradoxically worsened the acidemia in the dogs with chronic metabolic acidosis. *Source*: From Ref. 49.

H^+ secretion is difficult to discern because of other contributing factors. For example, H^+ secretion is stimulated by sustained respiratory acidosis and at the same time the filtered load is increased. As discussed below, HCO_3^- delivery is a major determinant of the rate of H^+ secretion, making it difficult to determine the extent to which the increase in filtered HCO_3^- or the increase in PCO_2 is responsible for the increase in overall renal H^+ secretion (54). In sustained respiratory alkalosis, the opposite occurs; filtered load falls at the same time that H^+ secretion is blunted (54). Given the direct effects of changes in PCO_2 on both H^+ secretion and net acid excretion, however, it is likely that changes in delivery only play a supporting role in respiratory acid–base disorders, allowing for changes in H^+ secretion to sustain differing levels of serum [HCO_3^-].

In metabolic acidosis, H^+ secretion is stimulated and net acid excretion increases (55–57). However, the fall in serum [HCO_3^-] engendered by the acidosis actually limits overall renal H^+ secretion, and the result is a

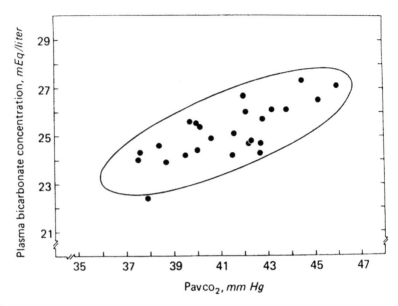

Figure 5   Relationship between PCO_2 in arterialized venous blood ($PAVCO_2$) and plasma [HCO_3^-] in normal human subjects. *Source*: From Ref. 52.

reduction compared to normal (57). Steady-state pH and serum [HCO_3^-] in metabolic acidosis appear to be influenced primarily by factors unrelated to acidemia, including the type of acid administered, mineralocorticoid levels, $PaCO_2$, ECF volume, distal Na^+ delivery and growth hormone (58–61). In metabolic alkalosis serum [HCO_3^-] is increased and as a result renal H^+ secretion is often increased above normal despite alkalemia, due in part to delivery dependence as well as to other factors (62). Steady-state pH and serum [HCO_3^-] in metabolic alkalosis are determined primarily by the state of Na^+, Cl^-, and K^+ balance, or by mineralocorticoid secretion, rather than by alkalemia (see section on metabolic alkalosis) (63–66).

Factors Not Related Directly to Acid–Base Homeostasis

As noted earlier, a host of factors can influence H^+ secretion in various portions of the nephron and many of these affect steady-state serum [HCO_3^-] (Tables 3 and 4). Most play a role in regulating Na^+ balance and ECF volume, and their effects on H^+ relate to the many linkages between Na^+ and H^+ transport along the nephron. These influences have been reviewed in detail elsewhere (1). In the following sections, only major influences are discussed.

Delivery Dependence

The rate of H^+ secretion along the nephron is tightly linked to HCO_3^- delivery in every segment of the nephron in which it has been studied (32,67–69). The close linkage between H^+ secretion and HCO_3^- delivery allows for efficient conservation of both filtered Na^+ and HCO_3^- in the face of variations in GFR and therefore in filtered load. Although this feature of renal H^+ transport serves to maintain a normal serum $[HCO_3^-]$, it can also contribute to the maintenance of metabolic alkalosis (see earlier). Delivery dependence can result in a sustained increase in serum $[HCO_3^-]$ if the filtered load of HCO_3^- is increased in the absence of changes in other factors (e.g., ECF volume) that influence H^+ secretion by the kidney. As an example, normal humans given an oral HCO_3^- supplement will increase their serum $[HCO_3^-]$ when ingesting a low salt diet (Fig. 6) (70). The increase occurs in the absence of a change in GFR, indicating that renal H^+ is increased due to an increase in filtered HCO_3^-. This effect is completely abrogated if the subjects are given salt, a treatment that increases ECF volume and blunts renal

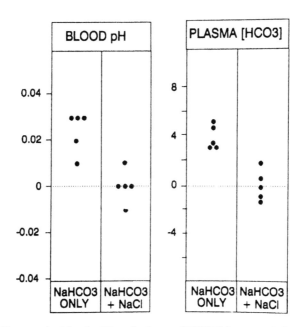

Figure 6 Changes in blood pH and plasma $[HCO_3^-]$ in normal human subjects given supplemental $NaHCO_3$, $2\,mEq/Kg$ body weight/day for 5 days. The subjects in the left-hand side of the graphs ($NaHCO_3$ only) were maintained on a severely restricted NaCl intake ($10\,mEq/day$), whereas the subjects on the right-hand side ($NaHCO_3 + NaCl$) were given NaCl $2\,mEq/Kg$ body weight in addition to the $NaHCO_3$. *Source*: From Ref. 70.

H^+ secretion (see later). Delivery dependence also contributes to sustaining metabolic alkalosis caused by diuretic administration or vomiting, and probably participates in the renal response to respiratory acidosis (54).

Extracellular Fluid Volume

Acute ECF volume expansion decreases renal HCO_3^- reabsorption in animal and human studies (71,72). Whether the effects seen in these acute experiments are due to the change in ECF volume per se or some other effect is difficult to discern. Acute saline loading has multiple effects, including changes in chloride delivery and in the secretion of many hormones known to influence renal H^+ secretion (see later). Moreover, the relevance of these acute observations to normal acid balance is difficult to assess because ECF volume was rapidly and massively expanded. Sustained ECF volume expansion appears to have no effect on serum $[HCO_3^-]$ in the absence of independent events that alter serum $[HCO_3^-]$. As an example, a sustained increase in ECF volume produced by the chronic administration of ADH and water results in no significant change in serum $[HCO_3^-]$, renal bicarbonate reabsorption or acid excretion (60). Although volume expansion appears to have no sustained effect on $[HCO_3^-]$ under normal conditions, it blocks the sustained increase in $[HCO_3^-]$ induced by acute or chronic alkali administration (Fig. 6) (70), and corrects the increase induced by the most common cause of metabolic alkalosis (64,73). Extracellular fluid volume depletion (induced by ingesting a very low salt intake or by hemorrhage) has no effect on serum $[HCO_3^-]$ in the absence of any superimposed changes in serum $[HCO_3^-]$ (74).

Aldosterone

Mineralocorticoid deficiency is associated with metabolic acidosis, and administration of mineralocorticoids to normal humans and experimental animals leads to a small but significant increase in serum $[HCO_3^-]$ (59,66,75,76). Aldosterone is the major endogenous mineralocorticoid hormone, and it stimulates renal H^+ secretion both indirectly by promoting Na^+ reabsorption (thereby facilitating H^+ secretion) and directly by upregulating the apical membrane H^+-ATPase in the intercalated cells of the collecting duct (77). Although some aldosterone is necessary to maintain normal acid balance, variations in extracellular fluid $[K^+]$ and volume are the primary signals for secretion of this hormone and its effects lead to appropriate renal adjustments to restore these variables to normal levels (77). Thus, the effect of aldosterone on H^+ appears to be a byproduct of its effects on Na^+ and K^+ transport. As an example, the increase in serum $[HCO_3^-]$ induced by mineralocorticoid administration is dependent on its ability to increase the Na^+ delivery to the distal nephron (59,76). Mineralocorticoid administration has no effect on serum $[HCO_3^-]$ in humans ingesting a very low salt diet, presumably because Na^+ delivery to and reabsorption in the collecting duct cannot be increased further in this setting (76). In humans, aldosterone probably plays no important role in acid–base homeostasis; complete mineralocorticoid deficiency only causes a minor decrement in serum $[HCO_3^-]$, 1–2 mEq/L, and administration of excess mineralocorticoid only causes a minor increase (66,75).

Parathyroid Hormone and Calcitriol

Parathyroid hormone (PTH) has small but readily demonstrable effects on serum $[HCO_3^-]$ in humans (78–80). Strikingly, however, the effects are opposite with acute and chronic exposures. Acutely, PTH administration inhibits H^+ secretion in the proximal tubule in experimental animals, by inhibiting apical membrane Na^+/H^+ exchange (81), and lowers serum $[HCO_3^-]$ notably in humans (79,80). When given as a chronic infusion over a period of days, by contrast, PTH causes a sustained 1–2 mEq/L increase in serum $[HCO_3^-]$ (78,79). The sustained effect of PTH may be related to the release of calcium and carbonate from bone, followed by a delivery-dependent (see earlier) increase in renal HCO_3^- reabsorption. No increase in net acid excretion occurs (78,79). Sustained calcitriol administration causes an identical increase in serum $[HCO_3^-]$ without a change in net acid excretion, and the increase is presumed to be due to similar effects on bone calcium dissolution (78).

Other Hormones (Table 4)

Angiotensin II stimulates renal H^+ in the proximal tubule, loop of Henle, and distal tubule, and blockade of this hormone decreases HCO_3^- reabsorption (37,82–84). The effects on proximal H^+ secretion appear to be biphasic, with low levels $(10^{-12}–10^{-10}\text{M})$ stimulating secretion and high levels $(10^{-8}\text{M}$ or higher) inhibiting it (85,86). Both stimulation and inhibition of H^+ secretion by angiotensin are mediated through changes in apical membrane Na^+/H^+ exchange activity (81). Despite the clear demonstration of effects on H^+ secretion in isolated tubule segments, physiological variations in angiotensin II have no discernible effect on systemic pH or $[HCO_3^-]$. This hormone may play a homeostatic role in the setting of ECF volume depletion, assuring adequate H^+ secretion to maintain body alkali stores in the face of decreased Na^+ delivery to the distal nephron.

Both renal nerve stimulation and norepinephrine increase Na^+/H^+ exchange in the proximal tubule (87). The increase in activity of this key H^+ transport protein occurs after agonist occupation of either the α_1- or α_2-adrenoreceptor, and the effect is additive when both are occupied (87). In intact animal studies, HCO_3^- reabsorption in the proximal tubule, loop of Henle, and surface distal tubules is decreased after renal denervation (37,84,88), and proximal tubular HCO_3^- reabsorption is stimulated by norepinephrine administration (89). Nonetheless, there is no evidence for any sustained effect on serum [HCO_3^-] related to changes in α-adrenergic activity. In contrast to α-adrenergic stimulation, dopamine causes a marked decrease in Na^+/H^+ activity in the proximal tubule, an effect mediated by activation of postsynaptic DA_1 receptors (81). Again, no sustained effect on serum [HCO_3^-] occurs.

Glucocorticoid administration increases Na^+/H^+ exchange activity in isolated proximal tubules and in membrane vesicles (90). In animal studies, HCO_3^- reabsorption is reduced in the proximal tubule and loop of Henle after adrenalectomy and restored toward normal by glucocorticoid replacement therapy (91,92). Despite these effects, there is little evidence in intact animals or humans that glucocorticoids increase serum [HCO_3^-], except when given in very large doses (93). Thyroid hormone stimulates Na^+/H^+ activity in cultured kidney cells and in brush border membrane vesicles (94,95), but has no effect on serum [HCO_3^-]. Atrial natriuretic peptide has no direct effect on H^+ secretion (96). It decreases HCO_3^- reabsorption indirectly by stimulating dopamine secretion (97). There is no effect of atrial natriuretic peptide on serum [HCO_3^-].

Growth hormone administration has no effect on serum [HCO_3^-] in humans under normal conditions but significantly ameliorates NH_4Cl-induced metabolic acidosis (98). The mechanism by which this occurs is unclear. A variety of other hormones, including nitric oxide, endothelin, calcitonin, and insulin-like growth factor appear to stimulate H^+ secretion by epithelial cells (Table 4), but their role in acid–base homeostasis is unknown.

Body K$^+$ Stores

Dietary K^+ restriction reduces body K^+ stores and produces a sustained increase in serum [HCO_3^-] (74,99). In humans ingesting adequate NaCl (see later), serum [HCO_3^-] increases by 2 mEq/L after a reduction in body K^+ of $\sim$400 mEq (serum [K^+] = 3.0 mEq/L) (Fig. 7) (74). With more severe depletion, serum [HCO_3^-] rises to as high as 35 mEq/L both in rats and humans (99–102). The rise in [HCO_3^-] is due to increased H^+ secretion by the kidney. Net acid excretion increases transiently and is followed by a sustained increase in renal HCO_3^- reabsorption (74,102). Potassium depletion increases proximal tubular H^+ secretion and stimulates K^+ reabsorption in the cortical collecting duct via the H^+/K^+ ATPase (103,104). In dogs, K^+ depletion paradoxically causes a decrease in serum [HCO_3^-] (101,105). This species difference appears to be due to more marked inhibition of aldosterone secretion by hypokalemia in dogs. If dogs are pretreated with mineralocorticoid, K^+ depletion increases serum [HCO_3^-] in this species as well (106).

The effect of K^+ depletion on HCO_3^- reabsorption (and on serum [HCO_3^-]) is modulated by concurrent dietary chloride intake (Fig. 7).

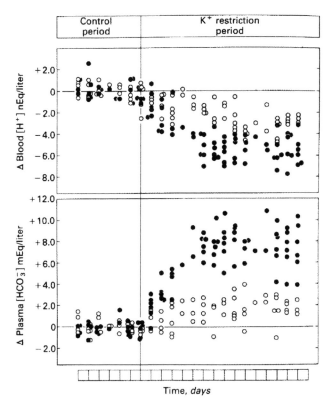

Figure 7 Influence of dietary Cl⁻ intake on the changes in blood [H⁺] and plasma [HCO₃⁻] induced by K⁺ depletion in normal human subjects. ●, data, in subjects on a severely restricted NaCl intake (10 mEq/day); ○, data in subjects ingesting a normal salt diet (1.8 mEq/Kg/day). *Source*: From Ref. 74.

In human subjects ingesting only 10 mEq of NaCl/day, serum [HCO₃⁻] increases by 8 mEq/L after a reduction in body K⁺ stores of 400 mEq, as opposed to only 2 mEq/L on a normal NaCl intake (74). The interplay between K⁺ and Cl depletion in modulating serum [HCO₃⁻] has generated an ongoing debate about the pathophysiology of metabolic alkalosis (see Chapter 16). In most clinical settings, K⁺ and Cl depletion occur concurrently, and both contribute to the sustained increase in serum [HCO₃⁻] that occurs.

In addition to its effects on HCO₃⁻ reabsorption, K⁺ depletion increases renal NH₄⁺ production and excretion notably (74,107). This increase is independent of dietary Cl⁻ intake, but when Cl⁻ intake is adequate it is counterbalanced by a fall in titratable acid excretion and thus no change in net acid excretion occurs (107,108). By contrast, when dietary

Cl^- is restricted, the increase in NH_4^+ excretion is not counterbalanced and net acid excretion increases, generating new HCO_3^- (74). The increase in NH_4^+ excretion is due in part to increased production, but also to increased secretion into the proximal tubule and to an increase in countercurrent NH_4^+ concentration in the loop of Henle. Stimulation of NH_4^+ production and excretion is one mechanism that likely contributes to the maintenance of metabolic alkalosis in hypokalemic patients (see Chapter 18).

In contrast to K^+ depletion, neither K^+ excess nor hyperkalemia has any sustained effect on renal HCO_3^- reabsorption or serum $[HCO_3^-]$ (109). However, hyperkalemia has been shown to suppress NH_4^+ excretion both in human and animal studies (109). In these studies, the fall in NH_4^+ excretion is balanced by an increase in titratable acid excretion with no net change in acid excretion. If phosphate intake is restricted and mineralocorticoid levels are fixed, titratable acid cannot increase and hyperkalemia causes a fall in serum $[HCO_3^-]$ (110). Hyperkalemia has been shown to inhibit renal NH_4^+ production slightly in some studies, but not in others (109). The mechanism by which hyperkalemia suppresses NH_4^+ excretion is unclear, but may be related to impairment of NH_4^+ uptake in the ascending loop of Henle's limb, preventing adequate countercurrent concentration and delivery to the medullary collecting duct.

Body Chloride Stores

Selective chloride loss from the body fluids (e.g., as a result of diuretic administration, vomiting, or nasogastric suction) generates new HCO_3^-, because it either is accompanied by H^+ loss (upper GI losses) or stimulates renal H^+ secretion (63,111). A similar change can be induced if Cl^- is removed and replaced by HCO_3^- using either peritoneal dialysis or hemofiltration (112,113). In all these settings, serum $[HCO_3^-]$ increases and the increase is maintained by renal mechanisms (see Chapter 17). The alkalosis seen in states of chloride depletion is maintained in part by a delivery-dependent increase in renal HCO_3^- reabsorption (62,114), in part by concomitant K^+ depletion and in part by changes in Cl^--dependent transport in the distal nephron (115). Chloride depletion is almost always accompanied by K^+ losses and the resultant K^+ depletion is known to promote HCO_3^- reabsorption and NH_4^+ excretion by the kidney (see above). Chloride depletion sustains the increase in $[HCO_3^-]$ induced by K^+ depletion by inhibiting HCO_3^- secretion and promoting H^+ secretion in the distal nephron (115,116). Bicarbonate secretion is linked directly to Cl^- reabsorption by the epithelial membrane Cl^-/HCO_3^- exchanger in the distal tubule and cortical collecting duct, and this transporter is activated by alkalemia (115–117). Chloride depletion limits distal Cl^- delivery, impeding distal HCO_3^- secretion and preventing correction of alkalosis (116,118,119). Chloride depletion also stimulates distal nephron H^+ secretion by limiting Cl^--dependent Na^+

reabsorption and increasing Na^+ delivery to sites where its reabsorption provides a driving force for H^+ secretion (see below).

Distal Sodium Delivery

Hydrogen ion secretion in the collecting ducts is not directly linked to Na^+ reabsorption, but the two processes are linked indirectly by charge balance. In order for H^+ secretion to increase significantly at this site in the nephron, Na^+ reabsorption must increase. This constraint is not a problem under most conditions, as sufficient Na^+ almost always reaches the distal nephron for adjustments in reabsorption to occur in response to changes in H^+ secretion. However, a severe limitation on distal Na^+ delivery can impair renal H^+ secretion. In human subjects or animals placed on a dietary Na^+ restriction of $10\,mEq/day$, for example, the increase in acid excretion and serum $[HCO_3^-]$ normally engendered by mineralocorticoid administration is completely blocked (59,76). In the clinical setting of sustained volume depletion, a limitation on Na^+ delivery has also been shown to impair distal acidification and cause metabolic acidosis (120). These examples represent extremes, and in most settings variations in distal Na^+ delivery caused by variations in ECF volume and dietary Na^+ intake have no notable effect on renal H^+ secretion and acid–base balance.

Phosphate Balance

Phosphate is ubiquitous in the foods we eat and is readily absorbed from the gut. Thus, body phosphate stores are easily maintained, and adequate phosphate is normally excreted in the urine to accomplish titratable acid excretion. Moreover, day-to-day variations in phosphate excretion do not influence net acid excretion (although titratable acid excretion may vary). Under experimental conditions, marked variations in phosphate excretion do influence titratable acid excretion and acid balance notably. These effects are probably not related to phosphate itself, however, but to other factors. Phosphate loading increases titratable acid excretion and phosphate depletion can reduce it to zero (121–123). In the former setting, serum $[HCO_3^-]$ increases but this is likely to be due to stimulation of parathyroid hormone secretion (see earlier) as well as to changes in Na^+ delivery to the distal nephron, rather than to changes in titratable acid excretion (124). Phosphate depletion impairs H^+ secretion directly and causes HCO_3^- wasting, effects that are likely responsible for the mild metabolic acidosis seen (122,125).

Overview

The pH, PCO_2, and $[HCO_3^-]$ of the body fluids are all maintained within remarkably narrow limits despite wide variations in acid generation, but no simple feedback system emerges as a control mechanism linking acid excretion to acid production. As discussed earlier, the prevailing $PaCO_2$ is the main determinant of steady-state serum $[HCO_3^-]$ through its effects on renal H^+ secretion (Fig. 5). This simple relationship, however, does not explain the kidney's ability to vary net acid excretion over a wide range to match net acid production precisely, as this response occurs without detectable changes in $PaCO_2$. Endogenous acid production has been varied from as low as 30 to as high as 150 mEq/day by altering dietary intake in human volunteers, also with no measurable effect on pH or serum $[HCO_3^-]$ (17,21).

Because of this disconnection between pH and net acid excretion, acid production has been proposed to signal changes in acid excretion not by changing systemic pH, but by altering the anion composition of the glomerular filtrate (43). According to this view, the HCO_3^- consumed in buffering strong acids produced by metabolism is replaced by the acid anion in the body fluids and glomerular filtrate. For each mmol of acid produced, 1 mmol of the anion (e.g., sulfate, phosphate, organic anions) thus enters the tubule urine and is excreted. The need to excrete these anions coupled with the constraints of Na^+ balance causes the Na^+ filtered with these anions to be reabsorbed, and its reabsorption (presumably in the distal nephron) stimulates the secretion of sufficient H^+ to match precisely the acid anions in the urine. This feedback mechanism requires a decrease in filtered HCO_3^- to match the increase in acid anions produced each day, however, and such a decrease is not observed. In addition, although there is much experimental evidence to support the role of anions in modulating net acid excretion and serum $[HCO_3^-]$ under conditions of severe dietary NaCl restriction, no such effects occur when NaCl intake is adequate (58). The kidney has different regulatory mechanisms for the absorption (and excretion) of each of the many anions (as well as for Na^+ itself), and it is difficult to imagine a regulatory system that combines and responds to all these signals to produce such tight control of acid excretion. Nonetheless, one cannot exclude the possibility that this non-pH mechanism contributes to the changes in acid excretion induced by variations in dietary intake.

A more plausible explanation for the failure to detect a relationship between pH and variations in day-to-day net acid production and excretion is that it is obscured by the influence of variations in $PaCO_2$ on serum $[HCO_3^-]$. Recall that individuals with a higher $PaCO_2$ have a higher serum $[HCO_3^-]$ in the steady state (see earlier). In normal humans ingesting diets with widely varying acid production rates, net acid excretion correlates with pH in the expected fashion when adjusted for the known effect of variations in $PaCO_2$ (21). In this study, 50% of the variation in serum $[HCO_3^-]$ was accounted for by variations in PCO_2, and 25% was accounted for by diet-induced changes in net acid production. One is left with the conclusion that acid balance is the result of a complex interplay among many influences, including strong ion balance, the prevailing PCO_2, variations in prevailing hormone levels and pH itself.

As amply demonstrated throughout this book, the normal equilibrium between variations in dietary intake and acid excretion is also easily disrupted. The causes of such disruptions are often unrelated to acid addition or loss, and include events such as hypokalemia, abnormalities in Cl and Na^+ balance as well as in the production and secretion of a variety of hormones. The easy disruption of normal acid balance is perhaps not surprising, because wide variations in $PaCO_2$ and $[HCO_3^-]$ and moderate variations in pH are quite compatible with life. Consider only the examples of humans living at high altitude and those with hereditary forms of renal tubular acidosis. From an evolutionary perspective, adaptability to alterations in acid–base equilibrium has perhaps diminished the necessity to have a more rigid control system for renal H^+ secretion. Clearly, changes in systemic pH can be limited much more quickly by changing ventilation to alter $PaCO_2$ than by changes in renal acid excretion. Moreover, the kidney's ability to be somewhat flexible about H^+ secretion allows this organ to devote its energy to the balance of other key ions such as Na^+ and K^+. The key to the kidney's ability to maintain alkali stores is its avid and high capacity for HCO_3^- reabsorption, a task accomplished primarily in the proximal tubule and loop of Henle. The fine-tuning of acid balance in the distal nephron is appropriately dependent on the interplay of forces necessary to maintain balance for all key cations and anions in the body fluids.

REFERENCES

1. Gennari FJ, Maddox DA. Renal regulation of acid–base homeostasis. Integrated response. In: Seldin DW, Giebisch G, eds. The Kidney. Physiology and Pathophysiology. Philadelphia: Lippincott Williams & Wilkins, 2000:2015–2053.
2. Adrogue HJ, Brensilver J, Cohen JJ, Madias NE. Influence of steady-state alterations in acid–base equilibrium on the fate of administered bicarbonate in the dog. J Clin Invest 1983; 71:867–883.
3. Swan RC, Pitts RF. Neutralization of infused acid by nephrectomized dogs. J Clin Invest 1955; 34:205–212.
4. Garella S, Dana CL, Chazan JA. Severity of metabolic acidosis as a determinant of bicarbonate requirements. N Engl J Med 1973; 289:121–126.
5. Bettice JA, Gamble JL Jr. Skeletal buffering of acute metabolic acidosis. Am J Physiol 1975; 229:1618–1624.
6. Burnell JM. Changes in bone sodium and carbonate in metabolic acidosis and alkalosis in the dog. J Clin Invest 1971; 50:327–331.
7. Lemann J Jr, Litzow JR, Lennon EJ. The effects of chronic acid loads in normal man: further evidence for the participation of bone mineral in the defense against chronic metabolic acidosis. J Clin Invest 1966; 45:1608–1614.

8. Bushinsky DA, Levi-Setti R, Coe FL. Ion microprobe determination of bone surface elements: effects of reduced medium pH. Am J Physiol 1986; 250:F1090–F1097.

9. Bushinsky DA, Lechleider RJ. Mechanism of proton-induced bone calcium release: calcium carbonate-dissolution. Am J Physiol 1987; 253:F998–F1005.

10. Bushinsky DA. Net calcium efflux from live bone during chronic metabolic, but not respiratory, acidosis. Am J Physiol 1989; 256:F836–F842.

11. Krieger NS, Sessler NE, Bushinsky DA. Acidosis inhibits osteoblastic and stimulates osteoclastic activity in vitro. Am J Physiol 1992; 262:F442–F448.

12. Bushinsky DA. Effects of parathyroid hormone on net proton flux from neonatal mouse calvariae. Am J Physiol 1987; 252:F585–F589.

13. Madias NE, Johns CA, Homer SM. Independence of the acute acid-buffering response from endogenous parathyroid hormone. Am J Physiol 1982; 243:F141–F149.

14. Bushinsky DA. Net proton influx into bone during metabolic, but not respiratory, acidosis. Am J Physiol 1988; 254:F306–F310.

15. Hood VL, Tannen RL. Protection of acid–base balance by pH regulation of acid production. N Engl J Med 1998; 339:819–826.

16. Harrington JT, Lemann J Jr. The metabolic production and disposal of acid and alkali. Med Clin North Am 1970; 54:1543–1554.

17. Lennon EJ, Lemann J Jr, Litzow JR. The effects of diet and stool composition on the net external acid balance of normal subjects. J Clin Invest 1966; 45:1601–1607.

18. Relman AS, Lennon EJ, Lemann J. Endogenous production of fixed acid and the measurement of the net balance of acid in normal subjects. J Clin Invest 1961; 40:1621–1630.

19. Oh MS. A new method for estimating GI absorption of alkali. Kidney Int 1993; 36:915–917.

20. Uribarri J, Douyon H, Oh MS. A re-evaluation of the urinary parameters of acid production and excretion in patients with chronic renal acidosis. Kidney Int 1995; 47:624–627.

21. Kurtz I, Maher T, Hulter HN, Schambelan M, Sebastian A. Effect of diet on plasma acid-base composition in normal humans. Kidney Int 1983; 24: 670–680.

22. Cohen RM, Feldman GM, Fernandez PC. The balance of acid, base and charge in health and disease. Kidney Int 1997; 52:287–293.

23. Oh MS. New perspective on acid–base balance. Semin Dial 2000; 13: 212–219.

24. Schwartz WB, Bank N, Cutler RWP. The influence of urinary ionic strength on phosphate $pK2$ and the determination of titratable acid. J Clin Invest 1959; 38:347–356.

25. Lemann J Jr, Bushinsky DA, Hamm LL. Bone buffering of acid and base in humans. Am J Physiol Renal Physiol 2003; 285:F811–F832.

26. Owen OE, Felig P, Morgan AP, Wahren J, Cahill GF Jr. Liver and kidney metabolism during prolonged starvation. J Clin Invest 1969; 48:574–583.

27. Hood VL, Danforth E Jr, Horton ES, Tannen RL. Impact of hydrogen ion on fasting ketogenesis: feedback regulation of acid production. Am J Physiol 1982; 242:F238–F245.

28. Atkinson DE, Bourke E. Metabolic aspects of the regulation of systemic pH. Am J Physiol 1987; 252:F947–F956.

29. Bean ES, Atkinson DE. Regulation of the rate of urea synthesis in liver by extracellular pH. A major factor in pH homeostasis in mammals. J Biol Chem 1984; 259:1552–1559.

30. Haussinger D, Sies H, Gerok W. Functional hepatocyte heterogeneity in ammonia metabolism. The intercellular glutamine cycle. J Hepatol 1985; 1:3–14.

31. Phromphetcharat V, Jackson A, Dass PD, Welbourne TC. Ammonia partitioning between glutamine and urea: interorgan participation in metabolic acidosis. Kidney Int 1981; 20:598–605.

32. Maddox DA, Gennari FJ. The early proximal tubule: a high-capacity delivery-responsive reabsorptive site. Am J Physiol 1987; 252:F573–F584.

33. Pitts RF, Alexander RS. The nature of the renal tubular mechanism for acidifying the urine. Am J Physiol 1945; 144:239.

34. Knepper MA, Packer R, Good DW. Ammonium transport in the kidney. Physiol Rev 1989; 69:179–249.

35. Halperin ML, Jungas RL. Metabolic production and renal disposal of hydrogen ions. Kidney Int 1983; 24:709–713.

36. Cohn DE, Klahr S, Hammerman MR. Metabolic acidosis and parathyroidectomy increase Na^+–H^+ exchange in brush border vesicles. Am J Physiol 1983; 245:F217–F222.

37. Capasso G, Unwin R, Ciani F, et al. Bicarbonate transport along the loop of Henle. II. Effects of acid–base, dietary, and neurohumoral determinants. J Clin Invest 1994; 94:830–838.

38. Jacobson HR. Effects of CO_2 and acetazolamide on bicarbonate and fluid transport in rabbit proximal tubules. Am J Physiol 1981; 240:F54–F62.

39. Levine DZ. An in vivo microperfusion study of distal tubule bicarbonate reabsorption in normal and ammonium chloride rats. J Clin Invest 1985; 75:588–895.

40. McFarlane-Anderson N, Alleyne GA. Transport of glutamine by rat kidney brush-border membrane vesicles. Biochem J 1979; 182:295–300.

41. Windus DW, Cohn DE, Klahr S, Hammerman MR. Glutamine transport in renal basolateral vesicles from dogs with metabolic acidosis. Am J Physiol 1984; 246:F78–F86.

42. Pitts RF. Production and excretion of ammonia in relation to acid–base regulation. In: Orloff J, Berliner RW, eds. Renal Physiology (Handbook of Physiology, Section 8). Bethesda: American Physiological Society, 1973: 455–496.

43. Schwartz WB, Cohen JJ. The nature of the renal response to chronic disorders of acid–base equilibrium. Am J Med 1978; 64:417–428.

44. Gennari FJ, Goldstein MB, Schwartz WB. The nature of the renal adaptation to chronic hypocapnia. J Clin Invest 1972; 51:1722–1730.

45. Schwartz WB, Brackett NC, Cohen JJ. The response of extracellular hydrogen ion concentration to graded degrees of chronic hypercapnia. J Clin Invest 1965; 44:291–301.

46. Krapf R, Beeler I, Hertner D, Hulter HN. Chronic respiratory alkalosis. The effect of sustained hyperventilation on renal regulation of acid–base equilibrium. N Engl J Med 1991; 324:1394–1401.

47. Chen LK, Boron WF. Acid extrusion in S3 segment of rabbit proximal tubule. I. Effect of bilateral CO_2/HCO_3. Am J Physiol 1995; 268:F179–F192.

48. Schwartz GJ, Al-Awqati Q. Carbon dioxide causes exocytosis of vesicles containing H^+ pumps in isolated perfused proximal and collecting tubules. J Clin Invest 1985; 75:1638–1644.

49. Cohen JJ, Madias NE, Wolf CJ, Schwartz WB. Regulation of acid–base equilibrium in chronic hypocapnia. Evidence that the response of the kidney is not geared to the defense of extracellular (H^+). J Clin Invest 1976; 57:1483–1489.

50. Madias NE, Schwartz WB, Cohen JJ. The maladaptive renal response to secondary hypocapnia during chronic HCl acidosis in the dog. J Clin Invest 1977; 60:1393–1401.

51. Madias NE, Adrogue HJ, Cohen JJ. Maladaptive renal response to secondary hypercapnia in chronic metabolic alkalosis. Am J Physiol 1980; 238:F283–9.

52. Madias NE, Adrogue HJ, Horowitz GL, Cohen JJ, Schwartz WB. A redefinition of normal acid–base equilibrium in man: carbon dioxide tension as a key determinant of normal plasma bicarbonate concentration. Kidney Int 1979; 16:612–618.

53. Madias NE, Adrogue HJ, Cohen JJ, Schwartz WB. Effect of natural variations in $PaCO_2$ on plasma [HCO_3^-] in dogs: a redefinition of normal. Am J Physiol 1979; 236:F30–F35.

54. Santella RN, Maddox DA, Gennari FJ. Delivery dependence of early proximal bicarbonate reabsorption in the rat in respiratory acidosis and alkalosis. J Clin Invest 1991; 87:631–638.

55. Sartorius OW, Roemmelt JC, Pitts RF. The renal regulation of acid–base balance in man. IV. The nature of the renal compensation in ammonium chloride acidosis. J Clin Invest 1949; 28:423–439.

56. Graber ML, Bengele HH, Mroz E, Lechene C, Alexander EA. Acute metabolic acidosis augments collecting duct acidification rate in the rat. Am J Physiol 1981; 241:F669–F676.

57. Santella RN, Gennari FJ, Maddox DA. Metabolic acidosis stimulates bicarbonate reabsorption in the early proximal tubule. Am J Physiol 1989; 257:F35–F42.

58. De Sousa RC, Harrington JT, Ricanati ES, Schelkrot JW, Schwartz WB. Renal regulation of acid–base equilibrium during chronic administration of mineral acid. J Clin Invest 1974; 53:465–476.

59. Harrington JT, Hulter HN, Cohen JJ, Madias NE. Mineralocorticoid-stimulated renal acidification: the critical role of dietary sodium. Kidney Int 1986; 30:43–48.

60. Lowance DC, Garfinkel HB, Mattern WD, Schwartz WB. The effect of chronic hypotonic volume expansion on the renal regulation of acid–base equilibrium. J Clin Invest 1972; 51:2928–2940.

61. Jehle S, Hulter HN, Krapf R. On the mechanism of growth hormone-induced stimulation of renal acidification in humans: effect of dietary NaCl. Clin Sci (Colch) 2000; 99:47–56.

62. Maddox DA, Gennari FJ. Load dependence of proximal tubular bicarbonate reabsorption in chronic metabolic alkalosis in the rat. J Clin Invest 1986; 77:709–716.

63. Kassirer JP, Schwartz WB. The response of normal man to selective depletion of hydrochloric acid. Am J Med 1966; 40:10–18.

64. Jacobson HR, Seldin DW. On the generation, maintenance, and correction of metabolic alkalosis. Am J Physiol 1983; 245:F425–F432.

65. Galla JH, Bonduris DN, Luke RG. Effects of chloride and extracellular fluid volume on bicarbonate reabsorption along the nephron in metabolic alkalosis in the rat. Reassessment of the classical hypothesis of the pathogenesis of metabolic alkalosis. J Clin Invest 1987; 80:41–50.

66. Kassirer JP, London AM, Goldman DM, Schwartz WB. On the pathogenesis of metabolic alkalosis in hyperaldosteronism. Am J Med 1970; 49:306–315.

67. Capasso G, Unwin R, Agulian S, Giebisch G. Bicarbonate transport along the loop of Henle. I. Microperfusion studies of load and inhibitor sensitivity. J Clin Invest 1991; 88:430–437.

68. Capasso G, Jaeger P, Giebisch G, Guckian V, Malnic G. Renal bicarbonate reabsorption in the rat. II. Distal tubule load dependence and effect of hypokalemia. J Clin Invest 1987; 80:409–414.

69. Richardson RM, Kunau RT Jr. Bicarbonate reabsorption in the papillary collecting duct: effect of acetazolamide. Am J Physiol 1982; 243:F74–F80.

70. Cogan MG, Carneiro AV, Tatsuno J, et al. Normal diet NaCl variation can affect the renal set-point for plasma pH- (HCO_3^-) maintenance. J Am Soc Nephrol 1990; 1:193–199.

71. Kurtzman NA. Regulation of renal bicarbonate reabsorption by extracellular volume. J Clin Invest 1970; 49:586–595.

72. Slatopolsky E, Hoffsten P, Purkerson M, Bricker NS. On the influence of extracellular fluid volume expansion and of uremia on bicarbonate reabsorption in man. J Clin Invest 1970; 49:988–998.

73. Cohen JJ. Selective Cl retention in repair of metabolic alkalosis without increasing filtered load. Am J Physiol 1970; 218:165–170.

74. Hernandez RE, Schambelan M, Cogan MG, Colman J, Morris RC Jr, Sebastian A. Dietary NaCl determines severity of potassium depletion-induced metabolic alkalosis. Kidney Int 1987; 31:1356–1367.

75. Sebastian A, Sutton JM, Hulter HN, Schambelan M, Poler SM. Effect of mineralocorticoid replacement therapy on renal acid–base homeostasis in adrenalectomized patients. Kidney Int 1980; 18:762–773.

76. Relman AS, Schwartz WB. The effect of DOCA on electrolyte balance in normal man and its relation to sodium chloride intake. Yale J Biol Med 1952; 24:540–558.

77. Stanton BA. Regulation of Na^+ and K^+ transport by mineralocorticoids. Semin Nephrol 1987; 7:82–90.

78. Hulter HN, Sebastian A, Toto RD, Bonner EL, Jr., Ilnicki LP. Renal and systemic acid-base effects of the chronic administration of hypercalcemia-

producing agents: calcitriol, PTH, and intravenous calcium. Kidney Int 1982; 21:445–58.

79. Hulter HN, Peterson JC. Acid–base homeostasis during chronic PTH excess in humans. Kidney Int 1985; 28:187–192.

80. Hellman DE, Au WYW, Bartter FC. Evidence for a direct effect of parathyroid hormone on urinary acidification. Am J Physiol 1965; 209:643–650.

81. Gesek FA, Schoolwerth AC. Hormonal interactions with the proximal Na(+)–H$^+$ exchanger. Am J Physiol 1990; 258:F514–F521.

82. Wang T, Giebisch G. Effects of angiotensin II on electrolyte transport in the early and late distal tubule in rat kidney. Am J Physiol 1996; 271:F143–F149.

83. Geibel J, Giebisch G, Boron WF. Angiotensin II stimulates both Na(+)–H$^+$ exchange and Na$^+$/HCO$_3^-$ cotransport in the rabbit proximal tubule. Proc Natl Acad Sci USA 1990; 87:7917–7920.

84. Liu FY, Cogan MG. Angiotensin II stimulation of hydrogen ion secretion in the rat early proximal tubule. Modes of action, mechanism, and kinetics. J Clin Invest 1988; 82:601–607.

85. Harris PJ, Young JA. Dose-dependent stimulation and inhibition of proximal tubular sodium reabsorption by angiotensin II in the rat kidney. Pflugers Arch 1977; 367:295–297.

86. Houillier P, Chambrey R, Achard JM, Froissart M, Poggioli J, Paillard M. Signaling pathways in the biphasic effect of angiotensin II on apical Na/H antiport activity in proximal tubule. Kidney Int 1996; 50:1496–1505.

87. Gesek FA, Strandhoy JW. Dual interactions between alpha 2-adrenoceptor agonists and the proximal Na(+)–H$^+$ exchanger. Am J Physiol 1990; 258:F636–F642.

88. Wang T, Chan YL. Neural control of distal tubular bicarbonate and fluid transport. Am J Physiol 1989; 257:F72–F76.

89. Chan YL. The role of norepinephrine in the regulation of fluid absorption in the rat proximal tubule. J Pharmacol Exp Ther 1980; 215:65–70.

90. Freiberg JM, Kinsella J, Sacktor B. Glucocorticoids increase the Na$^+$–H$^+$ exchange and decrease the Na$^+$ gradient-dependent phosphate-uptake systems in renal brush border membrane vesicles. Proc Natl Acad Sci USA 1982; 79:4932–4936.

91. Damasco MC, Malnic G. Effect of corticosteroids on proximal tubular acidification in the rat. Miner Electrolyte Metab 1987; 13:26–32.

92. Unwin R, Capasso G, Giebisch G. Bicarbonate transport along the loop of Henle effects of adrenal steroids. Am J Physiol 1995; 268:F234–F239.

93. Hulter HN, Licht JH, Bonner EL Jr, Glynn RD, Sebastian A. Effects of glucocorticoid steroids on renal and systemic acid–base metabolism. Am J Physiol 1980; 239:F30–F43.

94. Yonemura K, Cheng L, Sacktor B, Kinsella JL. Stimulation by thyroid hormone of Na$^+$–H$^+$ exchange activity in cultured opossum kidney cells. Am J Physiol 1990; 258:F333–F338.

95. Kinsella J, Sacktor B. Thyroid hormones increase Na$^+$–H$^+$ exchange activity in renal brush border membranes. Proc Natl Acad Sci USA 1985; 82: 3606–3610.

96. Baum M, Toto RD. Lack of a direct effect of atrial natriuretic factor in the rabbit proximal tubule. Am J Physiol 1986; 250:F66–F69.

97. Winaver J, Burnett JC, Tyce GM, Dousa TP. ANP inhibits Na(+)–H$^+$ antiport in proximal tubular brush border membrane: role of dopamine. Kidney Int 1990; 38:1133–1140.

98. Mahlbacher K, Sicuro A, Gerber H, Hulter HN, Krapf R. Growth hormone corrects acidosis-induced renal nitrogen wasting and renal phosphate depletion and attenuates renal magnesium wasting in humans. Metabolism 1999; 48:763–770.

99. Seldin DW, Welt LG, Cort JH. The role of sodium salts and adrenal steroids in the production of hypokalemic alkalosis. Yale J Biol Med 1956; 29:229–247.

100. Garella S, Chazan JA, Cohen JJ. Saline-resistant metabolic alkalosis or "chloride-wasting nephropathy". Report of four patients with severe potassium depletion. Ann Intern Med 1970; 73:31–38.

101. Garella S, Chang B, Kahn SI. Alterations of hydrogen ion homeostasis in pure potassium depletion: studies in rats and dogs during the recovery phase. J Lab Clin Med 1979; 93:321–331.

102. Capasso G, Kinne R, Malnic G, Giebisch G. Renal bicarbonate reabsorption in the rat. I. Effects of hypokalemia and carbonic anhydrase. J Clin Invest 1986; 78:1558–1567.

103. Doucet A, Marsy S. Characterization of K-ATPase activity in distal nephron: stimulation by potassium depletion. Am J Physiol 1987; 253:F418–F423.

104. Wingo CS. Active proton secretion and potassium absorption in the rabbit outer medullary collecting duct. Functional evidence for proton-potassium-activated adenosine triphosphatase. J Clin Invest 1989; 84:361–365.

105. Burnell JM, Teubner EJ, Simpson DP. Metabolic acidosis accompanying potassium deprivation. Am J Physiol 1974; 227:329–333.

106. Hulter HN, Sigala JF, Sebastian A. K$^+$ deprivation potentiates the renal alkalosis-producing effect of mineralocorticoid. Am J Physiol 1978; 235:F298–F309.

107. Jones JW, Sebastian A, Hulter HN, Schambelan M, Sutton JM, Biglieri EG. Systemic and renal acid–base effects of chronic dietary potassium depletion in humans. Kidney Int 1982; 21:402–410.

108. Tannen RL. The effect of uncomplicated potassium depletion on urine acidification. J Clin Invest 1970; 49:813–827.

109. Tannen RL. Effect of potassium on renal acidification and acid–base homeostasis. Semin Nephrol 1987; 7:263–273.

110. Hulter HN, Toto RD, Ilnicki LP, Sebastian A. Chronic hyperkalemic renal tubular acidosis induced by KCl loading. Am J Physiol 1983; 244:F255–F264.

111. Luke RG, Galla JH. Does chloride play an independent role in the pathogenesis of metabolic alkalosis?. Semin Nephrol 1989; 9:203–205.

112. Borkan S, Northrup TE, Cohen JJ, Garella S. Renal response to metabolic alkalosis induced by isovolemic hemofiltration in the dog. Kidney Int 1987; 32:322–328.

113. Galla JH, Bonduris DN, Dumbauld SL, Luke RG. Segmental chloride and fluid handling during correction of chloride-depletion alkalosis without volume expansion in the rat. J Clin Invest 1984; 73:96–106.

114. Wesson DE. Augmented bicarbonate reabsorption by both the proximal and distal nephron maintains chloride-deplete metabolic alkalosis in rats. J Clin Invest 1989; 84:1460–1469.

115. Gifford JD, Sharkins K, Work J, Luke RG, Galla JH. Total CO_2 transport in rat cortical collecting duct in chloride-depletion alkalosis. Am J Physiol 1990; 258:F848–F853.

116. Levine DZ, Iacovitti M, Harrison V. Bicarbonate secretion in vivo by rat distal tubules during alkalosis induced by dietary chloride restriction and alkali loading. J Clin Invest 1991; 87:1513–1518.

117. Star RA, Burg MB, Knepper MA. Bicarbonate secretion and chloride absorption by rabbit cortical collecting ducts. Role of chloride/bicarbonate exchange. J Clin Invest 1985; 76:1123–1130.

118. Wesson DE, Dolson GM. Enhanced HCO_3 secretion by distal tubule contributes to NaCl-induced correction of chronic alkalosis. Am J Physiol 1993; 264:F899–F906.

119. Wesson DE. Combined K^+ and Cl^- repletion corrects augmented H^+ secretion by distal tubules in chronic alkalosis. Am J Physiol 1994; 266:F592–F603.

120. Batlle DC, von Riotte A, Schlueter W. Urinary sodium in the evaluation of hyperchloremic metabolic acidosis. N Engl J Med 1987; 316:140–144.

121. Schiess WA, Ayer JL, Lottspeich WD, Pitts RF. The renal regulation of acid–base balance in man. II. Factors affecting the excretion of titratable acid in the normal human subject. J Clin Invest 1948; 27:57–64.

122. Gold LW, Massry SG, Arieff AI, Coburn JW. Renal bicarbonate wasting during phosphate depletion. A possible cause of altered acid–base homeostasis in hyperparathyroidism. J Clin Invest 1973; 52:2556–2561.

123. Krapf R, Glatz M, Hulter HN. Neutral phosphate administration generates and maintains renal metabolic alkalosis and hyperparathyroidism. Am J Physiol 1995; 268:F802–F807.

124. Bank N, Schwartz WB. The influence of anion penetrating ability on urinary acidification and the excretion of titratable acid. J Clin Invest 1960; 39:1516–1525.

125. Emmett M, Goldfarb S, Agus ZS, Narins RG. The pathophysiology of acid–base changes in chronically phosphate-depleted rats: bone–kidney interactions. J Clin Invest 1977; 59:291–298.

7

Gastrointestinal Influences on Hydrogen Ion Balance

Alan N. Charney

*NYU School of Medicine, Nephrology Section, VA Medical Center,
New York, New York, U.S.A.*

Mark Donowitz

*Hopkins Center for Epithelial Disorders, Johns Hopkins University School
of Medicine, Baltimore, Maryland, U.S.A.*

INTRODUCTION

The gastrointestinal tract plays an integral, though not obvious role in acid balance. Under normal circumstances, greater than 1000 mEq of H^+ and HCO_3^- are absorbed and secreted along the intestinal tract daily, associated with several hundred mmoles of dietary inorganic salts of organic cations and anions. Intestinal bacteria produce several hundred mmoles of organic acids that also may be absorbed or excreted in the stool (1–3). A complex relationship exists among these acid–base fluxes and the flux of other ions, involving many intestinal segmental and cellular control mechanisms (4). The size and nature of these fluxes and linkages are particularly relevant to acid balance following oral intake or in the presence of gastrointestinal disease.

Intestinal function markedly affects H^+ balance through absorption of dietary constituents. The nature of the diet, the degree of absorption and the stool excretion of metabolic products, all influence this balance. In addition, when the gastrointestinal tract is diseased, hundreds of mEq of H^+ or HCO_3^- may be lost, markedly disrupting acid–base balance. These losses

Table 1   Gastrointestinal Effects on Acid/Base Balance

I. Normal GI Tract
Diet
Drugs (e.g., diuretics, laxatives, milk alkali syndrome)
Therapy of acid/base disorders

II. Abnormal GI Tract
Vomiting (metabolic alkalosis)
Diarrhea (metabolic alkalosis or acidosis)
Fistulae (metabolic acidosis)
Surgery (metabolic alkalosis or acidosis)
Villous adenoma (metabolic alkalosis or acidosis)

---

can be caused by abnormalities in the enteric nervous system, by inflammatory mediators (including histamine, 5-hydroxytryptamine, eicosanoids, and nitric oxide) and by abnormal generation of the intracellular second messengers cAMP, cGMP, and calcium (5). Drugs, certain foods, and intestinal surgery and drainage may have similar effects. Finally, by absorbing orally administered medications, electrolytes and water, the intestine may be an important route for the development of or therapy for systemic acid–base disorders. The ways in which the normal and abnormal gastrointestinal tract relates to acid–base balance are summarized in Table 1.

THE INTESTINE IS NOT A KIDNEY

There are anatomic and physiologic parallels between the intestinal tract and the nephrons of the kidney. The structure of the gastrointestinal tract, divided into interacting but distinct regions with characteristic ion transport processes, is similar to the functional heterogeneity of the renal tubule. A major difference is the coordination of transport processes in the gastrointestinal tract by rich communicating networks formed by extensive endocrine, paracrine, and neural mediators. In both organ systems, H^+ and HCO_3^- transport influences and is influenced by the transmembrane and transepithelial transport of other ions such as Na^+ and Cl^-. This influence may be direct and affect cotransport or antiport processes, or may be indirect through effects on transmembrane or transepithelial electrical gradients. In both the kidney and the small and large intestine, the site of absorption and the rate of transport of Na^+ and Cl^- are influenced by changes in acid–base variables (pH, PCO_2, and $[HCO_3^-]$) (2,6–15). In contrast to the kidney, however, excretion of Na^+ and Cl^- in the stool is not affected by epithelial H^+ and HCO_3^- transport or by the systemic acid/base status (16–19). In further contrast to the kidney, acid secretion by the gastric parietal cell is not affected by systemic acid–base status. Systemic $[HCO_3^-]$ does influence ileal and colonic net HCO_3^- secretion (11,12,20), but the intestine exhibits only a transient and ultimately insignificant alteration in its excretion of base (in the form of HCO_3^- and organic anions) in the presence of metabolic acid/base disorders (2,14,16–19,21,22). Thus, the intestine shares none of the changes in electrolyte excretion that occur in the kidney in response to metabolic acid–base disorders. Similarly, there is no gastrointestinal response analogous to the renal response to respiratory disorders.

These differences between the kidney and gastrointestinal tract reflect different homeostatic roles with regard to solute, water, and acid–base physiology. The kidney regulates the volume, acidity, quantity, and concentration of the ionic constituents of the extracellular fluid through adjustments in reabsorption and excretion. The gastrointestinal tract exhibits none of these features. If the gastrointestinal tract is homeostatic in any sense, it is based on its role to provide the body with the constituents needed for survival (through regulated absorption). There is a homeostatic arrangement of sorts between the intestine and the kidney: the intestine is organized around efficient absorption; the kidney's role involves regulation by selective excretion.

BIOAVAILABILITY OF ORAL INTAKE

The most unique feature of the intestine as a transport organ is the nearly complete absorption of dietary constituents under normal conditions. The "bioavailability" of orally administered fluids, electrolytes, nutrients, and sources of acids and bases is nearly 100% (23). In adults eating a 2600 kcal Western diet, this amounts to 1–4 L of water, 400 g carbohydrate, 50–75 g protein, 75–100 g fat, 150 mEq Na^+, 100 mEq K^+, 200 mEq Cl^-, 50 mmol organic anions (e.g., citrate), and other nutrients (Table 2). Infants and children consume even greater quantities per kilogram body weight. This absorptive feat is remarkable when one considers the quantity of endogenous intestinal secretions: water: 7 L, Na^+: 650 mEq, K^+: 50 mEq, Cl^-: 500 mEq, and HCO_3^-: 200 mEq. Note that except for K^+, endogenous secretion of water and electrolytes by the gastrointestinal tract far exceeds oral intake. These secretions, which occur predominantly in response to dietary intake, are completely absorbed as well. Thus, aside from 10 mmol of organic anions, the normal stool contains less than 150 mL of water, less than 5 mEq each of Na^+, Cl^-, and HCO_3^-, and approximately 10 mEq of K^+.

The essentially complete absorption of water and solute is based on three distinct characteristics of the intestinal epithelium: a progressive increase in absorptive efficiency from jejunum to colon, excess transport capacity under normal conditions, and the capacity to adapt to altered or abnormal conditions (24–26). On a stable diet, the small and large intestines have the capacity to absorb a two- to three-fold greater quantity of fluid and

Table 2 Exogenous (Dietary) and Endogenous Input into the Gastrointestinal Tract

	Carbohydrates	Protein	Fat	Organic acids	Water (L/day)	$[Na^+]$	$[K^+]$	$[Cl^-]$	$[HCO_3^-]$	Organic anions (mmol/day)
		(gm/day)						(mEq/day)		
Exogenous (dietary)	400	50–75	75–100	<5	1–4	150	100	200	0	50
Endogenous	0	50	0	350	7	650	50	500	200	0
Total absorbed	400	100–125	75–100	350	8–11	800	140	700	200	40
Stool excretion	0	0	0	<5	0.1	<5	10	<5	<5	10

solutes than are usually presented to them following meals (27–30). This capacity is not affected by the frequency of food ingestion (31–33), the relative quantities of protein, fat, and carbohydrate (34), or the quantity of dietary constituents (35,36). Four-fold enrichment of dietary precursors of organic anions, for example, produces no changes in the fecal output of Na^+, K^+ and organic anions (37).

Changes in the intestinal excretion of Na^+ and K^+ in response to changes in dietary Na^+ and K^+ are minimal (27,38–40). The close link between diet and urine Na^+ and K^+ confirms that intestinal absorption or excretion of these ions cannot play an important role in their balance. Stool losses of solute and water are minimal over a wide range of dietary habits and conditions.

An important clinical application of near-100% bioavailability is that many electrolyte and acid–base disorders, even those generated by gastrointestinal disorders, can be treated by the oral route. Orally administered fluids, electrolytes, acids, and bases may be assumed to be completely absorbed. The effects of these remedies depend on the appropriateness of the treatment rather than on the extent of the remedy's absorption. As examples, hypokalemia is safely corrected by oral administration of potassium salts, and chronic metabolic acidosis may be treated by the oral administration of $NaHCO_3$ or bicarbonate-generating salts. The most dramatic example is oral rehydration therapy for ongoing secretory diarrhea. Clinical confidence in the efficiency of intestinal absorption is the basis of the gastrointestinal tract as a therapeutic route of choice.

IMPORTANCE OF DIET

The composition of the diet determines the nature and quantity of acids or bases that must be excreted daily by the kidney to maintain balance (2,41). Absorption of digested dietary proteins and to a lesser extent nucleic acids, carbohydrate and fat provides the substrates for metabolic acid production. These acids include sulfuric and phosphoric acids and various organic acids that cannot be further oxidized (e.g., uric acid, oxalic acid, glucuronic acid).

A less commonly recognized contribution of the diet to acid balance is the ingestion of inorganic salts of organic acids (e.g., potassium citrate). Approximately 40 mmol of organic anions are absorbed each day from an average Western diet. These anions consume H^+ ions (i.e., generate HCO_3^-) when metabolized in the liver (2,17,41). This diet-derived HCO_3^- increases renal organic anion excretion, suggesting an effect of diet on endogenous organic acid production (2,42). Approximately one-third of this urinary anion is citrate, which aids in the prevention of kidney stones. The diet also contains a small quantity (<5 mmol) of protonated organic acids (e.g., citric

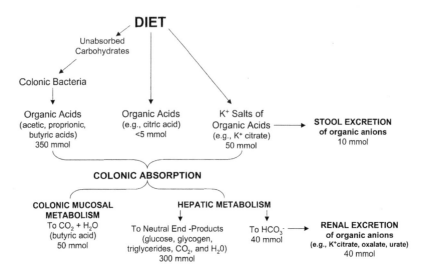

Figure 1   Absorption, metabolism, and excretion of short-chain fatty acids and anions. Indicated quantities, in mmols/day, are for the average Western diet.

acid); however, upon absorption they do not yield net H^+ ions because they are readily metabolized to neutral end products. A diagram of the sources, absorption, excretion and metabolism of organic acids and anions is presented in Fig. 1. Despite the large impact of diet on endogenous acid production and on renal acid excretion, wide variations in intake have little effect on systemic pH or $[HCO_3^-]$ (43) (see Chapters 6 and 8).

Role of Colonic Bacteria

Bacteria also produce organic acids in the colonic lumen, predominantly in the cecum. Carbohydrates (including nondigestible fiber, mono- and disaccharides, and starches) that fail to be absorbed more proximally may be metabolized by resident anaerobic bacteria to short chain fatty acids. These fatty acids contain from one (formic acid) to six (caproic acid) carbons and are ubiquitous in the colon. The three most plentiful are acetic (60%), propionic (25%), and butyric acids (15%) (44). Approximately 350 mmol of these acids are produced daily and as a group they may reach luminal concentrations of greater than 100 mmol/L. Absorption is nearly complete and serves to provide fuel for oxidative metabolism in colonic mucosal cells (1,3,45,46). The importance of short chain fatty acids (especially butyric acid) for nutrition of colonic epithelium is suggested by the colitis that results when the supply is diminished relative to metabolic demands (primarily of ion transport). Such a reduction in fatty acids may occur following antibiotic therapy or when the colon is bypassed and removed from the fecal stream (nutritional or diversion colitis) (46,47). Absorption of short chain fatty acids also stimulates Na^+, Cl^- and water absorption and this is evident in various diarrheal diseases when their concentrations are reduced and therefore their proabsorptive effects are lost (46,48).

Under normal conditions, these organic acids of bacterial origin, like those in the diet, do not affect acid–base balance when they are absorbed because the end products of their metabolism are neutral (Fig. 1). Each day, up to 50 mmol of butyric acid and lesser quantities of propionate and acetate are metabolized locally by the colonic mucosa to CO_2 and H_2O (1,45,46). Acetic, propionic and butyric acids are metabolized by the liver to triglycerides or CO_2 and H_2O, and propionic acid is metabolized to glucose or glycogen (1). Up to 5–10% of the energy needs of the body are provided for by these processes (46). Approximately 10 mmol of organic anions are excreted in the stool each day and, by their osmotic contribution, these anions are a determinant of stool water and volume (37). These anions are either ingested (see earlier) or are formed by the reaction of organic acids with luminal HCO_3^-: e.g., acetic acid $+ HCO_3^- \rightarrow$ acetate $+ H_2O + CO_2$. When considered together with the organic acids and HCO_3^- (<5 mEq) found in the stool, they comprise the net excretion of base by the intestine (Table 2).

Effects of Fasting

During the interprandial state, the intestine neither adds to nor subtracts H^+ and HCO_3^- ions from body fluids. The basal levels of gastric and small intestinal electrolyte and fluid secretion and small intestinal and colonic electrolyte and fluid absorption are almost exactly matched. These are not inconsequential quantities and volumes, but are a fraction of the output following food ingestion (Table 3). In either the fed or fasting state, stool losses of inorganic solutes and water are small. Fasting, if sufficiently prolonged and associated with decreased insulin levels, increases endogenous organic acid production as fat replaces carbohydrate as the major metabolic fuel. Ketoacidosis results, but compared with the process in diabetics, the acidosis is less severe (see later, gastrointestinal causes of metabolic acidosis).

Fasting or an equivalent absence of dietary precursors also reduces colonic production, stool excretion, and (presumably) absorption of organic anions (3,49). The effect this reduction has on systemic acid–base balance has not been studied. In fasting ketoacidosis, the absence of this source of potential base would presumably worsen the acidosis. During early fasting, ketonuria and associated natriuresis ensure a large urine volume, which aids the excretion of metabolic waste products and prevents uric acid stone formation when urine pH is low (50). During more prolonged fasting, increasing renal Na^+ avidity reduces urinary losses of Na^+ and water, both of which are in short supply during the fast. The reduction in diet-derived

Table 3   Rate of Flow and Electrolyte Concentrations of Gastrointestinal Fluids

	Volume (L/day)	[Na$^+$]	[K$^+$]	[Cl$^-$]	[HCO$_3^-$]
		(mEq/L)			
Saliva					
Unstimulated	0.2	10	30	10	15
Stimulated	1	50–90	20	50	60
Gastric fluid					
Unstimulated	0.5	80–100	5–10	100–120	10
Stimulated	1.5–2	10–20	5–15	130–160	0
Achlorhydria	1	50–120	5–10	100	20
Bile	1	135–155	5–10	85–110	40
Pancreatic fluid	2	120–160	5–10	30–75	70–120
Small intestinal fluid (succus entericus)	1	75–120	5–10	70–125	30
Ileostomy drainage					
New	1	115–140	5–15	95–125	30
Adapted	0.5	40–90	5	20	15–30
Colostomy	1	50–115	10–30	35–70	15–25
Normal stool	<0.15	20–30	55–75	15–25	30

Source: Adapted from Ref. 41.

organic anions further reduces urinary flow and decreases the inhibitory effect of these anions on renal tubular urate secretion. Despite these changes in urine flow and urate concentration, kidney stone formation is uncommon during prolonged fasting. This is in part because, as urine flow diminishes, decreased delivery of Na$^+$ to the distal nephron limits H$^+$ (and K$^+$) secretion, raises urinary pH toward 6, and thereby reduces the concentration of relatively insoluble uric acid (50).

INTESTINAL TRANSIT TIME

The transport function of the intestine is characterized by one feature that is unique among epithelial tissues: the transit time between segments may vary. The causes of this variation depend on the segments involved, although the most important influence is the luminal constituents themselves. Under normal conditions, changes in gastric and small intestinal motor activity are linked to segment-specific intestinal secretion by neural, paracrine, and endocrine mechanisms (51,52). This motor activity and secretion aid luminal mixing, digestion, and (in the small intestine) absorption. There is no evidence for motility-associated colonic secretion, but colonic motility by its nature slows the passage of the fecal mass and promotes absorption and bacterial growth.

Postprandial Alkaline Tide

One consequence of the variation in transit time in the proximal bowel is the generation of a transient postprandial increase in HCO_3^- stores, and the so-called "alkaline tide". The delay between gastric H^+ secretion in response to oral intake and the duodenal, pancreatic and biliary secretion of HCO_3^-, stimulated by gastric emptying, may range from several minutes to several hours. During this time, gastric venous $[HCO_3^-]$ rises (53,54) and is not immediately titrated by the relatively acidic venous outflow of the duodenum, pancreas, and gall bladder. The newly formed HCO_3^- is excreted by the kidney and urine pH rises (53,55). Loss of base is minimal when the delay is short, or when gastric acid secretion is minimal due to disease or pharmacologic inhibition of H^+ secretion (53). In all instances, the increase in blood $[HCO_3^-]$ is small (~ 1 mEq/L) and transient (56).

Patients with duodenal ulcer secrete excess acid as compared to normal individuals (see later). Patients with the Zollinger–Ellison syndrome have even more marked and uncontrolled gastric acid secretion (basal rate >15 mEq H^+/hr). However, urine base losses are not excessive in either disorder because of compensatory increases in fasting secretin and, as a consequence, in pancreatic HCO_3^- secretion (57). For this reason, metabolic acid–base disorders do not occur unless vomiting or diarrhea ensues. Unfortunately, the latter complications are common in patients with the Zollinger–Ellison syndrome, and invariably lead to significant metabolic alkalosis or acidosis.

Clinical Correlates of Altered Motility

Intestinal transit time may be shortened or lengthened by a variety of pathologic states involving serum electrolyte concentrations (e.g., K^+ or Ca^{2+}), the thyroid metabolic state, the presence of mechanical obstruction, dysfunction of the enteric nervous system, the presence of secretagogues, and invasive intestinal infections (58). The presence of watery diarrhea, a condition associated with fluid, electrolyte, and acid–base abnormalities, is commonly thought of as an imbalance between the ileocecal delivery of fluid and the colon's absorptive capacity (28,30,59). Shortened transit time should decrease the contact time between luminal contents and the absorptive epithelium, and increase fluid delivery to the colon. However, over a wide range of transit rates and for most segments of the small bowel, variations in transit time are not the primary cause of symptoms, or disturbances in acid–base, water, and electrolyte balance. Lengthened transit time is part of the mechanism of action of several antidiarrheal drugs and may favor bacterial overgrowth of the small intestine (1,60). Such overgrowth promotes organic acid overproduction, and in the special circumstance of a surgically produced intestinal blind loop or short bowel may result in metabolic acidosis (see later).

Surprisingly, colonic motility does not reliably correlate with the presence of most cases of diarrhea or constipation (61). However, decreased transit time due to increased colonic motility probably is an important component of the diarrhea associated with diabetes mellitus (62), hyperthyroidism (63), and irritable bowel syndrome (64). Even in these cases, other mechanisms of diarrhea are usually present including fat, bile acid, and glucose malabsorption and active electrolyte secretion (62–65). It appears that decreased intestinal transit time exacerbates rather than produces the diarrheal disorder (60).

CELLULAR TRANSPORT PATHWAYS OF H^+ AND HCO_3^-

Each gastrointestinal organ contributes to H^+ and HCO_3^- transport by either adding to or removing H^+ or HCO_3^- from the intestinal lumen or systemic circulation. The quantity of transported ions and water varies with the intestinal segment, the presence or suggestion (sham feeding) of food, and in certain cases by disease or drugs (Table 3). The functions served by H^+ and HCO_3^- transport and the resulting changes in luminal and cellular pH differ among the gastrointestinal organs. In general, these functions aid in the digestion, assimilation, and absorption of ingested foodstuffs, and are described in detail elsewhere (66,67).

The fluxes of H^+ and HCO_3^- considered here are transmembrane and transcellular (rather than paracellular) and are frequently linked to or are dependent on the fluxes of Na^+, K^+, and Cl^- ions. These processes include Na^+/H^+ exchange, Cl^-/HCO_3^- exchange, H^+/K^+ exchange, $Na^+/K^+/2Cl^-$ cotransport, membrane channels that conduct Na^+, K^+, Cl^-, or HCO_3^-, and ATP-driven exchange including Na^+/K^+ ATPase and H^+/K^+ ATPase. These transport proteins are found in apical or basolateral membrane locations depending on whether the cell absorbs H^+ and/or HCO_3^- from the lumen or secretes one or both species into the lumen. In some cases, the absorption of one species and secretion of the other takes place in separate cells. The net flux of H^+ in one direction (e.g., into the lumen) requires that HCO_3^- be transported in the opposite direction (e.g., into the blood). When H^+ and HCO_3^- are transported in the same direction at equivalent rates, there is no net transport of either species.

Some diseases affect all the transporting cells in a gastrointestinal segment (e.g., atrophic gastritis), while other diseases (e.g., *H. pylori* infection) and drugs (e.g., H^+/K^+ ATPase inhibitors) target specific transport processes and therefore the functions of specific cells. Systemic acid–base disorders do not result simply from the stimulation or inhibition of one or more of these transmembrane ion transport processes. As will be described below, gastrointestinal fluid must be lost from the body for systemic pH to be threatened. Nevertheless, the rates of specific transport processes are usually altered in association with fluid loss, and therefore are major determinants of the pathogenesis and therapy of the resulting acid–base disorder.

Salivary Glands

Salivary secretion is carried out by acini and duct cells of the parotid, sublingual, and submandibular glands under the influence of the sympathetic and parasympathetic nervous systems. As shown in Table 3, salivary secretion may total 1 L/day and contains approximately equal amounts of Cl^- and HCO_3^- (50 and 60 mEq/day, respectively). Because fluid (and therefore electrolyte) losses are relatively small, only a minimal effect on systemic acid–base balance would be expected when saliva is drained because of pharyngeal or esophageal pathology.

Esophagus

The squamous epithelium of the esophagus does not exhibit significant transport of water or electrolytes.

Stomach

The stomach parietal cell secretes H^+ into the lumen and HCO_3^- into the venous blood when food is ingested (Fig. 2) (66). Gastric secretion is a combination of HCl secretion from parietal cells and mucus cell secretion.

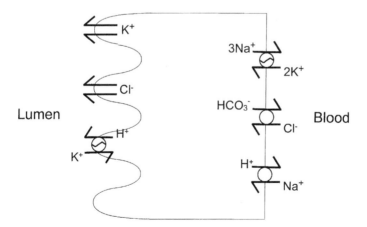

Gastric Parietal Cell

Figure 2 Gastric parietal cell plasma membrane ion transport processes under H^+-stimulated conditions. *Source*: Adapted from Ref. 66.

These cells secrete different solutions at different rates: parietal cells secrete a Na^+-poor solution of pH 1–2 at rates of 0.1–7 mL/min; mucus cells secrete an Na^+-rich solution at a rate of 1 mL/min (Table 3). The rate of parietal cell secretion is controlled by the neurohumoral response to food ingestion (or sham feeding) and may be stimulated or inhibited by disease and drugs. Under normal conditions, the basal rate of H^+ secretion averages 1–2 mEq/ hr and the maximal H^+ secretory rate is approximately 20 mEq/hr.

H^+ is secreted by the H^+/K^+ ATPase, a membrane-spanning protein which consists of a 100 kD α-subunit and 40 kD β-subunit (see Chapter 5). This ATPase is an electroneutral ion pump that has an active phosphorylated intermediate (E1E2 type) that exchanges H^+ for K^+ with 1:1 stoichiometry and uses one molecule of ATP per transport cycle. The H^+/K^+ ATPase is present in parietal cells on intracellular tubulovesicles under basal conditions. Following stimulation of acid secretion by gastrin, acetylcholine, or histamine (via H2 receptors), the tubulovesicles undergo exocytosis to fuse with the apical membrane and expand the apical surface area by 10-fold. H^+ secretion is terminated by somatostatin. The transport processes on the apical plasma membrane of parietal cells include K^+ and Cl^- channels and a variable amount of H^+/K^+ ATPase (Fig. 2). The basolateral membrane contains a Cl^-/HCO_3^- exchanger and several Na^+/H^+ exchangers (including isoforms NHE1, 2, and 4). Intracellular H^+ and HCO_3^- are produced by the action of carbonic anhydrase. The K^+ exchanged for H^+ across the apical membrane is recycled across the apical membrane by an apical membrane K^+ channel. Apical HCl secretion is electroneutral because both H^+ and Cl^- move from the cell into the lumen, the Cl^- moving through a still to be identified Cl^- channel. HCl secretion stops when the H^+/K^+ ATPase is removed from the apical membrane by endocytosis.

Pancreas

The pancreas secretes 1–2 L/day of isotonic fluid consisting of NaCl under basal (fasting) conditions and $NaHCO_3$ when stimulated (Fig. 3). Na^+ and K^+ are present at concentrations similar to those in blood under basal and stimulated conditions. Pancreatic duct secretion is primarily regulated by secretin, which acts through the adenylate cyclase-cAMP system. Ninety percent of secreted HCO_3^- is derived from the plasma. Bicarbonate secretion occurs against an electrochemical gradient energized by basolateral membrane Na^+/K^+ ATPase (68–70). An Na^+/H^+ exchanger transports intracellular H^+ ions, generated through the action of carbonic anhydrase, across the basolateral membrane. Cl^- crosses the apical membrane via the cystic fibrosis transmembrane regulator (CFTR) channel and is recycled by an apical membrane Cl^-/HCO_3^- exchanger. It is not known if HCO_3^- secretion occurs through the CFTR, which has a low but measurable permeability for HCO_3^-, or whether HCO_3^- is entirely secreted by apical anion

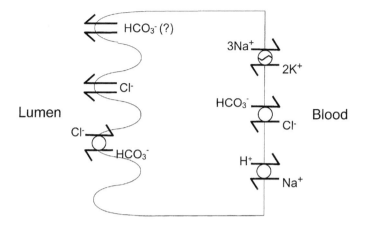

Pancreatic Duct Cell

Figure 3 Panceatic duct cell plasma membrane ion transport processes. *Source*: Adapted from Refs. 68–70.

exchange. The secreted anion is accompanied by paracellular transport of Na^+.

Duodenum

The major function of the duodenum is to allow for the osmotic equilibrium and pH adjustment of gastric effluent. No matter whether food is hypertonic, hypotonic, or isotonic to body fluids, the luminal contents are near isotonic and pH is 7.00 by the end of the duodenum. This is due to the movement of water and electrolytes through the relatively permeable duodenal mucosa and the isotonic secretion of HCO_3^- by Brunner's glands, duodenal crypt cells, pancreatic duct cells, and biliary cholangiocytes (71).

Jejunum and Ileum

In addition to its absorptive functions, the small intestine also secretes approximately 1 L/day of fluid containing 30 mEq of HCO_3^- and a variable amount of Cl^- (Table 3). The balance between Na^+ absorption and Cl^- secretion varies based on the stage of digestion. In the fasting state, the absorptive processes predominate, but immediately after eating, the reverse is true. Later in the digestive process, as diet-derived solute and HCO_3^--rich pancreatic secretions enter the small intestine, absorptive processes predominate again and secretory processes decline.

The Na^+ absorptive cell in the small intestine is the villus enterocyte (Fig. 4). In the absence of active transport, there is basal net water and

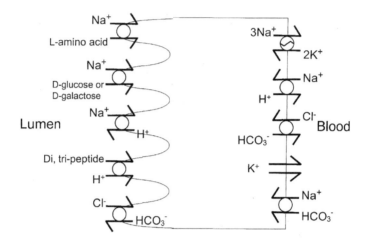

Small Intestine Na⁺ Absorptive Cell

Figure 4 Small intestinal Na^+ absorptive cell. Na^+–L-amino acids and Na^+ D-glucose or D-galactose refer to Na^+-linked substrate co-transporters that are linked to a Na^+ gradient. Di, tripeptide-H^+ co-transporters are linked to a H^+ gradient.

electrolyte secretion caused by tissue hydrostatic pressure. Basolateral membrane Na^+/K^+ ATPase generates an electrochemical gradient across the plasma membrane and a series of apical membrane Na^+ transport proteins use that gradient to energize lumen-to-cell Na^+ uptake. Several of these apical transport proteins take up products of digestion and include an Na^+-D-glucose/D-galactose transporter (SGLT1), a series of Na^+-L-amino acid transporters, and an H^+-dipeptide/tripeptide cotransporter. Another Na^+ uptake process is called electroneutral NaCl absorption. This process consists of an apical membrane Na^+/H^+ exchanger (NHE3 or NHE2, see Chapter 5) linked to an apical membrane Cl^-/HCO_3^- exchanger. This apical membrane anion exchanger has not yet been identified at a molecular level, but there is increasing evidence that it is the gene product of the downregulated-in-adenoma gene. The nature of the link between these exchangers is uncertain but may be a small local change in intracellular pH regulated by carbonic anhydrase activity. It also could involve a physical association via PDZ-domain proteins such as NHERF1 or NHERF2. The human jejunum has more Cl^-/HCO_3^- exchangers than Na^+/H^+ exchangers, and this disparity likely accounts for the lower level of neutral NaCl absorption in the jejunum than in the ileum. A basolateral K^+ channel helps maintain the transmembrane electrochemical gradient and recycles K^+ taken up from the interstitium by basolateral membrane Na^+/K^+ ATPase.

Chloride secretion is largely but not entirely restricted to the intestinal crypts (Fig. 5). A specialized Cl^- secretory cell exhibits Na^+/K^+ ATPase

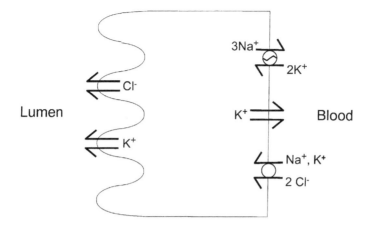

Small Intestinal Cl⁻ Secretory Cell

Figure 5 Small intestinal Cl⁻ secretory cell. *Source*: Adapted from Ref. 67.

activity, an $Na^+/K^+/2Cl^-$ co-transporter, and a K^+ channel along both the apical and basolateral membranes (67). The only transport processes along the apical membrane are a series of Cl^- channels including CFTR. It is unclear but likely that these apical Cl^- channels also transport HCO_3^-.

The major jejunal Na^+ absorptive process stimulated by meals is Na^+-substrate cotransport. In the ileum, luminal Na^+ stimulates apical membrane Na^+/H^+ exchange and neurohumoral and paracrine mediators stimulate electroneutral NaCl absorptive processes. Under basal (fasting) conditions, apical membrane anion channels in the Cl^- secretory cell are closed. In response to second messengers cAMP, cGMP, elevated intracellular Ca^{2+} and cell shrinkage, Cl^- channels open and basolateral membrane $Na^+/K^+/2Cl^-$ cotransport increases. Cholinergic, adrenergic, and locally released paracrine substances and NO appear to be major regulators of both electroneutral NaCl absorption and Cl^- secretion.

Colon

The pattern of colonic electrolyte transport is similar to that of the small intestine with active Na^+ transport present in surface and probably in some crypt cells, and active Cl^- secretion in crypt cells (72,73). Again, energy for all active electrolyte transport is spent at a basolateral membrane Na^+/K^+ ATPase. In Na^+ absorptive cells, the apical membrane Na^+ transport processes are electrogenic Na^+ absorption mediated by the epithelial Na^+ channel, ENaC, and electroneutral NaCl absorption (Fig. 6). The latter process consists, as in the ileum, of apical membrane Na^+/H^+ exchange and

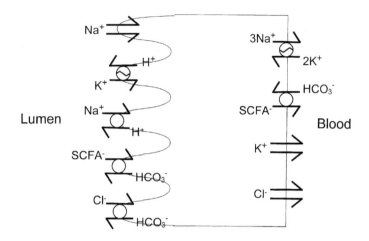

Distal Colonic Na⁺ Absorptive Cell

Figure 6   Distal colonic Na$^+$ absorptive cell.

Cl^-/HCO_3^- exchange. In addition, an apical membrane short chain fatty acid/anion exchanger linked to Na^+/H^+ antiporters (NHE3 and NHE2) and H^+/K^+ ATPase are present. It is not known how much H^+ is secreted by this H^+/K^+ ATPase. Stool pH (6.5–7.5) is similar to ileal luminal pH, suggesting that H^+ secretion into this poorly buffered medium is minimal. Na^+ absorptive cells have basolateral membrane K^+ and Cl^- channels as well. The colonic Cl^- secretory cell appears to have the same complement of transporters in the same locations as the small intestinal Cl^- secretory cell (Fig. 5).

GASTROINTESTINAL CAUSES OF ACID/BASE DISORDERS

The large quantity of water and electrolytes normally absorbed and secreted by the intestinal tract make this organ a prime source of metabolic acid–base and electrolyte disorders. Intestinal segments differ markedly with respect to fluid composition and secretory volume as shown in Table 3. In general, gastric fluid losses tend to cause metabolic alkalosis, and small intestinal fluid losses cause metabolic acidosis. A wide variety of clinical conditions may be responsible including intestinal inflammation, infections, tumors, and surgery (Table 4).

Not all intestinal fluid losses cause a clinically recognized acid–base disorder. The quantity of fluid lost, the type and quantity of oral or parenteral intake, and the metabolic and renal excretory capacity are all factors in determining the effect of gastrointestinal fluid losses on acid–base balance.

Table 4 Gastrointestinal Causes of Metabolic Alkalosis and Acidosis

---

A. Metabolic alkalosis
Vomiting, nasogastric suction, gastrostomy drainage
Inflammatory bowel disease (when colitis is present)
Osmotic diarrhea (lactose intolerance, laxatives and antacids)
Congenital chloride diarrhea, villous adenoma
Laxative abuse
Milk alkali syndrome, ingestion of HCO_3^- in renal failure

B. Metabolic acidosis
Secretory diarrhea
Fistulae
Villous adenoma
Ureteral diversion
Ileostomy
Jejunoileal bypass or blind loop

At the extremes, vomiting in a patient with the Zollinger–Ellison syndrome in whom basal gastric acid secretion is increased 10-fold will result in severe metabolic alkalosis, and diarrhea caused by cholera-induced net secretion in intestinal segments that normally absorb results in large fecal water losses and severe metabolic acidosis (48,74,75).

Importance of Gastrointestinal Na$^+$ and K$^+$ Losses

Essentially all gastrointestinal causes of metabolic acid–base disorders are associated with Na$^+$ and K$^+$ deficits. Sodium losses increase in direct proportion to the volume of gastric effluent or diarrheal water loss across a wide spectrum of causes (76,77). The resultant stimulation of Na$^+$ reabsorption by the kidney is proportional to the Na$^+$ deficit and a determinant of the severity of the acid/base disorder. Potassium losses also predictably accompany gastrointestinal fluid losses and like Na$^+$ losses are dependent on the volume lost, albeit to a smaller degree. The kidney is the predominant site of K$^+$ loss in metabolic alkalosis due to vomiting (see Chapters 17 and 18). Because K$^+$ loss may accompany both metabolic alkalosis and acidosis, other factors (described below) determine the nature of the acid–base disorder. Nevertheless, K$^+$ deficits are important in the pathogenesis of metabolic alkalosis, and affect the severity of both metabolic acid–base disorders by altering both cellular H$^+$ distribution and renal H$^+$ excretion (see Chapter 17).

Stimulation of collecting duct Na$^+$ reabsorption and urinary K$^+$ loss also accompany the abnormalities of acid–base balance caused by certain foods and orally administered drugs. The foods include licorice and some soft drinks containing glycyrrhetinic acid, an inhibitor of renal

11 β-hydroxysteroid dehydrogenase (78) (see Chapter 18). Inhibition of this enzyme causes an overabundance of cortisol at the mineralocorticoid receptor, and cortisol binds to and activates the receptor. The combination of mineralocorticoid-stimulated Na^+ reabsorption and K^+ wasting results in metabolic alkalosis. Various drugs may cause acid–base disorders even when prescribed and taken in accordance with their clinical indications. For example, diuretics may cause metabolic acidosis (e.g., acetazolamide) or metabolic alkalosis (e.g., hydrochlorothiazide) by promoting the urinary loss of Na^+, K^+, and HCO_3^- ions or Na^+, K^+, and Cl^- ions, respectively.

Metabolic Alkalosis

Gastric Fluid Loss

Loss of gastric acid through vomiting, nasogastric suction, or gastric drainage results in the direct addition of HCO_3^- to body fluids (79). Depletion of Cl^- and urinary losses of Na^+ and K^+ contribute to the generation and maintenance of the alkalosis (see Chapter 16). The volume and pH of the gastric fluid determine the severity of the alkalosis. Recurrent vomiting may occur in many intestinal diseases including obstruction of the intestine (at any level), pancreatitis, peritonitis, infectious and noninfectious gastroenteritis, and peptic ulcer disease. Nonintestinal diseases may cause vomiting as well: diabetic ketosis, uremia, various drugs, and central nervous system disorders. Vomiting in bulimia and/or anorexia (binge-purge syndrome) and the Zollinger–Ellison syndrome are two of the most common causes of severe metabolic alkalosis.

Urine pH and electrolyte concentrations reflect the pathogenesis of vomiting-induced alkalosis (Table 5). Acutely, urinary loss of HCO_3^- will produce a urine pH >7 and concomitant losses of Na^+ and K^+ ions. Because of the loss of Cl^-, the urine $[Cl^-]$ is very low ($<10\,mEq/L$). Not well recognized is the continued excretion of an alkaline, Na^+-rich urine if vomiting is persistent (80). When vomiting diminishes or ceases, urine pH

Table 5 Urinary Findings in Vomiting-Induced Metabolic Alkalosis

	Acute, or if vomiting continues (generation)	When vomiting diminishes or ceases (maintenance)
pH	>7	<6
$[Na^+]$	$>30\,mEq/L$	$<10\,mEq/L$
$[K^+]$	$>40\,mEq/L$	20–$40\,mEq/L$
$[HCO_3^-]$	$>30\,mEq/L$	$<5\,mEq/L$
$[Cl^-]$	$<10\,mEq/L$	$<10\,mEq/L$

Source: Adapted from Ref. 80.

and the concentrations of HCO_3^-, Na^+, and K^+ fall, producing the classic diagnostic findings of (established) metabolic alkalosis. The same findings occur during, and after discontinuation of gastric drainage.

Colonic Fluid Loss

Chloride-rich fluid losses in some diarrheal diseases can also cause metabolic alkalosis. In these cases, stool Cl^- losses are high and stool HCO_3^- losses are minimal, and the losses of Na^+, K^+, and water are sufficient to cause the same pathophysiologic sequence observed in vomiting: reduced glomerular filtration rate and stimulation of Na^+ reabsorption and H^+ secretion (Table 6). Diarrhea-associated causes of metabolic alkalosis are much rarer than vomiting or nasogastric drainage. They include congenital chloride diarrhea, and some cases of the chronic colitis of inflammatory bowel disease, osmotic diarrhea, laxative abuse, and 10–20% of cases of villous adenoma (Table 4). These causes have in common involvement of the colon (with or without involvement of the small intestine) with an abnormality in Cl^- absorption and/or frank Cl^- secretion (81–84). Characteristically, fecal $[Cl^-]$ is 50–150 mEq/L as compared to normal fecal $[Cl^-]$ of 15–25 mEq/L, and stool $[HCO_3^-]$ is less than 10 mEq/L. A striking example of the colonic role in metabolic alkalosis is the observation that, even though the severity of the diarrhea may be similar, patients with Crohn's enterocolitis or colitis may have this disorder but those with enteritis alone do not (85).

Ingestion of Base

Metabolic alkalosis may be caused by the ingestion of HCO_3^- or organic anions that generate HCO_3^- when metabolized. Because the renal capacity to excrete HCO_3^- is very great, clinically significant alkalosis is invariably associated with impairment of glomerular filtration. The classic triad of alkalosis, renal failure, and hypercalcemia is referred to as the milk alkali syndrome (86) (see Chapter 19). In this syndrome, ingestion of $CaCO_3$

Table 6 Rate of Flow and Electrolyte Concentrations of Diarrheal Fluid

Condition	Volume (L/day)	$[Na^+]$	$[K^+]$	$[Cl^-]$	$[HCO_3^-]$
		(mEq/L)			
Normal stool	<0.15	20–30	55–75	15–25	30
Inflammatory	1–3	50–100	15–20	50–100	10
Osmotic	1–5	5–20	20–30	5–20	10
Congenital Cl^- diarrhea	1–5	30–80	15–60	120–150	< 5
Secretory	1–20	40–140	15–40	25–105	20–75

Source: Adapted from Ref. 41.

results in hypercalcemia, impaired renal function, and metabolic alkalosis. Hypercalcemia-induced vomiting also may contribute to the alkalosis.

The oral administration of Mg(OH)$_2$ or Al(OH)$_3$ does not provide a sufficient quantity of base to body fluids to cause alkalosis although urine pH may rise. However, when ingested with a cation exchange resin (e.g., sodium polystyrene sulfonate) metabolic alkalosis may result. The mechanism involves the failure to form insoluble (Al)$_2$(CO$_3$)$_3$ or MgCO$_3$ in the presence of pancreatic HCO$_3^-$ secretion because of the formation of Al-polystyrene sulfonate or Mg-polystyrene sulfonate. The OH$^-$ of Mg(OH)$_2$ or Al(OH)$_3$ origin is absorbed rather than excreted as the insoluble CO$_3^{-2}$ salt, and in the presence of renal failure may accumulate. This scenario is unusual because, although cation exchange resins are used to manage hyperkalemia in patients with renal failure, Mg salts are contraindicated in these patients, and aluminum-containing antacids are now rarely used.

Metabolic Acidosis

If the metabolic acidoses are divided into those in which renal acid excretion is reduced (e.g., renal failure or renal tubular acidosis) and those in which the acid load is excessive, gastrointestinal causes should be included in the latter group (Table 4). Although the pathogenesis is often multifactorial, a reduction in renal acid excretion is not required for the acidosis to be manifest. Extracellular fluid volume depletion due to gastrointestinal losses can cause renal failure and lactic acidosis, and starvation ketoacidosis may complicate the clinical picture. The normal intestine also may participate in the production of metabolic acidosis by its efficient absorption of several alcohols and medications that upon metabolism may generate acid in large quantities and/or stimulate ketoacid or lactic acid production (see Chapter 12). The substances (and the organic acids produced) include ethanol (ketoacids and lactic acids), methanol (formic and lactic acids), ethylene glycol (lactic, glycolic, and oxalic acids), salicylates (various), and toluene (hippuric acid) (87).

Starvation Ketoacidosis

Fasting or starvation may cause metabolic acidosis because the fatty acids derived from adipose tissue are metabolized to β-hydroxybutyric and acetoacetic acids. The rate of production of these ketoacids may reach 1500 mmol/day in prolonged fasting as the contribution of fat to energy expenditure increases from 60% during the first days of starvation to about 80% (50,88). Fully developed acidosis does not usually occur for several weeks, and when it does occur it is mild (pH > 7.3, [HCO$_3^-$] > 17 mEq/L) (88). Although reduced serum insulin levels and an elevated glucagon-to-insulin ratio are responsible for the ketoacidosis (as in diabetic ketoacidosis), the low rate of insulin secretion is sufficient to prevent hyperglycemia and runaway ketone production. Starvation ketoacidosis responds rapidly to glucose administration.

Intestinal Fluid Loss

Loss of fluid from the small intestine usually causes metabolic acidosis because the normal secretions of the biliary and pancreatic systems, ileum and colon have a [HCO_3^-] greater than plasma (Table 3). Even in the absence of disease, biliary (40 mEq), pancreatic (200 mEq), and small intestinal fluids (30 mEq) together secrete more than 250 mEq of HCO_3^- a day. As a consequence, enterocutaneous fistulas or catheters draining any of these secretions commonly produces metabolic acidosis (Table 4). The rate of small intestinal fluid secretion may be greatly increased by various pathologic processes that produce secretory diarrhea or less commonly nonsecretory watery diarrhea (as is seen in 50% of cases with steatorrhea). Active secretion of Cl^- and HCO_3^- are characteristic and stool output is generally greater than is found in diarrheal diseases that cause metabolic alkalosis (Table 6). There are many causes of secretory diarrhea including infections, villous adenoma (80–90% of cases), various drugs and circulating hormones (e.g., vasoactive intestinal peptide of neoplastic origin) (58,84,89–91). The watery diarrhea and acidosis of colonic origin caused by unabsorbed bile salts (e.g., following ileal resection) characteristically disappears with fasting.

Secretory diarrhea usually causes acidosis without an increase in the serum anion gap (see Chapter 15). The gain of H^+ by body fluids due to stool losses of HCO_3^- is accompanied by an increase in [Cl^-] rather than by anions that are not readily excreted or metabolized. However, in some patients, extracellular volume depletion is severe and results in renal failure and lactic acidosis. If this occurs, the anion gap increases due to the retention of lactate, sulfate, phosphate, and retained anions of absorbed organic acids (of colonic bacterial origin) that have not been metabolized to neutral endproducts. Cholera-induced diarrhea is a prime example in this regard. In patients with cholera, the serum anion gap ranges from 20 to 30 mEq/L due in part to concomitant lactic acidosis and elevated serum phosphate and protein concentrations caused by volume contraction and renal failure (92,93). Vomiting, which often accompanies infectious causes of secretory diarrhea and potentially could correct the systemic pH, in fact tends to worsen extracellular fluid volume loss and thereby the acidosis.

Watery diarrhea itself and broad-spectrum antibiotic therapy have been shown to decrease colonic organic acid production. Decreased production may exaggerate intestinal electrolyte and fluid losses in the course of diarrhea and worsen the metabolic acidosis (48). This is because colonic absorptive capacity depends on the supply of metabolic fuel (i.e., short chain fatty acids—see earlier), and these organic acids ordinarily partially inhibit cAMP-mediated and cGMP-mediated Cl^- and HCO_3^- secretion (48,94,95).

Surgery-Induced Acidosis

In a surgically shortened small intestine, as in a jejunoileal bypass or blind loop, increased lactic acid production may on occasion cause metabolic acidosis. D-lactic acidosis occurs when colonic bacterial flora (primarily gram-positive anaerobes such as lactobacilli) have access to unabsorbed carbohydrate. In this setting, D-lactic acid is produced at rates beyond the metabolic capacity of the mammalian liver, which lacks D-lactic acid dehydrogenase (1,80,96). This relatively rare cause of metabolic acidosis also may occur when small bowel motility has been slowed by drugs or disease. Treatment may include antibiotics, provision of nonpathogenic anaerobic flora, reduction in dietary carbohydrate, and when possible, surgical revision of the bypassed or blind loop of intestine.

Surgical construction of an ileal conduit directs the drainage of urine destined for excretion into an ileal pouch or conduit. If urine dwells in the conduit for sufficient time, the ileum will efficiently absorb H^+, NH_4^+, K^+, and Cl^- ions (by the electrolyte transport pathways described above) and metabolic acidosis may result (97). Thus, long length and delayed emptying of the interposed segment predispose to acidosis. The ileum also secretes HCO_3^- and absorbs organic acids, but the quantities are too small to contribute to the acidosis. However, the proportionally greater urinary excretion of acid as titratable acid than as ammonium in the presence of an ileal conduit may exhaust urinary phosphate buffering capacity. For this reason, an unexpectedly severe acidosis may develop in the presence of urinary obstruction or renal failure, or in the presence of a modest acid load. Ureteral implantation into the cecum or sigmoid colon where dwell time is longer is an even more common cause of metabolic acidosis, but is now rarely performed because of an increased incidence of colon cancer.

A surgical ileostomy also has the potential of causing metabolic acidosis. As shown in Table 3, a new and in some cases an adapted ileostomy drains fluid relatively rich in HCO_3^-. However, the volume loss in a normally functioning ileostomy is relatively low (0.5–1 L/day) and metabolic acidosis occurs infrequently. A surgical colostomy drains fluid with a lower $[HCO_3^-]$ than an ileostomy and metabolic acidosis is not observed. In the presence of secretory diarrhea, however, ileostomy and sometimes colostomy drainage increases dramatically. When this occurs, marked fluid and electrolyte losses are often accompanied by metabolic acidosis. However, in this circumstance, the acidosis is due to a combination of HCO_3^- loss, lactic acid overproduction, and renal failure.

Respiratory Alkalosis and Acidosis

Intestinal causes of metabolic alkalosis and acidosis are sometimes complicated by primary respiratory acid–base disorders (Table 7). An example is the development of pneumonia following aspiration in a patient with

Table 7   Gastrointestinal Conditions Associated with Concomitant Metabolic and Respiratory Acid/Base Disorders

---

Hepatic failure or liver cirrhosis and ascites
Post-operative gastrointestinal surgery patients
Aspiration associated with vomiting or gastric drainage
Gastrointestinal infections
Hypokalemia or hypophosphatemia in patients with secretory diarrhea
   (or other gastrointestinal causes of metabolic acidosis or alkalosis)
Intestinal absorption of intoxicants (e.g., salicylates, ethanol, toluene)

---

vomiting or gastric drainage. These respiratory acid–base disorders may present therapeutic problems even in the absence of a metabolic acid–base disorder, but difficulty in diagnosis and management increase enormously when both metabolic and respiratory disorders coexist. Such concomitant clinical conditions are not unusual. Patients with liver cirrhosis and ascites (which may cause respiratory alkalosis) are often treated with thiazide diuretics or experience vomiting (both of which may cause metabolic alkalosis). Patients with secretory diarrhea (which may cause metabolic acidosis) may develop muscle weakness due to hypokalemia or hypophosphatemia (which may cause respiratory acidosis) (92). The management of primary respiratory acidosis and alkalosis is described in Chapters 20 and 21.

ROLE IN THERAPEUTICS

The intestine has an important therapeutic role in the management of acid/base disorders. The role derives from two aspects of its normal absorptive function: the absorption of dietary constituents that generate acids and bases upon metabolism, and the "near 100% bioavailability" of ingested solutes and water described above. Table 8 lists the various dietary changes, drugs and electrolytes that may be prescribed for patients with metabolic alkalosis and acidosis. Detailed descriptions of the indications, doses, and potential complications of these therapies are given in the chapters on metabolic acidosis and alkalosis.

Diet Modification

The diet is commonly modified to reduce endogenous acid production in patients with acute or chronic renal failure, renal tubular acidosis, or end-stage renal disease undergoing dialysis. In adults, protein may be restricted in such patients to <0.8 g/kg body weight per day as compared to the usual Western diet which contains 1–2 g/kg/day. Diet modification also may help prevent acidosis in patients with potential or recurrent D-lactic acidosis associated with jejunoileal bypass or a blind loop. Restriction of dietary carbohydrate to

Table 8   Oral Therapy of Metabolic Alkalosis and Acidosis

Metabolic alkalosis
KCl in Cl⁻-responsive alkalosis and/or hypokalemia
Ammonium chloride
Proton pump inhibitor or H_2 receptor blocker during continuous NG suction
Pernicious vomiting and congenital Cl⁻ diarrhea
Carbonic anhydrase inhibitor (e.g., acetazolamide)
K^+ sparing diuretics (e.g., spironolactone, triamterene, amiloride)

Metabolic acidosis
Dietary protein restriction (e.g., renal failure)
Dietary carbohydrate restriction in jejunoileal bypass or blind loop
$NaHCO_3$, $KHCO_3$, or metabolic base source (e.g., Na^+ citrate)
Antibiotics in jejunoileal bypass or blind loop
Rehydration solutions in secretory diarrhea

---

one-half the normal intake (of approximately 400 g/day) will minimize the substrate for D-lactic acid production by displaced colonic bacteria.

Absorption of Electrolytes

The efficient absorption of solutes and water by the normal gastrointestinal tract is the basis for the use of oral therapy for metabolic acid–base disorders. Administered electrolytes are rapidly absorbed by the proximal intestine. Absorption may be assumed to be complete, although the packaging of the medication (e.g., cellulose encapsulation of KCl) may intentionally increase the time and surface area of absorption. Complete assimilation of individual oral doses may not be evident for several hours regardless of the preparation. This is the case if metabolism is required (as when citrate is administered as a source of base), or when a change in renal function is required (as when a carbonic anhydrase inhibitor is administered to cause urinary HCO_3^- excretion). Of note, oral electrolyte solutions have been developed that by design are not absorbed by the intestine. These Na^+-sulfate-based, polyethylene glycol-containing solutions are used to cleanse the colon for diagnostic studies (98). Systemic acid–base balance is not affected by the ingestion of these solutions.

Although intestinal absorption of electrolytes and epithelial transport of H^+ and HCO_3^- ions are not directly affected by electrolyte or acid–base disorders, an important aspect of oral therapy, some changes in electrolyte and acid–base status may affect intestinal function. Examples include the antiperistaltic effects of hypokalemia, and vomiting caused by metabolic acidosis. Under these circumstances, or when oral intake is relatively contraindicated, parenteral therapy is recommended. When parenteral therapy is used, the dosing need not be altered but special attention should be given to the timing, site (peripheral venous vs. central venous) and concentration of administered treatment. In general, oral therapy is used for chronic disorders and in those acute disorders where the intestine is intact and functional, the degree of extracellular fluid volume depletion is moderate, and the rapidity of correction is not critical.

Oral Solutions for Treatment of Volume Depletion

Oral electrolyte solutions are extremely useful in the management of the fluid losses associated with secretory diarrhea (99). Oral rehydration solutions have been formulated that roughly correspond with anticipated losses, and contain Na^+ (50–90 mEq/L), K^+ (20–25 mEq/L), Cl^- (45–80 mEq/L) and HCO_3^- or a metabolic precursor of HCO_3^- (10–30 mEq/L). They are hypotonic which increases the hydrostatic driving force for absorption (100). The addition of glucose, rice flour or amylase-resistant starch also increases the rate of Na^+ absorption, but only the latter two appear to reduce stool water loss in severe diarrhea (75,90,91,93,100).

Oral intake of 75–100 mL/kg body weight in the first 4–6 hr is recommended initial therapy for mild to moderate extracellular fluid volume depletion in infants, children, and adults regardless of the etiology of the diarrhea (as suggested by World Health Organization) (75,90,92,101). Additional electrolyte solution is given for ongoing stool losses during and after repair of depleted extracellular fluid volume, and ad lib water and food intake (dilute formula or breast milk in infants) is encouraged. In adults, from 6 to 16 L may be required before the diarrhea abates. In some cases (as in persistent vomiting or stool losses >10 mL/kg/hr), oral therapy may be inadequate and intravenous fluids may be required (101).

Absorption of Drugs

Oral drug therapy for systemic acid–base disorders usually represents adjunctive rather than definitive treatment. Antibiotic therapy may be effective therapy for bacterial overgrowth in patients with D-lactic acidosis associated with jejunoileal bypass or a blind loop. However, surgical revision is usually required to prevent recurrence. Proton pump (H^+/K^+ ATPase) inhibitors or H_2 receptor blockers may be useful in the presence of ongoing gastric fluid losses to prevent or minimize metabolic alkalosis. KCl is often required as well despite the remarkable effectiveness of these drugs. Continuous nasogastric suction, persistent vomiting, and the presence of congenital Cl^- diarrhea are clinical examples of when one or another of these drugs may be effective. Other drugs useful in metabolic alkalosis act on the kidney rather than the intestine. Their lack of effect on the intestine, and rapid and reliable absorption insure that they will reach their site of action. As an example, carbonic anhydrase inhibitors may be prescribed in certain cases of metabolic alkalosis.

CONCLUDING COMMENTS

Homer Smith remarked that "... the composition of the body fluids is determined not by what the mouth takes in but by what the kidneys keep ..." (102). With regard to acid–base balance, the foregoing description of the normal and abnormal gastrointestinal tract, the importance of diet, and the efficient absorption of solutes and water in health and disease suggest otherwise. In a healthy adult, the primary determinant of the net acid or base that must be excreted each day to preserve acid–base balance is the diet. In addition, the digestion and absorption of dietary components involves the coordinated movement of a large volume of electrolyte-rich fluid into and out of the intestine. This feat is the more remarkable considering the strikingly intermittent timing of oral intake and its extremely varied composition.

As described herein, the essentially complete absorption of digestive fluids has two major clinical implications. First, if this fluid is not absorbed but is excreted (as in vomiting) marked disturbances of acid–base balance will result. If intestinal fluid secretion is increased by disease (as in secretory diarrhea), so much the worse. Second, the ready absorption of solutes and water provide for the oral therapy of acid–base, fluid, and electrolyte disorders. Indeed, oral therapy is based on the relative lack of effect of these disorders on intestinal function, and the preservation of absorptive function in the presence of active intestinal secretion. The intestine is both the most common source of acid–base disorders and the preferred route of therapy for these disorders. This functional paradox suggests that the internal milieu, and acid–base balance in particular, is determined as much or more by what is ingested and absorbed by the intestine as by what is kept by the kidney.

ACKNOWLEDGMENTS

This work was supported by the Office of Research and Development, Medical Research Service, Department of Veterans Affairs, and by National Institutes of Health Grants RO1 DK26523, PO1 DK44484, and the Hopkins Center for Epithelial Disorders.

The authors thank Drs. David S. Goldfarb, Mitchell L. Halperin, and Henry J. Binder for their scientific input, and Ms. Sharon Leu for her assistance in the preparation of the figures.

REFERENCES

1. Halperin ML, Kamel KS. D-Lactic acidosis: turning sugars into acids in the gastrointestinal tract. Kidney Int 1996; 49:1–8.
2. Cohen RM, Feldman GM, Fernandez PC. The balance of acid, base and charge in health and disease. Kidney Int 1997; 52:287–293.

3. Bugaut M. Occurrence, absorption and metabolism of short-chain fatty acids in the digestive tract of mammals. Comp Biochem Physiol 1987; 86B:439–472.

4. Cooke HJ. Role of the "little brain" in the gut in water and electrolyte homeostasis. FASEB J 1989; 3:127–138.

5. Cooke HJ. Neuroimmune signaling in regulation of intestinal ion transport. Am J Physiol (Gastrointest Liver Physiol.) 1994; 266(2 Pt 1):G162–G178.

6. Charney AN, Egnor RW. NaCl absorption in the rabbit ileum: effect of acid–base variables. Gastroenterology 1991; 100:403–409.

7. Charney AN, Dagher PC. Acid–base effects on colonic electrolyte transport revisited. Gastroenterology 1996; 111:1358–1368.

8. Dagher PC, Balsam L, Weber JT, Egnor RW, Charney AN. Modulation of chloride secretion in the rat colon by intracellular bicarbonate. Gastroenterology 1992; 103:120–127.

9. Dagher PC, Chawla H, Michael J, Egnor RW, Charney AN. Modulation of chloride secretion in the rat ileum by intracellular bicarbonate. Comp Biochem Physiol 1997; 118A(2):89–97.

10. Goldfarb DS, Egnor RW, Charney AN. Effects of acid–base variables on ion transport in rat colon. J Clin Invest 1988; 81:1903–1910.

11. Charney AN, Haskell LP. Relative effects of systemic pH, Pco_2, and HCO_3 concentration on colonic ion transport. Am J Physiol (Gastrointest Liver Physiol) 1984; 246(2 Pt 1):G159–G165.

12. Charney AN, Haskell LP. Relative effects of systemic pH, Pco_2 and bicarbonate concentration on ileal ion transport. Am J Physiol (Gastrointest Liver Physiol) 1983; 245(2):G230–G235.

13. Vaccarezza SG, Charney AN. Acid–base effects on ileal sodium chloride absorption in vitro. Am J Physiol (Gastrointest Liver Physiol) 1988; 254 (3 Pt 1):G329–G333.

14. Eherer AJ, Petritsch W, Berger J, Hinterleitner T, Charney AN, Krejs GJ. Effects of respiratory acidosis on electrolyte transport in human ileum. Eur J Clin Invest 1993; 23:206–210.

15. Crepeau R, Romeder JM, Plante GE. Effects of saline infusion and acute metabolic acidosis and alkalosis on water and electrolyte transport in the human colon. Can J Physiol Pharmacol 1977; 55:13–20.

16. Lemann J Jr, Litzow JR, Lennon EJ. The effects of chronic acid loads in normal man: further evidence for the participation of bone mineral in the defense against chronic metabolic acidosis. J Clin Invest 1966; 45:1608–1614.

17. Relman AS, Lennon EJ, Lemann JJ. Endogenous production of fixed acid and the measurement of the net balance of acid in normal subjects. J Clin Invest 1961; 70:1621–1630.

18. Goodman AD, Lemann J Jr, Lennon EJ, Relman AS. Production, excretion, and net balance of fixed acid in patients with renal acidosis. J Clin Invest 1965; 44:495–506.

19. Lemann J Jr, Lennon EJ, Goodman AD, Litzow JR, Relman AS. The net balance of acid in subjects given large loads of acid or alkali. J Clin Invest 1965; 44:507–517.

20. Feldman GM, Charney AN. Effect of acute metabolic alkalosis and acidosis on intestinal electrolyte transport in vivo. Am J Physiol (Gastrointest Liver Physiol) 1980; 239(5):G427–G436.
21. Charney AN, Goldfarb DS. Bicarbonate transport. In: Lebenthal E, Duffey M, eds. Textbook of Secretory Diarrhea. New York: Raven Press, 1990: 95–107.
22. Lemann J Jr, Lennon EJ. Role of diet, gastrointestinal tract and bone in acid–base homeostasis. Kidney Int 1972; 1:275–279.
23. Charney AN. Intestinal "bioavailability" of solutes and water: we know how but not why. Yale J Biol Med 1996; 69:329–335.
24. Diamond J, Karasov WH. Adaptive regulation of intestinal nutrient transporters. Proc Nat Acad Sci USA 1987; 84:2242–2245.
25. Ferraris RP, Diamond JM. Substrate-dependent regulation of intestinal nutrient transporters. Ann Rev Physiol 1989; 51:125–141.
26. Karasov WH, Diamond JM. Adaptive regulation of sugar and amino acid transport by vertebrate intestine. Am J Physiol (Gastrointest Liver Physiol) 1983; 245(4):G443–G462.
27. Agarwal R, Afzalpurkar R, Fordtran JS. Pathophysiology of potassium absorption and secretion by the human intestine. Gastroenterology 1994; 107:548–571.
28. Debongnie JC, Phillips SF. Capacity of the human colon to absorb fluid. Gastroenterology 1978; 74:698–703.
29. Rubens RD, Lambert HP. Homeostatic function of the colon in acute gastroenteritis. Gut 1972; 13:915–919.
30. Phillips SF, Giller J. The contribution of the colon to electrolyte and water conservation in man. J Lab Clin Med 1973; 81:733–746.
31. Sladen GE, Dawson AM. Interrelationships between the absorptions of glucose, sodium and water by the normal human jejunum. Clin Sci 1969; 36: 119–132.
32. Modigliani R, Bernier JJ. Absorption of glucose, sodium, and water by the human jejunum studied by intestinal perfusion with a proximal occluding balloon and at variable flow rates. Gut 1971; 12:184–193.
33. Turnberg LA, Bieberdorf FA, Morawski SG, Fordtran JS. Interrelationships of chloride, bicarbonate, sodium and hydrogen transport in the human ileum. J Clin Invest 1970; 49:557–567.
34. Fordtran JS, Locklear TW. Ionic constituents and osmolality of gastric and small-intestinal fluids after eating. Am J Digest Dis 1966; 11:503–521.
35. Hammer J, Phillips SF. Fluid loading of the human colon: effects on segmental transit and stool composition. Gastroenterology 1993; 105:988–998.
36. Proano M, Camilleri M, Phillips SF, Thomforde GM, Brown ML, Tucker R. Unprepared human colon does not discriminate between solids and liquids. Am J Physiol (Gastrointest Liver Physiol) 1991; 260(1 Pt 1):G13–G16.
37. Fernandez LB, Gonzalez E, Marzi A, Ledesma De Paolo MI. Fecal acidorrhea. N Engl J Med 1971; 284:295–298.
38. Squires RD, Huth EJ. Experimental potassium depletion in normal human subjects. J Clin Invest 1959; 38:1134–1148.

39. Dempsey EF, Carrol EL, Albright F, Henneman PH. A study of factors determining fecal electrolyte excretion. Metabolism 1958; 7:108–118.
40. Finkel Y, Jenkins HR, Booth IW. The adaptive response of rectal electrolyte absorption to impaired sodium balance in young children. J Pediatr Gastro Nutr 1991; 13:182–185.
41. Charney AN, Feldman GM. Internal exchanges of hydrogen ions: gastrointestinal tract. In: Seldin DW, Giebish G, eds. The Regulation of Acid–Base Balance. New York: Raven Press, 1989:89–105.
42. Packer RK, Curry CA, Brown KM. Urinary organic anion exchange in response to dietary acid and base loading. J Am Soc Nephrol 1985; 5: 1624–1629.
43. Kurtz I, Maher T, Hutler HN. Effect of diet on plasma acid–base composition in normal humans. Kidney Int 1983; 24:670–680.
44. Cummings JH, Branch WJ. Fermentation and production of short-chain fatty acids in human large intestine. In: Vahouny GB, Kritchevesky D, eds. Dietary Fiber: Basic and Clinical Aspects. New York: Plenum Press, 1990:131–152.
45. Roediger WEW. Utilization of nutrients by isolated epithelial cells of the rat colon. Gastroenterology 1982; 83:424–429.
46. Mortensen PB, Clausen MR. Short-chain fatty acids in the human colon: relation to gastrointestinal health and disease. Scand J Gastroenterol Suppl 1996; 216:132–148.
47. Harig JM, Soergel KH, Komorowski RA, Wood CM. Treatment of diversion colitis with short-chain-fatty acid irrigation. N Engl J Med 1989; 320:23–28.
48. Ramakrishna BS, Mathan VI. Colonic dysfunction in acute diarrhoea: the role of luminal short chain fatty acids. Gut 1993; 34:1215–1218.
49. Rubinstein R, Howard AV, Wrong OM. In vivo dialysis of faeces as a method of stool analysis. Clin Sci 1969; 37:549–564.
50. Kamel KS, Lin SH, Cheema-Dhadli S, Marliss EB, Halperin ML. Prolonged total fasting: a feast for the integrative physiologist. Kidney Int 1998; 53: 531–539.
51. Harris MS, Ramaswamy K, Kennedy JG. Induction of neurally mediated NaHCO$_3$ secretion by luminal distension in rat ileum. Am J Physiol (Gastrointest Liver Physiol) 1989; 257(2 Pt 1):G191–G197.
52. Frieling T, Wood JD, Cooke HJ. Submucosal reflexes: distension-evoked ion transport in the guinea pig distal colon. Am J Physiol (Gastrointest Liver Physiol) 1992; 263(1 Pt 1):G91–G96.
53. Johnson CD, Rai AS. Urine acid output as a test of completeness of vagotomy. Br J Surg 1990; 77(4):417–420.
54. Niv Y, Asaf V. Abolition of postprandial alkaline tide in arterialized venous blood of duodenal ulcer patients with cimetidine and after vagotomy. Am J Gastroenterol 1995; 90(7):1135–1137.
55. Vaziri ND, Byrne C, Ryan G, Wilson A. Preservation of urinary postprandial alkaline tide despite inhibition of gastric acid secretion. Am J Gastroenterol 1980; 74(4):328–331.
56. Johnson CD, Mole DR, Pestridge A. Postprandial alkaline tide: does it exist?. Digestion 1995; 56(2):100–106.

57. Straus E, Yalow RS. Hypersecretinemia associated with marked basal hyper-chlorhydria in man and dog. Gastroenterology 1977; 72:992–994.
58. Donowitz M, Kokke FT, Saidi R. Evaluation of patients with chronic diarrhea. N Engl J Med 1995; 332:725–729.
59. Read NW. Diarrhea: the failure of colonic salvage. Lancet 1982; 2:481–483.
60. Chang EB, Rao MC. Intestinal water and electrolyte transport. Mechanisms of physiological and adaptive responses. In: Johnson LR, ed. Physiology of the Gastrointestinal Tract. New York: Raven Press, 1994:2032–2034.
61. Hammer J, Pruckmayer M, Bergmann H, Kletter K, Gangl A. The distal colon provides reserve storage capacity during colonic fluid overload. Gut 1997; 41:658–663.
62. Falchuk KR. Motor and absorptive abnormalities of the gastrointestinal tract. New York State J Med 1982; 82:914–917.
63. Culp KS, Piziak VK. Thyrotoxicosis presenting with secretory diarrhea. Ann Intern Med 1986; 105:216–217.
64. Camilleri M, Prather CM. The irritable bowel syndrome: mechanisms and a practical approach to management. Ann Intern Med 1992; 116:1001–1008.
65. Galatola G. The Italian 75SeHCAT Multicentre Study Group. The prevalence of bile acid malabsorption in irritable bowel syndrome and the effect of cholestyramine: an uncontrolled open multicenter study. Eur J Gastroenterol Hepatol 1992; 103:702–704.
66. DelValle J, Lucey MR, Yamada T. Gastric secretion. In: Yamada T, ed. Textbook of Gastroenterology. Philadelphia: J.B. Lippincott Co., 1995:295–326.
67. Kaunitz JD, Barrett KE, McRoberts JA. Electrolyte secretion and absorption: small intestine and colon. In: Yamada T, ed. Textbook of Gastroenterology. New York: J.B. Lippincott Co., 1995:326–361.
68. Lee MG, Choi JY, Ljuo X, Strickland E, Thomas PJ, Muallem S. Cystic fibrosis transmembrane conductance regulator regulates luminal Cl/HCO_3 exchange in mouse submandibular and pancreatic ducts. J Biol Chem 1999; 274:14,670–14,677.
69. Ishiguro H, Steward MC, Lindsay AR, Case RM. Accumulation of intracellular HCO_3 by $Na–HCO_3$ cotransport in interlobular ducts from guinea-pig pancreas. J Physiol 1996; 495:169–178.
70. Zhao H, Star R, Muallem S. Membrane localization of H and HCO_3 transporters in the rat pancreatic ducts. J Gen Physiol 1994; 104:57–85.
71. Spirli C, Granato A, Zsembery A, Anglani F, Okolicsanyi L, LaRusso NF, et al. Functional polarity of Na/H and Cl/HCO_3 exchangers in a rat cholangiocyte cell line. Am J Physiol (Gastrointest Liver Physiol) 1998; 275 (6 Pt 1):G1236–G1245.
72. Rajendran VM, Binder HJ. Apical membrane Cl-butyrate exchange: mechanism of short chain fatty acid stimulation of active chloride absorption in rat distal colon. J Membr Biol 1994; 141:51–58.
73. Singh SK, Binder HJ, Boron WF, Geibel JP. Fluid absorption in isolated perfused colonic crypts. J Clin Invest 1995; 96:2373–2379.
74. Schiller LR, Santa Ana CA, Porter J, Fordtran JS. Glucose-stimulated sodium transport by the human intestine during experimental cholera. Gastroenterology 1997; 112:1529–1535.

75. Ramakrishna BS, Venkataraman S, Srinivasan P, Dash P, Young GP, Binder HJ. Amylase-resistant starch plus oral rehydration solution for cholera. N Engl J Med 2000; 342:308–313.

76. Smith JD, Perazella MA, DeFronzo RA. Hypokalemia. In: Arieff AI, DeFronzo RA, eds. Fluid, Electrolyte, and Acid–Base Disorders. New York: Livingstone Inc., 1995:393–395.

77. Fordtran JS. Speculations on the pathogenesis of diarrhea. Fed Proc 1967; 26(5):1405–1414.

78. Farese RV, Biglieri EG, Schackleton CH, Irony I, Gomez-Fontes R. Licorice-induced hypermineralocorticoidism. N Engl J Med 1991; 325:1223–1227.

79. Galla JH. Metabolic alkalosis. J Am Soc Nephrol 2000; 11:369–375.

80. Perez GO, Oster JR, Rogers A. Acid–base disturbances in gastrointestinal disease. Dig Dis Sci 1997; 32(9):1033–1043.

81. Bieberdorf FA, Gorden P, Fordtran JS. Pathogenesis of congenital alkalosis with diarrhea. Implications for the physiology of normal ileal electrolyte absorption and secretion. J Clin Invest 1972; 51:1958–1968.

82. Holmberg C, Perheentupa J, Launiala K. Colonic electrolyte transport in health and congenital chloride diarrhea. J Clin Invest 1975; 56:302–310.

83. Turnberg LA. Abnormalities in intestinal electrolyte transport in congenital chloridorrhoea. Gut 1971; 12:544–551.

84. Babior BM. Villous adenoma of the colon. Study of a patient with severe fluid and electrolyte disturbances. Am J Med 1966; 41:615–621.

85. Caprilli R, Vernia P, Latella G, Frieri G. Consequence of colonic involvement on electrolyte and acid–base homeostasis in Crohn's disease. Am J Gastro-enterol 1985; 80:509–512.

86. Fiorino AS. Hypercalcemia and alkalosis due to the milk-alkali syndrome: a case report and review. Yale J Biol Med 1996; 69(6):517–523.

87. Gabow PA. Disorders associated with an altered anion gap. Kidney Int 1985; 27:472–483.

88. Oster JR, Epstein M. Acid–base aspects of ketoacidosis. Am J Nephrol 1984; 4:137–151.

89. Hyams JS. Sorbitol intolerance: an unappreciated cause of functional gastro-intestinal complaints. Gastroenterology 1983; 84:30.

90. Pizzaro D, Posada G, Sandi L, Moran JR. Rice-based oral electrolyte solutions for the management of infantile diarrhea. N Engl J Med 1991; 324:517–521.

91. Molla AM, Rahman M, Sarker SA, Sack DA, Molla A. Stool electrolyte content and purging rates in diarrhea caused by rotavirus, enterotoxigenic *E. coli* and *V. cholerae* in children. J Pediatr 1981; 98:835–838.

92. Cieza J, Sovero L, Estremadoyro L. Electrolyte disturbances in elderly patients with severe diarrhea due to cholera. J Am Soc Nephrol 1995; 6:1463–1467.

93. Wang F, Butler T, Rabbani GH, Jones PK. The acidosis of cholera. Contributions of hyperproteinemia, lactic acidemia and hyperphosphatemia to an increased serum anion gap. N Engl J Med 1986; 315:1591–1595.

94. Dagher PC, Egnor RW, Taglietta-Kohlbrecher A, Charney AN. Short chain fatty acids inhibit cAMP-mediated chloride secretion in rat colon. Am J Physiol (Cell Physiol) 1996; 271(6 Pt 1):C1853–C1860.

95. Charney AN, Giannella RA, Egnor RW. Effect of short-chain fatty acids on cyclic 3′,5′-guanosine monophosphate-mediated colonic secretion. Comp Biochem Physiol A Mol Integr Physiol 1999; 124:169–178.

96. Oh MS, Phelps KR, Traube M, Barbosa-Saldivar JL, Boxhill C, Carroll HJ. D-Lactic acidosis in a man with the short-bowel syndrome. N Engl J Med 1979; 301:249–252.

97. Koch MO, McDougal WD. The pathophysiology of hyperchloremic metabolic acidosis after urinary diversion through intestinal segments. Surgery 1985; 98:561–570.

98. Fordtran JS, Santa Ana CA, Cleveland M. A low-sodium solution for gastrointestinal lavage. Gastroenterology 1990; 98:11–16.

99. Hirschhorn N, Kinzie JL, Sachar DB, Northrup RS, Taylor JO, Ahmed SZ, et al. Decrease in net stool output in cholera during intestinal perfusion with glucose-containing solutions. N Engl J Med 1968; 279:176–181.

100. Farthing MJ. Oral rehydration therapy. Pharmacol Ther 1994; 64:477–492.

101. Alam NH, Majumder RN, Fuchs GJ. The CHOICE Study Group. Efficacy and safety of oral rehydration solution with reduced osmolarity in adults with cholera: a randomised double-blind clinical trial. Lancet 1999; 354:296–299.

102. Smith HW. From Fish to Philosopher. The Story of Our Internal Environment. CIBA Edition ed. Boston: Little, Brown & Co., 1959.

8

An Evolutionary Perspective on the Acid–Base Effects of Diet

Anthony Sebastian, Lynda A. Frassetto, Renée L. Merriam, Deborah E. Sellmeyer, and R. Curtis Morris, Jr.

Department of Medicine, University of California San Francisco, San Franciso, California, U.S.A.

It is more important that a proposition be interesting than that it be true... But of course a true proposition is more apt to be interesting than a false one.

—Alfred North Whitehead (1,2)

Nothing in biology makes sense except in the light of evolution.

—Theodosius Dobzhansky (3)

...our DNA is a coded description of the worlds in which our ancestors survived.

—Richard Dawkins (4)

INTRODUCTION

We describe here acid–base physiology in humans who eat typical modern American diets (5,6), and argue that, owing to the nature of those diets and the effects of aging, many otherwise healthy adults suffer chronically from a state of progressively worsening, pathogenically significant, low-grade hyperchloremic metabolic acidosis* (7–10). We argue also that the same individuals suffer chronically from the *absence* of a low-grade diet-induced potassium-replete *metabolic alkalosis* for which natural selection has genetically adapted them but for which the modern diet does not nutritionally enable (11,12). In due course will emerge a redefinition of "metabolic acidosis" and "metabolic alkalosis."

The tonic metabolic acidosis induced by the modern diet results from an imbalance in the supply of nutrient precursors of HCO_3^- and H^+, resulting in the net delivery of H^+ to the systemic circulation each day. Specifically, it results from insufficient endogenous generation of HCO_3^- from the metabolism of dietary inorganic salts of organic acids (e.g., potassium citrate)—insufficient to keep pace with the body's daily generation of H^+ from noncarbonic acids (e.g., sulfuric acid, citric acid). The body produces noncarbonic acids either as end products of metabolism of ingested acid precursors (e.g., amino acids that produce sulfuric acid), or as incompletely oxidized dietary supplied or metabolically produced organic acids (e.g., citric acid). The systemic H^+/HCO_3^- imbalance produced by the modern diet reflects an inadequate supply of HCO_3^--precursor-rich plant foods (11).

The kidney mitigates the severity of the acidemia and hypobicarbonatemia induced by eating the modern diet (see Chapter 6). That renal mitigation, however, diminishes as renal function declines progressively with age, resulting in progressively worsening acidemia and hypobicarbonatemia (8). Accordingly, the modern-diet-dependent metabolic acidosis qualifies partly as an "acid load, base deficiency" acidosis and partly as a "renal" acidosis.

We argue that the modern diet's induced metabolic acidosis reflects a shift from a preagricultural hunter–gatherer-type net base-producing diet (11,13) to a modern agriculturally based net acid-producing diet (6,11), a diet in which the most common plant food ingested—cultivated cereal grains—happens to yield net acid on metabolism (11,14–16). We argue that humans remain genetically adapted to the ancestral hunter–gatherer-type diet, an adaptation that developed over millions of years of hominid evolution (13). The dietary shift, beginning with the invention of agriculture ~10,000 years ago, occurred too recently for natural selection to have had time to make substantial adjustments in human genetically determined metabolic machinery (17–21). From an evolutionary perspective, we consider the biologically natural and presumably optimal acid–base status of humans as a mild metabolic alkalosis, which one

---

*Though we focus on modern American diets, European diets and the diets of many Westernized and industrialized countries share the characteristics of American diets relevant to the issues discussed this chapter.

would expect to result from the daily delivery to the body of a dietary net load of base (22).

Those considerations compel us to judge the severity of the modern diet's induced metabolic acidosis against a reference point of plasma acid–base composition set by a diet with a substantially greater yield of HCO_3^- precursors than H^+ precursors (11). Because dietary HCO_3^- precursors consist predominantly of K^+ salts (e.g., K^+-citrate), we consider that both the chronic acidosis and the absent alkalosis produced by the modern diet cooccur with a state of chronic nutritional deficiency of K^+ as well as of HCO_3^- (23,24).

We will discuss some pathologies that have resulted from the pre- to postagricultural dietary shift (24–26). We will argue that diet-induced age-amplified low-grade metabolic acidosis, and the absence of diet-induced low-grade metabolic alkalosis, coupled with an unavoidably suboptimal dietary K^+, contribute to the pathogenesis of age-related disorders, including osteoporosis, sarcopenia, nephrolithiasis, hypertension, stroke, and renal insufficiency.

DEFINITIONS OF METABOLIC ACIDOSIS AND ALKALOSIS

Somewhat surprisingly, we cannot define "metabolic acidosis" and "metabolic alkalosis" simply and unambiguously. Clinicians define them as disorders initiated by primary changes in plasma $[HCO_3^-]$ (decreased in metabolic acidosis; increased in metabolic alkalosis)(see Chapters 9, 16, and 28). We point out, however, that in individual cases, clinicians have no unambiguous reference point against which to judge whether increases or decreases in serum $[HCO_3^-]$ have occurred within the wide range of clinically accepted "normal" values. Although one can easily target for diagnosis and management large deviations in plasma $[HCO_3^-]$—values falling outside the clinically defined "normal range"—the wide range of such "normal" values does not permit ready detection of potentially pathophysiologically significant chronic deviations within that range in individual cases (7–9,27,28).

Why We Need to Reconsider the Reference Point for the Diagnosis of Metabolic Acid–Base Disturbances

The need to reconsider the reference point for diagnosing metabolic acid–base disturbances emerges from studies in humans which indicate that, depending on diet composition and a person's age, healthy individuals have differing degrees of blood acidification and bicarbonate reduction, though their blood $[H^+]$ and plasma $[HCO_3^-]$ remain largely within the clinically defined "normal" range (7,8). To put this in perspective, below we discuss the determinants of the set-point at which the body regulates blood $[H^+]$ and plasma $[HCO_3^-]$.

DETERMINANTS OF THE SET-POINT AT WHICH BLOOD ACIDITY AND PLASMA $[HCO_3^-]$ REGULATE IN "NORMAL" SUBJECTS

Respiratory Determinants

In normal subjects ingesting self-selected diets, blood $[H^+]$ differs by as much as $10\,nEq/L$ (7,29). Those interindividual differences in blood acidity result in part from differences in the level at which the respiratory system regulates blood PCO_2 in response to factors other than those entrained by changes in blood acidity itself (7,29). Blood $[H^+]$ varies directly with PCO_2, not negatively as one might expect if blood $[H^+]$ determined PCO_2, given that acidemia stimulates alveolar ventilation. Confirming the primacy of PCO_2, plasma $[HCO_3^-]$ also varied *directly* with PCO_2 among individuals. In effect, normal individuals have differing degrees of mild respiratory acidosis or alkalosis depending on the set-point where the respiratory system regulates PCO_2.

Metabolic Determinants

Net endogenous acid production (NEAP) among individuals eating self-selected diets differs nearly tenfold, from about 20 to $120\,mEq/24\,hr$ (8,30,31), due to differences in diet composition. We know that plasma $[H^+]$ regulates at an increased level, and plasma $[HCO_3^-]$ at a decreased level, in clinical conditions that result in a sustained large increases in NEAP (e.g., lactic acidosis, diabetic ketoacidosis), as well as in experimental conditions that maintain greatly increased NEAPs with exogenous acid loads (32–34). Importantly, smaller differences in NEAP caused by differences in diet composition also play a role in determining interindividual differences in blood $[H^+]$ and plasma $[HCO_3^-]$ in normal subjects (7,8,30). In effect, they have differing degrees of low-grade metabolic acidosis depending on the magnitude of the diet-determined NEAP.

Estimating Diet Net Acid Load

We can quantify NEAP in normal humans by quantifying the inorganic constituents of diet, urine, and stool, and the total organic anion content of the urine (see Chapter 6). However, such studies require considerable labor, time, and expense. In the steady state, renal net acid excretion (RNAE) provides a reliable index of NEAP, because under those conditions a highly predictable relationship exists between the two variables (7,30,35) (Fig. 1). We can measure RNAE much more readily than NEAP.

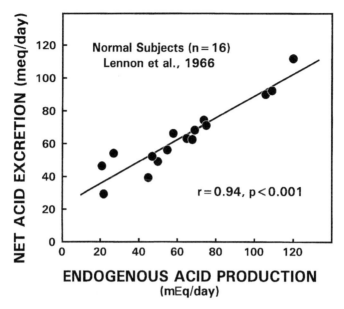

Figure 1 Relation between steady-state renal net acid excretion and net endogenous acid production in normal subjects ingesting one of three different diets. Each data point represents the mean steady-state value observed in one individual. Because the slope of the curve approximates one with a strong correlation, steady-state renal net acid excretion provides a reasonable estimate of net endogenous acid production. *Source*: Data plotted from tabular data in Ref. 30.

Effect of Differences in Diet Net Acid Load on Plasma Acid–Base Composition in Healthy Humans: Cross-Sectional Observations

In normal humans fed diets producing steady-state RNAEs ranging from 14 to 154 mEq/day, we observed a direct relationship between blood $[H^+]$ and RNAE, and an inverse relationship between plasma $[HCO_3^-]$ and RNAE, adjusting the variations in plasma $[H^+]$ and $[HCO_3^-]$ for the effects of interindividual differences in PCO_2 (7) (Fig. 2). Higher values of RNAE accompanied both lower values of plasma $[HCO_3^-]$ and higher values of blood $[H^+]$, consistent with the expected directional effect of NEAP on the titration of body buffers. Those findings indicate that normal subjects eating typical net acid-producing diets have a low-grade metabolic acidosis, the severity of which depends on the magnitude of the diet-determined NEAP.

Frassetto et al. (8) extended those findings to a substantially larger number of individuals eating a wider variety of diets (Fig. 3), with blood $[H^+]$ varying directly with RNAE ($=\sim$NEAP) even without adjusting for

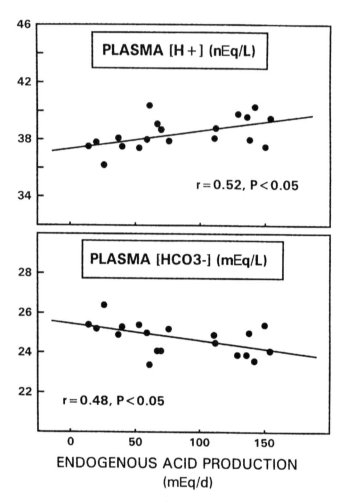

Figure 2   Relation between plasma [H$^+$] and net endogenous acid production, and between plasma [HCO$_3^-$] and net endogenous acid production, in the steady state, in 19 studies of 16 normal subjects ingesting one of three different diets. Endogenous acid production taken as the steady-state renal net acid excretion rate. Each data point represents the mean value observed in one individual. To adjust for differences at which the respiratory system regulates the set-point of blood carbon dioxide tension independently of blood acidity, we adjusted values to a common PCO$_2$ (38 mmHg). Note that with an increase in net endogenous acid production of 100 mEq/day, plasma [H$^+$] and [HCO$_3^-$] shift by ~1 nEq/L and ~1 mEq/L, respectively, in the acid direction. *Source*: Adapted from Ref. 7.

PCO$_2$ differences. The study provided quantitative data for determining deviations from the expected values of blood [H$^+$] and plasma [HCO$_3^-$] for a given PCO$_2$ and NEAP.

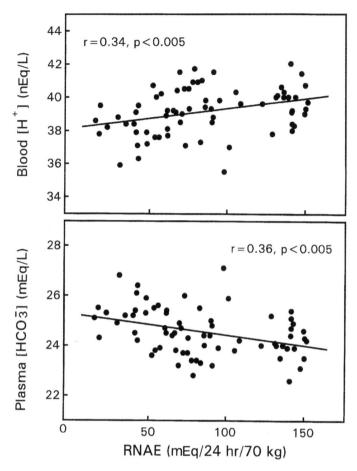

Figure 3 Relation between blood [H^+] and renal net acid excretion (RNAE), and between plasma [HCO_3^-] and renal net acid excretion and, in 64 normal subjects (ages 17–74 years) ingesting one of nine different typical American diets. Each data point represents the mean steady-state values in a single individual. We adjusted all values of blood hydrogen ion concentration and plasma bicarbonate concentration to a constant blood PCO_2 and GFR. Steady-state RNAE taken as an index of steady-state net endogenous acid production (NEAP). *Source*: Adapted from Ref. 8.

Effect of Changing the Diet Acid Load on Plasma
Acid–Base Composition in Healthy Subjects:
Interventional Studies

However physiologically predictable the observed relationship between plasma acid–base composition and RNAE among differing diets, the correlation does not establish it as cause–effect. Studies of the acid–base effect of different net acid-producing diets *in the same individuals* have not yet appeared. We can approach the cause–effect question, however, by examining the effect of changing NEAP in a given individual by administration of a small acid or base supplement to the diet, while otherwise maintaining the diet constant.

We performed such a study in postmenopausal women eating a constant typical net acid-producing diet. We supplemented the diet with potassium bicarbonate ($KHCO_3$) in amounts just sufficient to reduce NEAP (measured as RNAE) to the lower limits of the range observed with ordinary diets (36). Initially, we noted blood pH, 7.39, plasma [HCO_3^-], 23.7 mEq/L, and RNAE, 71 mEq/day. When we added $KHCO_3$ (60–120 mmol/day) for 18 days, pH increased by 0.02, [HCO_3^-] increased by 1.8 mEq/L, and RNAE decreased to 13 mEq/day (Fig. 4). The changes in plasma [HCO_3^-] correlated (inversely) with the changes in RNAE, despite the absolute values remaining within the clinically accepted normal range. After stopping $KHCO_3$, all measures returned to pre-$KHCO_3$ levels (Fig. 4). Those observations support the view that systemic acid–base equilibrium adjusts its set-point in response to differences in diet net acid load within the range of net acid loads observed with ordinary diets. Because blood [H^+] decreased and plasma [HCO_3^-] increased when NEAP decreased to the lower range of normal, the preexisting diet-determined NEAP in the higher range of normal clearly had influenced the set-point of systemic acid–base equilibrium, in effect causing a low-grade metabolic acidosis.

Definitions Revisited

From the above, we conclude that otherwise healthy humans who habitually eat ordinary net acid-producing diets typically sustain a chronic low-grade metabolic acidosis, the severity of which varies directly with the magnitude of the diet-determined NEAP. Accordingly, the blood [H^+] and plasma [HCO_3^-] at which a healthy person would have neither metabolic acidosis nor metabolic alkalosis manifests when the diet yields a zero net acid load. We therefore propose the plasma acid–base composition at zero NEAP as the reference point for the diagnosis of metabolic acid–base disturbances.

Some investigators refer to diet-induced metabolic acidosis as "eubicarbonatemic metabolic acidosis" (9,27,37), a term that emphasizes that one cannot rule out a potentially clinically significant metabolic acidosis by the routine laboratory finding of a plasma [HCO_3^-] within the clinically accepted normal range.

Effect of Age on Plasma Acid–Base Composition in Healthy Humans

Cross-Sectional Observations

The kidney contributes critically to the stability and set-point of systemic acid–base equilibrium (see Chapter 6) by adjusting daily net acid excretion

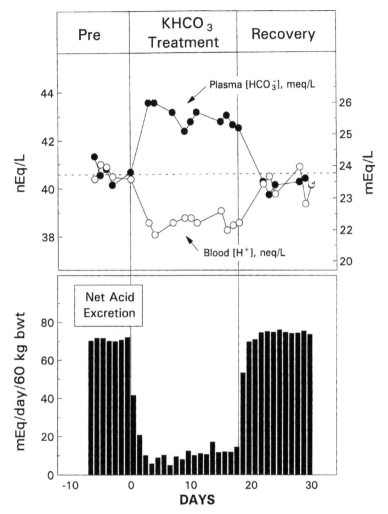

Figure 4 Effect of potassium bicarbonate ($KHCO_3$) administration (60–120 mEq/ day, 18 days) on blood [H^+], plasma [HCO_3^-], and renal net acid excretion in healthy postmenopausal women ($n = 18$ subjects). Lower panel: Sustained administration of $KHCO_3$ reduced net acid excretion to nearly zero, and therefore presumably neutralized nearly all of the daily net endogenous acid production. Upper panel: Concurrently with the elimination of the endogenous acid load, blood [H^+] decreased and plasma [HCO_3^-] increased, suggesting that the normal endogenous acid load before $KHCO_3$ administration sufficed to acidify the extracellular fluid compartment. When renal net acid excretion returned to its initial values following discontinuation of $KHCO_3$ administration, the pretreatment low-grade metabolic acidosis returned. *Source*: Adapted from Ref. 36.

in response to diet-induced differences in net acid load. Because renal function declines with age (over years), blood $[H^+]$ increases and plasma $[HCO_3^-]$ decreases with age for any given diet net acid load, exacerbating the already present low-grade diet-induced metabolic acidosis (8).

Blood acid–base measurements assembled from multiple individual published reports of normal values in adults show that with increasing age, steady-state blood $[H^+]$ increases, and plasma $[HCO_3^-]$ decreases (28). Measurements of blood $[H^+]$, PCO_2 and plasma $[HCO_3^-]$, RNAE, and 24-hr creatinine clearance in healthy adults over a wide range of ages, each of whom remained in a steady state on a constant diet while residing in a clinical research center, confirm age as a significant determinant of the blood acid–base composition in adult humans eating typical net acid-producing diets (8). From young adulthood to old age (17–74 years), otherwise healthy men and women develop a progressive increase in blood $[H^+]$ and decrease in plasma $[HCO_3^-]$, indicative of an increasing worsening of their diet-dependent low-grade metabolic acidosis (Fig. 5).

Age and diet net acid load (reflected in steady-state RNAE) *independently* codetermined the degree of metabolic acidosis. Over their respective ranges (17–74 years, 15–150 mEq/day), age had ~1.6 times greater effect on blood $[H^+]$ and plasma $[HCO_3^-]$ than diet net acid load (8). Age therefore substantially amplifies diet-induced metabolic acidosis.

Role of Age-Related Renal Functional Decline in the Age-Amplification of Diet-Induced Metabolic Acidosis

One might have predicted that advancing age would progressively worsen diet-induced acidosis, inasmuch as with age a state of chronic renal insufficiency often develops (38). Renal insufficiency induces metabolic acidosis, variably due to reduced conservation of filtered HCO_3^- and reduced excretion of acid (see Chapter 14) (39,40). Older humans have impaired acid-excretory ability in response to acute exogenous acid loading (41–43), and with more prolonged acid loading, a more severe degree of metabolic acidosis occurs and persists (44).

Indeed, when we substitute GFR for age, we found GFR a significant determinant of blood $[H^+]$ and plasma $[HCO_3^-]$ (8) (Fig. 6). Because the impact of GFR on plasma $[HCO_3^-]$ exceeded that of the diet net acid load by ~1.8 times, we know that age-related renal insufficiency (indexed by GFR reduction) substantially amplifies the chronic low-grade metabolic acidosis induced by diet.

When we consider GFR and age together as independent predictors, along with blood PCO_2 and NEAP, the age effect remains significant with GFR held constant, but not vice versa. Conceivably, nonrenal age-related factors [e.g., base release by bone (45,46)] also influence plasma acid–base composition.

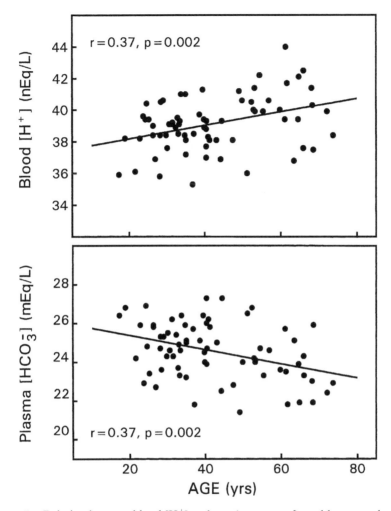

Figure 5 Relation between blood [H⁺] and age (*upper panel*), and between plasma [HCO₃⁻] and age (*lower panel*), in healthy normal subjects ($n = 64$). Each data point represents the steady-state value in an individual eating a constant diet. *Source*: From Ref. 8.

ACIDOSIS VS. ACID RETENTION

The Question of External H⁺ Balance in Normal Humans Eating Ordinary Net Acid-Producing Diets

Conceding that a low-grade metabolic acidosis persists in normal humans eating ordinary net acid-producing diets, one might still argue that no serious problems would occur so long as the kidneys excrete the daily net

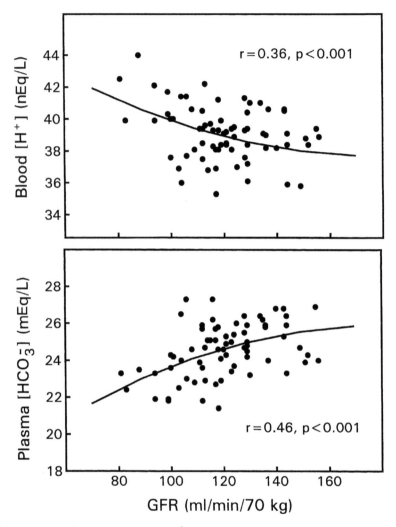

Figure 6 Relation between blood [H$^+$] and GFR (*upper panel*), and between plasma [HCO$_3^-$] and GFR (*lower panel*), in healthy normal subjects (*n* = 64). Each data point represents the steady-state value in an individual eating a constant diet. *Source*: From Ref. 8.

H$^+$ load. A small steady-state shift in systemic acid–base equilibrium in the acid direction might remain relatively benign so long as H$^+$ does not continually accumulate in the body.

To address this issue, Lennon, Lemann, and Litzow measured net acid balance (NEAP minus RNAE) in normal subjects ingesting diets yielding NEAP values ranging from 20 to 120 mEq/day, the typical range of ordinary American diets (30,31). They found H^+ balance (net acid balance) averaging zero, in contrast to patients with renal acidosis (39) and normal subjects experimentally administered large acid loads (32), who had decidedly positive H^+ balances.

On closer inspection of the data, however, we found positive values of net acid balance in about one-half of the subjects studied and, more importantly, a significant positive correlation between net acid balance and NEAP, indicating more net acid retention with higher NEAPs in the normal range (7) (Fig. 7). Importantly, the data points relating H^+ balance and NEAP fell on the regression line defined by the relationship between H^+ balance and NEAP in subjects given large supplements of acid and alkali (Fig. 8) (30,32), revealing a transition from base-retention to acid-retention within the range of NEAP for ordinary diets. For those reasons, we consider it unlikely that that the positive values for net acid balance among subjects eating unsupplemented ordinary diets reflect random variations around zero.

The data suggest that well over 50% of normal humans who consume diets that produce ≥ 40 mEq of NEAP per day continuously retain a fraction of their daily NEAP (7) (Fig. 7). Since the average NEAP of Americans

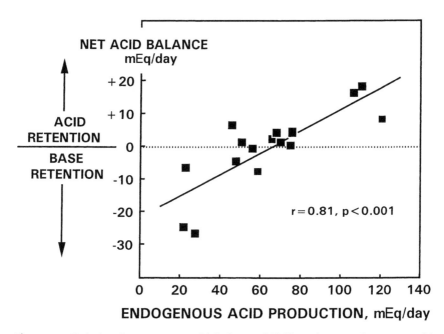

Figure 7 Relation between net acid balance (NAB) and net endogenous acid production (NEAP) in normal subjects ($n = 16$). Each data point represents the steady-state value in an individual eating a constant diet. The range of NEAP of the study subjects accords with that of free-living subjects eating typical diets. *Source*: Replotted from tabular data in Ref. 30.

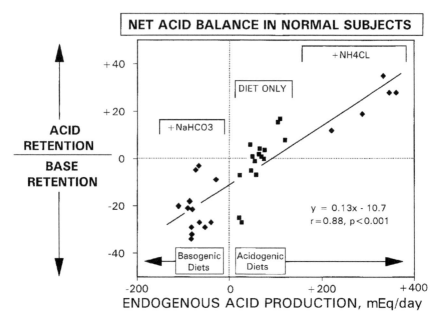

Figure 8 Relation between NAB and NEAP in normal subjects eating a constant diet with or without supplemental acid (NH₄Cl) or base (NaHCO₃) loading. Each data point represents the steady-state value in an individual. *Source*: Replotted from tabular data in Refs. 30, 32.

approximates 40–50 mEq/day (31,47), a substantial fraction of the American population may continuingly retain a fraction of their NEAP (Fig. 9). The findings suggest that above some near mid-level of NEAP within the range of NEAPs produced by ordinary diets, equality of NEAP and RNAE does not always obtain, and that when the steady-state NEAP exceeds about 40 mEq/day, external H^+ balance likely remains persistently positive (Fig. 9).

Do Current Methods of Measuring External H^+ Balance Have Sufficient Accuracy to Warrant the Above Conclusions?

Oh and coworkers (48–50) express skepticism about the accuracy the conventional methods for estimating net acid balance. In considering the results of such measurements in patients with chronic renal insufficiency (39,48,51), they argue that the reported findings indicating average positive net acid balance values of 10–20 mEq/day likely grossly overestimate reality (see Chapters 6 and 14). As their calculations show, the measured high rates of net acid balance would predict complete exhaustion of skeletal calcium salts within a few years. They believe this unlikely scenario predicates on errors in the measurements of NEAP and RNAE (see also Chapters 6 and 14).

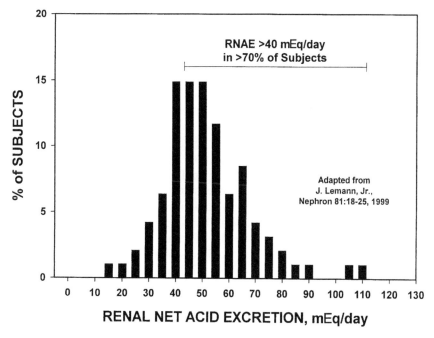

Figure 9 Frequency distribution of 24-hr renal net acid excretion (RNAE) rates in free-living men and women. Each bar represents a 5 mEq/day interval, with tick labels designating the upper limit of the interval. Fewer than 30% of subjects had RNAE values less than or equal to 40 mEq/day. *Source*: Data replotted from Ref. 31.

The considerations of Oh et al. urge caution interpreting the magnitude of net acid balance when the results compute as large and positive. They do not disallow, however, that H^+ balance can remain finitely, if only moderately, positive continuously in subjects with chronic acid-input metabolic acidosis—in particular, in healthy individuals eating net acid-producing diets. We will develop that point more fully below, in discussing the pathophysiologic sequelae of the chronic diet-induced low-grade metabolic acidosis in normal humans.

PATHOPHYSIOLOGICAL CONSEQUENCES OF DIET-INDUCED, AGE-AMPLIFIED METABOLIC ACIDOSIS IN HUMANS

Understandably most clinicians find it difficult to think "metabolic acidosis" when plasma acid–base composition falls in the range traditionally considered normal. Clinicians think of metabolic acidosis as a "disorder" that results from the buffering of excess noncarbonic acid in the systemic circulation, or from abnormal bicarbonate losses. Its presence implies pathophysiologic sequelae. If diet-induced acidosis had no such sequelae, one might rightly remain skeptical about using the term despite the arguments presented above. But in fact many acidosis-induced pathophysiological sequelae do develop as consequences of the normal diet acid load, indicated by their improvement on neutralizing the diet net acid load with small amounts of exogenous base (36,52–54).

In conditions causing metabolic acidosis, the severity of acidosis, as reflected in plasma acid–base composition, may underestimate the severity of the tissue injury attributable to the acidosis (9,27,37). With diet-dependent chronic metabolic acidosis, homeostatic adaptations occur that serve to minimize disturbances in extra- and intracellular $[H^+]$ and $[HCO_3^-]$. Those adaptations at the same time have detrimental "trade-off" effects when operating over long periods of time. The adaptations include decreased renal citrate excretion (53,55), dissolution of bone (56), hypercalciuria and hyperphosphaturia (57,58), skeletal muscle protein catabolism (59–63), reduction in intracellular K^+ (64), and renal proliferative and hypertrophic growth (65). The negative "trade-offs" include increased risks for renal calcification and stone formation, osteoporosis, muscle wasting, sequelae of K^+ depletion, and progression of renal disease (66–69).

Chronic Metabolic Acidosis and Bone Wasting

Metabolic acidosis reduces bone mass (10,70,71). Bone serves as an ion exchange reservoir that can release K^+ and Na^+ in exchange for H^+ (70,72–76). Bone also provides a large reservoir of base in the form of alkaline salts of calcium (phosphates, carbonates), which it releases into the systemic circulation in response to acid loads (32,51,57,70,77–87). The liberated base mitigates the severity of the acidosis, and thus contributes to systemic acid–base homeostasis. The liberated calcium and phosphorus disappear into the urine, without compensatory increase in gastrointestinal absorption, and thus bone mineral content declines (51,57,88,89).

Extensive studies in a variety of in vitro models demonstrate the response of bone to acute acidosis (10). Those studies reveal prompt initiation of a physicochemical process that results in titration of H^+ by bone carbonate, with attendant release of Na^+, K^+, and Ca^{2+} (75,79,80,87,90). In vivo, when acid loading continues (days to weeks), bone base continues to titrate H^+, helping to stop an otherwise progressive shift in systemic acid–base equilibrium in the acid direction, to its own detriment (32,51,57,91). Mobilization of bone base persists, and the bone minerals (calcium and phosphorus) accompanying that base continue disappearing into the urine, without compensatory increases in intestinal absorption (91,92). With chronicity of the acidosis, bone mineral content and bone mass progressively decline (56,78,93–97), and osteoporosis develops (56,71,93–96,98–100).

The skeleton's homeostatic contribution in titrating chronic net acid loads operates not solely as a passive physicochemical dissolution of bone mineral by an acidic extracellular fluid, but also as an active process involving cell-mediated bone resorption and reduced cell-mediated bone formation signaled by increased extracellular fluid H^+ and decreased HCO_3^- (71,101–108) (Fig. 10). Extracellular acidification (acidemia with hypobicarbonatemia) increases the activity of the bone-resorbing osteoclasts (102–105,107), and suppresses the activity of the bone-forming osteoblasts (102,103).

In humans, urinary hydroxyproline excretion increases, providing evidence that organic bone matrix resorption increases during acid loading (36,57,109). One can view inhibition of bone formation (102,103) as contributing to acid-base homeostasis, since it results in less utilization of extracellular base for bone formation.

Evidence That Chronic Diet-Induced Low-Grade Metabolic Acidosis Chronically Mobilizes Skeletal Base

Two lines of evidence indicate that chronic low-grade diet-induced acidosis imposes a chronic drain on bone: (a) stability of blood acid–base equilibrium in the face of continuing positive external balance of acid (7,30) (Figs. 7 and 9), and, (b) amelioration of negative calcium and phosphorus

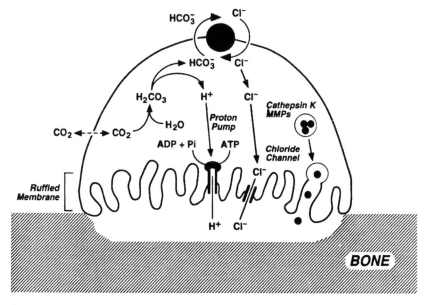

Figure 10 Acid–base components of osteoclastic bone resorption. *Source*: From Ref. 108.

balances, reduction of bone resorption, and stimulation of bone formation attendant to short-term neutralization of the dietary acid load (36) (Fig. 4). Longer-term (3 months) partial neutralization of the diet net acid load with potassium citrate also reduces bone resorption (54), and long-term (3 years) administration of potassium bicarbonate causes a persisting reduction in urine calcium excretion (110).

With decades-long metabolic acidosis, in order to account for acidosis-induced bone wasting, one need not postulate the release of large amounts of bone base per day relative to the ongoing NEAP. Bone base cannot continue for decades to contribute in large amounts (e.g., $>10\,mEq/day$) to the titration of endogenous acid, inasmuch as the bone reservoir does not contain enough base to last more than a few years at those rates. Nevertheless, we should not construe the latter point as arguing against a role for decades-long metabolic acidosis in stimulating bone wasting. Retention of only 1 or $2\,mEq$ of H^+ each day, undetectable by present measurement techniques, titrated by skeletal base over decades would result in a major depletion of bone mineral. For example, only $1\,mEq/day$ of base loss from bone as calcium hydroxyapatite over 40 years would equal $14,600\,mEq$ of base, equivalent to nearly $32,000\,mEq$ of calcium, or somewhat over 50% of total bone calcium content, much more than normally occurs with age-related bone loss. Yet, $1\,mEq/day$ per day of base release would titrate only about 2% of endogenous acid production in Americans eating their usual diets (31,47). Thus, the daily net acid retention needed to sustain skeletal demineralization in the long run needs only amount to a very small fraction of the daily diet net acid load—an amount that might easily escape detection by current methodologies for determining net acid balance.

Unlike chemical buffers, which exist *internal* to the system and serve as readily reversible temporary H^+ *banks*, one may regard bone and kidney as *external* H^+ *sinks* by virtue of their ability to generate *new* base for input to the circulation. The two sinks (bone and kidney) operate in parallel. When the body generates net acid endogenously, the acidified blood reaches bone and kidney concurrently, and both respond by adding new base to the systemic circulation, each according to its sensitivity and capacity. To whatever extent bone supplies base in response to its encounter with the acid-loaded blood, to that extent the kidney sees less acid (as reflected by lesser blood acidity and higher plasma $[HCO_3^-]$), and therefore, in the steady state, the kidney does not receive the full signal to generate new HCO_3^- equal to the full rate of endogenous acid production. Not surprising then the kidney does not "keep up" with endogenous acid production. Thus, if bone responds at all to the acid-loaded blood, however small a fraction of endogenous acid production it contributes base input to the systemic circulation, to that extent acid excretion in the urine will lag behind endogenous acid production, and *external* H^+ balance will compute as positive, correctly reflecting the reality of H^+ accumulation in the body. As discussed above, bone need contribute base at no more than 2% of endogenous acid production to substantially demineralize itself over decades of adult life. Many investigators have recognized this potential cumulative effect, over decades (46,86,111), and others have provided confirming clinical data in older women, with bone mineral density and fracture incidence directly related to the magnitude of diet-induced NEAP (112,113).

One might argue that as the kidney generates new HCO_3^- through net acid excretion, it will redeposit base into bone, and therefore bone base need not progressively deplete nor H^+ balance remain positive. But chronic acid loading titrates bone base by dissolution of the alkaline salts of calcium in the bone matrix, with subsequent disposal of the dissolved calcium in the urine. The kidney cannot generate *new* calcium with the *new* $HCO3^-$ generated, or even conserve the skeletally mobilized calcium, whose steady-state excretion rate in the urine among subjects varies directly with the net acid load of the diet (Fig. 11). Nor would one expect to find relief of the acidosis-induced activation of cell-mediated bone resorption, since acid excretion always plays catch-up with NEAP, and never catches-up. Interdicting

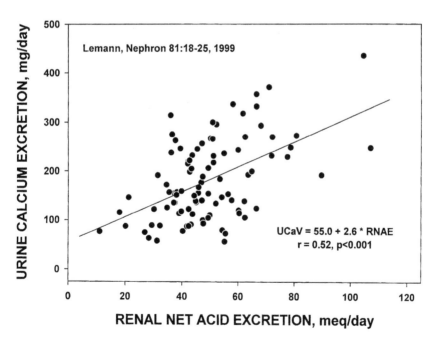

Figure 11 Relation between daily urine calcium excretion and daily renal net acid excretion in healthy free-living American women and men. Each data point represents the average of three 24-hr urine collections in a different individual. Group means: urine calcium, 180 ± 81 mg/day; renal net acid excretion, 49 ± 17 mEq/day. *Source*: Adapted from Ref. 31.

progressive loss of base from the skeletal reservoir requires relieving the chronic acidosis-induced inhibition of renal calcium reabsorption and activation of cell-mediated bone calcium resorption. One can achieve those effects only by neutralizing the diet net acid load.

Given that the calcium liberated from bone with acidosis-mediated base efflux escapes into the urine, not surprisingly urinary calcium excretion correlates positively with net acid excretion (read NEAP) in individuals eating typical net acid-producing diets (31) (Fig. 11), and not surprisingly those individuals commonly show a negative calcium balance, despite average dietary calcium intake (~800 mg/day) (114,115). Individuals eating diets containing substantially higher amounts of calcium do not show a negative calcium balance (114), but the NEAP engendered by such diets, possibly too low to sustain net bone base efflux, remains unknown. High calcium diets may keep NEAP low by displacement of higher for lower net acid producing foods (e.g., milk and/or calcium-rich plant foods substituting for meat and cereal grains) and/or by increasing dietary base input (e.g., organic anions in calcium-rich plant foods.). The most common forms of dietary calcium supplements (calcium citrate and calcium carbonate) also supply base. This base supply may critically determine the beneficial skeletal effects of dietary calcium supplementation (70,114).

We can test whether bone loss occurs in response to chronic low-level diet-induced metabolic acidosis by examining the effect of sustained neutralization of the diet net acid load by addition of exogenous base. Potassium bicarbonate, when administered in doses that nearly completely neutralize the diet net acid load, reduces urinary wasting of calcium and phosphorus (Fig. 12), improves preexisting negative balances of calcium and phosphorus and, as indicated by biochemical markers, reduces the rate of bone resorption and stimulates the rate of bone formation (36). Other investigators have also demonstrated significant improvement in calcium and phosphorus balances with neutralization of the diet net acid load by potassium bicarbonate administration in healthy humans (116), and with potassium citrate, reductions in bone resorption rates (54,117).

Evidence That Diet-Induced Metabolic Acidosis Contributes to the Pathogenesis of Clinical Osteoporosis

If chronic diet-induced metabolic acidosis imposes a chronic drain on bone, one might find that bone mass among groups of individuals relate to differences in their habitual diet NEAP. Frassetto et al. (118) approached this by using indirect estimates of the differences in diet net acid load among the groups, and relating those to differences in bone mass. They accomplished that by using food consumption data compiled by the United Nation's Food and Agricultural Organization (FAO) and computing indirect estimates of diet net acid load. For each of some 130 countries, FAO tables report consumption of vegetable and animal foods in units of per capita vegetable and

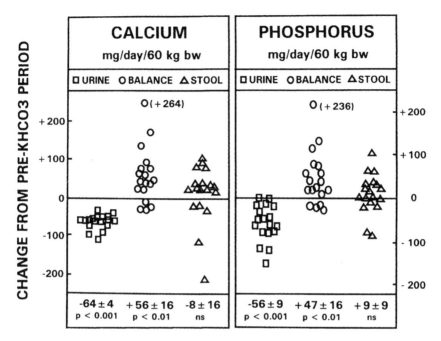

Figure 12 Effect of potassium bicarbonate supplementation on calcium and phosphorus excretion in urine, external calcium and phosphorus balance, and calcium and phosphorus excretion in stool, in 18 healthy postmenopausal women. The values at the bottom of the figure represent the average (±SD) of the potassium bicarbonate-induced changes from the control period (before supplementation). Values reflect comparisons between the control period and the supplementation period. *Source*: From Ref. 36.

animal protein consumed daily. Vegetable foods typically contain abundant K^+ salts of organic anions (119) that the body metabolizes to HCO_3^-, which reduces NEAP (11,14,15,120,121). By comparison, animal foods have a low content of K^+ per unit protein content. Because organic anion content of foods parallels that of K^+ (Fig. 13), the content of base precursors in vegetable foods also substantially exceeds that in animal foods. For a given total protein intake, therefore, the ratio of vegetable-to-animal protein consumed can provide a rough index for comparison of the base- to acid-generating potential of the diet.

One can approximate differences in bone mass among countries, based on published reports of the incidence of hip fractures in women over the age of 50 years. Hip fracture incidence provides a good index of bone mass because bone mass to a large extent determines the incidence of fractures of bone in older individuals (118). If chronic low-level diet-induced metabolic acidosis imposes a chronic, clinically significant drain on bone mass,

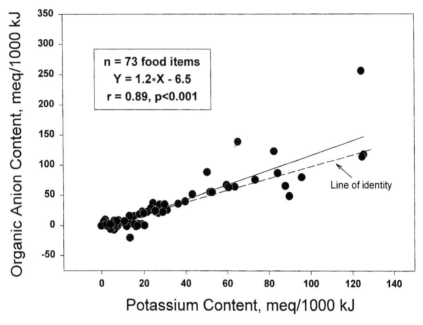

Figure 13   Relationship between net organic anion content and potassium content in common food items. Net organic anion content was calculated as the difference between the contents of inorganic cations and anions. *Source*: Data from Ref. 122.

one might observe differences in hip fracture incidence among countries related to differences in the ratio of vegetable-to-animal protein consumed.

Figure 14 depicts such an analyses for the 33 countries that provided the relevant data (118). Note the strong nonlinear reduction in fracture incidence with increasing ratio of vegetable-to-animal protein consumed. The ratio of base-generating (vegetable) to acid-generating (animal) foods consumed accounted for over two-thirds ($r^2 = 0.70$) of the total variability in hip fracture incidence among countries. Countries with the lowest ratio of vegetable-to-animal protein intake have the highest incidence of hip fracture, and vice versa. Though hip fracture differences among countries may relate in part to differences in genetically related determinants of bone mass (blacks) or hip architecture (Asians), a reanalysis of the largest homogenous subgroup (Caucasians, $n = 23$ countries) yielded results similar to those for the group as a whole (Fig. 15) (118).

The relationship between the ratio of vegetable-to-animal food intake and hip fracture rates in a more homogeneous group in a single country—elderly white American women—showed similar results (124). Further, hip bone loss rates achieved the highest values in the women with the lowest vegetable-to-animal food intake ratio. That study assumes importance

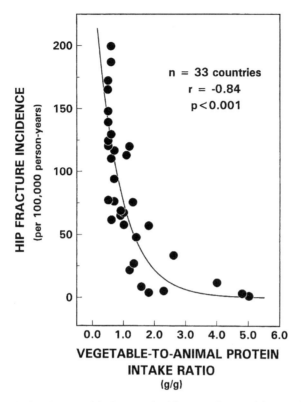

Figure 14 Relation between hip fracture incidence and vegetable-to-animal protein intake ratio in women over the age of 50 years in 33 countries. Each data point represents age-adjusted values for one country. *Source*: From Ref. 118.

because it eliminated the confounding effects of racial and cultural factors on hip fracture risk.

Those studies of Frassetto et al. and Sellmeyer et al. add to the weight of evidence implicating habitual ingestion of a net acid-producing diet as a determinant of age-related bone mass decline.

Using a less indirect index of NEAP, namely the ratio of dietary protein-to-potassium (Fig. 16), New et al. studied NEAP's effect on bone density and fracture incidence in elderly Scottish women (97,112,113). Those studies revealed lower values for lumbar spine mass and higher values of urinary excretion of bone resorption markers in women in the highest quartile of net acid load, compared to those in the lowest quartile. Further, the women who had sustained fractures during the observation period had significantly higher NEAPs, compared to those who had not. These studies extend the previous work demonstrating a positive association of lifelong fruit and vegetable intake (i.e., K^+ and base intake) on bone mineral density in women (126–128).

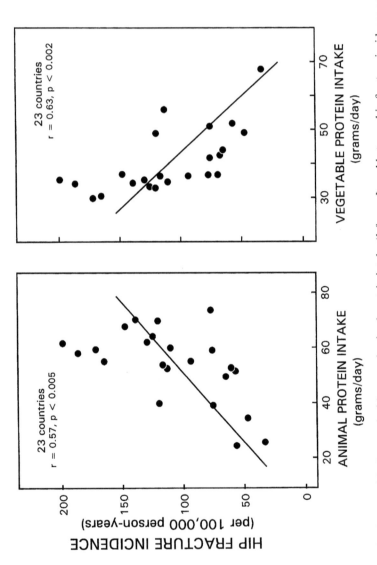

Figure 15 Relation between hip fracture incidence and animal protein intake (*left panel*), and between hip fracture incidence and vegetable protein intake, in women over the age of 50 years in 23 countries representing predominantly Caucasian populations. *Source:* From Ref. 118.

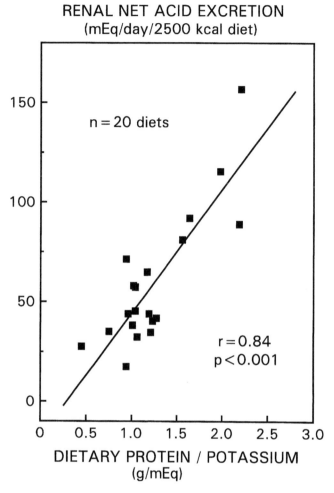

RENAL NET ACID EXCRETION
(mEq/day/2500 kcal diet)

n = 20 diets

r = 0.84
p < 0.001

DIETARY PROTEIN / POTASSIUM
(g/mEq)

Figure 16 The relation between steady-state RNAE, as an index of NEAP, and the ratio of dietary protein (Pro, g/day·10,460 kJ) to potassium (mEq/day 10,460 kJ) content for 20 different whole-food diets. RNAE $= -17.9 + 62.1$ (Pro/K) ($r = 0.84$, $R^2 = 0.71$, $P < 0.001$). Note that, for net acid-producing diets, in the steady tate, the ratio of dietary protein-to-potassium well predicts RNAE. *Source*: From Ref. 125.

Effect on Bone of Chronic Low-Grade Metabolic Acidosis
Caused by Urinary Diversion to a Surgically Created
Intestinal Bladder

Another line of evidence that chronic low-grade metabolic acidosis increases resorption of bone mineral and matrix comes from patients who have had their urine output diverted to a surgically created intestinal bladder, and who, as a result, develop a chronic low-grade metabolic acidosis (129,130). Such patients have increased rates of bone resorption, decreased bone mineral density of the spine and hip, and rates of bone turnover that correlate positively with the degree of their low-grade acidemia (129).

Effect on Bone of Chronic Low-Grade Metabolic Acidosis in the Setting of So-Called Incomplete Renal Tubular Acidosis

Additional evidence for the adverse skeletal effects of chronic low-grade metabolic acidosis comes from studies of patients with the so-called incomplete renal tubular acidosis (RTA). Low bone mass, histologically consistent with osteoporosis, occurs in patients with classic distal RTA (131), but it also appears to occur in patients with chronic low-grade metabolic acidosis in the setting of incomplete RTA (132,133). The diagnosis of incomplete RTA traditionally applies to patients judged *not* to have acidemia or hypobicarbonatemia by clinical criteria, but who nevertheless have a renal acidification defect like that of classic distal RTA in response to acid challenge. That such patients do not have acidemia or low plasma [HCO_3^-] requires skeptical interpretation, because excluding low-grade metabolic acidosis requires reference to the magnitude of the patients' typically positive diet net acid load. Indeed, several investigators have recognized that patients otherwise thought to have incomplete RTA manifest a low-grade metabolic acidosis (132–134).

Patients with nephrolithiasis diagnosed with incomplete RTA have fasting plasma [HCO_3^-] values lower than patients with nephrolithiasis without apparent renal acidification defect, and evidence hypercalciuria and increased bone matrix turnover (i.e., increased serum osteocalcin and urine hydroxyproline) more frequently (134). In patients preselected for osteoporosis (reduced bone density, vertebral fractures), a subgroup with impaired renal acidification exhibited slightly lower values of blood pH and plasma [HCO_3^-] compared to similarly osteoporotic patients without impaired renal acidification (133). The low plasma [HCO_3^-] in at least some patients diagnosed as incomplete RTA accompanies clinically diagnosed osteoporosis (132). Although the diagnosis of osteoporosis did not employ morphological criteria in any of these studies, morphologically identifiable osteoporosis has occurred in some patients with classic distal RTA (131), including one study of a large group of patients with RTA, in over half of which the investigators diagnosed incomplete RTA (135).

If most patients diagnosed as incomplete RTA will on critical evaluation have at least some degree of metabolic acidosis, two observations stand out for our present consideration: (a) incomplete RTA occurs with substantial frequency in patients preselected for osteoporosis (136), and (b) in the patients who have reduced bone mineral density, chronic alkali therapy by itself can lead to substantial improvement of the bone density, accompanying correction of hypercalciuria and improvement in external calcium balance (137).

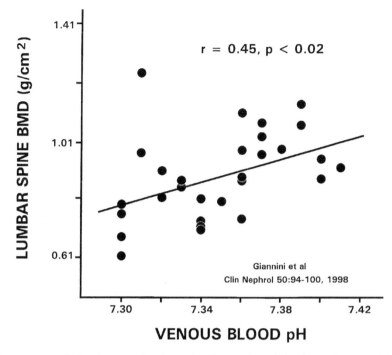

Figure 17 Relation between lumbar spine bone mineral density and venous blood pH in patients with idiopathic fasting hypercalciuria. As venous blood pH averages about 0.03 pH units lower than that of arterial blood pH, most of the pH values fall within the clinically accepted normal range. *Source*: Replotted from Ref. 138.

Another study reveals an inverse correlation between bone mineral density and blood acidity within the clinically adjudged normal range in renal stone formers with "fasting hypercalciuria" (138). Bone mineral density and blood pH, both regulating lower than in control subjects, correlated positively (138) (Fig. 17). Clinicians diagnose incomplete RTA with considerable frequency in patients with idiopathic hypercalciuria, in particular those with "fasting hypercalciuria." Whatever the cause of the low-grade metabolic acidosis in the patients studied in Fig. 17, its severity correlated with the degree of their bone loss (138).

Chronic Metabolic Acidosis and Muscle Wasting

Effect of Metabolic Acidosis on Skeletal Muscle Nitrogen Metabolism and Renal Nitrogen Excretion

In diseases that cause chronic metabolic acidosis, protein degradation in skeletal muscle accelerates (59–61,139), inducing negative nitrogen balance (61). These effects result from the acidosis itself, not its cause, nor from sequelae of the underlying acidosis-producing disorder, because they occur with widely differing acidosis-producing conditions (60,61,63,140–144) and because alkali administration reverses them (145–150).

Acidosis-induced proteolysis serves acid–base homeostasis, just as acidosis-induced osteolysis does. With increased skeletal release of amino acids, including glutamine and amino acids the liver converts to glutamine (the major source for renal synthesis of ammonia [NH_3]), the kidney can greatly increase excretion of H^+ (as ammonium ions [NH_4^+]) (see Chapter 6) (60,61,151,152). As part of an integrated acid–base homeostatic mechanism, chronic metabolic acidosis also causes an adaptive increase in renal glutamine extraction and NH_3 production (153), and accelerates hepatic production of glutamine, thereby helping to sustain the acidosis-augmented rates of renal glutamine extraction and utilization for NH_3 production and NH_4^+ excretion (142,154–156).

Effect of Chronic Diet-Induced Metabolic Acidosis on Renal Nitrogen Excretion in Humans

Given that acidosis–proteolysis connection, we tested whether renal nitrogen wasting might occur even with the low-grade metabolic acidosis caused by eating typical net acid-producing diets (157). In women given $KHCO_3$ to correct their diet-related low-grade metabolic acidosis, urinary NH_4^+ excretion decreased, as expected (Fig. 18). A sustained reduction in urea nitrogen excretion occurred, indicating that the higher pretreatment urea nitrogen excretion rates resulted from acidosis-induced nitrogen wasting (Fig. 18). Reduced urea and NH_4^+ excretion contributed about equally to the nitrogen-sparing effect of correcting the diet-related acidosis. In addition, with reduced renal NH_3 production, a reduction in NH_3 ammonia delivery to the systemic circulation contributes indirectly to improvement in nitrogen balance by limiting substrate (NH_3) availability for hepatic urea production (158). A reduction of urea excretion has been observed during alkali administration also in other acidotic states (145,146).

Quantitative Significance of Nitrogen Wasting from Chronic Diet-Induced Metabolic Acidosis

From the known usual rate of age-related loss of lean body mass in women (159), we can compute that the observed $KHCO_3$-induced nitrogen sparing in the women we studied (Fig. 18). We found that it potentially could prevent all ongoing losses of muscle mass and restore accrued deficits (157).

Chronic Metabolic Acidosis and Renal Injury

The question has arisen whether the metabolic acidosis that typically occurs during chronic progressive renal diseases in turn accelerates the progression of renal injury and functional decline (9,66,160,161). We believe the

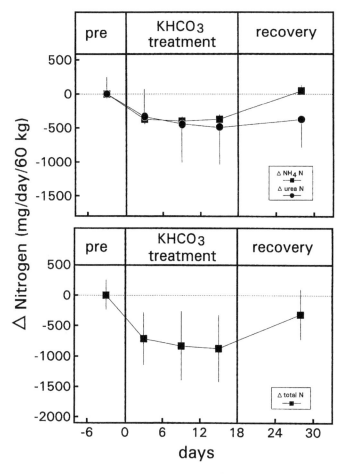

Figure 18 Effect of potassium bicarbonate administration on urinary excretion of ammonium and urea in healthy postmenopausal women. *Source*: From Ref. 157.

question germane because it prompts the question whether chronic diet-induced metabolic acidosis contributes to the pathogenesis of the renal structural and functional decline that occurs normally with aging.

Chronic metabolic acidosis contributes to the progression of renal disease putatively by at least five potential acidosis-inducible renal pathologies (161): (a) intrarenal calcium salt deposition (skeletal calcium mobilization and reduced renal citrate concentrations) (162); (b) renal cellular hypertrophy (metabolic sequelae of acidosis) (65,163); (c) intrarenal complement-induced cytotoxicity initiated and sustained by increased local concentrations of NH_3; (d) amino acid-induced hemodynamic injury (accelerated protein catabolism) (164); and, (e) intrarenal oxidant damage (hypermetabolism)

(165,166). Noting that two studies in experimentally induced renal disease in rats showed conflicting results of benefit from sustained alkali (sodium bicarbonate) therapy, one extensive review of the topic concluded that "there is little empirical evidence to support aggressive correction of metabolic acidosis as a tool to slow the progression of renal disease" (161). More recently, investigators have shown mitigation of reduced glomerular filtration rate and of renal tissue injury with systemic alkalinizing doses of calcium citrate in rats with experimental progressive renal insufficiency (167).

Yet in humans the question remains alive, as no one has yet carried out a clinical trial of sustained correction of acidosis either in patients with renal disease or in healthy subjects to determine if the rate of decline of glomerular filtration rate slows or stops. We consider intriguing the finding that glomerular filtration rate decline greatly attenuates with chronic alkali therapy in patients with classic distal renal tubular acidosis (168), and the finding in such patients that, despite the presumed primacy of dysfunction of the renal tubule, the degree of glomerular insufficiency and degree of acidosis correlate positively (169).

DIET-INDUCED POTASSIUM-REPLETE CHLORIDE-SUFFICIENT CHRONIC LOW-GRADE METABOLIC ALKALOSIS AS THE NATURALLY SELECTED OPTIMAL SYSTEMIC ACID–BASE STATE OF HUMANS

In this section, we shift attention from diet-induced low-grade metabolic acidosis to diet-induced low-grade metabolic alkalosis. We argue that natural selection designed humans for an "optimal" systemic acid–base status of low-grade chronic metabolic alkalosis, characterized by mild alkalemia and hyperbicarbonatemia, induced by habitual ingestion of a K^+-rich, Na^+- and Cl^--meager diet that supplies HCO_3^- precursors substantially in excess of H^+ precursors. We support this argument with a quantitative analysis indicating that the hunter–gatherer-based diet of our Paleolithic human ancestors—which diet resembled the diet that their hominid ancestors developed genetic adaptations to during the many million years of evolution leading to *Homo sapiens*—supplies a substantial net load of base (11). We show that the magnitude of the estimated net base input of the Paleolithic diet suffices to induce and sustain a low-grade metabolic alkalosis characterized by detectable alkalemia and hyperbicarbonatemia (22).

Estimation of the Diet Net Acid Load of the Ancestral Human Diet

Paleoanthropologists can trace human ancestry back 5–7 million years before encountering an ancestor who also qualified as an ancestor of humanity's nearest living relatives, the pongids (e.g., chimpanzees, gorillas). *Homo sapiens* emerged from hominid ancestors sometime during the last 3–5% of that period. *Homo sapiens's* hominid ancestors lived as hunter–gatherers, eating a diverse, plant-based diet with variable amounts of meat in increasing proportion as hunting technology progressed (13,170–174). The nutrient content of that diet counts as a major component of the environment influencing the genetic evolution of the hominid lineage leading to *Homo sapiens*. With the emergence of *Homo sapiens* about 200,000 years ago, the hunter–gatherer lifestyle continued, until the invention of agriculture about 10,000 years ago, when the composition of the human diet underwent a revolutionary change, with major acid–base implications.

Before agriculture began, *Homo sapiens* habitually ate exclusively a hunter–gatherer diet similar to the one to which natural selection had fitted their genome. The agricultural era of the last 10,000 years comprises too short a time on an evolutionary scale for natural selection to generate major genetic adaptations in response to the profound changes in the nutrient composition of the diet that resulted from the switch to the modern agricultural-based diet. From a nutritional point of view (17,21,175), and incidentally also from a psychological (176) and sociobiological (177) point of view, contemporary humans differ little genetically from stone age hunter–gatherers.

From data on the diets of existing hunter–gatherer societies, and from inferences about the Paleolithic environment, we can reconstruct the Paleolithic diet and the probable daily nutrient intakes of Paleolithic humans (13). In an estimated 3000 kcal diet, meat constituted 35% of the diet by weight and plant foods, 65%. Total protein intake estimates as 251 g/day, of which animal protein estimates as 191 g/day, and plant proteins, 60 g/day. By contrast, contemporary humans consume less than one-half that amount of animal protein, and only about one-third that amount of plant protein, per kilocalorie of diet (6). Na^+ intake estimates at about 29 mEq/day, and K^+ intake, in excess of 280 mEq/day. By contrast, contemporary humans consume between 100 and 300 mEq of Na^+ per day, and about 80 mEq of K^+ per day. Thus, in the switch to the modern diet, the K^+/Na^+ ratio reversed, from 1 to 10, to more than 3 to 1. Since food Na^+ exists largely in the form of Cl^- salts, and food K^+ largely in the form of HCO_3^--generating organic acid salts, the Cl^-/HCO_3^- ratio of the diet likewise reversed.

In computing the potential net acid (or base) load of the Paleolithic diet, one needs to consider the animal-to-plant food energy intake ratio, animal food fat energy density, and, the distribution of plant food energies among plant food groups. The potential net acid load of lean meats varies little by animal source (15), presumably reflecting the similarity of protein composition of skeletal muscle across vertebrate species. However, the potential net base load among plant foods varies greatly (11,14,15), with some foods supplying substantial amounts of net base in mEq per gram protein or per kcal food item (e.g., leafy-green and root vegetables), some substantially smaller amounts (e.g., legumes), while some supply a net acid load (e.g., cereal grains). While all plant foods contain protein, in those plant foods that produce net base, the amount of K^+-associated HCO_3^- precursors (e.g., potassium citrate) exceeds the amount of protein-dependent H^+ precursors. Thus, one cannot accurately predict the potential net acid (or base) load of the diet solely from knowledge of its total animal and vegetable content alone (11,178).

Using numerous plausible animal-to-plant food energy intake ratios, animal food fat energy densities, and distributions of plant food energies among plant food groups for ancestral hominids, and using established computational methods for estimating systemic sulfuric and organic acid and HCO_3^- yields from individual food items, adjusting for fractional intestinal absorption, we computed the diet-dependent NEAP for 159 preagricultural diets and compared those with computed and measured values for typical American diets (11). We found that 87% (139/159) of the diets computed as net base-producing, with NEAP averaging -88 mEq/day (Fig. 19). Using the same computational model, the average American diet,

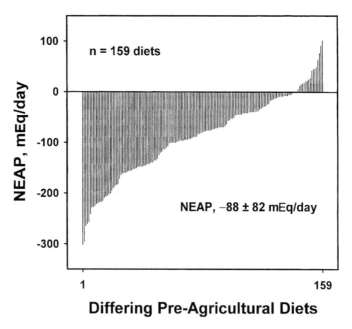

Figure 19 Estimations of net endogenous acid production rates (NEAP) for 159 retrojected diets likely to have been consumed by prehistoric, preagricultural *Homo sapiens* and their hominid ancestors. *Source*: From Ref. 11.

per composition reported in the most recent U.S. National Health and Examination Survey (NHANES III) (5,6), computed as net acid-producing, averaging +48 mEq/day, matching within a few percent the average estimated from steady-state renal net acid excretion rates in free-living Americans (31,47).

Why Do Contemporary Diets Yield Net Acid?

Although the modern diet has a substantially lower protein content and ratio of animal to plant protein than does the Paleolithic diet (6,13), that did not prevent the transition from the Paleolithic diet's net base production rate to the contemporary diet's net acid production rate. That transition occurred because the distribution of plant foods in the modern diet has shifted from high base-yielding plant foods (roots, tubers, leafy greens, and fruit) to a predominance of low base-yielding legumes and net acid-producing cereal grains (16). Cereal grains, one of the few plant food groups that yield net acid on metabolism—as predicted from their composition (11,15,16) and demonstrated by feeding (14)—constitute approximately 65% of plant food energy intake and supply over 50% of the plant protein ingested in the modern American diet (6). By contrast, cereal grains rarely contribute to hunter–gatherer diets, and contributed virtually nothing in prehistoric diets (179).

In addition to displacement of high HCO_3^--yielding plant foods by net acid-yielding cereal grains and low base-yielding legumes, displacement of high HCO_3^--yielding plant foods by energy-dense nutrient-poor foods (e.g., separated fats, vegetable oils, refined sugars) contribute to the negative-to-positive shift in NEAP. While removing cereal grains from the diet and substituting fruits and vegetables reduces NEAP nearly to zero, removing energy-dense nutrient-poor foods as well, and substituting fruits and vegetables, renders the diet substantially net base-producing (11). In other words, the mistakenly adjudged "high" protein intakes of the modern diet does not make it net acid-producing; rather it becomes net acid-producing because of "low" intakes of high base-yielding plant foods in preference to "high" intakes of cereal grains, legumes, and energy-dense nutrient-poor foods do (11,16).*

---

*Indeed, high protein intakes have desirable effects, for example an anabolic effect on bone, owing to substrate (amino acid) provision for building bone matrix, and a stimulatory effect that increases the bone growth-promoting factor, insulin-like growth hormone-I (180,181). Since metabolic alkalosis also has anabolic effects on bone (182) and since metabolic acidosis reduces serum IGF-I levels (183), the combination of a net base-producing/alkalosigenic diet and a high protein diet might optimize peak bone mass achievement and eliminate age-related declines in bone mass.

Has Natural Selection Genetically Adapted Us to a Net Base-Producing Diet?—Implications of Crossing the Acid–Base Neutral Zone

Considering that the hominid ancestors of *Homo sapiens* habitually ingested a net base-producing diet during millions of years of evolution, we cannot ignore that natural selection may have genetically adapted the metabolic machinery of *Homo sapiens* to a more or less sustained dietary net input of HCO_3^-. The genes of a species (e.g., *Homo sapiens*) encode a description of it ancestors' environment (4).

The switch from the ancestral net base-producing diet to the modern net acid-producing diet imposed a double jeopardy on modern humans, one due to a loss of potentially beneficial base input to the body, another due to a net addition of pathogenic acid to the body—crossing the neutral zone from base- to acid-land. In considering the acid–base effects of diet, we need to consider not only the potential negative effects of chronic diet-induced *metabolic acidosis* but also loss of the potential positive effects of chronic diet-induced *metabolic alkalosis*.

Is the Net Base Input of the Ancestral Human Diet Sufficiently Large to Produce a Detectable Signal for Inducing Potentially Beneficial Metabolic and Physiological Effects?

The human kidney excretes chronic K^+ and HCO_3^- loads with prodigious facility and capacity (184–187). One might then ask whether the habitual ingestion of the moderate dietary net base load characteristic of the human ancestral diet (20–100 mEq/day) can detectably reset systemic acid–basic equilibrium. We answered that question affirmatively in normal humans ingesting a low NaCl diet who received small net base-producing loads of sodium bicarbonate (188). In follow-up, we found that moderate chronic dietary net base loads (20–100 mEq/day) induced by administering $KHCO_3$ to normal humans, without chloride restriction, significantly perturbed plasma acid–base composition in the direction of metabolic alkalosis (22). The degree of metabolic alkalosis, moreover, correlated directly with the magnitude of the negative values of NEAP. Although blood $[H^+]$ and plasma $[HCO_3^-]$ remained within the broad range clinically judged as "normal," the magnitude of the changes permitted detection, and they persisted. Therefore, they potentially could provide a system-wide signal for possible beneficial metabolic and physiologic effects.

From an evolutionary nutritional perspective, then, it appears that the optimal diet of humans supplies an excess of HCO_3^--generating precursors relative to H^+-generating precursors. Likewise, from that perspective, given that hominids for millions of years before *Homo sapiens* emerged habitually ingested such a diet, natural selection had ample opportunity to eliminate individuals disadvantaged by habitually eating such a diet, and conversely had little opportunity to generate adaptations for habitually eating a nonbase-producing diet. We may then regard a stone age-type net base-producing diet as the evolutionary optimal human diet From this perspective, diet-induced chronic low-grade K^+-replete metabolic alkalosis would constitute the natural and optimal systemic acid–base state of humans.

Potential Health Benefits of Diet-Induced Low-Grade Metabolic Alkalosis in Humans

Clinicians may express skepticism that K^+-replete alkali-loading metabolic alkalosis, however mild, confers optimal systemic acid–base status. Clinicians view metabolic alkalosis as a "disorder," caused by pathological conditions, in which the associated alkalemia and hyperbicarbonatemia injure the body. However, the adverse effects of metabolic alkalosis depend on the severity of the accompanying alkalemia and increase in plasma $[HCO_3^-]$, and the associated state of body K^+ stores. No problems accompany decreases in blood $[H^+]$ and increases in plasma $[HCO_3^-]$ within the vicinity of the range of clinically adjudged "normal" values, but potential beneficial effects do, as we provide evidence and arguments for below. Clinicians often (if unintentionally) induce sustained low-grade metabolic alkalosis, for example, with thiazide treatment of hypertension or calcium nephrolithiasis, and do not consider it imperative to treat the low-grade alkalosis, though they sometimes do indirectly, by administering KCl when overt hypokalemia coexists. In thiazide treatment of calcium nephrolithiasis, some clinicians recommend supplementing dietary K^+ with its alkalinizing salts (e.g., potassium citrate), which sustains the low-grade metabolic alkalosis (189–191). Alkalinizing salts of potassium have the advantage of both increasing urinary citrate excretion (an inhibitor of stone formation) (189–191) and amplifying the thiazide reduction of urinary calcium excretion (47).

Independently of thiazides, inducing and sustaining a mild metabolic alkalosis with chronic alkali loading is recommended in treatment for calcium nephrolithiasis in patients with idiopathic hypocitraturia (192). Clinicians also induce mild metabolic alkalosis with alkali loading as standard treatment for patients on chronic hemodialysis, to minimize or prevent the diet-induced metabolic acidosis that ordinarily occurs between dialysis sessions (193).

Alkali-loading with K^+–alkali differs from the metabolic alkaloses that co-occur with K^+ and Cl^- depletion (see Chapter 16). It distinguishes itself also by its minimal perturbation of systemic acid-base equilibrium (22,191). Chronic net base loads substantially larger even than $50–100\,mEq/day$ produce only small decreases in blood $[H^+]$ and increases in plasma $[HCO_3^-]$, owing to the efficiency of renal HCO_3^- excretion (22,187) That efficiency, undoubtedly genetically determined, presumably represents a naturally selected adaptation to habitual dietary net base during the multimillion years of hominid evolution. Only with extraordinarily large alkali loads (many hundreds of mEq/day) and factors restricting renal HCO_3^- excretion, such as renal failure or hypercalcemia, does clinically important metabolic alkalosis result from alkali loading.

Several lines of evidence support the proposition that moderate net base loads, in the absence of K^+ and Cl^- depletion, may have beneficial metabolic and physiological effects.

Bone

As discussed earlier, in vitro studies (10,111) reveal that metabolic acidosis leads to bone resorption. Metabolic alkalosis, by contrast, reduces calcium efflux from bone, and both suppresses osteoclastic bone resorption and stimulates osteoblastic bone formation (182). Those effects occur linearly with medium pH values above 7.40 (effected by increasing medium $[HCO_3^-]$), suggesting that even minimal degrees of alkalosis show anabolic and antiresorptive effects. Those in vitro findings also suggest that inducing and sustaining a low-grade systemic metabolic alkalosis with appropriate amounts of dietary base might amplify the antiosteoporotic effects of simply neutralizing the diet net acid load with smaller amounts of base. Alkalosis-producing base input may augment bone also through renal conservation of calcium. Reduced urinary calcium excretion produced by alkali loading linearly correlates with the alkali load over a broad range (unpublished observations).

Those considerations have potential implications for treatment and prevention of osteoporosis. Bone mass declines progressively after it peaks in young adulthood because bone formation fails to keep pace with bone resorption. A small increase in the ratio of osteoblastic bone formation to osteoclastic bone resorption, such as might accompany low-grade K^+ alkali-loading metabolic alkalosis (36,54), might tip the scales just enough to equalize the unfavorable formation–resorption coupling and prevent bone mass decline, or tip them enough even to increase bone mass.

Observations on the skeletal remains of stone age humans provide some clues. Ancestral *Homo* species exhibit increased cortical thickness of their femurs, relative to body mass, and strength or rigidity (194). Prehistoric hunter–gatherer femurs show greater density than those from prehistoric periodic agriculturalists, and bone density in the hunter–gatherers remained relatively stable with age compared to the agriculturalists (195). Age-related bone mineral content in a strictly hunter–gatherer prehistoric population consistently showed slower rates of bone loss with age than in a prehistoric agriculturalist group (196). Although many lifestyle factors may have contributed to the stone agers' higher bone mass and lower rates of bone mass decline with age, the acid–base perspective we present precludes us from ignoring the potential role of habitual dietary net base input.

A more favorable bone formation–resorption coupling ratio secondary to chronic dietary net base input might also facilitate acquisition of bone during growth and development, leading to higher peak bone mass. Consider the finding that very large intermittent doses of alkali given to children with HCO_3^--wasting renal tubular acidosis, required to sustain complete correction of metabolic acidosis, greatly accelerated bone growth (197). Yet, to sustain correction of acidosis with intermittent doses of alkali in an HCO_3^--wasting disorder, one must overcorrect the acidosis throughout the interval between doses. Conceivably then the acceleration of bone growth resulted from repeated extended periods of low-grade metabolic alkalosis.

Nephrologists often administer acidosis-overcorrecting intermittent doses of alkali to prevent metabolic acidosis in the treatment of patients with end-stage renal disease requiring intermittent hemodialysis. To sustain correction of acidosis such that plasma acid–base composition does not reach acidotic levels between treatments, they induce metabolic alkalosis during dialysis by sufficiently increasing dialysis bath HCO_3^- concentration, which results in a sustained low-grade metabolic alkalosis during most of the interval between dialysis treatments (198,199). This practice reportedly yields superior results in ameliorating secondary hyperparathyroidism and osteodystrophy in the patients (198).

Skeletal Muscle

In children with HCO_3^--wasting renal tubular acidosis treated with large amounts of alkali (see above), bone growth accompanied a generalized growth acceleration, including skeletal muscle (197). Investigators seem not to have specifically tested the effect of alkali-loading metabolic alkalosis on skeletal muscle protein synthesis and catabolism. As discussed earlier, renal nitrogen losses accompanying low-grade diet-induced metabolic acidosis decreased on administration of supplemental $[HCO_3^-]$, suggesting that base supplementation reduces the age-related decline in muscle mass that occurs normally in adult humans eating net acid-producing diets (157). To completely prevent age-related declines in muscle mass might require restoring the diet to its Paleolithic net base-producing state, with its associated low-grade metabolic alkalosis. Administration of alkalosis-producing doses of exogenous base in humans can greatly reduce renal excretion of urea while concomitantly decreasing serum urea concentration, suggesting that alkali-loading alkalosis increases body nitrogen stores, of which skeletal muscle owns the lion's share (187).

Nephrolithiasis

Hypercalciuria increases the risk of formation of calcium-containing kidney stones, occurring $\sim$50% of stone formers (31). In patients with no identifiable cause of hypercalciuria, clinicians refer to the condition as idiopathic hypercalciuria. Treatments that reduce urinary calcium excretion in such patients can reduce or eliminate stone recurrence.

Whatever the precise mechanisms underlying idiopathic hypercalciuria, we need to consider the potential role of NEAP in determining its expression (Fig. 11) (31,36,88,200–202). Urinary calcium excretion in idiopathic hypercalciuria varies directly with NEAP in the acid range (measured by RNAE), as it does in healthy control subjects (31). For any given NEAP, however, calcium excretion remains higher in the patients, and never decreases low enough to prevent supersaturation of urine for calcium stone formation. Thus, idiopathic hypercalciuria seems to result in abnormally high urinary excretion rates of calcium, whatever the NEAP in the acid range. The lowest values of NEAP never reached negative values, however, and therefore we can draw no conclusions about the effect of negative NEAP (i.e., a dietary net base load) on calcium excretion. Conceivably, at net acid excretion rates in the range of -50 to $-100\,mEq/day$, calcium excretion might fall low enough to unsaturate the urine for calcium stone formation. Because of the exaggerated slope of the relationship between calcium excretion and acid load reported in some of these patients (203), one might find the calcium-lowering effect of base loading most impressive. Sustained negative NEAP might completely eliminate hypercalciuria and stone formation in idiopathic hypercalciuria.

In addition to a direct effect on renal handling of calcium, base loading, when accompanied by K^+, influences renal handling of phosphorus. Even small dietary loads of $KHCO_3$ can induce renal retention of phosphorus, increase serum phosphorus concentration, and reduce circulating calcitriol levels (204,205). Larger, moderately alkalosis-producing potassium HCO_3^- loads therefore might completely eliminate hypercalciuria by entraining effects on the putative hypercalciuria-causing underlying defects in phosphorus and calcitriol metabolism in patients with idiopathic hypercalciuria (31).

By inducing a low-grade metabolic alkalosis without associated K^+ depletion, moderate dietary net base loading (e.g., with $KHCO_3$ or fruits and vegetables) also would be expected to increase excretion of citrate (53), which by chelating calcium reduces its availability for stone formation. We predict that by both greatly increasing citrate excretion and greatly decreasing total calcium excretion, habitual ingestion of a moderate net base-producing potassium-rich diet (e.g., 50–100 mEq endogenous net base production and 200–250 mEq potassium intake per day) will completely prevent expression of the underlying defect(s) in patients with idiopathic hypercalciuria, both as hypercalciuria and as recurrent stone formation.

SUMMARY AND IMPLICATIONS FOR FURTHER RESEARCH

For the past century, studies of renal acid–base physiology focused overwhelmingly on mechanisms of urinary acidification and net acid excretion.

During human evolution, natural selection undoubtedly conserved those mechanisms because of their adaptive value in responding to metabolic acidosis-producing conditions experienced presumably intermittently by early humans and their hominid ancestors: food shortage (starvation ketoacidosis and autoproteolytic sulfuric acidosis); meat feasting (sulfuric acidosis); feasting on certain plant foods that are net acid producing (e.g., plums, cranberries); prolonged intense physical activity (lactic acidosis); and, infectious or toxic diarrhea (fecal HCO_3^- wasting). Given the episodic nature of those conditions, we need not suppose that natural selection designed the renal mechanisms promoting net acid excretion to operate *tonically* during an individual's lifetime. We have argued in this chapter that under the more usual day-to-day conditions of eating a typical hunter–gatherer-type diet, early humans and their hominid ancestors most often experienced a net load of base, and that natural selection directed renal regulation of systemic acid–base equilibrium over a lifetime predominantly to regulation of urinary alkalinization and net base excretion.

The ancestral human diet yielded net base because base input from plant-source foods exceeded acid input from animal-source foods. Diets rich in base-producing plant foods contain abundant K^+. Indeed, we estimate the K^+ content of ancestral hominid diets as three or four times greater than that of contemporary diets (13,23,206). Although we know much about the mechanisms of renal adaptation to chronic K^+ loads, and somewhat less about the mechanisms of renal adaptation to chronic base loads, we know little about the overall physiology of the kidney under the combined conditions of habitual dietary K^+ and base loads at levels likely supplied by the ancestral diet. Considering that high K^+ and HCO_3^- systemic loads prevailed during the 5+ million years of hominid evolution that eventuated in *Homo sapiens*, and that they prevailed in each generation throughout the growth, development, and reproductive period of each individual, our current norms for human renal physiology may be off base.

Beyond the kidney, a similar argument applies to our current perspective on what constitutes "normal" human physiology and metabolism in general. If our genes "describe" the environment of our ancestors (4), the genetic determinants of the many extrarenal metabolic and physiological functions influenced by acid–base and K^+ status may not realize their naturally selected design advantage to human health until the nutrient environment returns to its ancestral dietary K^+- and base-rich state. As Dawkins (207) puts it:

> Living organisms are beautifully built to survive and reproduce in their environments. Or that is what Darwinians say. But actually it isn't quite right. They are beautifully built for survival in their ancestors' environments. It is because their ancestors survived— long enough to pass on their DNA—that our modern animals

[including humans] are well-built. For they inherit the very same successful DNA. The genes that survive down the generations add up, in effect, to a description of what it took to survive back then. And that is tantamount to saying that modern DNA is a coded description of the environments in which ancestors survived. A survival manual is handed down the generations. A Genetic Book of the Dead.

ACKNOWLEDGMENTS

Many of the studies reported on in this chapter we performed in, or utilized resources provided by the UCSF Moffitt/MZ General Clinical Research Center (GCRC)(NIH MO1 RR00079). The authors thank the following colleagues for fruitful discussions: Uriel S. Barzel, Loren Cordain, S. Boyd Eaton, F. John Gennari, Robert P. Heaney, Jacob Lemann Jr., Susan A. New, Man S. Oh, and Karen M. Todd. The authors greatly appreciate the support of Annette Robinson in all stages of preparation of the manuscript.

REFERENCES

1. Auden WH, Kronenberger L. The Viking Book of Aphorisms. New York: The Viking Press, 1981.
2. Allman WF. The Stone Age Present: How Evolution Has Shaped Modern Life: from Sex, Violence, and Language to Emotions, Morals, and Communities. New York: Simon & Schuster, 1994.
3. Dobzhansky TG. Nothing in biology makes sense except in the light of evolution. The American Biology Teacher 1973; 35:125–129.
4. Dawkins R. Unweaving the Rainbow: Science, Delusion and the Appetite for Wonder. New York: Houghton Mifflin Company, 1998.
5. Kant AK. Consumption of energy-dense, nutrient-poor foods by adult Americans: nutritional and health implications. The Third National Health and Nutrition Examination Survey, 1988–1994. Am J Clin Nutr 2000; 72:929–936.
6. Smit E, Nieto FJ, Crespo CJ, Mitchell P. Estimates of animal and plant protein intake in US adults: results from the Third National Health and Nutrition Examination Survey, 1988–1991. J Am Diet Assoc 1999; 99:813–820.
7. Kurtz I, Maher T, Hulter HN, Schambelan M, Sebastian A. Effect of diet on plasma acid–base composition in normal humans. Kidney Int 1983; 24:670–680.
8. Frassetto L, Morris RC Jr, Sebastian A. Effect of age on blood acid–base composition in adult humans: role of age-related renal functional decline. Am J Physiol 1996; 271:1114–1122.
9. Alpern RJ, Sakhaee S. The clinical spectrum of chronic metabolic acidosis: homeostatic mechanisms produce significant morbidity. Am J Kidney Dis 1997; 29:291–302.

10. Bushinsky DA. Acid–base imbalance and the skeleton. In: Burckhardt P, Dawson-Hughes B, Heaney RP, eds. Nutritional Aspects of Osteoporosis. Berlin: Springer, 1998:208–217.
11. Sebastian A, Frassetto LA, Sellmeyer DE, Merriam RL, Morris RC Jr. Estimation of the net acid load of the diet of ancestral preagricultural *Homo sapiens* and their hominid ancestors. Am J Clin Nutr 2002; 76:1308–1316.
12. Frassetto LA, Sebastian A. Diet-induced potassium-replete chloride-sufficient chronic low-grade metabolic alkalosis as the naturally-selected optimal systemic acid–base state of humans: Implications for humans. The First Bay Area Clinical Research Symposium Book of Abstracts 2003; 1:65.
13. Eaton SB, Konner M. Paleolithic nutrition. A consideration of its nature and current implications. N Engl J Med 1985; 312:283–289.
14. Blatherwick NR. The specific role of foods in relation to the composition of the urine. Arch Int Med 1914; 14:409–450.
15. Remer T, Manz F. Potential renal acid load of foods and its influence on urine pH. J Am Diet Assoc 1995; 95:791–797.
16. Sebastian, Frassetto, Sellmeyer Morris Jr. Acid-grain: why contemporary diets are net acid-producing. J Am Soc Nephrol 2001; 12:140A.
17. Eaton SB, Konner M, Shostak M. Stone agers in the fast lane: chronic degenerative diseases in evolutionary perspective. Am J Med 1988; 84:739–749.
18. Eaton SB, Nelson DA. Calcium in evolutionary perspective. Am J Clin Nutr 1991; 54:281S–287S.
19. Tobian L. The Volhard lecture: potassium and sodium in hypertension. J Hypertens 1988; 6(suppl 4):S12–S24.
20. Tobian L. The protective effects of high potassium diets in hypertension, and the mechanisms by which high-NaCl diets produce hypertension. In: Laragh JH, Brenner BM, eds. Hypertension: Pathophysiology, Diagnosis, and Management. New York: Raven Press, 1995:299–312.
21. Eaton SB, Cordain L. Evolutionary aspects of diet: old genes, new fuels. Nutritional changes since agriculture. World Rev Nutr Diet 1997; 81:26–37.
22. Sebastian Frassetto, Sellmeyer Morris RC. Diet-induced potassium-replete chloride-sufficient chronic low-grade metabolic alkalosis as the naturally-selected optimal systemic acid–base state of humans. J Am Soc Nephrol 2001; 12:140A.
23. Sebastian Frassetto, Sellmeyer Morris Jr. The natural dietary potassium intake of humans exceeds current intakes minimally by a factor of four. J Am Soc Nephrol 2001; 12:40A.
24. Morris RC Jr, Frassetto LA, Schmidlin O, Forman A, Sebastian A. Expression of osteoporosis as determined by diet-disordered electrolyte and acid–base metabolism. In: Burckhardt P, Dawson-Hughes B, Heaney RP, eds. Nutritional Aspects of Osteoporosis. San Diego: Academic press, 2001:357–378.
25. Frassetto L, Morris RC Jr, Sellmeyer DE, Todd K, Sebastian A. Diet, evolution and aging—the pathophysiologic effects of the post-agricultural inversion of the potassium-to-sodium and base-to-chloride ratios in the human diet. Eur J Nutr 2001; 40:200–213.
26. Sebastian A. Evolution, diet, acid–base, and bone. GCRC J 2004; Fall/Winter 2003/2004:8–11.

27. Alpern RJ. Trade-offs in the adaptation to acidosis. Kidney Int 1995; 47:1205–1215.
28. Frassetto L, Sebastian A. Age and systemic acid–base equilibrium: analysis of published data. J Gerontol 1996; 51A:B91–B99.
29. Madias NE, Adrogue HJ, Horowitz GL, Cohen JJ, Schwartz WB. A redefinition of normal acid–base equilibrium in man: carbon dioxide as a key determinant of normal plasma bicarbonate concentration. Kidney Int 1979; 16:612–618.
30. Lennon EJ, Lemann J Jr, Litzow JR. The effect of diet and stool composition on the net external acid balance of normal subjects. J Clin Invest 1966; 45:1601–1607.
31. Lemann J Jr. Relationship between urinary calcium and net acid excretion as determined by dietary protein and potassium: a review. Nephron 1999; 81(suppl 1):18–25.
32. Lemann J Jr, Lennon EJ, Goodman AD, Litzow JR, Relman AS. The net balance of acid in subjects given large loads of acid or alkali. J Clin Invest 1965; 44:507–517.
33. Lemann J Jr, Relman AS. The relation of sulfur metabolism to acid–base balance and electrolyte excretion: the effects of dl-methionine in normal man. J Clin Invest 1959; 38:2215–2223.
34. Coe FL, Firpo JJJ, Hollandsworth DL, Segil L, Canterbury JM, Reiss E. Effect of acute and chronic metabolic acidosis on serum immunoreactive parathyroid hormone in man. Kidney Int 1975; 8:262–272.
35. Relman AS, Lennon EJ, Lemann J Jr. Endogenous production of fixed acid and the measurement of net balance of acid in normal subjects. J Clin Invest 1961; 40:1621–1630.
36. Sebastian A, Harris ST, Ottaway JH, Todd KM, Morris RC Jr. Improved mineral balance and skeletal metabolism in postmenopausal women treated with potassium bicarbonate [see comments]. N Engl J Med 1994; 330: 1776–1781.
37. Krapf R, Seldin DW, Alpern RJ. Clinical syndromes of metabolic acidosis. In: Seldin DW, Giebisch G, eds. The Kidney: Physiology and Pathophysiology. Philadelphia: Lippincott Williams & Wilkins, 2000:2073–2130.
38. Lindeman RD. Anatomic and physiologic age changes in the kidney. Exp Gerontol 1986; 21:379–406.
39. Goodman AD, Lemann J Jr, Lennon EJ, Relman AS. Production, excretion, and net balance of fixed acid in patients with renal acidosis. J Clin Invest 1965; 44:495–506.
40. Schwartz WR, Hall PW, Hays RM, Relman AS. On the mechanism of acidosis in chronic renal disease. J Clin Invest 1959; 38:39–52.
41. Adler S, Lindeman RD, Yiengst MJ, Beard E, Shock NW. Effect of acute acid loading on urinary acid excretion by the aging human kidney. J Lab Clin Med 1969; 72:278–289.
42. Agarwal BN, Cabebe FG. Renal acidification in elderly subjects. Nephron 1980; 26:291–295.
43. Nakhoul Zinger, Winaver Better. Impaired urinary acidification in the elderly. J Am Soc Nephrol 1994; 5:370.

44. Hilton JG Jr, Goodbody M, Kruesi OR. The effect of prolonged administration of ammonium chloride on the blood acid–base equilibrium of geriatric subjects. J Am Geriatr Soc 1955; 3:697–703.
45. Green J, Kleeman CR. The role of bone in regulation of systemic acid–base balance. Kidney Int 1991; 39:9–26.
46. Lemann J Jr, Bushinsky DA, Hamm LL. Bone buffering of acid and base in humans. Am J Physiol Renal Physiol 2003; 285:F811–F832.
47. Frassetto LA, Nash E, Morris RC, Sebastian A. Comparative effects of potassium chloride and bicarbonate on thiazide-induced reduction in urinary calcium excretion [in process citation]. Kidney Int 2000; 58:748–752.
48. Uribarri J, Douyon H, Oh MS. A re-evaluation of the urinary parameters of acid production and excretion in patients with chronic renal acidosis. Kidney Int 1995; 47:624–627.
49. Oh MS, Carroll HJ. External balance of electrolytes and acids and alkali. In: Seldin DW, Giebisch G, eds. The Kidney: Physiology and Pathophysiology. Philadelphia: Lippincott Williams & Wilkins, 2000:33–59.
50. Oh MS. Irrelevance of bone buffering to acid–base homeostasis in chronic metabolic acidosis. Nephron 1991; 59:7–10.
51. Litzow JR, Lemann J Jr, Lennon EJ. The effect of treatment of acidosis on calcium balance in patients with chronic azotemic renal disease. J Clin Invest 1967; 46:280–286.
52. Frassetto, Morris Jr, Sebastian. Potassium bicarbonate increases serum growth hormone concentrations in postmenopausal women. J Am Soc Nephrol 1996; 7:1349.
53. Sakhaee K, Williams RH, Oh MS, Padalino P, Adams-Huet B, Whitson P, et al. Alkali absorption and citrate excretion in calcium nephrolithiasis. J Bone Miner Res 1993; 8:789–794.
54. Marangella M, Di Stefano M, Casalis S, Berutti S, D'Amelio P, Isaia GC. Effects of potassium citrate supplementation on bone metabolism. Calcif Tissue Int 2004; 74:330–335.
55. Gordon EE. Effect of acute metabolic acidosis and alkalosis on acetate and citrate metabolism in the rat. J Clin Invest 1963; 42:137–142.
56. Barzel US, Jowsey J. The effects of chronic acid and alkali administration on bone turnover in adult rats. Clin Sci 1969; 36:517–524.
57. Lemann J Jr, Litzow JR, Lennon EJ. The effects of chronic acid loads in normal man: further evidence for participation of bone mineral in the defense against chronic metabolic acidosis. J Clin Invest 1966; 45:1608–1614.
58. Krapf R, Vetsch R, Vetsch W, Hulter HN. Chronic metabolic acidosis increases the serum concentration of 1,25-dihydroxyvitamin D in humans by stimulating its production rate. Critical role of acidosis-induced renal hypophosphatemia. J Clin Invest 1992; 90:2456–2463.
59. Garibotto G, Russo R, Sofia A, Sala MR, Sabatino C, Moscatelli P, et al. Muscle protein turnover in chronic renal failure patients with metabolic acidosis or normal acid–base balance. Miner Electrolyte Metab 1996; 22:58–61.
60. May RC, Kelly RA, Mitch WE. Metabolic acidosis stimulates protein degradation in rat muscle by a glucocorticoid-dependent mechanism. J Clin Invest 1986; 77:614–621.

61. Williams B, Layward E, Walls J. Skeletal muscle degradation and nitrogen wasting in rats with chronic metabolic acidosis. Clin Sci 1991; 80:457–462.
62. Mitch WE, Medina R, Grieber S, May RC, England BK, Price SR, et al. Metabolic acidosis stimulates muscle protein degradation by activating the adenosine triphosphate-dependent pathway involving ubiquitin and proteasomes. J Clin Invest 1994; 93:2127–2133.
63. May RC, Kelly RA, Mitch WE. Mechanisms for defects in muscle protein metabolism in rats with chronic uremia. Influence of metabolic acidosis. J Clin Invest 1987; 79:1099–1103.
64. Perez GO, Oster JR, Vaamonde CA. Serum potassium concentration in acidemic states. Nephron 1981; 27:233–243.
65. Lotspeich WD. Renal hypertrophy in metaboic acidosis and its relation to ammonia excretion. Am J Physiol 1965; 208:1135–1142.
66. Nath KA, Hostetter MK, Hostetter TH. Pathophysiology of chronic tubulo-interstitial disease in rats. Interactions of dietary acid load, ammonia, and complement component C3. J Clin Invest 1985; 76:667–675.
67. Clark EC, Nath KA, Hostetter MK, Hostetter TH. Role of ammonia in tubulointerstitial injury. Miner Electrolyte Metab 1990; 16:315–321.
68. Tolins JP, Hostetter MK, Hostetter TH. Hypokalemic nephropathy in the rat. Role of ammonia in chronic tubular injury. J Clin Invest 1987; 79:1447–1458.
69. Nath KA, Salahudeen AK, Clark EC, Hostetter MK, Hostetter TH. Role of cellular metabolites in progressive renal injury. Kidney Int Suppl 1992; 38:S109–S113.
70. Barzel US. The skeleton as an ion exchange system: implications for the role of acid–base imbalance in the genesis of osteoporosis. J Bone Miner Res 1995; 10:1431–1436.
71. Kraut JA, Mishler DR, Singer FR, Goodman WG. The effects of metabolic acidosis on bone formation and bone resorption in the rat. Kidney Int 1986; 30:694–700.
72. Bergstrom WH, Wallace WM. Bone as a sodium and potassium reservoir. J Clin Invest 1954; 33:867–873.
73. Post M, Shoemaker W. Bone electrolyte response to intravenous acid loads. Surg Gynecol Obstet 1962; 115:749–756.
74. Bettice JA, Gamble JL Jr. Skeletal buffering of acute metabolic acidosis. Am J Physiol 1975; 229:1618–1624.
75. Bushinsky DA, Levi-Setti R, Coe FL. Ion microprobe determination of bone surface elements: effects of reduced medium pH. Am J Physiol 1986; 250:F1090–F1097.
76. Bushinsky DA, Gavrilov K, Chabala JM, Featherstone JD, Levi-Setti R. Effect of metabolic acidosis on the potassium content of bone. J Bone Miner Res 1997; 12:1664–1671.
77. Bettice JA. Skeletal carbon dioxide stores during metabolic acidosis. Am J Physiol 1984; 247:F326–F330.
78. Burnell JM. Changes in bone sodium and carbonate in metabolic acidosis and alkalosis in the dog. J Clin Invest 1971; 50:327–331.
79. Bushinsky DA, Lechleider RJ. Mechanism of proton-induced bone calcium release: calcium carbonate dissolution. Am J Physiol 1987; 253:F998–F1005.

80. Bushinsky DA, Lam BC, Nespeca R, Sessler NE, Grynpas MD. Decreased bone carbonate content in response to metabolic, but not respiratory, acidosis. Am J Physiol 1993; 265:F530–F536.

81. Bushinsky DA. Internal exchanges of hydrogen ions: bone. In: Seldin DW, Giebisch G, eds. The Regulation of Acid–Base Balance. New York: Raven Press, 1989:69–88.

82. Lemann J Jr, Litzow JR, Lennon EJ. Studies of the mechanism by which chronic metabolic acidosis augments urinary calcium excretion in man. J Clin Invest 1967; 46:1318–1328.

83. Yoshimura H, Fujimoto M, Okumura O, Sugimoto J, Kuwada T. Three-step-regulation of acid–base balance in body fluid after acid load. J Clin Invest 1961; 40:109–125.

84. Eiam-Ong S, Kurtzman NA. Metabolic acidosis and bone disease. Miner Electrolyte Metab 1994; 20:72–80.

85. Bushinsky DA, Chabala JM, Gavrilov KL, Levi-Setti R. Effects of in vivo metabolic acidosis on midcortical bone ion composition. Am J Physiol 1999; 277:F813–F819.

86. Wachman A, Bernstein DS. Diet and osteoporosis. Lancet 1968; 1:958–959.

87. Bushinsky DA, Smith SB, Gavrilov KL, Gavrilov LF, Li J, Levi-Setti R. Chronic acidosis-induced alteration in bone bicarbonate and phosphate. Am J Physiol Renal Physiol 2003; 285:F532–F539.

88. Breslau NA, Brinkley L, Hill KD, Pak CYC. Relationship of animal protein-rich diet to kidney stone formation and calcium metabolism. J Clin Endocrinol Metab 1988; 66:140–146.

89. Gafter U, Kraut JA, Lee DBN, Silis V, Walling MW, Kurokawa K, et al. Effect of metabolic acidosis on intestinal absorption of calcium and phosphorus. Am J Physiol 1980; 239:G480–G484.

90. Bushinsky DA, Wolbach W, Sessler NE, Mogilevsky R, Levi-Setti R. Physicochemical effects of acidosis on bone calcium flux and surface ion composition. J Bone Miner Res 1993; 8:93–102.

91. Adams ND, Gray RW, Lemann J Jr. The calciuria of increased fixed acid production in humans: evidence against a role for parathyroid hormone and 1,25OH)2-vitamin D. Calcif Tissue Int 1979; 28:233–238.

92. Weber HP, Gray RW, Dominguez JH, Lemann J Jr. The lack of effect of chronic metabolic acidosis on 25-OH-vitamin D metabolism and serum parathyroid hormone in humans. J Clin Endocrinol Metab 1976; 43:1047–1055.

93. Barzel US. The effect of excessive acid feeding on bone. Calcif Tissue Res 1969; 4:94–100.

94. Delling G, Donath K. Morphometric, electron microscopic and physico-chemical investigation in experimental osteoporosis induced by chronic acidosis in the rat. Virchows Arch Abt A Path Anat 1973; 358:321–330.

95. Barzel US. Acid-induced osteoporosis: an experimental model of human osteoporosis. Calcif Tissue Res 1976; 21(suppl):417–422.

96. Myburgh KH, Noakes TD, Roodt M, Hough FS. Effect of exercise on the development of osteoporosis in adult rats. J Appl Physiol 1989; 66:14–19.

97. New SA, Macdonald HM, Grubb DA, Reid DM. Positive association between net endogenous noncarbonic acid production (NEAP) and bone

health: further support for the importance of the skeleton to acid-base balance. 1st Joint Meeting of the "International Bone and Mineral Society" and the "European Calcified Tissue Society", June 5–10, 2001, Madrid, Spain. http://www.salixhost.co.uk/madrid/sc.htm#SC17 [Last accessed 03.01.05].

98.   Upton PK, L'Estrange JL. Effects of chronic hydrochloric and lactic acid administrations on food intake, blood acid–base balance and bone composition of the rat. Quart J Exp Physiol 1977; 62:223–235.

99.   Jaffe HL, Bodansky A, Chandler JP. Ammonium chloride decalcification, as modified by calcium intake. The relation between generalized osteoporosis and osteitis fibrosa. J Exp Med 1932; 56:823–834.

100. Newell GK, Beauchene rE. Effects of dietary calcium level, acid stress, and age on renal, serum, and bone responses of rats. J Nutr 1975; 105:1039–1047.

101. Kraut JA, Mishler DR, Kurokawa K. Effect of colchicine and calcitonin on calcemic response to metabolic acidosis. Kidney Int 1984; 25:608–612.

102. Krieger NS, Sessler NE, Bushinsky DA. Acidosis inhibits osteoblastic and stimulates osteoclastic activity in vitro. Am J Physiol 1992; 262: F442–F448.

103. Bushinsky DA. Stimulated osteoclastic and suppressed osteoblastic activity in metabolic but not respiratory acidosis. Am J Physiol 1995; 268:C80–C88.

104. Arnett TR, Dempster DW. Effect of pH on bone resorption by rat osteoclasts in vitro. Endocrinology 1986; 119:119–124.

105. Goldhaber P, Rabadjija L. H^+ stimulation of cell-mediated bone resorption in tissue culture. Am J Physiol 1987; 253:E90–E98.

106. Blair HC, Teitelbaum SL, Ghiselli R, Gluck S. Osteoclastic bone resorption by a polarized vacuolar proton pump. Science 1989; 245:855–857.

107. Teti A, Blair HC, Schlesinger P, Grano M, Zambonin-Zallone A, Kahn AJ, et al. Extracellular protons acidify osteoclasts, reduce cytosolic calcium, and promote expression of cell-matrix attachment structures. J Clin Invest 1989; 84:773–780.

108. Ross FP, Teitelbaum SL. Osteoclast biology. In: Marcus R, Feldman D, Kelsey J, eds. Osteoporosis. San Diego: Academic Press, 2001:73–105.

109. Bernstein DS, Wachman A, Hattner RS. Acid base balance in metabolic bone disease. In: Barzel US, ed. Osteoporosis. New York: Grune & Stratton, 1970:207–216.

110. Frassetto L, Morris RC Jr, Sebastian A. Long-term persistence of the urine calcium-lowering effect of potassium bicarbonate in postmenopausal women. J Clin Endocrinol Metab 2005; 90:831–834.

111. Bushinsky DA, Frick KK. The effects of acid on bone. Curr Opin Nephrol Hypertens 2000; 9:369–379.

112. New SA, Macdonald HM, Campbell MK, Martin JC, Garton MJ, Robins SP, et al. Lower estimates of net endogenous non-carbonic acid production are positively associated with indexes of bone health in premenopausal and perimenopausal women. Am J Clin Nutr 2004; 79:131–138.

113. New SA. Acid–base homeostasis and the skeleton: is there a fruit and vegetable link to bone health?. In: New SA, Bonjour J-P, eds. Nutritional Aspects of Bone Health. London: Royal Society of Chemistry, 2003.

114. Heaney RP, Recker RR, Saville PD. Calcium balance and calcium requirements in middle-aged women. Am J Clin Nutr 1977; 30:1603–1611.

115. Recker RR, Heaney RP. The effect of milk supplements on calcium metabolism, bone metabolism and calcium balance. Am J Clin Nutr 1985; 41:254–263.

116. Lemann J Jr, Gray RW, Pleuss JA. Potassium bicarbonate, but not sodium bicarbonate, reduces urinary calcium excretion and improves calcium balance in healthy men. Kidney Int 1989; 35:688–695.

117. Sellmeyer DE, Schloetter M, Sebastian A. Potassium citrate prevents increased urine calcium excretion and bone resorption induced by a high sodium chloride diet. J Clin Endocrinol Metab 2002; 87:2008–2012.

118. Frassetto LA, Todd KM, Morris RC Jr, Sebastian A. Worldwide incidence of hip fracture in elderly women: relation to consumption of animal and vegetable foods. J Gerontol A Biol Sci Med Sci 2000; 55:M585–M592.

119. Souci SW, Fachmann W, Kraut H. Food Composition and Nutrition Tables. Stuttgart: Wissenschaftliche Verlagsgesellschaft mbH, 1986.

120. Hu J-F, Zhao X-H, Parpia B, Campbell TC. Dietary intakes and urinary excretion of calcium and acids: a cross-sectional study of women in China. Am J Clin Nutr 1993; 58:398–406.

121. Halperin ML. Metabolism and acid–base physiology. Artif Organs 1982; 6:357–362.

122. Holland B, Welch AA, Unwin ID, Buss DH, Paul AA, Southgate DAT. McCance and Widdowson's the Composition of Foods: Fifth Revised and Extended Edition. 5th ed. Cambridge, UK: The Royal Society of Chemistry and Ministry of Agriculture, Fisheries and Food, 1991.

123. Faulkner KG. Bone matters: are density increases necessary to reduce fracture risk? J Bone Miner Res 2000; 15:183–187.

124. Sellmeyer DE, Stone KL, Sebastian A, Cummings SR. A high ratio of dietary animal to vegetable protein increases the rate of bone loss and the risk of fracture in postmenopausal women. Study of Osteoporotic Fractures Research Group. Am J Clin Nutr 2001; 73:118–122.

125. Frassetto LA, Todd KM, Morris RC Jr, Sebastian A. Estimation of net endogenous noncarbonic acid production in humans from diet potassium and protein contents. Am J Clin Nutr 1998; 68:576–583.

126. New SA, Bolton-Smith C, Grubb DA, Reid DM. Nutritional influences on bone mineral density: a cross-sectional study in premenopausal women. Am J Clin Nutr 1997; 65:1831–1839.

127. New SA, Robins SP, Campbell MK, Martin JC, Garton MJ, Bolton-Smith C, et al. Dietary influences on bone mass and bone metabolism: further evidence of a positive link between fruit and vegetable consumption and bone health? Am J Clin Nutr 2000; 71:142–151.

128. Tucker KL, Hannan MT, Chen H, Cupples LA, Wilson PWF, Kiel DP. Potassium, magnesium, and fruit and vegetable intakes are associated with greater bone mineral density in elderly men and women. Am J Clin Nutr 1999; 69:727–736.

129. Fujisawa M, Nakamura I, Yamanaka N, Gotoh A, Hara I, Okada H, et al. Changes in calcium metabolism and bone demineralization after orthotopic intestinal neobladder creation. J Urol 2000; 163:1108–1111.

130. Giannini S, Nobile M, Sartori L, Aragona F, Ruffato A, Dalle CL, et al. Bone density and skeletal metabolism in patients with orthotopic ileal neobladder. J Am Soc Nephrol 1997; 8:1553–1559.

131. Domrongkitchaiporn S, Pongsakul C, Stitchantrakul W, Sirikulchayanonta VV, Ongphiphadhanakul B, Radinahamed P, et al. Bone mineral density and histology in distal renal tubular acidosis. Kidney Int 2001; 59:1086–1093.

132. Sanchez A, Libman J. Renal acidification mechanism disorders in patients with osteoporosis. Medicine 1995; 55:197–202.

133. Weger M, Deutschmann H, Weger W, Kotanko P, Skrabal F. Incomplete renal tubular acidosis in 'primary' osteoporosis. Osteoporosis Int 1999; 10:325–329.

134. Osther PJ, Bollerslev J, Hansen AB, Engel K, Kildeberg P. Pathophysiology of incomplete renal tubular acidosis in recurrent renal stone formers: evidence of disturbed calcium, bone and citrate metabolism. Urol Res 1993; 21: 169–173.

135. Harrington TM, Bunch TW, Van Den Berg CJ. Renal tubular acidosis. A new look at treatment of musculoskeletal and renal disease. Mayo Clin Proc 1983; 58:354–360.

136. Weger W, Kotanko P, Weger M, Deutschmann H, Skrabal F. Prevalence and characterization of renal tubular acidosis in patients with osteopenia and osteoporosis and in non-porotic controls. Nephrol Dial Transplant 2000; 15:975–980.

137. Preminger GM, Sakhaee K, Pak CYC. Hypercalciuria and altered intestinal calcium absorption occurring independently of vitamin D in incomplete distal renal tubular acidosis. Metabolism 1987; 36:176–179.

138. Giannini S, Nobile M, Sartori L, Calo L, Tasca A, Dalle CL, et al. Bone density and skeletal metabolism are altered in idiopathic hypercalciuria. Clin Nephrol 1998; 50:94–100.

139. Mitch WE. Mechanisms causing loss of lean body mass in kidney disease. Am J Clin Nutr 1998; 67:359–366.

140. Vazquez JA, Adibi SA. Protein sparing during treatment of obesity: ketogenic versus nonketogenic very low calorie diet. Metabolism 1992; 41:406–414.

141. Bell JD, Margen S, Calloway DH. Ketosis, weight loss, uric acid, and nitrogen balance in obese women fed single nutrients at low caloric levels. Metabolism 1969; 18:193–208.

142. Welbourne TC, Joshi S. Enteral glutamine spares endogenous glutamine in chronic acidosis. J Parenteral Enteral Nutr 1994; 18:243–247.

143. Reaich D, Channon SM, Scrimgeour CM, Goodship THJ. Ammonium chloride-induced acidosis increases protein breakdown and amino acid oxidation in humans. Am J Physiol 1992; 263:E735–E739.

144. May RC, Bailey JL, Mitch WE, Masud T, England BK. Glucocorticoids and acidosis stimulate protein and amino acid catabolism in vivo. Kidney Int 1996; 49:679–683.

145. Papadoyannakis NJ, Stefanidis CJ, McGeown M. The effect of the correction of metabolic acidosis on nitrogen and potassium balance of patients with chronic renal failure. Am J Clin Nutr 1984; 40:423–627.

146. Hannaford MC, Leiter LA, Josse RG, Goldstein MB, Marliss EB, Halperin ML. Protein wasting due to acidosis of prolonged fasting. Am J Physiol 1982; 243:E251–E256.
147. Gougeon-Reyburn R, Lariviere F, Marliss EB. Effects of bicarbonate supplementation on urinary mineral excretion during very low energy diets. Am J Med Sci 1991; 302:67–74.
148. Gougeon-Reyburn R, Marliss EB. Effects of sodium bicarbonate on nitrogen metabolism and ketone bodies during very low energy protein diets in obese subjects. Metabolism 1989; 38:1222–1230.
149. Reaich D, Channon SM, Scrimgeour CM, Daley SE, Wilkinson R, Goodship THJ. Correction of acidosis in humans with CRF decreases protein degradation and amino acid oxidation. Am J Physiol 1993; 265:E230–E235.
150. Graham KA, Reaich D, Channon SM, Downie S, Goodship TH. Correction of acidosis in hemodialysis decreases whole-body protein degradation. J Am Soc Nephrol 1997; 8:632–637.
151. Guder WG, Haussinger D, Gerok W. Renal and hepatic nitrogen metabolism in systemic acid base regulation. J Clin Chem Clin Biochem 1987; 25:457–466.
152. Cersosimo E, Williams PE, Radosevich PM, Hoxworth BT, Lacy WW, Abumrad NN. Role of glutamine in adaptations in nitrogen metabolism during fasting. Am J Physiol 1986; 250:E622–E628.
153. Pitts RF. Production and excretion of ammonia in relation to acid–base balance. In: Orloff J, Berliner RW, eds. Handbook of Physiology. Section 8. Washington, DC: American Physiological Society, 1973:455–496.
154. Haussinger D. Organization of hepatic nitrogen metabolism and its relation to acid-base homeostasis. Klin Wochenschr 1990; 68:1096–1101.
155. Oliver J, Koelz AM, Costello J, Bourke E. Acid–base induced alterations in glutamine metabolism and ureogenesis in perfused muscle and liver of the rat. Eur J Clin Invest 1977; 7:445–449.
156. Almond MK, Iles RA, Cohen RD. Hepatic glutamine metabolism and acid–base regulation. Miner Electrolyte Metab 1992; 18:237–240.
157. Frassetto L, Morris RC Jr, Sebastian A. Potassium bicarbonate reduces urinary nitrogen excretion in postmenopausal women. J Clin Endocrinol Metab 1997; 82:254–259.
158. Cheema-Dhadli S, Jungas RL, Halperin ML. Regulation of urea synthesis by acid–base balance in vivo: role of NH_3 concentration. Am J Physiol 1987; 252:F221–F225.
159. Forbes GB. The adult decline in lean body mass. Hum Biol 1976; 48:161–173.
160. Nath KA, Hostetter MK, Hostetter TH. Increased ammoniagenesis as a determinant of progressive renal injury. Am J Kidney Dis 1991; 17:654–657.
161. Gennari FJ. Is metabolic acidosis a risk factor in the progression of renal insufficiency? In: Koch KM, Stein G, eds. Pathogenetic and Therapeutic Aspects of Chronic Renal Failure. New York: Marcel Dekker, Inc, 1997:33–44.
162. Kramer HJ, Meyer-Lehnert H, Mohaupt M. Role of calcium in the progression of renal disease: experimental evidence. Kidney Int 1992; 41(suppl 36):S2–S7.
163. Hostetter TH. Progression of renal disease and renal hypertrophy. Annu Rev Physiol 1995; 57:263–278.

164. Brenner BM, Meyer TW, Hostetter TH. Dietary protein intake the the
      progressive nature of kidney disease: the role of hemodynamically mediated
      glomerular injury in the pathogenesis of progressive glomerular sclerosis in
      aging, renal ablation, and intrinsic renal disease. N Engl J Med 1982;
      307:652–659.
165. Schrier RW, Harris DCH, Chan L, Shapiro JI, Caramelo C. Tubular hyper-
      metabolism as a factor in the progression of chronic renal failure. Am J
      Kidney Dis 1988; 12:243–249.
166. Haugen E, Nath KA. The involvement of oxidative stress in the progression of
      renal injury. Blood Purif 1999; 17:58–65.
167. Gadola L, Noboa O, Marquez MN, Rodriguez MJ, Nin N, Boggia J, et al.
      Calcium citrate ameliorates the progression of chronic renal injury. Kidney
      Int 2004; 65:1224–1230.
168. Sebastian A, McSherry E, Morris RC Jr. Metabolic acidosis with special refer-
      ence to the renal acidoses. In: Brenner BM, Rector FC Jr, eds. The Kidney.
      Philadelphia: W. B. Saunders, 1976:615–660.
169. Caruana RJ, Buckalew VM Jr. The syndrome of distal (type 1) renal tubular
      acidosis. Clinical and laboratory findings in 58 cases. Medicine 1988; 67:
      84–99.
170. Gaulin SJC, Konner M. On the natural diet of primates, including humans.
      In: Wurtman R, Wurtman J, eds. Nutrition and the Brain. New York: Raven
      Press, 1977:1:1–86.
171. Gaulin SJ. A Jarman/Bell model of primate feeding niches. Hum Ecol 1979;
      7:1–20.
172. Boyd R, Silk JB, Boyd R, Silk JB, eds. How Humans Evolved. 2nd ed. New
      York: W. W. Norton and Company, 2000.
173. Cordain L, Miller JB, Eaton SB, Mann N, Holt SH, Speth JD. Plant-animal
      subsistence ratios and macronutrient energy estimations in worldwide hunter–
      gatherer diets [see comments]. Am J Clin Nutr 2000; 71:682–692.
174. Mann N. Dietary lean red meat and human evolution. Eur J Nutr 2000;
      39:71–79.
175. Eaton SB, Eaton III SB, Konner MJ. Paleolithic nutrition revisited. In:
      Trevathan WR, Smith EO, McKenna JJ, eds. Evolutionary Medicine.
      New York: Oxford University Press, Inc, 1999:313–332.
176. Cosmides L, Tooby J, Barkow JH. The Adapted Mind: Evolutionary Psychol-
      ogy and the Generation of Culture. New York: Oxford University Press, 1992.
177. Wilson EO. Consilience: the Unity of Knowledge. 1st New York: Knopf,
      1998.
178. Sebastian A. Estimating diet net acid load: reply to T Remer and F Manz. Am
      J Clin Nutr 2003; 78:803–804.
179. Cordain L. Cereal grains: humanity's double-edged sword. In: Simopoulos AP,
      ed. Evolutionary Aspects of Nutrition and Health. Basel: Karger, 1999:19–73.
180. Schurch MA, Rizzoli R, Slosman D, Vadas L, Vergnaud P, Bonjour JP.
      Protein supplements increase serum insulin-like growth factor-I levels and
      attenuate proximal femur bone loss in patients with recent hip fracture. A
      randomized, double-blind, placebo-controlled trial [see comments]. Ann
      Intern Med 1998; 128:801–809.

181. Allen NE, Appleby PN, Davey GK, Kaaks R, Rinaldi S, Key TJ. The associations of diet with serum insulin-like growth factor I and its main binding proteins in 292 women meat-eaters, vegetarians, and vegans. Cancer Epidemiol Biomarkers Prev 2002; 11:1441–1448.

182. Bushinsky DA. Metabolic alkalosis decreases bone calcium efflux by suppressing osteoclasts and stimulating osteoblasts. Am J Physiol 1996; 271:F216–F222.

183. Brungger M, Hulter HN, Krapf R. Effect of chronic metabolic acidosis on the growth hormone/IGF-1 endocrine axis: new cause of growth hormone insensitivity in humans. Kidney Int 1997; 51:216–221.

184. Hene RJ, Koomans HA, Boer P, Dorhout Mees EJ. Adaptation to chronic potassium loading in normal man. Miner Electrolyte Metab 1986; 12:165–172.

185. Rabelink TJ, Koomans HA, Hene RJ, Dorhout Mees EJ. Early and late adjustment to potassium loading in humans. Kidney Int 1990; 38:942–947.

186. Witzgall H, Behr J. Effects of potassium loading in normal man on dopaminergic control of mineralocorticoids and renin release. J Hypertens 1986; 4:201–205.

187. Van Goidsenhoven GMT, Gray OV, Price AV, Sanderson PH. The effect of prolonged administration of large doses of sodium bicarbonate in man. Clin Sci 1954; 13:383–401.

188. Cogan MG, Carneiro AV, Tatsuno J, Colman J, Krapf R, Morris RC Jr, et al. Normal diet NaCl variation can affect the renal set-point for plasma pH-(HCO_3^-) maintenance [see comments]. J Am Soc Nephrol 1990; 1:193–199.

189. Nicar MJ, Peterson R, Pak CYC. Use of potassium citrate as potassium supplement during thiazide therapy of calcium nephrolithiasis. J Urol 1984; 131:430–433.

190. Pak CYC, Peterson R, Sakhaee K, Fuller C, Preminger G, Reisch J. Correction of hypocitraturia and prevention of stone formation by combined thiazide and potassium citrate therapy in thiazide-unresponsive hypercalciuric nephrolithiasis. Am J Med 1985; 79:284–288.

191. Odvina CV, Preminger GM, Lindberg JS, Moe OW, Pak CY. Long-term combined treatment with thiazide and potassium citrate in nephrolithiasis does not lead to hypokalemia or hypochloremic metabolic alkalosis. Kidney Int 2003; 63:240–247.

192. Asplin JR, Favus MJ, Coe FL. Nephrolithiasis. In: Brenner BM, ed. The Kidney. Philadelphia: W. B. Saunders Company, 2000:1774–1819.

193. Gennari FJ. Acid–base balance in dialysis patients. Semin Dial 2000; 13: 235–239.

194. Ruff CB, Trinkaus E, Walker A, Larsen CS. Postcranial robusticity in Homo. I: temporal trends and mechanical interpretation. Am J Phys Anthropol 1993; 91:21–53.

195. Nelson D. Bone density in three archaeological populations. Am J Phys Anthropol 2000; 63:198.

196. Perzigian AJ. Osteoporotic bone loss in two prehistoric Indian populations. Am J Phys Anthropol 1973; 39:87–95.

197. McSherry E, Morris RC Jr. Attainment and maintenance of normal stature with alkali therapy in infants and children with classic renal tubular acidosis. J Clin Invest 1978; 61:509–527.

198. Lefebvre A, De Vernejoul MC, Gueris J, Goldfarb B, Graulet AM, Morieux C. Optimal correction of acidosis changes progression of dialysis osteodystrophy. Kidney Int 1989; 36:1112–1118.

199. Oettinger CW, Oliver JC. Normalization of uremic acidosis in hemodialysis patients with a high bicarbonate dialysate [see comments]. J Am Soc Nephrol 1993; 3:1804–1807.

200. Lemann J Jr, Adams ND, Gray RW. Urinary calcium excretion in human beings. N Engl J Med 1979; 301:535–541.

201. Licata AA, Bou E, Bartter FC, Cox J. Effects of dietary protein on urinary calcium in normal subjects and in patients with nephrolithiasis. Metabolism 1979; 28:895–900.

202. Trinchieri A, Zanetti G, Curro A, Lizzano R. Effect of potential renal acid load of foods on calcium metabolism of renal calcium stone formers. Eur Urol 2001; 39(suppl 2):33–36.

203. Houillier P, Normand M, Froissart M, Blanchard A, Jungers P, Paillard M. Calciuric response to an acute acid load in healthy subjects and hypercalciuric calcium stone formers. Kidney Int 1996; 50:987–997.

204. Sebastian A, Hernandez RE, Portale AA, Colman J, Tatsuno J, Morris RC Jr. Dietary potassium influences kidney maintenance of serum phosphorus concentration. Kidney Int 1990; 37:1341–1349.

205. Lemann J Jr, Pleuss JA, Gray RW. Potassium causes calcium retention in healthy adults. J Nutr 1993; 123:1623–1626.

206. Eaton SB, Eaton SB III, Konner MJ. Paleolithic nutrition revisited: a twelve-year retrospective on its nature and implications [see comments]. Eur J Clin Nutr 1997; 51:207–216.

207. Dawkins R. Science and Sensibility: Queen Elizabeth Hall Lecture, London, 24th March 1998. Series title: Sounding the Century ('What will the Twentieth Century leave to its heirs?'). http://www.world-of-dawkins.com/science_and_sensibility.htm

9

Metabolic Acidosis: General Considerations

Michael Emmett

Baylor University Medical Center, Dallas, Texas, U.S.A.

INTRODUCTION

Metabolic acidosis is a pathologic disturbance that reduces serum bicarbonate concentration ($[HCO_3^-]$) and generates acidemia, defined as an arterial blood pH < 7.35. Metabolic acidosis triggers hyperventilation and this secondary response reduces arterial carbon dioxide tension ($PaCO_2$). Uncomplicated metabolic acidosis thus results in a low $[HCO_3^-]$, $PaCO_2$, and pH. Metabolic acidosis can also occur in combination with other acid–base disturbances, producing a mixed disturbance in which the values for pH, $PaCO_2$, and $[HCO_3^-]$ may be low, normal, or even high (see Chapters 22 and 28).

SECONDARY RESPIRATORY RESPONSE TO METABOLIC ACIDOSIS

In 1874, Kussmaul (1) pointed out that decompensated diabetic patients hyperventilate ("Kussmaul ventilation"). The signal that leads to this hyperventilation is acidemia. The fall in systemic pH engendered by metabolic acidosis activates peripheral chemoreceptors in the aorta and carotid arteries as well as central chemoreceptors located on the ventral surface of the brain stem. Stimulation of these receptors increases the depth and rate of ventilation and thereby decreases $PaCO_2$ (2). The central chemoreceptors are more important than the peripheral chemoreceptors in this response to metabolic acidosis (3,4).

When hyperventilation develops in response to metabolic acidosis, the resultant decrease in $PaCO_2$ increases the $[HCO_3^-]/PaCO_2$ ratio driving the pH back toward the normal range, as defined by the Henderson–Hasselbalch equation:

$$pH = 6.1 + \log([HCO_3^-] \downarrow\downarrow /0.03 \times PaCO_2\downarrow) \qquad (1)$$

The down arrows in this equation are inserted to emphasize that in metabolic acidosis, the primary event is a reduction in the numerator ($[HCO_3^-]$) and the secondary response is a reduction in the denominator ($PaCO_2$), which is insufficient to restore pH to the pre-acidosis value.

The $PaCO_2$ begins to fall within 1–2 hr after onset of metabolic acidosis and should reach a steady–state value by 12–24 hr. This secondary response is an integral component of the metabolic acidosis and is not considered a "respiratory alkalosis" that has developed in response to the metabolic acidosis. If an adequate respiratory response (see below) has not developed within 12–24 hr after onset of metabolic acidosis, primary hypoventilation is present and a diagnosis of respiratory acidosis, in addition to metabolic acidosis, is made (see Chapters 22 and 28). In this case, a diagnosis of mixed metabolic acidosis and respiratory acidosis is preferred to the term "uncompensated metabolic acidosis." Conversely, if hyperventilation is excessive and reduces $PaCO_2$ below the expected range, then respiratory alkalosis complicating metabolic acidosis is diagnosed. When such mixed acid–base disorders exist, the prevailing pH may be acidic, physiologically neutral, or alkaline depending on the severity of each disturbance (5).

Normal Response

The normal range for the secondary respiratory response to metabolic acidosis has been determined by studying patients with various forms of uncomplicated metabolic acidosis and normal individuals with experimentally induced metabolic acidosis (6,7). The response is predictable and linearly related to serum $[HCO_3^-]$ between 24 and $\sim$8 mEq/L (7) (Fig. 1). The first formula derived to describe this relationship, based on the observations shown in Fig. 1, is known as "Winters' equation":

$$\text{Expected } PaCO_2 = (1.5 \times (\text{Measured } [HCO_3^-]) + 8) +/- 2\,\text{mmHg} \qquad (2)$$

According to this equation, a patient with simple metabolic acidosis with a serum $[HCO_3^-]$ of 10 mEq/L should have a $PaCO_2$ between 21 and 25 mmHg. If the patient's $PaCO_2$ is <21 or >25 mmHg, the secondary respiratory response is not appropriate for the level of metabolic acidosis and a second acid–base diagnosis should be considered—respiratory

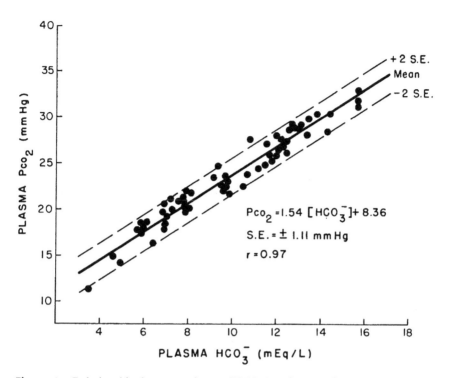

Figure 1 Relationship between plasma [HCO₃] and PCO₂ in 60 patients with established, untreated, and uncomplicated metabolic acidosis. *Source:* From Ref. 7.

alkalosis (if $PCO_2 < 21$) or respiratory acidosis (if $PCO_2 > 25$). The respiratory response is independent of the specific cause of the metabolic acidosis.

The relationship between $PaCO_2$ and serum [HCO₃] in uncomplicated chronic metabolic acidosis that is used in Chapters 28 and 29 of this book is based on a compilation of many studies (including the Winters study) (6). It predicts that $PaCO_2$ will decrease by 1.2 mmHg for each 1 mEq/L fall in plasma [HCO₃]. For the example above, this relationship predicts that the expected $PaCO_2$ for a serum [HCO₃] of 10 mEq/L is 23 mmHg, consistent with the value calculated using Winters' equation. Another formula almost as reliable as the above equations, yet simpler to remember and use, is:

$$PaCO_2 = [HCO_3^-] + 15. \tag{3}$$

This equation predicts a $PaCO_2$ of 25 mmHg for the patient with a serum [HCO₃] of 10 mEq/L. The $PaCO_2$ in patients with metabolic acidosis also approximates the last two digits of their measured arterial pH (8). When metabolic acidosis reduces serum [HCO₃] to 10 mEq/L, for example, $PaCO_2$ should fall to ~ 23 mmHg, with the resulting pH being 7.23.

The pitfalls and limitations of these rules are discussed in Chapter 28. Two key limitations are their failure to consider the time course of the response and their lack of applicability when serum [HCO_3^-] is < 6–7 mEq/L.

Potential Adverse Effects of the Fall in $PaCO_2$

Sustained hyperventilation in chronic metabolic acidosis can potentially have an adverse effect on pH in metabolic acidosis (9). A chronic reduction in $PaCO_2$ (respiratory alkalosis) elicits a reduction in plasma [HCO_3^-] as a result of a period of bicarbonaturia and depressed renal net acid excretion. This change in renal HCO_3^- reabsorption and acid excretion is largely responsible for the expected secondary metabolic response to chronic respiratory alkalosis (see Chapter 21). A similar renal response also develops when chronic metabolic acidosis causes a secondary fall in $PaCO_2$ (9). A "maladaptive cycle" then ensues, beginning with a primary reduction in serum [HCO_3^-], a secondary fall in $PaCO_2$, and a subsequent additional decrement in serum [HCO_3^-] in response to the chronic hyperventilation. This secondary reduction diminishes the degree to which arterial pH is protected by the respiratory adaptation acutely. In dogs with severe metabolic acidosis, this maladaptation actually results in more severe acidemia than would occur in the complete absence of secondary hyperventilation (9). In studies in humans, however, acidemia is not worsened (10).

PLASMA ELECTROLYTE PROFILE AND DIFFERENTIAL DIAGNOSIS

Metabolic acidosis is usually caused by one or more of the following three pathophysiological mechanisms:

1. Loss of $NaHCO_3$ (or loss of a Na^+ salt derived from the reaction of $NaHCO_3$ with organic acids such as acetoacetic or lactic acid) from the body at an abnormally rapid rate.
2. Impairment in renal acid excretory capacity.
3. Addition of relatively strong acids, endogenous or exogenous in origin, to the body fluids at an abnormally rapid rate.

In order to understand these pathophysiologies, the anion gap (described below and in Chapter 28) is used as a first step in analyzing the disorder.

USE OF ANION GAP IN METABOLIC ACIDOSIS

The ionic profile of normal serum is depicted in Fig. 2. The law of electroneutrality states that all solutions contain equal concentrations of positively and negatively charged ions. Consequently, if the concentration of every ion

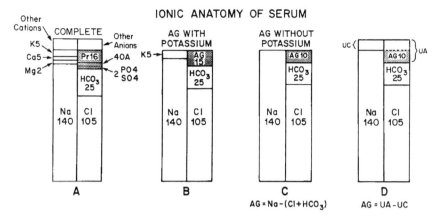

Figure 2 Cations and anions in normal serum. The complete profile is shown in panel (**A**). The anion gap (AG), calculated with and without potassium, is shown in panels (**B**) and (**C**), respectively. The relationship between the anion gap and the difference between all unmeasured anions and unmeasured cations is shown in panel (**D**).

dissolved in serum is expressed in electrical charge units (mEq/L), the sum of the anions must equal that of the cations. If such an analysis considers only the quantitatively most important serum electrolytes, Na^+, Cl^-, and HCO_3^-, then $[Na^+]$ normally exceeds the sum of $[Cl^-] + [HCO_3^-]$. The arithmetic difference $[Na^+] - ([Cl^-] + [HCO_3^-])$, normally about $12 \pm 4\,mEq/L$ ($\pm 2SD$) (11), is called the anion gap [AG]. However, each laboratory must establish its own normal range because various analytical techniques for each of these electrolytes yield different normal ranges (12).

The anion gap does not represent a specific ionic constituent. It includes the normal negative protein charge (primarily due to albumin), inorganic phosphate, sulfate, organic anions, and multiple other anions. Because albumin is a major contributor to the unmeasured anions, changes in pH and albumin concentration affect the magnitude of the AG (see Chapter 28). The effect of these changes, however, is not large under most circumstances. The AG is a helpful tool for classifying the metabolic acidosis, because it increases when certain types of metabolic acidosis develop but remains within the normal range with others.

Pathophysiology and Anion Gap

When metabolic acidosis increases $[H^+]$ in the extracellular fluid (ECF), it is virtually all buffered by the following reaction:

$$H^+ + HCO_3^- \rightarrow H_2CO_3 \rightarrow CO_2 + H_2O \qquad (4)$$

Consequently, if a given quantity of H^+ enters the ECF, a nearly equimolar fall in $[HCO_3^-]$ occurs (Fig. 3). If H^+ is added as HCl, the decrease in $[HCO_3^-]$ is associated with an equivalent increase in $[Cl^-]$. In this case, the [AG] does not change notably. If the added H^+ is not HCl (e.g., lactic, acetoacetic, phosphoric, or sulfuric acid), then its addition to the ECF decreases the $[HCO_3^-]$ and increases the [AG]. Although it is easy to understand how the administration of HCl generates a hyperchloremic acidosis, most clinical disorders associated with a normal AG, or hyperchloremic, acidosis do not develop this way. Most often, hyperchloremic acidosis is

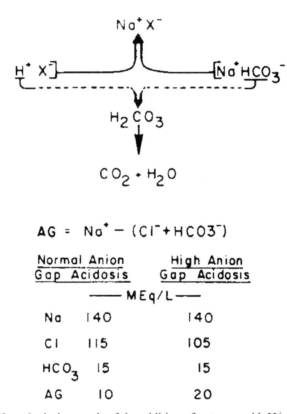

Figure 3 Hypothetical example of the addition of a strong acid, $H^+ X^-$ (left side of upper part of the figure) to the body fluids. If 10 mEq/L of this acid is added, it reacts with HCO_3^-, resulting in a 10 mEq/L reduction in $[HCO_3^-]$ and a 10 mEq/L increase in $[X^-]$. If the strong acid is HCl, the decrease in $[HCO_3^-]$ is counterbalanced by an equal increase in $[Cl^-]$, as shown in the bottom part of the figure, and the [AG] remains relatively stable. If the strong acid is not HCl (e.g., lactic, acetoacetic, phosphoric, or sulfuric acids), then the reduction in $[HCO_3^-]$ is counterbalanced by an equivalent increase in the [AG]. *Source*: From Ref. 11.

caused by the loss of fluids with a high concentration of NaHCO₃, or a salt derived from the reaction of NaHCO₃ with organic acids.

Consider the hypothetical situation shown in Fig. 4: 1 L of an isotonic solution of NaHCO₃ (140 mEq/L) is lost from the ECF. The ECF [Na⁺] will not change because the [Na⁺] in the lost fluid is the same as in the ECF. However, the [HCO₃⁻] in the lost fluid is much higher than the ECF [HCO₃⁻] (140 mEq/L vs. 25 mEq/L). Consequently ECF [HCO₃⁻] falls. Simultaneously, the ECF volume shrinks as a result of the loss of an isotonic Na⁺ solution. The [Cl⁻] increases because no Cl⁻ was lost and ECF Cl⁻ is now distributed in a smaller ECF volume. There is a minimal change of the anion gap (13).

The fluid losses that produce hyperchloremic acidosis in clinical disorders typically contain NaHCO₃, or NaHCO₃-equivalent salts, at a concentration greater than 25 mEq/L but generally much lower than the 150 mEq/L used in the example. Nonetheless, the mechanism is the same as the one described, albeit with diminished magnitude. The kidney avidly reabsorbs dietary chloride in these patients due to ECF volume contraction,

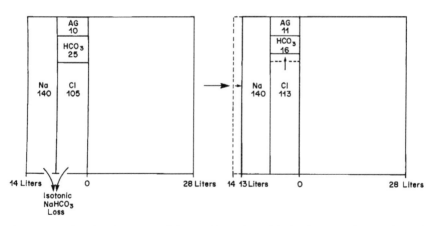

Figure 4 The development of hyperchloremic acidosis due to selective loss of NaHCO₃ from the extracellular fluid (ECF). In each diagram, the ECF is depicted on the left-hand side of the 0 and the intracellular fluid on the right-hand side. In this example, 1 L of isotonic NaHCO₃ (NaHCO₃ = 150 mEq/L) is lost from the ECF (*left-hand panel*). As shown in the right-hand panel, ECF [Na⁺] does not change because [Na⁺] in the lost fluid = ECF [Na⁺]. ECF [HCO₃⁻] falls, however, because [HCO₃⁻] in the lost fluid is much higher than that in the ECF (140 mEq/L vs. 24 mEq/L). ECF volume shrinks from 14 to 13 L as a result of the 1 L loss, and therefore ECF [Cl⁻] increases because no Cl⁻ was lost and this anion is now distributed in a smaller volume. There is a minimal change of the anion gap. *Source*: From Ref. 13.

sustaining the hyperchloremia. As already noted, salts generated from the reaction of $NaHCO_3$ with organic acids are often lost rather than $NaHCO_3$ itself. Sodium acetate, lactate, citrate, and β-hydroxybutyrate are examples. Loss of these salts is equivalent to the loss of $NaHCO_3$ (see Chapters 7 and 15). Salts containing organic anions represent a major portion of the alkali lost in the stool with severe diarrhea.

The causes of hyperchloremic (normal [AG]) and high [AG] metabolic acidoses are listed in Table 1. This separation helps narrow the diagnostic possibilities, although some patients develop both high anion gap and hyperchloremic acidosis. This may occur in patients with mild to moderate renal disease (see Chapter 14, and Fig. 5). Another condition that often generates mixed hyperchloremic-high [AG] acidosis is diabetic ketoacidosis (DKA). The production and accumulation of β-hydroxybutyric acid and acetoacetic acid in this disorder initially produces a high [AG] metabolic acidosis. However, saline administration promotes the renal excretion of Na^+ salts containing acetoacetate and β-hydroxybutyrate, and replacement with chloride, converting the high [AG] acidosis into a hyperchloremic acidosis (see Chapter 10) (14).

PLASMA POTASSIUM CONCENTRATION IN METABOLIC ACIDOSIS

Metabolic acidosis is accompanied by movement of some H^+ from the ECF into cells where it combines with a variety of intracellular buffers. This movement accounts for a distribution space of infused acids of about 50% of body weight (see Chapter 6). Movement of H^+ into cells mandates either an equimolar movement of an anion or exchange with an intracellular cation (such as K^+). In fact, either event can occur, depending on the nature of the acid administered. As a result, the change in serum $[K^+]$ that occurs in acute metabolic acidosis is highly dependent on the anion that accompanies the added H^+. Infusions of HCl, or the HCl precursor NH_4Cl, predictably increase serum $[K^+]$, but infusions of organic acids, such as lactic acid or β-hydroxybutyric acid, result in little if any change in $[K^+]$ (15). These differences are likely due to differing volumes of distribution of chloride compared with organic anions. Because chloride is largely restricted to the ECF, infusions of HCl generate a greater K^+ shift than infusions of organic acids whose anions can more readily penetrate cell membranes together with H^+. The electrolyte profile of patients with acute lactic acidosis provides evidence for the absence of a transcellular K^+ shift. Despite the development of marked lactic acidosis following seizures, plasma $[K^+]$ does not change (16).

Serum $[K^+]$ in patients with organic acidoses reflects overall K^+ balance, renal function, and transcellular shifts due to factors such as hyperglycemia, insulin deficiency, and catecholamine levels, which are all unrelated

Table 1   Causes of Metabolic Acidosis

1. *Hyperchloremic (normal anion gap) metabolic acidosis*
  Gastrointestinal loss of HCO_3
    Diarrhea
    Ureterosigmoidostomy
  Renal loss of HCO_3^-
    Proximal renal tubular acidosis (RTA)
      Isolated—sporadic, familial
      Fanconi syndrome
        Familial
        Cystinosis
        Tyrosinemia
        Multiple myeloma
        Wilson's disease
        Ifosfamide
        Osteopetrosis
    Carbonic anhydrase inhibitors
    Ileal bladder
  Reduced renal H^+ secretion
    Distal RTA (classic, Type 1)
      Familial
      Hypercalcemic/hypercalcuric states
      Sjögren syndrome
      Autoimmune diseases
      Amphotericin
      Renal transplants
    Type 4 RTA
      Hyporeninemic-hypoaldosteronism
      Tubulointerstitial disease
      Non-steroidal anti-inflammatory drugs
    Defective mineralocorticoid (MC) synthesis or secretion
      Addison disease
      Acquired adrenal enzymatic defects—chronic heparin therapy
      Congenital adrenal enzymatic defects—adrenal hyperplasia
    Inadequate renal response to MC
      Sickle cell disease
      Systemic lupus erythematosis
      Potassium sparing diuretics
      Pseudohypoaldosteronism Type 1 and Type 2
    Early uremia
  HCl/HCl precursor ingestion/infusion
    HCl
    NH_4Cl
    Arginine HCl

(Continued)

Table 1   (*Continued*)

Other
    Recovery from sustained hypocapnia
    Treatment of diabetic ketoacidosis
    Toluene inhalation with good kidney function
2. *High anion gap metabolic acidosis*
    Organic acidoses
        Lactic acidosis
        Diabetic ketoacidosis
        Alcoholic ketoacidosis
        D-Lactic acidosis
    Ingestions/poisonings
        Methanol
        Ethylene glycol
        Salicylates
    Uremia

---

to pH. In hyperchloremic metabolic acidosis as well, serum $[K^+]$ is dependent on factors unrelated to pH. The hyperkalemia in the hyperkalemic hyperchloremic acidosis encountered clinically in patients with chronic kidney disease (see Chapter 13) is due to impaired renal K^+ excretion rather than transcellular K^+ shifts. The most common cause of hyperchloremic acidosis, diarrhea, is associated with hypokalemia as a result of stool K^+ losses (see Chapter 15). Patients with classic distal renal tubular acidosis develop hypokalemic hyperchloremic metabolic acidosis due to increased renal K^+ excretion (see Chapter 13). In consequence, transcellular K shifts in response to ECF pH generally play a relatively minor role in serum K concentration derangements which develop in patients with metabolic acidosis.

CLINICAL MANIFESTATIONS OF METABOLIC ACIDOSIS

Pulmonary and Cardiovascular Effects

Because metabolic acidosis stimulates ventilation, some patients may develop labored breathing and complain of dyspnea. Acidemia directly depresses cardiac function and dilates peripheral arterioles but simultaneously activates the sympathetic nervous system and increases systemic catecholamine levels; the latter effects generally counterbalance the direct effects of acidemia (17,18).

    However, severe acidemia (pH < 7.2) blunts the effectiveness of sympathetic/catecholamine activation and when this occurs, cardiac function deteriorates, peripheral arteries dilate, and cardiovascular collapse may ensue (19). In contrast, acidemia directly constricts systemic veins and may act additively or synergistically with the sympathetic nervous system

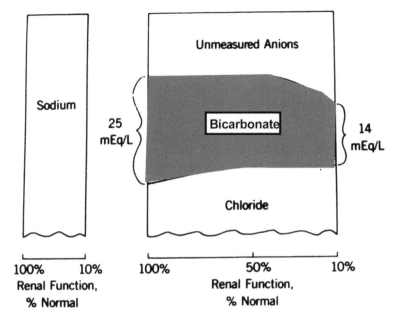

Figure 5 Early kidney disease produces a hyperchloremic acidosis, as serum [Cl⁻] rises to match the fall in [HCO₃⁻]. As kidney function deteriorates over time, the metabolic acidosis evolves into a high [AG] form because the anions of the strong acids produced by metabolism (e.g., phosphoric, sulfuric) can no longer be excreted. *Source*: From Ref. 51.

to produce venoconstriction (17,20). This venoconstriction increases central blood volume and can produce pulmonary edema. Pulmonary vascular resistance also increases sharply in response to acute metabolic acidosis (21). Severe acidemia is arrhythmogenic and reduces the cardiac fibrillation threshold (22).

Acute acidemia reduces hemoglobin's affinity for oxygen thereby enhancing tissue O_2 unloading (the acute Bohr effect) (23). However, acidemia that persists for more than 6–12 hr causes the red blood cell concentration of 2,3-diphosphoglycerate to fall, opposing the acute Bohr effect and restoring the oxyhemoglobin dissociation curve toward its baseline status (24).

Gastrointestinal Effects

Nausea and vomiting often occur in patients with metabolic acidosis, but the role of acidemia per se vs. that of the underlying clinical disorder remains uncertain. For example, uremic acidosis is frequently associated with nausea and vomiting, but this is probably due to uremic toxicity rather than acidosis. Similarly, nausea and vomiting occur frequently in patients with ketoacidosis but the contribution of hepatic swelling, gastroparesis, and hyperglycemia are probably as important, or more important, than metabolic acidosis (25).

Skeletal Effects

Bone mineral is largely comprised of alkaline calcium-phosphate salts. Synthesis of mineralized bone generates an acid load that must be excreted. Conversely, dissolving bone mineral releases alkali into the body's fluid spaces. The adult skeleton contains more than 25,000 mEq of alkali that can potentially be used to buffer acid loads. In fact, participation of bone calcium salts in buffering acid has been demonstrated both in intact human subjects and in bone taken from animals and studied in vitro (see Chapters 6 and 14) (26,27). In human studies, acid retention is associated with negative calcium balance, providing support for the role of bone dissolution in buffering retained H^+ (27). Measurements of bone carbonate have revealed reduced levels in patients with chronic kidney disease and metabolic acidosis (28).

Although calcium release from bone clearly contributes to buffering retained acid in experimental short-term metabolic acidosis, the magnitude of this response and its role in maintaining a stable plasma [HCO_3^-] in the long-term metabolic acidosis characteristic of chronic renal insufficiency remains an area of controversy (see Chapter 14) (27,29,30). The main argument against a sustained role for calcium release is that the buffering response required (if the amount of acid retained in the studies cited earlier is correct) would require virtual complete dissolution of the skeleton over a period of 3–4 years. This obviously does not occur, and thus the amount of acid retained and buffered by bone in long-term metabolic acidosis must be much less than previously reported. Nonetheless chronic metabolic acidosis contributes to the development of osteoporosis, osteomalacia, and renal osteodystrophy (27,28), and correction of acidosis by alkali administration rapidly reverses negative calcium balance (27). One group of investigators proposes that even in patients with normal renal function, H^+ retention increases in direct relation to the rate of endogenous acid production (see Chapter 8).

Muscle Protein Metabolism

Metabolic acidosis has a wide range of effects on muscle protein metabolism and general nutritional status. It has been observed for centuries that chronic kidney disease leads to weight loss and cachexia. This response has been attributed to various uremic "toxin." One of the uremic "toxins" potentially responsible for malnutrition may be chronic metabolic acidosis (31). Metabolic acidosis accelerates catabolism of muscle proteins, leading to muscle atrophy (32). This adverse effect is due to stimulation of protein catabolic pathways at several sites (33). The normal protein turnover rate in adults is 4–6 g/kg/day and most of this turnover occurs within muscle cells.

Although several muscle protein catabolic pathways have been identified, ATP-dependent ubiquitin–proteasome catabolism, a tightly regulated protein degradation reaction sequence, is most important. Through this pathway, the protein destined for destruction is modified by addition of a string of five or more small ubiquitin protein molecules. Ubiquitinization causes unfolding of the protein and the unfolded protein then enters one end of a hollow cylindrical intracellular structure, the proteasome, to be degraded within its core. The resultant small peptides exiting from the proteasome are largely hydrolyzed to their constituent amino acids.

The activity of the ubiquitin–proteasome pathway is increased in a number of catabolic states such as advanced cancer, burns, sepsis, and uremia (33). The synthesis and muscle content of both ubiquitin and proteasomes also increase markedly in uremic animals with metabolic acidosis (34). Correction of the metabolic acidosis restores activity of the ubiquitin–proteasome pathway to the normal range (34).

In addition to activation of ubiquitin–proteasome catabolism, metabolic acidosis increases the activity of other catabolic enzymes responsible for oxidizing amino acids. The essential branched-chain amino acids (valine, leucine, and isoleucine) make up about 18–20% of muscle protein. After these branched-chain amino acids are released from muscle protein, many donate their α-amino group to α-ketoglutarate, forming glutamate and the branched-chain keto analog of the amino acid (Fig. 6). These branched-chain keto acids are then oxidized via branched-chain ketoacid dehydrogenase (BCKAD). Activity of the enzyme BCKAD, which is the rate-limiting step in this sequence, is sharply increased by metabolic acidosis (and by glucocorticoids) (35). The glutamate generated via this series of reactions is converted to glutamine and transported to the kidney. Here, the enzymes glutaminase and glutamine dehydrogenase release glutamine's amino groups to generate two molecules of ammonium. The net effect of this process, which is activated by metabolic acidosis, is the mobilization and catabolism of muscle protein to provide glutamine to the kidney where its deamination supplies ammonium to increase net acid excretion.

Normal subjects with experimentally induced metabolic acidosis increase their protein catabolic rate and their rate of amino acid oxidation, develop negative nitrogen balance, and reduce their albumin synthetic rate (36,37). The accelerated rates of muscle proteolysis and amino acid oxidation, and the negative nitrogen balance of patients with renal failure, are all ameliorated by correction of their metabolic acidosis with exogenous NaHCO₃ (36–38). These observations support the suggestion over 170 years ago by Bright (39) that alkali salts might be of benefit to uremic patients.

Despite the evidence that chronic metabolic acidosis in patients with kidney failure is a major factor contributing to accelerated protein catabolism and malnutrition, several large cross-sectional studies have not shown

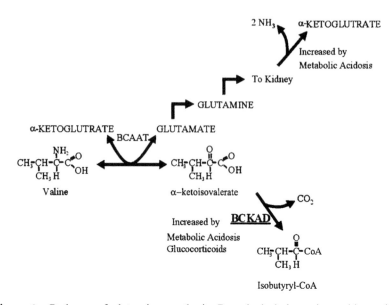

Figure 6 Pathway of glutamine synthesis. Branched chain amino acids, such as valine, are released from muscle proteins and donate their α-amino group to α-ketoglutarate (via branched chain α-amino transferase—BCAAT), forming glutamate and the branched chain keto amino acid analog. This keto analogue is oxidized via branched chain ketoacid dehydrogenase (BCKAD). Activity of BCKAD, which is the rate-limiting step in this sequence, is increased by metabolic acidosis (together with glucocorticoids). Glutamate is converted to glutamine and transported to the kidney where its amino groups are utilized for NH_4^+ excretion.

the expected correlation between the degree of metabolic acidosis and several nutritional markers in this population (40). This initially surprising finding may be due to the fact that better nourished and "healthier" dialysis patients ingest more dietary protein. They, therefore, generate a greater dietary acid load, and as a result have lower steady-state serum $[HCO_3^-]$. This relationship may confound the cross-sectional results (41).

EFFECTS OF METABOLIC ACIDOSIS ON THE KIDNEY

Hypertrophy

Metabolic acidosis increases H^+ secretion in both the proximal and distal tubule, and increases the renal synthesis and excretion of NH_4^+ (42). These acid excretory processes are increasingly activated when metabolic acidosis persists and becomes chronic. Stimulation of acid excretion requires increased activity of a number of energy generating processes as well as ion transporting proteins and enzymes. Metabolic acidosis increases the synthesis of both the apical membrane Na^+/H^+ antiporter and the basolateral $Na^+/HCO_3^-/CO_3^-$ symporter in the proximal tubule that mediate H^+ secretion and $NaHCO_3$ reclamation (42). The enzymes that deaminate glutamine and then metabolize the resulting α-ketoglutarate are activated by chronic metabolic acidosis (43). In the distal tubule, the activity of type-A intercalated cells (H^+ secreting) increases while the activity of type-B intercalated cells (HCO_3^- secreting) falls (44).

This wide ranging stimulation of the kidney's acid excretory mechanisms is associated with generalized renal growth and hypertrophy (44). Stimulation of kidney growth by chronic metabolic acidosis seems paradoxical because as described above chronic metabolic acidosis leads to muscle wasting, negative nitrogen balance, and generalized growth retardation. However metabolic acidosis and high renal NH_4^+ levels activate kidney growth via protein kinase C signaling and by increasing the activity of a series of renal "immediate early genes" that promote organ and cell growth (44).

Although renal hypertrophy in response to metabolic acidosis enhances net acid excretion, and this response is beneficial with regard to the maintenance of acid–base balance, hypertrophy may have deleterious consequences in individuals with renal insufficiency. This principle has been most clearly demonstrated in a rodent model of polycystic kidney disease. Metabolic acidosis accelerates cyst growth and renal dysfunction while correction of acidosis with oral alkali salts improves renal function (45,46). Under certain conditions, acidosis may even contribute to the de novo development of renal cysts. Another deleterious effect of chronic metabolic acidosis in patients with already damaged kidneys may be the acceleration of interstitial damage. Metabolic acidosis increases kidney NH_4^+ synthesis resulting in high renal interstitial NH_4^+ concentrations. These levels of NH_4^+ activate complement and may trigger complement-mediated tissue damage (47). In a rodent model, correction of the acidosis ameliorates the degree of kidney damage (47).

Nephrocalcinosis and Nephrolithiasis

Chronic metabolic acidosis is also associated with nephrocalcinosis and nephrolithiasis. These effects are most likely due to the fact that metabolic acidosis causes a sharp reduction in urine citrate excretion (48). Reduced citrate excretion helps to conserve body alkali stores, but can adversely affect the solubility of calcium in the urine. Low urine citrate concentration is a major risk factor for the development of renal parenchymal calcification and calcium stones. The nephrocalcinosis and nephrolithiasis that occur in patients with distal RTA are largely due to hypocitraturia. Patients with incomplete distal RTA (subclinical metabolic acidosis, alkaline urine pH, and high urine NH_4^+ excretion) also have reduced urine citrate excretion and a high frequency of nephrolithiasis. Treatment of patients with classic or incomplete distal RTA with $NaHCO_3$ raises their plasma $[HCO_3^-]$ and urine citrate excretion, reducing the frequency of kidney stones.

Patients with other causes of chronic metabolic acidosis, such as those with chronic diarrhea, also have low urine citrate excretion and may develop kidney stones as a result of the same mechanism. In addition, patients with diarrhea are at risk to develop other urine chemical abnormalities that predispose to kidney stone formation. For a variety of reasons, patients with steatorrhea and ileal disease, or ileal resection, increase gut absorption of dietary oxalate and develop hyperoxaluria (49). This abnormality interacts with the hypocitraturia to markedly increase the likelihood of calcium oxalate stones. The fluids lost with diarrhea also reduce urine volumes and increase urine solute concentrations. In contrast to patients with distal RTA, patients with diarrhea can generally acidify their urine. If patients excrete small volumes of concentrated and acidic urine, these changes predispose them as well to uric acid kidney stone formation (50).

SUMMARY

Metabolic acidosis is a disorder of acid–base equilibrium that is initiated by a primary reduction in serum $[HCO_3^-]$ and, when uncomplicated, manifested by a low serum $[HCO_3^-]$, PCO_2, and pH. The low PCO_2 in metabolic acidosis is a secondary response and is the result of hyperventilation, stimulated directly by acidemia. The fall in PCO_2 engendered by metabolic acidosis is directly related to the magnitude of the reduction in $[HCO_3^-]$ caused by this disorder, and assessment of this response is an important step in diagnosis and management. Metabolic acidosis is caused by one or more of the following pathophysiological mechanisms:

1. The loss of bicarbonate or the salts of organic anions from the body (e.g., diarrhea states),
2. The rapid addition of strong (or relatively strong) acids to the body fluids (e.g., diabetic ketoacidosis or lactic acidosis),
3. Impairment of renal acid excretion (e.g., renal insufficiency).

The pathophysiology, differential diagnosis, and management of metabolic acidoses are aided by an understanding of the anion gap, that is, the difference between the concentration of sodium and the sum of the chloride and bicarbonate concentrations in the serum. Chronic metabolic acidosis produces few symptoms, but has adverse effects on cardiovascular function, and on bone and muscle metabolism, which are all ameliorated by alkali administration. It is associated with renal hypertrophy, nephrocalcinosis, and nephrolithiasis, and may contribute to progressive renal damage in patients with renal insufficiency.

REFERENCES

1. Kussmaul A. Zur lehre vom diabetes mellitus. Uber eine eigentumlichte tode-sartmbei diabetikern.. Deutche Arch Klin Med 1874; 14:1.
2. Fencl V, Miller TB, Pappenheimer JR. Studies on the respiratory response to disturbances of acid–base balance, with deductions concerning the ionic composition of cerebral interstitial fluid. Am J Physiol 1966; 210:459–472.
3. Javaheri S, Clendening A, Papadakis N, Brody JS. Changes in brain surface pH during acute isocapnic metabolic acidosis and alkalosis. J Appl Physiol 1981; 51:276–281.
4. Kaehny WD, Jackson JT. Respiratory response to HCl acidosis in dogs after carotid body denervation. J Appl Physiol 1979; 46:1138–1142.
5. Narins RG, Emmett M. Simple and mixed acid–base disorders: a practical approach. Medicine (Baltimore) 1980; 59:161–187.
6. Bushinsky DA, Coe FL, Katzenberg C, Szidon JP, Parks JH. Arterial PCO_2 in chronic metabolic acidosis. Kidney Int 1982; 22:311–314.
7. Albert MS, Dell RB, Winters RW. Quantitative displacement of acid–base equilibrium in metabolic acidosis. Ann Intern Med 1967; 66:312–322.
8. Fulop M. A guide for predicting arterial CO_2 tension in metabolic acidosis. Am J Nephrol 1997; 17:421–424.
9. Madias NE, Schwartz WB, Cohen JJ. The maladaptive renal response to secondary hypocapnia during chronic HCl acidosis in the dog. J Clin Invest 1977; 60:1393–1401.
10. Krapf R, Beeler I, Hertner D, Hulter HN. Chronic respiratory alkalosis. The effect of sustained hyperventilation on renal regulation of acid–base equilibrium. N Engl J Med 1991; 324:1394–1401.
11. Emmett M, Narins RG. Clinical use of the anion gap. Medicine (Baltimore) 1977; 56:38–54.
12. Winter SD, Pearson JR, Gabow PA, Schultz AL, Lepoff RB. The fall of the serum anion gap. Arch Intern Med 1990; 150:311–313.
13. Emmett M, Seldin DW. Evaluation of acid–base disorders from plasma composition. In: Seldin DW, Giebisch G, eds. The Regulation of Acid–Base Balance. New York: Raven Press, 1989:213–263.
14. Adrogue HJ, Eknoyan G, Suki WK. Diabetic ketoacidosis: role of the kidney in the acid–base homeostasis re-evaluated. Kidney Int 1984; 25:591–598.
15. Adrogue HJ, Madias NE. Changes in plasma potassium concentration during acute acid–base disturbances. Am J Med 1981; 71:456–467.
16. Orringer CE, Eustace JC, Wunsch CD, Gardner LB. Natural history of lactic acidosis after grand-mal seizures. A model for the study of an anion-gap acidosis not associated with hyperkalemia. N Engl J Med 1977; 297:796–799.
17. Mitchell JH, Wildenthal K, Johnson RL Jr. The effects of acid–base disturbances on cardiovascular and pulmonary function. Kidney Int 1972; 1:375–389.
18. Gonzalez NC, Clancy RL. Inotropic and intracellular acid–base changes during metabolic acidosis. Am J Physiol 1975; 228:1060–1064.
19. Marsh JD, Margolis TI, Kim D. Mechanism of diminished contractile response to catecholamines during acidosis. Am J Physiol 1988; 254:H20–H27.

20. Sharpey-Schafer EP, Semple SJ, Halls RW, Howarth S. Venous constriction after exercise; its relation to acid–base changes in venous blood. Clin Sci 1965; 29:397–406.
21. Bergofsky EH, Lehr DE, Fishman AP. The effect of changes in hydrogen ion concentration on the pulmonary circulation. J Clin Invest 1962; 41: 1492–1502.
22. Orchard CH, Cingolani HE. Acidosis and arrhythmias in cardiac muscle. Cardiovasc Res 1994; 28:1312–1319.
23. Perutz MF, Muirhead H, Mazzarella L, Crowther RA, Greer J, Kilmartin JV. Identification of residues responsible for the alkaline Bohr effect in haemoglobin. Nature 1969; 222:1240–1243.
24. Benesch RE, Benesch R, Yu CI. The oxygenation of hemoglobin in the presence of 2,3-diphosphoglycerate. Effect of temperature, pH, ionic strength, and hemoglobin concentration. Biochemistry 1969; 8:2567–2571.
25. Barrett EJ, Sherwin RS. Gastrointestinal manifestations of diabetic ketoacidosis. Yale J Biol Med 1983; 56:175–178.
26. Bushinsky DA, Frick KK. The effects of acid on bone. Curr Opin Nephrol Hypertens 2000; 9:369–379.
27. Lemann J Jr, Bushinsky DA, Hamm LL. Bone buffering of acid and base in humans. Am J Physiol Renal Physiol 2003; 285:F811–F832.
28. Bushinsky DA. The contribution of acidosis to renal osteodystrophy. Kidney Int 1995; 47:1816–1832.
29. Oh MS. Irrelevance of bone buffering to acid–base homeostasis in chronic metabolic acidosis. Nephron 1991; 59:7–10.
30. Uribarri J, Douyon H, Oh MS. A re-evaluation of the urinary parameters of acid production and excretion in patients with chronic renal acidosis. Kidney Int 1995; 47:624–627.
31. Bailey JL, Mitch WE. Metabolic acidosis as a uremic toxin. Semin Nephrol 1996; 16:160–166.
32. May RC, Kelly RA, Mitch WE. Metabolic acidosis stimulates protein degradation in rat muscle by a glucocorticoid-dependent mechanism. J Clin Invest 1986; 77:614–621.
33. Mitch WE, Goldberg AL. Mechanisms of muscle wasting. The role of the ubiquitin–proteasome pathway. N Engl J Med 1996; 335:1897–1905.
34. Bailey JL, Wang X, England BK, Price SR, Ding X, Mitch WE. The acidosis of chronic renal failure activates muscle proteolysis in rats by augmenting transcription of genes encoding proteins of the ATP-dependent ubiquitin–proteasome pathway. J Clin Invest 1996; 97:1447–1453.
35. May RC, Hara Y, Kelly RA, Block KP, Buse MG, Mitch WE. Branched-chain amino acid metabolism in rat muscle: abnormal regulation in acidosis. Am J Physiol 1987; 252:E712–E718.
36. Ballmer PE, McNurlan MA, Hulter HN, Anderson SE, Garlick PJ, Krapf R. Chronic metabolic acidosis decreases albumin synthesis and induces negative nitrogen balance in humans. J Clin Invest 1995; 95:39–45.
37. Reaich D, Channon SM, Scrimgeour CM, Goodship TH. Ammonium chloride-induced acidosis increases protein breakdown and amino acid oxidation in humans. Am J Physiol 1992; 263:E735–E739.

38. Papadoyannakis NJ, Stefanidis CJ, McGeown M. The effect of the correction of metabolic acidosis on nitrogen and potassium balance of patients with chronic renal failure. Am J Clin Nutr 1984; 40:623–627.
39. Bright R. Reports of Medical Cases selected with a View to Illustrating the Symptoms and Cure of Diseases by a Reference to Morbid Anatomy. London: Longman 1831:2.
40. Brady JP, Hasbargen JA. A review of the effects of correction of acidosis on nutrition in dialysis patients. Semin Dial 2000; 13:252–255.
41. Louden JD, Roberts RR, Goodship TH. Acidosis and nutrition. Kidney Int Suppl 1999; 73:S85–S88.
42. Preisig PA, Alpern RJ. Chronic metabolic acidosis causes an adaptation in the apical membrane Na/H antiporter and basolateral membrane Na(HCO$_3$)$_3$ symporter in the rat proximal convoluted tubule. J Clin Invest 1988; 82: 1445–1453.
43. Curthoys NP, Gstraunthaler G. Mechanism of increased renal gene expression during metabolic acidosis. Am J Physiol Renal Physiol 2001; 281:F381–F390.
44. Alpern RJ. Trade-offs in the adaptation to acidosis. Kidney Int 1995; 47: 1205–1215.
45. Torres VE, Mujwid DK, Wilson DM, Holley KH. Renal cystic disease and ammoniagenesis in Han:SPRD rats. J Am Soc Nephrol 1994; 5:1193–1200.
46. Tanner GA. Potassium citrate/citric acid intake improves renal function in rats with polycystic kidney disease. J Am Soc Nephrol 1998; 9:1242–1248.
47. Nath KA, Hostetter MK, Hostetter TH. Increased ammoniagenesis as a determinant of progressive renal injury. Am J Kidney Dis 1991; 17:654–657.
48. Hamm LL. Renal handling of citrate. Kidney Int 1990; 38:728–735.
49. Dobbins JW, Binder HJ. Importance of the colon in enteric hyperoxaluria. N Engl J Med 1977; 296:298–301.
50. Riese RJ, Sakhaee K. Uric acid nephrolithiasis: pathogenesis and treatment. J Urol 1992; 148:765–771.
51. Widmer B, Gerhardt RE, Harrington JT, Cohen JJ. Serum electrolyte and acid–base composition. The influence of graded degrees of chronic renal failure. Arch Intern Med 1979; 139:1099–1102.

10

Diabetic and Other Forms of Ketoacidosis

Horacio J. Adrogué

Baylor College of Medicine, VA Medical Center, Houston, Texas, U.S.A.

Nicolaos E. Madias

Department of Medicine, Caritas St. Elizabeth's Medical Center,
Tufts University School of Medicine, Boston, Massachusetts, U.S.A.

INTRODUCTION

Ketosis is an abnormal state of nutrient metabolism that develops when the rate of production of ketones exceeds their removal; as a result, ketones accumulate in body fluids as reflected by high blood and urine levels (1–4). Because ketones are largely organic acids (e.g., β-hydroxybutyric and acetoacetic acid) that dissociate almost completely at the pH of the body fluids, they produce H^+ which consumes HCO_3^- and causes metabolic acidosis. Hence the designation of ketoacidosis. The term ketosis is used to describe a mild form of the disturbance, reserving the term ketoacidosis for the full-blown condition that features substantial metabolic acidosis (5).

PATHOPHYSIOLOGY—GENERAL CONSIDERATIONS

The mechanisms underlying ketoacidosis are essentially the same whether it develops as an acute complication of diabetes mellitus or in nondiabetic subjects (e.g., starvation ketosis, alchoholic ketoacidosis). Abnormal levels or action of insulin and glucagon are required for the development of ketosis (5–8). Insulin deficiency or resistance impairs glucose utilization in skeletal muscle and increases adipose tissue and muscle breakdown, thereby augmenting delivery of glycerol and alanine (gluconeogenic substrates) to the liver. Hepatic gluconeogenesis, in turn, is stimulated by insulin deficiency and, more importantly, by glucagon excess. The fatty acids released from the enhanced lipolysis are converted to ketones by the hepatocytes under the influence of glucagon excess. Pancreatic β-cell destruction is largely responsible for the hormonal imbalance observed in most cases of diabetic ketoacidosis. Conversely, insulin deficiency in the presence of normal β-cells plays a major role in ketosis associated with fasting, starvation, ethanol ingestion, and some liver diseases.

DIABETIC KETOACIDOSIS

Diabetic ketoacidosis (DKA) is a disease state characterized by the presence of hyperglycemia and hyperosmolality, metabolic acidosis due to ketoacid accumulation, extracellular and intracellular fluid depletion, and varying degrees of electrolyte deficiency, particularly of potassium and phosphate (7–9).

Roles of Insulin and Glucagon

The abnormal metabolism of carbohydrates and lipids observed in DKA is largely caused by a rise in the molar ratio of glucagon/insulin in plasma. The two hormones are metabolic antagonists with respect to fuel production and utilization but their primary effects occur on different tissues. Insulin acts on muscle and adipose tissue augmenting glucose transport and inhibiting lipolysis. Glucagon acts primarily on the liver increasing glycogenolysis, gluconeogenesis, and ketogenesis. Insulin's action on the hepatocyte is essentially that of an antiglucagon hormone, as it has minimal hepatic effects in the absence of glucagon-induced metabolic changes. Insulin decreases glucagon release from α cells in the pancreatic islets and inhibits a glucagon-activated, cAMP-dependent protein kinase in the hepatocyte (5). Beyond the critical role of glucagon in ketone body production, other hormones, including catecholamines, cortisol, growth hormone, and thyroid hormones increase hepatic ketogenesis and may participate in the pathogenesis of DKA (10) (Fig. 1).

In fasting individuals, the major source of glucose (approximately 90%) is the liver, through glycogenolysis and gluconeogenesis. The kidney contributes the remaining 10% through synthesis of glucose from three-carbon precursors (gluconeogenesis). After a meal, glucose absorption increases the plasma glucose level. The resultant hyperglycemia-induced stimulation of insulin secretion suppresses hepatic glucose production, largely through inhibition of glycogenolysis, and stimulates glucose uptake by the liver, the gut, and peripheral tissues, including skeletal muscle.

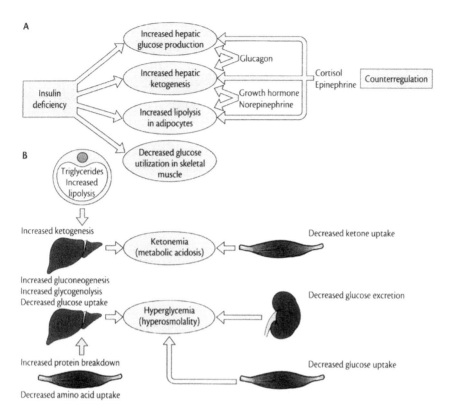

Figure 1 Role of insulin deficiency, counter-regulatory hormones, and various tissues and organs in the pathogenesis of hyperglycemia and ketosis in DKA. (**A**) Metabolic processes affected by insulin deficiency, on the one hand, and excess of glucagon, cortisol, epinephrine, norepinephrine, and growth hormone, on the other. (**B**) The roles of the adipose tissue, liver, skeletal muscle, and kidney in the pathogenesis of hyperglycemia and ketonemia. Excessive hepatic production of glucose and impairment of glucose utilization are the main determinants of hyperglycemia. Increased hepatic production of ketones and their reduced utilization by peripheral tissues account for the ketonemia. *Source*: From Ref. 10.

Pathophysiology

Hyperglycemia

In uncontrolled diabetes, hyperglycemia is caused by increased hepatic and renal glucose production and decreased glucose utilization in muscle and adipose tissue. Decreased glucose utilization, once considered the major contributor to hyperglycemia in uncontrolled diabetes, is currently believed to play a smaller role than excessive glucose production. Figure 2 depicts the

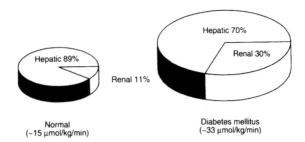

Figure 2   Contributions of the liver and the kidney to endogenous glucose production in conscious normal and diabetic dogs. Total glucose production is indicated in parentheses. *Source*: From Ref. 11.

hepatic and renal contribution to endogenous glucose production in conscious normal and diabetic dogs (11). The rise in the glucagon/insulin ratio in plasma characteristic of uncontrolled diabetes activates key enzymes that accelerate the rates of both glycogenolysis and gluconeogenesis. The increased ratio also promotes glucose overproduction by modulating the effects of other hormones, availability of substrate, and rates of fatty acid oxidation (Fig. 1). Volume depletion secondary to hyperglycemia-induced osmotic diuresis reduces the urinary loss of glucose, thereby worsening hyperglycemia.

An important contributor to the development of hyperglycemia in uncontrolled diabetes may be the prevailing acidemia (12–14). In dogs with acidemia induced by hypercapnia, a substantially smaller glucose infusion rate maintains euglycemia as compared to dogs without respiratory acidosis during constant insulin infusion, reflecting less glucose entry into cells for a given insulin level (15) (Fig. 3). Although the sympathetic surge characteristic of acidemia undoubtedly contributes to glucose intolerance, adrenergic blockade during acute respiratory acidosis does not prevent the disturbed glucoregulation. Nor does plasma insulin fall during acute respiratory acidosis. In fact, acidemia reduces tissue extraction of insulin and, more specifically, insulin uptake by the liver (15). Although plasma glucagon levels increase during metabolic or respiratory acidosis, the glucagon/insulin ratio in the portal circulation remains unchanged, thereby reducing the possible role of glucagon in the hyperglycemia of acidemic states. The hyperglycemia of acidemia is most likely mediated by a reduction of insulin binding to its receptor and decreased tissue sensitivity to the hormone (15,16).

Metabolic Acidosis

Although the metabolic acidosis of DKA is mostly caused by the overproduction of β-hydroxybutyric and acetoacetic acids, additional acids, including lactic acid, free fatty acids, and other organic acids can contribute to the fall in plasma [HCO_3^-] (5). Insulin deficiency, coupled with counterregulatory hormone excess (largely glucagon), activates cAMP, which in turn leads to phosphorylation and

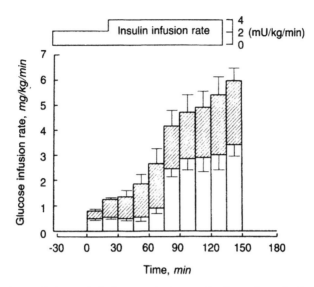

Figure 3 Rate of glucose infusion required to maintain euglycemia during insulin infusion studies in normal and acidemic dogs (respiratory acidosis, arterial pH = 7.18). Open area in each column represents the value in acidemic dogs; the entire column is the value in normal dogs. *Source*: From Ref. 11.

activation of lipase in adipocytes, thereby promoting lipolysis (17,18). Lipolysis of triglyceride stores in the adipocyte provides long-chain fatty acids, which are the principal substrate for hepatic ketogenesis (19,20). However, hepatic triglycerides might also serve as a source of fatty acids in the presence of fatty liver, a not uncommon condition in patients with diabetes (5).

Role of Fatty Acid Oxidation: In addition to augmented substrate in the form of long-chain fatty acids, development of substantial ketogenesis by the hepatocyte mitochondria requires a major increase in fatty acid oxidation. A transport system, the carnitine shuttle, is needed for long-chain fatty acids to enter the mitochondrial matrix. This carrier system consists of two carnitine palmitoyl-transferases (CPT)—an outer CPT I and an inner CPT II—and carnitine/acyl-carnitine translocase. The key regulatory step for fatty acid oxidation takes place in a transesterification reaction catalyzed by CPT I (19,21). This enzyme controls the entry of acyl-coenzyme A (CoA) esters, which are derived from the long-chain fatty acids, from the cytosol into the mitochondria (Fig. 4). In the normal fed state and in well-controlled diabetes, CPT I is inhibited such that fatty acids cannot enter the mitochondria for oxidation and ketoacid formation, but are re-esterified to triglycerides and transported out of the cytosol as very-low-density plasma lipoproteins. Inhibition of CPT I is provided by malonyl-CoA, a metabolite whose level is dependent on adequate glycolysis and activity of acetyl-CoA

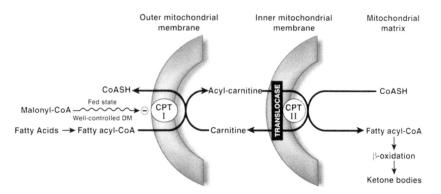

Figure 4 Regulation of hepatic ketogenesis. Synthesis of ketones in the liver depends on transfer of fatty acyl-CoA into the mitochondria by carnitine palmitoyl-transferase I (CPT I). In the fed state and in well-controlled diabetes, CPT I activity is inhibited by cytoplasmic malonyl CoA. During fasting and in patients with uncontrolled diabetes, the increase in the glucagon/insulin molar ratio suppresses malonyl CoA synthesis, allowing for increased transfer of fatty acyl-CoA into the mitochondria and increased ketogenesis. *Source*: From Ref. 5.

carboxylase (22,23). The concentration of malonyl-CoA is maximal in the fed state, but it sharply decreases with fasting and uncontrolled diabetes. In these conditions, an increase in the glucagon/insulin ratio blocks glycolysis and inhibits acetyl-CoA carboxylase, two processes that lead to a major drop in malonyl-CoA levels. Consequently, CPT I activity is enhanced, allowing conversion of the acyl-CoA esters of long-chain fatty acids to acyl-carnitines that can be transported toward the interior of mitochondria (24). The transesterification to acyl-carnitine is then reversed by CPT II, which works in conjuction with the translocase, allowing the release of fatty acyl-CoA in the mitochondrial matrix. The capacity of the hepatocytes for fatty acid oxidation is large and most of the fatty acyl-CoA molecules entering the mitochondria are oxidized to ketone bodies.

The Anion Gap: During the development of DKA, ketoacids released into the body fluids are titrated by HCO_3^- and other body buffers (25–27). As a result of this buffering process, HCO_3^- ions are replaced by ketoanions in the extracellular fluid producing the characteristic increase in plasma unmeasured anions (the so-called "anion gap") that is seen in diabetic ketoacidosis. In uncomplicated DKA, the increment in the anion gap (AG) above its normal value should be approximately equal to the decrement in plasma $[HCO_3^-]$ (25,26). Thus, the ratio of excess AG (i.e., measured AG minus normal AG) in mEq/L to the decrement in $[HCO_3^-]$ (i.e., normal plasma $[HCO_3^-]$ minus measured plasma $[HCO_3^-]$) should be approximately 1.0. In fact, this pattern is seen in most patients with DKA (26,28–31). As can be seen in Table 1, the decrement in plasma $[HCO_3^-]$ is essentially equal

Table 1 Comparison of Admission Data in Diabetic Ketoacidosis (DKA)

	Danowski et al. (112) (N=8, [])	Seldin et al. (128) (N=10, [])	Nabarro et al. (28) (N=7, [])	Shaw et al. (129) (N=30, [])	Assal et al. (29) (N=9, [])	Oh et al. (30) (N=35, [])	Adrogué et al. (26) (N=150, [])[a]
Blood (pH)					7.06 ± 0.03	7.07 ± 0	7.06 ± 0.0
$[Na]_p$, (mEq/L)	130 ± 3.2	129 ± 3.7	136 ± 0.5	131 ± 1.4	146 ± 3.0	136 ± 1.6	132 ± 0.6
$[K]_p$, (mEq/L)	4.9 ± 0.5	4.7 ± 0.2	5.7 ± 0.2	5.8 ± 0.3	5.6 ± 0.3		5.7 ± 0.1
$[Cl]_p$, (mEq/L)	94 ± 2.8	94 ± 3.5	93 ± 1.0	96 ± 1.3	106 ± 3.0	101 ± 1.4	98 ± 0.6
$[HCO_3]_p$, (mEq/L)	7.0 ± 0.8	7.4 ± 1.0	7.5 ± 1.1	5.0 ± 0.6[a]	5.6 ± 1.0	9.6 ± 0.3	6.2 ± 0.2[a]
Anion gap, (mEq/L)	34.3 ± 1.3	32.1 ± 1.5	40.8 ± 2.1	36.7 ± 1.7	40.0	25.0 ± 1.2[b]	33.5 ± 0.6
$\Delta[HCO_3]_p$, (mEq/L)[c]	17.0 ± 0.8	16.6 ± 1.0	16.5 ± 1.1	22.0 ± 0.6[a]	18.4	14.4 ± 0.3	20.8 ± 0.2
ΔAnion gap (mEq/L)[d]	18.3 ± 1.3	16.1 ± 1.5	24.8 ± 2.1	20.7 ± 1.7	24.0	13.0 ± 0.9	17.5 ± 0.6

[a]TCO_2 was measured.
[b]The value was calculated with $[K]_p$.
[c]The values were derived using a baseline value of either 24 mEq/L or 27 mmol/L depending on whether $[HCO_3]_p$ or TCO_2 were measured, respectively.
[d]The values were derived using a baseline value of 16 mEq/L.

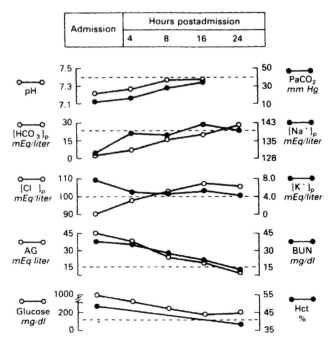

Figure 5 Laboratory data on admission and follow-up values in a patient admitted for diabetic ketoacidosis and featuring pure AG acidosis. Each symbol represents a single measurement. *Source*: From Ref. 31.

to the excess AG in most reported studies (in two studies, $\overline{\Delta}$ AG actually exceeds Δ [HCO$_3^-$] by 6–8 mEq/L, most likely due to a pre-existing metabolic alkalosis—see later).

Figure 5 charts the course of treatment in a patient with DKA. In this patient, the decrement in plasma [HCO$_3^-$] was essentially equal to the increase in AG before treatment was begun. During the course of therapy, plasma [HCO$_3^-$] increased as the AG fell, and serum [Cl$^-$] rose concomitantly. By 16 hr after admission, serum [HCO$_3^-$] was 16 mEq/L, and blood pH was almost normal. Of note, the BUN was increased on admission, reflecting a prerenal fall in renal function, which was corrected by treatment (see later).

Although most patients with DKA have an increased AG, one occasionally encounters a patient with pure hyperchloremic metabolic acidosis (32,33). The presenting data and course of treatment in such a patient are depicted in Fig. 6 (31). Severe metabolic acidosis, accompanied by the appropriate respiratory response, was present on admission, but the decrement in plasma [HCO$_3^-$] was not associated with an increase in the AG (AG = 16 mEq/L in this example, which includes [K$^+$] in the calculation).

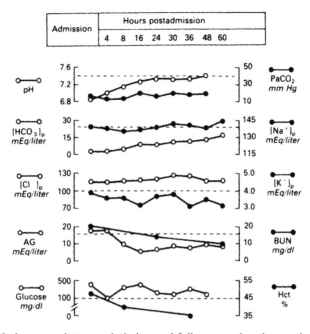

Figure 6 Laboratory data on admission and follow-up values in a patient admitted for diabetic ketoacidosis but featuring pure hyperchloremic acidosis. Each symbol represents a single measurement. *Source*: From Ref. 31.

A notable additional feature is that the blood urea nitrogen (BUN) concentration is within normal limits. Despite standard treatment, 60 hr elapsed before the serum [HCO$_3^-$] rose to 17 mEq/L. Serum [Cl$^-$], although elevated on admission, increased further during treatment, and was associated with a reciprocal decrement in the AG. The fall in the AG, was due, at least in part, to a major reduction in the serum protein concentration. Thus, two differences are noteworthy in patients with DKA and a normal AG. The first is that there is less evidence of impairment of renal function, and the second is a slower recovery from metabolic acidosis compared with patients presenting with an increased AG. Considering that the DKA patient is unable to properly metabolize ketoacids, whether ketoanions are retained in the ECF or are wasted in the urine should have no major effect on the severity of the acid–base disorder.

The representative cases depicted in Figs 5 and 6 portray the extremes of the acid–base patterns observed on admission for uncomplicated DKA (31). In fact, most patients have elements of both increased AG and hyperchloremic acidosis with one element being dominant (Table 1). Although various factors could potentially alter the stoichiometric relationship between the increment in AG and the decrement in plasma [HCO$_3^-$], the level of renal function appears to be the major determinant of the type of metabolic acidosis encountered on admission for DKA (Fig 7).

Additional conditions might alter the ratio of excess AG/bicarbonate deficit in patients with DKA, including hyperproteinemia, vomiting or exogenous bicarbonate therapy, and hypocapnia. Differences in the apparent distribution volume of HCO_3^- and ketone anions have also been proposed to explain the hyperchloremic acidosis of DKA; this hypothesis, however, has not been verified experimentally (26).

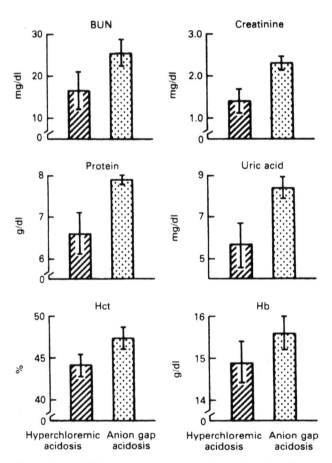

Figure 7   Comparison of laboratory data on admission for diabetic ketoacidosis in patients presenting with hyperchloremic acidosis (*left side of each panel*) and those presenting with anion gap acidosis (*right side of each panel*). Patients were classified according to the excess anion gap/bicarbonate deficit ratio values. Hyperchloremic acidosis was arbitrarily defined to exist when the excess anion gap/bicarbonate deficit ratio was below 0.8 [80%]. Each bar depicts mean values ± 1 SE. *Source:* From Ref. 31.

Role of the Kidney in Modulating the AG: Because renal reabsorption of filtered plasma ketoanions is limited and the production of ketoacids can reach levels as high as 1000 to 2000 mEq/day, the urinary excretion of Na^+ and K^+ salts of the ketoacid anions can be enormous (28,34,35). The renal "wasting" of ketone salts in association with glucosuria-induced osmotic diuresis, poor fluid intake, and vomiting, result in ECF volume depletion and a reduction in renal function. Renal blood flow and GFR both fall during DKA, with recovery to normal values following the episode (36,37). Increased urea production from enhanced catabolism of amino acids in patients with DKA also contributes to the elevation of BUN levels.

Patients with DKA who develop substantial volume depletion, will tend to present with an increased AG metabolic acidosis because of their limited ability to excrete ketone salts. Conversely, patients with DKA who are able to maintain salt and water intake, thereby minimizing ECF volume depletion, will tend to present with variable degrees of hyperchloremic acidosis, due to urinary excretion of ketone salts and retention of chloride (26,31).

Effect of Treatment on AG: Volume replacement with saline infusions during treatment of DKA causes dilution of both ketones and HCO_3^-; thus, the AG decreases due to replacement of an unmeasured anion (ketones) with a measured anion (Cl^-). Additionally, correction of K^+ depletion (see later) with its Cl^- salt results in the cellular uptake of K^+ in exchange for H^+, while most of the Cl^- remains in the ECF. Because the H^+ extruded is titrated by HCO_3^-, the net effect is the development of hyperchloremic acidosis.

Renal Response to Ketoacidosis: Diabetic ketoacidosis causes a several-fold increase in net acid excretion. A voltage-dependent stimulus for H^+ secretion exists in the distal nephron whenever Na^+ is absorbed without an accompanying anion (see chapter 4). In DKA, a substantial electrical gradient favoring distal H^+ secretion develops as a result of increased distal Na^+ delivery (ketonuria and osmotic diuresis), avid Na^+ reabsorption (ECF volume contraction), and the presence of poorly reabsorbable anions (ketones). As a result, acid excretion, as titratable acid and ammonium, can attain levels as high as 250 and 500 mEq per day, respectively (35). Although this vigorous response suggests that the kidney very effectively defends acid–base homeostasis in the course of DKA, such a conclusion is untenable. Maximal stimulation of renal acidification in DKA does not suffice to compensate for the large urinary loss of HCO_3^- precursors in the form of salts of ketoacids. In fact, experimental studies have shown that despite maximal stimulation of urinary acidification, for each mmol of β-hydroxybutyrate excreted, the kidney could salvage only about 0.5 mEq of potential base (38). Although ketones have been shown to inhibit the rate of renal ammoniagenesis in the experimental animal, this effect most probably plays only a minor role in humans, as a large increment in urinary ammonium excretion is present in DKA (39).

Effect of Treatment on Renal Response: Balance studies carried out in the early period after admission for DKA reveal that correction of volume depletion results in massive urinary losses of HCO_3^- precursors (salts of ketoacids) that exceed urinary titratable acidity and ammonium excretion (Table 2) (31). Thus, in the initial period after admission, the kidneys behave in a maladaptive fashion relevant to the systemic acid–base composition (31). Only when the plasma ketones have fallen substantially, is stimulation of urinary excretion of titratable acidity and ammonium capable of generating sufficient new HCO_3^- to begin to correct the ketoacidosis.

Sodium and Water

The hyperglycemia-induced increase in effective osmotic pressure of the ECF triggers a shift of water out of cells, most prominently skeletal muscle, which reduces serum $[Na^+]$. An increase of 100 mg/dL [5.6 mmol/liter] in the glucose concentration decreases serum $[Na^+]$ by approximately 1.7 mEq/L, the end result being a rise in serum osmolality of approximately 2.0 mOsm/kg H_2O (40,41). The resulting expansion of the ECF compartment is, however, brief due to simultaneous renal and extrarenal loss of fluids. The hyperglycemia-induced increase in the filtered load of glucose exceeds the renal tubular reabsorptive capacity resulting in substantial glucosuria—one of the hallmarks of DKA. In turn, glucosuria causes osmotic

Table 2   Role of the Kidney in the Acid–Base Defense in Normal Subjects and During Recovery from Diabetic Ketoacidosis

Post-admission	Normal subjects[a] $TA + NH_4 - HCO_3^-$		Diabetic ketoacidosis[b] $TA + NH_4 - HCO_3^-$ [c]	
	Balance mEq	Cum. balance mEq	Balance mEq	Cum. balance mEq
0 to 4 hr	12.7	12.7	-45.0 ± 8.2	-45.0 ± 8.2
4 to 8 hr	12.7	25.4	-10.3 ± 13.5	-55.3 ± 20.8
8 to 12 hr	12.7	38.1	1.8 ± 6.8	-53.5 ± 27.1
12 to 16 hr	12.7	50.8	16.5 ± 2.0	-37.0 ± 28.3
16 to 20 hr	12.7	63.5	14.3 ± 2.3	-22.7 ± 28.9
20 to 24 hr	12.7	76.2	21.2 ± 4.8	-1.5 ± 31.2

[a]Estimate based on net acid excretion equal to 1.25 mEq/kg body weight/day and body weight equal to that of the diabetic patient (61 kg).
[b]The values presented are means ±1 SE of four studies.
[c]Actual plus potential bicarbonate is shown; ketone salts other than ammonium represent potential bicarbonate.

diuresis that results in urinary losses of 75–150 mL/kg of water and 4–10 mEq/kg of Na^+ and Cl^- over an entire episode of DKA.

Because the total of the Na^+ and K^+ concentrations in the urine falls short of that in serum, osmotic diuresis elevates serum $[Na^+]$ and $[Cl^-]$; moderation of hyponatremia or frank hypernatremia can ensue (42). However, other factors also act to modify the serum $[Na^+]$ and $[Cl^-]$ (43). Some Na^+ enters into cells replacing cellular K^+ losses, thereby decreasing serum $[Na^+]$. Urinary losses of Na^+ as ketone salts tend to increase serum $[Cl^-]$, whereas selective Cl^- depletion during vomiting tends to cause hypochloremia. Further, the intake of fluid and electrolytes (sodium, potassium, and chloride) influences serum $[Na^+]$ and $[Cl^-]$. Differences in the magnitude of these phenomena from one patient to another account for the variability in serum electrolyte composition observed at presentation. Table 3 reviews the admitting laboratory values of patients with DKA. Note that serum $[Na^+]$ is usually depressed; the rare presence of hypernatremia is indicative of a profound water depletion, usually seen in the most critically ill patients.

Prerenal azotemia due to volume depletion is almost always present (see earlier) and is usually reversible, but occasionally it can progress to acute tubular necrosis (44). As previously discussed, the levels of urea nitrogen, creatinine, total protein, uric acid, hematocrit, and hemoglobin can all be elevated on admission, a reflection of ECF volume contraction and/or renal dysfunction, but they normalize swiftly after volume repletion.

Potassium

Diabetic ketoacidosis is usually accompanied by varying degrees of K^+ depletion that results from multiple causes, including large kaliuresis (due to osmotic diuresis and ketoacid anion excretion), decreased intake, and frequent vomiting (1–3). Despite depletion of body K^+ stores in DKA, serum $[K^+]$ is rarely low at the time of presentation, ranging in most instances from normal to high levels, and occasionally attaining dangerously elevated values (Table 3).

The relative or absolute increase in serum $[K^+]$ had been classically attributed to the concomitant acidemia causing a shift of K^+ out of cells in exchange for H^+ moving intracellularly (45–48). However, acidosis-induced transcellular K^+ movement in DKA is not an important cause of hyperkalemia. Indeed, ketoacidemia induced by ketoacid infusion in normal animals fails to increase serum $[K^+]$, as a result of the associated stimulation of insulin secretion (49,50).

Insulin deficiency, coupled with hypertonicity, is the main mediator of the relatively high serum $[K^+]$ despite a substantial K^+ deficit (51). Increased serum osmolality translocates potassium-rich cell water to the extracellular compartment (52). Hyperglycemia produces hyperkalemia in insulin-deficient diabetics, especially when hypoaldosteronism is also present (53). By contrast, hyperglycemia in nondiabetic individuals causes a fall in serum

Table 3   Salient Laboratory Abnormalities on Admission for Diabetic Ketoacidosis (DKA)

Parameter	Value				Comments
Glucose	350–750 mg/dl				Values below 200 mg/dl ("euglycemic DKA") can be seen, especially in alcoholics or pregnant insulin-dependent diabetics; also, values above 1000 mg/dl can be seen, especially in severe volume contraction leading to renal failure and interruption of glucosuria; glucose concentration not related to severity of DKA
Blood ketones	Positive in plasma diluted 1:1 or greater				Nitroprusside reagent (Ketostix, Acetest) does not react with β-hydroxybutyrate; color reaction is mostly (>80%) due to acetoacetate
Bicarbonate	<15 mmol/l				Always reduced in DKA unless complicated by co-existing metabolic alkalosis
pH	<7.30				Always reduced in DKA unless complicated by co-existing metabolic alkalosis or respiratory alkalosis
		Plasma concentration			
		Low	*Normal*	*High*[a]	
Sodium		67	26	7	Body stores depleted
Chloride		33	45	22	
Potassium		18	43	39	Body stores depleted
Magnesium		7	25	68	
Phosphate		11	18	71	Body stores depleted
Calcium		28	68	40	
BUN, creatinine	High				Because creatinine can be spuriously elevated (crossreaction with acetoacetate), BUN can better reflect renal function
White blood cell count	Usually high				Not necessarily indicative of infection; associated with lymphopenia and eosinopenia
Hemocrit, total protein	Frequently increased				Due to intravascular volume depletion
SGOT, SGPT, LDH, CPK	High (20–65%)				Partially due to interference of acetoacetate with colorimetric assays; elevated CPK might be related to phosphate depletion and possible associated rhabdomyolysis
Amylase	Often increased				Isoenzyme evaluation reveals that site of origin is pancreas (50%), salivary glands (36%) or mixed (14%)

[a]Data from Kreisberg (Ref. 2).

Abbreviations: SGOT, serum glutamic-oxaloacetic transaminase; SGPT, serum glutamic-pyruvic transaminase; LDH, lactate dehydrogenase; CPK, creatine phosphokinase.

[K$^+$] due to stimulation of insulin release. Insulin enhances the uptake of K$^+$ in the liver, muscles, and adipose tissue; this uptake is only partially dependent on glucose entry into cells, and other glucose-independent mechanisms have been implicated (54). Thus, insulin deficiency/resistance is the main culprit in the increase in serum [K$^+$] characteristic of DKA.

Glucagon might also play a contributory role (53,55). This hormone causes an increased K$^+$ output from the liver that is usually transient because of the counter-regulatory enhancement of insulin secretion. However, increments in plasma glucagon in the presence of impaired insulin secretion might result in sustained hyperkalemia (55). The sympathetic nervous system may be another contributor.

Phosphate

The osmotic diuresis of hyperglycemia leads to decreased renal reabsorption of phosphate accounting for phosphate depletion in DKA (56). Nonetheless, serum phosphate levels are usually normal or increased at presentation (Table 3). The initial serum phosphate correlates positively with serum osmolality, glucose, and anion gap. Insulin deficiency and metabolic acidosis induce a shift of phosphate from cells to the extracellular compartment thereby masking phosphate depletion. Insulin therapy shifts phosphate back into cells, rapidly lowering the serum levels (57,58).

Diagnosis

The diagnosis is made by recognition of characteristic symptoms and signs, coupled with biochemical features that include hyperglycemia and ketosis (59). A commonly used but more restrictive diagnostic criterion of DKA includes a triad of hyperglycemia (plasma glucose > 250 mg/dL), ketosis (serum ketones 4+ positive by the nitroprusside reaction in a dilution 1:1 or greater), and metabolic acidosis (plasma bicarbonate < 15 mEq/L, blood pH < 7.30). However, the hypobicarbonatemia and acidemia might be absent in DKA because of the co-existence of additional acid–base disorders (60).

Clinical Aspects

Diabetic ketoacidosis is a medical emergency most often observed in type 1 diabetes. Less frequently, DKA is the presenting condition in obese patients with newly diagnosed type 2 diabetes. In patients with uncontrolled type 2 diabetes, DKA can be observed in combination with nonketotic hyperglycemia. The risk of developing DKA in type 1 diabetics is approximately 1–2% each year (61). The morbidity associated with DKA is dependent on the severity of the acid–base and electrolyte disturbances present. Despite advances in treatment, the mortality rate for DKA remains approximately 7% in the US (62).

Precipitating Events

Omission of insulin doses, various forms of stress, and dietary indiscretions (especially a large alcohol intake) represent the most common precipitating events of DKA (63,64). In young individuals with type 1 diabetes, emotional stress can trigger repeated episodes of DKA over short intervals. Infectious illnesses often precipitate DKA and must be aggressively treated if the ketoacidosis is to be controlled. Common such etiologies include seemingly trivial viral infections as well as pneumonia, pyelonephritis, and septicemia (32). Pregnancy, myocardial infarction, cerebrovascular accident, intra-abdominal catastrophes including pancreatitis, K^+ depletion, and drugs such as corticosteroids, can also precipitate DKA (59).

Symptoms and Signs

Weakness, malaise, air hunger, thirst, polyuria, vomiting, and altered sensorium are commonly observed (1–3). Severe abdominal pain secondary to ketosis (possibly a hypertriglyceridemia-induced pancreatitis) can be observed, and these patients sometimes are mistakenly triaged to surgery (5). However, the abdominal pain can represent an independent process, such as acute appendicitis (that requires surgery) or pyelonephritis, which in turn may have precipitated DKA. Increased rate and depth of respirations, the so-called Kussmaul breathing, is an almost constant finding. Signs of volume depletion, including orthostatic hypotension, tachycardia, decreased skin turgor, and soft eyeballs, can be evident on physical examination (65). Although DKA is sometimes referred to as diabetic coma, only 10% of patients are unconscious at presentation and about 20% are alert (5). The majority of patients present, however, with a clouded sensorium. Severe obtundation, coma, or convulsions, rarely seen in pure DKA, are prominent manifestations of severe nonketotic hyperglycemia. The patient's temperature is often decreased but the presence of hypothermia does not rule out an infectious process. Conversely, if fever is present, the likelihood of infection is high. A search for tooth or skin infection, perirectal abscess, or other infectious precipitating event is most important. Patients might describe experiencing the distinct taste and smell of ketones, and the examiner might notice a fruity odor in the subject's breath.

Serum Ketones

The clinical diagnosis of DKA depends on semi-quantitative assessment of serum ketones with reagent sticks or tablets; reagent tablets should be powdered before use. A "large" reading [4+ reaction] for ketones in plasma diluted 1:1 or greater is diagnostic of DKA; such a reading in a urine sample is not diagnostic of DKA, however, as it can be observed in other conditions, including ordinary fasting, fasting induced by an illness that has precipitated lactic acidosis or nonketotic hyperglycemia, or nonketotic hyperglycemia itself (5). The low renal threshold for ketones accounts for the possible development of a sufficiently high urine ketone concentration in all ketotic states to be detected as a "large" test response [4+ reaction].

The semi-quantitative test for ketones measures only acetoacetate and acetone (a product derived from nonenzymatic decarboxylation of acetoacetate); it does not detect β-hydroxybutyrate. The latter ketoacid is formed from the reduction of acetoacetate in a reaction utilizing NADH. A plasma ketone level of at least 6 mmol/L is required to achieve a "large" test reading in an undiluted sample. Therefore, a "large" test reading in plasma diluted 1:1 or greater indicates a ketone concentration of at least 12 mmol/L, a level found in DKA but rarely present in other ketotic states (66,67). Exceptions include a short-term fast in late pregnancy, lactating women, and some alcoholic patients (68–70).

The β-hydroxybutyrate concentration in all ketotic states is at least 2–3 times higher than that of acetoacetate. This ratio is increased further by alterations in the redox state of hepatocytes that occur with tissue hypoxia, ethanol ingestion, or with high rates of fatty acid oxidation. Under these conditions, the semi-quantitative essay is less reliable for detection of ketosis. Sulfhydryl drugs, including captopril, can produce a false-positive ketone test (71). An interaction of the colorimetric assay for creatinine with acetoacetate (chromogen) results in higher measured serum creatinine levels on admission for DKA, followed by large decreases after insulin's lowering effects on ketone levels. Table 3 presents a summary of salient abnormalities of blood measurements in patients presenting with DKA.

Differential Diagnosis

The differential diagnosis of DKA includes conditions with symptoms and signs related to the neurologic, gastrointestinal, or respiratory systems. Neurologic disorders include metabolic diseases (e.g., hypoglycemia, uremia, nonketotic hyperglycemia, lactic acidosis), toxic encephalopathies (e.g., ethanol, methanol, ethylene glycol, opium derivatives, other narcotics), head trauma, cerebrovascular accident, meningitis, and encephalitis. Gastroenteritis (abdominal pain, nausea, vomiting) and pneumonia (dyspnea) can also resemble DKA.

Therapy

The main therapeutic goals of the successful management of DKA include repletion of fluid deficit and securing an adequate circulation, reversal of the altered intermediary metabolism, correction of the electrolyte and acid–base imbalance, and treatment of the initiating event (72–75). To accomplish these objectives, a number of requirements must be fulfilled. These include continuous physician availability, 24-hr access to laboratory facilities, equipment and drugs for handling medical emergencies, and maintenance of a flowchart documenting vital signs, mental condition, serum chemistries, urine tests, insulin dosing, fluid administration (intravenous and oral), urine output, electrolyte intake, and other medications (Table 4).

Fluids

Intravenous saline should be started at once to correct the impaired hemodynamic status and the renal dysfunction; in addition, it lowers plasma glucose levels by enchancing glucosuria and decreasing counter-regulatory hormone release (catecholamines) (76,77). Isotonic saline should be infused at the fastest rate possible in patients in circulatory shock. Patients who do not have an extreme volume deficit should receive about 500 mL/hr for the first four hours followed by 250 mL/hr for the next four hours. More rapid administration is not recommended, as it can delay correction of acidemia (see earlier) and increase the risk of cerebral edema (77). Some experts prefer

Table 4   Procedures/Studies for Diagnosis, Management, and Monitoring of Diabetic Ketoacidosis (DKA) and Nonketotic Hyperglycemia (NKH)[a]

Bedside procedures/studies	Laboratory procedures/studies
	Blood
Body weight	Glucose (hourly by test strip until < 250 mg/dl, then every 2 hr; confirm in laboratory every 2–4 hr)
Blood glucose (test strips)	Electrolytes (every 2–4 hr)
Blood and urine ketones (test strips or tablets)	pH, $PaCO_2$, PaO_2 (every 2–4 hr)
Blood pressure and heart rate (every 30 min for 4 hr, hourly for next 4 hr, then every 2–4 hr)	Urea nitrogen, creatinine
Mental status (hourly)	Osmolality
Urine output (hourly for 6 hr, every 4 hr thereafter)	Hb, WBC, and differential
CVP or peripheral venous pressure (hourly during the initial 4–8 hr of high-rate fluid infusion)	Cultures
Body temperature (every 2 hr for 6 hr and every 6 hr thereafter)	*Urine*
Electrocardiogram	Microscopy and cultures
Chest x-ray	Glucose, ketones

[a]The frequency of repeat tests indicated above represents general guidelines that might require adjustments depending on the patient's presentation and response to treatment.

lactated Ringer's solution to minimize the increase in serum $[Cl^-]$, but there is no evidence that such a practice is of benefit (5). Further, it has the potential of inducing rebound metabolic alkalosis as it loads the patient with the HCO_3^- precursor, lactate. Once the patient is hemodynamically stable, the use of half-isotonic saline with the addition of 20–40 mEq of K^+ per liter is appropriate for K^+ repletion. Patients presenting with extreme volume depletion can require a fluid infusion of as much as 5–10 L within the first 24 hr (5). Fluid challenges of this magnitude demand that the patient receive careful monitoring for signs of pulmonary edema. Central venous or pulmonary artery catheterization may be required in some patients to accurately monitor intravascular volume.

It is unwise to allow oral fluid intake in the early phase of DKA because vomiting is common, especially if acute gastric distention is present. Although efforts should be made to avoid routine bladder catheterization in patients with DKA to prevent the development or exacerbation of a urinary tract infection, a catheter may be required if the patient is stuporous or urine output cannot be monitored reliably.

Insulin

All patients with DKA require insulin to reverse the ketoacidosis and correct hyperglycemia (78,79). Insulin suppresses ketone and glucose production in the liver through its antiglucagon effect. Of lesser importance is insulin-induced enhancement of glucose utilization in muscle and adipose tissue and inhibition of lipolysis. Regular insulin should be given, if possible, intravenously (5).

Mild insulin resistance is virtually a constant finding, although occasionally it may be extreme (80). Consequently, insulin requirements in DKA are always several-fold higher than in normal persons. A loading dose of 15–30 units given as a bolus on arrival is recommended to secure binding of insulin to anti-insulin antibodies that might be present in patients who have been previously treated with animal insulin, and to assure saturation of insulin receptors (81). In patients who are markedly volume depleted, insulin therapy should be withheld for the initial 30–60 min to allow some repletion of the ECF volume with isotonic saline. In the absence of saline, insulin can exacerbate ECF volume depletion by translocating glucose into cells, thereby causing a fall in ECF tonicity and a shift of water to the ICF compartment. In fact, fluid repletion alone in the absence of insulin administration reduces plasma glucose concentration by 35–70 mg/dL per hour (82).

The initial insulin bolus should be followed by 10–20 units/hr (but only 3–8 units/hr if plasma glucose is 150–300 mg/dL) until the patient is able to eat, at which time subcutaneous insulin administration is resumed (83–85). Although continuous intravenous insulin infusion is most

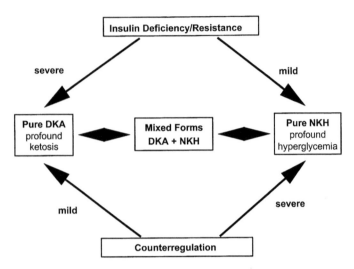

Figure 8 Diabetic ketoacidosis (DKA) and nonketotic hyperglycemia (NKH) are different forms of the same disease process. *Source*: From Ref. 10.

commonly used, intramuscular or subcutaneous administration appears to be as effective in correcting hyperglycemia and ketoacidosis (57). Plasma glucose concentration should fall at approximately 5–10% per hour. As the glucose level approaches 300 mg/dL, 5% dextrose in water at 50 ml/hr should be included in the intravenous fluids and the plasma glucose concentration should be followed closely.

A solution containing 100 units of insulin in 100 mL of isotonic saline is commonly used, adjusting the infusion rate to secure the insulin dosage desired. Because some patients are very resistant to insulin, much larger doses might be required. In all cases, the hourly dose should be doubled if the expected reduction in the plasma glucose is not observed within a few hours. Monitoring serum ketones during therapy is unnecessary since it does not help in the adjustment of insulin dosage (86).

Alkali

Bicarbonate administration should be unnecessary (at least in patients with predominantly increased AG acidosis) because ketones, when finally metabolized to CO_2 and H_2O, regenerate HCO_3^- (1–3). In support of this view, several studies have shown that HCO_3^- administration did nothing to improve the recovery of patients with DKA who presented with very severe acidemia (arterial pH of 6.90–7.10) (87,88). The administration of HCO_3^- in DKA may also have some potentially deleterious effects because it can augment hepatic ketogenesis and lead to worsening of the CNS acidosis, hypokalemia, and rebound metabolic alkalosis (87–89). The potential

Table 5 Potential Advantages and Disadvantages of Bicarbonate Administration in the Management of Diabetic Ketoacidosis (DKA)

Advantages

Improves hemodynamic status if shock persists after volume repletion and severe metabolic acidosis is present

Increases myocardial contractility and enhances cardiac and vascular responsiveness to catecholamines

Aids correction of hyperkalemia, especially in patients with prerenal azotemia

Prevents a rapid fall in CSF osmolality and therefore might decrease risk of cerebral edema

Aids correction of cell metabolism and function (including CNS), impaired by severe acidosis

Improves acidosis-induced glucose intolerance and insulin resistance

Disadvantages

Induces or worsens hypokalemia, leading to cardiac arrhythmias (especially in digitalized patients) and/or dysfunction of respiratory muscles (respiratory failure)

Produces ECF volume expansion that can cause pulmonary edema

Reduces cerebral blood flow (pH effect) and O_2 delivery to the brain

Worsens hypophosphatemia due to cellular uptake of phosphate and depresses O_2 delivery to tissues (increased affinity of Hb for O_2)

Produces hypernatremia and increased serum osmolality

Decreases further CSF pH, leading to worsening of CNS function

Induces overshoot (rebound) alkalosis once conversion of ketone salts to bicarbonate takes place

Aggravates ketogenesis and lactic acidosis

Predisposes to tetany resulting from hypocalcemia and alkalemia

---

advantages and disadvantages of HCO_3^- administration are summarized in Table 5. The controversy regarding its utility is based on variable assessment of the associated risks and benefits by different workers (59,89–91).

Table 6 summarizes our recommendations in terms of indications, goals, and dose estimation for HCO_3^- administration in DKA (91,92). After weighing the arguments, it appears that judicious administration of HCO_3^- to severely acidemic patients, especially those with predominant hyperchloremic metabolic acidosis, confers net benefit; the goal is to support the arterial pH at 7.10–7.20 and serum $[HCO_3^-]$ at approximately 10 mEq/L. Bicarbonate should be added to an IV infusion, if possible, instead of administering by intravenous bolus, unless hyperkalemia is present, because of the risk of severe hypokalemia.

Potassium

The typical patient with DKA has a K^+ deficit of 4–8 mEq/kg body weight at the time of admission, yet the initial serum $[K^+]$ will usually be normal or

Table 6 Indications, Goals, and Dose Estimation for Bicarbonate Administration in the Management of Diabetic Ketoacidosis (DKA)

Indications

Extreme metabolic acidosis (pH < 7.00, TCO_2 < 5 mmol/L), independent of prevailing hemodynamic status

Severe metabolic acidosis (pH < 7.15, TCO_2 < 10 mmol/L) in association with one or more of the following:

- Shock unresponsive to volume repletion
- Persistence or worsening of acidemia after several hours of therapy
- Predominant hyperchloremic acidosis instead of the usual high anion gap acidosis
- Worsening of mental status and CNS depression

Severe hyperkalemia ($[K^+]_p$ > 7 mEq/L)

Goals and dose estimation

If TCO_2 < 5 mmol/L (indication 1), it should be increased to no more than 8–10 mmol/L

If TCO_2 is 5 to 10 mmol/L (indication 2), it should be increased to no more than 13–15 mmol/L

Dose estimation: (desired plasma TCO_2 − current plasma TCO_2) × b.wt (kg) × 0.5^a

Calculated bicarbonate dose can be added to IV infusion (1–2 ampules or 44–88 mEq $NaHCO_3$ per liter) or given by IV bolus (50% of estimated dose immediately, and the rest within 2–4 hr provided that hypokalemia is not present or is simultaneously treated and that evidence of pulmonary edema is not found)

Monitor blood acid-base status every 30–60 min (for 2–4 hr) after initiation of bicarbonate therapy to adjust dose to patient's needs

---

[a]Derives from the "apparent space of distribution" of bicarbonate (retained HCO_3^- in mEq/kg divided by the $\Delta[HCO_3^-]_p$ from preinfusion) that is 50% of body weight in normal subjects but higher in hypobicarbonatemic states. Thus, this formula purposefully underestimates bicarbonate requirements to avoid the risk of overcorrection.

elevated (see earlier and Table 3). Serum $[K^+]$ decreases with therapy because of insulin-mediated uptake by cells, dilution due to volume repletion by intravenous fluids, correction of metabolic acidosis, and urinary K^+ losses. Thus, K^+ supplementation is required (1–3). Specifically, after the initial fluid challenge has restored the urinary output and assuming that serum $[K^+]$ is below 5.0 mEq/L, an intravenous infusion of 10–20 mEq/hr should be started and continued until the DKA is controlled and serum $[K^+]$ is 4.0–5.0 mEq/L. Serum $[K^+]$ should be monitored periodically and the K^+ infusion rate adjusted, as needed. Details about K^+ supplementation are provided in Table 7.

Phosphate

Because phosphate administration is of unproven clinical utility and potentially dangerous (i.e., it might result in hypocalcemia and hypomagnesemia),

Table 7 Potassium Supplementation (KCl) in the Management of Diabetic Ketoacidosis (DKA) and Nonketotic Hyperglycemia (NKH)

KCl should not be added to the initial 2 liters of IV infusion to avoid hyperkalemia because
  * Urinary output is initially unknown
  * Initial $[K^+]_p$ is usually normal or high
Exception to the above rule on K^+ supplementation: add K^+ to the initial 2 liters of IV fluids if
  * Initial $[K^+]_p$ < 4.0 mEq/l and
  * Adequate diuresis is secured
KCl should be added to the third liter of IV infusion and subsequently if
  * Urinary output is adequate (should be at least 30–60 ml/hr) and
  * $[K^+]_p$ < 5.0 mEq/l
Rate of IV K^+ supplementation:
  20–30 mEq/hr if $[K^+]_p$ < 4.0 mEq/l
  10–20 mEq/hr if $[K^+]_p$ > 4.0 mEq/l
Concentration of K^+ in IV infusions:
  20 mEq/l when IV supplementation is started and subsequently
  if $[K^+]_p$ < 4.0 mEq/l, and IV infusion rate is ≥1 liter/hr
  40 mEq/l (maximum) if $[K^+]_p$ < 4.0 mEq/l and IV infusion rate is < 1 liter/hr
Monitoring of K^+ supplementation is accomplished by
  $[K^+]_p$ every 2–4 hr during the initial 12–24 hr of therapy
  ECG every 30–60 min during the initial 4–6 hr (i.e., only lead II)

---

it should not be infused unless the serum phosphate is < 0.5 mg/dL; in those circumstances, 10–30 mmol of potassium phosphate might be added to the intravenous infusion and repeated if necessary to correct persistent hypophosphatemia. The hypophosphatemia of DKA may have serious consequences (e.g., impaired myocardial and/or skeletal muscle contractility) if it occurs in undernourished patients, such as chronic alcoholics. In this population, parenteral phosphate replacement of 60–120 mmol administered over a 24 hr period is recommended.

Cerebral Edema and Other Complications

Patients with DKA may be admitted with a relatively normal mental status and become unconscious within the first 12 hr of therapy, despite a partial or complete correction of the hyperglycemia and ketoacidosis (93). These patients are typically, but not exclusively, children or young adults, and their morbidity and mortality is relatively high (94). Often, the fatal outcome is unexpected, as these patients do not have the underlying vascular, cardiac, and renal abnormalities found in older diabetics. At autopsy, cerebral edema is consistently present (94). Although cerebral edema leading to death or chronic sequelae (e.g., isolated growth hormone deficiency) is fortunately rare, a milder form occurs often in the course of treatment of DKA (5,95,96).

The pathogenesis of this condition is poorly understood (97,98). Osmotic disequilibrium between brain cells and the CSF is often cited as the principal cause. In response to hyperglycemia, brain cells increase their osmolality to match that of the CSF within hours and thus defend themselves against shrinkage. Once this cellular adaptation to hypertonicity has occurred, a sudden decrease in CSF tonicity, due to hypotonic fluid infusions or a fall in plasma glucose, may cause swelling of these adapted cells and produce cerebral edema. Insulin administration also activates the plasma membrane Na^+/H^+ exchanger (NHE-1), which promotes sodium entry in brain cells, facilitating development of cerebral edema. The effects of rapid crystalloid volume loading in diabetics with DKA and the resulting dilutional hypoalbuminemia have been shown to produce some degree of brain swelling or increase in CSF pressure (99–101). Alterations in CSF pH and oxygen tension following HCO_3^- administration may also contribute to the development of cerebral edema. These mechanisms are only hypotheses, however, and the pathogenesis remains uncertain. Still, it seems prudent in treating DKA (and nonketotic hyperglycemia) to avoid excessively aggressive volume replacement, sudden changes in the patient's serum glucose and [Na^+], and excessive use of HCO_3^-.

A number of additional life-threatening complications can develop in the course of DKA in spite of adequate medical care (Table 8). Shock of cardiac origin or resulting from sepsis or volume depletion, as well as cerebral thrombosis/edema, are among the most serious complications (102).

NONKETOTIC HYPERGLYCEMIA

Nonketotic hyperglycemia (NKH) (59), is a syndrome characterized by the presence of severe hyperglycemia (usually >800 mg/dL) and the absence of

Table 8 Complications of Diabetic Ketoacidosis (DKA) and Nonketotic Hyperglycemia (NKH)

Hypoglycemia
Hypokalemia and hyperkalemia
Fluid overload (pulmonary edema)
Cerebral edema (with possible neurologic sequelae or death)
Acute gastric dilatation, erosive gastritis
Infection: urinary tract, pneumonia, mucormycosis
Venous and arterial thrombosis
Acute tubular necrosis (renal failure)

---

clinically significant ketosis (see Table 10). The DKA and NKH share the same general pathogenesis—insulin deficiency/resistance and excessive counter-regulation (the most important element being high glucagon levels), but the importance of each of these endocrine abnormalities appears to differ (103). Pure DKA, which features profound ketosis, might emanate from severe insulin deficiency/resistance, with milder abnormalities in counter-regulation (Fig. 8). By contrast, NKH, which features marked hyperglycemia without ketosis, might be caused by relatively mild insulin deficiency/resistance but more intense counter-regulation. The most important clinical distinction, however, is that the severity of the fluid deficit and secondary renal dysfunction is greater in NKH than in DKA. This finding in NKH plays a critical pathogenetic role in the profound hypertonicity observed (104–106). In some instances, a large exogenous source of glucose can be of great importance in the development of this condition (11) (Table 9).

Table 9 Fluid Deficit and Glucose Load as Precipitating Factors of Nonketotic Hyperglycemia (NKH) in Diabetes Mellitus

Condition	Physiologic derangement	Clinical setting
Fluid deficit	Poor water intake	
	Relatively preserved CNS function	Elderly, nursing home patients
	Major CNS abnormality	Cerebrovascular accident; subdural hemorrhage
	Urinary fluid loss	Large osmotic diuresis; diuretics
	Extrarenal fluid loss	
	Gastrointestinal	Gastroenteritis, peptic ulcer disease, gastrointestinal bleeding, pancreatitis
	Skin	Heat stroke, burns
Glucose load	Increased glucose intake	Highly sweetened drinks, enteral or tube-feeding, hyperalimentation, peritoneal dialysis
	Increased endogenous glucose production	
	Stress	Psychologic/physical trauma
	Infection	Pneumonia, pyelonephritis, sepsis
	Major illness	Myocardial infarction
	Medication	Corticosteroids, phenytoin, calcium-channel blockers.

Hypertonicity and Renal Dysfunction

Renal dysfunction, most commonly caused by volume depletion, must be present to generate and sustain the extreme hyperglycemia observed in most patients with NKH (11). Fluid deficit can be caused by poor fluid intake (e.g., in patients who are frail and unable to perceive or respond to thirst because of sedation, stroke, or other causes) and/or abnormal fluid losses due to osmotic diuresis, vomiting, diarrhea, fever, or diuretics. A simple calculation demonstrates the virtual impossibility of maintaining plasma glucose levels substantially higher than 400 mg/dL in the presence of normal renal function, because of the magnitude of obligatory glucosuria (11). In a patient with a plasma glucose of 400 mg/dL and a normal GFR, for example, the amount of glucose that escapes reabsorption (difference between plasma glucose and the "renal threshold concentration," 180 mg/dL) is approximately 400 g/day. Glucose is also removed by cellular metabolism; whole-body glucose utilization is approximately 200 g/day under euglycemic conditions, and increases in proportion to the glucose concentration even in the absence of insulin. In patients with severe hyperglycemia and adequate renal function, therefore, substantial glucose removal, on the order of 600–1000 g/day, would result both from glucosuria and internal disposal. An equal amount of new glucose must enter the circulation to satisfy these demands in steady-state, severe hyperglycemia. Thus, unless the patient has an exceptionally high level of endogenous glucose production (in excess of three times the normal rate in the fasting state) or an extremely large exogenous source of glucose is present, severe hyperglycemia cannot be sustained in the absence of renal failure. Exogenous sources of glucose include tube-feeding solutions, parenteral hyperalimentation, or peritoneal dialysis with a high glucose concentration in the dialysate. Table 9 summarizes the role of fluid deficit and glucose load as precipitating factors of NKH (11).

Absence of Ketosis

There are several theories to account for the absence of substantial ketosis in NKH (107). It has been proposed that in NKH there is sufficient insulin to inhibit lipolysis but not enough to stimulate peripheral glucose uptake. This explanation is based on the presumed less severe insulin deficit of patients with NKH, and the known inhibition of ketosis by relatively low insulin levels. Because hypertonicity has been shown to inhibit lipolysis in vitro, it may also be partly responsible for the absence of substantial ketoacidosis in NKH (108). A more recent explanation offered for the absence of ketosis is hepatic resistance to glucagon such that malonyl-CoA levels do not decrease as much as in DKA (109,110).

Diagnosis

Typically, patients with this disorder are elderly with Type 2 diabetes, and present with a depressed sensorium, progressing to obtundation and finally coma. They may be oliguric or anuric. Patients with "pure" NKH have no acid–base abnormalities, no clinically significant ketonemia, a markedly elevated blood glucose concentration, and elevated BUN and creatinine concentrations. The diagnosis is based on the presence of severe hyperglycemia (glucose levels >800 mg/dL), hypertonicity (>340 mOsm/kg H_2O), absence of significant ketosis, and profound volume depletion (59). The salient clinical and biochemical features that distinguish DKA from NKH are shown in Tables 10 and 11. Many patients exhibit a mixed pattern with clinical and biochemical features of both DKA and NKH. These patients should be diagnosed as having DKA–NKH (111).

Clinical Manifestations

Depression of the sensorium, somnolence, obtundation, and coma are prominent manifestations of NKH, and the degree of CNS depression correlates with the severity of serum hypertonicity (104). Water loss from the central nervous system with brain shrinkage has been documented within 1 hr of severe hyperglycemia in experimental animals, but brain volume recovers at 4–6 hr. Neither ketosis nor metabolic acidosis, features that are consistently present in DKA but usually absent in NKH, produce extreme depression of the sensorium (104). In fact, a serum tonicity (i.e., effective osmolality) of 340 mOsm/kg H_2O or higher appears to be

Table 10 Contrasting Clinical Features of Pure Forms of Diabetic Ketoacidosis (DKA) and Nonketotic Hyperglycemia (NKH)[a]

Feature	Pure DKA	Mixed forms	Pure NKH
Incidence	5–10 times higher	⇔	5–10 times lower
Mortality	5–10%	⇔	10–60%
Onset	Rapid (< 2 days)	⇔	Slow (> 5 days)
Age of patient	Usually < 40 years	⇔	Usually > 40 years
Type 1 diabetes	Common	⇔	Rare
Type 2 diabetes	Rare	⇔	Common
First indication of diabetes	Often	⇔	Rare
Volume depletion	Mild/moderate	⇔	Severe
Renal failure (most commonly of pre-renal nature)	Mild	⇔	Severe
Subsequent therapy with insulin	Always	⇔	Occassional

[a]Mixed forms of DKA–NKH have intermediate features denoted by the symbol ⇔.

Table 11 Contrasting Biochemical Features of Pure Diabetic Ketoacidosis (DKA) and Nonketotic Hyperglycemia (NKH)[a]

Plasma levels	Pure DKA	Mixed forms	Pure NKH
Glucose	< 800 mg/dL	⇔	> 800 mg/dL
Ketone bodies	4+ in 1:1 dilution	⇔	not 4+ in 1:1 dilution
Effective osmolality	< 340 mOsm/kg	⇔	> 340 mOsm/kg
pH	Decreased	⇔	Normal
[HCO$_3^-$]	Decreased	⇔	Normal
[Na$^+$]	Low or normal	⇔	Normal or high
[K$^+$]	Variable	⇔	Variable

[a]Mixed forms of DKA–NKH have intermediate features denoted by the symbol ⇔.

necessary for the development of coma, and such levels are commonly observed in NKH but not in DKA (59,104). Circulatory collapse secondary to profound volume depletion can be observed in NKH. All other symptoms and signs previously described for patients in DKA (except for dyspnea and Kussmaul respiration that arise from metabolic acidosis) may also be observed in NKH.

Assessment of Effective Osmolality

To estimate serum tonicity (effective osmolality), one should calculate its value, using only the sodium and glucose concentrations (effective osmolality $= 2 \times$ [Na$^+$] + glucose/18). Not infrequently, a comatose diabetic patient is found to have a measured osmolality of 350 mOsm/kg H$_2$O but the calculated effective osmolality of, for example, 350 mOsm/kg H$_2$O; in this case, the patient's coma is more likely to be due to conditions other than NKH (e.g., alcohol, uremia, cerebrovascular accident). Conversely, a comatose diabetic patient who is admitted with a calculated effective osmolality of 350 mOsm/kg H$_2$O most likely has NKH encephalopathy. Nonetheless, one should always exclude other causes of coma. Sometimes it is difficult to establish whether a neurologic finding is a cause or effect. For example, stroke can lead to NKH, and conversely NKH can cause a cerebrovascular accident (5,97). Rapid reversal of the neurological syndrome with therapy for NKH indicates that it was not the cause but the result of this metabolic disorder.

Therapy

Management of NKH is similar to that previously described for DKA (59). Despite claims to the contrary, patients in NKH are not more sensitive to insulin than those in DKA (84). Because a precipitous fall in extracellular tonicity might trigger cerebral edema with secondary worsening of the patient's condition, treatment should aim at decreasing plasma glucose by no more than 200 mg/dL per hour. Considering that metabolic acidosis is generally absent in these patients, bicarbonate therapy is not indicated (111).

Because the fluid deficit is generally severe in NKH patients, many of whom have heart disease and are elderly, central venous pressure and/or pulmonary capillary wedge pressure should be closely monitored during fluid replacement. Potassium supplementation represents a most important aspect in the management of these patients, because a large total body K^+ deficit is a constant finding (see Table 7 for guidelines for K^+ administration). The complications of therapy of NKH are generally similar to those observed in the management of DKA (112–115), but the prognosis is substantially worse, as evidenced by their higher mortality (Table 10).

STARVATION KETOSIS

The mechanisms responsible for the development of starvation ketosis in nondiabetic subjects are similar to those outlined for DKA, with one exception—the availability of insulin (116,117). In fact, the presence of insulin during fasting prevents progression of ketosis to full-blown ketoacidosis (117).

During the postprandial state, the plasma glucose gradually falls. As a result, the pancreas decreases insulin release and increases glucagon secretion, thereby preventing development of hypoglycemia. When normal or obese subjects fast for periods longer than 2 or 3 days, glycogen stores become depleted and energy requirements are satisfied increasingly by catabolism of fat; therefore, a state of ketosis develops (111). Decreased insulin secretion during fasting leads to release of free fatty acids from adipocytes, which then become the energy source in most tissues except the brain; the shift towards lipid degradation and consumption in the fasting state "spares" glucose for its continued use by the brain, an organ that is unable to oxidize fatty acids (117). A fraction of the mobilized fatty acids are taken up by hepatocytes, transformed into ketones (about 80% of which is β-hydroxybutyric acid), and released into the circulation (117). Ketones are efficiently oxidized by extrahepatic tissues, including the central nervous system, providing a backup substrate for the brain should hepatic glucose production be inadequate. Chronically emaciated subjects whose adipose stores have been depleted to less than 10% of normal might be unable to mount a fasting ketosis.

During prolonged starvation the concentration of ketones increases by only 2–4 mmol/L, because both fatty acids and ketones stimulate insulin release, which in turn imposes substrate limitation. In addition, ketones might have a small, direct inhibitory effect on lipolysis. Consequently, plasma [HCO_3^-] falls by 2–4 mEq/L within a few days of fasting and reaches levels no lower than 17–18 mEq/L even after several weeks of total starvation (118).

Intense ketonuria but only a weakly positive serum test is characteristically found in starvation ketosis. Because ketoacids and uric acid compete for renal transport sites, prolonged fasting might lead to clinically significant hyperuricemia, including the development of acute gouty arthritis and urate nephrolithiasis. Resumption of food intake results in prompt restoration of normal acid–base equilibrium.

ALCOHOLIC KETOACIDOSIS

Alcohol ingestion combined with poor dietary intake leads to alcoholic ketoacidosis (117,119–121). The resulting metabolic acidosis can be relatively severe (70). Most subjects are chronic ethanol abusers who have experienced a recent binge. Alcoholic ketoacidosis appears to be more common in diabetic than in nondiabetic subjects.

Pathogenesis

The pathogenesis involves ethanol itself, starvation, insulin deficiency, glucagon and catecholamine excess, and vomiting (120). Ethanol inhibits gluconeogenesis and stimulates lipolysis. Acute starvation, a near constant feature in alcoholic ketoacidosis, causes depletion of hepatic glucagon stores. The end result is increased glucagon/insulin molar ratio, and stimulation of lipolysis and hepatic ketogenesis.

Ethanol is metabolized to acetaldehyde in a reaction catalyzed by an alcohol dehydrogenase; acetaldehyde is then oxidized to acetic acid. These reactions are associated with the reduction of NAD^+ to NADH, which then promotes conversion of pyruvate to lactate and of acetoacetate to β-hydroxybutyrate (122). Acetic acid derived from ethanol metabolism provides substrate for ketogenesis and contributes to the enhanced endogenous acid load. Blood ethanol levels are usually undetectable or only mildly elevated.

Vomiting due to gastritis, pancreatitis, or other processes is commonly observed and can lead to volume depletion, increased counter-regulatory hormone secretion (i.e., catecholamines, cortisol, growth hormone), and prerenal azotemia. It might culminate in circulatory collapse and lactic acidosis.

Clinical Manifestations

The clinical features are very similar to those of DKA. An important exception is that plasma glucose is usually normal or only mildly elevated and may even be low in alcoholic ketoacidosis. Not surprisingly, glucosuria is rarely seen (70). Nausea, vomiting, abdominal pain, mental confusion, and Kussmaul breathing are commonly observed. Some patients also exhibit acute withdrawal symptoms, including delirium tremens, or mild jaundice caused by alcoholic hepatitis. A severe alteration in mental status is not observed in the absence of ethanol intoxication or withdrawal, hypoglycemia, or a serious infectious illness.

Laboratory Features

The acid–base status of patients with alcoholic ketoacidosis is variable depending on the relative contribution of several processes, including ketoacidosis with the expected increased serum anion gap; hyperchloremic metabolic acidosis due to the urinary loss of ketoacid anions; lactic acidosis secondary to circulatory failure or alcoholic pancreatitis; primary hypocapnia resulting from underlying liver disease, abdominal pain, or delirium tremens; and metabolic alkalosis caused by concurrent vomiting. Accordingly, blood pH levels can vary widely from the severely acidic to the alkaline range (123). Markedly depressed $PaCO_2$ and serum [HCO_3^-] levels are observed when primary respiratory alkalosis accompanies alcoholic ketoacidosis.

The ratio of serum levels of β-hydroxybutyrate to acetoacetate is usually higher in patients with alcoholic ketoacidosis than in those with diabetic ketoacidosis. The significance of the predominant increase in serum β-hydroxybutyrate is that patients with alcoholic ketoacidosis might not have strongly positive nitroprusside reactions in both serum and urine, a finding that could lead to an erroneous diagnosis (124). In fact, a weakly positive nitroprusside test in association with high AG acidosis might also be seen in lactic acidosis and in methanol or ethylene glycol intoxication (see Chapter 12). An elevated serum osmolal gap is often seen in alcoholic ketoacidosis that reflects, in part, acetone accumulation and the possible presence of ethanol (125). Serum urate levels are commonly elevated due to impaired renal excretion as a result of volume depletion and the decrease in tubular secretion of urate caused by competition with the increased serum ketoacids.

Diagnosis

Because up to 90% of circulating ketones in alcoholic ketoacidosis are in the form of β-hydroxybutyrate, the nitroprusside reaction is often negative or only weakly positive, complicating recognition of the disease (126). Adding a few drops of hydrogen peroxide to a urine specimen converts β-hydroxybutyrate into acetoacetate, a ketoacid that is detectable by nitroprusside. Alternatively, direct measurement of blood β-hydroxybutyrate levels with commercially available diagnostic kits (e.g., KetoSite® system) can circumvent the problem.

Diabetic alcohol abusers can develop DKA or a mixture of DKA and alcoholic ketoacidosis. In cases of uncertainty with respect to the possible presence of DKA in a patient with alcoholic ketoacidosis, insulin should be included in the treatment regimen. Lactic acidosis can be a concurrent acid–base abnormality or the only disorder in an ethanol abuser.

Measurement of serum levels of suspected toxins and urinalysis for evaluation of calcium oxalate crystals is required to rule out an exogenous intoxication.

Treatment

Therapy of alcoholic ketoacidosis involves correction of the fluid, electrolyte, and metabolic abnormalities, and management of any concomitant illness (127). The main elements of treatment are parenteral administration of saline, dextrose, K^+, and thiamine. Saline infusion will repair the fluid deficit and inhibit sympathetic discharge and counter-regulatory hormones, thereby depressing lipolysis and ketogenesis. Dextrose infusion will increase insulin and reduce glucagon secretion, correcting the main determinants of the ketoacidosis. Administration of K^+ and thiamine will repair the commonly existing deficits in ethanol abusers.

REFERENCES

1. Felig P. Diabetic ketoacidosis. N Engl J Med 1974; 290:1360–1363.
2. Kreisberg RA. Diabetic ketoacidosis: new concepts and trends in pathogenesis and treatment. Ann Int Med 1978; 88:681–695.
3. Adrogué HJ, Maliha G. Diabetic ketoacidosis. In: Adrogué HJ, ed. Acid-Base and Electrolyte Disorders. Contemporary Management in Critical Care. New York: Churchill Livingstone, 1991:21–35.
4. Karam JH, Salber PR, Forsham PH. Pancreatic hormones and diabetes mellitus. In: Greenspan FS, Forsham PH, eds. Basic and Clinical Endocrinology. East Norwalk: Lange Medical Publications, 1986:523–574.
5. Foster DW, McGarry JD. Acute complications of diabetes mellitus: ketoacidosis, hyperosmolar coma, and lactic acidosis. In: DeGroot LJ, Jameson JL, eds. Endocrinology. 4th ed. Philadelphia: WB Saunders, 2001:908–920.
6. Skillman TG. Diabetes mellitus. In: Mazzaferri EL, ed. Endocrinology. New York: Medical Examination Publishing, 1986:595–665.
7. Felts PW. Ketoacidosis. Med Clin North Am 1983; 67:831–843.
8. Fleckman AM. Diabetic ketoacidosis. Endocr Metab Clin North Am 1993; 22:181–207.
9. Foster DW, McGarry JD. The metabolic derangements and treatment of diabetic ketoacidosis. N Engl J Med 1983; 309:159–169.
10. Adrogué HJ, Madias NE. Disorders of acid-base balance. In: Schrier RW, Berl T, Bonventre JV, eds. Atlas of Diseases of the Kidney. Boston: Current Medicine, Blackwell, 1999:6.20–6.28.
11. Adrogué HJ. Glucose homeostasis and the kidney. Kidney Int 1992; 42:1266–1282.
12. Cuthbert C, Alberti KGMM. Acidemia and insulin resistance in the diabetic ketoacidotic rat. Metabolism 1978; 27:1903–1916.
13. Walker BG, Phear DN, Martin FIR, Baird CW. Inhibition of insulin by acidosis. Lancet 1963; 2:964–965.

14. Misbin RI, Pulkkinen AJ, Loften SA, Merimee TJ. Ketoacids and the insulin receptor. Diabetes 1978; 27:539–542.
15. Adrogué HJ, Chap Z, Okuda Y, Michael L, Hartley C, Entman M, Field JB. Acidosis-induced glucose intolerance is not prevented by adrenergic blockade. Am J Physiol 1988; 255:E812–E823.
16. Van Putten JPM, Wieringa T, Krans HMJ. Low pH and ketoacids induce insulin receptor binding and postbinding alterations in cultered 3T3 adipocytes. Diabetes 1985; 34:744–750.
17. Dobbs R, Sakurai H, Sasaki H, Faloona G, Valverde I, Baetens D, Orci L, Unger R. Glucagon: role in the hyperglycemia of diabetes mellitus. Science 1975; 187:544–547.
18. Unger RH, Orci L. Glucagon and the A cell: physiology and pathophysiology. N Engl J Med 1981; 304:1518–1524, 1575–1580.
19. McGarry JD, Foster DW. Regulation of hepatic fatty acid oxidation and ketone body production. Annu Rev Biochem 1980; 49:395–420.
20. Foster DW. From glycogen to ketones—and back. Diabetes 1984; 33: 1188–1199.
21. McGarry JD, Woeltje KF, Kuwajima M, Foster DW. Regulation of ketogenesis and the renaissance of carnitine palmitoyltransferase. Diabetes Metab Rev 1989; 5:271–284.
22. McGarry JD, Leatherman GF, Foster DW. Carnitine palmitoyltransferase I: the site of inhibition of hepatic fatty acid oxidation by malonyl-CoA. J Biol Chem 1978; 253:4128–4136.
23. McGarry JD, Brown NF. The mitochondrial carnitine palmitoyltransferase system—from concept to molecular analysis. Eur J Biochem 1997; 244:1–14.
24. Murphy MSR, Pande SV. Mechanism of carnitine acylcarnitine translocase-catalyzed import of acylcarnitines into mitochondria. J Biol Chem 1984; 259:9082–9089.
25. Adrogué HJ, Wesson DE. Blackwell's Basics of Medicine. Acid–Base. Boston: Blackwell Scientific Publications, 1994.
26. Adrogué HJ, Wilson H, Boyd AE, Suki WN, Eknoyan G. Plasma acid–base patterns in diabetic ketoacidosis. N Engl J Med 1982; 307:1603–1610.
27. Kleeman CR, Narins RG. Diabetic acidosis and coma. In: Maxwell MH, Kleeman CR, eds. Clinical Disorders of Fluid and Electrolyte Metabolism. New York: McGraw-Hill, 1980:1339–1377.
28. Nabarro JDN, Spencer AG, Stowers JM. Metabolic studies in severe diabetic ketosis. Q J Med 1952; 21:225–248.
29. Assal JP, Aoki TT, Manzano FM, Kozak GP. Metabolic effects of sodium bicarbonate in management of diabetic ketoacidosis. Diabetes 1974; 23: 405–411.
30. Oh MS, Carroll HJ, Goldstein DA, Fein IA. Hyperchloremic acidosis during the recovery phase of diabetic ketoacidosis. Ann Intern Med 1978; 89: 925–927.
31. Adrogué HJ, Eknoyan G, Suki WN. Diabetic ketoacidosis: role of the kidney in the acid–base homeostasis reevaluated. Kidney Int 1984; 25:591–598.
32. Adrogué HJ, Barrero J, Ryan JE, Dolson GM. Diabetic ketoacidosis: a practical approach. Hospital Practice 1989; 24:83–112.

33. Adrogué HJ, Barrero J, Dolson GM. Diabetic ketoacidosis. In: Suki WN, Massry SG, eds. Therapy of Renal Diseases and Related Disorders. 2nd ed. Boston: Martinus Nijhoff Publishers, 1991:193–206.
34. Pitts RF. The renal regulation of acid base balance with special reference to the mechanism for acidifying the urine. Science 1945; 102:49–54.
35. Pitts RF. Acid–base regulation by the kidneys. Am J Med 1950; 9:356–372.
36. Bernstein LM, Foley EF, Hoffman WS. Renal function during and after diabetic coma. J Clin Invest 1952; 31:711–716.
37. Reubi FC. Glomerular filtration rate, renal blood flow and blood viscosity during and after diabetic coma. Circ Res 1953; 1:410–413.
38. Guest GM, Rapoport S. Electrolytes of blood plasma and cells in diabetic acidosis and during recovery. Proc Am Diabetes Assn 1947; 7:97–115.
39. Pitts RF. Renal regulation of acid–base balance. Physiology of the Kidney and Body Fluids. Chicago: Year Book, 1974;198–241.
40. Adrogué HJ, Wesson DE. Blackwell's Basics of Medicine. Vol. 3: Salt & Water. Blackwell Scientific Publications, 1994.
41. Gennari FJ. Hypo-hypernatraemia: disorders of water balance. Oxford Textbook of Clinical Nephrology. 2d ed. Oxford:Oxford University Press, 1998: 175–200.
42. Adrogué HJ, Madias NE. Hyponatremia. N Engl J Med 2000; 342:1581–1589.
43. Roscoe JM, Halperin ML, Rolleston FS, Goldstein MB. Hyperglycemia-induced hyponatremia: metabolic considerations in calculation of serum sodium depression. Can Med Assoc J 1975; 112:452–453.
44. Linton AL, Kennedy AC. Diabetic ketosis complicated by acute renal failure. Posgrad Med J 1963; 39:364–366.
45. Adrogué HJ, Madias NE. Changes in plasma potassium concentration during acute acid-base disturbances. Am J Med 1981; 71:456–467.
46. Adrogué HJ. Mechanisms of transcellular potassium shifts in acid–base disorders. In: Hatano M, ed. Proceedings of the. XIth International Congress of Nephrology. Tokyo: Springer-Verlag 1991;252–261.
47. Adrogué HJ, Wesson DE. Blackwell's Basic of Medicine. Potassium. Boston: Blackwell Scientific Publications, 1994.
48. Fraley DS, Adler S. Isohydric regulation of plasma potassium by bicarbonate in the rat. Kidney Int 1976; 9:333–343.
49. Adrogué HJ, Chap Z, Ishida T, Field JB. Role of the endocrine pancreas in the kalemic response to acute metabolic acidosis in conscious dogs. J Clin Invest 1985; 75:798–808.
50. Goldfarb S, Cox M, Singer I, Goldberg M. Acute hyperkalemia induced by hyperglycemia: hormonal mechanisms. Ann Int Med 1976; 84:426–432.
51. Adrogué HJ, Lederer ED, Suki WN, Eknoyan G. Determinants of plasma potassium levels in diabetic ketoacidosis. Medicine 1986; 65:163–172.
52. Makoff DL, DaSliva JA, Rosenbaum BJ, Levy SE, Maxwell MH. Hypertonic expansion: acid–base and electrolyte changes. Am J Physiol 1970; 218: 1201–1207.
53. DeFronzo RA, Sherwin RS, Dillingham M, Hendler R, Tamborlane WV, Felig P. Influence of basal insulin and glucagon secretion on potassium and sodium metabolism. J Clin Invest 1978; 61:472–479.

54. Clausen T, Kohn PG. The effect of insulin on the transport of sodium and potassium in rat soleus muscle. J Physiol (Lond) 1977; 265:18–42.
55. Massara F, Martelli S, Cagliero E, Camanni F, Molinatti GM. Influence of glucagon on plasma levels of potassium in man. Diabetologia 1980; 19: 414–417.
56. Kebler R, McDonald FD, Cadnapaphornchai P. Dynamic changes in serum phosphorus levels in diabetic ketoacidosis. Am J Med 1985; 79:571–576.
57. Fisher JN, Shahshahani MN, Kitabchi AE. Diabetic ketoacidosis: Low-dose insulin therapy by various routes. N Engl J Med 1977; 297:238–241.
58. Pfeifer MA, Samols E, Wolter CF, Winkler CF. Low-dose versus high-dose insulin therapy for diabetic ketoacidosis. Southern Med J 1979; 72:149–154.
59. Alberti KGMM. Diabetic acidosis, hyperosmolar coma, and lactic acidosis. In: Becker KL, ed. Principles and Practice of Endocrinology and Metabolism. Philadelphia: JB Lippincott, 1990:1175–1187.
60. Cronin JW, Kroop SF, Diamond J, Rolla AR. Alkalemia in diabetic keto-acidosis. Am J Med 1984; 77:192–194.
61. Wetterhall SF, Olson DR, DeStafano F, Stevenson JM, Ford ES, German RR, Will JC, Newman JM, Sepe SJ, Vinicor F. Trends in diabetes and diabetic complications. Diabetes Care 1992; 15:960–967.
62. Clements RS, Vourganti B. Fatal diabetic ketoacidosis: major causes and approaches to their prevention. Diabetes Care 1978; 1:314–325.
63. Morris AD, Boyle DIR, McMahon AD, Greene SA, MacDonald TM, Newton RW. Adherence to insulin treatment, glycaemic control, and keto-acidosis in insulin-dependent diabetes mellitus. Lancet 1997; 350:1505–1510.
64. Tattersall R. Brittle diabetes. Clin Endocrinol Metab 1977; 6:403–419.
65. Beigelman PM. Severe diabetic ketoacidosis (diabetic "coma"): 482 episodes in 257 patients; experience of three years. Diabetes 1971; 20:490–500.
66. Cahill GF, Herrera MG, Morgan AP, Soeldner JS, Steinke J, Levy PL, Richard GA, Kipnis DM. Hormone–fuel interrelationships during fasting. J Clin Invest 1966; 45:1751–1769.
67. Owen OE, Morgan AP, Kemp HG, Sullivan JM, Herrera MG, Cahill CF. Brain metabolism during fasting. J Clin Invest 1967; 46:1589–1595.
68. Mahoney CA. Extreme gestational starvation ketoacidosis: case report and review of pathophysiology. Am J Kidney Dis 1992; 20:276–280.
69. Chernow B, Finton C, Rainey TG, O'Brian JT. "Bovine ketosis" in a nondia-betic postpartum woman. Diabetes Care 1982; 5:47–49.
70. Wren KD, Slovis CM, Minion GE, Rutkowski R. The syndrome of alcoholic ketoacidosis. Am J Med 1991; 91:119–128.
71. Csako G, Elin RJ. Unrecognized false-positive ketones from drugs containing free-sulfhydryl groups (letter). JAMA 1993; 269:1634.
72. Taylor AL. Diabetic ketoacidosis. Postgrad Med 1980; 68:161–173.
73. Kitabchi AE, Matteri R, Murphy MB. Optimal insulin delivery in diabetic ketoacidosis (DKA) and hyperglycemic hyperosmolar nonketotic coma (HHNC). Diabetes Care 1982; 5(suppl 1):78–87.
74. Beigelman PM. Severe diabetic ketoacidosis. In: Beigelman PM, Kumar D, eds. Diabetes Mellitus for the Houseofficer. Baltimore: Williams & Wilkins, 1986:23–36.

75. Ellemann K, Soerensen JN, Pedersen L, Edsberg B, Andersen OO. Epidemiology and treatment of diabetic ketoacidosis in a community population. Diabetes Care 1984; 7:528–532.

76. Waldhäusl W, Kleinberger G, Korn A, Dudczak R, Bratusch-Marrain P, Nowotny P. Severe hyperglycemia: effects of rehydration on endocrine derangements and blood glucose concentration. Diabetes 1979; 28:577–584.

77. Adrogué HJ, Barrero J, Eknoyan G. Salutary effects of modest fluid replacement in the treatment of adults with diabetic ketoacidosis. JAMA 1989; 262:2108–2113.

78. Kozak GP, Rolla AR. Diabetic comas. In: Kozak GP, ed. Clinical Diabetes Mellitus. Philadelphia: WB Saunders, 1982:109–145.

79. Unger RH, Foster DW. Diabetes mellitus. In: Wilson JD, Foster DW, Kronenberg HM, Larsen PR, eds. Williams' Textbook of Endocrinology, 9th ed. Philadelphia: WB Saunders, 1998:973–1059.

80. Barrett EJ, DeFronzo RA, Bevilacqua S, Ferrannini E. Insulin resistance in diabetic ketoacidosis. Diabetes 1982; 31:923–928.

81. Flier JS. Lilly lecture: syndromes of insulin resistance. From patient to gene and back again. Diabetes 1992; 41:1207–1219.

82. Luzi L, Barrett EJ, Groop LC, Ferrannini E, DeFronzo RA. Metabolic effects of low-dose insulin therapy on glucose metabolism in diabetic ketoacidosis. Diabetes 1988; 37:1470–1477.

83. Barrett EJ, DeFronzo RA. Diabetic ketoacidosis: diagnosis and treatment. Hosp Pract (Off Ed) 1984; 19(4):89–95, 99–104.

84. Rosenthal NR, Barrett EJ. An assessment of insulin action in hyperosmolar hyperglycemic nonketotic diabetic patients. J Clin Endocrinol Metab 1985; 60:607–612.

85. Padilla AJ, Loeb JN. "Low dose" versus "high dose" insulin regimens in the management of uncontrolled diabetes. A survey. Am J Med 1977; 63:843–848.

86. Fulop M, Murthy V, Michilli A, Nalamati J, Qian Q, Saitowitz A. Serum beta-hydroxybutyrate measurement in patients with uncontrolled diabetes mellitus. Arch Intern Med 1999; 159:381–384.

87. Bureau MA, Begin R, Berthiaume Y, Shapcott D, Khoury K, Gagnon N. Cerebral hypoxia from bicarbonate infusion in diabetic acidosis. J Pediatrics 1980; 96:968–973.

88. Lever E, Jaspan JB. Sodium bicarbonate therapy in severe diabetic ketoacidosis. Am J Med 1983; 75:263–268.

89. Okuda Y, Adrogué HJ, Field JB, Nohara H, Yamshita K. Counterproductive effects of sodium bicarbonate in diabetic ketoacidosis. J Clin Endocrinol Metab 1996; 81:314–320.

90. Morris LR, Murphy MB, Kitabchi AE. Bicarbonate therapy in severe diabetic ketoacidosos. Ann Intern Med 1986; 105:836–840.

91. Narins RG, Cohen JJ. Bicarbonate therapy for organic acidosis: the case for the continued use. Ann Intern Med 1987; 106:615–618.

92. Adrogué HJ, Brensilver J, Cohen JJ, Madias NE. Influence of steady-state alterations in acid–base equilibrium on the fate of administered bicarbonate in the dog. J Clin Invest 1983; 71:867–883.

93. Clements RS, Morrison AD, Blumenthal SA, Winegard AI. Increased cerebrospinal-fluid pressure during treatment of diabetic ketosis. Lancet 1971; 2:671–675.

94. Young E, Bradley RF. Cerebral edema with irreversible coma in severe diabetic ketoacidosis. N Engl J Med 1967; 276:665–669.

95. Keller RJ, Wolfsdorf JI. Isolated growth hormone deficiency after cerebral edema complicating diabetic ketoacidosis. N Engl J Med 1987; 316:857–859.

96. Krane EJ, Rockoff MA, Wallman JK, Wolfsdorf JI. Subclinical brain swelling in children during treatment of diabetic ketoacidosis. N Eng J Med 1985; 312:1147–1151.

97. Guisado R, Arieff AI. Neurologic manifestations of diabetic comas: correlation with biochemical alterations in the brain. Metabolism 1975; 24:665–679.

98. Winegrad AI, Kern EFO, Simmons DA. Cerebral edema in diabetic ketoacidosis. N Engl J Med 1985; 312:1184–1185.

99. Fein IA, Rackow EC, Sprung CL, Grodman R. Relation of colloid osmotic pressure to arterial hypoxemia and cerebral edema during crystalloid volume loading of patients with diabetic ketoacidosis. Ann Intern Med 1982; 96: 570–575.

100. Durr JA, Hoffman WH, Sklar AH, El Gamal T, Steinhart CM. Correlates of brain edema in uncontrolled IDDM. Diabetes 1992; 41:627–632.

101. Silver SM, Clark EC, Schroeder BM, Sterns RH. Pathogenesis of cerebral edema after treatment of diabetic ketoacidosis. Kidney Int 1997; 51: 1237–1244.

102. Bryan CS, Reynolds KL, Metzger WT. Bacteremia in diabetic patients: comparison of incidence and mortality with nondiabetic patients. Diabetes Care 1985; 8:244–249.

103. Davidson MB. Diabetic ketoacidosis and hyperosmolar nonketotic syndrome. In: Davidson MB, ed. Diabetes Mellitus, Diagnosis and Treatment. New York: Churchill Livingstone, 1991:175–212.

104. Fulop M, Rosenblatt A, Kreitzer SM, Gerstenhaber B. Hyperosmolar nature of diabetic coma. Diabetes 1975; 24:594–599.

105. Gerich JE, Martin MM, Recant L. Clinical and metabolic characteristics of hyperosmolar nonketotic coma. Diabetes 1971; 20:228–238.

106. Matz R. Uncontrolled diabetes mellitus: diabetic ketoacidosis and hyperosmolar coma. In: Bergman M, ed. Principles of Diabetes Management. New York: Medical Examination Publishing, 1987:109–121.

107. Joffe BI, Goldberg RB, Krut LH, Seftel HC. Pathogenesis of nonketotic hyperosmolar diabetic coma. Lancet 1975; 1:1069–1071.

108. Gerich J, Panhaus JC, Gutman RA, Recant L. Effect of dehydration and hyperosmolarity on glucose, free fatty acid and ketone body metabolism in the rat. Diabetes 1973; 22:264–271.

109. Azain MJ, Fukuda N, Chao F-F, Yamamoto M, Ontko JA. Contributions of fatty acid and sterol synthesis to triglyceride and cholesterol secretion by the perfused rat liver in genetic hyperlipemia and obesity. J Biol Chem 1985; 260:174–181.

110. Begin-Heick N. Absence of the inhibitory effect of guanine nucleotides on adenylate cyclase activity in white adipocyte membranes of the ob/ob mouse: effect of the ob gene. J Biol Chem 1985; 260:6187–6193.

111. Adrogué HJ, Tannen RL. Ketoacidosis, hyperosmolar states, and lactic acidosis. In: Tannen RL, Kokko JP, eds. Fluids and Electrolytes. 3rd ed. Philadelphia: WB Saunders, 1996:643–674.

112. Danowski TS, Nabarro JDN. Hyperosmolar and other types of nonketoacidotic coma in diabetes. Diabetes 1965; 14:162–165.

113. Jackson WPU, Forman R. Hyperosmolar nonketotic diabetic coma. Diabetes 1966; 15:714–721.

114. Johnson RD, Conn JW, Dykman CJ, Pek S, Starr JI. Mechanisms and management of hyperosmolar coma without ketoacidosis in the diabetic. Diabetes 1969; 18:111–116.

115. Arieff AI, Carroll HJ. Nonketotic hyperosmolar coma with hyperglycemia: clinical features, pathophysiology, renal function, acid–base balance, plasma-cerebrospinal fluid equilibria and the effects of therapy in 37 cases. Medicine 1972; 51:73–94.

116. Grey N, Karl L, Kipnis DM. Physiologic mechanisms in the development of starvation ketosis in man. Diabetes 1975; 24:10–16.

117. Cahill GF. Ketosis. Kidney Int 1981; 20:416–425.

118. Owen OE, Reichard GA. Human forearm metabolism during progressive starvation. J Clin Invest 1971; 50:1536–1545.

119. Cooperman MT, Davidoff F, Spark R, Pallotta J. Clinical studies of alcoholic ketoacidosis. Diabetes 1974; 23:433–439.

120. Jenkins DW, Eckel RE, Craig JW. Alcoholic ketoacidosis. JAMA 1971; 217:177–183.

121. Fulop M, Hoberman HD. Phenformin-associated metabolic acidosis. Diabetes 1976; 25:292–296.

122. Lefevre A, Adler H, Lieber CS. Effect of ethanol on ketone metabolism. J Clin Invest 1970; 49:1775–1782.

123. Harrington JR, Cohen JJ. Metabolic acidosis. In: Cohen JJ, Kassirer JP, eds. Acid Base. Boston: Little, Brown, 1982:121–225.

124. Marliss EB, Ohman JL, Aoki TT, Kozak GP. Altered redox state obscuring ketoacidosis in diabetic patients with lactic acidosis. N Engl J Med 1970; 283:978–980.

125. Schelling JR, Howard RL, Winter SD, Linas SL. Increased osmolal gap in alcoholic ketoacidosis and lactic acidosis. Ann Intern Med 1990; 113:580–582.

126. Rose BD, Post TW. Clinical Physiology of Acid–Base and Electrolyte Disorders. New York: McGraw-Hill, 2001:801–803.

127. Miller PD, Heinig RE, Waterhouse C. Treatment of alcoholic acidosis. The role of dextrose and phosphorus. Arch Intern Med 1978; 138:67–72.

128. Seldin DW, Tarail R. The metabolism of glucose and electrolytes in diabetic ketoacidosis. J Clin Invest 1950; 29:552–565.

129. Shaw CE, Hurwitz GE, Schmukler M, Brager SH, Bessman SP. A clinical and laboratory study of insulin dosage in diabetic ketoacidosis: comparison with small and large doses. Diabetes 1962; 11:23–30.

11

Lactic Acidosis

Virginia L. Hood

University of Vermont College of Medicine, Burlington, Vermont, U.S.A.

INTRODUCTION

Lactic acidosis is not a disease but an epiphenomenon that occurs in association with a number of serious disorders, which cause considerable morbidity and mortality. The production of lactic acid is not pathological. Rather, it is a vital source of necessary ATP both at its site of production and for distant tissues. Lactic acidosis occurs when an imbalance between the generation and utilization of lactic acid results in an increase in circulating lactate with accompanying bicarbonate consumption. There is no general agreement about the level of hyperlactatemia required to qualify as lactic acidosis, but patients with plasma lactate concentrations of greater than 4 mmol/L usually have a clinically significant metabolic acidosis (1) or a mixed acid–base disorder (see Chapters 9 and 22).

PHYSIOLOGY AND PATHOPHYSIOLOGY

Normal Lactate Metabolism

Synthesis

Lactic acid is generated as an intermediate step in the conversion of glucose to CO_2 and water. For each mole of glucose metabolized via the glycolytic pathway, 2 mol of lactic acid are generated; the hydrogen ions are buffered yielding lactate anions. The only synthetic pathway for lactate production within cells is the conversion of pyruvate to lactate catalyzed by the enzyme

351

lactate dehydrogenase (LDH). Lactate utilization is also entirely dependent on the conversion of lactate to pyruvate with NAD^+ as an obligate cofactor (1). These processes take place in the cytoplasm. The concentration of lactate in the cell is determined by the concentration of pyruvate and the relative amounts of NAD^+ and NADH (2).

The major determinant of lactate generation is the amount of pyruvate, a central metabolite in both carbohydrate and fat metabolism (Fig. 1). Pyruvate is the primary end product of the glycolytic pathway, a series of reactions that convert 1 mol of glucose to 2 mol of pyruvate while generating 2 mol of ATP. The entire series of reactions occurs in the cytoplasm and can proceed in the absence of oxygen. Intracellular ATP serves as a negative feedback regulator of the pathway with ATP-inhibiting and ADP-stimulating phosphofructokinase (PFK), one of the rate-limiting steps (3,4).

Pyruvate is also generated by the deamination of alanine in the liver and glutamine in the kidney. Although these amino acids are an important source of gluconeogenesis, particularly within the liver, they are a quantitatively less important source of pyruvate than glycolysis.

Pyruvate is metabolized within the mitochondria either by pyruvate dehydrogenase (PDC) to acetyl CoA, and hence to CO_2 and H_2O via the tricarboxylic acid (TCA) cycle, or to a lesser extent by pyruvate carboxylase (PC) to oxaloacetate and into the gluconeogenic pathway. The majority of pyruvate generated is metabolized through the TCA cycle, which produces 18 mol of ATP per mole pyruvate. Pyruvate carboxylase is present only in the liver and kidney, the two organs with the capacity to produce glucose. Both these pathways of pyruvate metabolism require mitochondrial oxidative capacity. Under normal circumstances, pyruvate is metabolized as quickly as it is generated, so intracellular levels remain low.

The other determinant of cell lactate concentration is the cytoplasmic ratio of $NADH/NAD^+$. For any given cellular concentration of pyruvate, the ratio of $NADH/NAD^+$ will determine the fraction of pyruvate converted to lactate. With normal mitochondrial function, $NADH/NAD^+$ is generally low and lactate/pyruvate approximately 10. During states of impaired mitochondrial function, due to hypoxia or other factors, $NADH/NAD^+$ ratio is greatly increased. In this setting where cellular pyruvate concentrations rise as the result of decreased mitochondrial ATP generation causing increased glycolytic activity by disinhibition of PFK, pyruvate conversion to lactate is stimulated outside the mitochondria thus resulting in large increases in lactate generation (2).

Although increased lactic acid production is commonly considered to be a negative consequence of anaerobic metabolism (see later), increases in lactic acid generation can occur in a variety of cells, including red blood, vascular smooth muscle, neuronal, and skeletal muscle cells, with intact oxidative capacity (5). Increased Na^+/K^+ ATPase activity leads to increased

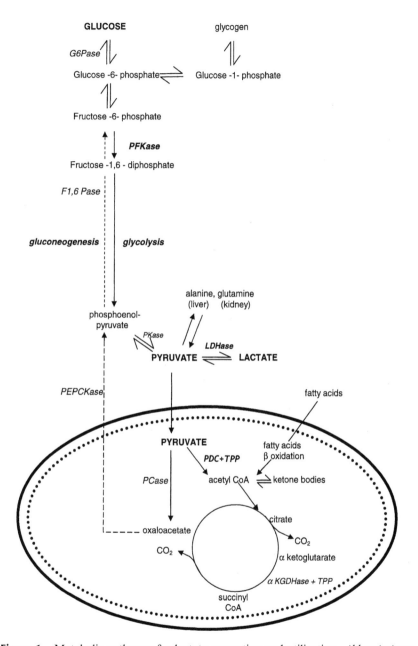

Figure 1 Metabolic pathways for lactate generation and utilization. *Abbreviations*: G6Pase, glucose-6-phosphatase; PFKase, phosphofructokinase (acidosis inhibits, alkalosis stimulates); F1,6,Pase, fructose-1,6-diphosphatase; PKase, pyruvate kinase; LDHase, lactate dehydrogenase; PEPCKase, phosphoenolpyruvate carboxykinase; PDC, pyruvate dehydrogenase complex; TPP, thiamine pyrophosphate (absent in thiamine deficiency); PCase, pyruvate carboxylase; α KGDHase, α ketoglutarate dehydrogenase.

lactic acid generation under fully oxygenated conditions in several cell types (5). Thus, it has been postulated that glycolysis, in some settings, is not evidence of impaired oxidative metabolism but reflects intracellular coupling of ATP production from glycolysis and ATP consumption by ion pumps in the same intracellular compartment (6).

All cells are capable of generating lactate and adding it to the circulation. Under normal circumstances, generation occurs primarily in the brain, red cells, skeletal muscle, and skin (Table 1). Skeletal muscle contributes only small amounts of lactate to the circulation under basal conditions, but during strenuous exercise, generalized motor seizures (7), or shock (8), this amount may be greatly increased. Immediately following a generalized convulsion, serum lactate concentrations have been measured as high as 16 mmol/L (7).

Utilization

Although all cells except red blood cells can use lactate, the liver and kidney are the primary sites for lactate consumption (9–11). Both organs convert lactate to pyruvate using LDH. Pyruvate is then either metabolized to glucose or oxidized through the TCA cycle to CO_2 and water. During these processes, 1 mol of H^+ is consumed with each mole of lactate. Of the two organs, the liver plays the more important role quantitatively. This interaction between lactate generation via glycolysis in red cells, brain, and skin and utilization via gluconeogenesis in liver and kidney (Cori cycle) provides a required glucose supply to these organs during fasting states (2).

Table 1 Daily Basal Generation and Utilization of Hydrogen Ions (mmol)

Proton source	Generation		Utilization/excretion	
	Tissue	Amount	Tissue	Amount
CO_2	All cells	15,000	Lungs	15,000
Lactic acid	Total	1,290	Total	1,290
	Skin	350	Liver	722
	RBC	302	Kidney	386
	Brain	235	Heart	80
	Muscle	218	Other	102
	GI mucosal	115		
	WBC, platelets	70		
Ketoacids	Liver	450	Brain, muscle, kidney, heart	450
Net organic/ inorganic acid	Diet	70	Kidney (excretion)	70

Source: Modified from Refs. 137,138.

pH and Lactate Metabolism

Despite the relatively large quantity of lactate and H^+ generated each day, their rapid utilization results in no net gain or loss of acid, an extracellular lactate concentration of 1–2 mmol/L, and a stable pH. However, it has also been appreciated for many years that the prevailing pH can influence lactate metabolism (12,13). Acidosis inhibits, whereas alkalosis stimulates glycolysis, and this effect is mediated, at least in part, by the pH sensitivity of the key rate-limiting glycolytic enzyme, PFK (4,12). Furthermore, a variety of studies in normal animals and humans indicate that alkalosis elevates, whereas acidosis decreases blood lactate levels. The magnitude of the change is small (1–3 mmol/L) under basal conditions, but is accentuated in humans and in animals in settings where blood lactate is increased (13,14). Furthermore, administration of sodium bicarbonate, as well as hypocapnia, increases lactate production and blood lactate concentrations in animals and humans with experimental and clinical lactic acidosis, whereas superimposed metabolic or respiratory acidosis decreases blood lactate concentrations in these settings (13–15). Similar pH effects have been noted under conditions of ketoacidosis. Alkalosis stimulates ketoacid production, whereas acidosis is inhibitory (13,16,17). In view of the similar impact that pH has on endogenous acid generation in both types of clinically significant endogenous acidosis, i.e., lactic acidosis and ketoacidosis, it has been proposed that these effects represent a defense mechanism to protect against severe acidosis (13) (Fig. 2). By reducing the rate of excessive endogenous acid production, acidosis serves to mitigate its own severity. The converse

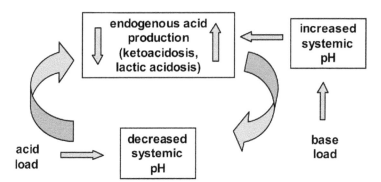

Figure 2 Negative feedback control of endogenous acid production. Increased production of lactic acid or ketoacids reduces systemic pH, which in turn inhibits the rate of endogenous acid production. Other exogenous or endogenous acid loads also suppress endogenous acid production. Base loads or therapy accentuates the production of lactic acid or ketoacids and thus interferes with feedback regulation of acid–base balance.

of this paradigm is that alkali administration in these settings will increase the rate of either lactic acid or ketoacid generation and, thereby, the blood levels of these anions (13).

Pathophysiology

The key to understanding the development and maintenance of lactic acidosis is to realize that both result from an imbalance between generation and utilization. Hence, factors disproportionately increasing production and/or decreasing utilization cause lactic acid accumulation (Tables 1 and 2).

Basal lactic acid production averages 1300 mmol/day (Table 1). Increased production occurs when ATP is low and PFK activity increased facilitating increased glycolysis, which provides excess pyruvate and increased NADH. The kidney and liver are the major users of lactate, so the development of imbalance is likely to occur more frequently when there is compromised liver or renal function. Utilization requires adequate tissue oxygen supply as well as mitochondrial enzyme and cofactor availability and function for optimal TCA cycle operation. Changes in utilization contribute to lactic acid accumulation in most of the common settings.

In the group of conditions known as congenital lactic acidosis (CLA), a variety of inherited and acquired enzymatic defects (Table 3) affecting both production and oxidation pathways can produce clinically significant lactic acidosis. The biggest subgroup involves reduced pyruvate oxidation by various mechanisms and hence increased conversion of pyruvate to lactate. In two animal models of acquired lactic acidosis [the induction of lactic acidosis by intravenous infusion of phenformin into diabetic animals and the induction of lactic acidosis by severe hypoxia (18,19)], overproduction

Table 2 Pathogenesis of Lactic Acidosis

Increased lactic acid generation
  Tissue hypoxia
    Reduced oxygen delivery (hypotension, shock)
    Reduced arterial oxygen content (hypoxemia, anemia, carbon monoxide
      poisoning)
    Increased tissue demand (exercise, seizures)
  Catecholamines
  Alkalosis
Decreased utilization
  Liver dysfunction
    Reduced perfusion, reduced mass, cellular dysfunction
  Enzymatic or cofactor deficiency
    Inherited
    Acquired

Table 3 Inherited or Acquired Enzymatic Defects in Metabolic Pathways

Defects in gluconeogenesis
   Type 1 glycogenesis (G6Pase deficiency)
   Fructose1,6-diphosphatase deficiency
   Phosphoenolpyruvate carboxykinase deficiency
   Pyruvate carboxylase deficiency (biotin deficiency)
Defects in pyruvate oxidation
   Pyruvate dehydrogenase complex (PDC) deficiency (thiamine deficiency)
   Mitochondrial myopathies
      Electron transport chain
      TCA cycle
      Pyridine nucleotide shuttle
      Adenine nucleotide transporter
      Oligomysin sensitive ATPase
Cofactor deficiencies
   Thiamine (PDC activity)
   Biotin (PC activity)
Others
   Methylmalonic academia

of lactate by both muscle and gut, as well as decreased hepatic extraction, play prominent pathophysiological roles. In addition, conversion from renal lactate extraction to generation has been found in hypoxia-induced lactic acidosis. Thus, combined overproduction and underutilization of lactate underlie the development of lactic acidosis in experimentally induced lactic acidosis. These factors also operate in humans (see Discussion of Section "Etiology").

METABOLIC CONSEQUENCES OF LACTIC ACID ACCUMULATION

The major concern with lactic acid accumulation is metabolic acidosis. Acidosis is considered the most life-threatening consequence of conditions associated with lactic acid accumulation. Mencken (20), the famous essayist, who wrote for the Baltimore Sun in the early 20th century, became concerned about the problem of acidosis and alerted the general public to this problem, stating that life was a battle against acidosis (20). He got the idea from Dr George Crile, who said that death was acidosis—that it was caused by the failure of the organism to maintain the alkalinity necessary for its normal functioning. But even though death may be acidosis, the question remains, when is acidosis death?

Severe acidosis in the absence of significant organ failure is rarely lethal. There are many recorded cases of survivors with systemic pH as low as 6.50 (21), and most clinicians have seen patients presenting to the emergency room or the intensive care unit with pH < 7.10 but with adequate blood pressure and tissue perfusion. There is only very scant evidence that acidosis alone causes tissue injury. Most sources refer to studies of shock, where the contributions of the components of hypoperfusion, hypoxia, and acidosis were not examined separately. In fact, cardiac myocyte injury occurs during reperfusion and not as the result of tissue hypoxia or acidosis (22,23). Indeed, extracellular acidosis, by limiting toxic Ca^{2+} accumulation in cells, has been shown to be protective during reperfusion in isolated cells and perfused heart studies (24).

Oxygen delivery to tissues is enhanced in acute acidosis but hindered in chronic acidosis. During vigorous exercise, decreased pH helps to maintain tissue oxygenation by increasing capillary blood flow, which increases oxygen delivery and aids removal of accumulating CO_2, as well as increasing O_2 extraction (Bohr effect) (25). Also, aggressive correction of chronic acidosis in the presence of respiratory or cardiac dysfunction can worsen tissue oxygenation because ventilation and regional perfusion may be unable to compensate for higher oxygen binding affinity of hemoglobin resulting from reduced red cell DPG (26).

The main concern about acidosis is that it impairs myocardial function (27). Both in vitro and in vivo studies in animals have demonstrated impaired cardiac function when pH is less than 7.2. However, in intact animals, the depressant effect seems to be counterbalanced by catecholamine stimulation until pH is less than 7.1 (28). Nevertheless, infusions of lactic acid into experimental animals have been shown to decrease systemic blood pressure and cardiac output prior to the development of a severe acidosis (29).

There is no direct experimental information about the effects of lactic acid accumulation on cell function in humans, as acidosis does not occur in the absence of the other potentially life-threatening conditions that either cause or accompany clinical lactic acidosis. In a study of treatment of acquired lactic acidosis in adults (see later), arterial pH was a strong and independent predictor of survival. However, this association neither confirms causality nor provides evidence that correction of the acidosis can improve outcomes (30).

CLINICAL MANIFESTATIONS

In most instances, lactic acidosis is part of a larger clinical syndrome with the signs and symptoms of the underlying condition(s) dominating the clinical picture. When lactic acidosis is associated with tissue hypoxia, patients are almost always severely ill and overt shock is usually present. The consequences of tissue hypoxia may be worsened by the development of lactic acidosis, because acidosis, if severe enough, can result in decreased cardiac output and hypotension (26). As with any serious metabolic acidosis, compensatory hyperventilation may be the first indication of lactic acidosis. Lactic acidosis associated with drugs or toxins, and tumor-associated lactic acidosis is frequently slow in onset. Patients may have very few systemic symptoms and usually show no cardiovascular impairment (1). Although malaise, weakness, nausea, vomiting, abdominal pain, and progressive mental clouding can occur, hyperventilation may be the only clinical symptom. Congenital lactic acidosis most often presents with the signs and symptoms of the progressive neurodegeneration and growth retardation that results from the defects in mitochondrial oxidative metabolism that lead to lactate accumulation (31,32). Up to half of the patients may present with renal abnormalities (33), including bicarbonaturia, phosphaturia, hypercalciuria, proteinuria, or impaired renal function. d-Lactic acidosis may present with unexplained neurological symptoms in association with symptoms and signs of malabsorption (34).

DIAGNOSIS

Lactic acidosis is rarely diagnosed from clinical symptoms or signs but most often suspected by the presence of a metabolic acidosis with an increased anion gap (see Chapter 9). The degree of acidosis and increase in anion gap that are required to make the diagnosis are not well established. Historically, the anion gap ($[Na^+]-[HCO_3^-]-[Cl^-]$) was generally noted to be greater than $16\,mmol/L$ (1), but with newer autoanalyzer measurement techniques anion gaps above $9\ mmol/L$ may be abnormal. In addition, it is now recognized that both a low-serum albumin concentration and an acid pH can significantly lower the anion gap (see Chapter 28), countervailing any increase due to lactate accumulation. Thus, an increased anion gap is not a sensitive indicator of the presence of hyperlactatemia. In one series, half of those with blood lactate levels between 2.5 and 9.9 mmol/L had anion gaps less than $12\,mEq/L$ (35). Nevertheless, as lactic acid can accumulate without causing overt acidemia if a metabolic or respiratory alkalosis coexists, an increased anion gap may be the only clue that hyperlactatemia is present. The diagnosis of hyperlactatemia in the presence of an increased anion gap can be made by exclusion if neither ketosis nor uremia is present and toxicology screens are negative, but it is now made most commonly simply by blood lactic acid measurement. It should be noted that the elevated anion gap accompanying methanol, ethylene glycol, paraldehyde, or salicylate poisoning can result from increased lactate along with the accumulation of other unmeasured anionic metabolites. In addition, in states of chronic hyperlactatemia, lactate anions are excreted more readily than chloride and are replaced by this anion, before the kidney can regenerate bicarbonate. This sequence of events results in a clinical picture with neither a very high blood lactate level nor increased anion gap. An analogous situation has been well documented in diabetic ketoacidosis where, during ECF volume repletion with isotonic saline, the increased anion gap acidosis is replaced by a hyperchloremic acidosis as ketoanions are excreted in the urine (see Chapter 10).

The diagnosis of lactic acidosis is confirmed by direct measurement of blood or plasma lactate concentration. Patients with metabolic acidosis, a decreased serum [HCO_3^-], an increased anion gap, and plasma lactate concentration of greater than 4–5 mmol/L can be reliably diagnosed as having lactic acidosis. For lactate measurement, blood should be quickly processed or deproteinized to prevent spurious increases in lactate due to glycolytic activity of the red blood cells. Particular care should be taken with venous samples to avoid stasis of blood during venipuncture (1). Venous lactate concentrations are approximately 50–100% higher than arterial concentrations, but either can be used for clinical assessment. Normal arterial blood lactate concentration is < 1.5 mmol/L and venous blood lactate is < 2.0 mmol/L.

In the rare instances where the lactic acid is produced in the D(–) form by bacteria in short-bowel syndromes (see later), it will not be detected by the standard enzymatic technique, which uses an L(+)-LDH enzyme. In this situation, the diagnosis can be made by substituting the D(–) form of the enzyme in the assay.

Associated laboratory findings can include hyperphosphatemia, from increased release from cells (36) and hyperuricemia, a consequence of competitive inhibition of tubular urate secretion by lactate (37). Serum [K^+] is usually normal (see Chapter 9).

ETIOLOGY

There is no ideal or agreed upon classification for the causes of lactic acidosis. Traditionally, the classification was based on presumed pathogenic processes. The disorders have been divided into two categories, types A and B, depending on the presence or absence of evidence of poor tissue oxygenation (38). Type A included conditions associated with tissue hypoxia, and type B, a wide variety of disorders in which overt hypoperfusion or tissue hypoxia was not thought to be an issue (1) but oxygen utilization appeared to be compromised (39). Type B encompassed the effects of various congenital enzymatic defects as well as conditions such as diabetes mellitus, liver failure, multiple organ failure, sepsis, neoplastic diseases, and a variety of drug- or toxin-induced metabolic defects. This has proved a useful classification for studying factors important in the pathogenesis of lactic acidosis, but in clinical practice the factors contributing to both type A and type B conditions often occur simultaneously. A more recent attempt to use pathological processes as a basis for classification identifies disorders associated with defects in oxygen delivery and those with defects in oxygen utilization. However, this division does not provide distinctive categories, as here too, both sets of pathological processes operate in many common clinical settings. In addition, there appears to be instances where lactic acid accumulates in cells with intact oxidative capacity (6,40), thus not reflecting disorders of either reduced oxygen delivery or utilization but increased aerobic glycolysis (see Sepsis). Moreover, other pathogenic processes, such as superimposed hypoglycemia (41) or alkalosis (13) can contribute to lactate accumulation in a variety of conditions.

A pathogenic classification is shown in Table 2. As clinical disorders associated with lactic acidosis do not fall neatly into this pathogenic classification, they will be discussed under the headings noted in Table 4.

Tissue Hypoxia

Tissue hypoxia is common to all patients with cardiopulmonary failure, hypotension, hemorrhage, severe anemia, carbon monoxide poisoning, seizures, and exhaustive exercise. The resultant lactic acidosis sometimes precedes overt hypotension by several hours, but if the underlying disorder is untreated, shock inevitably follows. This disorder almost invariably resulted in death and once carried the diagnosis of idiopathic lactic acidosis (42). With better diagnostic techniques, a reason for the tissue hypoxia can almost always be recognized, and the term "idiopathic lactic acidosis" is no longer used. By identifying and correcting the cause, progression of shock and lactic acidosis can often be prevented. When the cause is not immediately obvious, the index of suspicion for unrecognized sepsis or splanchnic ischemia should always be high.

Common Disorders with More than One Pathogenic Process

Sepsis/Systemic Inflammatory Response Syndrome

The cause of hyperlactatemia in sepsis/systemic inflammatory response syndrome (SIRS) is multifactorial (Table 2) (43), its usefulness for monitoring the course or as a prognostic indicator is limited (44), and treatment remains that of the underlying condition. One or more of the anaerobic or aerobic mechanisms determine its presence and severity. Reduced O_2 delivery in shock leads to increased anaerobic metabolism and thus increased lactic acid production. Increases in intracellular H^+ and lactate concentrations can activate K^+–ATP channels in vascular smooth muscle cells, contributing to the pathological vasodilation characteristic of sepsis and other forms of vasodilatory shock (45), further impairing tissue perfusion. Reduced lactate consumption can occur as the result of defective mitochondrial pyruvate oxidation (46). Activation of these mechanisms may not be entirely detrimental to cell function. Lactate is the preferred substrate for cardiac

Table 4 Predisposing Conditions or Disorders Causing Lactic Acidosis

Tissue hypoxia
  Cardiopulmonary failure
  Severe anemia
  Shock (hemorrhage, sepsis)
  Carbon monoxide poisoning
  Seizures
  Exercise
Common disorders
  Sepsis/SIRS
  Diabetes mellitus
  Malignancy (lymphoma, leukemia, sarcoma, carcinoma)
  HIV/AIDS
  Liver disease
  Renal failure
  Multiple organ failure
  Other conditions (asthma, pheochromocytoma, malaria)
Specific disorders
  Drugs/toxins
    Biguanides (phenformin, metformin)
    Ethanol, methanol, isopropyl alcohol
    Ethylene glycol, propylene glycol
    Fructose, sorbitol, xylitol
    Salicylates
    Catecholamines, pheochromocytoma
    Cyanide, nitroprusside
    Cocaine
    Isoniazid
  Streptozotocin
    Paraldehyde
    Diethyl ether
    Dithiazanine
    Nucleoside analogues (didanosine, zidovudine, stavudine, zalcitabine, fialuridine)
  D-Lactic acidosis
  Hereditary or acquired enzymatic defects or cofactor deficiencies

metabolism in sepsis and hepatic lactate extraction is increased two to three times above baseline (40). These and other observations suggest that global cellular ischemia is not the only or even major mechanism for increased lactate levels in sepsis. One working hypothesis is that increased aerobic glycolysis, perhaps stimulated by epinephrine-induced increased Na^+/K^+ ATPase activity, may explain continuing hyperlactatemia in sepsis after adequate resuscitation measures have been implemented (6).

In sepsis, both lactate levels and clearance have been correlated with mortality (47) although the causality of these associations is still a point of contention (6). Nevertheless, in the absence of more sensitive indicators, lactate levels are still considered a useful measure of impaired global cellular metabolism in critically ill patients (44).

Diabetes Mellitus

Patients with diabetes mellitus are at increased risk for developing lactic acidosis associated with hypoxemia because of underlying atherosclerosis and microvascular disease. They may be also more likely than nondiabetic persons to develop tissue hypoxia in major stress situations such as sepsis or myocardial infarction. In addition, abnormalities in both lactate oxidation (48) and production (49) have been described that could predispose those with diabetes to lactic acidosis given appropriate precipitating factors. Interestingly, it is uncommon for significant lactic acidosis to accompany ketoacidosis possibly because the acidosis associated with excess ketogenesis inhibits PFK thus limiting glycolysis.

Hepatic and Multiple Organ Failure

While reduced liver metabolism of lactate has been implicated as the major contributor to the lactate accumulation in animal models of lactic acidosis (18), it may only be part of the explanation in humans. Blood lactate levels can be increased in those with severe liver disease but serious lactic acidosis is unusual (50). In patients with parenchymal liver disease but without fulminant acute hepatic failure, shock was the major factor for precipitating all instances of lactic acidosis (51). Factors such as reduced PDC activity (52), hypoglycemia (53), or respiratory alkalosis (54) may also contribute to lactate accumulation in patients with liver disease.

Lactic acidosis that occurs with multiple organ failure is also multifactorial; tissue hypoxia from shock, hypercatabolic state, and the metabolic defects described for the coexisting liver and renal dysfunction and/or systemic inflammatory response all contribute to upsetting the balance between utilization and production.

Malignancy

Lactic acidosis occurs with many neoplasms, including lymphoma, leukemias, and carcinoma (lung, breast, pancreas, and colon) (55–57). Both increased production of lactic acid by tumor cells with intrinsically high anaerobic glycolysis and reduced utilization by reduced liver mass due to metastases play roles of varying importance in individual cases. Hypoglycemia is frequently present (55). Bicarbonate therapy increases acid production and lactate excretion while having no impact on serum [HCO_3^-] (56,57). Reducing tumor mass can reduce lactic acidosis (55).

HIV/AIDS

Lactic acidosis has been reported in patients with HIV in the absence of systemic hypoxemia or tissue hypoxia (58). Hyperlactatemia is now recognized to occur frequently in persons taking antiviral nucleoside analogue reverse transcriptase inhibitors, previously noted to be associated with mitochondrial dysfunction (59), with a spectrum ranging from symptomatic hyperlactatemia with hepatic steatosis to chronic or intermittent low-grade hyperlactatemia without acidosis (60). In a cross-sectional study of 880 patients with HIV over a 1-month period, 8.3% had blood lactate levels > 1.1 times the upper limit of normal (97.5 percentile of the normal range) and 1% had levels > 2.2 times the upper limit of normal. The odds ratio for hyperlactatemia using regimens containing stavudine with or without didanosine compared to zidovudine-containing regimens was 2.7 (95% CI 1.5–4.8). The major risk factors were treatment with, and the length of time receiving, stavudine. There were also associations with lipoatrophy, hyperlipidemia, and hyperglycemia (61). In vitro studies comparing mitochondrial toxicity of the nucleoside analogues suggest that relative toxicities are zalcitabine $>$ stavudine $>$ didanosine (62). As with many situations where hyperlactatemia develops, this complication in HIV patients is likely to be multifactorial, with mitochondrial dysfunction and/or hepatic steatosis contributing.

Renal Failure and Renal Replacement Therapies

Lactic acid production is increased with renal replacement therapy although this process does not result in acidosis. During a hemodialysis session, blood lactate levels do not decrease as would be expected given lactate's dialysance (63), indicating increased production (63). The increased production most likely results from stimulation of lactic acid generation by the alkalinization that occurs during dialysis. This explains both the lack of acidosis and also the lack of alkalosis that would be expected given the large transfer of bicarbonate during the standard dialysis session (63).

In most forms of peritoneal dialysis (PD), lactate is used as the base replacement. Lactate is absorbed at a rate of 14–25 mmol/hr over the 24-hr period of PD (63,64). When metabolized, lactate consumes H^+ thereby correcting the acidosis of renal failure. However, should there be circumstances when lactate cannot be metabolized (liver impairment) or its production is increased [concurrent treatment with metformin (65)], lactate can accumulate, becoming ineffective as base replacement, and potentially impairing cardiac function independently of the pH (66).

A similar problem can arise in those patients treated with continuous renal replacement therapies (CRRT) where lactate containing solutions are used as replacement fluids (67). Hence, when there is reason to believe that lactate utilization is impaired or its generation increased, the use of lactate-containing replacement solutions should be avoided.

Organ Transplantation

Hyperlactatemia occurs in 10% of heart transplant recipients but usually resolves rapidly. Lactate levels as high as 14 mmol/L have been reported and are highly correlated with the dose of inotropic agents used for circulatory support (68). During liver transplantation, hyperlactatemia is an expected occurrence. In one study, plasma lactate concentration began rising soon after surgery commenced and then more rapidly so during the anhepatic period; it peaked at 7.3 (± 0.41, SE) mmol/L in the first 60 min after graft reperfusion and remained elevated for the subsequent 2 hr before returning to baseline (69). Acidosis is rarely a concern in this setting as HCO_3^- is given when pH is less than 7.3. Commonly, within 30 min of graft reperfusion, an alkalosis occurs as lactate starts being utilized by the functioning liver. The intraoperative rise in lactate can be ameliorated by pretransplant treatment with dichloroacetate (DCA) (69). PDH activity has been shown to be reduced in cirrhotic livers and can be increased by treatment with DCA (52) although this is not usually needed as plasma lactate levels prior to transplantation are generally within the normal range (69).

Other Disorders Precipitating Lactic Acidosis

Lactic acidosis can occur following grand mal seizures (7), in patients with pheochromocytoma (70), cocaine intoxication (71), and severe asthma (72,73). Although all these conditions can be associated with impaired O_2 delivery to tissues, there are many reports where both O_2 delivery and cellular oxygenation appear adequate. Under these conditions, one common finding is increased β-adrenergic stimulation. Epinephrine stimulation of Na^+/K^+ ATPase may be linked to local lactic acid production, which serves as an ATP source (6). In asthma, coexisting respiratory alkalosis may also play a role (72).

Specific Disorders

Drugs and Toxins

Biguanides: The most notorious group of drugs is the biguanides, including phenformin (74–76) and metformin (76). Although lactic acidosis occurs less frequently with metformin (77,78), it is still a serious problem in patients with impaired renal function, a condition that allows the drug to accumulate. These drugs inhibit hepatic uptake and oxidation of lactate, and increase lactic acid production. Whereas phenformin accumulates in the mitochondrial membranes where its influence on oxidative metabolism can be significant, metformin concentrates in the cell cytoplasm (79). The incidence of phenformin associated lactic acidosis was 40–64/100,000 patient years prior to its withdrawal from use, whereas metformin-associated lactic acidosis occurs much less frequently, 9/100,000 patient years (77,80). Pooled data from 176 comparative trials of metformin and other hypoglycemic agents found no cases of fatal or nonfatal lactic acidosis in 35,619 patient years of metformin use, nor any in the 30,002 patient years of the nonmetformin use group (80). The cause of metformin-associated lactic acidosis is often multifactorial being as much the consequence of conditions causing circulatory collapse and renal failure as the accumulation of the drug (81). Furthermore, in individuals, prognosis is more dependent on the severity of the underlying condition than the severity of the presenting lactic acidosis or metformin level. Patients at increased risk include those with impaired renal, hepatic, or cardiac function (76,79).

Nucleoside Analogues: A second group of drugs of growing importance for precipitating lactic acidosis is the antiviral nucleoside analogue reverse transcriptase inhibitors (see HIV/AIDS section). These important agents for the treatment of HIV/AIDS inhibit mitochondrial DNA polymerase γ causing both lactic acidosis and hepatic steatosis. Fialuridine, a nucleoside analogue that has been used in the treatment of hepatitis B, causes defective mitochondrial DNA and lactic acidosis (82).

Ethanol: By impairing conversion of lactate to glucose in the liver, ethanol ingestion can cause small increases in blood lactate (83). Also, as dehydrogenation of ethanol to acetaldehyde and acetate depletes NAD^+, there is increased conversion of pyruvate to lactate. Serious lactic acidosis is rare, though it has been described in association with nondiabetic ketoacidosis and concurrent respiratory alkalosis (84).

Methanol, Isopropyl Alcohol: The toxic metabolites of methanol, formaldehyde and formic acid, inhibit mitochondrial oxidation leading to increased lactic acid production. Isopropyl alcohol intoxication is associated with lactic acid accumulation (85) thought to be the consequence of its metabolism via alcohol dehydrogenase as described for ethanol and the glycols.

Ethylene Glycol, Propylene Glycol: Lactic acid accumulation can be a quantitatively significant contributor to the increased anion gap acidosis that accompanies ethylene glycol intoxication (86). Although glycolate, a metabolite of ethylene glycol, can cause large artifactual elevations in plasma l-lactate if measured by analyzers using l-lactate oxidase (87), lactic acid accumulation does occur with ethylene glycol intoxication (86). The mechanism for the lactate accumulation is thought to be the increased $NADH/NAD^+$ that occurs during the metabolism of ethylene glycol via alcohol dehydrogenase that shunts pyruvate away from the TCA cycle and into lactate.

Propylene glycol is used as a solvent in numerous pharmaceuticals and as a preservative in processed foods. There have been a series of case reports linking episodes of lactic acidosis with high levels of propylene glycol resulting from lorazepam (88–90) or nitroglycerin infusions (91) or silver sulfadiazine topical applications (92). Lactate accumulation is thought to result from the oxidation of propylene glycol to lactic acid as well as the increased ratio of $NADH/NAD^+$ that occurs with its metabolism by alcohol dehydrogenase.

Salicylates: The late component of metabolic acidosis that develops with salicylate intoxication is due to lactic acidosis, which is almost certainly exacerbated by the concomitant respiratory alkalosis that results from salicylate-induced hyperventilation (93,94).

Lactic acid accumulation is common in patients with acute liver failure caused by drug toxicity from *acetaminophen* (95) and *fialuridine* (123).

Catecholamines: Epinephrine increases glycolysis and inhibits pyruvate oxidation. Norepinephrine and epinephrine in very high concentrations cause vasoconstriction of skin, skeletal muscle, and splanchnic vessels resulting in increased anaerobic metabolism and reduced hepatic extraction of lactate. Catecholamines infused for circulatory support in shock states can exacerbate hyperlactatemia by both increasing production and decreasing utilization. Lactic acidosis can be the presenting finding in patients with pheochromocytoma (70,96). As mentioned above, the effects of endogenously produced catecholamines may contribute to the hyperlactatemia that occurs with vigorous exercise, asthma, septic and hemorrhagic shock, and burns (6), under both aerobic and anaerobic conditions.

A variety of other agents have been reported to cause lactic acidosis. These are listed in Table 4.

Thiamine Deficiency

Thiamine is essential for normal glucose metabolism. After phosphorylation in the small bowel, it becomes the cofactor for pyruvate dehydrogenase (PDC), alpha ketoglutarate dehydrogenase, and transketolase. When PDC is inhibited, acetyl CoA cannot form nor enter the citric acid cycle, leaving pyruvate to accumulate and driving its conversion into lactate. Instances of thiamine deficiency causing lactic acidosis have been described in those receiving total parenteral nutrition (TPN) without micronutrient replacement (97,98), as well as in fulminant beri beri (99), and may contribute to the lactic acidosis that can accompany acute alcoholic liver injury.

D-Lactic Acidosis

D-Lactic acidosis is an entity well known to veterinarians but less familiar to physicians. The condition occurs in patients with jejunal bypass and with other short-bowel syndromes (34,100). D-Lactic acid is a normal metabolite of the glycolytic pathway in some bacteria but not in humans who lack the D(–)-lactic dehydrogenase enzyme. In patients with defects in small bowel function, excess carbohydrate is delivered to the colon where D-lactic acid is produced by an abnormal bacterial flora. Once absorbed, it is poorly metabolized and presents as an increased anion gap metabolic acidosis.

A clinically important distinguishing feature of d-lactate accumulation is the accompanying neurological disorder characterized by episodes of confusion, slurred speech, ataxia, weakness, and sometimes unusual behavior that is not a feature of other metabolic acidosis of equivalent severity. A high-calorie diet may exacerbate the condition (34). As only L(+)-lactate is measured in standard lactate determinations, blood lactate concentrations in d-lactic acidosis are normal. The diagnosis is made by substituting the D(–)-LDH enzyme in the standard lactate assay. Alternatively, a lactic acid peak can be seen with proton nuclear magnetic resonance spectroscopy (101). Although a rare condition, it is treatable by eradicating the gut bacteria with nonabsorbable antibiotics, such as neomycin or vancomycin, and/or correcting the anatomic bowel defect.

Hereditary Defects and Congenital Lactic Acidosis

Lactic acidosis occurs as the result of a variety of inherited defects in enzymes important for mitochondrial energy metabolism, including gluconeogenesis, pyruvate oxidation, and electron transport. It has been postulated that mitochondrial DNA is very susceptible to mutation because of its small size, rapid turnover rate, high intramitochondrial free radicals, and lack of adequate DNA repair processes (102). Hence, multiple enzymatic defects have been described and form the basis for a variety of clinical syndromes (Table 3). The numerous disorders of mitochondrial metabolism may have implications beyond CLA, including the development or manifestations of such disorders as aging, diabetes mellitus, and even ischemia (102).

Several enzymes are large complexes of subunits encoded by multiple genes complicating analysis of specific mutations, although the molecular pathology of several defects has been described (103). Defects in the pyruvate dehydrogenase multienzyme complex (PDC) (31,32) produce cells unable to oxidize pyruvate in the mitochondria, thereby reducing it to lactate in the cytoplasm. Hence, lactate accumulates in blood, cerebrospinal fluid, and urine. These disorders account for 10–15% of CLA. Because the CNS is dependent on oxidative phosphorylation of glucose for energy, progressive neurodegeneration and its clinical consequences are present in most children with CLA. CNS findings vary in both severity and age of onset. Other organs with high oxidative energy needs such as heart muscle, skeletal muscle, and kidney are also at risk. Renal abnormalities, including decreased GFR, proteinuria, bicarbonaturia, phosphaturia, or Fanconi syndrome are common and may be the first sign of the condition (33).

The diagnosis of specific syndromes is made by clinical assessment of skeletal muscle, heart, hepatic and neurological function, blood and CSF levels of lactate, plasma amino acids, and plasma and urinary carnitine. Specific enzyme defects can be identified in cultured skin fibroblasts, lymphocytes, and/or muscle biopsies in specialized laboratories (103). Treatment is generally unsatisfactory although DCA has been used with some success in some instances (see Section Treatment).

CLINICAL COURSE

The clinical course of patients with lactic acidosis is for the most part that of the underlying condition which initiated the accumulation of lactic acid. In one study of patients with lactate $> 5 \, \text{mmol/L}$, mortality was 41% at 24 hr, and 83% at 30 days with only 17% being discharged from the hospital. Only 10% of those with systolic blood pressure $< 90 \, \text{mmHg}$ and none with an APACHE score > 30 survived (30,104). Although the probability of survival was also inversely proportional to the lactate concentration, the strongest predictors of survival were APACHE II score, arterial pH (highly correlated with $[HCO_3^-]$), and systolic blood pressure (Table 5). Treatment with $NaHCO_3$ did not affect arterial lactate, arterial pH, or survival. The likelihood of resolution of the lactic acidosis in 72 hr was inversely proportional to the baseline arterial lactate concentration.

TREATMENT

The treatment of any disease or disorder revolves around identifying the cause, reversing the consequences, and preventing reoccurrence. With lactic acidosis, the cause and the consequences overlap. Lactic acidosis is rarely a disease by itself (except for D-lactic acidosis and CLA) and can be better considered as a reflection of the severity of its associated underlying disorder(s).

As the real cause of lactic acidosis (the accumulation of lactic acid in the tissues and circulation) is an imbalance between the generation and utilization of lactic acid as a consequence of some disorders, treatment involves removing the underlying condition, thereby reversing the imbalance.

Table 5 Predictors of Mortality at 24 hr

Clinical index	Survived ($n = 74$)	Died ($n = 52$)	p
Age	55 (18)	58 (16)	0.410
Lactate (mmol/L)	9.2 (4.9)	12.2 (5.9)	0.004
Arterial pH	7.29 (0.10)	7.18 (0.15)	< 0.001[a]
Arterial O_2 sat	96.5 (2.8)	90.3 (13.8)	0.002
Heart rate	116 (22)	106 (27)	0.028
Systolic BP	114 (27)	88 (25)	< 0.001[a]
APACHE II score	16 (6.9)	23.9 (7.4)	< 0.001[a]

Predictors of survival in logistic regression.
( ) Standard deviation.
[a]*Source*: Modified from Ref. 30.

The principles of management involve four strategies. Circulatory support is most important because, when the circulation is impaired, it is usually at least a component of both the cause and life-threatening consequences. Disease-specific measures are essential to reduce production and increase utilization of lactic acid. Containing the acidosis, the most controversial aspect of care, must be considered. Pharmacological measures to increase lactate utilization may be instituted.

Circulatory Support

Correcting volume depletion and optimizing cardiac function are important for lactate removal via the liver as well as for preventing or correcting tissue hypoxia and reducing production. Maintenance of adequate circulatory support and ventilation improves tissue oxygenation, reducing the demand for anaerobic metabolism, and allows for optimal liver and kidney perfusion to promote lactate utilization. Peripheral vasoconstrictors for the purpose of increasing blood pressure should be used with caution. Both epinephrine and dopamine improve arterial pressure, cardiac output, and oxygen consumption in persons with infection-induced lactic acidosis. However, when compared, most patients given epinephrine did not complete treatment because of worsening lactic acidosis, whereas those treated with dopamine showed improvement, manifested by an increase in pH, a decrease in blood lactate, and a positive correlation between O_2 consumption and delivery (105). Patients treated in the first 7 hr to attain a central venous pressure of 8–12 mmHg, mean arterial pressure > 65 mmHg, urine output > 0.5 mL/min, and a central venous O_2 saturation $> 70\%$, have lower lactate levels and less acidosis during the subsequent 65 hr, and less organ damage and a 42% reduction in mortality (106).

Disease-Specific Measures

After resuscitation, identifying, removing, and/or modifying the cause is the cornerstone of treatment. Disease-specific measures include administering appropriate antibiotics for sepsis and d-lactic acidosis; discontinuing drugs, such as metformin or antiviral nucleoside analogues; monitoring blood concentrations of nitroprusside closely especially in those with renal failure; giving insulin, glucose, and thiamine in appropriate situations; and removing toxins and tumor mass, if possible.

Containing the Acidosis

Treating the acidosis itself is the most controversial aspect of management, because the degree of acidosis usually reflects the severity of the underlying condition rather than being the cause of it. As discussed above, the most important step for containing the acidosis is circulatory support. The second step is to identify and correct, where possible, other coincidental causes of

Table 6 Therapies for Containing the Acidosis

	Advantages	Disadvantages
Sodium bicarbonate		
Bolus	Rapid effect	Hypertonicity
		CO_2 production
Isotonic infusion	Slow effect	Volume excess
		CO_2 production
Renal replacement	Rapid effect	Requires RRT access
therapy	Provides unlimited base	Increases lactic
		acid production
	No hypertonicity	
	No volume excess	
	CO_2 removed in dialysate	
Carbicarb	Less CO_2 production	Same volume issues
		as $NaHCO_3$
THAM	No increase in CO_2	Depresses respiration
		Hypoglycemia
		Hyperkalemia

the low pH, such as accumulation of other organic acids and/or CO_2. If a life-threatening acidosis persists, base must be administered. Base is usually provided in the form of $NaHCO_3$ but can be given as Carbicarb® or *tris*-hydroxymethyl aminomethane (THAM) (see below). Base should not be given as lactate or acetate for obvious reasons. The risks and benefits for base administration are outlined in Table 6.

Rationale for Base Administration

There are advantages and disadvantages to giving base to treat an endogenous acidosis. The key issue is whether treatment beneficially influences the outcome and, if so, whether this benefit outweighs the risks. In ventilated, very sick patients given NaCl and $NaHCO_3$ in random order, cardiac output, pulmonary wedge pressure, and blood pressure were not different. Even in subjects who had a pH < 7.20 at presentation, there was no demonstrable

Table 7 Therapies for Increasing Pyruvate Oxidation

	Advantages	Disadvantages
Improve liver persuion/functon		
Dichloroacetate	Reduces plasma lactate	No effect on survival
	Reduces acidosis	No effect on BP, CO
Thiamine (if deficient)	Improves PDC activity	
	Improves α KGDH activity	

hemodynamic benefit of $NaHCO_3$ administration (107). In a subsequent study, $NaHCO_3$ treatment did not alter survival (108).

Sodium Bicarbonate

Concerns (Table 6): If large amounts of $NaHCO_3$ are given, Na^+ accumulation can lead to volume overload or hypertonicity. Too rapid delivery can cause an alkalosis that may depress ventilation and worsen hypoxemia. In addition, CO_2 generated by HCO_3^- buffering of H^+ may paradoxically lower pH, particularly if poor tissue perfusion or poor lung function limits CO_2 removal. Base administration can also increase lactic acid production with potentially adverse consequences on energy availability. In animals, $NaHCO_3$ administration can decrease cardiac output, blood pressure, and survival (109). How important are these concerns? Volume overload and hypertonicity are largely dependent on the amount of isotonic or hypertonic solutions used and the presence of impaired renal function. Paradoxical intracellular acidosis as a result of base therapy is of theoretical and not practical importance. $NaHCO_3$ administration decreases intracellular pH transiently in animal and human hepatocytes as a result of increased CO_2 generation (110,111) but this effect is not relevant in clinical situations (112). Base administration increases lactic acid production in malignancy and with renal replacement therapies (see above). The consequences of increased lactic acid production under these circumstances are not fully understood. However, ongoing lactate generation and its loss into urine or dialysate could tax already limited energy stores in severely ill persons, where glycolysis becomes dependent on glucose generated via gluconeogenesis at the expense of increased catabolism of body protein (57). These issues and their relevance to human lactic acidosis management are discussed in detail elsewhere (21,113–115). Most of the adverse consequences of $NaHCO_3$ administration can be minimized by the route, rate, and amount given.

Routes of Bicarbonate Administration: The commonly used method for estimating HCO_3^- replacement assumes a HCO_3^- space of 50% of body weight and no ongoing net acid production. Using this set of assumptions, the amount required to return serum $[HCO_3^-]$ to $10\,mEq/L$ is: [10 – serum $[HCO_3^-]] \times (0.5 \times$ body weight in kg). If there is ongoing lactic acid accumulation, sufficient additional HCO_3^- must be given to offset this load. A reasonable goal is to maintain serum $[HCO_3^-] > 10\,mEq/L$ and pH > 7.20 if there is myocardial dysfunction, or pH > 7.10 and $[HCO_3^-] > 5\,mEq/L$ in other situations while the cause of the lactic acidosis is being addressed. In critically ill patients with multiple organ failure and ongoing lactic acid production, the only effective way to deliver enough HCO_3^- is via CRRT (116,117). The advantages of CRRT are the ability to deliver large amounts of HCO_3^- while avoiding volume overload and hypertonicity, and the simultaneous removal of lactate and other "toxins." In fact, CRRT may improve outcomes in critically ill patients with lactic acidosis in septic shock syndromes (111,118). Controlled trials are needed to clarify the true effect of this approach.

Carbicarb

The buffer known as Carbicarb (International Medication Systems, South El Monte, CA) (119,120) was developed to overcome the problem of excess CO_2 production that occurs when HCO_3^- is added to the highly buffered solutions that comprise the body fluids. Carbicarb is a mixture of 0.33 M Na_2CO_3 and 0.33 M $NaHCO_3$. When Na_2CO_3 is added to a solution in which CO_2 and H_2O are freely available, one CO_2 molecule is consumed for every two HCO_3^- molecules produced. When these HCO_3^- molecules titrate H^+ from nonbicarbonate buffers, two molecules of CO_2 are generated. Hence, Carbicarb has the same alkalinizing capacity in physiological situations as $NaHCO_3^-$ but produces only two-thirds the amount of CO_2. When Carbicarb is administered under conditions in which relatively little HCO_3^- is likely to be titrated, CO_2 will be consumed, whereas when endogenous acid production is heightened and/or systemic acidosis is severe, CO_2 will be generated, but in lesser amounts than with an equivalent buffering load of $NaHCO_3^-$. Despite this theoretical advantage, Carbicarb has only a limited place as a base replacement, because the extra CO_2 generated by $NaHCO_3$ as compared to Carbicarb is trivial and is readily excreted by the lungs.

tris-Hydroxymethyl Aminomethane [$(CH_2OH)_3$ C–NH_2]

tris-Hydroxymethyl aminomethane is a biologically inert amino alcohol of low toxicity that buffers CO_2 and acids (121). It rapidly distributes through the extracellular space, slowly enters cells except hepatocytes and erythrocytes, and is excreted by the kidney in its protonated form (122). It supplements the buffering capacity of HCO_3^- by accepting a proton without producing CO_2, and can actually reduce PCO_2 by accepting a proton from carbonic acid and thereby producing a new HCO_3^-. Because of its capacity to raise HCO_3^- without increasing PCO_2, it has become a popular choice for treating the mixed metabolic and respiratory acidosis (123) commonly seen in patients with multiple organ failure or acute lung injury (123). There have been no controlled trials to compare its effectiveness with other base replacement strategies. Its adverse effects include respiratory depression, hypoglycemia, and hyperkalemia. It is administered as a 0.3 M solution in a dose of (0.3 × body weight (kg) × (desired HCO_3^- – observed HCO_3^-) mmol.

Increasing Lactate Utilization (Table 7)

Dichloroacetate

Dichloroacetate is a potent stimulator of pyruvate dehydrogenase (PDC), the rate-limiting enzyme for the aerobic oxidation of pyruvate, lactate, and glucose. When given parenterally, it acts within minutes. It increases pyruvate dehydrogenase activity by maintaining it in its unphosphorylated, catalytically active form (124). Thus, it enhances pyruvate oxidation and facilitates the removal of lactate and alanine (125). It has numerous other metabolic effects, described in an excellent review (126). In humans, DCA transiently reduces blood lactate concentrations (125,127), increases cardiac index, decreases peripheral vascular resistance, and increases O_2 availability (127). Similar effects occur in subjects with angina and coronary artery disease (128). However, despite limiting the increase in blood lactate concentrations during exercise, DCA neither increased muscle blood flow or oxygen availability, nor improved exercise tolerance in subjects with heart failure (129). Dichloroacetate has been used successfully in the treatment of both experimental and clinical lactic acidosis. In animals with type A or B lactic acidosis, DCA decreased production and increased hepatic extraction of lactate as well as improving blood pressure (130–132). Dichloroacetate lowers blood lactate concentrations in patients with several forms of CLA (133,134) and also in acquired forms associated with sepsis, cancer, hepatic or renal disease, or multiple disorders (135,136). Following an observational study of DCA in which 80% of patients had a decreased blood lactate in 6 hr, a controlled trial was undertaken in patients with lactate > 5 mmol/L and pH < 7.35 or base deficit > 6 mEq/L (104). Dichloroacetate was given in two doses 50 mg/kg over 30 min 2 hr apart. Blood lactate was reduced and blood pH increased in those given DCA. Of those with blood lactate > 8.9 mmol/L, the DCA group had 58% and control group 43% resolution. However, there was no effect on systolic blood pressure, cardiac output, or survival in either normotensive or hypotensive patients. Seventy percent of those with presenting blood pressure < 90 mmHg were dead within 24 hr. Although arterial pH was improved in the treatment group, there was no impact on survival. These findings reinforce the view that the acidosis is a marker of the severity of the condition, not the cause of it, and that it is not the primary determinant of outcome.

Dichloroacetate has been tested in a randomized controlled trial of children with plasma lactate > 5 mmol/L in association with severe malaria. Although there was no difference in survival, plasma lactate decreased promptly in the DCA group and remained lower than the control group for the first 4 hr. Dichloroacetate was also used in a controlled trial to prevent the lactic acidosis that accompanies liver transplantation. Two doses of 40 mg/kg, one after anesthesia and one 4 hr later, attenuated the rise in blood lactate, reduced the bicarbonate requirements, and incidence of hypernatremia. It has been used in some situations in CLA.

Although chronic use of DCA has resulted in serious neurological side effects (131), this does not appear to be a problem in the management of acute lactic acidosis. The most commonly used dosage for acute treatment in adults is 50 mg/kg mixed in 50 ml of isotonic saline and infused intravenously over 30 min. Repeat doses can be given to responders at 2 and 4 hr and then at 12-hr intervals as long as the blood lactate concentration remains above 5 mmol/L.

Treatment Summary

The principles of management involve treatment of causes, reversal of consequences, and prevention of recurrence by ensuring adequate oxygen delivery to tissues, prompt recognition and correction of the underlying conditions including addressing disease-specific issues, containing the acidosis, and considering pharmacological measures to increase lactate utilization. If containing the acidosis becomes necessary, base can be given as intravenous infusions of isotonic $NaHCO_3$ or THAM when small quantities are required. Intermittent or CRRT provide a very efficient way to deliver large quantities of base, until the underlying disorder is resolved, while maintaining normal tonicity and volume as well as removing anions and other toxins, even though this strategy will usually result in continued lactic acid generation. Of all the treatments available, CRRT appear to be the most useful although systematic testing of these therapies has not yet occurred.

REFERENCES

1. Kreisberg RA. Lactate homeostasis and lactic acidosis. Ann Intern Med 1980; 92:227–237.
2. Kreisberg RA. Glucose–lactate interrelations in man. N Engl J Med 1972; 287:132.
3. Halperin ML. Factors that control the effect of pH on glycolysis in leukocytes. J Biol Chem 1969; 244:4110.
4. Trivedi B, Danforth WH. Effect of pH on the kinetics of frog muscle phosphofructokinase. J Biol Chem 1966; 241:4110–4112.
5. James JH, Fang CH, Schrantz SJ, Hasselgren PO, Paul RJ, Fischer JE. Linkage of aerobic glycolysis to sodium–potassium transport in rat skeletal muscle. Implications for increased muscle lactate production in sepsis. J Clin Invest 1996; 98:2388–2397.
6. James JH, Luchette FA, McCarter FD, Fischer JE. Lactate is an unreliable indicator of tissue hypoxia in injury or sepsis. Lancet 1999; 354:505–508.
7. Orringer CE, Eustace JC, Wunsch CD, Gardner LB. Natural history of lactic acidosis after grand-mal seizures. A model for the study of an anion-gap acidosis not associated with hyperkalemia. N Engl J Med 1977; 297:796–799.
8. Daniel AM, Shizgal HM, MacLean LD. The anatomic and metabolic source of lactate in shock. Surg Gynecol Obstet 1978; 147:697–700.
9. Rowell LB, Kraning KK II, Evans TO, Kennedy JW, Blackmon JR, Kusumi F. Splanchnic removal of lactate and pyruvate during prolonged exercise in man. J Appl Physiol 1966; 21:1773–1783.
10. Berry MN. The liver and lactic acidosis. Proc R Soc Med 1967; 60:52.

11. Hermansen L, Stensvold I. Production and removal of lactate during exercise in man. Acta Physiol Scand 1972; 86:191–201.
12. Relman AS. Metabolic consequences of acid–base disorders. Kidney Int 1972; 1:347–359.
13. Hood VL, Tannen RL. Protection of acid–base balance by pH regulation of acid production. N Engl J Med 1998; 339:819–826.
14. Hood VL, Tannen RL. Regulation of acid production in ketoacidosis and lactic acidosis. Diabetes Metab Rev 1989; 5:393–409.
15. Jones NL, Sutton JR, Taylor R, Toews CJ. Effect of pH on cardiorespiratory and metabolic response to exercise. J Appl Physiol 1977; 43:959–964.
16. Hood VL, Danforth E Jr, Horton ES, Tannen RL. Impact of hydrogen ion on fasting ketogenesis: feedback regulation of acid production. Am J Physiol 1982; 242:F238–F245..
17. Hood VL, Keller U, Haymond MW, Kury D. Systemic pH modifies ketone body production rates and lipolysis in humans. Am J Physiol 1990; 259:E327–E334.
18. Arieff AI, Park R, Leach WJ, Lazarowitz VC. Pathophysiology of experimental lactic acidosis in dogs. Am J Physiol 1980; 239:F135–F142.
19. Arieff AI, Graf H. Pathophysiology of type A hypoxic lactic acidosis in dogs. Am J Physiol 1987; 253:E271–E276.
20. Mencken HL. Prejudices. Exeunt Omnes. New York: Borzoi, 1920:180–193.
21. Stacpoole PW. Lactic acidosis: the case against bicarbonate therapy. Ann Intern Med 1986; 105:276–279.
22. Allen DG, Orchard CH. Myocardial contractile function during ischemia and hypoxia. Circ Res 1987; 60:153–168.
23. Vanden Hoek TL, Shao Z, Changqing LI, Zak R, Schumacker PT, Becker LB. Reperfusion injury in cardiac myocytes after simulated ischemia. Am Physiol Soc 1996; 270:1334–1341.
24. Levitsky J, Gurell D, Frishman WH. Sodium ion/hydrogen ion exchange inhibition: a new pharmacologic approach to myocardial ischemia and reperfusion injury. J Clin Pharmacol 1998; 38:887–897.
25. Wasserman K. Coupling of external to cellular respiration during exercise: the wisdom of the body revisited. Am J Physiol 1994; 266:E519–E539.
26. Mitchell JH, Wildenthal K, Johnson RL Jr. The effects of acid–base disturbances on cardiovascular and pulmonary function. Kidney Int 1972; 1: 375–389.
27. Kraut JA, Kurtz I. Use of base in the treatment of severe acidemic states. Am J Kidney Dis 2001; 38:703–727.
28. Wildenthal K, Mierzwiak DS, Myers RW, Mitchell JH. Effects of acute lactic acidosis on left ventricular performance. Am J Physiol 1968; 214: 1352–1359.
29. Teplinsky K, O'Toole M, Olman M, Walley KR, Wood LD. Effect of lactic acidosis on canine hemodynamics and left ventricular function. Am J Physiol 1990; 258:H1193–H1199.
30. Stacpoole PW, Wright EC, Baumgartner TG, et al. Natural history and course of acquired lactic acidosis in adults. DCA–Lactic Acidosis Study Group. Am J Med 1994; 97:47–54..

31. Robinson BH. The metabolic and molecular bases of inherited disease. In: Shriver CR, Beaudet AL, Sly WS, Valle D, eds. Lactic Acidemia (Disorders of Pyruvate Carboxylase, Pyruvate Dehydrogenase). New York: McGraw-Hill, 1995:1479–1499.

32. Shoffner JM, Wallace DC. The metabolic and molecular bases of inherited disease. In: Scriver CR, Beaudet AL, Sly, WS, Valle D, eds. Oxidative Phosphorylation Diseases. New York: McGraw-Hill, 1995:1535–1609.

33. Neiberger RE, George JC, Perkins LA, Theriaque DW, Hutson AD, Stacpoole PW. Renal manifestations of congenital lactic acidosis. Am J Kidney Dis 2002; 39:12–23.

34. Dahlquist NR, Perrault J, Callaway CW, Jones JD. D-Lactic acidosis and encephalopathy after jejunoileostomy: response to overfeeding and to fasting in humans. Mayo Clin Pro 1984; 59:141–145.

35. Iberti TJ, Leibowitz AB, Papadakos PJ, Fischer EP. Low sensitivity of the anion gap as a screen to detect hyperlactatemia in critically ill patients. Crit Care Med 1990; 18:275–277.

36. O'Connor LR, Klein KL, Bethune JE. Hyperphosphatemia in lactic acidosis. N Engl J Med 1977; 297:707–709.

37. Yu T. Effect of sodium lactate infusion on urate clearance in man. Proc Soc Exp Biol Med 1957; 96:809.

38. Cohen RD. Clinical and biochemical aspects of lactic acidosis. Oxford: Blackwell Scientific Publications, 1976.

39. Kreisberg RA. Pathogenesis and management of lactic acidosis. Annu Rev Med 1984; 35:181–193.

40. Hotchkiss RS, Karl IE. Reevaluation of the role of cellular hypoxia and bioenergetic failure in sepsis. J Am Med Assoc 1992; 267:1503–1510.

41. Medalle R, Webb R, Waterhouse C. Lactic acidosis and associated hypoglycemia. Arch Intern Med 1971; 128:273–278.

42. Huckabee WE. Abnormal resting blood lactate: II lactic acidosis. Am J Med 1961; 30:840.

43. Kirschenbaum LA, Astiz ME, Rackow EC. Interpretation of blood lactate concentrations in patients with sepsis. Lancet 1998; 352:921–922.

44. Koch T, Geiger S, Ragaller MJ. Monitoring of organ dysfunction in sepsis/systemic inflammatory response syndrome: novel strategies. J Am Soc Nephrol 2001; 12(suppl 17):S53–S59.

45. Landry DW, Oliver JA. The pathogenesis of vasodilatory shock. N Engl J Med 2001; 345:588–595.

46. Vary TC, Siegel JH, Rivkind A. Clinical and therapeutic significance of metabolic patterns of lactic acidosis. Perspect Crit Care 1988; 1:85–132.

47. Abramson D, Scalea TM, Hitchcock R, Trooskin SZ, Henry SM, Greenspan J. Lactate clearance and survival following injury. J Trauma 1993; 35:584–588; discussion 588–589.

48. DiMuetter RC, Shreeve WW. Converstion of ddl-lactate-2-C_{14} or -3-C_{14} pyruvate-2-C_{14} to blood glucose in humans: effects of diabetes, insulin, tolbutamide, and glucose load. J Clin Invest 1963; 42:525–533.

49. Wahren J, Hagenfeldt, L, Felig P. Splanchnic and leg exchange of glucose, amino acids and free fatty acids during exercise in diabetes mellitus. J Clin Invest 1975; 55:1303–1314.

50. Mulhausen R, Eichenholz A, Blumentals A. Acid–base disturbances in patients with cirrhosis of the liver. Medicine (Baltimore) 1967; 46:185–189.

51. Kruse JA, Zaidi SA, Carlson RW. Significance of blood lactate levels in critically ill patients with liver disease. Am J Med 1987; 83:77–82.

52. Shangraw RE, Rabkin JM, Lopaschuk GD. Hepatic pyruvate dehydrogenase activity in humans: effect of cirrhosis, transplantation, and dichloroacetate. Am J Physiol 1998; 274:G569–G577.

53. Heinig RE, Clarke EF, Waterhouse C. Lactic acidosis and liver disease. Arch Intern Med 1979; 139:1229–1232.

54. Record CO, Iles RA, Cohen RD, Williams R. Acid–base and metabolic disturbances in fulminant hepatic failure. Gut 1975; 16:144–149.

55. Sillos EM, Shenep JL, Burghen GA, Pui CH, Behm FG, Sandlund JT. Lactic acidosis: a metabolic complication of hematologic malignancies: case report and review of the literature. Cancer 2001; 92:2237–2246.

56. Fraley DS, Adler S, Bruns FJ, Zett B. Stimulation of lactate production by administration of bicarbonate in a patient with a solid neoplasm and lactic acidosis. N Engl J Med 1980; 303:1100–1102.

57. Fields AL, Wolman SL, Halperin ML. Chronic lactic acidosis in a patient with cancer: therapy and metabolic consequences. Cancer 1981; 47:2026–2029.

58. Chattha G, Arieff AI, Cummings C, Tierney LM Jr. Lactic acidosis complicating the acquired immunodeficiency syndrome. Ann Intern Med 1993; 118:37–39.

59. Mhiri C, Baudrimont M, Bonne G, et al. Zidovudine myopathy: a distinctive disorder associated with mitochondrial dysfunction. Ann Neurol 1991; 29:606–614..

60. Miller KD, Cameron M, Wood LV, Dalakas MC, Kovacs JA. Lactic acidosis and hepatic steatosis associated with use of stavudine: report of four cases. Ann Intern Med 2000; 133:192–196.

61. Boubaker K, Flepp M, Sudre P, et al. Hyperlactatemia and antiretroviral therapy: the Swiss HIV Cohort Study. Clin Infect Dis 2001; 33:1931–1937.

62. Medina DJ, Tsai CH, Hsiung GD, Cheng YC. Comparison of mitochondrial morphology, mitochondrial DNA content, and cell viability in cultured cells treated with three anti-human immunodeficiency virus dideoxynucleosides. Antimicrob Agents Chemother 1994; 38:1824–1828.

63. Gennari FJ. Acid–base homeostasis in end-stage renal disease. Semin Dial 1996; 9:404–411.

64. Dixon S, McKean WI, Pryor JE, Irvine ROH. Changes in acid–base balance during peritoneal dialysis with fluid containing lactate ions. Clin Sci 1970; 39:51–60.

65. Khan IH, Catto GRD, MacLeod AM. Severe lactic acidosis in patient receiving continuous ambulatory peritoneal dialysis. BMJ 1993; 307:1056–1057.

66. Cross H, Clarke K, Opie LH, Radda GK. Is lactate-induced myocardial ischaemic injury mediated by decreased pH or increased intracellular lactate? J Mol Cell Cardiol 1995; 27:1369–1381.

67. Druml W. Metabolic aspects of continuous renal replacement therapies. Kidney Int Suppl 1999; 72:S56–S61.
68. Mohacsi P, Pedrazzinia G, Tanner H, Tschanz HU, Hullin R, Carrel T. Lactic acidosis following heart transplantation: a common phenomenon? Eur J Heart Fail 2002; 4:175–179.
69. Shangraw RE, Winter R, Hromco J, Robinson ST, Gallaher EJ. Amelioration of lactic acidosis with dichloroacetate during liver transplantation in humans. Anesthesiology 1994; 81:1127–1138.
70. Madias NE, Goorno WE, Herson S. Severe lactic acidosis as a presenting feature of pheochromocytoma. Am J Kidney Dis 1987; 10:250–253.
71. Jonsson S, O'Meara M, Young JB. Acute cocaine poisoning. Importance of treating seizures and acidosis. Am J Med 1983; 75:1061–1064.
72. Appel D, Rubenstein R, Schrager K, Williams MH Jr. Lactic acidosis in severe asthma. Am J Med 1983; 75:580–584.
73. Prakash S, Mehta S. Lactic acidosis in asthma: report of two cases and review of the literature. Can Respir J 2002; 9:203–208.
74. Steiner D, Williams RH. Respiratory inhibition and hypoglycemia by biguanides and decamethylenediguanide. Biochim Biophys Acta 1958; 30:329.
75. Dembo AJ, Marliss EB, Halperin ML. Insulin therapy in phenformin-associated lactic acidosis; a case report, biochemical considerations and review of the literature. Diabetes 1975; 24:28–35.
76. Phillips PJ, Scicchitano R, Clarkson AR, Gilmore HR. Metformin associated lactic acidosis. Aust N Z J Med 1978; 8:281–284.
77. Stang M, Wysowski DK, Butler-Jones D. Incidence of lactic acidosis in metformin users. Diabetes Care 1999; 22:925–927.
78. Misbin RI, Green L, Stadel BV, Gueriguian JL, Gubbi A, Fleming GA. Lactic acidosis in patients with diabetes treated with metformin. N Engl J Med 1998; 338:265–266.
79. Cusi K, DeFronzo RA. Metformin: a review of its metabolic effects. Diabetes Rev 1998; 6:89–131.
80. Salpeter S, Greyber E, Pasternak G, Salpeter E. Risk of fatal and nonfatal lactic acidosis with metformin use in type 2 diabetes mellitus (Cochrane Review). Cochrane Database Syst Rev 2002; 2.
81. Lalau JD, Christian Lacroix, Patricia Compagnon, Bertrand de Cagny, Jean P. Rigaud, et al. Role of metformin accumulation in metformin-associated lactic acidosis. Diabetes Care 1995; 18:779–784.
82. McKenzie R, Fried MW, Sallie R, et al. Hepatic failure and lactic acidosis due to fialuridine (FIAU), an investigational nucleoside analogue for chronic hepatitis B. N Engl J Med 1995; 333:1099–1105.
83. Kreisberg RA, Owen WC, Siegel AM. Ethanol-induced hyperlactic-acidemia: inhibition of lactate utilization. J Clin Invest 1971; 50:166–174.
84. Fulop M. Alcoholism, ketoacidosis, and lactic acidosis. Diabetes Metab Rev 1989; 5:365–378.
85. Lacouture PG, Wason S, Abrams A, Lovejoy FH Jr. Acute isopropyl alcohol intoxication. Diagnosis and management. Am J Med 1983; 75:680–686.
86. Gabow PA, Clay K, Sullivan JB, Lepoff R. Organic acids in ethylene glycol intoxication. Ann Intern Med 1986; 105:16–20.

87. Morgan TJ, Clark C, Clague A. Artifactual elevation of measured plasma L-lactate concentration in the presence of glycolate. Crit Care Med 1999; 27: 2177–2179.
88. Cate JCT, Hedrick R. Propylene glycol intoxication and lactic acidosis. N Engl J Med 1980; 303:1237.
89. Kelner MJ, Bailey DN. Propylene glycol as a cause of lactic acidosis. J Anal Toxicol 1985; 9:40–42.
90. Parker MG, Fraser GL, Watson DM, Riker RR. Removal of propylene glycol and correction of increased osmolar gap by hemodialysis in a patient on high dose lorazepam infusion therapy. Intensive Care Med 2002; 28:81–84.
91. Demey HE, Daelemans RA, Verpooten GA, et al. Propylene glycol-induced side effects during intravenous nitroglycerin therapy. Intensive Care Med 1988; 14:221–226.
92. Fligner CL, Jack R, Twiggs GA, Raisys VA. Hyperosmolality induced by propylene glycol. A complication of silver sulfadiazine therapy. J Am Med Assoc 1985; 253:1606–1609.
93. Gabow PA, Anderson RJ, Potts DE, Schrier RW. Acid–base disturbances in the salicylate-intoxicated adult. Arch Intern Med 1978; 138:1481–1484.
94. Eicherholz A, Mulhauser RO, Redlead PS. Nature of acid–base disturbance in salicylate intoxication. Metabolism 1963; 12:164–174.
95. Bernal W, Donaldson N, Wyncoll D, Wendon J. Blood lactate as an early predictor of outcome in paracetamol-induced acute liver failure: a cohort study. Lancet 2002; 359:558–563.
96. Keller U, Mall T, Walter M, Bertel O, Mihatsch JM, Ritz R. Phaeochromocytoma with lactic acidosis. Br Med J 1978; 2:606–607.
97. Velez RJ, Myers B, Guber MS. Severe acute metabolic acidosis (acute beriberi): an avoidable complication of total parenteral nutrition. JPEN J Parenter Enteral Nutr 1985; 9:216–219.
98. Romanski SA, McMahon MM. Metabolic acidosis and thiamine deficiency. Mayo Clin Proc 1999; 74:259–263.
99. Attas M, Hanley HG, Stultz D, Jones MR, McAllister RG. Fulminant beriberi heart disease with lactic acidosis: presentation of a case with evaluation of left ventricular function and review of pathophysiologic mechanisms. Circulation 1978; 58:566–572.
100. Oh MS, Phelps KR, Traube M, Barbosa-Saldivar JL, Boxhill C, Carroll HJ. D-Lactic acidosis in a man with the short-bowel syndrome. N Engl J Med 1979; 301:249–252.
101. Traube M, Bock JL, Boyer JL. D-Lactic acidosis after jejunoileal bypass: identification of organic anions by nuclear magnetic resonance spectroscopy. Ann Intern Med 1983; 98:171–173.
102. Stacpoole PW. Lactic acidosis and other mitochondrial disorders. Metabolism 1997; 46:306–321.
103. Kerr DS. Lactic acidosis and mitochondrial disorders. Clin Biochem 1991; 24:331–336.
104. Stacpoole PW, Wright EC, Baumgartner TG, et al. A controlled clinical trial of dichloroacetate for treatment of lactic acidosis in adults. The Dichloroacetate–Lactic Acidosis Study Group. N Engl J Med 1992; 327:1564–1569.

105. Day NP, Phu NH, Bethell DP, et al. The effects of dopamine and adrenaline infusions on acid–base balance and systemic haemodynamics in severe infection. Lancet 1996; 348:219–223.

106. Rivers E, Nguyen B, Havstad S, et al. Early goal-directed therapy in the treatment of severe sepsis and septic shock. N Engl J Med 2001; 345:1368–1377.

107. Cooper DJ, Walley KR, Wiggs BR, Russell JA. Bicarbonate does not improve hemodynamics in critically ill patients who have lactic acidosis. A prospective, controlled clinical study. Ann Intern Med 1990; 112:492–498.

108. Mathieu D, Neviere R, Billard V, Fleyfel M, Wattel F. Effects of bicarbonate therapy on hemodynamics and tissue oxygenation in patients with lactic acidosis: a prospective, controlled clinical study. Crit Care Med 1991; 19: 1352–1356.

109. Graf H, Leach W, Arieff AI. Evidence for a detrimental effect of bicarbonate therapy in hypoxic lactic acidosis. Science 1985; 227:754–756.

110. Levraut J, Labib Y, Chave S, Payan P, Raucoules-Aime M, Grimaud D. Effect of sodium bicarbonate on intracellular pH under different buffering conditions. Kidney Int 1996; 49:1262–1267.

111. Levraut J, Giunti C, Ciebiera JP, et al. Initial effect of sodium bicarbonate on intracellular pH depends on the extracellular nonbicarbonate buffering capacity. Crit Care Med 2001; 29:1033–1039.

112. Cuhaci B, Lee J, Ahmed Z. Sodium bicarbonate and intracellular acidosis: myth or reality? Crit Care Med 2001; 29:1088–1090.

113. Madias NE. Lactic acidosis. Kidney Int 1986; 29:752–774.

114. Narins RG, Cohen JJ. Bicarbonate therapy for organic acidosis: the case for its continued use. Ann Intern Med 1987; 106:615–618.

115. Forsythe SM, Schmidt GA. Sodium bicarbonate for the treatment of lactic acidosis. Chest 2000; 117:260–267.

116. Gudis SM, Mangi S, Feinroth M, Rubin JE, Friedman EA, Berlyne GM. Rapid correction of severe lactic acidosis with massive isotonic bicarbonate infusion and simultaneous ultrafiltration. Nephron 1983; 33:65–66.

117. Hilton PJ, Taylor J, Forni LG, Treacher DF. Bicarbonate-based haemofiltration in the management of acute renal failure with lactic acidosis. QJM 1998; 91:279–283.

118. Honore PM, Jamez J, Wauthier M, et al. Prospective evaluation of short-term, high-volume isovolemic hemofiltration on the hemodynamic course and outcome in patients with intractable circulatory failure resulting from septic shock. Crit Care Med 2000; 28:3581–3587.

119. Filley GF, Kindig NB. Carbicarb, an alkalinizing ion-generating agent of possible clinical usefulness. Trans Am Clin Climatol Assoc 1984; 96:141–153.

120. Bersin RM, Arieff AI. Improved hemodynamic function during hypoxia with Carbicarb, a new agent for the management of acidosis. Circulation 1988; 77:227–233.

121. Nahas GG, Sutin KM, Fermon C, et al. Guidelines for the treatment of acidaemia with THAM. Drugs 1998; 55:191–224.

122. Brasch H, Thies E, Iven H. Pharmacokinetics of *tris* (hydroxymethyl-)aminomethane in healthy subjects and in patients with metabolic acidosis. Eur J Clin Pharmacol 1982; 22:257–264.

123. Luchsinger PC. The use of 2-amino-2hydroxymethyl-1,3-propanediol in the management of respiratory acidosis. Ann N Y Acad Sci 1961; 92:743–750.

124. Whitehouse S, Randle PJ. Activation of pyruvate dehydrogenase in perfused rat heart by dichloroacetate. Biochem J 1973; 134:651.

125. Wells PG, Moore GW, Rabin D, Wilkinson GR, Oates JA, Stacpoole PW. Metabolic effects and pharmacokinetics of intravenously administered dichloroacetate in humans. Diabetologia 1980; 19:109–113.

126. Stacpoole PW. The pharmacology of dichloroacetate. Metabolism 1989; 38: 1124–1144.

127. Ludvik B, Peer G, Berzlanovich A, Stifter S, Graf H. Effects of dichloroacetate and bicarbonate on haemodynamic parameters in healthy volunteers. Clin Sci (Colch) 1991; 80:47–51.

128. Wargovich TJ, MacDonald RG, Hill JA, Feldman RL, Stacpoole PW, Pepine CJ. Myocardial metabolic and hemodynamic effects of dichloroacetate in coronary artery disease. Am J Cardiol 1988; 61:65–70.

129. Wilson JR, Mancini DM, Ferraro N, Egler J. Effect of dichloroacetate on the exercise performance of patients with heart failure. J Am Coll Cardiol 1988; 12:1464.

130. Park R, Arieff AI. Treatment of lactic acidosis with dichloroacetate in dogs. J Clin Invest 1982; 70:853–862.

131. Crabb DW, Yount EA, Harris RA. The metabolic effects of dichloroacetate. Metabolism 1981; 30:1024–1039.

132. Graf H, Leach W, Arieff AI. Effects of dichloroacetate in the treatment of hypoxic lactic acidosis in dogs. J Clin Invest 1985; 76:919–923.

133. Aynsley-Green A, Weindling AM, Soltesz G, Ross B, Jenkins PA. Dichloroacetate in the treatment of congenital lactic acidosis. J Inherit Metab Dis 1984; 7:26.

134. Kuroda Y, Ito M, Toshima K, et al. Treatment of chronic congenital lactic acidosis by oral administration of dichloroacetate. J Inherit Metab Dis 1986; 9:244–252.

135. Stacpoole PW, Harman EM, Curry SH, Baumgartner TG, Misbin RI. Treatment of lactic acidosis with dichloroacetate. N Engl J Med 1983; 309:390–396.

136. Stacpoole PW, Lorenz AC, Thomas RG, Harman EM. Dichloroacetate in the treatment of lactic acidosis. Ann Intern Med 1988; 108:58–63.

137. Cohen RD. Some acid problems. J R Coll Physicians Lond 1982; 16:69.

138. Park R, Arieff AI. Lactic acidosis. Adv Intern Med 1980; 25:33–68.

Toxin-Induced Metabolic Acidosis

Man S. Oh

Department of Medicine, State University of New York, Health Science Center at Brooklyn, Brooklyn, New York, U.S.A.

Mitchell L. Halperin

Division of Nephrology, St.Michael's Hospital, University of Toronto, Toronto, Canada

INTRODUCTION

In this chapter, we discuss metabolic acidosis caused by drugs and toxins. Because drugs become toxins when their unwanted side effects become a clinical problem, the distinction between drugs and toxins is not always clear. Recommended doses can be toxic to some while being therapeutic to others. Some of the chemicals included in this chapter, such as ethylene glycol, methanol, and toluene, are clearly toxins because they have no approved therapeutic utility for humans. On the other hand, some chemicals, such as salicylic acid, are drugs approved for human use. They become toxins only when an excessive amount is given. Ethanol is not included in this chapter even though metabolic acidosis can occur when excessive amounts are consumed. Alcoholic ketoacidosis is discussed in Chapter 10.

The majority of the chemicals to be discussed belong to the alcohol family. One nonalcohol chemical, toluene, is oxidized to form an alcohol soon. On the basis of their relative frequency of use and morbidity, five toxins are discussed in some detail: salicylic acid, ethylene glycol, methanol, toluene, and acetaminophen. The remainder will be discussed briefly in two groups: toxins associated with lactic acidosis and uncommon

Table 1 Toxin-Associated Acid–Base Disorders

Toxins	Acid–base disorder	Putative metabolites/ causes
Salicylate	Respiratory alkalosis High anion gap metabolic acidosis	Effects on CNS, β-hydroxybutyric acid, L-lactic acid
Ethylene glycol	High anion gap metabolic acidosis	Glycolic acid, L-lactic acid
Methanol	High anion gap metabolic acidosis	Formic acid, L-lactic acid
Toluene	Hyperchloremic metabolic acidosis	Hippuric acid, benzoic acid
Acetaminophen	High anion gap metabolic acidosis	L-lactic acid, pyroglutamic acid
Nucleoside analogs	High anion gap metabolic acidosis	L-lactic acid
Isoniazid	High anion gap metabolic acidosis	L-lactic acid
Tricyclic antidepressants	High anion gap metabolic acidosis	L-lactic acid
Benzyl alcohol	Hyperchloremic metabolic acidosis	Hippuric acid, benzoic acid
Propylene glycol	High anion gap metabolic acidosis	L-lactic acid, D-lactic acid
Diethylene glycol	High anion gap metabolic acidosis	2-hydroxyethoxyacetic acid, L-lactic acid
Paraldehyde	High anion gap metabolic acidosis	β-hydroxybutyric acid, L-lactic acid

toxins. A summary of the toxins discussed in this chapter is presented in Table 1.

MAJOR TOXINS

Salicylic Acid

Salicylic acid can only be used externally in its natural form (Fig. 1). The most widely used salicylate derivative is aspirin (acetylsalicylic acid), which is an acetyl ester of the phenolic group (molecular weight 180 Da). The pK of aspirin is 3.5, and that of salicylic acid 3.0 (1).

Pharmacology

Salicylate is absorbed for the most part in the upper small bowel (1,2). Its absorption occurs primarily by passive diffusion of undissociated salicylic

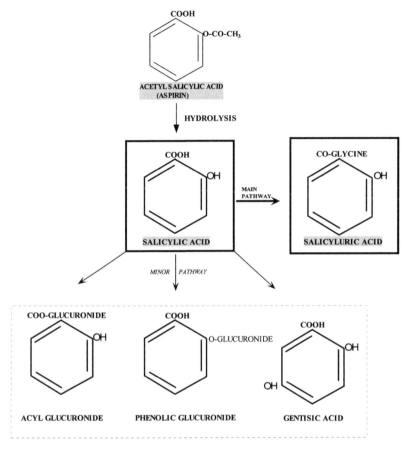

Figure 1 Metabolism of salicylate. Acetylsalicylic acid (ASA) can be absorbed intact. It is rapidly hydrolyzed by esterases and the acetyl moiety acetylates (AC) proteins in platelets or COX, inhibiting production of prostaglandins. Much of ASA is hydrolyzed before entering the systemic circulation. The main pathway of the metabolism of salicylic acid is a conjugation reaction with glycine to form salicyluric acid, which is rapidly excreted by the kidney. This pathway is saturated in toxicity. A conjugation reaction with glucuronide is a minor pathway.

acid. Substantial absorption occurs in the intestine (2). Rectal absorption is slower than oral absorption. It is also absorbed through the intact skin (3). The anti-inflammatory effects of aspirin are mediated through inhibition of cyclo-oxygenase (COX), caused by acetylation of specific amino acids on the enzyme, thereby inhibiting prostaglandin synthesis (4–6). As a result, most of the pharmacological effects attributed to salicylate derivatives, such as the antipyretic and antiplatelet actions, are expected only with aspirin, which contains the acetyl ester (Fig. 1). The antipyretic effect of salicylates also depends on the ability to inhibit prostaglandin synthesis, and hence binding to prostaglandin E receptor subtype EP3 (9). Acetylsalicylate is rapidly hydrolyzed to salicylate by esterases in the gastrointestinal mucosa, liver, and plasma (2) (Fig. 1). Inhibition of cyclo-oxygenease in platelets prevents thromboxane synthesis (6).

Excretion of salicylate occurs largely in the form of a conjugate product with glycine (salicyluric acid) (75%). The availability of glycine does not appear to be a limiting factor in salicyluric acid formation. About 10% of salicylate is excreted as free salicylate (2). Salicylate is extensively bound to plasma proteins primarily to albumin. The volume of distribution of salicylate is about 0.2 L/kg body weight, except at high doses because of saturation of binding sites on plasma proteins, especially albumin (1,2).

The plasma half-life of salicylate at low doses is 2–3 hr, 12 hr at therapeutic doses, and 15–30 hr at toxic levels (2). Administration of 2.4 g of aspirin per day results in excretion of 67% as salicyluric acid; with 7.2 g administered, only 40% appears as salicyluric acid (1). Clearance of salicyluric acid, salicylic acid glucuronide, and salicylic phenolic glucuronide is close to that of para-aminohippurate (PAH) (2); these clearances are reduced by probenecid.

Unbound salicylate is filtered freely by the glomerulus. Reabsorption appears to occcur by nonionic diffusion of the undissociated acid. As a result, reabsorption decreases as urine pH rises. At a urine pH < 6.0, clearance of salicylate is 5–15% of creatinine clearance; at a urine pH of 8.0, salicylate clearance rises to 180% of creatinine clearance, indicating tubular secretion (2).

Transcellular movement of salicylate occurs by diffusion of undissociated salicylic acid. At equilibrium, the concentration of this form is equal in the cell and in the extracellular fluid (ECF) compartment (7). Metabolic acidosis increases intracellular salicylate concentration, presumably by favoring entry of the undissociated form into cells, thereby increasing its toxicity (Fig. 2).

Metabolic Effects

Uncoupling Oxidative Phosphorylation: Salicylate acts like the well-known uncoupler of oxidative phosphorylation, 2,4-dinitro phenol, reducing ATP production per O_2 consumed (8). Hypoglycemia is common with salicylate intoxication (9), an effect likely due to increased glucose utilization by the brain and/or impaired gluconeogenesis (10). In response to brain hypoglycemia, counter-regulatory hormones are released, stimulating glycogenolysis and gluconeogenesis. Systemic hypoglycemia occurs after the glycogen store in the liver is exhausted. In one case report (11), 125 g of glucose were administered over 5 hr to treat hypoglycemia, suggesting that glucose consumption by the brain could increase as much as five-fold. Salicylate, while an antipyretic, can cause fever, probably because of its

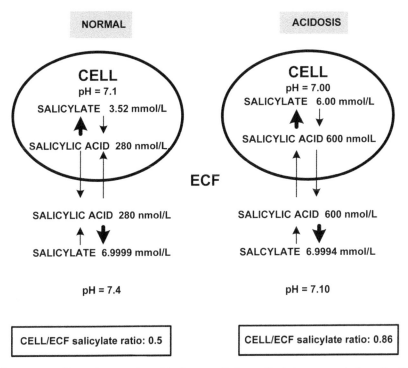

Figure 2 Effect of systemic acidosis on cellular salicylate accumulation. In the example shown, salicylate concentration in the ECF is 7 mmol/L. At the pH of the body fluid, only a tiny fraction is in the form of undissociated salicylic acid (note the concentrations of this species are in nanomoles per liter). This is the form that diffuses across cell membranes and at equilibrium its concentration in cells equals that in the ECF. In the cell, protons from salicylic acid are immediately buffered, and the quantity of intracellular salicylate depends on intracellular pH. Because the ICF pH is 0.3 pH unit lower than the ECF pH under normal conditions (*left side of the figure*), the intracellular salicylate is only one-half that in the ECF at equilibrium. In the presence of metabolic acidosis (*right side of the figure*), the difference between the ECF and ICF pH is reduced and the concentration of undissociated salicylic acid rises, both events leading to increase in intracellular salicylate concentration.

uncoupling effect that increases heat production. In this regard, 2,4 dinitrophenol can also cause a fever accompanied by profuse sweating for heat dissipation (Fig. 3).

Actions on the Krebs Cycle: Salicylate inhibits the Krebs cycle at two steps, the conversion of α-ketoglutarate to succinate and the conversion of succinate to fumarate, by inhibiting α-ketoglutarate dehydrogenase and succinate dehydrogenase, respectively. Inhibition of Krebs cycle would stimu-

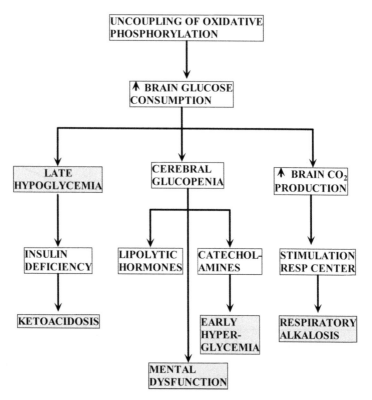

Figure 3 Pathogenesis of salicylate toxicity mediated through uncoupling of oxidative phosphorylation. If the uncoupling effect were most pronounced in the brain, it could lead to cerebral glucopenia before systemic hypoglycemia, which in turn may produce mental dysfunction as well as ketoacidosis through stimulation of the release of lipolytic hormones. Increased glucose consumption in the brain may produce cerebral respiratory acidosis while it leads to systemic respiratory alkalosis.

late lipolysis and thereby ketogenesis, and anaerobic glycolysis. Mild increases in lactic acid and ketoacid production may occur in certain patients, especially in children (12).

Acid–Base Changes

Respiratory Alkalosis: Respiratory alkalosis is the most common acid–base disorder in salicylate poisoning in adults (13,14). In one series, 78% of patients with salicylate poisoning had this disorder alone or in combination with metabolic acidosis (14). Although salicylate is thought to stimulate the central respiratory center directly (15), uncoupling of oxidative phosphorylation would increase CO_2 production and stimulate ventilation by creating a local respiratory acidosis.

Metabolic Acidosis: Children have a higher incidence of acidemia and ketonemia than adults, although adults commonly have metabolic acidosis combined with respiratory alkalosis (12–14). The pathogenesis of the metabolic acidosis is not clear. The anion gap is increased, but the contribution of salicylate anion is modest (13,14). For example, ingestion of 50 (325 mg) aspirin tablets provides only 90 mEq of H^+. Increases in lactate and ketone anions are also typically modest (13). Lactic acidosis may reflect a response to respiratory alkalosis (16). Increased ketoacid levels occur with salicylate poisoning, but rarely in excess of 5 mEq/L. A low plasma volume may increase the serum anion gap due to a higher concentration of albumin. The low serum $[HCO_3^-]$ is partly due to the secondary renal response to a low $PaCO_2$ (see Chapter 21).

Renal Urate Excretion

Although salicylate was thought to affect renal urate reabsorption and secretion depending on its concentration (Fig. 4), more recent data indicate that salicylate only affects urate reabsorption (17). When the salicylate con-

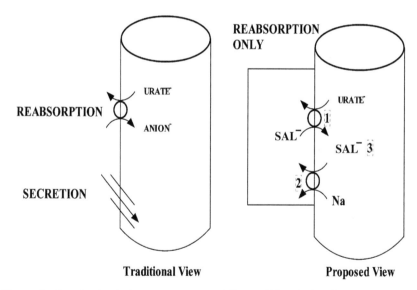

Figure 4 Proximal tubule urate transport. The traditional view is that salicylates affect both urate reabsorption and secretion (*pathways shown on left*). At low concentrations, secretion is inhibited, and at higher concentrations, reabsorption is inhibited. More recent data indicate that salicylates affect only urate reabsorption (*pathway shown on right*). At low luminal concentrations, salicylates promote urate reabsorption by acting as the organic counteranion (**3**). At high luminal concentrations, salicylates compete with urate on the anion exchanger (**1**), because reabsorption by the Na-organic anion cotransporter (**2**) is saturated.

centration in the proximal tubule epithelial cells is higher than in the proximal tubule lumen, urate reabsorption is facilitated by coupling with salicylate secretion via a specific urate-organic anion countertransporter, resulting in reduced urate excretion. When salicylate concentration is higher in the tubule lumen, by contrast, it competes with urate binding to the same urate/anion countertransporter, and thereby urate reabsorption is inhibited, resulting in increased urate excretion (Fig. 4).

Other Manifestations

Hearing loss and tinnitus are common in salicylate poisoning, but are usually completely reversed within a few days (18). Noncardiogenic pulmonary edema develops primarily in the elderly and in smokers (19); it can lead to pulmonary or cerebral edema through mechanisms yet to be defined. Death due to salicylate poisoning is caused most often by asystole or ventricular fibrillation (20). In a series of 97 patients with salicylate poisoning, 7 died; 5 due to asystole and 2 with ventricular fibrillation (21). Uncoupling of oxidative phosphorylation in the cardiac conduction system was suggested as the cause. Delayed presentation, coma, hyperpyrexia, pulmonary edema, older age, and acidemia are all associated with poor prognosis (22).

Diagnosis

Salicylate intoxication is usually suspected from the history and symptoms. Tinnitus, deafness, and hyperventilation are useful clues. Fever occurs most often in small children. Late manifestations of toxicity include lethargy progressing to confusion, coma, and seizures. Salicylate poisoning may also be caused by the application of topical salicylates because its absorption is enhanced by diseases of the skin. Urine screening for salicylates (e.g., the Trinder test) is highly sensitive but false positive tests can occur therefore it should be used with caution (23). Measurement of serum salicylate levels is now readily available and confirms the diagnosis.

Treatment

Cardiac monitoring should be instituted promptly in severe salicylate poisoning, because cardiac arrhythmias are the greatest risk to the patient (21). The goal of treatment is to reduce the intracellular concentration of salicylate by preventing gut absorption and promoting removal of any absorbed salicylate.

Remove Salicylate from the Gut: Gastric lavage along with instillation of activated charcoal can effectively remove unabsorbed salicylate from the gut. Because of delayed gastric emptying induced by aspirin and delayed absorption of enteric-coated aspirin, the stomach contents should be aspirated even 6–12 hr after ingestion (24). At the same time, activated charcoal (1 g/kg body weight) should be given. Multiple dose-activated charcoal

(MDAC) is recommended because unabsorbed salicylate can be removed by binding to charcoal when the drug enters the intestine (25). Obviously, an MDAC is without effect if absorption of salicylate is complete.

Increase Renal Excretion: Increasing urine volume and pH facilitates salicylate excretion (26,27). Forced diuresis alone has little effect, but alkaline diuresis is effective (27). The recommended treatment is to infuse 1.5 L of a 150 mEq/L $NaHCO_3$ solution over 4 hr. This therapy results in less fluid retention than saline. One should be cautious about increasing arterial pH because of continued hyperventilation; blood pH should be kept below 7.50, if possible. Sodium bicarbonate increases pH in the proximal tubule fluid and thereby diminishes the concentration of undissociated salicylic acid, reducing its reabsorption. Acetazolamide also increases salicylate excretion, even though it decreases the pH in the proximal tubule. A potential danger of acetazolamide is reduction in protein-binding of salicylate, increasing free salicylate concentration. As a result, acetazolamide is not recommended for treatment.

Remove Salicylate by Hemodialysis or Hemoperfusion: Clearances by hemoperfusion and hemodialysis are quite comparable; both are limited by protein-binding of salicylate (28). Hemodialysis is recommended when serum salicylate concentration is > 100 mg/dL, or if renal failure, fluid overload or clinical deterioration is present. Peritoneal dialysis is not effective.

Ethylene Glycol

Ethylene glycol ($OH-CH_2-CH_2-OH$) has a molecular weight of 62 Da. It is a slightly viscous, clear, and colorless liquid with a sweet taste. It has a low vapor pressure (0.05 mm Hg at 20°C). Ethylene glycol is widely used as antifreeze, in hydraulic brake fluids, as a solvent in the paint and plastics industries, and in the formulation of printers' inks, stamp pad inks, and inks for ball point pens (29).

Toxicology

Ethylene glycol poisoning occurs in suicide attempts and in accidental ingestions. The lethal dose is usually $\sim$1.4 mL/kg body weight (about 100 mL for an average size adult) (30), but survival after drinking much larger amounts has been reported (31). Ingested ethylene glycol is readily absorbed and distributes throughout body water. When its metabolism is prevented by an ethanol infusion, the half-life is approximately 17 hr (32).

Metabolism and H^+ Production

Ethylene glycol is both metabolized (Fig. 5) and excreted unchanged in the urine (32). Its low vapor pressure minimizes pulmonary excretion or loss via the skin. Ethylene glycol is converted to glycoaldehyde by alcohol dehydro-

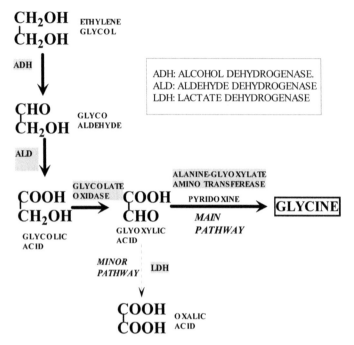

Figure 5 Metabolism of ethylene glycol. The main acid that accumulates is glycolic acid, which can be further metabolized to glyoxylic acid and then to glycine. A tiny fraction of ethylene glycol is metabolized to oxalic acid.

genase in the liver. Its affinity to this enzyme is 100-fold lower than for ethanol (33), and thus the rate of metabolism is rapid only when its concentration is high.

Glycoaldehyde is further metabolized to glycolic acid by hepatic aldehyde dehydrogenase, and glycolic acid is the main toxin that accumulates in ethylene glycol poisoning (34). Glycolic acid is converted to glyoxylic acid by glycolate oxidase, reducing NAD^+ to NADH (35). The ratio of NADH to NAD^+ is the main determinant of this reaction. Usually, the concentration of glycolate is about 10-fold greater than glyoxylate. Metabolic clearance of glycolate is quite rapid, with a half-life of ~7 hr (36,37). One percent or less of glyoxylate is converted to oxalic acid, mainly by the action of LDH. To a lesser extent, glycolate oxidase converts glyoxylate to oxalate (35). Virtually, all oxalate produced is precipitated as calcium oxalate, contributing to acute renal failure and hypocalcemia.

Oxalic and glycolic acids have different effects on the net H^+ load. If 100 mL (112 g) of ethylene glycol were metabolized to glycolic acid, 1800 mEq of H^+, a lethal acute load, would be produced. In fact, the fraction converted to glyoxylate is further converted to glycine by alanine-glyoxylate amino-transferase, resulting in removal of H^+ (35). To the extent that oxalate is produced, this substance is precipitated with Ca^{++} released from bone, also removing part of the H^+ load as alkali is released from the skeleton along with Ca^{++}. Elevated lactate levels are often observed in ethylene glycol toxicity probably because of the increased $NADH/NAD^+$ ratio (38).

Clinical Manifestations

Central nervous system (CNS) symptoms such as inebriation, ataxia, and slurred speech are the effects of ethylene glycol itself (29,30). At this stage, the serum osmolal gap (see below) is high. After a latent period of about 4–12 hr, patients develop nausea, vomiting, hyperventilation, elevated blood pressure, tachycardia, tetany, and convulsions. At this point, an increased anion gap metabolic acidosis is present (34,39). The tetany is due to hypocalcemia, possibly due to deposition of calcium oxalate crystals (36,40–43). Leukocytosis of an unknown mechanism is invariably present (29,36).

Renal failure is common and usually develops 36–48 hr after ingestion (29,30); glycoaldehyde and glyoxylic acid appear to be the main culprits (44). In patients who survive, calcium oxalate crystals can persist in the kidney for months (29). Cranial nerve palsies may be seen (45). Pathologic lesions at autopsy show calcium oxalate deposition in the vessels and meninges of the brain and kidney tubules.

Diagnosis

The diagnosis is made from the history and clinical findings as well as laboratory manifestations. Early on, CNS symptoms and increased serum osmolal gap suggest the diagnosis. Later, a high anion gap metabolic acidosis, leukocytosis, and hypocalcemia are characteristic. Calcium oxalate crystals and acute renal failure are additional clues. The kidneys might be enlarged (29) and painful on palpation. Measurements of ethylene glycol in the serum or urine confirm the diagnosis. Because enzymatic assays have false positives on rare occasions, mass spectrometry is the best way to measure ethylene glycol (46,47). A search for calcium oxalate crystals in the urine may be negative early on after ingestion (41). When present, the calcium oxalate crystals are not the usual envelope-shaped dihydrates, but rather are primarily needle-shaped monohydrates, described as spindle, cigar, hemp seed-, or prism-shaped (Fig. 6). In many reports, calcium oxalate crystals were not recognized because they were mistakenly called either uric acid or hippurate crystals (38,40–43).

The serum osmolal gap (see Chapter 28) is usually high (>10 mOsmols/kg H_2O), but may be normal if the measurement is made after ethylene glycol is almost completely metabolized (48). At that point, however, metabolic acidosis with a high anion gap is invariably present. Concomitant ingestion of alcohol (ethanol or isopropyl alcohol) delays the onset of

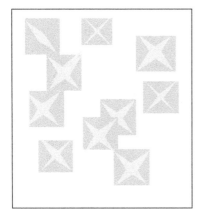 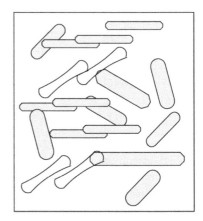

Figure 6 Calcium oxalate crystala. On the left are schematic depictions of calcium oxalate *dihydrate* crystals, which have a typical Maltese Cross appearance. On the right are depictions of calcium oxalate *monohydrate* crystals, which have an elongated appearance of either a cigar or dumbbell shape. The latter are the main crystal shapes that appear in the urine of patients with ethylene glycol poisoning.

acidosis by inhibiting ethylene glycol metabolism but will also increase the osmolal gap (49).

Treatment

Treatment is aimed at inhibiting the conversion of ethylene glycol to its toxic metabolites and removing it from the body. Its metabolism is blocked by inhibiting alcohol dehydrogenase with 4-methylpyrazole (fomepizole) (30,50), or by providing ethanol to saturate the enzyme. Ethylene glycol is removed very effectively by hemodialysis.

Fomepizole: The target level of fomepizole in humans is 100–300 µmol/L (8.6–24.6 mg/L). The loading dose is 15 mg/kg, followed by 10 mg/kg q12h for 4 doses, then 15 mg/kg q12h (because of P-450 enzyme induction) thereafter until ethylene glycol levels fall below 20 mg/dL (3 mmol/L). If fomepizole is given within 6 hr of the start of dialysis, no extra fomepizole need be given. If it is given more than 6 hr before the start of dialysis, an additional dose of fomepizole should be administered. Fomepizole is removed by hemodialysis and the dosing should be increased to q4h during treatment.

Ethanol: Maintenance of a plasma ethanol level of about 100 mg/dL (20 mmol/L; 3 mmol/L) inhibits ethylene glycol metabolism nearly completely. Administration of a bolus of 0.6 g of ethanol per kg of body weight increases its plasma level by 1 mg/mL (100 mg/dL). The maintenance dose should be equal to the expected metabolic rate, about 0.11 g/kg body weight

(51). In alcoholic patients, the rate of ethanol metabolism is about 50% higher. Clearance of ethanol by hemodialysis is about equal to that of urea. Thus, at urea clearance of 200 mL/min, the ethanol clearance would be 12 L/hr. At a plasma ethanol concentration of 100 mg/dL (22 mmol/L), dialysis would remove 12 g of ethanol hourly, which is the amount that should be added to the basic infusion rate.

Removal of Ethylene Glycol: A reduction in the level of ethylene glycol in plasma can be achieved by enhanced renal excretion through a forced diuresis, but hemodialysis (performed as a continuous therapy in the intensive care unit until the plasma level is < 20 mg/dL) is preferred because renal failure is common (37). If dialysis is not available or contraindicated, one can partially block the metabolism of ethylene glycol, with administration of 1/10 the usual dose of ethanol (0.06 g/kg), to slow its conversion to glycolic acid and then rely on subsequent conversion to glyoxylic acid, and then to glycine. Because conversion to glycine requires the enzyme alanine-glyoxylate amino-transferase with pyridoxine as a cofactor (35), supplements of vitamin B_6 (50 mg i.v. q6h) should be used (29).

Removal of Glycolate: Glycolate is concentrated in the tubular fluid (36). The possibility of "ion trapping" to enhance its excretion as with salicylate has been suggested (36). Removal of glycolate by hemodialysis is quite high (51).

Methanol

Methanol (CH_3OH), also known as methyl alcohol, carbinol, wood spirit, and wood alcohol, has a molecular weight of 32 Da, and a specific gravity of 0.79. It is used as antifreeze, as an additive to gasoline and diesel oil, and as a solvent for the manufacture of various drugs. The main source of methanol poisoning in the United States is windshield wiper fluids (52). Pure methanol has a slight alcoholic odor; crude material has a repulsive, pungent odor. Methanol has a vapor pressure of 126 mm Hg at 25°C, and 760 mm Hg at 64.8°C (its boiling point). The high vapor pressure allows elimination by evaporation through the lung and the skin, but also allows poisoning by inhalation. Ingested methanol is rapidly absorbed and distributes throughout the body water (53).

Toxicity

Methanol itself is not very toxic but its metabolic products, formaldehyde and formic acid, are. The extremely rapid metabolism to formic acid limits the accumulation of formaldehyde (54). Unmetabolized formaldehyde rapidly binds to tissue proteins (55). The usual fatal dose of methanol is 80–150 mL (64–120 g or 2.0–3.75 mol) (56). The maximal safety limit to inhalation exposure of methanol set by EPA is 200 parts per million (ppm) for 8 hr. The amount of methanol contained in 1 ppm is $1.43\,mg/m^3$ ($1.43\,mg/1000\,L$). At a minute ventilation rate of $5\,L/min$ and a methanol content of 200 ppm, the amount of methanol inhaled in 8 hr would be ($2400\,L/1000$) $\times$ 200 $\times$ 1.43 = 686 mg (21.5 mmol).

Excretion of Methanol

Pulmonary clearance of methanol of $5.6\,mL/min$ has been reported (57), but a calculation based on Henry's law and partial pressure at body temperature predicts a ventilatory loss of $< 2\,mL/min$. The main nonrenal clearance is dermal insensible loss. Methanol is distributed throughout the body fluids and has a high vapor pressure, so that loss of water from any source must be accompanied by a loss of methanol. Because water loss from the skin is two- to three-fold greater than the lung, methanol loss from the skin must also be greater than ventilatory loss. At a urine output of $2\,L/day$, methanol clearance is about $1.4\,mL/min$.

Metabolism and H^+ Production

Methanol is convereted to formaldehyde by alcohol dehydrogenase in the liver (Fig. 7) by first order kinetics at low concentrations and at zero order kinetics when the concentration is high. The formaldehyde is rapidly converted to formic acid by aldehyde dehydrogenase. Each step converts NAD^+

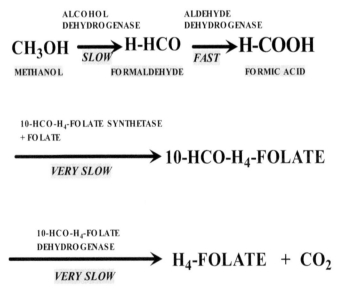

Figure 7 Metabolism of methanol. Formic acid is the main acid that accumulates in methanol poisoning, but the bulk of ingested methanol is slowly metabolized to CO_2.

to NADH. The latter step is much faster so formaldehyde levels are only slightly increased, yet still are in a toxic range (54). Formic acid is further metabolized slowly to *N*-10-formyl tetrahydrofolate (58,59), and then to tetrahydrofolate (60). Humans have a greater susceptibility than rats to methanol toxicity, which has been attributed to low levels of folate and low activity of *N*-10-formyl tetrahydrofolate dehydrogenase in human liver (60). In the rhesus monkey, pretreatment with folate reduced plasma formate by 50% after methanol administration, whereas folate deficiency increased the plasma formate level about three-fold (61). Thus, folate deficient malnourished alcoholics likely to have an increased susceptibility to methanol toxicity.

The metabolic acidosis of methanol poisoning is an increased anion gap type, accounted for by formate and lactate (62–64). The lactate level often exceeds that of formate (63,64). The lactic acidosis is due to inhibition of cytochrome oxidase by formate (65) and the increased $NADH/NAD^+$ ratio caused by methanol metabolism. When formate is metabolized to neutral end products, HCO_3^- ions are regenerated. Filtered formate is reabsorbed in the proximal tubule via the formate-chloride exchanger, and thus its excretion in the urine is low.

Clinical Signs and Symptoms

Early on, symptoms of intoxication (e.g., inebriation, ataxia, and slurred speech) dominate. Later, blurred vision, blindness, abdominal pain, malaise, headache, and vomiting develop (56). Funduscopic examination may reveal papilledema. Visual impairment is related to metabolism of methanol in the retina via retinal dehydrogenase (66). In one report, all of the 115 patients who were frankly acidotic on admission suffered from visual impairment (56,62). Fixed and dilated pupils might be due to reduced light perception caused by papilledema. Seven of the 32 survivors in a Toronto series had visual sequelae (22%) (67). Degeneration of ganglion cells with sparing of optic nerves and tracts was seen on ocular examination (56). Necrosis of the putamen and basal ganglia is frequent (68,69). Abdominal pain and tenderness are often due to acute pancreatitis. In one report, 13 of 17 autopsies, pancreatic necrosis was observed (56). Kussmaul respiration is not common even when the acidosis is severe, probably because of central depressive effects of methanol. Only 25% of patients with serum $[HCO_3^-] < 10\,mEq/L$ had Kussmaul respirations (56). The mortality rate from methanol poisoning is correlated with the degree of acidosis, coma, or seizures at presentation. The cause of death is a peculiar cessation of respiration of unknown mechanism, described below:

> "As coma deepened, respiration became shallow and less frequent. Gradually tonic contracture of the limbs appeared, the patient suddenly went into opisthotonos and, at the end of a tremendous single

gasp, the chest locked in a position of full inspiration. Manual artificial respiration was not possible at this stage because of complete immobility of the chest wall. Tracheostomy and respirators were not effective. The tonic muscle contractions were not affected by intravenous sodium amytal." (56).

Diagnosis

On presentation, the most characteristic finding is visual impairment. Signs of acute pancreatitis are also often present. The serum osmolal gap is increased, if osmolality is measured by freezing point depression. Vapor pressure osmometry does not detect methanol. The serum anion gap is increased with metabolic acidosis unless methanol metabolism is inhibited by ethanol or isopropyl alcohol, or when a condition for a decreased serum anion gap coexists (70). Confirmation requires direct measurement of serum methanol levels.

Treatment

Sodium bicarbonate should be infused in doses appropriate to maintain arterial pH above 7.20. Another goal at the same time is to reduce the concentrations of methanol, formaldehyde, and formate in blood. This can be achieved by inhibiting hepatic alcohol dehydrogenase with fomepizole or ethanol (71,72). The same principles apply as discussed earlier for ethylene glycol.

Because renal clearance and dermal loss are too slow, hemodialysis is necessary (53,73,74); plasma methanol concentration falls by 50% in 2–3 hr of treatment (53). The indications for hemodialysis include ingestion of at least 30 mL of absolute methanol, a blood methanol level of > 50 mg/dL (15 mmol/L), high anion-gap metabolic acidosis, and papilledema. Because brain infarction is quite common (68), hemodialysis should be done without heparin. If hemodialysis is unavailable or contraindicated, forced diuresis should be tried (53), and dermal loss increased by raising the skin temperature. Supplementation with folic acid or folinic acid (5-formyl tetrahydrofolic acid; Leucovorin) (61) might accelerate formate metabolism. The usual recommended dose is 1–2 mg/kg body weight every 4–6 hr intravenously.

Toluene

Chemistry and Toxicology

Toluene, also known as methylbenzene or phenylmethane, has a molecular weight of 92 Da. It is commonly used as an industrial solvent, and is found in transmission fluid, gasoline, acrylic paints, varnishes, paint thinners, adhesives, glues, rubber cement, airplane glue, and shoe polish (75,76). Toluene levels of 100 ppm are considered safe; 150 ppm acceptable for short periods (less than 8 hr); and 200 ppm dangerous to health and life (77).

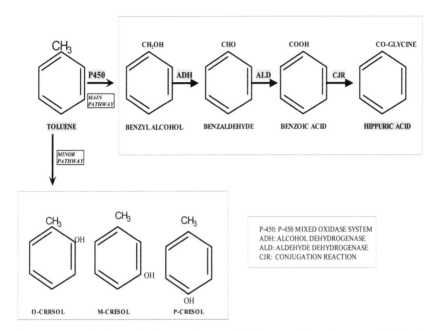

Figure 8 Metabolism of toluene. The rate-limiting step in toluene metabolism is conversion to benzyl alcohol through cytochrome P-450 in the liver. Benzyl alcohol is further metabolized to benzaldehyde, then to benzoic acid, and then ultimately to hippuric acid through conjugation with glycine. Conversion to cresol is a minor pathway.

Metabolism and H$^+$ Production

Toluene is metabolized to benzyl alcohol by hepatic cytochrome P-450 with NADPH as a cofactor (78,79) (Fig. 8). Chronic toluene abusers develop metabolic acidosis more readily than acute users, because of induction of the P-450 enzyme system, the rate-limiting enzyme in toluene metabolism (80). Benzyl alcohol is metabolized to benzylaldehyde by alcohol dehydrogenase, and then to benzoic acid by aldeyhyde dehydrogenase (89). Each of these steps produces one mole of NADH per mole of benzyl alcohol metabolized. Ethanol inhibits the metabolism of benzyl alcohol by competing with it for oxidation by alcohol dehydrogenase (80). Because of rapid renal excretion, hippurate levels in plasma are usually only modestly elevated (81). With a lower GFR, a higher circulating level of benzoate is found, and in renal failure, hippurate and benzoate accumulate in the plasma (82).

Pathogenesis of Metabolic Acidosis in Toluene Poisoning

Typically, toluene poisoning leads to hyperchloremic metabolic acidosis, often accompanied by profound hypokalemia (83–85). In a few cases, urine

PCO_2 is not appropriately elevated in response to HCO_3^- loading, suggesting impaired H^+ secretion in the collecting duct (85). Based on these findings and in vitro studies on the turtle bladder (85), the metabolic acidosis was attributed to distal renal tubular acidosis (see Chapter 13) (83–85). Some patients had Fanconi syndrome (86). An alternative possibility is an organic acidosis due to overproduction of hippuric acid (80). The absence of an increased serum anion gap in most cases can be attributed to the rapid renal excretion of hippurate. Hypokalemia is often severe ($[K^+] < 1.5\,mEq/L$) (87), and is attributed to low K^+ intake and increased excretion due to Na^+ delivery to the distal nephron with poorly absorbable hippurate and benzoate anions rather than Cl^- (88). Toluene abusers are often chronically malnourished, and overproduction of hippuric acid might cause disproportionally low blood urea nitrogen (BUN).

Causes of Intoxication and Prevalence

Poisoning occurs most commonly from deliberate inhalation to induce euphoria (83), but it can occur accidentally (89). Toluene abuse has become widespread worldwide among children and adolescents, because it is readily available and inexpensive. It is estimated that 3–4% of American teenagers engage in sniffing on a regular basis and that 7–12% of high school students have tried sniffing at least once (90).

Clinical Features

Toluene intoxication has a similar clinical presentation to alcohol intoxication before electrolyte and acid–base abnormalities develop. The primary effects are on the CNS causing euphoria, dizziness, confusion, stupor, and coma (75,83). Chronic abuse of toluene can lead to neuropsychosis, cerebral cortex atrophy, cerebellar degeneration and ataxia, optic and peripheral neuropathies, decreased cognitive ability, blindness, and deafness (85). Toluene can also cause bronchospasm, and aspiration pneumonia or asphyxia can result from CNS depression. Toluene crosses the placenta readily (80,91), and has teratogenic effects. It causes GI symptoms, and hypoxia may result from prolonged breathing into a plastic bag and/or respiratory depression (92). Renal failure occurs, and is attributed to acute tubular necrosis caused by hypotension or possibly rhabdomyolysis (84). Of note, the increase in BUN is low relative to the increase in serum creatinine (80,83,84).

Diagnosis

The diagnosis is usually based on a history of exposure to toluene, confirmed by measurement of toluene in the serum. Blood toluene levels $> 2.5\,mcg/mL$ correlate with illness. Levels of $50\,mcg/mL$ are associated with a very high mortality rate. Detection of hippurate in the urine will also suggest the diagnosis.

Treatment

Patients should be given supportive care, including intravenous saline to re-expand the ECF volume and KCl, to treat the hypokalemia. Ventilation therapy may be needed, especially if there is a superimposed respiratory acidosis. There is no specific drug therapy for toluene poisoning (76).

Acetaminophen (Paracetamol)

Acetaminophen is one of the most widely used nonprescription analgesics. Two organic acidoses have been associated with its use: lactic acidosis and pyroglutamic acidosis (93). The production of a toxic metabolite of acetaminophen, N-acetyl-p-benzoquinone-imine (NAPBQI), is responsible for both types of acidosis. Acetaminophen is normally metabolized mainly to nontoxic glucuronide and sulfate conjugates. Less than 5% is metabolized to NAPBQI, which reacts with glutathione. An NAPBQI toxicity results from glutathione depletion (94–97). Under these conditions, NAPBQI combines with sulfhydryl groups of macromolecules, and reactive oxygen species (ROS) can accumulate and cause tissue damage (95). The fraction of NAPBQI produced from acetaminophen depends on the activity of P-450 enzyme systems. Thus, activation of the enzyme by certain drugs or chronic use of ethanol increases production of NAPBQI, and a usual dose of acetaminophen may result in toxicity (98).

One of the toxic effects of an NAPBQI is inhibition of mitochondrial respiration, resulting in lactic acidosis (94–97). Thus, lactic acidosis can occur before severe liver damage develops (99–102), but it also occurs in late stages of toxicity as a nonspecific effect of liver injury. Until 1990, when the causal relationship between acetaminophen and pyroglutamic acidosis was first identified (103,104), lactic acidosis was the only type of metabolic acidosis thought to be associated with acetaminophen. Now, it appears that pyroglutamic acidosis is more important.

Pyroglutamic acidosis occurs because NAPBQI decreases the concentration of reduced glutathione, thereby increasing the synthesis of γ-glutamylcysteine, leading to the formation of pyroglutamic acid (Fig. 9). Reduced glutathione (GSH) normally inhibits this first step in the synthesis of glutathione.

A hereditary defect in glutathione synthase causes overproduction of γ-glutamylcysteine and hence pyroglutamic acidosis by a similar mechanism. Certain drugs such as the antibiotic flucloxacillin and the anticonvulsant vigabatrin (105,106) may impair metabolism of pyroglutamic acid and thereby cause pyroglutamic acidosis.

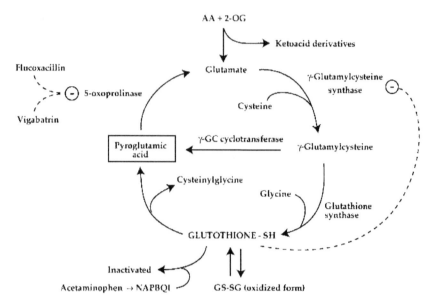

Figure 9 Production of the reduced form of glutathione. The pathway begins with glutamate, a key intermediate in transamination reactions. When reduced glutathione levels are low (e.g., due to combination with a metabolite of acetaminophen), γ-glutamylcysteine synthetase is stimulated. If γ-glutamylcysteine accumulates, pyroglutamic acid accumulates as well. In addition, if γ-oxyprolinease is inhibited, pyroglutamic acid will also accumulate. As described in the text, the diminished ability to detoxify an ROS in this setting is likely to be more important than the acidosis.

TOXINS LEADING TO THE PRODUCTION OF LACTIC ACID

Antiretroviral Drugs

Lactic acidosis has been reported in patients with HIV infection treated with nucleoside analogue reverse transcriptase inhibitors, most commonly with zidovudine, but also with zalcitabine, didanosine, stavudine, lamivudine, and indinavir (107–111) (see Chapter 11). All these drugs are associated with mitochondrial myopathy as well as hepatic steatosis (112). Either the muscle or the liver involvement could, in theory, explain the lactic acidosis, but liver involvement appears necessary as the disorder can occur without skeletal muscle involvement (109). The lactic acidosis has been treated with thiamine (113), as thiamine deficiency is quite prevalent in this malnourished population (114).

Isoniazid (INH) Overdose

An overdose of isoniazid (INH), whether accidental or intentional, commonly results in intractable seizures followed by lactic acidosis (115–119).

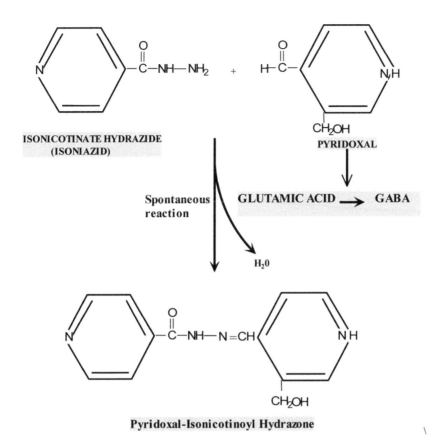

Pyridoxal-Isonicotinoyl Hydrazone

Figure 10 Mechanism of seizure in INH poisoning. Isoniazid forms a pyridoxalisonicotinoyl hydrazone complex by combining with pyridoxal in a nonenzymatic reaction. The resulting acute pyridoxal deficiency leads to acute GABA deficiency and hence a seizure disorder because pyridoxal is a necessary cofactor for the production of GABA.

The mechanism of seizure and lactic acidosis is thought to be the formation of an isonicotinoyl hydrazide, vitamin B_6 complex, pyridoxal isonicotinoyl hydrazone (Fig. 10), rapidly inducing a vitamin B_6 deficiency state (120). Vitamin B_6 is a critical cofactor in the formation of gamma amino butyric acid (GABA), and therefore B_6 deficiency leads to GABA deficiency. The GABA is an inhibitory neurotransmitter, and GABA deficiency results in increased excitability and seizure activity (121). The INH-associated seizures and lactic acidosis can almost invariably be reversed rapidly by administering a large dose of intravenous vitamin B_6 (119). Patients on chronic hemodialysis are at increased risk of INH-induced toxicity because they tend to be deficient of vitamin B_6, as hemodialysis removes this vitamin quite efficiently (122).

Tricyclic Antidepressants

Patients consuming a diet poor in B vitamins and taking tricyclic antidepressants can develop a chronic lactic acidosis. The lactic acidosis is presumed to be due to inhibition by this class of drugs of an ATP-dependent kinase that activates riboflavin to form key metabolites that are components of the mitochondrial electron transport system, the pathway that regenerates ATP (123). Adding a large of dose riboflavin to the diet leads to a prompt reversal of the metabolic acidosis (124,125).

UNCOMMON TOXINS

Benzyl Alcohol

Benzyl alcohol is an aromatic alcohol that is used as a preservative in parenteral medications (126). Severe poisoning with metabolic acidosis has occurred only in infants and children when this alcohol is used to clear intravenous lines, probably because the drug dosage per weight is greater for a smaller person. Also, metabolism of this alcohol is slower in infants. Premature infants had higher plasma levels of benzoic acid and greater urinary excretion of benzoic acid and benzyl alcohol than full-term infants (127).

Benzyl alcohol is metabolized to benzylaldehyde by hepatic alcohol dehydrogenase, and then to benzoic acid by aldehyde dehydrogenase (Fig. 11). Each step converts NAD^+ to NADH. Benzoic acid is conjugated by glycine to hippuric acid (80%) and in a small amount by glucuronic acid (20%). Metabolic acidosis is due to the production of hippuric acid and, to a

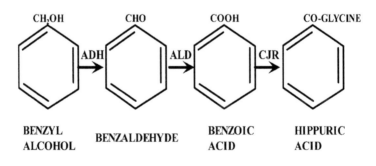

Figure 11 Metabolism of benzyl alcohol. The metabolic pathways are identical to those of toluene except that the initial step begins with alcohol dehydrogenase.

smaller extent, benzoic acid. The acidosis is sometimes accompanied by hypotension with hepatic and renal failure. This complication appears to be a toxic effect of benzyl alcohol rather than its metabolites. Discontinuation of benzyl alcohol-containing solutions has improved survival of premature infants (128,129).

Propylene Glycol

Propylene glycol (1,2 propanediol) is a common diluent for many injectable medications. It is metabolized to lactaldehyde by alcohol dehydrogenase, and subsequently to lactic acid by aldehyde dehydrogenase. At each step NADH is produced (Fig. 12) (130). Clinical manifestations of propylene glycol toxicity include CNS dysfunction such as disorientation, nystagmus, depression, ataxia, stupor, and seizure; and cardiac effects, such as hypotension, widening of QRS complex, and cardiac arrhythmias including asystole (131–134). The metabolic acidosis that develops clinically appears to be due to L-lactic acid accumulation, but experimental observations in animals have shown that the principal acid is D-lactic acid (135).

Isopropyl Alcohol

Isopropyl alcohol (isopropanol, 2-propanol, $CH_3–CH–OH–CH_3$) has a molecular weight of 62 Da. It is widely available as rubbing alcohol, and is also present in toiletries, disinfectants, window-cleaning solutions, antifreeze, paint removers, and industrial solvents. It is rapidly absorbed from the intestine and skin, and also through the lung by inhalation. It is distributed

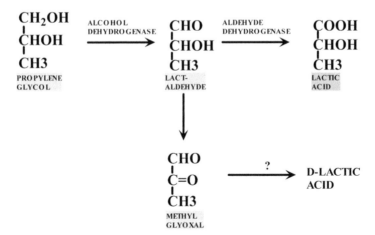

Figure 12 Metabolism of propylene glycol. The main pathway is conversion to L-lactic acid, but an additional pathway is conversion to methylglyoxal, which can be converted to D-lactic acid.

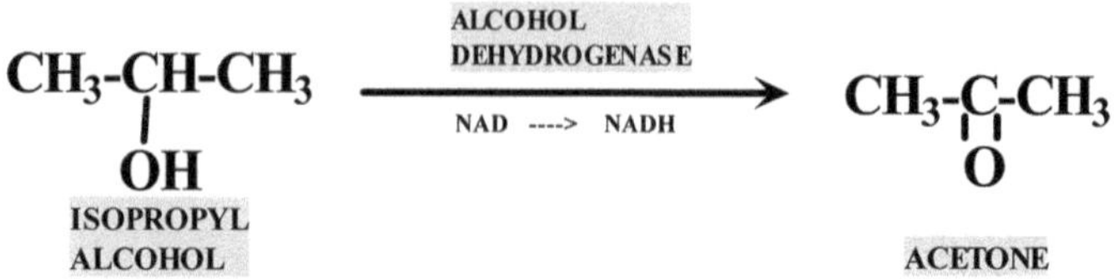

$$CH_3\text{-}\underset{\underset{\displaystyle OH}{|}}{CH}\text{-}CH_3 \xrightarrow[\text{NAD} \text{----> } \text{NADH}]{\text{ALCOHOL} \atop \text{DEHYDROGENASE}} CH_3\text{-}\underset{\displaystyle O}{\overset{\displaystyle |\,|}{C}}\text{-}CH_3$$

ISOPROPYL
ALCOHOL
ACETONE

Figure 13 Metabolism of isopropyl alcohol. Isopropyl alcohol is rapidly converted to acetone through the action of alcohol dehydrogenase. Acetone is not an acid, but gives a positive reaction to the ketone test.

throughout total body water. Isopropyl alcohol is metabolized by alcohol dehydrogenase to acetone by first-order kinetics (Fig. 13), and has a blood half-life of about 2.5–3 hr (136). A small amount is excreted unmetabolized by the kidney, and some by the lung. Because acetone is the end-product of metabolism, this alcohol causes acetonemia but not metabolic acidosis. The alcohol itself and, to a lesser extent, acetone are CNS depressants, and might cause hypotension. An isopropyl alcohol level in excess of 400 mg/dL implies a poor prognosis, and should be treated with hemodialysis, particularly if coma and hypotension are present (137,138). Isopropyl alcohol removal by dialysis is extremely efficient. Isopropyl alcohol poisoning is very unlikely if the serum acetone test is negative 30 min after ingestion of the alcohol. In such instances, concomitant ethanol ingestion should be considered.

Diethylene and Triethylene Glycol

Diethylene glycol (106 Da) is used as an antifreeze for sprinkler systems, a water seal for gas tanks, and as a lubricating and finishing agent. Diethylene glycol was used as a solvent in sulfanilamide elixir and resulted in 105 deaths in 1937. This accidental poisoning led the U.S. Congress to pass the 1938 Federal Food, Drug and Cosmetic Act (139). Despite the ban on its use as a diluent, mass poisoning accidents have occurred in Haiti (140), Bangladesh (141), South Africa (142), and Nigeria (143). This agent is absorbed transdermally, and intoxication has occurred after topical application (144).

Diethylene glycol intoxication resembles that of ethylene glycol. The patients develop progressive inebriation, anion gap metabolic acidosis, renal failure, hepatitis, pancreatitis, coma, and death. Acute renal failure is the most common manifestation (140,143). Metabolism of diethylene glycol requires the actions of alcohol dehydrogenase and aldehyde dehydrogenase. Metabolic acidosis is not as predictable as with ethylene glycol poisoning, and the offending acid is 2-hydroxyethoxyacetic acid (145). When this glycol was given to rats, about 80% was excreted in the urine unmetabolized, and the remainder was excreted as 2-hydroxyethoxyacetic acid (Fig. 14).

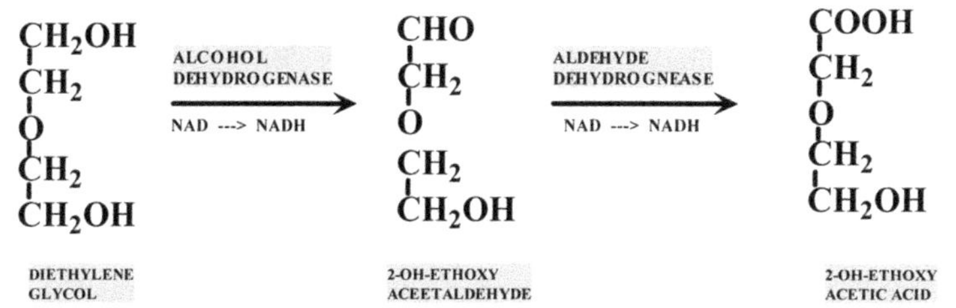

Figure 14 Metabolism of diethylene glycol. The main acid that accumulates is 2-OH-ethoxyacetic acid through the successive actions of alcohol and aldehyde dehydrogenases.

Triethylene glycol is produced from ethylene oxide and ethylene glycol and has a molecular weight of 150 Da. It is used in various plastics to increase pliability, in air disinfection, and in brake fluid. Poisoning causes metabolic acidosis and coma. The pathway for its metabolism is not known, but it does require alcohol dehydrogenase (33). Accordingly, its metabolism is decreased by inhibition of alcohol dehydrogenase (146). Triethylene glycol poisoning has also been treated successfully with ethanol infusion (147).

Paraldehyde

Paraldehyde is a tricyclic polymer of acetaldehyde that has been used as a sedative for more than a century. It was used widely for the treatment of delirium tremens, but its use was gradually replaced by the safer and more effective benzodiazepine sedatives (148,149). About 20–30% of paraldehyde is excreted unchanged through the lung, and the remainder is metabolized to acetaldehyde and then to acetic acid. Liver disease retards this oxidation, and drugs such as metronidazole and disulfiram inhibit it. Unmetabolized acetaldehyde is rapidly eliminated through the lung, because it is extremely volatile (boiling point, 21°C).

Paraldehyde-induced acidosis was first reported in 1957 (149). The offending acid has not been identified, but acetate, pyruvate, L-lactate, and acetoacetate have been excluded. β-hydroxybutyric acid was not measured in these patients. Acetaldehyde gives a false-positive nitroprusside reaction (pseudoketosis), and this should be borne in mind when ketoacidosis is considered as the cause of acidosis (150).

REFERENCES

1. Levy G. Clinical pharmacokinetics of aspirin. Pediatrics 1978; 62:867–872.
2. Davison C. Salicylate metabolism in man. Ann NY Acad Sci 1971; 179:249–268.
3. Brubacher JR, Hoffman RS. 1996 Salicylism from topical salicylates: review of the literature. J Toxicol Clin Toxicol 1997; 34:431–443.

4. Rowlinson SW, Crews BC, Goodwin DC, Schneider C, Gierse JK, Marnett LJ. Spatial requirements for 15-(R)-hydroxy-5Z,11Z, 13E-eicosatetraenoic acid synthesis within the cyclooxygenase active site of murine COX-2. Why acetylated COW-1 does not synthesize 15-(R)-hete. J Biol Chem 2000; 275:6586–6591.

5. Schneider C, Brash AR. Stereospecificity of hydrogen abstraction in the conversion of arachidonic acid to 15R-HETE by aspirin-treated cyclooxygenase-2. Implications for the alignment of substrate in the active site. J Biol Chem 2000; 275:4743–4746.

6. Lecomte M, Laneuville O, Ji C, DeWitt DL, Smith WL. Acetylation of human prostaglandin endoperoxide synthase-2 (cyclooxygenase-2) by aspirin. J Biol Chem 1994; 269:13207–13215.

7. Hill JB. Experimental salicylate poisoning: observation of the effects of altering blood pH on tissue and plasma salicylate concentrations. Pediatrics 1971; 47:658–665.

8. Miyahara JT, Karler R. Effect of salicylate on oxidative phosphorylation and respiration of mitochondria fragments. Biochem J 1965; 97:194–198.

9. Seltzer HS. Drug-induced hypoglycemia: a review based on 473 cases. Diabetes 1972; 21:955–966.

10. Thurston JH, Pollock PG, Warren SK, Jones EM. Reduced brain glucose with normal plasma glucose in salicylate poisoning. J Clin Invest 1970; 49: 2139–2145.

11. Sainsbury SI. Fatal salicylate toxicity from bismuth subsalicylate. West J Med 1991; 55:637–739.

12. Singer RB. The acid–base disturbances in salicylate intoxication. Medicine (Baltimore) 1954; 33:1–15.

13. Winters RW, White IS, Hughes MC, Ordway NK. Disturbances of acid–base equilibrium in salicylate intoxication. Pediatrics 1959; 23:260–272.

14. Gabow PA, Anderson R, Potts DL, Schrier RW. Acid–base disturbances in the salicylate intoxicated adult. Arch Intern Med 1978; 138:1481–1484.

15. Alexander JK, Spalter HF, West JR. Modification of the respiratory response to carbon dioxide by salicylate. J Clin Invest 1955; 34:533–537.

16. Halperin ML, Connors HP, Relman AS, Karnovsky ML. Factors that control the effect of pH on glycolysis in leukocytes. J Biol Chem 1969; 244:384–390.

17. Roch-Ramel F, Guisan B. Renal transport of urate in humans. News Physiol Sci 1999; 14:80–84.

18. Myeres EN, Bernstein JM, Forstiropolous G. Salicylate ototoxicity. N Engl J Med 1965; 273:587–590.

19. Heffiner JE, Sahn SA. Salicylate-induced pulmonary edema. Ann Intern Med 1981; 95:405–409.

20. Berk WA, Anderson JC. Salicylate-associated asytole: report of two cases. Am J Med 1989; 86:505–506.

21. Chapman BJ, Proudfoot AT. Adult salicylate poisoning: deaths and outcome in patients with high plasma salicylate concentrations. Q J Med 1989; 72: 699–707.

22. Proudfoot AT, Brown SS. Acidemia and salicylate poisoning in adults. BMJ 1969; 2:547–553.

23. King JA, Storrow AB, Finkelstein JA. Urine Trinder spot test: a rapid salicylate. Ann Emerg Med 1995; 26:330–333.
24. Pierce RP, Gazewood J, Blake RL Jr. Salicylate poisoning from enteric coated aspirin: delayed absorption may complicate management. Postgrad Med 1991; 89:61–68.
25. Johnson D, Eppler J, Giesbrecht E. Effect of multiple-dose activated charcola on the clearance of high-dose intravenous aspirin in a porcine. Ann Emerg Med 1995; 26:569–574.
26. Lawson AAH, Proudfoot AT, Brown SS. Forced diuresis in the treatment of acute salicylate poisoning in adults. Q J Med 1969; 38:31–38.
27. Prescott LF, Balali-Mood M, Critchley JAJH. Diuresis or urinary alkalinzation for salicylate poisoning? Br Med J 1982; 285:1383–1386.
28. Jacobsen D, Wilk-Larsen E, Bredesen JE. Hemodialysis of hemoperfusion in severe salicylate poisoning? Hum Toxical 1988; 7:161–163.
29. Parry MF, Wallach R. Ethylene glycol poisoning. Am J Med 1974; 57: 143–150.
30. Barceloux DG, Krenzelok EP, Olson K, Watson W. American Academy of Clinical Toxicology Practice Guidelines on the treatment of ethylene glycol poisoning. J Toxicol Clin Toxicol 1999; 37:537–560.
31. Johnson B, Meggs WJ, Bentzel CJ. Emergency department hemodialysis in a case of severe ethylene glycol poisoning. Ann Emerg Med 1999; 33:108–110.
32. Vasavada N, Williams C, Hellman RN. Ethylene glycol intoxication: case report and pharmacokinetic perspectives. Pharmacotherapy 2003; 23(12): 1652–1658.
33. Herold DA, Keil K, Bruns DE. Oxidation of polyethylene glycols by alcohol dehydrogenase. Biochem Pharmacol 1989; 38:73–76.
34. Clay KL, Murphy RC. On the metabolic acidosis of ethylene glycol intoxication. Toxicol Appl Pharmacol 1977; 39:39–49.
35. Poore RE, Hurst CH, Assimos DG, Holmes RP. Pathways of hepatic oxalate synthesis and their regulation. Am J Physiol 1997; 272:289–294.
36. Jacobsen D, Hewlett TP, Webb R, Brown ST, Ordinaro AT, McMartin KE. Ethylene glycol intoxication: evaluation of kinetics and crystalluria. Am J Med 1988; 84:145–152.
37. Moreau CL, Kerns W II, Tomaszewski CA, McMartin KE, Rose SR, Ford MD, Brent J, Group MS. Glycolate kinetics and hemodialysis clearance in ethylene glycol poisoning. J Toxicol Clin Toxicol 1998; 36:659–666.
38. Gabow PA, Clay K, Sullivan JB, Lepoff R. Organic acids in ethylene glycol intoxication. Ann Intern Med 1986; 105:16–19.
39. Jacobsen D, Bredesen JE, Eide I, Ostborg J. Anion and osmolal gaps in the diagnosis of methanol and ethylene glycol poisoning. Acta Med Scand 1982; 212:17–23.
40. Godolphin W, Meagher EP, Sanders HD, Frohlich J. Unusual calcium oxalate crystals in ethylene glycol poisoning. Clin Toxicol 1980; 16:479–486.
41. Jacobsen D, Akesson J, Shefter E. Urinary calcium oxalate monohydrate crystals in ethylene glycol poisoning. Scand J Clin Lab Invest 1982; 42:231–234.
42. Huhn KM, Rosenberg FM. Critical clue to ethylene glycol poisoning. CMAJ 1995; 15:193–195.

43. Paulsen D, Kronborg J, Borg EB, Hagen T. Cigar-like oxalate crystals in ethylene glycol poisoning. Tidsskr Nor Laegeforen 1994; 114:435–436.

44. Poldelski V, Johnson A, Wright S, Rosa VD, Zager RA. Ethylene glycol-mediated tubular injury: identification of critical metabolites and injury pathways. Am J Kidney Dis 2001; 38(2):339–348.

45. Spillane L, Roberts JR, Meyer AE. Multiple cranial nerve deficits after ethylene glycol poisoning. Ann Emerg Med 1991; 20:208–210.

46. Eder AF, McGrath CM, Dowdy YG. Ethylene glycol poisoning: toxicokinetic and analytical factors affecting laboratory diagnosis. Clin Chem 1998; 44: 168–177.

47. Jones AW, Nilsson L, Gladh SA, Karlsson K, Beck-Friis J. 2,3-Butanediol in plasma from an alcoholic mistakenly identified as ethylene glycol by gas-chromatographic analysis. Clin Chem 1991; 37:1453–1455.

48. Darchy B, Abruzzese L, Pitiot O, Figueredo B, Domart Y. Delayed admission for ethylene glycol poisoning: lack of elevated serum osmol gap. Intensive Care Med 1999; 25:859–861.

49. Ammar KA, Heckerling PS. Ethylene glycol poisoning with a normal anion gap caused by concurrent ethanol ingestion: Importance of the osmolal gap. Am J Kidney Dis 1996; 27:130–133.

50. Scalley RD, Ferguson DR, Piccaro JC, Smart ML, Archie TE. Treatment of ethylene glycol poisoning. Am Fam Physician 2002; 66(5):807–812.

51. Peterson CD, Collins AJ, Himes JM, Bullock ML, Keane WF. Ethylene glycol poisoning: pharmacokinetics during therapy with ethanol and hemodialysis. N Engl J Med 1981; 304:21–23.

52. Davis LE, Hudson A, Benson BE, Jones Easom LA, Coleman JK. Methanol poisoning exposures in the United States: 1993–1998. J Toxicol Clin Toxicol 2002; 40(4):499–505.

53. Jacobsen D, Ovrebo S, Sejersted OM. Toxicokinetics of formate during hemodialysis. Acta Med Scand 1983; 214:409–412.

54. Eells JT, McMartin KE, Black K. Formaldehyde poisoning: rapid metabolism in formic acid. JAMA 1981; 246:1237–1238.

55. Matsumoto K, Moriya F, Nanikawa R. The movement of blood formaldehyde in methanol intoxication. II. The movement of blood formaldehyde and its metabolism in the rabbit. Nippon Hoigaku Zasshi 1990; 44:205–211.

56. Bennett IL, Cary FH, Mitchell GE, Cooper MN. Acute methyl alcohol poisoning: a review based on experiences in an outbreak of 323 cases. Medicine (Baltimore) 1953; 32:431–463.

57. Jacobsen D, Ovrebo S, Arnesen E, Paus PN. Pulmonary excretion of methanol in man. Scand J Clin Lab Invest 1983; 43:377–379.

58. Himes RH, Rabinowitz JC. Formyltetrahydrofolate synthetase. II. Characteristics of the enzyme and the enzyme reaction. J Biol Chem 1962; 237: 2903–2914.

59. Himes RH, Rabinowitz JC. Formyltetrahydrofolate synthetase. III. Characteristics of the enzyme and the enzyme reaction. J Biol Chem 1962; 237:2915–2925.

60. Johnlin FC, Fortman CS, Nghiem DD, Tephly TR. Studies on the role of folic acid and folate-dependent enzymes in human methanol poisoning. Mol Pharmacol 1987; 31:557–561.
61. McMartin KE, Martin-Amat G, Makar AB, Tephley TR. Methanol poisoning. V. Role of formate metabolism in the monkey. J Pharmacol Exp Therap 1977; 201:564–572.
62. Sejersted O, jacobsen D, Ovrebo S, Jansen H. Formate concentration in plasma from patients poisoned with methanol. Acta Med Scand 1983; 213:105–110.
63. Shahangian S, Ash KO. Formic and lactic acidosis in a fatal case of methanol intoxication. Clin Chem 1986; 32:395–396.
64. Smith SR, Snith SJM, Buckley BM. Combined formate and lactate acidosis in methanol poisoning. Lancet 1981; 2:1295–1296.
65. Leisivuori J, Savolainen H. Methanol and formate acid toxicity. Biochemical mechanisms. Pharmacol Toxicol 1991; 69:157–163.
66. Eells JT, Henry MM, Lewandowski MF, Seme MP, Murray TG. Development and characterization of a rodent model of methanol induced retinal and optic nerve toxicity. Neurotoxicology 2000; 21:321–330.
67. Liu JJ, Daya MR, Carrasquillo O, Kales SN. Prognostic factors in patients with methanol poisoning. J Toxicol Clin Toxicol 1998; 36:175–181.
68. Kuteifan K, Oesterle H, Tajahmady T, Gutbub AM, Laplatte G. Necrosis and haemorrhage of the putamen in methanol poisoning shown on MRI. Neurocardiology 1998; 40:158–160.
69. Chen JC, Schneiderman JF, Wortzman G. Methanol poisoning: bilateral putaminal and cerebellar cortical lesions on CT and MR. J Comput Assist Tomogr 1991; 15:522–524.
70. Haviv YS, Rubinger D, Zamir E, Safadi R. Pseudo-normal osmolal and anion gaps following simultaneous ethanol and methanol ingestion. Am J Nephrol 1998; 18:436–438.
71. Mycyk MB, Leikin JB. Antidote review: fomepizole for methanol poisoning. Am J Ther 2003; 10:68–70.
72. Barceloux DG, Bond GR, Krenzelok EP, Cooper H, Vale JA. American Academy of Clinical Toxicology Ad Hoc Committee on the Treatment Guidelines for Methanol Poisoning. American Academy of Clinical Toxicology practice guidelines on the treatment of methanol poisoning. J Toxicol Clin Toxicol 2002; 40(4):415–446.
73. Osterloh JD, Pond SM, Grady S, Becker CE. Serum formate concentration in methanol intoxication as a criterion for hemodialysis. Ann Intern Med 1986; 104:200–203.
74. McCoy HG, Gipole RJ, Ehlers SM. Severe methanol poisoning. Application of a pharmacokinetic model for ethanol therapy and hemodialysis. Am J Med 1979; 67:804–807.
75. Ellenhorn MJ, Schonwald S, Ordog G. Inhalant Abuse. Ellenhorn's Medi Toxicol 1997; 2:1493–1495.
76. Anderson CE, Loomis GA. Recognition and prevention of inhalant abuse. Am Fam Physician 2003; 68(5):869–874.

77. Oettingen WF, Donahue DD. The toxicity and potential danger of toluene. JAMA 1942; 118:579–585.
78. Blake RC II, Coon MJ. On the mechanism of action of cytochrome P-450. Evaluation of homolytic and heterolytic mechanisms of oxygen–oxygen bond cleavage during substrate hydroxylation by peroxides. J Biol Chem 1981; 256:12127–12133.
79. Blake RC, Coon MJ. On the mechanism of action of cytochrome P-450. Role of peroxy spectral intermediates in substrate hydroxylation. J Biol Chem 1981; 256:5755–5773.
80. Carlisle EJF, Donnelly SM, Vasuvattakul S, Kamel KS, Tobe S, Halperin ML. Glue-sniffing and distal renal tubular acidosis: sticking to the facts. J Am Soc Nephrol 1991; 1:1019–1027.
81. Smith HW, Finfelstein N, Aliminosa L, Crawford B, Graber M. The renal clearances of substituted hippuric acid derivitives and other aromatic acids in dogs and man. J Clin Invest 1945; 24:388–404.
82. Jone CM, Wu AH. An unusual case of toluene-induced metabolic acidosis. Clin Chem 1988; 34:2596–2599.
83. Streicher H, Gabow P, Moss A, Kono D, Kaehny W. Syndromes of toluene sniffing in adults. Ann Intern Med 1981; 94:758–762.
84. Fichman CM, Oster JR. Toxic effects of toluene. A new cause of high anion gap metabolic acidosis. JAMA 1979; 241:11713–11715.
85. Batlle DC, Sabatini S, Kurtzman N. On the mechanism of toluene-induced renal tubular acidosis. Nephron 1988; 49:210–218.
86. Kamijima M, Nakazawa Y, Yamakawa M, Shibata E, Hisanaga N, Ono Y, Toida M, Takeuchi Y. Metabolic acidosis and renal tubular injury due to pure toluene inhalation. Arch Environ Health 1994; 49:410–413.
87. Gerkin RD Jr, LoVecchio F. Rapid reveral of life-threatening toluene-induced hypokalemia with hemodialysis. J Emerg Med 1998; 16:723–725.
88. Carlisle E, Donnelly S, Ethier J, Quaggin S, Kaiser U, Kamel K, Halperin M. Modulation of the secretion of potassium by accompanying anions in humans. Kidney Int 1991; 39:1206–1212.
89. Shibata K, Yoshita Y, Matsumoto H. Extensive chemical burns from toluene. Am J Emerg Med 1994; 12:353–355.
90. Litovitz TL, Klein-Schwartz W, Caravati EM, Youniss J, Crouch B, Lee S. 1998 annual report of the American Association of Poison Control Centers Toxic Exposure Surveillance System. Am J Emerg Med 1999; 17:435–487.
91. Hass U, Lung SP, Hougaard KS. Developmental neurotoxicity after toluene inhalation exposure in rats. Neurotoxicol Teratol 1999; 21:349–357.
92. Einav S, Amitai Y, Reichman J, Geber D. Bradycardia in toluene poisoning. Clin Toxicol 1997; 35:295–298.
93. Steelman R, Goodman A, Biswas S, Zimmerman A. Metabolic acidosis and coma in a child with acetaminophen toxicity. Clin Pediatr (Phila) 2004; 43(2):201–203.
94. Ramsay RR, Rashed MS, Nelson SD. In vitro effects of acetaminophen metabolites and analogs on the respiration of mouse liver mitochondria. Arch Biochem Biophys 1989; 272:449–457.

95. Erstline RL, Ray SD, Ji S. Reversible and irreversible inhibition of hepatic mitochondrial respiration by acetaminophen and its toxic metabolites, *N*-acetyl-p-benzoquinoeneimine (NAPQI). Arch Biochem Biophys 1989; 38: 2387–2390.

96. Burcham PC, Harman AW. Acetaminophen toxicity results in site-specific mitochondrial damage in isolated mouse hepatocytes. J Biol Chem 1991; 266:5049–5054.

97. Landin JS, Cohen SD, Khairalla EA. Identification of a 54-kDa mitochondrial acetaminophen-binding protein as a aldehyde dehydrogenase. Toxicol Appl Pharmacol 1996; 141:299–307.

98. Lee WM. Acute liver failure in the United States. Semin Liver Dis 2003; 23(3):217–226.

99. Lee SP. Severe metabolic acidosis early in paracetamol poisoning. Brit Med J 1982; 285:851–852.

100. Roth B, Woo O, Blanc P. Early metabolic acidosis and coma after acetaminophen ingestion. Ann Emerg Med 1999; 33:452–456.

101. Koulouris Z, Tierney MG, Jones G. Metabolic acidosis and coma following a severe acetaminophen overdose. Ann Pharmacotherap 1999; 33:1191–1193.

102. Gray TA, Buckley BM, Vale JA. Hyperlactataemia and metabolic acidosis following paracetamol poisoning. Quart J Med 1987; 65:811–821.

103. Pitt JJ, Brown GK, Clift V, Christodoulou J. Atypical pyroglutamic aciduria: possible role of paracetamol. J Inher Metab Dis 1990; 13:755–756.

104. Pitt JJ. Association between paracetamol and pyroglutamic aciduria. Clin Chem 1990; 36:173–174.

105. Bonham JR, Rattenbury JM, Meeks A, Pollitt RJ. Pyroglutamic aciduria from vigabatrin. Lancet 1989; 1:1452–1453.

106. Dempsey GA, Lyall HJ, Corke CF, Scheinkestel CD. Pyroglutamic acidemia: a cause of high anion gap metabolic acidosis. Crit Care Med 2000; 28:1803–1807.

107. Freiman J, Helfert K, Hamrell M, Stein D. Hepatomegaly with severe steatosis in HIV-seropositive patients. AIDS 1993; 7:379–385.

108. Sundar K, Suarez M, Banogon PE, Shapiro JM. Zidovudine-induced fatal lactic acidosis and hepatic failure in patients with acquired immunodeficiency syndrome: report of two patients and review of the literature. Crit Care Med 1997; 25:1425–1430.

109. Olano JP, Borucki MJ, Wen JW, Haque AK. Massive hepatic steatosis and lactic acidosis in a patient with AIDS who was receiving zidovudine. Clin Infect Dis 1995; 21:973–976.

110. Chattha G, Arieff AL, Cummings C, Tierney LM. Lactic acidosis complicating the acquired immunodeficiency syndrome. Ann Intern Med 1993; 118: 37–39.

111. Boubaker K, Flepp M, Sudre P, et al. Hyperlactatemia and antiretroviral therapy: the Swiss HIV cohort study. Clin Infect Dis 2001; 33:1931–1937.

112. Gopinath R, Hutcheson M, Cheema-Dhadli S, Halperin ML. Chronic lactic acidosis in a patient with acquired immunodeficienct syndrome and mitochondrial myopathy: biochemical studies. J Am Soc Nephrol 1992; 3:1212–1219.

113. Schramm C, Wanitschke R, Galle PR. Thiamine for the treatment of nucleo-side analogue-induced severe lactic acidosis. Eur J Anaesthesiol 1999; 16: 733–735.
114. Jamieson CP, Obeig OA, Powell-Tuck J. The thiamin, riboflavin and pyridox-ine status of patients on emergency admission to hospital. Clin Nutri 1999; 18:87–91.
115. Nolan CM, Elarth AM, Barr HW. Intentional isoniazid overdosage in young Southeast Asian refugee women. Chest 1988; 93:803–806.
116. Martinjak-Dvorsek I, Gorjup V, Horvat M, Noc M. Acute isoniazid neuro-toxicity during preventive therapy. Crit Care Med 2000; 28:567–568.
117. Sullivan EA, Geoffroy P, Weisman R, Hoffman R, Frieden TR. Isoniazid poisonings in New York city. J Emerg Med 1998; 16:57–59.
118. Shah BR, Santucci K, Sinert R, Steiner P. Acute isoniazid neurotoxicity in an urban hospital. Pediatrics 1995; 95:700–704.
119. Alvarez FG, Guntupalli KK. Isoniazid overdose: four case reports and review of the literature. Intensive Care Med 1995; 21:641–644.
120. Mayes PA. Structure and function of the water-soluble vitamins. In: Murray RK, Granner DK, Mayes PA, Rodwell VW, eds. Harper's Biochemistry. New York: McGraw-Hill, 1999:627–641.
121. Chin L, Sievers ML, Herrier RN, Picchioni AL. Convulsions as the etiology of lactic acidosis in acute isoniazid toxicity in dogs. Toxicol Appl Pharmacol 1979; 49:377–384.
122. Siskind MS, Thienemann D, Kirlin L. Isoniazid-induced neurotoxicity in chronic dialysis patients: report of three cases and a review of the literature. Nephron 1993; 64:303–306.
123. Pinto J, Huang YP, Rivlin RS. Inhibition of riboflavin metabolism in rat tissues by chlorpromazine, imipramine, and amitriptyline. J Clin Invest 1981; 67:1500–1506.
124. Luzzati R, Del Bravo P, Di Perri G, Luzzani A, Concia E. Riboflavine and severe lactic acidosis. Lancet 1999; 353:901–902.
125. Fouty B, Frerman F, Reves R. Riboflavin to treat nucleoside analogue-inducing lactic acidosis. Lancet 1998; 352:291–292.
126. Lopez-Herce J. Benzyl alcohol poisoning following diazepam intravenous infusion. Ann Pharmacother 1995; 29:632.
127. LeBel M, Ferron L, Masson M, Pichette J, Carrier C. Benzyl alcohol metabo-lism and elimination in neonates. Dev Pharmacol Ther 1988; 11:347–356.
128. Gershanik J, Boecler B, Ensley H, McCloskey S, George W. The gasping syn-drome and benzyl alcohol poisoning. N Engl J Med 1982; 307:1384–1388.
129. Menon PA, Thach BT, Smith CH, Landt M, Roberts JL, Hillman RE, Hillman LS. Benzyl alcohol toxicity in a neonatal intensive care unit: Inci-dence, symptomatology, and mortality. Am J Perinatol 1984; 1:288–292.
130. Kehlner MJ, Bailey DN. Propylene glycol as a cause of lactic acidosis. J Anal Toxicol 1985; 9:40–42.
131. Woycik DL. Correction and comment possible toxicity from propylene glycol in injectible drug preparations. Ann Pharmacother 1997; 31:1413.
132. Seay RE. Comment possible toxicity from propylene glycol in lorazepam infusion. Ann Pharmacother 1997; 31:647–648.

133. McConnel JR. Propylene glycol toxicity following continuous etomidate infusion for the control of refractory cerebral edema. Neurosurgery 1996; 38: 232–233.
134. Brooks DE, Wallace KL. Acute propylene glycol ingestion. J Toxicol Clin Toxicol 2002; 40(4):513–516.
135. Christopher MM, Eckfeldt JH, Eaton JW. Propylene glycol ingestion causes D lactic acidosis. Lab Invest 1990; 62:114–118.
136. Rich J, Scheife RT, Katz N, Caplan LR. Isopropyl alcohol intoxication. Arch Neurol 1990; 47:322–324.
137. Rosansky SJ. Isopropyl alcohol poisoning treated with hemodialysis: kinetics of isopropyl alcohol and acetone removal. J Toxicol Clin Toxicol 1982; 19:265–271.
138. King LH Jr, Bradley KP, Shires DL Jr. Hemodialysis for isopropyl alcohol poisoning. JAMA 1970; 211:1855.
139. Wax PM. Elixirs, diluents, and the passage of the 1938. Federal Food, Drug and Cosmetic Act. Ann Intern Med 1995; 122:456–461.
140. O'Brien KL, Selanikio JD, Hecdivert C, et al. Epidemic of pediatric deaths from acute renal failure caused by diethylene glycol poisoning: acute renal failure investigation team. JAMA 1998; 279:1175–1180.
141. Hanif M, Mobarak MR, Ronan A, Rahman D, Donova JJ Jr, Bennish ML. Fatal renal failure caused by diethylene glycol in paracetamol elixir: the Bangladesh epidemic. BMJ 1995; 311:88-91.
142. Bowie MD, McKenzie D. Diethylene glycol poisoning in children. S A Med J 1972; 46:931–934.
143. Okuonghae HO, Ighogboja IS, Lawson JO, Nwana EJ. Diethylene glycol poisoning in Nigerian children. Ann Torp Paediatr 1992; 12:235–238.
144. Cantarell MC, Fort J, Camps J, Sans M, Piera L. An acute intoxication due to topical application of diethylene glycol. Ann Intern Med 1987; 106:478–479.
145. Wiener HL, Richardson KE. Metabolism of diethylene glycol in male rats. Biochem Pharmacol 1989; 38:539–541.
146. Borron SW, Baud FJ, Garnier R. Intravenous 4-methylpyrazole as an antidote for diethylene glycol and triethylene glycol poisoning: a case report. Vet Hum Toxicol 1997; 39:26–28.
147. Vassiliadis J, Graudins A, Dowsett RP. Triethylene glycol poisoning treated with intravenous ethanol infusion. J Toxicol Clin Toxicol 1999; 37:733–736.
148. Thompson WL, Johnson AD, Maddrey WL. Diazepam and paraldehyde for treatment of severe delirium tremens. A controlled trial. Ann Intern Med 1975; 82:175–180.
149. Gutman RA. Paraldehyde acidosis. Am J Med 1967; 42:435–440.
150. Hadden JW. Pseudoketosis and hyperacetaldehydemia in paraldehyde acidosis. Am J Med 1969; 47:642–647.

—————————— 13 ——————————

Renal Tubular Acidosis

K. M. L. S. T. Moorthi and Daniel Batlle

Division of Nephrology, Northwestern University Feinberg School of Medicine, Chicago, Illinois, U.S.A

INTRODUCTION

The human body fuelled by a typical western diet, rich in protein, generates about 1 mmol of mineral acid per kg body weight each day. To maintain body alkali stores, the kidney must excrete an equivalent amount of acid each day (see Chapter 6). This excess nonvolatile acid is excreted by titrating filtered buffers (e.g., phosphates and creatinine) and by excreting ammonium (NH_4^+). Renal acid excretion can be inadequate as a result of either impaired NH_4^+ and titratable acid excretion or inadequate HCO_3^- reabsorption. Both defects can develop as a result of impaired H^+ secretion along the renal tubules.

The renal tubular acidosis (RTA) syndromes encompass a disparate group of tubular transport defects that have in common the inability to secrete H^+, a defect that is disproportionately large in relation to any reduction in the glomerular filtration rate (GFR) (1–15). This inability results in failure to excrete acid in the form of NH_4^+ and titratable acids or to recapture all filtered HCO_3^-, and leads to chronic metabolic acidosis.

Broadly, five general types of RTA have been described (Table 1). The initial classification of tubular defects in urinary acidification was designed to separate those involving the distal nephron from those affecting the proximal nephron. Distal RTA is characterized by inability to lower urine pH despite severe acidemia and minimal bicarbonate wastage. Proximal RTA (type II), by contrast, is characterized by marked HCO_3^- wastage, but preserved ability

Table 1   General Types of Renal Tubular Acidosis

Distal RTA (classic or Type I RTA)
Proximal RTA (bicarbonate wastage or Type II RTA)
Distal RTA with bicarbonate wastage (Type III RTA)
Hyperkalemic RTA associated with aldosterone deficiency (Type IV RTA)
Hyperkalemic distal RTA without aldosterone deficiency

---

to lower urine pH when plasma [HCO_3^-] (and therefore filtered HCO_3^-) is below a certain level. Distal RTA was the first RTA recognized, and thus the terms "type I" and "classic RTA" are sometimes used to describe this form of RTA. The term "type III RTA" is used to describe patients, in whom HCO_3^- wastage coexists with failure to lower urine pH despite profound acidemia, thus demonstrating a mixed pattern of tubular dysfunction (1).

When aldosterone deficiency was described as a cause of metabolic acidosis and hyperkalemia, the term "type IV RTA" was coined to describe this type of tubular acidosis (12). Unlike patients with type I RTA, patients with aldosterone deficiency are able to lower urine pH below 5.5 and, unlike those with type II RTA, these patients do not have significant HCO_3^- wastage. Thus, the tubular dysfunction associated with aldosterone deficiency is clearly distinguishable from that associated with either proximal or distal RTA. Later, however, it was recognized that some patients with metabolic acidosis and hyperkalemia could not lower urine pH despite acidosis or after an infusion of sodium sulfate (13–15). In these patients, metabolic acidosis and hyperkalemia result from impairment in both H^+ and K^+ secretion, and the defect was not primarily the result of aldosterone deficiency. This distinct pattern of impaired H^+ and K^+ secretion was ascribed to a voltage-defect similar to that produced by amiloride (16–19).

Some of the genetic defects associated with the hereditary types of both proximal and distal RTA have been identified and are the subject of a number of reviews (7,11,20–22). These genetic advances have expanded our understanding of the molecular mechanisms that lead to proximal and distal RTA.

PROXIMAL RENAL TUBULAR ACIDOSIS

Pathophysiology

Proximal RTA (type II RTA) is characterized by a defect in the ability to reabsorb HCO_3^- in the proximal tubule. Bicarbonate is freely filtered, and its concentration in the glomerular filtrate is equal to that in plasma. The majority of the filtered HCO_3^- (>70%) is reabsorbed in the proximal tubule and the remaining 30% is reclaimed by the loop of Henle, distal tubules, and collecting tubules (see Chapters 4 and 6). In an individual with a GFR of

Table 2 Serum [HCO_3^-], and Urine pH and [HCO_3^-] in Proximal Renal Tubular Acidosis

	Urine pH	Urine [HCO_3^-]
Normal [HCO_3^-]	>6.4	High
Acidosis*	<5.5	Low

*serum [HCO_3^-] below its renal threshold (usually 15–20 mEq/L).

$100\,mL/min$, approximately $2500\,mEq$ of HCO_3^- is filtered daily, and virtually all of this HCO_3^- is reabsorbed so that essentially none appears in the urine. The finding of considerable amounts of HCO_3^- in the urine in the absence of alkali loading, therefore, is indicative of a defect in HCO_3^- reabsorption. Because the vast majority of HCO_3^- is normally recaptured in the proximal tubule, the presumption is that renal HCO_3^- wastage involves a defect in proximal HCO_3^- reabsorption.

This presumption is supported by the knowledge that HCO_3^- reabsorptive capacity is more limited in the distal nephron. Thus, if there is a major defect in HCO_3^- reabsorption in the proximal tubule, a larger quantity of filtered HCO_3^- is delivered to the distal segments, including the thick ascending limb, overwhelming the distal system and resulting in urinary HCO_3^- wastage. For patients with proximal RTA to reabsorb HCO_3^- completely, the filtered load must be reduced to a critical level, usually achieved when plasma [HCO_3] is $<20\,mEq/L$. This plasma level is termed the renal threshold, below which HCO_3^--free urine can be produced (23,24). At normal or even slightly reduced plasma [HCO_3^-] levels above this threshold, urine pH is typically high (>6.4), but when plasma [HCO_3^-] falls to or below the threshold, urine pH falls to <5.5 (Table 2).

Patients with proximal RTA often are hypokalemic and display urinary K^+ wastage. The K^+ wastage is almost certainly due to increased delivery of Na^+ and HCO_3^- to the distal nephron, because K^+ excretion is proportional to the amount of Na^+ and also HCO_3^- delivered to the distal nephron. This relationship explains the fact that as the acidosis is corrected by HCO_3^- administration, K^+ losses increase because of increased delivery of the administered HCO_3^- to the cortical collecting tubule. Mild secondary hyperaldosteronism may also contribute to the urinary K^+ wastage.

Clinical Features and Causes of Proximal RTA

Proximal RTA can be seen as an isolated defect in HCO_3^- transport (that is, in H^+ secretion, see Chapter 4), termed isolated proximal RTA, or in association with multiple defects in tubular transport (22–24). Generalized proximal tubule dysfunction, also known as Fanconi's syndrome, is the more common type. A list of the many conditions associated with proximal RTA is given in Table 3.

Table 3   Causes of Proximal Renal Tubular Acidosis

Isolated proximal RTA
Primary
  Sporadic
  Autosomal Dominant
  Autosomal Recessive
Carbonic anhydrase deficiency
  Carbonic anhydrase II deficiency with osteopetrosis
  Carbonic anhydrase inhibitors

Proximal RTA with generalized tubular dysfunction
Primary or idiopathic
  Sporadic
  Genetically transmitted
Secondary to inherited diseases
  Cystinosis
  Tyrosinosis
  Hereditary fructose intolerance
  Lowe's syndrome
  Wilson's disease
  Pyruvate carboxylase deficiency
  Metachromatic leukodystrophy
  Galactosemia
Drugs and toxic agents
  Heavy metal toxicity
  Outdated tetracyclines
  L-arginine and L-lysine
  Streptozotocin
  G-mercaptopurine
  Toluene
  Sulfanilamide
  Valproic acid
  Gentamicin
  Ifosfamide
Miscellaneous
  Hyperparathyroidism
  Multiple myeloma
  Sjogren's syndrome
  Amyloidosis
  Nephrotic syndrome
  Renal transplantation
  Hypervitaminosis D
  Vitamin D deficiency or resistance
  Chronic active hepatitis
  Paroxysmal nocturnal hemoglobinuria
  Balkan nephropathy
  Renal vein thrombosis in newborns

Isolated Proximal RTA

Isolated proximal RTA is a rare disorder (2) and is divided into three subcategories: autosomal dominant, autosomal recessive, and sporadic (Table 4). Autosomal dominant proximal RTA has been reported in a single Costa Rican family. The clinical features include mild growth retardation and reduced bone density. The autosomal recessive type is associated with severe growth retardation, ocular abnormalities such as glaucoma, cataracts and band keratopathy, and mental retardation (22). Sporadic isolated proximal RTA is a nonfamilial transient disorder that has been reported during infancy. Patients with this disorder have defective renal and intestinal bicarbonate reabsorption. Recurrent vomiting during infancy and growth retardation are common clinical findings (23,25). The etiology of the bone abnormalities seen with isolated proximal RTA is not completely known.

Lemann et al. (26) examined the bone densities and net balances of fixed acid and minerals in two members of the Costa Rican family with hereditary isolated proximal RTA and short stature. In these two patients, net acid production was normal, net acid excretion matched production, and calcium balance was ~zero despite persistent metabolic acidosis. However, their bone densities were significantly lower than expected for their age and sex, and their iliac cortices were thinner than those of their unaffected brother. The histomorphometric analysis did not reveal any evidence of osteomalacia or osteitis fibrosa (26). From this study, it appears that there is no net bone loss in this form of isolated proximal RTA. The growth retardation may be due to reduced bone stores of HCO_3^-/CO_3^- or total body HCO_3^- deficit. Growth hormone inhibition by acidosis likely plays a role in impaired growth in all types of RTA. Autosomal dominant and autosomal recessive proximal RTA are usually permanent and require life-long alkali therapy. In contrast, sporadic isolated proximal RTA is transient and alkali therapy can be discontinued after several years.

Table 4 Genetics of Isolated Proximal Renal Tubular Acidosis

Syndrome	Gene localization	Locus symbol	Gene product
Autosomal dominant	?	?	?
Autosomal recessive	4q21	SLC4A4	NBC-1
Sporadic in infancy	–	–	Immaturity of NHE3 ?

$NBC-1 = Na^+/HCO_3^-$ Cotransporter.
$NHE3 = Na^+/H^+$ Exchanger.

Proximal RTA with Associated Defects (Fanconi's Syndrome)

The second category of proximal RTA, known as Fanconi's syndrome, is characterized by multiple proximal renal tubular defects. This syndrome is manifested by HCO_3^- wastage, accompanied by excessive urinary losses of glucose, phosphate, amino acids, uric acid and, to a lesser degree, Na^+, Ca^{++}, and K^+ (27). The exact nature of the defect underlying the HCO_3^- wastage is still not known. Reabsorption of all the substances involved, HCO_3^-, glucose, phosphate, and amino acids, is driven by the Na^+ gradient across the apical membrane.

Mechanisms of Proximal RTA

In the proximal tubule, HCO_3^- is reabsorbed in a four-step process, illustrated in Figure 1:

   i. H^+ ions are secreted into the tubule lumen both by the Na^+/H^+ exchanger (NHE3 isoform)and the H^+ ATPase pump on the apical membrane of the epithelial cells.
   ii. The secreted H^+ ions react with filtered HCO_3^- to form CO_2 and H_2O, a process facilitated by luminal carbonic anhydrase (CA IV isoform).

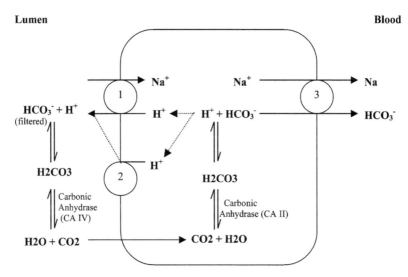

Figure 1   Schematic representation of HCO_3^- reabsorption in the proximal convoluted tubule. The Na^+ H^+ exchanger (NHE-3) **(1)** and the H^+ ATPase pump **(2)** secrete H^+ ions at the luminal membrane. The Na^+-HCO_3^- cotransporter (NBC-1) **(3)** provides the exit pathway for HCO_3^- in the basolateral membrane. Cytoplasmic carbonic anhydrase (CA II) and membrane-bound carbonic anhydrase (CA IV) are necessary to reabsorb HCO_3^-.

iii. CO_2 enters the cell by diffusion and recombines with H_2O, a process facilitated by cytosolic carbonic anhydrase (CA II isoform), thereby regenerating H^+ and HCO_3^-.

iv. HCO_3^- exits across the basolateral membrane via the Na^+-HCO_3^- cotransporter (NBC) (see Chapters 4 and 5).

Theoretically, proximal RTA could occur if there is a defect in any of these steps. The following section reviews the defects that could lead to or are known to cause proximal RTA.

Defects in Na^+-HCO_3^- Cotransporter (kNBC)

Three isoforms of NBC have been identified in the kidney (kNBC-1, -2 and -3) (28–31). In the kidney, kNBC works in the HCO_3^- efflux mode and is necessary for adequate HCO_3^- reabsorption, while NBC in some other tissues (i.e., the liver and pancreas) works in HCO_3^- influx mode and leads to cell alkalinization. The stoichiometry of kNBC is three equivalents of HCO_3^- for every Na^+ while in other tissues it is two equivalents of HCO_3^- for every Na^+(32). The isoform kNBC-1, is found in the basolateral membrane of the proximal tubule and is electrogenic (Fig. 1). The isoform kNBC-3, is found in the inner renal medulla and the brain and is electroneutral (33). The function of kNBC-1 appears to be coordinated with the apical Na^+/H^+ exchanger (NHE-3). The activity of both kNBC-1 and NHE3 increase during chronic metabolic acidosis, respiratory acidosis, chronic hyperfiltration, and after administration of angiotensin II (34,35).

In two patients with isolated proximal RTA, short stature, mental retardation, bilateral glaucoma, cataracts, and band keratopathy, two different homozygous missense mutations (R298S, R510S)in the *SLC4A4* gene, which encodes kNBC-1, have been described. In another patient with isolated proximal RTA, short stature, mental retardation, and bilateral glaucoma, a homozygous nonsense Q29X mutation in the *SLC4A4* gene was identified (36). This patient did not have cataracts or band keratopathy. Figure 2 illustrates these mutations and the associated clinical manifestations. Both kNBC-1 and pNBC-1 are similar, except that pNBC-1 has a unique 5′-end (37). The Q29X mutation causes a loss of kNBC-1 function, while the R298S and R510S mutations cause a loss of both kNBC-1 and pNBC-1 function. Complete loss of kNBC-1 function alone may lead to proximal RTA, short stature, mental retardation, and bilateral glaucoma, whereas band keratopathy and cataracts may require loss of both kNBC-1 and pNBC-1.

Defects in the Na^+/H^+ Exchanger

One of the eight isoforms of the Na^+/H^+ exchanger, NHE3, encoded by the gene *SLC9A3*, is expressed on the apical membrane of proximal tubular cells and in intestinal epithelial cells (38–41). In an NHE-3 knockout mouse

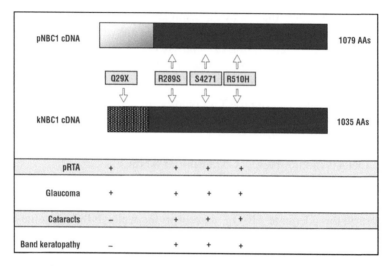

Figure 2 Known mutations of NBC-1 and associated clinical manifestations in patients with proximal RTA and ocular abnormalities. kNBC 1, kidney-typeNa$^+$-HCO$_3^-$ cotransporter; pNBC 1, pancreatic-type Na$^+$-HCO$_3^-$ cotransporter; AAs, amino acids. *Source*: From Ref. 22.

model, HCO$_3^-$ absorption falls by 61% compared to wild type mice, and small decreases in plasma pH and [HCO$_3^-$] occur, suggesting that defects in NHE3 could cause a proximal RTA (42). If one extrapolates from the NHE3 knockout data to humans, a defect in NHE3 should result not only in proximal RTA but also in significant renal Na$^+$ wastage and hypotension (42). Despite this evidence, no mutations in the gene encoding NHE3 have been identified in patients with isolated proximal RTA.

Defects in Carbonic Anhydrase (CA)

An isolated defect of proximal tubular HCO$_3^-$ reabsorption could also be caused by carbonic anhydrase deficiency. The kidney has at least two forms of carbonic anhydrase, CA II and CA IV. Also present in red blood cells, CA II is found in the cell cytoplasm of both proximal and distal tubules, whereas CA IV is mainly found in the brush border of the proximal tubule and is the isoform of CA involved in facilitating apical HCO$_3^-$ reabsorption (Fig. 1). Sly et al. (43) reported three siblings with RTA, osteopetrosis, cerebral calcification, and mental retardation with inherited deficiency of CA II in red blood cells. These patients had features of both proximal and distal RTA (Type III RTA) (44). A derangement in CA IV expression or function could specifically lead to impairment of proximal HCO$_3^-$ reabsorption, but, to our knowledge, CA IV deficiency has not been demonstrated in any patients with isolated proximal RTA.

Other Defects in Proximal RTA

Defects in the function or expression of apical Cl^-/base exchangers in the kidney could also lead to proximal RTA. Several isoforms of these apical anion exchangers have been identified in proximal tubule and cortical collecting duct epithelial cells (see Chapter 5) (45). Included among these are the Cl^-/formate, Cl^-/oxalate, and Cl^-/hydroxyl exchangers in proximal tubule and the Cl^-/HCO_3^- exchanger in the cortical collecting duct. Chloride/ formate exchange, which was first identified in kidney proximal tubule, works in parallel with the apical Na^+/H^+ exchanger, and is thought to reabsorb the majority of filtered Cl^- (see Chapters 4 and 5) (45). To date, no such defects have been identified in patients with proximal RTA.

The generalized proximal tubular dysfunction in Fanconi's syndrome could be a result of a generalized defect of Na^+-coupled apical membrane transporters, a defect in basolateral Na^+/K^+-ATPase, or metabolic disorders that lower intracellular concentrations of ATP. The defect in HCO_3^- reabsorption in this syndrome may be secondary to a defect in basolateral Na^+/K^+-ATPase activity (46). A model of Fanconi's syndrome has been produced by administering maleic acid to rats and dogs, and in this model renal cortical Na^+/K^+-ATPase activity is markedly diminished (47). The relevance of these observations to human Fanconi's syndrome remains to be determined.

Fructose administration to patients with hereditary fructose intolerance induces a proximal RTA (48). Patients with this disorder lack the enzyme fructose 1-phosphate aldolase and thus are unable to convert fructose 1-phosphate into intracellular phosphate. High intracellular concentrations of fructose 1-phosphate and low concentrations of ATP, GTP and adenine nucleotides are found in cells in the proximal tubule in a rat model of this disease, and this is the only segment of the kidney that possesses the enzyme fructokinase (49). These findings suggest that in inherited metabolic disorders, proximal RTA may be caused by an inadequate supply of ATP to transport systems, particularly to basolateral Na^+-K^+-ATPase.

Diagnosis of Proximal RTA

The diagnosis of proximal RTA is established by the presence of a hyperchloremic metabolic acidosis and HCO_3^- wastage. Patients with proximal RTA have an intact ability to lower urine pH <5.5 when the plasma $[HCO_3^-]$ is less than the renal threshold (usually $<20\,mEq/L$) (Table 2). Traditionally, a fractional HCO_3^- excretion of 15% or higher is said to be needed to establish the diagnosis of proximal RTA (1,2). Given the large capacity of the distal nephron to reabsorb HCO_3^-, however, even minor degrees of HCO_3^- wastage (i.e., fractional HCO_3^- excretion $\sim$5%)are, in our opinion, sufficient for the diagnosis (50). The most definitive way to diagnose proximal RTA is to assess HCO_3^- excretion when plasma $[HCO_3^-]$

is increased by intravenous administration of $NaHCO_3$ (HCO_3^- titration test). When this condition is present, a marked increase in urinary HCO_3^- excretion and urine pH occurs as plasma $[HCO_3^-]$ rises above the renal threshold and can easily be appreciated. Urine PCO_2, measured after HCO_3^- infusion, is normal in patients with proximal RTA (i.e., above 70 mmHg, see later) indicating that distal H^+ secretion is intact (51). Hypokalemia and renal potassium wasting are also usually present in patients with proximal RTA. Glucosuria in the face of normal blood glucose, aminoaciduria, hyperphosphaturia, and hyperuricosuria characterize the presence of Fanconi's syndrome (27,52).

Therapy of Proximal RTA

Patients with proximal RTA should be given HCO_3^- supplements (23,53). In children, in particular, HCO_3^- replacement therapy is critical for the prevention of growth retardation due to acidosis (53). The magnitude of the bicarbonaturia that occurs when serum $[HCO_3^-]$ is normalized requires that large amounts of HCO_3^- be administered (5-15 meq/kg body weight). By adding a thiazide diuretic (e.g., hydrochlorothiazide 25–50 mg daily), the amount can be minimized. Thiazides enhance proximal tubule and loop HCO_3^- reabsorption by reducing extracellular volume and this effect allows for a reduction in the amount of bicarbonate to be given daily.

Both sodium bicarbonate and thiazide administration unfortunately aggravate hypokalemia by promoting K^+ secretion in the collecting duct, and therefore plasma $[K^+]$ must be carefully monitored when these therapies are used. A mixture of sodium and potassium salts is usually needed. We recommend Polycitra (K-Shohl solution, a mixture of sodium and potassium citrate). This oral solution contains 1 mEq of K^+ and 1 mEq of Na^+ per mL, and the citrate, when metabolized, is equivalent to 2 mEq of HCO_3^- per mL.

In patients with Fanconi's syndrome, serum (phosphorus) should also be corrected as needed to avoid bone disease. In untreated Fanconi's syndrome, the skeletal abnormalities typically found are rickets in children and osteomalacia in adults, likely due to chronic hypophosphatemia or Vitamin D deficiency (54,55).

DISTAL RENAL TUBULAR ACIDOSIS (DISTAL RTA)

Distal RTA can present with either low or high plasma $[K^+]$. The defects leading to these two types, and the corresponding clinical features, are quite different and we will consider these two entities separately. The diagnosis and treatment of both entities, however, will be discussed together at the end of this chapter for the sake of simplicity and convenience.

Classic Distal RTA (Type I)

Pathophysiology

Excretion of sufficient nonvolatile acid to match daily endogenous production is accomplished in the distal nephron by H^+ secretion (see Chapter 4). Secretion of H^+ at this site results in acid excretion by titrating filtered buffers destined for excretion, such as phosphate, creatinine and uric acid, and by combining with NH_3 to form NH_4^+, thereby "trapping" it in the urine. In the absence of these buffers, secretion of H^+ would quickly produce a limiting transtubular $[H^+]$ gradient in the collecting tubule. In humans this gradient (a minimum urine pH of 4.5) would only allow the excretion of only $0.03\,mEq$ of H^+/L of urine. Thus, the presence of urinary buffers is essential to excrete the 50–$70\,mEq$ of H^+ needed daily to maintain acid balance. A defect in distal H^+ secretion is present in Type I RTA, reducing the maximal transtubular $[H^+]$ gradient. This defect, in turn, results in a decrease in both NH_4^+ and titratable acid excretion. These changes reduce net acid excretion, lead to a positive acid balance and result in the development of a hyperchloremic metabolic acidosis.

An inability to secrete H^+ and thus lower urine pH normally (i.e., <5.5) in the face of spontaneous acidemia, no matter how severe, is the hallmark of Type I RTA. An incomplete form of Type I RTA is manifested by the inability to lower urine pH maximally after acid loading, in subjects in whom metabolic acidosis does not develop spontaneously (see later) (4–6,56).

Associated Abnormalities: Patients with type I RTA often present with nephrocalcinosis and kidney stones or both. A decrease in citrate excretion and an increase in calcium excretion are the predisposing factors for these complications. They also typically present with hypokalemia, which results from excessive urinary K^+ losses. The precise cause of the urinary K^+ wasting remains unclear. A defect in H^+/K^+-ATPase function in the apical membrane of collecting tubule epithelial cells would provide an explanation for both K^+ wastage and impaired H^+ secretion (57). The finding of gastric parietal cell hypoacidity in some patients with Type I RTA suggests that a common defect in the H^+/K^+-ATPase of both gastric parietal cells and renal collecting tubule cells (58). Administration of vanadate, a nonspecific inhibitor of the H^+/K^+-ATPase, to rats also results in a hypokalemic metabolic acidosis similar to that seen in patients with Type I RTA (57). We administered vanadate to rats and found marked inhibition of H^+/K^+-ATPase in collecting ducts from both K^+-repleted and K^+-depleted rats (59). Our rats did not develop overt hypokalemia or metabolic acidosis, but urine NH_4^+ excretion was reduced suggesting impaired distal acidification (Batlle et al. unpublished data). An argument against the H^+/K^+-ATPase hypothesis is the finding that severe hypokalemia occurs in hereditary types of RTA where the genetic defect does not affect H^+/K^+ ATPase activity. For instance, patients with mutations in two different sub-units of the H^+-ATPase pump often have severe hypokalemia (see later, hereditary distal RTA). A role of the H^+/K^+-ATPase in causing distal RTA, with severe hypokalemia, in our opinion, remains an attractive possi-bility but requires more direct evidence, which is currently lacking.

Clinical Features and Causes of Classic Distal RTA

Classic distal RTA may occur as a primary entity or may be acquired as a result of renal tubule involvement in a variety of renal diseases, systemic conditions, or drugs. In children, distal RTA usually occurs as a primary entity, whereas in adults it is frequently an acquired disease. Table 5 lists the causes of distal RTA. Hypergammaglobulinemia, autoimmune disorders with renal involvement, and disorders of calcium metabolism are among the most common causes of acquired distal RTA. The primary type of distal RTA can present sporadically, but often is inherited in a dominant or reces-sive pattern, as discussed below.

Acquired Distal RTA: The acquired form of classic distal RTA is seen in a variety of conditions. This disorder may develop in up to 50% of patients with Sjogren's syndrome and hyperglobulinemic purpura (60,61). The mechanism by which hyperglobulinemia causes distal RTA is not known, but it is independent of the class or quantity of abnormal circu-lating globulin (61). In patients with Sjogren's syndrome, high levels of serum gamma globulin, serum protein, and serum β-2 microglobulin are the best predictors of the development of classic distal RTA (62). Classic dis-tal RTA has also been reported in patients with cryoglobulinemia (63), fibrosing alveolitis (64), thyroiditis and Grave's disease (65), systemic lupus erythematosis (66,67), primary biliary cirrhosis (68), chronic active hepatitis (69–73), and multiple myeloma (74). Distal RTA is also seen in patients with chronic renal allograft rejection (75–77).

Patients with primary hyperparathyroidism appear to develop distal RTA only after they develop nephrocalcinosis (78,79). Similarly, patients with Vitamin D intoxication, hyperthyroidism, idiopathic hypercalciuria, medullary sponge kidney, and Fabry's disease who do not have nephrocal-cinosis do not develop distal RTA (80–85). Deposition of calcium in the renal medulla and in the cortical regions adjacent to the collecting ducts appears to be the primary mechanism causing impaired distal acidification in disorders of calcium metabolism (86–88).

Among drugs that cause distal RTA, amphotericin B is a classic exam-ple (see later under mechanisms of distal RTA). Lithium causes distal RTA in animals but in humans usually results in a mild and incomplete type of distal RTA (89). Distal RTA has also been considered as a complication of toluene intoxication. It was initially suggested that toluene caused distal

Table 5 Causes of Distal RTA

Primary or hereditary
  Autosomal dominant
    (Mutations in the anion exchanger isoform AE-1)
  Autosomal recessive with deafness
    (Mutations in the B1 subunit of H^+ ATPase)
  Autosomal recessive with relatively well preserved hearing
    (Mutations in the a4 subunit of H^+ ATPase)
Acquired
Associated with nephrocalcinosis
  Primary nephrocalcinosis
  Idiopathic hypercalciuria
  Hyperthyroidism
  Excess vitamin D
  Hyperparathyroidism
  Urolithiasis
  Fabry's disease
  Medullary sponge kidney
  Sarcoidosis
Associated with systemic diseases
  Multiple myeloma
  Systemic lupus erythematosis
  Chronic active hepatitis
  Primary biliary cirrhosis
  Sjogren's syndrome
  Hypergammaglobulinemias
  Thyroiditis
  Grave's disease
  Renal transplant rejection
Drug/toxin induced
  Amphotericin
  Toluene
  Vanadate (?)

RTA by causing back-leak of H^+ in the collecting tubule in a manner similar to amphotericin. However, toluene is metabolized to hippuric acid, and the levels of this organic acid can be as high as $30\,mg/mL$ during daily toluene inhalations by individuals addicted to this compound (90). Thus, it seems likely that much of the acidosis that develops in such patients is the result of an organic acid production and accumulation (see also Chapter 12) (90,91). A reversible distal acidification defect, however, has been documented in some patients (90). In the northeastern part of Thailand, endemic cases of severe hypokalemic distal RTA have been reported (92). This area has been found to have high levels of vanadium, an inhibitor of H^+/K^+-

ATPase (as well as Na^+/K^+-ATPase), in the soil and well water, and the local population has a higher than normal concentration of vanadium in urine and tissue (92).

Inherited Distal RTA: Both autosomal dominant and recessive patterns of inheritance occur in patients with hereditary distal RTA, and the mode of inheritance affects the clinical presentation and severity (Table 6). Autosomal recessive distal RTA occurs early in life and is frequently associated with a family history of consanguinity (7). The phenotypic features include osteopetrosis, deafness and mental retardation, and typically the clinical phenotype is more severe than autosomal dominant distal RTA. Hypokalemia, metabolic acidosis, nephrocalcinosis, renal calculi, and growth retardation are seen in both autosomal recessive and dominant distal RTA, but tend to be more severe and more common in patients with autosomal recessive distal RTA.

Metabolic acidosis is the key determinant of delayed growth. If metabolic acidosis occurs early in life and is untreated, significant growth retardation can be seen in both autosomal dominant and recessive distal RTA. As the genetic defects responsible for autosomal dominant and autosomal recessive distal RTA are better characterized, it may be possible to establish clinical correlates with each of the specific genetic defects.

Incomplete Distal RTA: Incomplete Type 1 RTA is a syndrome manifested by an inability to maximally lower urinary pH after acid loading in patients in whom metabolic acidosis does not develop spontaneously (51,56). It has been described with both hereditary and acquired types of distal RTA. For instance, relatives of patients with identified autosomal dominant distal RTA caused by mutations in the *AE1* gene (see later) often have an

Table 6 Comparison of Clinical Features of Autosomal Recessive and Dominant Distal RTA

Clinical feature	Autosomal recessive	Autosomal dominant
Age of presentation	Early in life	Adulthood
Parent consanguinity	Common	Rare
Severity of dRTA	Severe	Mild to moderate
Hypokalemia	Severe	Mild to moderate
Bone disease	Common	Rare
Growth retardation	Common	Rare
Nephrocalcinosis	Common	Rare
Mental retardation	May be present	Absent
Cerebral calcification	Common	Absent
Deafness	Common	Absent

incomplete distal RTA (93). Chronic interstitial nephritis, kidney stones, medullary sponge kidney, and lithium therapy are a few causes of acquired incomplete distal RTA. Ammonium excretion is normal or only slightly reduced and these patients also may have low urinary citrate excretion. The cause of the low urinary excretion of citrate has been ascribed to enhanced proximal tubule reabsorption driven by the presence of subclinical acidosis.

In patients on chronic lithium therapy, HCO_3^- administration fails to raise urine PCO_2, a sign of impaired collecting duct H^+ secretion (see later), even though they retained the ability to lower urine pH after NH_4Cl loading (89). These patients usually do not develop a metabolic acidosis, indicating that their defect in H^+ secretion is mild. Lithium therapy, at therapeutic plasma levels, consistently causes this type of incomplete distal RTA (89). A similar pattern is described in patients with a variety of disorders, who thus appear to have an "incomplete form" of incomplete distal RTA (94).

Mechanisms of Classic Distal RTA

Pathophysiology

Normal collecting duct function. As a background to understanding the possible defects in H^+ secretion in the collecting duct, a brief review of H^+ secretion in this part of the distal nephron is in order (for more detail, see Chapters 4 and 5). The collecting duct has three distinct functional segments: cortical, outer medullary and inner medullary. The cortical collecting duct has the capacity for both H^+ and HCO_3^- secretion. The outer medullary collecting duct has the highest capacity for H^+ secretion, whereas the inner medullary collecting duct has a lower capacity. Throughout the collecting duct, H^+ secretion is accomplished by active transport, provided by H^+-ATPase and H^+/K^+-ATPase. Both transporters are located in the apical membrane of α-intercalated cells (Fig. 3). Apical H^+ secretion generates HCO_3^- inside the intercalated cell, which exits via a Cl^-/HCO_3^- exchanger (AE1) on the basolateral membrane (see Chapters 4 and 5). Polypeptides on HCO_3^- exchange transporters are encoded by at least two gene families, *SLC4* and *SLC26* (95). The *SLC4* gene family includes at least three Na^+-independent Cl^-/HCO_3^- exchanger genes and multiple Na^+-HCO_3^- cotransporter and Na^+-dependent anion exchanger genes. The most extensively studied among them are the Na^+-independent anion exchangers, AE1, AE2, and AE3, all of which are expressed in kidney. The *AE1* gene encodes eAE1 (band 3), the major intrinsic protein of the erythrocyte, as well as kAE1, the basolateral Cl^-/HCO_3^- exchanger of the acid-secreting α-intercalated cell. Mutations in AE1 are responsible for some forms of heritable distal RTA. The widely expressed AE2 anion exchanger participates in recovery from alkaline loads and in regulatory cell volume increase following shrinkage (95).

Intercalated cells constitute 40% of the cells in the distal nephron, and exist in two forms: one secretes H^+ using H^+-ATPase (α type) and the other

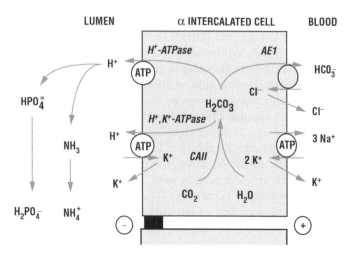

Figure 3 Collecting duct α-intercalated cell showing the H^+ ATPase and the H^+/K^+ ATPase pumps on the apical membrane and the anion exchanger (AE-1 or Cl^-/HCO_3^- exchanger) and Na^+/K^+ ATPase on the basolateral membrane. Under normal conditions the H^+ ATPase is the major pump secreting H^+ into the tubule lumen, where it combines with phosphate and ammonia to accomplish acid excretion.

is involved in HCO_3^- secretion (β type). The α-intercalated cell is abundant in the outer medullary collecting duct, but is also present in the cortical collecting duct. The α-intercalated cell has an H^+-ATPase in the apical membrane and a Cl^-/HCO_3^- exchanger (AE1) in the basolateral membrane (Fig. 4). The β-intercalated cell, found only in the cortical collecting tubule, secretes HCO_3^- into the tubule lumen via a Cl^-/HCO_3^- exchanger in the apical membrane and has an H^+-ATPase on the basolateral membrane (96–100). The identity of the luminal Cl^-/HCO_3^- exchanger has been a matter of debate. It has been proposed that an isoform of the anion exchanger, AE4, performs this function in the rabbit kidney and that pendrin accomplishes this function in the mouse (101). The expression and possibly the function of AE4 is species specific. In rats and in mice, AE4 functions as a Cl^-/HCO_3^- exchanger in the basolateral membrane of α-intercalated cells, whereas in rabbits AE4 is localized to the apical and lateral membranes and may contribute to HCO_3^- secretion (101). Pendrin is an apical Cl^-/HCO_3^- exchanger encoded by the *PDS* gene (45,102) and may have an essential role in Cl^- reabsorption and HCO_3^- secretion (45). So far no mutations in the pendrin gene have been identified in patients with proximal or distal RTA. It is reasonable to postulate that some patients with pendrin mutations, who usually present with goiter (103), may have a mild renal phenotype that will require provocative tests of urinary acidification for its identification.

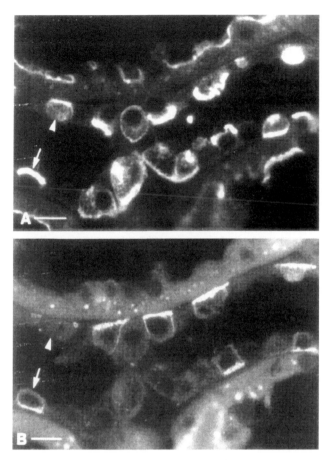

Figure 4 (A) Immunofluorescence demonstrating H^+-ATPase in the apical membrane of the α-intercalated cell. (B) Immunofluorescence demonstrating AE-1 in the basolateral membrane of the α-intercalated cell. *Source*: From Alper et al. Proc. Natl Acad. Sci USA 1989;86:5429–5433.

Principal cells constitute 60% of the cells in the distal tubule and collecting tubules and are involved in water and Na^+ reabsorption, and K^+ secretion (104). The lumen-negative transepithelial potential created by Na^+ reabsorption via the apical membrane Na^+ channel (EnaC) then promotes either passive Cl^- reabsorption through the paracellular pathway or K^+ secretion through K^+ channels (primarily ROMK) in the apical membrane. The lumen-negative potential generated by Na^+ reabsorption in principal cells also favors H^+ secretion by neighboring α-intercalated cells.

Carbonic anhydrase. Unlike the proximal tubule, the collecting duct contains only the type II isoenzyme (CA II) in the cytosol of intercalated cells. As noted earlier, this isoform is also found in the cytosol of proximal tubule cells, as well as in bone, brain, and retina (43,105,106). Defects in cytosolic CA II have been reported to cause a mixed type of RTA (see "CA II Gene Mutations" below) (43).

Defective H$^+$ Secretion: Potential mechanisms underlying distal RTA are summarized in Table 7 and are outlined below.

H$^+$-ATPase defects. Defects in H$^+$-ATPase have long been postulated as the key mechanism for distal RTA (3–7,11–13). This hypothesis is supported by the demonstration of the absence of apical H$^+$-ATPase staining in renal biopsies from patients with distal RTA associated with Sjogren's syndrome (107,108). In one of these reports, physiologic tests were consistent with a secretory defect type of distal RTA (107). In fact, genetic defects in H$^+$-ATPase have now been identified in hereditary distal RTA, discussed later (under molecular pathogenesis) (109–111).

Rate-dependent defects. The term "rate dependent" defect is used to designate abnormalities in H$^+$ secretion that are secondary to abnormalities in the transport of other ions in the collecting duct. For example, a decrease in the ability to generate a negative lumen potential, as a result of either impaired Na$^+$ reabsorption or enhanced Cl$^-$ reabsorption, will decrease H$^+$ secretion in this segment of the nephron. Such a defect is likely to

Table 7 Potential Mechanisms of Distal RTA

Type	Example
Secretory defects	
a. Diffuse H$^+$ pump defect	Kidney transplant rejection
b. Medullary collecting duct H$^+$ pump defect	Nephrocalcinosis
c. Diffuse H$^+$ pump failure and K$^+$ secretory defect	Obstructive nephropathy
d. Medullary H$^+$/K$^+$ ATPase defect?	vanadate?
Rate-dependent defects	
a. Voltage-dependent defect	Amiloride
b. Enhanced chloride transport	Gordon's syndrome
c. Reduced urinary buffer	Hyperkalemia
d. Aldosterone deficiency	Selective aldosterone deficiency
e. Aldosterone resistance	Pseudohypoaldosteronism
f. Reduced intracellular H$^+$	Cytosolic carbonic anhydrase deficiency
g. Reduced H$^+$ conductance	Toluene
Permeability defects	
a. H$^+$ back-leak	Amphotericin B
b. Enhanced HCO$_3^-$ secretion	Unknown

decrease K^+ secretion as well (see hyperkalemic distal RTA), and is unlikely to be responsible for Type I RTA. The availability of buffers (e.g., NH_3, HPO_4^-) is critically important for the secretion of the H^+ to be effective in excreting adequate amounts of acid. Thus, reduction in a urinary buffer such as NH_3, as seen in chronic hyperkalemic states, limits the rate of H^+ excretion and results in a form of hyperkalemic distal RTA or contributes to it. The H^+-ATPase is also responsive to aldosterone, and thus aldosterone deficiency can slow the rate of H^+ secretion by this transporter leading to a rate dependent form of RTA.

Back-leak. An abnormal increase in H^+ permeability in the apical membrane of collecting duct cells, resulting in back-leak of secreted H^+, is a postulated mechanism for distal RTA that was once widely accepted. Administration of amphotericin, however, provides the only known model for such a defect (112). In the turtle urinary bladder and in mammalian collecting tubules, application of amphotericin to the mucosal (or apical membrane) side results in H^+ back-diffusion (lumen to blood) (113). The drug also increases K^+ permeability but not HCO_3^- permeability. Toluene was initially felt to cause a permeability defect as well. Unlike amphotericin, however, toluene does not reduce the pH gradient generated across the turtle bladder, suggesting that it does not cause H^+ back-diffusion (90). In humans exposed to toluene, urine PCO_2 does not increase normally after $NaHCO_3$ loading, indicating a diminished rate of H^+ secretion by the collecting tubules (90). Another mechanism that could mimic a permeability defect is mistargeting of the Cl^-/HCO_3^- exchanger to the apical rather than basolateral membrane of the α-intercalated cell. This would cause the α-intercalated cell to operate as a β type cell with enhanced HCO_3^- secretion (see "*AE1* mutations" below).

Molecular Pathogenesis: The hereditary form of distal RTA, although rare, has received increased attention recently because of dramatic advances in the understanding of its genetic basis (93,114–117). Mutations have been identified in the genes encoding the anion exchanger (AE1), cytosolic carbonic anhydrase enzyme (CA II), and H^+-ATPase (B_1 and A_4 subunits).

AE1 Gene mutations. The *AE1* gene was targeted as a potential candidate gene for hereditary distal RTA because H^+ secretion by the α-intercalated cell requires simultaneous HCO_3^- exit through the basolateral membrane, via the Cl^-/HCO_3^- exchanger (most likely AE1 in humans, Fig. 3). Malfunction of AE1 could result in a decrease in H^+ secretion in the collecting duct. The AE1 knockout mouse lacks AE1 immunostaining in α-intercalated cells, a finding consistent with a role for AE1 defects as a potential cause of a distal RTA (118). Functional studies revealing impaired distal acidification or even the presence of metabolic acidosis, however, have not been reported in this mouse model.

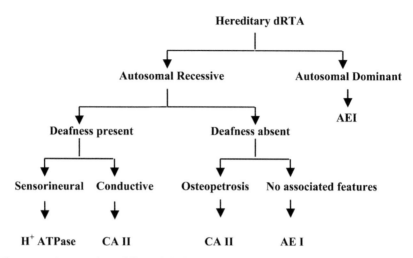

Figure 5 Approach to differential diagnosis of hereditary distal RTA (dRTA) using deafness as a key feature. At the bottom of each branch of the tree are the key transporters (H⁺ ATPase or AEI) or enzymes (CA II, type II isoform of carbonic anhydrase) that have been identified to have loss of function mutations with each abnormality. AEI mutations causing recessive dRTA are rare and so far have been reported in patients from Southeast Asia.

The *AE* gene family has at least three members, with the *AE1* (also known as *band 3, SCL4A1, or EPB3*)gene being the most abundant. In the collecting duct, the basolateral Cl^-/HCO_3^- exchanger protein is encoded by the *AE1* gene, present on chromosome 7, and this same gene gives rise to the erythrocyte Cl^-/HCO_3^- exchanger. The kidney form of *AE1* differs from the erythrocyte form in that it is truncated at the amino terminus, lacking exons 1–3 (119).

Mutations in the gene encoding the erythrocyte Cl^-/HCO_3^- exchanger have been described in autosomal dominant distal RTA (93,114–116). The *AE1* mutation most frequently found in affected members was a single base change resulting in a missense mutation (Arg → His) at codon 589 (R589S). A second mutation at codon 589, R589H, was found in the several unrelated families with autosomal dominant distal RTA (93,116). The exact mechanism by which the *AE1* mutations R589H and R589S cause autosomal dominant distal RTA remains to be elucidated (7,120). Insertion of the HCO_3^-/Cl^- exchanger into the apical, rather than the basolateral membrane (i.e., mistargeting)could negate the H⁺ ions pumped by the H⁺-ATPase or H^+/K^+-ATPase (119). Among individuals with autosomal dominant distal RTA, correlation between genotype and phenotype has not been apparent. A family with R589C mutation has been reported in which the father had severe nephrocalcinosis and lithiasis and isosthenuria but no metabolic acidosis (20). By contrast, the patient's daughter was acidotic, hypokalemic, and hypercalciuric, but without nephrocalcinosis. Thus, the clinical phenotype can be altered by (still undefined) modifier genes, some of which themselves may be RTA genes. Deafness has not been reported with dominant distal RTA and *AE1* gene mutations, which makes it a useful distinguishing clinical feature.

From these studies, it appears that *AE1* gene mutations are responsible for the autosomal dominant type of distal RTA. Mutations in *AE1* also cause hereditary spherocytosis and ovalocytosis. However, these conditions are usually not associated with distal RTA and conversely distal RTA is not associated with abnormal red cell fragility (21). Mutations in *AE1* have also been identified as a major cause of autosomal recessive distal RTA in southern Asia (121), but not as yet in the Western hemisphere. Compound heterozygosity of *AE1* mutations has been associated with Southeast Asian ovalocytosis (SAO)and distal RTA, and homozygosity of *AE1* mutations has been associated with distal RTA and hemolytic anemia.

CA II gene mutations. The CA II gene is located at q22 on chromosome 8. At least 12 different mutations have been identified so far in different kindreds with distal RTA (122–125). The syndrome of CA II deficiency, caused by these mutations, has a varied phenotypic presentation and has been diagnosed in a variety of ethnic backgrounds. It is particularly common in Arab populations of the Middle East. More than 70% of the reported cases of CA II deficiency syndrome are from these populations, probably the result of both a high rate of consanguineous marriages and an increased frequency of the CA II deficiency allele (122).

Deficiency of CA II is also the primary defect underlying the autosomal recessive syndrome of osteopetrosis, renal tubular acidosis, and cerebral calcification (43,69). In this disorder, it causes a mixed pattern of proximal and distal RTA (type III RTA). Early onset of hypokalemia, paroxysmal muscle weakness, moderate to severe mental retardation, and growth retardation are the other associated manifestations.

H^+*-ATPase gene mutations.* A defect in H^+-ATPase function has long been implicated as a likely cause of both hereditary and acquired distal RTA (8,9). In patients with hereditary distal RTA, mutations in the genes encoding this key enzyme were only recently uncovered. Karet et al. (109) studied 31 unrelated kindreds with a recessive form of hereditary distal RTA associated with sensorineural hearing loss, screening for mutations in the *ATP6V1B1* gene, which encodes the B_1 subunit of H^+-ATPase. This gene was found to be defective in 19 of the 31 total kindreds. None of these mutations were found among 36 unaffected control subjects. The finding of 15 independent mutations showing specificity for distal RTA and cosegregating with the disease constitutes proof that mutations in *ATP6V1B1* cause recessive distal RTA. These *ATP6B1* mutations are likely to disrupt the structure or abrogate the production of the normal B_1 subunit protein (109).

The results of genetic analysis for *ATP6B1* mutations in 13 kindreds with hereditary recessive distal RTA with normal hearing were also reported by the same group (126). No mutations at this gene locus were associated with distal RTA in these kindreds. A genome-wide linkage search revealed a new locus, however, at chromosome 7q33–34, in 9 of the 13 kindreds (126). A gene, *ATP6V0A4,* encoding a novel kidney-specific H^+-ATPase pump accessory subunit, the A_4 subunit, was shown to be involved. These 9 kindreds were screened, and 8 were found to have different homozygous mutations in the *ATP6V0A4* gene (110). Other kindreds with this form of RTA did not show linkage to either *ATP6V0A4* or to *ATP6V1B1,* which implies the existence of additional mutations at different loci in this disorder. More recently, the same group investigated 26 new kindreds with recessive distal RTA and reported 7 novel *ATP6V0A4* mutations (111). They also reported the development of mild hearing loss, usually in the young adulthood, as opposed to the severe hearing loss that usually occurs in childhood in *ATP6V1B1* mutations (111).

Expression studies demonstrated the *ATP6V0A4* gene product in α-intercalated cells in the kidney (110) and within the human inner ear (111). Although the involvement of the A_4 subunit in distal RTA shows that it must be essential for proper H^+-ATPase pump function in the kidney, its role within the multisubunit pump structure remains unclear. In yeast, some mutations showed that this subunit is important for the assembly of the H^+-ATPase, whereas other mutations had greater effects on ATPase activity and H^+ transport.

The foregoing shows that *ATP6V1B1* mutations are associated with recessive distal RTA and severe deafness in childhood, whereas *ATP6V0A*4 mutations are associated with mild hearing loss that develops later, in early adulthood. Some families with primary recessive distal RTA do not link to either *ATP6V1B1* or *ATP6V0A4.* There are numerous other candidate genes for recessive distal RTA including the genes for all known subunits of the H^+-ATPase or genes whose products are required for the trafficking of ths transporter to the apical membrane (21).

Deafness and the Diagnosis of Hereditary Distal RTA: Deafness is an important feature in some of the hereditary forms of distal RTA(7). The age at which hearing impairment develops varies from as early as 8 months to 15 years, although most patients have hearing impairment before 12 years of age. The presence or absence of deafness and the type of deafness, conductive vs. sensorineural, aids in the differential diagnosis of the various forms of hereditary distal RTA (7). Figure 5 depicts a diagnostic approach to hereditary distal RTA using deafness as a key feature. The H^+-ATPases are ubiquitous in nature and some subunits can be found both in the inner ear and in the kidney. Endolymph pH is maintained near 7.40 in the cochlea, but is lower in the endolymphatic sac, indicating an active acidification process.

An H^+-ATPase containing the B_1 subunit is present in the human cochlea (109). Normal auditory function relies on a proper pH within the endolymphatic system, and this H^+-ATPase presumably is responsible for the maintenance of this pH. Thus, *ATP6V1B1* mutations resulting in loss of H^+-ATPase function could cause hearing impairment as well as distal RTA.

Bilateral sensorineural hearing loss occurs in the majority of patients with *ATP6V1B1* mutations and distal RTA. In a minority of distal RTA kindreds without *ATP6V1B1* mutations, however, sensorineural hearing loss was also present (21). It will be interesting to find out what types of gene mutations are found in these individuals. *ATP6V1B1* null mice models have been created, but have not helped to evaluate the contribution of the B_1 subunit in the ear or genital tract, as these animals have normal hearing and fertility. These mice are not spontaneously acidotic, but do display a urinary acidification defect when challenged (127).

Patients with CA II deficiency syndrome and those with H^+-ATPase mutations have many features in common. Both forms of distal RTA often present with hypokalemia, nephrocalcinosis, and both have a pattern of recessive transmission often with a history of consanguinity. The type of deafness is useful in separating these two genetic lesions clinically. Conductive deafness is seen in patients with CA II deficiency, some have middle ear effusions and some ossicle ankylosis (128). Dense cartilage calcification in the endochondrial layer of the otic capsule and ossicles has been found in patients with a recessive form of osteopetrosis (129). The calcification causes narrowing of the eustachian tube predisposing these patients for serous otitis media and ossicle ankylosis which may result in conductive deafness. Cranial nerve deficits due to bony encroachment have also been noted and the hearing deficits reported were generally mild (130).

DISTAL RENAL TUBULAR ACIDOSIS WITH HYPERKALEMIA

Pathophysiology

A hyperkalemic form of distal RTA can be caused by of any of the following abnormalities (Table 8):

i. Selective aldosterone deficiency,
ii. Inability to generate a normal electrical potential (lumen-negative) in the cortical collecting duct or a generalised defect involving both H^+ and K^+ secretion
iii. A combination of i–ii and
iv. Failure of the collecting duct to respond to the actions of aldosterone.

In addition, hyperkalemia (regardless of its etiology) suppresses NH_4^+ excretion, and may contribute to the development of hyperchloremic metabolic acidosis (131).

Table 8 Mechanisms and Causes of Distal RTA with Hyperkalemia

Mechanism	Example
Aldosterone deficiency	Hyporeninemic hypoaldosteronism
Voltage dependent defects	
– Interference with Na^+ reabsorption	Amiloride, trimethoprim chronic obstructive uropathy
– Enhanced Cl^- transport	Pseudohypoaldosteronism Type II
H^+-ATPase defect + Aldosterone deficiency	Chronic obstructive uropathy
Aldosterone resistance	Pseudohypoaldosteronism Type I

In adults with underlying renal disease two pathogenic subtypes of hyperkalemic distal RTA are frequently encountered (8–10). One subtype, which corresponds to the animal model of selective aldosterone deficiency (SAD), is characterized by hyperkalemic hyperchloremic metabolic acidosis associated with low plasma and urinary aldosterone levels, reduced NH_4^+ excretion, and preserved ability to lower urine pH below 5.5 (8–10,12–15). This constellation of findings is often referred to as type IV RTA. In these subjects, impaired acid excretion is felt to be secondary to reduced urinary buffer availability. Indeed NH_4^+ formation can be suppressed as a result of both hyperkalemia and aldosterone deficiency (132–134). The rate of H^+ secretion, however, in the inner medullary collecting tubule has also been shown to be reduced in an experimental model of SAD (135). This reduction in the rate of H^+ secretion does not interfere with the ability to lower urine pH below 5.5 in either adrenalectomized rats or patients with aldosterone deficiency (10).

In the other subtype of hyperkalemic RTA, NH_4^+ excretion is also reduced but, characteristically, urine pH cannot be lowered below 5.5 not only during acidemia, but also after stimulation of Na^+-dependent distal acidification by either sodium sulfate or furosemide administration (8,13). Plasma aldosterone levels may be normal or elevated but are more often reduced (8,9,13). The term hyperkalemic distal RTA is used to designate this type and has been well characterized in some patients with obstructive uropathy, sickle cell disease, and other types of interstitial nephritis of various etiologies (13). The finding of low aldosterone level suggests the existence of a combined defect, that is, SAD combined with a tubular defect that interferes with the ability to maximally lower urine pH (13).

Hyperkalemic distal RTA has been attributed to a failure to generate a favorable transtubular voltage gradient (lumen-negative)in the collecting duct (13–17). This voltage gradient is generated, at least in part, by secondary active Na^+ reabsorption (136,137). A defect in Na^+ reabsorption at this site impairs formation of an optimal electrochemical gradient for both H^+ and K^+ secretion, and this defect is manifested by the inability both to lower urinary pH and excrete K^+ in a normal fashion. The existence of such a defect was inferred by analogy from the pattern of altered acidification produced experimentally by amiloride both in the turtle urinary bladder (16,17) and in the rabbit cortical collecting duct (19). Further, when amiloride is administered to humans, urinary pH cannot be lowered below 5.5 and K^+ excretion is impaired, suggesting that these features are characteristic of a voltage-dependent defect (8). Impairment in both H^+ and K^+ secretion can also occur when distal Na^+ delivery is markedly reduced. The term "voltage-dependent defect" is used to describe the alteration in urinary acidification that ensues as a result of impaired Na^+ reabsorption in the cortical collecting duct, despite adequate Na^+ delivery and sufficiently high luminal $[Na^+]$. The coexistence of a defect in the H^+-ATPase pump and a K^+ secretory defect could also cause this type of hyperkalemic distal RTA (10).

Patients with either SAD or hyperkalemic distal RTA have inappropriately low NH_4^+ excretion. Low NH_4^+ excretion in patients with SAD has been attributed to hyperkalemia because acidosis is ameliorated and NH_4^+ excretion increases following correction of hyperkalemia in some patients with this disorder (107). However, administration of fludrocortisone also increases NH_4^+ excretion and ameliorates acidosis in these patients (12). The increase in NH_4^+ excretion may be a direct result of the lowering of serum $[K^+]$, although aldosterone deficiency per se may interfere with ammoniagenesis and NH_4^+ excretion directly. It seems likely that both hyperkalemia and aldosterone deficiency contribute to the low NH_4^+ excretion characteristic of patients with SAD.

Patients with either SAD or hyperkalemic distal RTA also have abnormally low K^+ excretion. In addition, these patients fail to respond to stimuli that normally augment K^+ excretion, such as mineralocorticoid administration, sodium sulfate (an agent that increases luminal electronegativity in the distal nephron), and acetazolamide, a diuretic that increases K^+ excretion by increasing distal Na^+ delivery and urinary flow rates (14).

Clinical Features and Causes

Patients with hyperkalemic distal RTA present with clinical findings that often are indistinguishable from those with SAD. Unlike patients with classic distal RTA, patients with either form of hyperkalemic RTA have normal urinary excretion of calcium and citrate (138,139). Hence, nephrolithiasis and kidney stones are not a part of the clinical spectrum. The major differences in the clinical features of the hyperkalemic and classic distal RTA are presented in Table 9.

Patients with RTA caused by either SAD or hyperkalemic distal RTA are usually middle-aged or elderly, have cardiovascular disease and have moderate renal insufficiency (i.e., serum creatinine concentrations 2–5 mg/dl).

Table 9 Comparison of Clinical Features of Distal RTA with Hypokalemia and with Hyperkalemia

Clinical feature	Hypokalemia	Hyperkalemia
Serum $[K^+]$	Normal or decreased	Increased
Net acid excretion	Decreased	Decreased
K^+ excretion	Increased	Decreased
Calcium excretion	Increased	Normal
Citrate excretion	Decreased	Normal
Urinary $[HCO_3^-]$ with normal serum $[HCO_3^-]$	<5 mEq/L	<5 mEq/L
Urine-blood PCO_2^*	Decreased	Decreased
Nephrocalcinosis	Yes	No
Rickets	Yes	No
Growth failure	Yes	No
Daily alkali requirement	1–4 mEq/kg/day	0.5–1 mEq/kg/day

*Difference between urine and blood PCO_2 under conditions of $NaHCO_3$ loading.

Asymptomatic hyperchloremic metabolic acidosis with elevated plasma $[K^+]$ is by far the most common presentation of RTA in adults (13,14). Patients with this disorder usually have stable moderate hyperkalemia (5.5–6.5 mEq/L) without electrocardiographic abnormalities. At times, however, severe hyperkalemia can develop with typical electrocardiographic changes. The hyperkalemia can also be intermittent and some patients may have a normal glomerular filtration rate.

Selective Aldosterone Deficiency

Patients with selective aldosterone deficiency have decreased aldosterone production but normal glucocorticoid production. Angiotensin II, Na^+ intake, and plasma $[K^+]$ regulate aldosterone secretion from the zona glomerulosa of the adrenal cortex (140,141). Other minor regulators of aldosterone release include adrenocorticotropin (ACTH), natriuretic peptides, and hyponatremia (142). Low aldosterone production is usually, but not always, associated with low plasma renin activity (PRA) (143). Other clinical conditions that may be associated with reduced plasma aldosterone despite normal PRA include heparin administration, Addison's disease, angiotensin-II-converting enzyme inhibitors, and the rare syndrome of corticosterone methyloxidase deficiency (144).

Selective aldosterone deficiency is typically, but not always, accompanied by low plasma renin levels (hyporeninemic hypoaldosteronism) (144–153). Aldosterone is present but in a reduced amount which appears inappropriately low for the degree of hyperkalemia, leading to a state of relative hypoaldosteronism (144). Table 10 lists the causes of SAD. The

Table 10 Causes of Selective Aldosterone Deficiency (SAD)

Low renin
Obstructive uropathy
Renal transplant (early)
Amyloidosis, myeloma
Sickle cell nephropathy
Systemic lupus erythematosus
Interstitial renal disease
Diabetic nephropathy
Prostaglandin synthesis inhibitors (NSAIDs)
Pentamidine
Normal or high renin
Heparin therapy
Angiotensin-II-converting enyzme inhibitors
Addison's disease (or any adrenal gland failure)
21-hydroxylase deficiency
Normoreninemic hypoaldosteronism of critically ill patients
Corticosterone methyloxidase deficiency

---

development of hyperkalemic hyperchloremic metabolic acidosis in these patients is very common and is present in about 75% of cases. The use of chronic nonsteroidal antiinflammatory drugs (NSAIDs) and pentamidine has also been associated with hyporeninemic hypoadosteronism (154–157).

In the majority of cases of hypoaldosteronism, some degree of chronic renal impairment is present. Patients with diminished GFR require an increased amount of aldosterone to maintain K^+ homeostasis. It has been suggested that the levels of circulating aldosterone increase with progressive loss of GFR, facilitating the adaptive increase in K^+ secretion per nephron. In patients with chronic renal insufficiency, particularly in those with tubulointerstitial damage involving the juxtaglomerular apparatus (the site of renin production), the resultant impairment in renin secretion may explain the frequent development of SAD.

Hyperkalemic Distal RTA

Obstructive nephropathy is a major cause of this form of hyperkalemic distal RTA. Originally, the development of distal RTA in patients with obstructive nephropathy was attributed to a voltage-dependent defect (13). More recent clinical studies, however, suggest that H^+-ATPase failure is involved, based on the finding of a normal antikaliuretic response to amiloride (9). In the rabbit, moreover, H^+ secretion is decreased in the medullary collecting tubule after the relief of ureteric obstruction (158,159), and this defect is accompanied by a decrease in H^+-ATPase activity in both cortical and medullary collecting ducts (160). After ureteral obstruction in the rat,

H^+-ATPase staining in collecting duct intercalated cells is discontinuous, particularly in the inner medulla.

Because SAD does not affect the ability to achieve highly acidic urine during systemic acidosis, the presence of a urine pH >5.5 in the face of hyperkalemia and a hyperchloremic metabolic acidosis, by definition, is diagnostic for hyperkalemic distal RTA. A patient with hyperkalemic metabolic acidosis, by this definition, who also has a low serum or urinary aldosterone has a combined defect—hyperkalemic distal RTA and SAD (13–15).

Iatrogenic Causes of Hyperkalemic RTA: Sodium channel inhibitors, like trimethoprim and pentamidine, can cause hyperkalemia often with only mild to moderate metabolic acidosis. The calcineurin inhibitors cyclosporine and tacrolimus can cause hyperkalemic distal RTA (161–163). Treatment with cyclosporine A and tacrolimus decreases both urinary K^+ and H^+ excretion (163–165). Cyclosporine and tacrolimus both inhibit renal Na^+/K^+-ATPase activity, and this effect may be responsible for both the acidosis and hyperkalemia (167). Another possible mechanism whereby cyclosporine could cause hyperkalemia is direct inhibition of apical membrane K^+ channels in collecting duct principal cells (168). Cyclosporine suppresses plasma renin activity, which could result in hypoaldosteronism. In addition, this agent may cause insensitivity of the collecting duct to aldosterone, which could also impair K^+ excretion (162,164).

Trimethoprim (TMP) is a recognized cause of hyperkalemia, associated with a decrease in K^+ excretion unrelated to renal failure, adrenal insufficiency, or tubulointerstitial disease (169–171). Patients with preexisting renal dysfunction are much more likely to develop clinically significant hyperkalemia than patients with normal renal function (169). Trimethoprim, like amiloride, blocks the apical membrane Na^+ channel (ENaC) in the collecting duct (171,172). As a result, transepithelial voltage is reduced and K^+ secretion is diminished. TMP also appears to inhibit renal Na^+/K^+-ATPase activity (173). Acidosis is not a prominent feature of hyperkalemic patients receiving TMP, but has occasionally been reported to occur (169–179). The antiparasitic drug, pentamidine, is clinically associated with hyperkalemia, and this drug has also been shown to block ENaC (157,180). Additionally, an aldosterone mediated effect has been noted in some hyperkalemic patients receiving this drug (157).

Aldosterone Resistance: Pseudohypoaldosteronism

Aldosterone resistance is manifested by the clinical features of aldosterone deficiency (hyperkalemia, acidosis) despite normal or elevated levels of aldosterone. Moreover, the administration of exogenous mineralocorticoids fails to correct these abnormalities. Aldosterone resistance is an inherited disorder that produces two clinical syndromes, referred to as type I and type II pseudohypoaldosteronism (PHA). Although both result in hyperkalemia and metabolic acidosis, the clinical presentation and genetic basis for these two types differ notably (Table 11). In addition to these inherited disorders, some degree of resistance to aldosterone's effect in the collecting duct has been described in patients with chronic renal disease, particularly in those with tubulointerstitial nephropathies (13).

Pseudohypoaldosteronism Type I (PHA I)

Usually PHA I occurs during infancy and is associated with normal renal and adrenal function (181). The clinical presentation varies from severely affected patients who die in infancy, to asymptomatic carriers (182). Infants with this disorder typically have weight loss, dehydration, hypotension, failure to thrive, high urine Na^+ excretion despite hypotension, a hyperchloremic metabolic acidosis, and hyperkalemia. Aldosterone levels and renin activity are both elevated (183).

Pseudohypoaldosteronism Type I can be inherited in either an autosomal dominant or autosomal recessive mode (Table 11). The autosomal dominant form (type IA)is usually mild and many of these individuals are asymptomatic carriers. The autosomal recessive form, by contrast, is characterized by severe Na^+ wasting, hyperkalemia, failure to thrive, and if left untreated, can lead to death. Treatment of patients with PHA I requires dietary salt supplementation, and sometimes K^+ binding resins (183). Clinical improvement is normally seen within 10–14 days of treatment.

Mutations in the *MLR* gene encoding the mineralocorticoid receptor protein have been identified, in hereditary dominant and some sporadic cases, that lead to failure to respond to the actions of aldosterone in the target tissue (termed target tissue resistance) (184,185). The recessive forms of PHA I are associated with mutations in the amiloride-sensitive epithelial Na^+ channel (ENaC) (186,187). Mutations have been described in the genes encoding all three subunits of the channel (α, β, and γ subunits). Defects in ENaC lead to decreased Na^+ reabsorption and hence urinary Na^+ wasting.

The presence of a mild form of PHA I and subsequent improvement in patients with *MLR* mutations but not in those with the ENaC mutations, suggests that the mineralocorticoid receptor either remains partially functional or that the requirement for aldosterone to maintain Na^+ balance diminishes after infancy. Patients with congenital hypoaldosteronism due to aldosterone synthase deficiency also improve as they grow older, providing support for a decreased need for aldosterone with maturation (188,189). Patients with ENaC mutations clearly have a more serious defect in Na^+ balance, as this transporter is necessary for adequate Na^+ reabsorption regardless of dietary Na^+intake.

Pseudohypoaldosteronism Type II (Gordon Syndrome)

Pseudohypoaldosteronism type II (PHA II), similar to PHA I, presents with hyperkalemia and hyperchloremic metabolic acidosis. Although neonates

Table 11 Genetics and Clinical Features of Pseudohypoaldosteronism

Syndrome	Mode of inheritance	Gene localization	Locus symbol	Gene product	Clinical features
Pseudo-hypoaldosteronism Type IA	Dominant	4q31.1	MLR	Mineralocortocoid receptor	Milder phenotype, may resolve with time
Pseudo-hypoaldosteronism Type IB	Recessive	16p12	SNCC1B, SNCC1G	β and γ subunits of ENaC	Severe phenotype
		12p13	SNCCAA	α subunit of ENaC	
Pseudo-hypoaldosteronism Type II (Gordon's Syndrome)	Dominant	12p13.3 17p11-q21	WNK1 WNK4	WNK1 kinase WNK4 kinase	Hypertension, short stature, responsive to thiazides

have been reported (190), PHA II patients typically develop clinical manifestations in adolescence or adulthood. In contrast to PHA I, these include hypertension, short stature, and low or normal renin and aldosterone levels (191). This difference is accounted for by the fact that patients with PHA II retain Na^+ avidly (urine $[Na^+] < 10 \, mEq/L$), whereas those with PHA I typically waste this cation (192). Patients with PHA II demonstrate renal resistance to the effects of mineralocorticoids, as they remain hyperkalemic even with prolonged mineralocorticoid administration.

Pseudohypoaldosteronism type II is predominantly inherited in an autosomal dominant fashion, and loci have been identified on chromosomes 1, 12, and 17 (193,194). The primary defect appears to be increased reabsorption of Cl^- in the distal tubule, termed a "chloride shunt" (195,196). Because of increased Cl^--coupled Na^+ reabsorption at this site in the nephron, extracellular fluid volume increases resulting in hypertension and suppression of renin and aldosterone. The combination of decreased Na^+ delivery to the collecting duct and suppressed aldosterone levels causes hyperkalemia and metabolic acidosis.

Patients diagnosed with PHA II respond to treatment with thiazide diuretics, sometimes in combination with a low Na^+ diet. Furosemide treatment also appears to correct the disorder, although patients appear to be more responsive to thiazides. Discontinuation of therapy results in recurrence of hypertension, metabolic acidosis, and hyperkalemia. Diuretics presumably work by increasing Na^+ delivery to the collecting duct and thereby promoting K^+ secretion. In a single patient with PHA II, dietary salt restriction alone normalized blood pressure and corrected both the hyperkalemia and acidosis. It is not clear how salt restriction improved the hyperkalemia in this patient.

Mutations in WNK kinases have been identified in Gordon's syndrome (196). WNK kinases belong to the family of serine-threonine kinases and are found exclusively in the distal nephron. Two genes have been identified that encode for WNK kinases 1 and 4 on chromosomes 12 and 17, respectively and mutations in these genes appear to produce a gain of function (197). How the mutations in these genes lead to the clinical manifestations of Gordon's syndrome is not fully known.

DIAGNOSTIC EVALUATION OF DISTAL RTA

The diagnosis of distal RTA should be suspected whenever a hyperchloremic metabolic acidosis is present without any obvious cause (i.e., diarrhea)in the setting of relatively normal GFR. With appropriate suspicion, all that is usually needed for confirmation is an inappropriately low rate of acid excretion and information on urine pH. Ammonium is the most important component of acid excretion in the presence of metabolic acidosis, and thus one has either to measure it directly or estimate it by calculating the urine anion gap (see below) (198). The urine pH is typically inappropriately high in the classic form (distal or type I RTA) and it is low in type IV distal RTA (i.e., SAD). We use the urinary anion gap as the initial diagnostic test. An algorithm summarizing our approach for the diagnosis of hypokalemic and hyperkalemic RTA is presented in Fig. 6.

Urine Anion Gap

In patients with a hyperchloremic acidosis, the urine anion gap is helpful in determining whether the acidosis is due to a renal or extrarenal etiology, with the caveats discussed below (198). The principle is similar to that of the plasma anion gap, namely, that the sum of all cations and anions must be equal. Thus,

$$[Cl^-] + [HCO_3^-] + [\text{unmeasured anions}] = [Na^+] + [K^+]$$
$$+ [\text{unmeasured cations}]$$

The unmeasured anions include sulfate, phosphate, and organic anions. Cations not routinely measured include NH_4^+, Ca^{++}, and Mg^{++}.

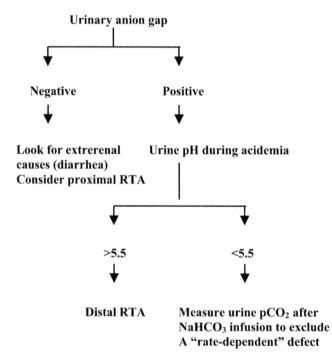

Figure 6 Diagnostic approach to hyperchloremic metabolic acidosis with low or normal serum potassium concentration.

Of these, NH_4^+ is by far the predominant species when metabolic acidosis is present. The urine anion gap can be calculated from the urine electrolytes by the formula:

Urine anion gap $= [Na^+] + [K^+] - [Cl^-]$ if urine pH is < 6.5 or:

Urine anion gap $= [Na^+] + [K^+] - ([Cl^-] + [HCO_3^-])$ if the urine pH is > 6.5.

The urine anion gap will be low (usually a negative value)if there is a decrease in unmeasured anions or an increase in unmeasured cations (e.g., NH_4^+). The urine anion gap will be increased (usually a positive value) if there is an increase in unmeasured anions or a decrease in unmeasured cations. Because the concentrations of unmeasured anions in the urine do not change notably and because NH_4^+ is the major unmeasured cation in the presence of metabolic acidosis, the urine anion gap is a useful estimate of urine $[NH_4^+]$ in this setting. Patients with an acidification defect typically have a positive gap (because NH_4^+ excretion is inappropriately low), whereas in diarrheal states (providing that distal Na^+ delivery is adequate) the gap is negative, reflecting the fact that NH_4^+ excretion is not impaired (198). In proximal RTA, the urine anion gap is negative (provided plasma $[HCO_3^-]$ is low) because distal acidification is normal.

Minimal Urine pH and Maximal Acid Excretion During Metabolic Acidosis

Along with measurement of urine electrolytes and calculation of the anion gap, urine pH should be measured to assess the ability of the collecting duct to acidify the urine. Urine pH can be evaluated during spontaneous metabolic acidosis or after administration of an acidifying salt. It can also be assessed by the infusion of sodium sulfate or after giving furosemide (see later for details of these tests). If systemic acidosis is present, urine pH should be <5.5. The finding of a urine pH <5.5 is consistent with appropriate urinary acidification and, by definition, excludes distal RTA. The finding of a urinary pH >5.5 in the face of acidosis is usually diagnostic of distal RTA, provided that distal Na^+ delivery is adequate. One must recall, however, that some patients with RTA have urine pH values <5.5 during acidosis, and yet have impaired distal acidification. Some of these patients have defects in NH_4^+ excretion, and many have hyperkalemia and/or aldosterone deficiency.

Urine pH should be measured in a freshly voided sample in the morning and ideally collected under mineral oil. Mild acidosis is sufficient to evaluate urine acidification; it is not necessary to induce severe acidosis. Urine pH is influenced by the patient's position and urine flow. Because the recumbent position may increase the urine pH, it is preferable to ask the patient to void in the upright position (199).

Ammonium Chloride Loading Test

If systemic acidosis is not present, ammonium chloride can be given orally in a dose of 0.1 g/kg of body weight daily for 3–5 days. Alternatively, a single dose of the same amount may be given. Urine is then collected hourly from two to eight hours. In our experience, the 3-day test gives more reliable results, and we prefer it because it allows time for a maximal increase in NH_4^+ excretion. The urine pH in normal subjects falls below 5.5 (usually below 5.0) by the first day and remains low thereafter. Ammonium excretion increases at least 3–5 fold by the third day. An alternative acidifying agent is calcium chloride (2 mEq/kg of body weight orally). This substance gives results similar to ammonium chloride and can be used in patients who cannot tolerate the latter treatment because of nausea and vomiting or in patients with liver disease in whom NH_4Cl is contraindicated. A complete scheme of the laboratory workup of a patient suspected of having distal RTA is presented in Table 12.

Table 12 Laboratory Workup to Evaluate Patients Suspected of Having dRTA

Test	Comments
Urine pH	Freshly voided urine collected in mineral oil.
	Knowledge of acid-base status needed.
	Knowledge of urine [Na^+] needed because urine pH does not fall maximally when urine [Na^+] < 20 mEq/L.
	If urine pH < 6.3, urine contains little HCO_3^- and proximal RTA unlikely.
	If urine pH is less than 5.5, the classic forms of distal RTA can be excluded but not other types such as type IV RTA and some rate-dependent defects.
Urine Na^+, K^+, Cl^-	Calculate urine anion gap.[a] A negative value suggests that NH_4^+ excretion is not reduced and tends to rule out distal RTA.[b]
Net acid excretion[b]	Calculated as NH_4^+ excretion + titratable acidity – HCO_3 excretion.
Other provocative tests[c]	Urine pCO_2 after bicarbonate loading.
	Urine pH and acid excretion after furosemide or Na_2SO_4 administration.
	Urine pH and urine K^+ excretion after amiloride.

[a]Urine [Na^+] + [K^+] – [Cl^-].
[b]Blood pH should be 7.35 or lower. If metabolic acidosis is not present, give NH_4Cl (0.1 g/kg) for 2 to 3 days.
[c]These tests usually are not needed if diagnosis is clear from history and above tests.

Provocative Tests

Provocative tests involving the use of sodium sulfate or furosemide to assess Na^+-dependent acidification can provide additional useful mechanistic information (8,9). These agents increase distal Na^+ delivery, thereby enhancing the negative transepithelial potential in the collecting duct and stimulating H^+ and K^+ secretion. A reduction in urine pH and an increase in K^+ excretion after the administration of either of these agents indicate a normal response to this enhanced electronegativity. It must be recognized, however, that the evidence obtained from these maneuvers is indirect and may be sometimes subject to different interpretations (see below).

Sodium Sulfate Infusion: Normal subjects can lower urine pH maximally, provided that distal Na^+ delivery is adequate and that collecting duct Na^+ reabsorption is adequately stimulated (8,10,200,201). Administration of sodium sulfate insures adequate distal Na^+ delivery. The second requirement can be accomplished by placing the subject on a low Na^+ diet (i.e., 20 mEq daily)for 3 days, which, in turn, stimulates aldosterone release and enhances distal Na^+ reabsorption. Alternatively, sodium sulfate infusion can be performed following the administration of fludrocortisone (1 mg orally over the 12 hr preceding the sodium sulfate infusion) (201).

The sodium sulfate test, properly performed, results in a fall of urine pH below 5.5 (usually below 5.0) regardless of whether or not systemic acidosis is present. It should be pointed out that urine collections should continue for 2–3 hr after the infusion is discontinued because some subjects have a late response. Patients with chronic renal insufficiency also respond normally to sodium sulfate despite their inability to retain Na^+ maximally. The increase in acid excretion that follows sodium sulfate infusion is mainly in the form of NH_4^+ (200,201). The kaliuretic response to sodium sulfate administration is also useful in assessing distal K^+ secretory capacity. In contrast to patients with classic distal RTA, patients with hyperkalemic distal RTA usually do not increase K^+ excretion normally (8,10).

Furosemide or Bumetanide Test: Loop diuretics increase Na^+ delivery to the collecting duct by blocking NaCl reabsorption in the loop of Henle. A portion of this excess Na^+ is reabsorbed in the collecting duct, establishing a favorable transepithelial voltage for H^+ and K^+ secretion (8,10). This conclusion is buttressed by the finding that the fall in urine pH and the increase in acid excretion caused by this manuever are obliterated by amiloride. Amiloride also lessens the kaliuretic effect of furosemide. The difference in K^+ excretion observed at comparable urine flow rates when furosemide is given alone and when it is given with amiloride portrays to a large extent the contribution of the amiloride-sensitive (i.e., Na^+-dependent) component of distal H^+ and K^+ secretion.

The furosemide test is performed by first collecting a urine sample and then giving 40–80 mg of furosemide orally (8). Alternatively, oral bumetanide (1–2 mg) can be given (9). Urine samples are then collected hourly for 4 hours. Normal individuals and patients with pure aldosterone deficiency should be able to lower their urine pH below 5.5. Patients who fail to lower urine pH < 5.5 have either an H^+ pump defect or a voltage-dependent defect (9,202). These possibilities can be evaluated further by the amiloride test described below.

Amiloride Test: Amiloride at low doses blocks apical Na^+ channels in the cortical collecting duct. Administration of amiloride predictably leads to an increase in urine pH and a decrease in urine K^+ excretion in normal individuals and in individuals with renal insufficiency. In patients with a complete voltage-dependent defect, amiloride should not increase urine pH or decrease K^+ excretion further. A normal response to amiloride (i.e., an increase in urine pH and a decrease in K^+ excretion)indicates that the voltage-dependent mechanism of H^+ and K^+ excretion is intact (9). The test is performed by giving 20 mg of amiloride by mouth after a baseline urine collection. Urine is then collected hourly for measurement of pH and electrolyte excretion (9).

Urine PCO_2 as an Index of Distal Acidification: Sodium bicarbonate loading increases urine PCO_2 to values considerably higher than in blood because of delayed dehydration of the carbonic acid formed when H^+ is secreted into collecting duct fluid that is rich in HCO_3^- (202–205). Secreted H^+ ions react with HCO_3^- in the tubule lumen to form carbonic acid (H_2CO_3) and, because carbonic anhydrase is not present in the collecting duct lumen, this acid is carried into the urine before it can spontaneously dehydrate to form CO_2 and H_2O. Thus, the degree to which urine PCO_2 rises is a measure of the stimulation of distal H^+ secretion in response to increased HCO_3^- delivery. Normally, urine PCO_2 rises to >70 mm Hg after maximal alkalinization of the urine (urine pH of 7.8 or higher), provided that urine $[HCO_3^-]$ is sufficiently high (i.e., >80 mEq/L)(89,90).

The correlation between urine $[HCO_3^-]$ and PCO_2 suggested that part of the high CO_2 tension in highly alkaline urine may be due solely to the concentration of the urine rather than enhanced distal H^+ secretion (204). A major contribution attributable solely to acidification, however, can clearly be demonstrated by observing the urine PCO_2 at high levels of urine $[HCO_3^-]$ in subjects with impaired distal acidification. In these subjects, urine PCO_2 is significantly lower than in normal subjects despite having the same urine $[HCO_3^-]$.

All patients with classic distal RTA who have been tested have subnormal values of urine PCO_2 after sodium bicarbonate loading, with the exception of experimental distal RTA secondary to amphotericin (89,90). In amphotericin-induced distal RTA, urine PCO_2 rises normally because H^+

secretion is intact; the acidification defect is due to back leak of H^+, which is minimized when the tubule fluid is alkaline (205,206). In all other patients with distal RTA, the subnormal urine PCO_2 indicates that the net rate of distal H^+ secretion is decreased, but it does not disclose the mechanisms responsible for decreased distal acidification.

The sensitivity of urine PCO_2 to detect a decrease in the distal capacity for H^+ secretion is particularly useful in evaluating patients suspected of having abnormal urinary acidification, but in whom urine pH during acidosis is appropriately low. A subnormal rise in urine PCO_2, for example, occurs in patients with incomplete distal RTA (75,76,89).

Another tool to evaluate distal H^+ ion secretion is assessment of urine PCO_2 after the infusion of neutral sodium phosphate. Urine PCO_2 is critically dependent on urine phosphate concentration when the pH of the urine is close to 6.8, the pK of the phosphate buffer system. Under these conditions, phosphate rather than HCO_3^- is responsible for generating CO_2 in the urine. By contrast, in the highly alkaline urine (pH greater than 7.8) produced by sodium bicarbonate loading, phosphate plays no role in the generation of urine PCO_2 (3,75,76). This test is performed by infusing neutral phosphate (1 mmol/L total body water in 180 cc of normal saline) slowly at a rate of 1 mL/min for 3 hours. This maneuver usually results in a two- to three-fold increase in plasma phosphate concentration. Similar results have been reported using oral phosphate loading (207). Urine phosphate concentration must increase to about 20 mmols/L in two or three successive urine collections after the beginning of the phosphate infusion (75,76). Under these conditions, urine PCO_2 rises consistently above 80 mmHg both in normal subjects and in patients with renal insufficiency.

THERAPY OF DISTAL RTA

The aims of treatment of classic RTA are not only to correct the biochemical abnormalities, but also to improve growth in children, and to prevent kidney stones and the skeletal abnormalities associated with the disease. Another aim is to prevent the progression of nephrocalcinosis, which in rare cases leads to chronic renal failure. In the hyperkalemic types the primary focus is the correction of hyperkalemia and metabolic acidosis (see Chapter 14).

Alkali therapy should provide adequate base to balance daily acid production. Because children have a higher rate of acid production, they require higher doses of alkali. A mixture of sodium and potassium citrate salts is recommended (Table 13). All patients with classic distal RTA have associated hypocitraturia, but children with this disorder also have calcium oxalate and calcium phosphate excretion rates that approach saturation, which makes them more susceptible to nephrolithiasis. Citrate salts correct

Table 13 Recommended Solutions for Alkali Therapy With or Without Potassium

Shohl solution	Comments
Sodium citrate and citric acid	Contains 1 mEq Na^+/ml and is equivalent to 1 mEq of HCO_3^- per ml
Polycitra (K-Shohl solution) Sodium citrate, potassium citrate and citric acid	Contains 1 mEq K^+ and 1 mEq Na^+/ml and is equivalent to 2 mEq HCO_3^- per ml

the hypocitraturia and prevent nephrolithiasis (208). This organic anion also corrects the metabolic acidosis, thereby decreasing urine calcium excretion. Infants require as much as 5–8 mEq per kg of citrate or HCO_3^- per kg body weight, whereas adults require only about 0.5 1 mEq per kg body weight. Patients with hereditary distal RTA require lifetime treatment. The prognosis is excellent if the diagnosis is made early and appropriate amounts of alkali are continuously administered. However, alkali therapy has no effect on hearing impairment in those patients who have either sensorineural or conductive deafness (209).

REFERENCES

1. Mcsherry E, Sebastian A, Morris RCJ. Renal tubular acidosis in infants: the several kinds, including bicarbonate wasting, classic renal tubular acidosis. J Clin Invest 1972; 51:499–514.
2. Edelman CMJR, Rodriguez-Soriano J, Boichis H. An isolated defect in renal bicarbonate reabsorption as a cause of hyperchloremic acidosis. J Pediatr 1965; 67:946.
3. Arruda JAL, Kurtzman NA. Mechanisms and classification of deranged distal urinary acidification. Am J Physiol 1980; 239:F515–F523.
4. Batlle DC, Kurtzman NA. Distal renal tubular acidosis: Pathogenesis and classification. Am J Kidney Dis 1982; 1:328–344.
5. Batlle D, Flores G. Underlying defects in distal renal tubular acidosis: new understandings. Am J Kidney Dis 1996; 27:896–915.
6. Kurtzman NA. Renal tubular acidosis: a constellation of syndromes. Hosp Pract 1987; 22:173–178, 181.
7. Batlle D, Ghanekar H, Jain S, Mitra A. Hereditary distal renal tubular acidosis: new understandings. Ann Rev Med; 52:471–484.
8. Batlle DC. Segmental characterization of defects in collecting tubule acidification. Kidney Int 1986; 30:546–554.
9. Schlueter W, Keilani T, Hizon M, Kaplan B, Batlle DC. On the mechanism of impaired distal acidification in hyperkalemic renal tubular acidosis— evaluation with amiloride and bumetanide. J Am Soc Nephrol 1992; 3: 953–964.

10. Batlle DC. Sodium dependent urinary acidification in patients with aldosterone deficiency and in adrenalectomized rates: effect of furosemide. Metabolism 1986; 35:852–860.

11. Rodriguez Soriano J. Renal tubular acidosis: the clinical entity. J Am Soc Nephrol 2002; 13:2160–2170.

12. Sebastian A, Schambelan M, Lindenfeld S. Amelioration of metabolic acidosis with fludrocortisone therapy in hyporeninemic hypoaldosteronism. N Engl J Med 1977; 197:576–583.

13. Batlle DC, Arruda JA, Kurtzman NA. Hyperkalemic distal renal tubular acidosis associated with obstructive uropathy. N Engl J Med 1981; 304:373–380.

14. Batlle DC. Hyperkalemic hyperchloremic metabolic acidosis associated with selective aldosterone deficiency and distal renal tubular acidosis. Semin Nephrol 1981; 1:260–273.

15. Batlle DC, Itsarayoungyen K, Arruda JA. Hyperkalemic hyperchloremic metabolic acidosis in sickle cell hemoglobinopathies. Am J Med 1982; 72:188–192.

16. Kurtzman NA. "Short circuit" renal tubular acidosis. J Lab Clin Med 1980; 95:633–636.

17. Arruda JAL, Subbarayudu K, Dytko G, Mola R, Kurtzman NA. Voltage dependent distal acidification defect induced by amiloride. J Lab Clin Med 1980; 95:407–416.

18. Hulter HN, Ilnicki LP, Licht JH, Sebastian A. On the mechanism of diminished urinary carbon dioxide tension caused by amiloride. Kidney Int 1982; 21:8–13.

19. Stoner LC, Burg MB, Orloff J. Ion transport in cortical collecting tubule—effect of amiloride. Am J Physiol 1974; 227:453–459.

20. Alper SL. Genetic diseases of acid base transporters. Ann Rev Physiol 2002; 64:899–923.

21. Karet FE. Inherited distal renal tubular acidosis. J Am Soc Nephrol 2002; 13:2178–2184.

22. Igarashi T, Sekine T, Inatomi J, Seki G. Unraveling the molecular pathogenesis of isolated proximal renal tubular acidosis. J Am Soc Nephrol 2002; 13:2171–2177.

23. Nash MA, Torrado AD, Greifer I. Renal tubular acidosis in infants and children. J Pediatr 1972; 80:738–748.

24. Rodriguez-Soriano J, Boichis H, Edelman CMJR. Bicarbonate reabsorption and hydrogen ion excretion in children with renal tubular acidosis. J Pediatr 1967; 71:802–813.

25. Rodriguez-Soriano J, Boichis H, Stark H. Proximal renal tubular acidosis: a defect in bicarbonate reabsorption with normal urinary acidification. Pediatr Res 1967; 1:81–98.

26. Lemann J, Adams ND, Wilz DR, Brenes LG. Acid and mineral balances and bone in familial proximal renal tubular acidosis. Kidney Int 2000; 58:1267–1277.

27. Morris RCJ, Sebastian A. Renal tubular acidosis and the Fanconi syndrome. In: Stanbury JB, Wyngaarden JB, Frederickson DS, eds. The Metabolic Basis of Inherited Disease. New York: 1983.

28. Abuladze N, Lee I. Axial heterogeneity of sodium bicarbonate cotransporter expression in the rabbit proximal tubule. Am J Physiol 1998; 274:F628–F633.

29. Burnham CE, Amlal H, Wang ZH, Shull GE, Soleimani M. Cloning and functional expression of a human kidney Na^+/HCO_3^- cotransporter. J Biol Chem 1997; 272:19111–19114.
30. Pushkin A, Abuladze N, Lee I. Cloning, tissue distribution, genomic organization, and functional characterization of NBC3, a new member of the sodium bicarbonate cotransporter family. J Biol Chem 1999; 274:16569–16575.
31. Romero MF, Hediger MA, Boulpaep EL. Expression cloning and characterization of a renal electrogenic Na^+/HCO_3^- cotransporter. Nature 1997; 387:409–413.
32. Soleimani M, Grassl SM, Aronson PS. Stoichiometry of the Na^+/HCO_3^- cotransporter in basolateral membrane vesicles isolated from rabbit renal cortex. J Clin Invest 1987; 79:1276–1280.
33. Wang A, Conforti L, Petrovic S. Mouse Na^+/HCO_3^- cotransporter isoform NBC3 (kNBC3): cloning, expression and renal distribution. Kidney Int 2001; 59:1405–1414.
34. Preisig PA, Alpern RJ. Increased Na^+/H^+ Antiporter and Na^+/HCO_3^- symporter activities in chronic hyperfiltration—a model of cell hypertrophy. J Gen Physiol 1991; 97:195–217.
35. Geibel J, Giebisch G, Boron WF. Angiotensin II stimulates both Na^+/HCO_3^- exchange and Na^+/HCO^{3-} cotransport in the rabbit proximal tubule. Proc Natl Acad Sci USA 1990; 87:7917–7920.
36. Igarashi T, Inatomi J, Sekine T. Novel nonsense mutation in the Na^+/HCO_3^- cotransporter gene (SCL4A4) in a patient with permanent proximal renal tubular acidosis. J Am Soc Nephrol 2001; 12:713–718.
37. Abuladze N, Song M, Pushkin A, Newman D, Lee I, Nicholas S, Kurtz I. Structural organization of the human NBCl gene: kNBCl is transcribed from an alternative promoter in intron 3. Gene 2000; 251:109–122.
38. Amemiya M, Loffing J, Lotscher M, Kaissling B, Alpern RJ, Moe OW. Expression of NHE3 in the apical membrane of rat renal proximal tubule and thick ascending limb. Kidney Int 1995; 48:1206–1215.
39. Biemesderfer D, Pizzonia J, Abu-Alfa A, Exner M, Reilly R, Igarashi P, Aronson PS. NHE3: a Na^+/H^+ exchanger isoform of renal brush border. Am J Physiol 1993; 265:F736–F742.
40. Bookstein C, Depaoli AM, Xie Y, Niu P, Musch MW, Rao MC, Chang EB. Na^+/H^+ exchangers, NHE-1 and NHE-3, of rat intestine—expression and localization. J Clin Invest 1994; 93:106–113.
41. Hoogerwerf WA, Tsao SC, Devuyst O, Levine SA, Yun CHC, Yip JW, Cohen ME, Wilson PD, Lazenby AJ, Tse CM, Donowitz M. NHE2 and NHE3 are human and rabbit intestinal brush border proteins. Am J Physiol 1996; 270:G29–G41.
42. Schultheis PJ, Clarke LL, Meneton P, Miller ML, Soleimani M, Gawenis LR, Riddle TM, Duffy JJ, Doetschman T, Wang T, Giebisch G, Aronson PS, Lorenz JN, Shull GE. Renal and intestinal absorptive defects in mice lacking the NHE3 Na^+/H^+ exchanger. Nature Genet 1998; 19:282–285.
43. Sly WS, Hewett-Emmett D, Whyte MP, Yu YS, Tashian RE. Carbonic anhydrase II deficiency identified as the primary defect in the autosomal recessive

syndrome of osteopetrosis with renal tubular acidosis and cerebral calcification. Proc Natl Acad Sci USA 1983; 80:2752–2756.

44. Bridi GS, Brackett NC, Falcon PW, Still WJS, Sporn IN. Glomerulonephritis and renal tubular acidosis in a case of chronic active hepatitis with hyperimmunoglobulinemia. Am J Med 1972; 52:267–278.

45. Soleimani M. Molecular physiology of the renal chloride formate exchanger. Curr Opin Nephrol Hypertens 2001; 10:677–683.

46. Coor C, Salmon RF, Quigley R, Marver D, Baum M. Role of adenosine triphosphate (ATP) and Na^+/K^+ ATPase in the inhibition of proximal tubule transport with intracellular cystine loading. J Clin Invest 1991; 87: 955–961.

47. Albander HA, Weiss RA, Humphreys MH, Morris RC. Dysfunction of the proximal tubule underlies maleic acid induced type II renal tubular acidosis. Am J Physiol 1982; 243:F604–F611.

48. Morris RC. An experimental renal acidification defect in patients with hereditary fructose intolerance—its resemblance to renal tubular acidosis. J Clin Invest 1968; 47:1389–1398.

49. Burch HB, Choi S, Dence CN, Alvey TR, Cole BR, Lowry OH. Metabolic effects of large fructose loads in different parts of the rat nephron. J Biol Chem 1980; 255:8239–8244.

50. Batlle DC, Chan YL. Effect of L-arginine on renal tubular bicarbonate reabsorption by the rat kidney. Miner Electr Metab 1989; 15:187–194.

51. Batlle DC. Renal tubular acidosis. In: Seldin, Giebisch, eds. The Regulation of Acid–Base Balance. New York:, 1989:353–390.

52. Roth KS, Foreman JW, Segal S. The Fanconi syndrome and mechanisms of tubular transport dysfunction. Kidney Int 1981; 20:105–116.

53. Mcsherry E, Morris RCJ. Attainment and maintenance of normal stature with alkali therapy in infants and children with classic renal tubular acidosis. J Clin Invest 1978; 61:509–527.

54. Brenner RJ, Spring DB, Sebastian A, Mcsherry EM, Genant HK, Palubinskas AJ, Morris RC. Incidence of radiographically evident bone disease, nephrocalcinosis, and nephrolithiasis in various types of renal tubular acidosis. N Engl J Med 1982; 307:217–221.

55. Tieder M, Modai D, Samuel R, Arie R, Halabe A, Bab I, Gabizon D, Liberman UA. Hereditary hypophosphatemic rickets with hypercalciuria. N Engl J Med 1985; 312:611–617.

56. Tannen RL, Falls WFJ, Brackett NCJ. Incomplete renal tubular acidosis: some clinical and physiological features. Nephron 1975; 15:111–123.

57. Dafnis E, Spohn M, Lonis B, Kurtzman NA, Sabatini S. Vanadate causes hypokalemic distal renal tubular acidosis. Am J Physiol 1992; 262:F449–F453.

58. Sitprija V, Eiam-Ong S, Suvanapha R, Kullavanijaya P, Chinayon S. Gastric hypoacidity in distal renal tubular acidosis. Nephron 1988; 50:395–396.

59. Mujais SK, Chen Y, Batlle D. Profile of H^+/K^+ ATPase along the collecting duct: effect of K^+ depletion. Clin Res 1991; 39:F709A.

60. Marquez-julio A, Rapoport A, Wilansky DL, Rabinovich S, Chamberlain D. Purpura associated with hypergammaglobulinemia, renal tubular acidosis and osteomalacia. Can Med Assoc J 1977; 116:53–58.

61. Morris RCJ, Fudenberg HH. Impaired renal acidification in patients with hypergammaglobulinemia. Medicine (Baltimore) 1967; 46:57–69.
62. Pertovaara M, Korpela M, Pasternack A. Factors predictive of renal involvement in patients with primary Sjogren's syndrome. Clin Nephrol 2001; 56:10–18.
63. LoSpalluto J, Dorward B, Biller W. Cryoglobulinemia based on interaction between a gammamacroglobulin and 7S gamma globulin. Am J Med 1962; 32:142.
64. Mason AMS, McIllmur MB, Golding PL, Hughes DTD. Fibrosing alveolitis associated with renal tubular acidosis. Br Med J 1970; 4:596–599.
65. Mason AMS, Golding PL. Renal tubular acidosis and autoimmune thyroid disease. Lancet 1970; 2:1104–1107.
66. Jessop S, Eales L, Mumford G, Rabkin R. Renal tubular function in systemic lupus erythematosis. S Afr Med J 1972; 46:848.
67. Tu WH, Shearn MA. Systemic lupus erythematosus and latent renal tubular dysfunction. Ann Int Med 1967; 67:100–109.
68. Golding PL. Renal tubular acidosis in chronic liver disease. Postgrad Med J 1975; 51:550–556.
69. Shapira E, Benyosep Y, Eyal FG, Russell A. Enzymatically inactive red cell carbonic anhydrase B in a Family with renal tubular acidosis. J Clin Invest 1974; 53:59–63.
70. Cochrane AMG, Tsantoulos DC, Moussouros A, Mcfarlane IG, Eddleston ALWF, Williams R. Lymphocyte cytotoxicity for kidney cells in renal tubular acidosis of autoimmune liver disease. Br Med J 1976; 2:276–278.
71. Golding PL, Smith M, Williams R. Multisystem involvement in chronic liver disease—studies on incidence and pathogenesis. Am J Med 1973; 55:772–782.
72. Reade AE, Sherlock S, Harrison CV. Active "juvenile" cirrhosis considered as part of a systemic disease. Gut 1963; 4:378.
73. Seedat YK, Raine ER. Active chronic hepatitis associated with renal tubular acidosis and successful pregnancy. S Afr Med J 1965; 39:595–597.
74. Lazar GS, Feinstein DI. Distal renal tubular acidosis in multiple myeloma. Arch Int Med 1981; 141:655–657.
75. Batlle DC, Mozes MF, Manaligod J, Arruda JAL, Kurtzman NA. The pathogenesis of hyperchloremic metabolic acidosis associated with kidney transplantation. Am J Med 1981; 70:786–796.
76. Batlle DC, Sehy JT, Roseman MK, Arruda JAL, Kurtzman NA. Clinical and pathophysiologic spectrum of acquired distal renal tubular acidosis. Kidney Int 1981; 20:389–396.
77. Jordan M, Cohen EP, Roza A, Adams MB, Johnson C, Gluck SL, Bastani B. An immunocytochemical study of H^+ ATPase in kidney transplant rejection. J Lab Clin Med 1996; 127:310–314.
78. Cohen SI, Fitzgerald MG, Fourman P. Polyuria in hyperparathyroidism. Quart J Med 1957; 26:423.
79. Reynolds TB, Bethune JE. Renal tubular acidosis secondary to hyperparathyroidism. Clin Res 1966; 17:169.
80. Huth EJ, Mayock RL, Kerr RM. Hyperthyroidism associated with renal tubular acidosis. Am J Med 1959; 26:818.

81. Ferris T, Kashgarian M, Levitin H. Renal tubular acidosis and renal potassium wasting acquired as a result of hypercalcemic nephropathy. N Engl J Med 1961; 265:924–928.

82. Parfitt AM, Higgins BA, Nassim JR. Metabolic studies in patients with hypercalciuria. Clin Sci Mol Med 1964; 27:463–482.

83. Deck MDF. Medullary sponge kidney with renal tubular acidosis: a report of 3 cases. J Urol 1965; 94:330–335.

84. Morris RCJ, Yamauchi H, Palubinskas AJ. Medullary sponge kidney. Am J Med 1965; 38:883–892.

85. Yeoh SA. Fabry's disease with renal tubular acidosis. Singapore Med J 1967; 8:275–279.

86. Preminger GM, Sakhaee K, Skurla C, Pak CYC. Prevention of recurrent calcium stone formation with potassium citrate therapy in patients with distal renal tubular acidosis. J Urol 1985; 134:20–23.

87. Buckalew VM Jr, Purvis ML, Shulman MG, Herndon CN, Rudman D. Hereditary renal tubular acidosis. Report of a 64 member kindred with variable clinical expression including idiopathic hypercalciuria. Medicine (Baltimore) 1974; 53:229–254.

88. Reynolds TB. Observations on the pathogenesis of renal tubular acidosis. Am J Med 1958; 25:503–515.

89. Batlle D, Gaviria M, Grupp M, Arruda JA, Wynn J, Kurtzman NA. Distal nephron function in patients receiving chronic lithium therapy. Kidney Int 1982; 21:477–485.

90. Batlle DC, Sabatini S, Kurtzman NA. On the mechanism of toluene induced renal tubular acidosis. Nephron 1988; 49:210–218.

91. Carlisle EJ, Donnelly SM, Vasuvattakul S, Kamel KS, Tobe S, Halperin ML. Glue sniffing and distal renal tubular acidosis: sticking to the facts. J Am Soc Nephrol 1991; 1:1019–1027.

92. Nilwarangkur S, Nimmannit S, Chaovakul V, Susaengrat W, Ongajyooth S, Vasuvattakul S, Pidetcha P, Malasit P. Endemic primary distal renal tubular acidosis in Thailand. Quar J Med 1990; 74:289–301.

93. Bruce LJ, Cope DL, Jones GK, Schofield AE, Burley M, Povey S, Unwin RJ, Wrong O, Tanner MJ. Familial distal renal tubular acidosis is associated with mutations in the red cell anion exchanger (Band 3, AE1) gene. J Clin Invest 1997; 100:1693–1707.

94. Batlle DC, Grupp M, Gaviria M. Distal renal tubular acidosis with intact capacity to lower urinary pH. Am J Med 1982; 72:751–758.

95. Alper SL, Darman RB, Chernova MN, Dahl NK. The AE gene family of Cl^-/HCO^{3-} exchangers. J Nephrol 2002; 15(Suppl 5):S41–S53.

96. Alper SL, Natale J, Gluck S, Lodish HF, Brown D. Subtypes of intercalated cells in rat kidney collecting duct defined by antibodies against erythroid band 3 and renal vacuolar H^+ ATPase. Proc Natl Acad Sci USA 1989; 86:5429–5433.

97. Brown D, Hirsch S, Gluck S. An H^+ ATPase in opposite plasma membrane domains in kidney epithelial cell subpopulations. Nature 1988; 331:622–624.

98. Gluck SL, Underhil DM, Iyori M. Biochemical regulation of proton secretion by the vacuolar H^+ ATPase of renal epithelial cells. In: Santo NG, Capasso G,

eds. Acid–Base and Electrolyte Imbalance, Molecular, Cellular, and Clinical Aspects. Naple, Italy, 2002:30–42.

99. Nelson RD, Guo XL, Masood K, Brown D, Kalkbrenner M, Gluck S. Selectively amplified expression of an isoform of the vacuolar H^+ ATPase 56 kilodalton subunit in renal intercalated cells. Proc Natl Acad Sci USA 1992; 89:3541–3545.

100. Schwartz GJ, Barasch J, Al Awqati Q. Plasticity of functional epithelial polarity. Nature 1985; 318:368–371.

101. Ko SB, Luo X, Hager H, Rojek A, Choi JY, Licht C, Suzuki M, Muallem S, Nielsen S, Ishibashi K. AE4 is a DIDS-sensitive Cl^-/HCO^{3-} exchanger in the basolateral membrane of the renal CCD and the SMG duct. Am J Physiol 2002; 283:C1206–C1218.

102. Soleimani M, Greeley T, Petrovic S, Wang ZH, Amlal H, Kopp P, Burnham CE. Pendrin: an apical $Cl^-/OH^-/HCO^{3-}$ exchanger in the kidney cortex. Am J Physiol 2001; 280:F356–F364.

103. Kopp P. Perspective: genetic defects in the etiology of congenital hypothyroidism. Endocrinology 2002; 143:2019–2024.

104. Koeppen BM. Electrophysiological identification of principal and intercalated cells in the rabbit outer medullary collecting duct. Pflugers Archiv Eur J Physiol 1987; 409:138–141.

105. Kumpulainen T. Immunohistochemical localization of human carbonic anhydrase isozymes. Ann NY Acad Sci 1984; 429:359–368.

106. Sato S, Zhu XL, Sly WS. Carbonic anhydrase isozymes IV and II in urinary membranes from carbonic anhydrase II-deficient patients. Proc Natl Acad Sci USA 1990; 87:6073–6076.

107. Cohen EP, Bastani B, Cohen MR, Kolner S, Hemken P, Gluck SL. Absence of H^+ ATPase in cortical collecting tubules of a patient with Sjogren's syndrome and distal renal tubular acidosis. J Am Soc Nephrol 1992; 3:264–271.

108. Defranco PE, Haragsim L, Schmitz PG, Bastani B, Li JP. Absence of vacuolar H^+ ATPase pump in the collecting duct of a patient with hypokalemic distal renal tubular acidosis and sjogren's syndrome. J Am Soc Nephrol 1995; 6: 295–301.

109. Karet FE, Finberg KE, Nelson RD, Nayir A, Mocan H, Sanjad SA, Rodriguez-Soriano J, Santos F, Cremers CWRJ, di Pietro A, Hoffbrand BI, Winiarski J, Bakkaloglu A, Ozen S, Dusunsel R, Goodyer P, Hulton SA, Wu DK, Skvorak AB, Morton CC, Cunningham MJ, Jha V, Lifton RP. Mutations in the gene encoding B1 subunit of H^+ ATPase cause renal tubular acidosis with sensorineural deafness. Nature Genet 1999; 21:84–90.

110. Smith AN, Skaug J, Choate KA, Nayir A, Bakkaloglu A, Ozen S, Hulton SA, Sanjad SA, Al Sabban EA, Lifton RP, Scherer SW, Karet FE. Mutations in ATP6N1B, encoding a new kidney vacuolar proton pump 116-kD subunit, cause recessive distal renal tubular acidosis with preserved hearing. Nature Genet 2000; 26:71–75.

111. Stover EH, Borthwick KJ, Bavalia C, Eady N, Fritz DM, Rungroj N, Giersch AB, Morton CC, Axon PR, Akil I, Al Sabban EA, Baguley DMBianca S, Bakkaloglu A, Bircan Z, Chauveau D, Clermont MJ Guala A, Hulton SA, Kroes H, Li VG, Mir S, Mocan H, Nayir A, Ozen

S, Rodriguez SJ, Sanjad SA, Tasic V, Taylor CM, Topaloglu R, Smith AN, Karet FE. Novel ATP6V1B1 and ATP6V0A4 mutations in autosomal recessive distal renal tubular acidosis with new evidence for hearing loss. J Med Genet 2002; 39:796–803.

112. Steinmetz PR, Lawson LR. Defect in acidification induced in vitro by amphotericin B. J Clin Invest 1970; 49:596–601.

113. Rosen S. Turtle bladder. II. Observations on epithelial cytotoxic effect of amphotericin B. Exper Mol Pathol 1970; 12:297–305.

114. Inaba M, Yawata A, Koshino I, Sato K, Takeuchi M, Takakuwa Y, Manno S, Yawata Y, Kanzaki A, Sakai J, Ban A, Ono K, Maede Y. Defective anion transport and marked spherocytosis with membrane instability caused by hereditary total deficiency of red cell band 3 in cattle due to a nonsense mutation. J Clin Invest 1996; 97:1804–1817.

115. Jarolim P, Shayakul C, Prabakaran D, Jiang L, Stuart-Tilley A, Rubin HL, Simova S, Zavadil J, Herrin JT, Brouillette J, Somers MJ, Seemanova E, Brugnara C, Guay-Woodford LM, Alper SL. Autosomal dominant distal renal tubular acidosis is associated in three families with heterozygosity for the R589H mutation in the AE1 (band 3)gene. J Biol Chem 1998; 273: 6380–6388.

116. Karet FE, Gainza FJ, Gyory AZ, Unwin RJ, Wrong O, Tanner MJ, Nayir A, Alpay H, Santos F, Hulton SA, Bakkaloglu A, Ozen S, Cunningham MJ, di Pietro A, Walker WG, Lifton RP. Mutations in the chloride bicarbonate exchanger gene AE1 cause autosomal dominant but not autosomal recessive distal renal tubular acidosis. Proc Natl Acad Sci USA 1998; 95: 6337–6342.

117. Vasuvattakul S, Yenchitsomanus PT, Vachuanichsanong P, Thuwajit P, Kaitwatcharachai C, Laosombat V, Malasit P, Wilairat P, Nimmannit S. Autosomal recessive distal renal tubular acidosis associated with Southeast Asian ovalocytosis. Kidney Int 1999; 56:1674–1682.

118. Peters LL, Jindel HK, Gwynn B, Korsgren C, John KM, Lux SE, Mohandas N, Cohen CM, Cho MR, Golan DE, Brugnara C. Mild spherocytosis and altered red cell ion transport in protein 4.2 null mice. J Clin Invest 1999; 103:1527–1537.

119. Brosius FC III, Alper SL, Garcia AM, Lodish HF. The major kidney band 3 gene transcript predicts an amino terminal truncated band 3 polypeptide. J Biol Chem 1989; 264:7784–7787.

120. DuBose TD Jr. Autosomal dominant distal renal tubular acidosis and the AE1 gene. Am J Kidney Dis 1999; 33:1190–1197.

121. Bruce LJ, Wrong O, Toye AM, Young MT, Ogle G, Ismail Z, Sinha AK, McMaster P, Hwaihwanje I, Nash GB, Hart S, Lavu E, Palmer R, Othman A, Unwin RJ, Tanner MJA. Band 3 mutations, renal tubular acidosis, and South-east Asian ovalocytosis in Malaysia and Papua New Guinea: loss of up to 95% band 3 transport in red cells. Biochem J 2000; 351:839.

122. Fathallah DM, Bejaoui M, Lepaslier D, Chater K, Sly WS, Dellagi K. Carbonic anhydrase II (CA II)deficiency in Maghrebian patients: evidence for founder effect and genomic recombination at the CA II locus. Hum Genet 1997; 99:634–637.

123. Aramaki S, Yoshida I, Yoshino M, Kondo M, Sato Y, Noda K, Jo R, Okue A, Sai N, Yamashita F. Carbonic anhydrase II deficiency in three unrelated Japanese patients. J Inherit Metab Dis 1993; 16:982–990.

124. Hu PY, Ernst AR, Sly WS, Venta PJ, Skaggs LA, Tashian RE. Carbonic anhydrase II deficiency: single base deletion in exon 7 is the predominant mutation in Caribbean hispanic patients. Am J Hum Genet 1994; 54:602–608.

125. Hu PY, Lim EJ, Ciccolella J, Strisciuglio P, Sly WS. Seven novel mutations in carbonic anhydrase II deficiency syndrome identified by SSCP and direct sequencing analysis. Hum Mutat 1997; 9:383–387.

126. Karet FE, Finberg KE, Nayir A, Bakkaloglu A, Ozen S, Hulton SA, Sanjad SA, Al Sabban EA, Medina JF, Lifton RP. Localization of a gene for autosomal recessive distal renal tubular acidosis with normal hearing (rdistal RTA2)to 7q33–34. Am J Hum Genet 1999; 65:1656–1665.

127. Finberg KE. Generation and characterization of H^+ ATPase B1 subunit deficient mice. [Abstr]. J Am Soc Nephrol 2001; 12:3A–4A.

128. Zakzouk SM, Sobki SH, Mansour F, al Anazy FH. Hearing impairment in association with distal renal tubular acidosis among Saudi children. J Laryngol Otol 1995; 109:930–934.

129. Myers EN, Stool S. The temporal bone in osteopetrosis. Arch Otolaryngol 1969; 89:460–469.

130. Sly WS, Whyte MP, Sundaram V, Tashian RE, Hewettemmett D, Guibaud P, Vainsel M, Baluarte HJ, Gruskin A, Almosawi M, Sakati N, Ohlsson A. Carbonic anhydrase II deficiency in 12 families with the autosomal recessive syndrome of osteopetrosis with renal tubular acidosis and cerebral calcification. N Engl J Med 1985; 313:139–145.

131. Szylman P, Better OS, Chaimowitz C, Rosler A. Role of hyperkalemia in metabolic acidosis of isolated hypoaldosteronism. N Engl J Med 1976; 294:361–365.

132. Sastrasinh S, Tannen RL. Effect of potassium on renal NH_3 production. Am J Physiol 1983; 244:F383–F391.

133. Tannen RL. Relationship of renal ammonia production and potassium homeostasis. Kidney Int 1977; 11:453–465.

134. Welbourne TC, Francoeur D. Influence of aldosterone on renal ammonia production. Am J Physiol 1977; 233:E56–E60.

135. DuBose TD Jr, Caflisch CR. Effect of selective aldosterone deficiency on acidification in nephron segments of the rat inner medulla. J Clin Invest 1988; 82:1624–1632.

136. Koeppen BM, Helman SI. Acidification of luminal fluid by the rabbit cortical collecting tubule perfused in vitro. Am J Physiol 1982; 242:F521–F531.

137. Stokes JB. Potassium secretion by cortical collecting tubule: relation to sodium absorption, luminal sodium concentration, and transepithelial voltage. Am J Physiol 1981; 241:F395–F402.

138. Uribarri J, Oh MS, Carroll HJ. Clinical characteristics of patients with the syndrome of hyporeninemic hypoaldosteronism. Kidney Int 1981; 19:138.

139. Uribarri J, Oh MS. Hypocitraturia in renal stone formers. Kidney Int 1983; 23:139.

140. Cannon PJ, Ames RP, Laragh JH. Relation between potassium balance and aldosterone secretion in normal subjects and in patients with hypertensive or renal tubular disease. J Clin Invest 1966; 45:865–879.
141. White PC. Disorders of aldosterone biosynthesis and action. N Engl J Med 1994; 331:250–258.
142. Batlle DC, Kurtzman NA. Clinical disorders of aldosterone metabolism. Dis Mon 1984; 30:1–55.
143. Davenport MW, Zipser RD. Association of hypotension with hyperreninemic hypoaldosteronism in the critically ill patient. Arch Intern Med 1983; 143: 735–737.
144. Mitra A, Batlle D. Aldosterone deficiency and resistance. In: DuBose, Hamm, eds. Acid–base and Electrolyte Disorders. A companion to Brenner's and Rector's, the Kidney. Saunders, 2002:24:413–433.
145. Hudson JB, Chobanian AW, Relman AS. Hypo aldosteronism: a clinical study of a patient with an isolated adrenal mineralocorticoid deficiency, resulting in hyperkalemia and Stokes–Adams attacks. N Engl J Med 1957; 257:529.
146. Perez GO, Oster JR, Vaamonde CA. Renal acidosis and renal potassium handling in selective hypoaldosteronism. Am J Med 1974; 57:809–816.
147. Posner JB, Jacobs DR. Isolated analdosteronism: I. clinical entity with manifestations of persistent hyperkalemia, periodic paralysis, salt losing tendency, and acidosis. Metabolism 1964; 13:513–521.
148. Schambelan M, Stockigt JR, Biglieri EG. Isolated hypoaldosteronism in adults. A renin deficiency syndrome. N Engl J Med 1972; 287:573–578.
149. Schambelan M, Sebastian A, Biglieri EG. Prevalence, pathogenesis, and functional significance of aldosterone deficiency in hyperkalemic patients with chronic renal insufficiency. Kidney Int 1980; 17:89–101.
150. Skanse B, Hokfelt B. Hypoaldosteronism with otherwise intact adrenocortical function, resulting in a characteristic clinical entity. Acta Endocrinol 1958; 28:29.
151. Tan SY, Burton M. Hyporeninemic hypoaldosteronism. An overlooked cause of hyperkalemia. Arch Intern Med 1981; 141:30–33.
152. Vagnucci AH. Selective aldosterone deficiency. J Clin Endocrinol Metab 1969; 29:279–289.
153. Weidmann P, Reinhart R, Maxwell MH, Rowe P, Coburn JW, Massry SG. Syndrome of hyporeninemic hypoaldosteronism and hyperkalemia in renal disease. J Clin Endocrinol Metab 1973; 36:965–977.
154. Anggard E, Larsson C, Weber P. Interactions between the renal prostaglandins and the rennin–angiotensin system. Adv Prostaglandins Thromboxane Res 1976; 2:587–594.
155. Lijnen P, Staessen J, Fagard R, Amery A. Effect of prostaglandin inhibition by indomethacin on plasma active and inactive renin concentration in men. Can J Physiol Pharmacol 1991; 69:1355–1359.
156. Oates JA, Whorton AR, Gerkens JF, Branch RA, Hollifield JW, Frolich JC. Participation of prostaglandins in the control of renin release. Feder Proc 1979; 38:72–74.
157. Lachaal M, Venuto RC. Nephrotoxicity and hyperkalemia in patients with acquired immunodeficiency syndrome treated with pentamidine. Am J Med 1989; 87:260–263.

158. Ribeiro C, Suki WN. Acidification in the medullary collecting duct following ureteral obstruction. Kidney Int 1986; 29:1167–1171.

159. Laski ME, Kurtzman NA. Site of the acidification defect in the perfused postobstructed collecting tubule. Miner Electr Metab 1989; 15:195–200.

160. Sabatini S, Kurtzman NA. Enzyme activity in obstructive uropathy: basis for salt wastage and the acidification defect. Kidney Int 1990; 37:79–84.

161. Adu D, Turney J, Michael J, McMaster P. Hyperkalaemia in cyclosporin treated renal allograft recipients. Lancet 1983; 2:370–372.

162. Bantle JP, Nath KA, Sutherl DE, Najarian JS, Ferris TF. Effects of cyclosporine on the rennin–angiotensin–aldosterone system and potassium excretion in renal transplant recipients. Arch Intern Med 1985; 145:505–508.

163. Woo M, Przepiorka D, Ippoliti C, Warkentin D, Khouri I, Fritsche H, Korbling M. Toxicities of tacrolimus and cyclosporin A after allogeneic blood stem cell transplantation. Bone Mar Transplan 1997; 20:1095–1098.

164. Batlle DC, Gutterman C, Tarka J, Prasad R. Effect of short term cyclosporine A administration on urinary acidification. Clin Nephrol 1986; 25:S62–S69.

165. Kamel KS, Ethier JH, Quaggin S, Levin A, Albert S, Carlisle EJF, Halperin ML. Studies to determine the basis for hyperkalemia in recipients of a renal transplant who are treated with cyclosporine. J Am Soc Nephrol 1992; 2:1279–1284.

166. Alessiani M, Cillo U, Fung JJ, Irish W, Abuelmagd K, Jain A, Takaya S, Vanthiel D, Starzl TE. Adverse effects of FK 506 overdosage after liver transplantation. Transplan Proc 1993; 25:628–634.

167. Tumlin JA, Sands JM. Nephron segment specific inhibition of Na^+/K^+ ATPase activity by cyclosporine A. Kidney Int 1993; 43:246–251.

168. Ling BN, Eaton DC. Cyclosporin A inhibits apical secretory K^+ channels in rabbit cortical collecting tubule principal cells. Kidney Int 1993; 44:974–984.

169. Ellison DH. Hyperkalemia and trimethoprim-sulfamethoxazole. Am J Kidney Dis 1997; 29:959–965.

170. Marinella MA. Trimethoprim induced hyperkalemia: an analysis of reported cases. Gerontology 1999; 45:209–212.

171. Velazquez H, Perazella A, Wright FS. Renal mechanism of trimethoprim induced hyperkalemia. Ann Int Med 1993; 119:296–301.

172. Choi MJ, Frenandez PC, Patnaik A. Brief report: trimethoprim induced hyperkalemia in a patient with AIDS. N Engl J Med 1993; 328:703–706.

173. Eiam-Ong S, Kurtzman A, Sabatini S. Studies on the mechanism of trimethoprim induced hyperkalemia. Kidney Int 1996; 49:1372–1378.

174. Alappan R, Perazella MA, Buller GK. Hyperkalemia in hospitalized patients treated with trimethoprim–sulfamethoxazole. Ann Int Med 1996; 124:316–320.

175. Funai N, Shimamoto Y, Matsuzaki M. Hyperkalemia with renal tubular dysfunction by sulfamethoxazole–trimethoprim. Hematologia 1993; 25:137–141.

176. Perazella MA, Buller GK. Hyperkalemia and trimethoprim–sulfamethoxazole. Am J Kidney Dis 1997; 29:959–965.

177. Schlanger LE, Kleyman TR, Ling BN. K^+ sparing diuretic actions of trimethoprim: inhibition of Na^+ channels in A6 distal nephron cells. Kidney Int 1994; 45:1070–1076.

178. Sheehan MT, Wen SF. Hyperkalemic renal tubular acidosis induced by trimethoprim–sulfamethoxazole in an AIDS patient. Clin Nephrol 1998; 50:188–193.

179. Lin SH, Kuo AA, Yu FC. Reversible voltage-dependent distal renal tubular acidosis in a patient receiving standard doses of trimethoprim–sulfamethoxazole. Nephrol Dial Transplan 1997; 12:1031–1033.

180. Kleyman TR, Roberts C, Ling BN. A mechanism for pentamidine induced hyperkalemia: inhibition of distal nephron sodium transport. Ann Int Med 1995; 122:103–106.

181. Cheek DB, Perry JW. A salt wasting syndome in infancy. Arch Dis Child 1958; 33:252–256.

182. Kuhnle, U, Hinkel GK, Hubl W. Pseudohypoaldosteronism: family studies to identify asymptomatic carriers by stimulation of the renin–aldosterone system. Horm Res 1996; 46:124–129.

183. Zennaro MC, Borensztein P, Soubrier F. The enigma of pseudohypoaldosteronism. Steroids 1994; 94:96.

184. Geller DS, Rodriguez-Soriano J, Boado AV. Mutations in the mineralocorticoid receptor gene cause autosomal dominant pseudohypoaldosteronisim type I. Nat Genet 1998; 19:279–281.

185. Tajima T, Kitagawa H, Yokoya S, Tachibana K, Adachi M, Suwa S, Katoh S, Fujieda K. A novel missense mutation of mineralocorticoid receptor gene in one Japanese family with a renal form of pseudohypoaldosteronism. J Clin Endocrinol Metab 2000; 85:4690–4694.

186. Adachi M, Tachibana K, Asakura Y. Compound heterozygous mutations in the a subunit gene of ENaC (1627delG and1570-1- - > GA)in one sporadic Japanese patient with a systemic form of pseudohypoaldosteronism type 1. J Clin Endocrinol Metab 2001; 86:9–12.

187. Chang SS, Grunder S, Hanukoglu A, Rosler A, Mathew PM, Hanukoglu I, Schild L, Lu Y, Shimkets RA, NelsonWilliams C, Rossier BC, Lifton RP. Mutations in subunits of the epithelial sodium channel cause salt wasting with hyperkalaemic acidosis, pseudohypoaldosteronism type 1. Nature Genet 1996; 12:248–253.

188. Mitsuuchi Y, Kawamoto T, Miyahara K, Ulick S, Morton DH, Naiki Y, Kuribayashi I, Toda K, Hara T, Orii T, Yasuda K, Miura K, Yamamoto Y, Imura H, Shizuta Y. Congenitally defective aldosterone biosynthesis in humans—inactivation of the P-450C18 gene (Cyp11B2)due to nucleotide deletion in Cmo-I deficient patients. Biochem Biophys Res Comm 1993; 190:864–869.

189. Pascoe L, Curnow KM, Slutsker L, Rosler A, White PC. Mutations in the Human Cyp11B2 (aldosterone synthase)gene causing corticosterone methyloxidase II deficiency. Proc Natl Acad Sci USA 1992; 89:4996–5000.

190. Gereda JE, BonillaFelix M, Kalil B, Dewitt SJ. Neonatal presentation of Gordon syndrome. J Pediatr 1996; 129:615–617.

191. Gordon RD. Syndrome of hypertension and hyperkalemia with normal glomerular filtration rate. Hypertension 1986; 8:93–102.

192. Throckmorton DC, Bia MJ. Pseudohypoaldosteronism—case report and discussion of the syndrome. Yale J Biol Med 1991; 64:247–254.

193. Disse-Nicodeme S, Achard JM, Desitter I, Houot AM, Fournier A, Corvol P, Jeunemaitre X. A new locus on chromosome 12p13.3 for pseudohypoaldosteronism type II, autosomal dominant form of hypertension. Am J Hum Genet 2000; 67:302–310.

194. Mansfield TA, Simon DB, Farfel Z, Bia M, Tucci JR, Lebel M, Gutkin M, Vialettes B, Christofilis MA, KauppinenMakelin R, Mayan H, Risch N, Lifton RP. Multilocus linkage of familial hyperkalaemia and hypertension, pseudohypoaldosteronism type II, to chromosomes 1q31–42 and 17p11-q21. Nature Genet 1997; 16:202–205.

195. Schambelan M, Sebastian A, Rector FC. Mineralocorticoid resistant renal hyperkalemia without salt wasting (type II pseudo hypoaldosteronism)—role of increased renal chloride reabsorption. Kidney Int 1981; 19:716–727.

196. Take C, Ikeda K, Kurasawa T, Kurokawa K. Increased chloride reabsorption as an inherited renal tubular defect in familial type II pseudohypoaldosteronism. N Engl J Med 1991; 324:472–476.

197. Wilson FH, Disse-Nicodeme S, Choate KA, Ishikawa K, Nelson-Willams C, Desitter I, Gunel M, Milford DV, Lipkin GW, Achard JM, Feely MP, Dussol B, Berland Y, Unwin RJ, Mayan H, Simon DB, Farfel Z, Jeunemaitre X, Lifton RP. Human hypertension caused by mutations in WNK kinases. Science 2001; 293:1107–1112.

198. Batlle DC, Hizon M, Cohen E, Gutterman C, Gupta R. The use of the urinary anion gap in the diagnosis of hyperchloremic metabolic acidosis. N Engl J Med 1988; 318:594–599.

199. Wrong O. Distal renal tubular acidosis—the value of urinary pH, PCO_2 and NH^{4+} Measurements. Pediatr Nephrol 1991; 5:249–255.

200. Morris RC, Piel CF, Audioun E. Renal tubular acidosis—effects of sodium phosphate and sulfate on renal acidification in two patients with renal tubular acidosis. Pediatrics 1965; 36:899–904.

201. Shinoda T, Shiigai T. Sodium sulfate and furosemide loading tests for the diagnosis of renal tubular acidosis. Nippon Rinsho 1985; 43:1849–1854.

202. Donckerwolcke RA, Valk C, Vanwijngaardenpenterman MJG, Vanstekelenburg GJ. The diagnostic value of the urine to blood carbon dioxide tension gradient for the assessment of distal tubular hydrogen secretion in pediatric patients with renal tubular disorders. Clin Nephrol 1983; 19:254–258.

203. Dubose TD. Hydrogen ion secretion by the collecting duct as a determinant of the urine to blood PCo_2 gradient in alkaline urine. J Clin Invest 1982; 69: 145–156.

204. Arruda JAL, Nascimento L, Mehta PK, Rademacher DR, Sehy JT, Westenfelder C, Kurtzman NA. Critical importance of urinary concentrating ability in generation of urinary carbon dioxide tension. J Clin Invest 1977; 60: 922–935.

205. Garg LC. Lack of effect of amphotericin-B on urine blood PCo_2 gradient in spite of urinary acidification defect. Pflugers Archiv Eur J Physiol 1979; 381:137–142.

206. Julka NK, Arruda JAL, Kurtzman NA. Mechanism of amphotericin induced distal acidification defect in rats. Clin Sci 1979; 56:555–562.

207. Vallo A, Rodriguezsoriano J. Oral phosphate loading test for the assessment of distal urinary acidification in children. Miner Electr Metab 1984; 10: 387–390.

208. Domrongkitchaiporn S, Khositseth S, Stitchantrakul W, Tapaneya-olarn W, Radinahamed P. Dosage of potassium citrate in the correction of urinary abnormalities in pediatric distal renal tubular acidosis patients. Am J Kidney Dis 2002; 39:383–391.

209. Bajaj G, Quan A. Renal tubular acidosis and deafness: report of a large family. Am J Kidney Dis 1996; 27:880–882.

14

Metabolic Acidosis in Chronic Renal Insufficiency

F. John Gennari

University of Vermont College of Medicine, Burlington, Vermont, U.S.A.

INTRODUCTION

Metabolic acidosis is a common, but not invariable, feature of chronic kidney disease. Serum [HCO_3^-] varies widely, but the average value typically falls as serum creatinine concentration rises (Fig. 1) (1,2). Metabolic acidosis is not confined to advanced renal insufficiency; serum [HCO_3^-] often is below normal in individuals with creatinine values of only $2\,mg/dL$ (1,2). As serum creatinine concentration rises to $>4\,mg/dL$, however, serum [HCO_3^-] typically falls to 16–20 mEq/L in most patients. This chapter addresses the nature and causes of this metabolic acidosis and reviews its potentially deleterious effects and management.

NORMAL REGULATION OF ACID–BASE HOMEOSTASIS

Each day strong acids are generated by metabolic events as a result of the diet normally ingested in Western culture. The H^+ produced by these acids is rapidly buffered by body alkali stores, which then are regenerated by H^+ excretion by the kidney. Under normal conditions, renal H^+ excretion is closely correlated with acid production, and this process maintains serum [HCO_3^-] stable within the normal range. The nature of this balance is

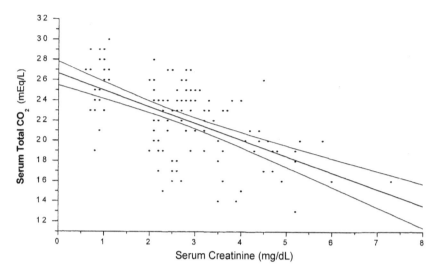

Figure 1 Relationship between serum creatinine concentration and total CO_2 in subjects with normal renal function (average serum creatinine 0.9 mg/dL, left-hand side of the data) and in patients with varying degrees of chronic renal insufficiency. Serum total CO_2 is inversely related to serum creatinine concentration: total CO_2 (mEq/L) = 26.6–1.64 × creatinine ($R = 0.58$, $P < 0.001$). The curved lines in the figure represent 95% confidence intervals for this relationship.

discussed in detail in Chapter 6, and only the key points with relation to chronic kidney disease reviewed here. The kidney has two tasks to accomplish in maintaining body HCO_3^- stores. First, all the filtered HCO_3^- must be reclaimed by the renal tubules, and second, H^+ must be excreted in the urine in order to create new HCO_3^- to replace that lost in the buffering process. These tasks are accomplished by H^+ and NH_4^+ secretion. In order for sufficient H^+ to be excreted each day, it must be linked with either phosphate, forming $H_2PO_4^-$ (titratable acid) or with ammonia to form NH_4^+. Ammonium ions are normally the major contributor to acid excretion, and are produced in the kidney by a metabolic process that is regulated by systemic pH (3). Excretion of NH_4^+ is complex, involving production and secretion in the proximal tubule, reabsorption and countercurrent multiplication in the loop of Henle, and diffusion of NH_3 into the medullary collecting ducts where it recombines with secreted H^+ (4). The structural integrity of the kidney is critical for this complex series of events, and it is not surprising that NH_4^+ excretion is impaired in chronic kidney disease (see below). By contrast, titratable acid excretion and HCO_3^- reclamation are maintained until renal damage is severe.

PATHOPHYSIOLOGY OF METABOLIC ACIDOSIS IN RENAL INSUFFICIENCY

Studies in Humans (Table 1)

In humans with advanced kidney disease, NH_4^+ excretion is universally decreased, accounting for <50% of net acid excretion, as compared to 75–85% in individuals with normal renal function (5–8). The reduction in excretion is associated with a decrease in renal NH_4^+ production (5). In some patients, impaired renal conservation of filtered HCO_3^- is present, manifested by the continued loss of HCO_3^- in the urine as serum $[HCO_3^-]$ falls to <20 mEq/L (7,9,10).

In addition to impaired acid excretion under baseline conditions, patients with renal insufficiency have an extremely limited ability to increase acid excretion in response to an acid load (6,7). This impairment is accounted for primarily by a limitation in the damaged kidney's ability to increase NH_4^+ excretion (6,7,11). Urine pH is appropriately low, indicating a normal capacity for H^+ secretion into the medullary and papillary collecting duct urine (6,7,11). Titratable acid excretion is either normal or increased, not surprisingly, given normal acidification and reduced NH_4^+ excretion. Hyperkalemia, a common finding in patients with renal insufficiency (12), is known to impair NH_4^+ production and excretion (13), but is unlikely to be responsible for the impairment in NH_4^+ excretion (see later).

Studies in Animals

The findings in humans have been reproduced in a model of kidney disease in animals, induced by partial removal of renal tissue (remnant kidney model). Animals with remnant kidneys develop a mild metabolic acidosis and have impaired NH_4^+ production and excretion, associated with normal renal acidification and normal or increased titratable acid excretion (14–17).

Table 1 Summary of Changes in Acid Excretion in Humans with Chronic Renal Insufficiency

Baseline conditions
Ammonium excretion decreased (<50% of total acid excretion)
Ammonium production decreased
Urine pH normal
Titratable acid excretion normal or increased
Response to acid load
Inability to increase acid excretion
Response to alkali administration
Impaired renal HCO_3^- conservation in some patients with advanced renal damage[a]

[a] GFR <10 mL/min.

Using this animal model, investigators have examined single nephron function to assess more specifically where the defect in acid excretion occurs (Table 2).

Ammonium Production/Excretion

In animals with remnant kidneys, NH_4^+ production and secretion in functioning proximal tubules are increased rather than decreased. Ammonium reabsorption in the loop of Henle and delivery to the distal nephron are also increased (14,15,17). The major difference from control animals is impaired re-entry of NH_4^+ into the papillary collecting duct (14). This impairment could not be accounted for by any changes in collecting duct pH. The collecting duct defect is associated with a reduction in NH_4^+ concentration in the medullary loops of Henle and in papillary osmolality, supporting the view that countercurrent concentration of NH_4^+ is impaired. Thus, despite increased production and secretion of NH_4^+ in functioning tubules, the reduction in overall renal mass limits total production and impairs countercurrent multiplication, reducing NH_4^+ delivery and entrapment in the papillary collecting duct. As a result, NH_4^+ excretion is impaired compared to animals with normal renal function. In this rat model, NH_4^+ excretion also fails to increase appropriately in response to an acid load (as in humans), presumably due to the same pathophysiology (17).

Table 2 Impairment of Net Acid Excretion in Renal Insufficiency—Pathophysiology

---

Ammonium
  $\downarrow$ Total NH_4^+ production due to $\downarrow$ in functioning nephrons
  Impaired countercurrent concentration due to $\downarrow$ in functioning nephrons
  $\uparrow$ Secretion in functioning proximal tubules
  Normal re-uptake in functioning loops of Henle
  $\downarrow$ Re-entry into papillary collecting ducts
  $\downarrow$ NH_4^+ excretion
H^+ secretion/HCO_3^- reabsorption
  Normal throughout nephron in animal models
  Increases normally in response to $\uparrow$ in single nephron GFR
  Impaired conservation in some instances when GFR $< 10\,\text{ml/min}$
Titratable acid excretion
  Normal or $\uparrow$
Other abnormalities
  Hypoaldosteronism may contribute, but not a requirement for $\downarrow$ NH_4^+ excretion
  Hyperkalemia can impair NH_4^+ production, but not a requirement
    for $\downarrow$ production

H^+ Secretion/HCO_3^- Reabsorption

Single nephron H^+ secretion is uniformly increased in the remnant kidney in all segments of functioning nephrons, including the proximal tubule, loop of Henle, distal tubule, and collecting duct (14,16,18–20). In the proximal tubule, H^+ secretion increases in direct relation to HCO_3^- delivery in a fashion indistinguishable from control animals (16). The rate of H^+ secretion is highest in animals fed a high protein diet, which in turn have the highest single nephron GFR. Although proximal tubular H^+ secretion increases appropriately, it is not "stimulated" enough to prevent an increase in distal delivery. The increase in distal HCO_3^- delivery results in increased H^+ secretion in the loop, distal tubule, and collecting duct. The urine remains essentially free of HCO_3^- (14,16,18,20).

Although HCO_3^- reabsorption is essentially complete in this animal model, it is possible that diversion of distal nephron H^+ secretion to recapturing the increased amount of HCO_3^- arriving at this site could impair the ability of H^+ to entrap NH_4^+ or titrate other buffers (14). This possibility cannot be excluded, but seems unlikely as distal H^+ secretion is sufficient not only to recapture this HCO_3^- but also to increase titratable acid excretion (14,15,17). Thus, impaired H^+ excretion appears to be limited to the component carried into the urine as NH_4^+.

Role of Hypoaldosteronism

Low aldosterone secretion rates, associated in most cases with low renin levels, have been implicated to contribute to the metabolic acidosis of chronic kidney disease (21,22). In one often-cited report, four patients with kidney disease and metabolic acidosis associated with hypoaldosteronism were treated with the oral mineralocorticoid agent, fludrocortisone (22). In these patients, NH_4^+ excretion and serum [HCO_3^-] increased after treatment. Despite these positive results, the role of aldosterone deficiency in the pathogenesis of the metabolic acidosis of renal insufficiency is uncertain. Hypoaldosteronism is a common finding in patients with chronic kidney disease (23), but this abnormality is only associated with metabolic acidosis in $\sim$50% of cases (21). moreover, when serum [HCO_3^-] values in patients with chronic kidney disease and low aldosterone levels are compared to patients with similar GFRs and normal aldosterone levels, no differences are noted (23).

Role of Hyperkalemia

Hyperkalemia is a common feature of chronic renal insufficiency (12), and this electrolyte abnormality has been implicated as a factor contributing to metabolic acidosis because it is known to inhibit NH_4^+ excretion (13). The major evidence against such a role is that hyperkalemia is not present in the rat remnant kidney model of renal insufficiency (16), and this model demonstrates the characteristic impairment in NH_4^+ excretion. In humans with renal insufficiency, serum $[K^+]$ shows no correlation with the degree of acidosis (1,2), also arguing against a role for hyperkalemia.

SUMMARY OF PATHOPHYSIOLOGY

In humans with chronic kidney disease, NH_4^+ excretion is low and does not increase normally in response to an acid load (Table 1). Urine pH and titratable acid excretion are unaffected. In some patients with advanced renal insufficiency (GFR <10 ml/min), renal conservation of filtered HCO_3^- is also impaired. In an animal model of renal insufficiency, NH_4^+ excretion is also reduced despite the finding that NH_4^+ production and secretion into the functioning cortical tubules are increased (Table 2). Secretion of H^+ is also increased in all segments of functioning tubules and all filtered HCO_3^- is recaptured. The major defect is impaired NH_4^+ delivery to the papillary collecting duct, limiting entrapment, and excretion of this cation. Animal studies show no evidence of HCO_3^- wasting, but this finding is not surprising because, in the absence of specific tubular defects, this abnormality is only seen in humans with advanced renal insufficiency. Hyperkalemia and hypoaldosteronism are common findings in patients with chronic kidney disease, but these abnormalities do not appear to be necessary for the impairment in renal acid excretion.

ACID BALANCE IN CHRONIC RENAL INSUFFICIENCY

Effect of Changes in Acid Production

Diet-induced changes in acid production have a small but significant effect on serum $[HCO_3^-]$ in individuals with normal renal function (24). As renal function declines and acid excretion is progressively impaired, this effect may well become more prominent. In humans ingesting a typical Western diet, in fact, serum [total CO_2] falls in direct relation to the decline in GFR that occurs with aging (see Chapter 8) (25). In the remnant kidney model in the rat, variations in protein intake (the major dietary contributor to endogenous acid production) also have a notable effect on acid base status. Steady state arterial pH and plasma $[HCO_3^-]$ are higher in animals eating a diet containing only 6% protein than in animals ingesting a diet containing 24% protein (7.42 and 24.5 mEq/L vs. 7.37 and 22.3 mEq/L) (16).

Although many studies of protein restriction have been carried out in humans with chronic kidney disease, there are surprisingly few observations correlating protein intake with steady-state serum [total CO_2]. In one study, the influence on serum $[HCO_3^-]$ of ingesting a very low protein diet (0.3 g/kg body weight), supplemented with keto-analogues of amino acids, was evaluated in patients with advanced kidney disease (creatinine clearances

<10 ml/min) (26). Serum [HCO_3^-] and pH were notably higher (7.39 and 21.7 mEq/L vs. 7.33 and 18.6 mEq/L) in the patients who complied with this diet as compared to those did not. In two smaller studies, serum [HCO_3^-] increased by 1–2 mEq/L when protein intake was reduced by approximately 50% (27,28).

Role of Acid Retention

Impaired acid excretion is clearly the major cause of metabolic acidosis in patients with chronic kidney disease. An unresolved issue, however, is whether retention of endogenously produced acid occurs or whether a new equilibrium is achieved at a lower serum [HCO_3^-], in which acid excretion equals production. The case for continuous acid retention is based upon two carefully performed balance studies in humans (9,10). The first of these studies used a specially prepared liquid formula diet to simplify measurement of endogenous acid production in seven patients with advanced renal insufficiency and one patient with renal tubular acidosis and normal renal function (9). The group had a mean daily acid retention of 19 mEq, which was highly significant and different from individuals with normal renal function who were in balance on the same diet. The inclusion of a subject with renal tubular acidosis and the unusual diet, however, limit the ability to generalize from these observations. The second study included eight subjects with chronic kidney disease ingesting a standard American diet (10). These patients retained 10 mEq of acid per day on average, but the value was not significantly different from zero. Correction of acidosis with oral $NaHCO_3$ improved acid balance in seven out of eight instances, a change that was statistically significant.

The implication of sustained acid retention with a stable serum [HCO_3^-] is that bone buffers (calcium salts) must be continuously released in order to prevent progressively severe metabolic acidosis. In fact, calcium balance is negative in patients with chronic kidney disease and metabolic acidosis, and correction of the acidosis improves calcium balance (10,29). When acid balance was measured simultaneously, mean calcium loss was ∼50% of the amount needed to balance the acid retention (10). Strikingly, alkali administration improves calcium balance even in individuals with normal renal function, suggesting that low-level acid retention may even occur in the absence of kidney disease (30).

The requirement for continuous bone calcium loss to maintain serum [HCO_3^-] led to a challenge of the results showing acid retention in chronic kidney disease (31,32). The reasoning behind this challenge is straightforward; there are insufficient bone calcium stores to buffer the 10–20 mEq of acid estimated to be retained each day for any extended period of time without complete bone dissolution (31). An alternative explanation, proposed by Oh and colleagues, is a systematic error in the acid balance measurements that only becomes apparent in subjects with metabolic acidosis and renal insufficiency (33). To test this hypothesis, these investigators re-examined acid balance in subjects with chronic kidney disease, using a new technique that assesses alkali absorption from the gut indirectly, by calculating the difference between all inorganic cations and anions in the urine (33). In contrast to the studies cited above, this technique includes calcium excretion (but not balance) in the assessment of acid balance. Calcium excretion reflects calcium release from internal sources (i.e., from bone) as well as calcium absorbed from the gut. Thus, if bone calcium release plays an important role in buffering retained H^+, this new approach should show either no net positive balance (any retained H^+ being counterbalanced by Ca^{2+} excretion) or at least a reduction in H^+ balance to the extent that calcium release from bone is buffering retained H^+.

Despite the inclusion of calcium, however, their results again showed a large positive acid balance (+16 mEq/day) in subjects with renal insufficiency and metabolic acidosis. In patients with a comparable degree of renal insufficiency but without metabolic acidosis, strikingly, positive acid balance was not observed. In the patients with acid retention, a positive charge balance ("cation gap") equal to H^+ retention was present (as would be expected). They concluded that such a cation gap was impossible, and therefore a systematic error must be occurring when acid balance is assessed in the presence of metabolic acidosis. They proposed that the most likely errors when acidosis is present are the loss of cationic amino acids in the urine, which are equivalent to acid excretion, and underestimation of titratable acid excretion (see Chapter 6) (32,33).

The interpretation proposed by these investigators has been challenged by Lemann, one of the investigators who authored the earlier studies, and colleagues (34). Their major criticism is that one cannot assess gut alkali absorption from urine electrolyte measurements because an unknown quantity of the inorganic cations and anions in urine come from internal sources, leading either to over- or underestimation of absorption from the gut. In the absence of clear steady-state conditions, moreover, they assert that one cannot either assess charge balance or accurately assess acid production because of transient ion fluxes. This latter criticism is particularly telling because the results reported by Oh and colleagues were based on a single urine collection. Lemann et al. (34) reviewed the measurements used in his earlier studies, and concluded it was very unlikely that any major systematic errors could be present. This analysis is likely correct, as it is quite a speculative stretch to imagine a measurement error that only is manifest in patients who are in positive acid balance, but the issue remains unresolved.

Although Lemann et al. (34) argue that the technique of Oh and co-workers do not accurately assess acid balance, they agree that acid retention in patients with chronic kidney disease must be much lower than 10–20 mEq/day, possibly only 1–2 mEq/day, because major progression of bone disease is not a feature of even long-standing metabolic acidosis in renal disease. It is also possible that sustained metabolic acidosis can cause the release of calcium from bone even in the absence of acid retention. In studies of bone metabolism in vitro, reducing bath [HCO_3^-] causes release of calcium from bone, and if sustained, promotes osteoclast activity and bone dissolution (35,36).

In closing this debate, it is possible that metabolic acidosis is actually a necessary adaptation in some patients with renal insufficiency, required to stimulate and thereby maximize renal H^+ secretion, in a manner analogous to the role of hyperkalemia in stimulating K^+ excretion when renal function is impaired (12). Metabolic acidosis is well recognized to stimulate H^+ secretion in all segments of the nephron (37). According to this hypothesis, serum [HCO_3^-] (and systemic pH) falls to the level necessary to stimulate renal H^+ secretion sufficiently to recapture all filtered HCO_3^- and to maximize NH_4^+ and titratable acid excretion. Such an adaptation could serve to restore a semblance of acid balance, minimizing acid retention and limiting bone calcium loss.

CLINICAL CHARACTERISTICS OF RENAL INSUFFICIENCY-ASSOCIATED METABOLIC ACIDOSIS

Laboratory Findings

Electrolytes

Serum [total CO_2] is typically reduced to 18–22 mEq/L in patients with mild to moderate chronic kidney disease (1,2). Figure 1 depicts the values obtained in patients with stable serum creatinine levels between 2 and 8 mg/dL, who were not receiving diuretics or other drugs that may influence serum [total CO_2] (Jaffery, Hood, Gennari, unpublished observations). A noteworthy feature in these patients, and in similar reports in the literature (1,2), is the marked variability in serum [total CO_2] at any given level of renal impairment. The cause of the greater variability in [total CO_2] in these patients (as compared to individuals with normal renal function) is unclear but could be due to differences in the capacity to excrete acid as well as to variations in endogenous acid production (see earlier).

In patients with renal insufficiency in whom arterial pH and PCO_2 have been measured, the low serum [HCO_3^-] is associated with a reduction both in arterial pH and PCO_2, confirming the presence of metabolic acidosis (10,22,29,38). The ventilatory response to the reduction in serum [HCO_3^-] is unaffected in renal insufficiency (39), and thus arterial pH falls within the expected range for uncomplicated metabolic acidosis. Because the acidosis is mild in most instances, arterial pH values of 7.30–7.37 are typical.

The metabolic acidosis is often though not always associated with hyperkalemia (12). Although there is considerable variability, serum [Cl^-] also increases significantly (1,2). Serum [Na$^+$] is normal. Table 3 presents the mean electrolyte values found in patients with less severe (creatinine 2–3.9 mg/dL) and more severe (creatinine 4 mg/dL or higher) renal insufficiency.

Anion Gap

Metabolic acidosis in renal insufficiency is usually subdivided into two types depending on the anion gap. Individuals with a normal anion gap are classified as having type 4 or hyperkalemic renal tubular acidosis (see Chapter 13), and individuals with an increased anion gap are classified as having "uremic" acidosis. Although this classification suggests two distinct disorders, the pathogenesis is the same (1,2). Both are characterized by impaired NH$_4^+$ excretion with normal urine acidification. The anion gap, moreover, is linearly related to serum creatinine concentration in patients with chronic kidney disease over a wide range, with no break point (2). The gradual increase is due to a progressive impairment in the ability to excrete the sulfate, phosphate, and other anions of the strong acids produced. Patients with an anion gap within the range of normal are able to excrete these anions, replacing them with Cl$^-$ in the tubule reabsorbate and producing hyperchloremia. Hyperchloremia is sustained as renal function declines and the anion gap increases, and only disappears when renal failure is severe (2).

Aldosterone

As noted earlier, low plasma aldosterone levels (usually accompanied by low renin levels) are common in patients with chronic kidney disease (22,23). This hormonal abnormality probably plays little role in the pathogenesis of the metabolic acidosis.

Table 3 Average Serum Values in Patients with Stable Chronic Renal Insufficiency[a]

Degree	N	Creatinine (mg/dL)	[Na$^+$]	[K$^+$]	[Cl$^-$]	[total CO$_2$]	AG[b]
					mEq/L		
Moderate	81	3.17 (1.04)	141 (2.7)	4.7 (0.5)[c]	107 (4.1)[c]	22.1 (3.3)[c]	11.7 (2.7)
Advanced	22	4.86 (0.77)	142 (2.0)	4.7 (0.5)[c]	110 (4.3)[c]	18.8 (2.9)[d]	13.2 (2.5)

[a]103 stable outpatients not on diuretics or bicarbonate supplements, with either moderate (creatinine values 2–3.9 mg/dL) or advanced (creatinine values ≥ 4.0 mg/dL) kidney disease (Jaffery, Hood, Gennari, unpublished observations). Data shown are mean values (± 1 SD).
[b]AG = anion gap, [Na$^+$] − ([total CO$_2$] + [Cl$^-$]).
[c]p < 0.05 compared to individuals with normal renal function.
[d]p < 0.05 compared to moderate renal insufficiency.

Urine pH

Some patients with advanced renal insufficiency and metabolic acidosis also have a component of HCO_3^- wasting (7,9,10). With the exception of these patients, urine pH is typically <5.5 (6,7).

Symptoms

The mild metabolic acidosis characteristic of chronic kidney disease is usually asymptomatic. When severe (serum $[HCO_3^-]$ <16 mEq/L), metabolic acidosis can be associated with nonspecific symptoms such as anorexia and malaise and, on occasion, shortness of breath.

DELETERIOUS EFFECTS OF METABOLIC ACIDOSIS

The sustained, often low grade, metabolic acidosis in chronic kidney disease has deleterious long-term effects on bone and muscle metabolism, and has been proposed to exacerbate renal damage (Table 4).

Bone Metabolism

Regardless of whether acid balance is achieved in patients with kidney disease, they clearly have reduced bone calcium stores (40). Moreover, bone calcium loss in these patients correlates with the severity of metabolic acidosis (41). These human observations were all made in patients who died of kidney failure, not surprisingly with severe acidosis, so it is difficult to extrapolate the results to patients with renal insufficiency and milder acidosis. Nonetheless they are supported by in vitro experiments in animal bone showing increased release of calcium, as well as activation of osteoclasts, when medium $[HCO_3^-]$ is reduced (35,36).

Although acidosis appears to be a major contributing factor to the reduction in bone calcium stores, other factors clearly participate in the demineralization (40). Deficiency of 1–25 dihydroxy vitamin D and hyperparathyroidism, for example, are known causes of bone demineralization (42).

Table 4 Morbid Effects of Chronic Metabolic Acidosis

Loss of calcium from bones
Increased muscle catabolism
Acceleration of renal damage by[a]:
Calcium deposition
Complement activation
Stimulation of growth factors
Oxidant damage

[a]Hypothesized effects (see text).

These abnormalities interact with metabolic acidosis. Metabolic acidosis appears either to promote parathyroid hormone release or to impair the inhibitory effects of calcitriol on its release (40,43). Despite these complexities, correction of acidosis by $NaHCO_3$ administration uniformly improves bone calcium stores and bone calcium turnover in patients with kidney disease (29,43,44). Perhaps the clearest rationale for correction of metabolic acidosis in patients with renal insufficiency is to improve bone mineral balance (see Chapters 6 and 8).

Muscle Metabolism

Studies in animals and humans with kidney disease have shown that concomitant metabolic acidosis promotes muscle protein catabolism (27,38,45–48). This catabolic effect is dependent on stimulation of glucocorticoids and is due to acidosis as opposed to other effects of renal insufficiency (47–49). Strikingly, increased muscle catabolism is evident in the presence of only mild reductions in serum $[HCO_3^-]$ (45,50). Normalization of serum $[HCO_3^-]$ improves muscle metabolism (27,38).

Progression of Renal Insufficiency

In addition to adverse effects on bone and muscle metabolism, metabolic acidosis has been hypothesized to accelerate the rate of progression of chronic kidney disease (51). The mechanisms proposed for this effect include stimulation of chronic inflammation and tubulointerstitial fibrosis by calcium deposition in the kidney, stimulation of complement activation by increased ammoniagenesis, and stimulation of growth factors and oxidant injury from hypermetabolism (52). Despite experimental evidence suggesting a role for each of these mechanisms, there is no evidence in humans, and conflicting evidence in animal studies, that metabolic acidosis affects the rate of progression of renal damage (53–55). Perhaps the strongest argument against an important effect of acidosis is the lack of progression to renal failure in patients with types 1 and 2 renal tubular acidosis.

DIAGNOSIS AND MANAGEMENT

The presence of a serum [total CO_2] or $[HCO_3^-] < 22\,mEq/L$ in a patient with chronic kidney disease should alert the clinician to the possibility of renal disease-associated metabolic acidosis. The low value is characteristically associated with hyperchloremia, regardless of whether the anion gap is normal or increased. Hyperkalemia is a common, but not invariable, associated feature. As in any individual with a low serum $[HCO_3^-]$, one must be certain that respiratory alkalosis is not the cause (see Chapter 28). This assessment can be made by measuring arterial pH and $PaCO_2$. Urine pH should be < 5.5, excluding renal acidification defects.

Although renal disease-associated metabolic acidosis has characteristic features, none are pathognomonic. Thus, one must always consider other causes, particularly those that are easily reversible (see Chapter 9). Although hypoaldosteronism is not a key factor in the pathogenesis of renal insufficiency-associated acidosis, drugs that interfere with aldosterone synthesis or effect may exacerbate the acidosis. These drugs include spirono-lactone, triamterene, amiloride, heparin, nonsteroidal anti-inflammatory drugs, ACE inhibitors, and angiotensin receptor blockers. Severe volume depletion can mimic the metabolic acidosis of renal insufficiency, by limiting distal Na^+ delivery (56).

Treatment

When metabolic acidosis is severe (serum $[HCO_3^-] < 18\,mEq/L$) or symptomatic, alkali therapy should be undertaken to increase body alkali stores (Table 5). Because the cause is impaired acid excretion rather than impaired HCO_3^- reabsorption in most patients, serum $[HCO_3^-]$ can be usually be increased by relatively modest dosages of oral sodium bicarbonate. Estimating acid production to be $\sim 1\,mEq/kg$ body weight and assuming some renal acid excretion, a maintenance dose of as little as $30\,mEq/day$ (two $600\,mg$ tabs twice a day) should be sufficient to increase serum $[HCO_3^-]$ to $>20\,mEq/L$. An alternative therapy is sodium citrate. This liquid preparation provides $5\,mEq$ of the HCO_3^- precursor, citrate, per teaspoon. Neither preparation is ideal. Sodium bicarbonate therapy involves large number of pills each day, and citrate promotes aluminum absorption from the gut. Calcium carbonate can also provide some alkali, to the extent that bicarbonate is formed and absorbed in the stomach, but is unlikely to be sufficient on its own to fully correct acidosis.

Although the mild metabolic acidosis commonly seen in renal insufficiency (serum $[HCO_3^-]$ $19–24\,mEq/L$) is usually asymptomatic and is not associated with increased morbidity and mortality, data are accumulating to support the use of supplemental alkali to minimize bone disease and muscle catabolism (38,40,47). The risks of alkali therapy are minimal. In

Table 5 Treatment of Metabolic Acidosis in Renal Insufficiency

Administration of alkali supplements	
Sodium bicarbonate	$7\,mEq$ HCO_3^- per/tablet
Sodium citrate	$5\,mEq$ citrate per teaspoon
Calcium carbonate	$10\,mmol$ of CO_3^{2-} per $500\,mg$ tablet[a]
Diet modification	
Reduce intake of foods containing acid-generating proteins	

[a]Only a fraction of this CO_3^{2-} is converted to HCO_3^- and absorbed as such.

contrast to NaCl intake, $NaHCO_3$ ingestion does not lead to Na^+ retention or to ECF volume expansion (58). To the extent that the acidosis is overcorrected, it is conceivable that alkalemia may promote calcium phosphate precipitation in the body. No adverse effects have been reported in multiple studies in humans receiving supplemental alkali, however, some for as long as 18 months (30,38,40,43).

Another approach to treating hypobicarbonatemia, as yet untested, is diet modification. A change in diet away from grain and animal products (bread, meat, and milk) to vegetables could also improve body alkali stores (see Chapter 8). Unfortunately, such a diet increases K^+ intake and this may be a problem for patients with chronic kidney disease. An additional concern is the potential for malnutrition caused by coping with a special diet limited in protein and grain content coupled with the anorexia commonly present in these patients. If protein intake is $>1\,g/kg$ body weight, it should be reduced in any case.

SUMMARY

Metabolic acidosis is a common feature of renal insufficiency, presenting early with a normal anion gap and progressing to an increased anion gap late in its course. The primary cause is impaired NH_4^+ production and excretion by the damaged kidney. Acidosis is usually asymptomatic, but has deleterious effects on bone and muscle metabolism. Treatment is recommended when serum $[HCO_3^-]$ is $<18\,mEq/L$, but may be beneficial even when the acidosis is milder.

REFERENCES

1. Widmer B, Gerhardt RE, Harrington JT, Cohen JJ. Serum electrolyte and acid base composition. The influence of graded degrees of chronic renal failure. Arch Intern Med 1979; 139:1099–1102.
2. Hakim RM, Lazarus JM. Biochemical parameters in chronic renal failure. Am J Kidney Dis 1988; 11:238–247.
3. Tannen RL. Ammonia and acid-base homeostasis. Med Clin North Am 1983; 67:781–798.
4. Knepper MA, Packer R, Good DW. Ammonium transport in the kidney. Physiol Rev 1989; 69:179–249.
5. Tizianello A, De Ferrari G, Garibotto G, Gurreri G, Robaudo C. Renal metabolism of amino acids and ammonia in subjects with normal renal function and in patients with chronic renal insufficiency. J Clin Invest 1980; 65:1162–1173.
6. Wrong O, Davies HEF. The excretion of acid in renal disease. Quart J Med 1959; 28:259–313.
7. Schwartz WB, Hall PW, Hays RM, Relman AS. On the mechanism of acidosis in chronic renal disease. J Clin Invest 1959; 38:39–52.

8. Van Slyke DD, Linder GC, Hiller A, Leiter L, Macintosh JF. The excretion of ammonia and titratable acid in nephritis. J Clin Invest 1926; 2:255–288.

9. Goodman AD, Lemann J, Lennon EJ, Relman AS. Production, excretion, and net balance of fixed acid in patients with renal acidosis. J Clin Invest 1965; 44: 495–506.

10. Litzow JR, Lemann J Jr, Lennon EJ. The effect of treatment of acidosis on calcium balance in patients with chronic azotemic renal disease. J Clin Invest 1967; 46:280–286.

11. Welbourne T, Weber M, Bank N. The effects of glutamine administration on urinary ammonium excretion in normal subjects and patients with renal disease. J Clin Invest 1972; 51:1852–1860.

12. Gennari FJ, Segal AS. Hyperkalemia: an adaptive response in chronic renal insufficiency. Kidney Int 2002; 62:1–9.

13. Tannen RL. Effect of potassium on renal acidification and acid-base homeostasis. Semin Nephrol 1987; 7:263–273.

14. Buerkert J, Martin D, Trigg D, Simon E. Effect of reduced renal mass on ammonium handling and net acid formation by the superficial and juxtamedullary nephron of the rat. Evidence for impaired reentrapment rather than decreased production of ammonium in the acidosis of uremia. J Clin Invest 1983; 71:1661–1675.

15. Schoolwerth AC, Sandler RS, Hoffman PM, Klahr S. Effects of nephron reduction and dietary protein content on renal ammoniagenesis in the rat. Kidney Int 1975; 7:397–404.

16. Maddox DA, Horn JF, Famiano FC, Gennari FJ. Load depedence of proximal tubular fluid and bicarbonate reabsorption in the remnant kidney of the Munich—Wistar rat. J Clin Invest 1986; 77:1639–1649.

17. MacClean AJ, Hayslett JP. Adaptive change in ammonia excretion in renal insufficiency. Kidney Int 1980; 17:595–606.

18. Kunau RT Jr, Walker KA. Distal tubular acidification in the remnant kidney. Am J Physiol 1990; 258:F69–F74.

19. Wong NL, Quamme GA, Dirks JH. Tubular handling of bicarbonate in dogs with experimental renal failure. Kidney Int 1984; 25:912–918.

20. Levine DZ, Iacovitti M, Buckman S, Hincke MT, Luck B, Fryer JN. ANG II-dependent HCO_3^- reabsorption in surviving rat distal tubules: expression/activation of H(+)-ATPase. Am J Physiol 1997; 272:F799–F808.

21. DeFronzo RA. Hyperkalemia and hyporeninemic hypoaldosteronism. Kidney Int 1980; 17:118–134.

22. Sebastian A, Schambelan M, Lindenfeld S, morris RC Jr. Amelioration of metabolic acidosis with fludrocortisone therapy in hyporeninemic hypoaldosteronism. N Engl J med 1977; 297:576–583.

23. Schambelan M, Sebastian A, Biglieri EG. Prevalence, pathogenesis, and functional significance of aldosterone deficiency in hyperkalemic patients with chronic renal insufficiency. Kidney Int 1980; 17:89–101.

24. Kurtz I, Maher T, Hulter HN, Schambelan M, Sebastian A. Effect of diet on plasma acid–base composition in normal humans. Kidney Int 1983; 24: 670–680.

25. Frassetto LA, Morris RC Jr, Sebastian A. Effect of age on blood acid–base composition in adult humans: role of age-related renal functional decline. Am J Physiol 1996; 271:F1114–F1122.
26. Barsotti G, Cupisti A, Ciardella F, Morelli E, Niosi F, Giovannetti S. Compliance with protein restriction: effects on metabolic acidosis and progression of renal failure in chronic uremics on supplemented diet. Contrib Nephrol 1990; 81:42–49.
27. Williams B, Hattersley J, Layward E, Walls J. Metabolic acidosis skeletal muscle adaptation to low protein diets in chronic uremia. Kidney Int 1991; 40:779–786.
28. Bernhard J, Beaufrere B, Laville M, Fouque D. Adaptive response to a low-protein diet in predialysis chronic renal failure patients. J Am Soc Nephrol 2001; 12:1249–1254.
29. Cochran M, Wilkinson R. Effect of correction of metabolic acidosis on bone mineralisation rates in patients with renal osteomalacia. Nephron 1975; 15:98–110.
30. Sebastian A, Harris ST, Ottaway JH, Todd KM, Morris RC Jr. Improved mineral balance and skeletal metabolism in postmenopausal women treated with potassium bicarbonate. N Engl J med 1994; 330:1776–1781.
31. Oh MS. Irrelevance of bone buffering to acid–base homeostasis in chronic metabolic acidosis. Nephron 1991; 59:7–10.
32. Oh MS. New perspective on acid–base balance. Semin Dial 2000; 13:212–219.
33. Uribarri J, Douyon H, Oh MS. A re-evaluation of the urinary parameters of acid production and excretion in patients with chronic renal acidosis. Kidney Int 1995; 47:624–627.
34. Lemann J Jr, Bushinsky DA, Hamm LL. Bone buffering of acid and base in humans. Am J Physiol Renal Physiol 2003; 285:F811–F832.
35. Krieger NS, Sessler NE, Bushinsky DA. Acidosis inhibits osteoblastic and stimulates osteoclastic activity in vitro. Am J Physiol 1992; 262:F442–F448.
36. Bushinsky DA. Net calcium efflux from live bone during chronic metabolic, but not respiratory, acidosis. Am J Physiol 1989; 256:F836–F842.
37. Gennari FJ, Maddox DA. Renal regulation of acid–base homeostasis: integrated response. In: Seldin DW, Giebisch G, eds. The Kidney. Physiology and Pathophysiology. Vol. 2. Philadelphia: Lippincott Williams & Wilkins, 2000:2015–2053.
38. Reaich D, Channon Sm, Scrimgeour Cm, Daley SE, Wilkinson R, Goodship TH. Correction of acidosis in humans with CRF decreases protein degradation and amino acid oxidation. Am J Physiol 1993; 265:E230–E235.
39. Bushinsky DA, Coe FL, Katzenberg C, Szidon JP, Parks JH. Arterial PCO_2 in chronic metabolic acidosis. Kidney Int 1982; 22:311–314.
40. Bushinsky DA. The contribution of acidosis to renal osteodystrophy. Kidney Int 1995; 47:1816–1832.
41. Mora Palma FJ, Ellis HA, Cook DB, et al. Osteomalacia in patients with chronic renal failure before dialysis or transplantation. QJM 1983; 52:332–348.
42. Hruska KA, Teitelbaum SL. Renal osteodystrophy. N Engl J med 1995; 333:166–174.
43. Lefebvre A, de Vernejoul mC, Gueris J, Goldfarb B, Graulet AM, Morieux C. Optimal correction of acidosis changes progression of dialysis osteodystrophy. Kidney Int 1989; 36:1112–1118.

44. Bishop mC, Ledingham JG. Alkali treatment of renal osteodystrophy. Br med J 1972; 4:529.
45. Garibotto G, Russo R, Sofia A, et al. Skeletal muscle protein synthesis and degradation in patients with chronic renal failure. Kidney Int 1994; 45: 1432–1439.
46. Mitch WE, Clark AS. Specificity of the effects of leucine and its metabolites on protein degradation in skeletal muscle. Biochem J 1984; 222:579–586.
47. Hara Y, May RC, Kelly RA, Mitch WE. Acidosis, not azotemia, stimulates branched-chain, amino acid catabolism in uremic rats. Kidney Int 1987; 32:808–814.
48. May RC, Kelly RA, Mitch WE. Mechanisms for defects in muscle protein metabolism in rats with chronic uremia Influence of metabolic acidosis. J Clin Invest 1987; 79:1099–1103.
49. May RC, Kelly RA, Mitch WE. Metabolic acidosis stimulates protein degradation in rat muscle by a glucocorticoid-dependent mechanism. J Clin Invest 1986; 77:614–621.
50. Bergstrom J, Alvestrand A, Furst P. Plasma and muscle free amino acids in maintenance hemodialysis patients without protein malnutrition. Kidney Int 1990; 38:108–114.
51. Hostetter TH. Progression of renal disease and renal hypertrophy. Annu Rev Physiol 1995; 57:263–278.
52. Schrier RW, Harris DC, Chan L, Shapiro JI, Caramelo C. Tubular hypermetabolism as a factor in the progression of chronic renal failure. Am J Kidney Dis 1988; 12:243–249.
53. Throssell D, Brown J, Harris KP, Walls J. Metabolic acidosis does not contribute to chronic renal injury in the rat. Clin Sci (Colch) 1995; 89:643–650.
54. Nath KA, Hostetter MK, Hostetter TH. Pathophysiology of chronic tubulointerstitial disease in rats. Interactions of dietary acid load, ammonia, and complement component C_3. J Clin Invest 1985; 76:667–675.
55. Gennari FJ. Is metabolic acidosis a risk factor in the progression of renal insufficiency? In: Koch KM, Stein G, eds. Pathogenetic and Therapeutic Aspects of Chronic Renal Failure. New York: Marcel Dekker, 1997:33–44.
56. Batlle DC, von Riotte A, Schlueter W. Urinary sodium in the evaluation of hyperchloremic metabolic acidosis. N Engl J med 1987; 316:140–144.
57. Kraut JA. The role of metabolic acidosis in the pathogenesis of renal osteodystrophy. Adv Ren Replace Ther 1995; 2:40–51.
58. Husted FC, Nolph KD, Maher JF. $NaHCO_3$ and NaCl tolerance in chronic renal failure. J Clin Invest 1975; 56:414–419.

15

Hyperchloremic Metabolic Acidosis Due to Intestinal Losses and Other Nonrenal Causes

Donald E. Wesson and Melvin Laski

Departments of Internal Medicine and Physiology, Texas Tech University Health Sciences Center, Lubbock, Texas, U.S.A

INTRODUCTION

Hyperchloremic metabolic acidosis (HCMA) results either from the loss of HCO_3^- or the retention of HCl or its equivalent (see Chapter 9), and is defined by the presence of a normal anion gap. In most instances, it is caused by disorders of the kidney or gastrointestinal (GI) tract. This chapter focuses on intestinal disorders and other nonrenal causes (Table 1).

Excessive loss of HCO_3^- from the lower GI tract due to diarrhea is by far the most common cause of HCMA, but intestinal losses may also be associated with other acid–base disorders as well. The specific disorder depends on: (1) the associated change in extracellular fluid (ECF) volume; (2) whether the volume loss has compromised hemodynamic status; (3) deficits of other electrolytes such as Cl^- and K^+; and/or (4) distinctive pattern of electrolyte losses such as those associated with villous adenoma. Even when diarrhea is the presenting symptom and the patient's serum $[HCO_3^-]$ is low and serum $[Cl^-]$ is high, the clinician must first determine whether HCMA is present because respiratory alkalosis can cause the same electrolyte profile. The specific cause can usually be determined with a careful history and critical evaluation of appropriate blood and urine studies.

Table 1 Hyperchloremic Metabolic Acidosis: Intestinal and Other
Nonrenal Causes

Intestinal
  Diarrhea
  Biliary drainage
  Pancreato-cutaneous fistula
  Entero-cutaneous fistula
  Villous adenoma
Other nonrenal causes
  Acid loading with NH_4Cl
  Parenteral nutrition

DIAGNOSIS

Measurement of arterial pH and $PaCO_2$ is necessary to confirm the presence
of metabolic acidosis and allow assessment of whether the ventilatory
response to this disorder is appropriate (see Chapter 28). The serum anion
gap, defined as serum $[Na^+]$ minus the sum of $[Cl^-]$ and $[HCO_3^-]$, is then calculated to demonstrate that it is normal, establishing the presence of
HCMA. In making this determination, one must take into account the
pH and albumin concentration of the serum, both of which affect the anion
gap through changes in the contribution of proteins to the unmeasured
anions (see Chapters 9 and 28). Although the usual normal value is taken
to be 12 mEq/L, for example, it can drop below 10 mEq/L when hypoalbuminemia and an acid pH are present. A normal gap is one that is within
4–5 mEq/L of the expected value.

   If the cause of the HCMA is not evident from history and physical
examination, the urine anion gap (UAG) can help discern between a renal
as opposed to an intestinal cause (see Chapters 13 and 28) (1,2). The
UAG is calculated as follows:

$$UAG = ([Na^+] + [K^+]) - [Cl^-] \qquad (15.1)$$

In the setting of metabolic acidosis (serum $[HCO_3^-]$ <20 mEq/L), the UAG
should be negative due to increased excretion of the unmeasured cation,
NH_4^+, if renal acid excretion is normal. Thus, a negative UAG in a patient
with HCMA suggests a nonrenal cause. Unusual circumstances may complicate interpretation of the UAG. Large urine concentrations of unmeasured
anions (ketones, certain antibiotics, and other organic anions) can yield a
positive UAG even when urine $[NH_4^+]$ is high. If the urine is very alkaline
(pH > 7), urine $[HCO_3]$ must be included in the calculation; otherwise,
UAG may be positive despite adequate NH_4^+ excretion. Large concentrations of other cations (e.g., Ca^{2+}) can also yield a more negative UAG,
and impair the relationship between UAG and urine $[NH_4^+]$.

PATHOPHYSIOLOGY OF METABOLIC ACIDOSIS IN DIARRHEA

The role of GI tract in acid–base balance is discussed in detail in Chapter 7. Here, the salient features are reviewed to assist in understanding the pathophysiology of the metabolic acidosis associated with abnormal intestinal losses (see Fig. 1). Gastrointestinal secretion of H^+ and HCO_3^- is largely

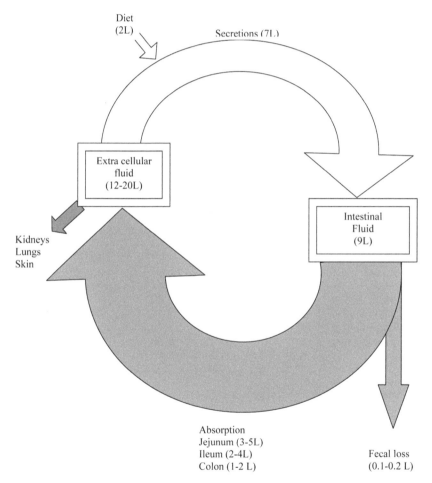

ENTEROSYSTEMIC CYCLE

Diet (2L)

Secretions (7L)

Extra cellular fluid (12-20L)

Intestinal Fluid (9L)

Kidneys
Lungs
Skin

Absorption
Jejunum (3-5L)
Ileum (2-4L)
Colon (1-2 L)

Fecal loss
(0.1-0.2 L)

Figure 1 Diagram of the normal enterosystemic fluid cycle. Approximately 9 L are added to the gut each day (two from dietary intake and seven from normal secretion into the GI tract in the process of digestion), almost all of which is absorbed and added back to the ECF. Final ECF volume is adjusted primarily by changes in renal salt and water excretion. *Source*: Adapted from Ref. 3.

unresponsive to acid–base status. Thus, the GI tract does not play a major regulatory role in acid–base balance but rather is an "agent provocateur" in causing acid–base disorders when its function is disturbed. Because large quantities of H^+ and HCO_3^- continuously cycle throughout the GI tract through secretion and absorption, excess losses of GI fluid can cause acidosis and/or alkalosis depending on the site or sites from which the fluid is lost. In addition, the GI tract transports Na^+, Cl^-, and K^+ and their losses or disturbed transport can modify the type and/or maintenance of acid–base disorders associated with GI fluid losses. In this chapter, we focus on the GI transport events that begin in the proximal small bowel and progress to the colon, as disordered function in this portion of the gut most commonly produces metabolic acidosis.

Water Losses (Tables 2 and 3)

The 8–10 L of isotonic fluid normally entering the proximal small bowel in humans is comparable in size to the entire ECF volume (Fig. 1) (3). More than 90% of this fluid is normally absorbed, thereby completing an efficient enterosystemic cycle. The small intestine absorbs >8 L and the colon 1–2 L of fluid per day (3). Maximal fluid absorptive capacity of the colon is 5–6 L/day provided that the inflow is steady rather than intermittent (4).

Table 2 Electrolyte Concentrations of Lower Gastrointestinal Fluids[a]

Site	Volume (L/day)	[Na⁺] (mEq/L)	[K⁺] (mEq/L)	[Cl⁻] (mEq/L)	[HCO₃⁻] (mEq/L)
Bile	1	135–155	5–10	85–110	40
Pancreatic fluid	2	120–160	5–10	30–75	70–120
Small intestine	1	75–120	5–10	70–125	30
Colon (colostomy)	1	50–115	10–30	35–70	15–25
Stool water	0.15	20–30	55–75	15–25	30[b]

[a]See also Table 3 in Chapter 7.
[b]Includes organic anions representing HCO_3^- losses in stool.

Table 3 Changes in Stool Water Volumes and Electrolytes in Diarrhea[a]

Condition	Volume (L/day)	[Na⁺] (mEq/L)	[K⁺] (mEq/L)	[Cl⁻] (mEq/L)	[HCO₃⁻] (mEq/L)
Normal	0.15	20–30	55–75	15–25	30
Inflammatory	1–3	50–100	15–20	50–100	10
Secretory	1–20	40–140	15–40	25–105	20–75

[a]See also Table 6 in Chapter 7.

Loss of this normally absorbed fluid can result in major electrolyte losses, particularly of Na^+. In some diarrheal states, such as cholera, excess electrolytes are secreted into bowel fluids (3), potentially making losses even more substantial.

Normal stool mass averages about 120 g/day in normal subjects and is 60–85% H_2O (3). This mass increases to about 500 g/day in inflammatory bowel disease (5) and can be increased to > 1 kg/day with osmotic cathartic laxatives (Tables 2 and 3). Adults with cholera and other secretory causes of diarrhea can lose many liters of stool per day, up to 1 L/hr in the case of adults with cholera (3,6).

The osmolality of stool water in normal subjects is the same or slightly higher than that of plasma, and is accounted for primarily by electrolytes (3,5), so there is no net H_2O loss in normal stool. The osmolality of stool water in diarrheal states also tends to be the same or higher than that of plasma (5,6) so that water losses do not exceed solute losses. As a result, serum $[Na^+]$ is either normal or slightly reduced in cholera, both in adults and children (5,7).

Electrolyte Losses (Tables 2 and 3)

Both Cl^-/HCO_3^- and Na^+/H^+ exchange occur in the ileum but the former predominates making for net HCO_3^- secretion (8). The amount added is dramatically increased with the rapid ileal transit times characteristic of most diarrheal states (see Chapter 7). Cyclic AMP in the ileum is upregulated by cholera toxins, increasing HCO_3^- secretion and enhancing stool losses. The ileum is a major affected site for the secretory diarrhea of cholera (6).

Under basal conditions, the small intestine delivers 600–1500 mL/day of a relatively HCO_3^--rich fluid to the colon (Table 2). Delivery of this HCO_3^- from the ileum along with that contributed by colonic HCO_3^- secretion helps to neutralize organic acids produced by colonic bacterial metabolism. The organic anions produced by this buffer reaction are lost in the stool and therefore represent alkali lost to the body (see Chapter 6). The concentration of these organic anions is either unchanged or decreased in diarrhea (5). The primary acid–base transporting activity of the colon is HCO_3^- secretion mediated by Cl^-/HCO_3^- exchange (see Chapter 7). Colonic HCO_3^- secretion is increased in secretory diarrheal diseases like cholera (9).

Excretion of HCO_3^- plus the secreted HCO_3^- consumed in titrating bacterial organic acids in the colon normally yields approximately 30 mEq of alkali loss each day. Even though the $[HCO_3^-]$ of diarrheal stool can vary between 30 and 80 mEq/L (9), the loss of 1 L of this fluid still contains only about two times the HCO_3^- normally lost in stool and this amount can be easily regenerated by the kidneys. Larger volume stool losses and/or persistent losses over many days, however, can lead to HCO_3^- losses that exceed the kidney's ability to regenerate new HCO_3^-, particularly when

PATHOGENESIS OF METABOLIC ACIDOSIS IN DIARRHEA

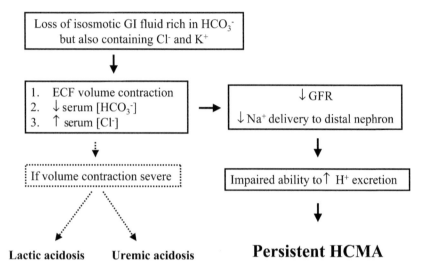

Figure 2 Pathophysiology of metabolic acidosis in diarrhea. HCMA = hyperchloremic metabolic acidosis. As the diagram indicates, HCMA is the more common occurrence, but if ECF volume depletion is severe enough, phosphate and sulfate retention can lead to uremic acidosis, or impaired tissue perfusion can lead to lactic acid overproduction and lactic acidosis.

associated ECF volume depletion limits the ability of the kidney to excrete acid (see Fig. 2 and Chapters 6 and 13). In this setting, HCMA develops. When the diarrhea ceases, correction of the acidosis requires regeneration of the lost HCO_3^- by increased renal acid excretion. This correction requires normal renal acidification, which in turn is dependent on restoration of an adequate ECF volume.

Potassium is normally the major cation in stool H_2O, with smaller contributions made by Na^+, Mg^{2+}, Ca^{2+}, and NH_4^+ (5,10). In diarrhea due to inflammatory bowel disease and to secretory causes like cholera, the K^+ concentration of stool water decreases and Na^+ concentration increases (5,6) (Table 3). Thus, diarrhea causes a relatively greater loss of Na^+ and a smaller loss of K^+ per liter of stool than does normal stool. Stool K^+ losses are also modest in experimental diarrhea in humans (11). As a result, serum $[K^+]$ may be normal or only modestly decreased in adults (6,12) and children (13) presenting with even severe diarrhea. Nevertheless, K^+ depletion can occur, both due to stool K^+ losses and inadequate K^+ intake (12). Because aldosterone promotes colonic K^+ secretion and serum aldosterone levels are increased in states of severe diarrhea associated with volume depletion (14), increased K^+ secretion combined with high intestinal fluid flow rates in diarrheal states could accelerate losses and promote K^+ depletion. High serum aldosterone levels may also increase renal K^+ excretion and thereby contribute to the K^+ depletion. Potassium depletion increases both renal ammoniagenesis and H^+ secretion (15), potentially facilitating correction of HCMA. As discussed in Chapter 18, K^+ depletion can also result in metabolic alkalosis if not corrected.

Effects on ECF Volume and Acid–Base Parameters

Because the $[Na^+]$ of stool water increases in diarrheal states (5,7), large volume diarrhea can cause profound Na^+ losses and therefore severe ECF volume depletion. In response to this Na^+ depletion, proximal tubule and loop Na^+ reabsorption increase in the kidney, reducing Na^+ delivery to the distal nephron. A reduction in Na^+ delivery may compromise H^+ secretion and, therefore, acid excretion (16,17). Reduced acid excretion related to Na^+ depletion impedes the correction of HCMA caused by diarrhea-induced HCO_3^- losses (Fig. 2). Extracellular fluid volume depletion is typically manifested by increased serum creatinine concentrations and sometimes with an increase in serum phosphate concentration and an associated increase in the anion gap. If ECF volume depletion is severe enough to compromise tissue perfusion, lactic acidosis can occur, producing a combined hyperchloremic and anion gap metabolic acidosis (Fig. 2). In this setting, HCO_3^- is both lost in the stool and titrated by lactic acid in the body fluids. Lactic acidosis is a serious complication and requires restoration of tissue perfusion (i.e., ECF volume repletion) to stop the excess lactic acid production. Infants with anion gap metabolic acidosis, compared to those with pure HCMA, have more prolonged diarrhea prior to presentation and evidence of more severe volume depletion (18).

In patients with diarrhea, ECF volume repletion facilitates correction of the metabolic acidosis (12,16–20). Although seen in infants, significant lactic acidosis almost never occurs in the setting of severe diarrhea in older children and adults (6,13). Instead, the anion gap acidosis that is frequently associated with severe diarrhea appears to be increased due to the concentration of plasma proteins associated with volume depletion.

MANAGEMENT OF HCMA DUE TO DIARRHEA

Patients with HCMA due to diarrhea need urgent evaluation of ECF fluid volume status and losses of electrolytes, determination of the cause of the diarrhea, and institution of fluid replacement. Intervention with nonspecific symptomatic therapy as well as appropriate antibiotic agents should be implemented concurrently (21).

Even though HCMA in severe diarrhea is due to HCO_3^- loss, patients with mild acidosis usually require only volume repletion to facilitate renal

H^+ excretion and thereby regenerate the lost HCO_3^- (12,16–20). With more severe acidosis, and particularly if the pH is < 7.1, intravenous $NaHCO_3$ replacement should be instituted.

Although severe K^+ depletion is not typically a feature, it is wise to determine K^+ status in a patient with diarrhea by assessing urine K^+ excretion, because plasma $[K^+]$ often fails to accurately reflect overall balance. Deficits should be corrected with oral K^+ if tolerated or intravenous administration if the oral route is not available or if cardiac arrhythmias are present, digitalis is being administered, or neuromuscular symptoms or signs are present.

If the ECF volume deficit is mild, oral electrolyte, and H_2O replacement is reasonable. If the oral route is unavailable and/or the volume deficit is severe, intravenous replacement with isotonic saline solutions will be required. Correction of any volume deficits is critical for optimizing renal acidification and correction of compromised tissue perfusion.

PANCREATIC AND BILIARY LOSSES

Bile from the liver and gallbladder contains HCO_3^- and its addition to the intestinal tract contributes to neutralization of gastric H^+ entering the upper small intestine (Table 2) (see Chapter 7). When the gallbladder is not stimulated, most of the secreted bile is reabsorbed and thus contributes to a small intrahepatic cycle of HCO_3^- secretion and reabsorption. By contrast, when the gallbladder is stimulated the majority of its contents, which may have a $[HCO_3^-]$ as high as 50–100 mEq/L, is rapidly emptied into the intestine. Approximately 1 L of bile is normally produced daily with a $[HCO_3^-]$ of 40 mEq/L (Table 2). Percutaneous drainage of biliary output thus can produce a modest daily HCO_3^- loss.

The exocrine pancreas secretes a HCO_3^--rich fluid that is primarily responsible for neutralizing the highly acidic fluid leaving the stomach (see Chapter 7). Bicarbonate concentration in pancreatic secretions varies from values comparable to plasma (20–25 mEq/L) to as high as 150 mEq/L under strong stimulation (Table 2). Normal secretions have a volume of up to 2 L/day, with $[HCO_3^-]$ varying from 70 to 120 mEq/L (Table 2). Food ingestion stimulates pancreatic HCO_3^- secretion, as does vasoactive intestinal peptide (VIP), secretin, cholecystokinin, and vagal stimulation. Under normal circumstances, excess HCO_3^- is added to the duodenum following eating, and the HCO_3^- not neutralized by H^+ is absorbed by intestinal mucosa. In severe diarrheal states HCO_3 secreted by the pancreas has reduced contact time with intestinal mucosa and contributes to stool alkali losses (6). Between 140 and 280 mEq of HCO_3^- may be lost each day in the presence of a draining pancreato-cutaneous fistula. The impact of such pancreatic HCO_3^- losses will be to generate HCMA, especially if GFR is decreased or renal H^+ secretion is impaired. Hyperchloremic metabolic acidosis caused by biliary drainage or pancreatic fistulae can be treated by the oral administration of alkali as Shohl's solution (sodium citrate) or by the intravenous administration of bicarbonate. The daily dose should match the prospective loss.

VILLOUS ADENOMA

Villous adenomas of the colon present with a variety of fluid and electrolyte abnormalities although the acid–base disorders have not been a particular focus of interest in most reports. Hyperchloremic metabolic acidosis is common (20) but marked chloride-depletion alkalosis also occurs (see Chapter 17). These tumors are usually found in the descending colon and rectum and reportedly have a marked tendency to undergo malignant transformation. Although the diarrhea produced due to secretion by the tumor has a Na^+ and Cl^- concentration similar to that of plasma, the mechanism by which one tumor presents with HCMA and another with chloride-depletion alkalosis is unknown. Severe volume depletion with circulatory collapse and lactic acidosis may also occur. Resection of the tumor provides definitive treatment.

STRONG ACID INGESTION OR ADMINISTRATION

Acidosis may also be produced by the administration or ingestion of acid or its equivalent. Early studies in dogs showed that the chronic ingestion of small amounts of mineral acids readily induced metabolic acidosis (22). There is no substantial clinical correlate, however, of this experimental model. The ingestion of a strong acid to attempt suicide is fortunately rare, and its most dire immediate consequence is the corrosive effect of acid on the upper GI tract. The effects of the burn, tissue necrosis, hemorrhage, and shock that follow such ingestions obscure the consumption of HCO_3^- and tissue buffers it causes. Most individuals who have ingested strong acids are likely to develop lactic acidosis related to shock, rather than HCMA.

Treatment of mineral acid ingestions should be directed at restoring ECF volume, as other critical interventions are ongoing to treat esophageal burns, necrosis, and hemorrhage. Bicarbonate should be administered only if arterial blood pH is below 7.1. A somewhat less corrosive, but also potentially deadly form of hydrochloric acid ingestion is the inhalation of chlorine gas. If the dose inhaled is not great enough to cause immediate death from respiratory damage, acidosis may occur due to the formation of hydrochloric acid from elemental chlorine and water in the body.

Ammonium chloride, although not an acid per se, causes HCMA because it dissociates to form NH_3 and HCl in the body fluids. The newly formed NH_3 is rapidly incorporated into glutamine or urea, leaving behind the strong acid, HCl (23). Because of this property, NH_4Cl is used for diagnostic tests of renal acidification (see Chapter 13). When limited NH_4Cl loads (10–15 g/day) are given, mild to moderate HCMA develops, and the change in renal acid excretion induced by this metabolic acidosis provides a quantitative measure of renal acidification capacity. At least one case of attempted suicide by NH_4Cl ingestion has been reported in the literature (24).

PARENTERAL NUTRITION

Total parenteral nutrition preparations have occasionally been associated with the development of HCMA, most commonly in neonates and young children (25–27). When analyzed, these cases were presumed to occur either with protein hydrolysate formulas, which are no longer used, or with synthetic amino acid mixtures that contained an excess of cationic amino acids relative to anionic amino acids. When one considers the relatively small amount of potential acid present even in older parenteral nutrition formulae, however, the load appears to be inadequate to produce a significant acidosis and therefore other factors must have contributed. Consistent with the relatively small acid load, the reported cases and studies largely involved hyperalimentation in pediatric and neonatal patients. Given the high capacity of the normal adult kidney to excrete acid, it is unlikely that parenteral nutrition in adults with normal renal function could cause acidosis from excess amino acid intake. If renal acidification is abnormal, however, the ammonium load provided by current amino acid solutions may induce acidosis. Hyperchloremic metabolic acidosis has been reported in patients receiving a potassium sparing diuretic while also receiving parenteral nutrition (28), but such agents are known to impair distal nephron H^+ secretion. Either the effect of the diuretic on acidification per se or the effect of hyperkalemia upon ammoniagenesis might be responsible. The clinician should be alert in the use of these agents.

   Metabolic acidosis may occur in adults receiving parenteral nutrition, but in most cases the clinical setting is so complex as to render a precise definition of the cause of acidosis impossible. Patients receive such therapy after trauma, burn, and in the presence of pancreatitis or sepsis. Alternatively, they may have inflammatory bowel disease or be postbowel resection with a chronic malabsorptive state. Because many of the patients have inadequate renal blood flow due to vascular disease, shock, or hypovolemia, the interpretation of metabolic acidosis must be made in the light of functional renal insufficiency. Those with bowel disease may also be losing excessive amounts of HCO_3^- in the stool. Any acidosis that develops in the patient receiving parenteral nutrition requires a full diagnostic evaluation to determine its cause.

Parenteral nutrition has been associated with other acid–base disorders, including lactic acidosis due to thiamine deficiency (29) and respiratory acidosis (30). The thiamine deficiency was caused by errors in compounding a vitamin supplement preparation, and with appropriate safeguards that should not be a problem. The respiratory acidosis resulted from high carbohydrate delivery in the setting of compromised pulmonary function. Metabolism of carbohydrates results in generation of considerably greater amounts of CO_2 than does metabolism of an isocaloric quantity of lipids. If the patient has chronic respiratory failure and is already unable to clear CO_2 effectively, a high carbohydrate load and subsequent excess CO_2 generation will worsen respiratory acidosis. Such high CO_2 loads must be considered when ventilator settings are adjusted. The patient with adult respiratory distress syndrome, high PEEP settings, and stiff lungs may develop respiratory acidosis if carbohydrate loads are excessive. Increasing the amount of lipid relative to the amount of carbohydrate in the preparation may be necessary.

REFERENCES

1. Goldstein MB, Bear R, Richardson RM, Marsden PA, Halperin ML. The urine anion gap: a clinically useful index of ammonium excretion. Am J Med Sci 1986; 292:198–202.
2. Batlle DC, Hizon M, Cohen E, Gutterman C, Gupta R. The use of the urinary anion gap in the diagnosis of hyperchloremic metabolic acidosis. N Engl J Med 1988; 318:594–599.
3. Phillips SF. Diarrhea: a current view of the pathophysiology. Gastroenterology 1972; 63:495–518.
4. Debongnie JC, Phillips SF. Capacity of the human colon to absorb fluid. Gastroenterology 1978; 74:698–703.
5. Vernia P, Gnaedinger A, Hauck W, Breuer RI. Organic anions and the diarrhea of inflammatory bowel disease. Dig Dis Sci 1988; 33:1353–1358.
6. Wang F, Butler T, Rabbani GH, Jones PK. The acidosis of cholera. Contributions of hyperproteinemia, lactic acidemia, and hyperphosphatemia to an increased serum anion gap. N Engl J Med 1986; 315:1591–1595.
7. Mahalanabis D, Wallace CK, Kallen RJ, Mondal A, Pierce NF. Water and electrolyte losses due to cholera in infants and small children: a recovery balance study. Pediatrics 1970; 45:374–385.
8. Turnberg LA, Bieberdorf FA, Morawski SG, Fordtran JS. Interrelationships of chloride, bicarbonate, sodium, and hydrogen transport in the human ileum. J Clin Invest 1970; 49:557–567.
9. Teree TM, Mirabal-Font E, Ortiz A, Wallace WM. Stool losses and acidosis in diarrheal disease of infancy. Pediatrics 1965; 36:704–713.
10. Binder HJ, Sandle GI. Electrolyte absorption and secretion in the mammalian colon. In: Johnson LR, ed. Physiology of the Gastrointestinal Tract. New York: Raven Press, 1987:1389–1418.

11. Agarwal R, Afzalpurkar R, Fordtran JS. Pathophysiology of potassium absorption and secretion by the human intestine. Gastroenterology 1994; 107:548–571.

12. Cieza J, Sovero Y, Estremadoyro L, Dumler F. Electrolyte disturbances in elderly patients with severe diarrhea due to cholera. J Am Soc Nephrol 1995; 6:1463–1467.

13. Hill LL, Morris CR, Williams RL. Role of tissue hypoxia and defective renal acid excretion in the development of acidosis in infantile diarrhea. Pediatrics 1971; 47(suppl 2):246+.

14. Schwarz KB, Ternberg JL, Bell MJ, Keating JP. Sodium needs of infants and children with ileostomy. J Pediatr 1983; 102:509–513.

15. Knepper MA, Packer R, Good DW. Ammonium transport in the kidney. Physiol Rev 1989; 69:179–249.

16. Izraeli S, Rachmel A, Frishberg Y, et al. Transient renal acidification defect during acute infantile diarrhea: the role of urinary sodium. J Pediatr 1990; 117:711–716.

17. Batlle DC, von Riotte A, Schlueter W. Urinary sodium in the evaluation of hyperchloremic metabolic acidosis. N Engl J Med 1987; 316:140–144.

18. Weizman Z, Houri S, Ben-Ezer Gradus D. Type of acidosis and clinical outcome in infantile gastroenteritis. J Pediatr Gastroenterol Nutr 1992; 14:187–191.

19. Elliott EJ, Walker-Smith JA, Farthing MJ. The role of bicarbonate and base precursors in treatment of acute gastroenteritis. Arch Dis Child 1987; 62:91–95.

20. Babior BM. Villous adenoma of the colon. Study of a patient with severe fluid and electrolyte disturbances. Am J Med 1966; 41:615–621.

21. Thielman NM, Guerrant RL. Clinical practice. Acute infectious diarrhea. N Engl J Med 2004; 350:38–47.

22. De Sousa RC, Harrington JT, Ricanati ES, Shelkrot JW, Schwartz WB. Renal regulation of acid–base equilibrium during chronic administration of mineral acid. J Clin Invest 1974; 53:465–476.

23. Sartorius OW, Roemmelt JC, Pitts RF. The renal regulation of acid–base balance in man IV. The nature of the renal compensation in ammonium chloride acidosis. J Clin Invest 1949; 28:423–439.

24. Relman AS, Shelburne PF, Talman A. Profound acidosis resulting from excessive ammonium chloride in previously healthy subjects. A study of two cases. N Engl J Med 1961; 264:848–852.

25. Chan JC. The influence of synthetic amino acid and casein hydrolysate on the endogenous production and urinary excretion of acid in total intravenous alimentation. Pediatr Res 1972; 6:789–796.

26. Chan JC. Letter: origin of acidosis in total parenteral nutrition: controversy. J Pediatr 1976; 88:157–160.

27. Heird WC, Dell RB, Driscoll JM Jr, Grebin B, Winters RW. Metabolic acidosis resulting from intravenous alimentation mixtures containing synthetic amino acids. N Engl J Med 1972; 287:943–948.

28. Kushner RF, Sitrin MD. Metabolic acidosis. Development in two patients receiving a potassium-sparing diuretic and total parenteral nutrition. Arch Intern Med 1986; 146:343–345.

29. From the Centers for Disease Control and Prevention. Lactic acidosis traced to thiamine deficiency related to nationwide shortage of multivitamins for total parenteral nutrition—United States, 1997. JAMA 1997; 278:109,111.

30. Covelli HD, Black JW, Olsen MS, Beekman JF. Respiratory failure precipitated by high carbohydrate loads. Ann Intern Med 1981; 95:579–581.

16

Metabolic Alkalosis: General Considerations

Robert G. Luke

Department of Medicine, University of Cincinnati College of Medicine, Cincinnati, Ohio, U.S.A.

INTRODUCTION

This chapter provides definitions, a general classification, and an overview of the epidemiologic, pathophysiologic, clinical, diagnostic and prognostic aspects that are common to all forms of metabolic alkalosis. The major general categories of metabolic alkalosis—based on their pathophysiology—are treated in detail in the subsequent three chapters: Cl^- depletion (Chapter 17), K^+ depletion (Chapter 18), and miscellaneous disorders (Chapter 19).

DEFINITIONS

Metabolic alkalosis is an acid–base disorder in which a primary disease process leads to the net accumulation of base within or the net loss of acid from the extracellular fluid (ECF). Although in strict terms of acid–base chemistry this occurs because of a decrease in the strong ion difference (see Chapter 1) (1), metabolic alkalosis, when it occurs as a simple acid–base disorder, is more commonly recognized as an increase in plasma $[HCO_3^-]$ and a consequent decrease in arterial $[H^+]$, as defined by their relationship in the Henderson equation. The decrease in $[H^+]$ is reported as an elevation in arterial blood pH, defined as alkalemia.

RESPIRATORY ADAPTATION

Unopposed by other primary acid–base disorders, the increase in arterial blood pH promptly and predictably depresses ventilation resulting in increased $PaCO_2$ and buffering of the magnitude of the alkalemia. The confidence bands for this secondary respiratory response are the widest and most deformed of the acid–base disorders; probably due to the patient populations or the model used to study the response (2). The most authoritative studies predict an increase in $PaCO_2$ of 0.6–0.7 mmHg for every 1.0 mEq/L increase in plasma $[HCO_3^-]$ (2). This response considerably buffers the change in arterial pH. For example, in chronic metabolic alkalosis with a plasma $[HCO_3^-]$ of 45 mEq/L, the arterial pH would be 7.70 if the $PaCO_2$ remained at 40 mmHg whereas it is only 7.54 with the secondary rise in $PaCO_2$ to 54 mmHg. Although a $PaCO_2 > 55$ mmHg is uncommon, secondary increases to 60 mmHg or higher have been documented in severe metabolic alkalosis (2–4).

Evidence now favors the concept that the magnitude of the compensatory increase in $PaCO_2$ is directly related to the extent of the alkalosis and the degree of elevation of the plasma $[HCO_3^-]$, irrespective of its etiology and of whether or not there is an intracellular acidosis (5). The signal for this respiratory response is an effect of alkalinization of the cerebral interstitial fluid on the medullary chemoreceptors (6). The respiratory response to the primary metabolic alkalosis is independent of hypoxia, hypokalemia, renal failure, and cause (2,5,7) and is usually not detectable clinically (8,9) as it is more dependent on a change in depth of ventilation rather than rate (8). Even in chronic lung disease with CO_2 retention, metabolic alkalosis is associated with a further elevation of $PaCO_2$ (4,10). Indeed, chronic respiratory acidosis (see Chapter 20) and metabolic alkalosis commonly occur together as a mixed acid–base disturbance, as patients with chronic lung disease and CO_2 retention often require diuretics for cor pulmonale and/or hypertension.

In severe metabolic alkalosis, $PaCO_2$ may increase to >60 mmHg in the rare circumstances when plasma $[HCO_3^-]$ exceeds plasma $[Cl^-]$—so-called "crossed anions"—in conditions of prolonged vomiting or nasogastric aspiration. It is obviously essential for the clinician to not misdiagnose such an elevation of $PaCO_2$ as a primary disturbance and to manage the patient as if they had respiratory failure. For example, in a situation in which artificial ventilation becomes necessary, setting the ventilator to reduce $PaCO_2$ in such a patient could result in life-threatening alkalemia with the creation of respiratory alkalosis to compound metabolic alkalosis (11). On the other hand, the clinician must also recognize that, in the presence of established metabolic alkalosis, absence of an increase in $PaCO_2$ represents a mixed acid–base disturbance: metabolic and respiratory alkalosis (see Chapter 22).

CLASSIFICATION

The major clinically and pathophysiologically relevant classification is based on whether or not the metabolic alkalosis is dependent on Cl^- depletion. The Cl^--depletion forms, also termed the Cl^--responsive alkaloses, are more common. The other major grouping, not related to Cl^- depletion, are the Cl^--resistant alkaloses, most of which are due to K^+ depletion with mineralocorticoid excess. Cl^--depletion metabolic alkalosis (CDA), by definition, can be corrected without K^+ repletion although a modest degree of K^+ depletion or, at least hypokalemia, is common in CDA both because the kidney in these circumstances tends to be "K^+-wasting" and because K^+ shifts into cells in exchange for H^+ [12]. Although experimental studies have shown that K^+ repletion is not essential to correct CDA (13), mixed K^+ and Cl^--depletion metabolic alkalosis also occurs in humans (14,15) and has been studied experimentally in animals (16). Several other relatively uncommon causes constitute the balance of etiologies of metabolic alkalosis (Table 1).

Disequilibrium occurs in acute or acute-on-chronic metabolic alkalosis when generation of HCO_3^- and resultant elevation of plasma $[HCO_3^-]$ exceeds the capacity of the renal tubule to reabsorb HCO_3^- (17). Transient bicarbonaturia with concomitant Na^+ or K^+ loss ensues until a new steady state is achieved and urinary HCO_3^- excretion ceases. In this regard, there is nothing paradoxical about the so-called "paradoxical aciduria" sometimes

Table 1 Causes of Metabolic Alkalosis

Cl^- depletion syndromes
GI losses: vomiting or nasogastric aspiration,[a] chloridorrhea, gastrocystoplasty, villous adenoma
Renal losses: chloruretic diuretics, posthypercapnia, severe K^+ depletion
Skin losses: cystic fibrosis
Potassium depletion syndromes
GI losses: laxative abuse
Renal losses: hyperaldosteronism, primary and secondary, other hypokalemic hypertensive syndromes, Bartter and Gitelman syndromes
Low GFR + base loading
Milk-alkali syndrome, ESRD and excess base, "nonreabsorbable" antacids with cation exchange resin
Transient
Multiple blood transfusions with citrate, "overshoot" alkalosis, extensive bony metastases, infant formulas with low Cl^- content
Miscellaneous
Recovery from starvation

---

[a]Even in the presence of achlorhydria.

described in stable chronic metabolic alkalosis; metabolic alkalosis is being maintained because urinary excretion of HCO_3^- is prevented by the effects of Cl^- or K^+ depletion to either diminish renal HCO_3^- secretion or increase renal HCO_3^- reabsorption. Recognition of the disequilibrium phase is important, especially in the presence of accompanying substantial renal impairment, because the clinician may be misled by a high urine $[Na^+]$ into believing that the patient has developed acute tubular necrosis (ATN). This misdiagnosis can be easily prevented by noting a low urine $[Cl^-]$ (<20 mEq/L) or by a urine pH >6.5. In contrast, in ATN, both $[Na^+]$ and $[Cl^-]$ are similarly elevated in the urine and urine pH is usually acidic.

The course of metabolic alkalosis can be divided into generation, maintenance, and recovery phases (17). Generation occurs by loss of H^+ from the ECF into the external environment or into the cells, or by gain of base by the oral or intravenous route or from the base stored in bone apatite. Important maintenance mechanisms are Cl^- depletion, mineralocorticoid excess and K^+ depletion, and states of low or absent glomerular filtration rate (GFR) associated with base excess. In some instances, mechanisms generating and maintaining alkalosis may be occurring simultaneously.

For the maintenance phase, the clinical question is always: why do this patient's kidneys not correct the elevated plasma $[HCO_3^-]$ by excretion of HCO_3^-? The possible answers are discussed in detail in subsequent chapters.

During the recovery or correction phase, excess HCO_3^- is excreted in Cl^--depletion alkalosis in exchange for administered Cl^- until plasma $[HCO_3^-]$ and $[Cl^-]$ are returned to normal. In K^+-depletion alkalosis, plasma $[HCO_3^-]$ may fall without urinary excretion of HCO_3^-, because administered K^+ enters cells to replete intracellular stores, and this K^+ entry is associated with H^+ movement from cells into the ECF causing downward titration of plasma $[HCO_3^-]$ (16,18,19).

Although these stages can be clearly delineated in animal models of metabolic alkalosis, in the clinical situation the genesis of the generation phase may be obscure, even after a careful history. This is especially true if the patient is concealing bulimia or diuretic or laxative abuse.

Much less commonly, patients can develop a metabolic alkalosis if they ingest alkali such as $NaHCO_3$ (e.g., baking soda) or calcium carbonate and cannot excrete the excess HCO_3^- because they have substantial chronic renal insufficiency, or end-stage renal disease and are treated with conventional hemodialysis with a high dialysate $[HCO_3^-]$.

PATHOPHYSIOLOGY

The pathophysiology of metabolic alkalosis has excited controversy during the past 50 years mainly to explain the maintenance phase. As always, hypotheses depend on the technology and knowledge of renal physiology extant at the time of study. Now, in the molecular era, new studies of the response of Na^+/H^+ exchangers, Na^+ HCO_3 cotransporters, anion $(Cl^--HCO_3^-)$ exchangers, H^+ pumps (H^+-ATPase and H^+/K^+-ATPase) and Cl^- channels to acid–base perturbations are illuminating our concepts of the complexity of electrolyte transport by the kidney. These studies suggest that the day-to-day control of acid and base excretion by the kidney is substantially dependent on the collecting duct with its heterogeneity of segments, cell types, and acid–base transporters (see Chapters 4 and 5).

A brief historical review is of interest to place the physiology and the pathophysiology in the context of the times. In 1920, MacCallum et al. (20) described an increase in the "alkali reserve" in a model of pyloric obstruction in dogs. The relationship of alkalemia with hypochloremia was noted in that study and in subsequent experimental models and in patients (21–23). In the 1950s, the role of K^+ in the genesis of metabolic alkalosis was studied extensively by Cooke et al. (24). In the 1960s, an important and illuminating series of meticulous experiments was carried out in dogs and humans by Schwartz and coworkers (13,25). These studies made it clear that Cl^- played an essential role in the correction of metabolic alkalosis, but the role of Cl^- was only regarded as permissive. Chloride was thought to be merely a "mendicant anion," allowing for Na^+ reabsorption without obligating H^+ secretion. The evidence of the importance of Cl^- channels and Cl^-/HCO_3^- exchangers in modulating HCO_3^- reabsorption and secretion was not yet available.

A fundamental problem in virtually all these experiments was that concomitant deficits of Na^+, K^+, Cl^-, and ECF volume coexisted, and that selective repletion to determine the single and necessary abnormality responsible for maintenance of metabolic alkalosis was difficult to establish and document (26). In this situation demonstration of renal correction of metabolic alkalosis, in the absence of administered H^+ but in the presence of *maintained deficits* of a particular ion or of ECF contraction, can prove that these deficits could not be responsible for maintenance of metabolic alkalosis (27,28). Thus, if correction of metabolic alkalosis associated with hypokalemia occurs without administration of exogenous K^+, then a K^+ deficit cannot be responsible for maintenance of the alkalosis (17). Likewise, if K^+ administration with HCO_3^-, but without Cl^-, corrects metabolic alkalosis and there is no decrease in renal acid excretion (excretion of HCO_3), then correction is not by a renal mechanism (16,18), but rather by a shift of H^+ from cells as the cellular deficit of K^+ is corrected. These concepts are further discussed in the next three chapters. In clinical practice, of course, deficits of Cl^-, Na^+, K^+, and ECF volume, which are present to varying degrees in most etiologies of metabolic alkalosis, are all usually repleted simultaneously.

The tight connection between K^+-independent and ECF volume-maintained metabolic alkalosis was thought by most previously and by some still today to be based on the thesis that net HCO_3^- reabsorption in the kidney was solely dependent on modulation of Na^+–H^+ exchange (25,29). Thus, the demands of Na^+ conservation were believed to require continued HCO_3^- reabsorption with Na^+ (via Na^+–H^+ exchange or electrical coupling) despite alkalemia until ECF volume was restored to normal. The intriguing concept then emerged of an intra-nephronal shift of reabsorption of filtered load of Na^+ in ECF volume depletion from the Cl^--rich reabsorption in the distal nephron to the HCO_3-rich reabsorption in the proximal tubule, though this hypothesis was not supported by segmental nephron micropuncture experiments (30).

Subsequently, demonstration of HCO_3^- secretion in the cortical collecting duct via luminal Cl/HCO_3^- exchange in specific epithelial cells (type B or β-intercalated cells) afforded the possibility of correction of metabolic alkalosis by a mechanism that was independent of Na^+ reabsorption. Subsequently, HCO_3^- secretion in the collecting duct was shown to occur during in vivo correction of Cl^- depletion metabolic alkalosis by Cl^- administration without Na^+ (see Chapter 17). Secretion of HCO_3^- into the collecting duct appears to be a more efficient mechanism of excreting HCO_3^- than a reduction in reabsorption of filtered HCO_3^- in the proximal tubule and in more distal segments. In support of these studies in mammals, Cl^-–HCO_3^- exchange in the turtle bladder has been shown to participate in HCO_3^- secretion in response to vasoactive intestinal peptide (VIP) as well as to neurogenic mechanisms (31). Poikilothermic reptiles that lack effective distal nephrons and eat large meals intermittently develop hypochloremic alkalosis for several days postprandially (32,33).

It is interesting to speculate that the "alkaline tide" that occurs after a meal may be due to secretion of HCO_3^- into the collecting duct via a signal related to gastric HCl secretion. In addition, HCO_3^- loading in the presence of low Cl^- intake in man results in mild metabolic alkalosis perhaps related to impaired Cl^-/HCO_3^- exchange in the collecting duct (see Chapter 7). The Cl^-/HCO_3^- exchanger appears to be upregulated in response to HCO_3^- loading.

Potassium depletion is usually associated with only *mild* metabolic alkalosis, and the latter may not occur at all if HCO_3^- loss via the kidney (as in renal tubular acidosis) or by the gut (as in severe diarrhea), is present (see Chapters 13 and 15). In such circumstances, metabolic acidosis may accompany hypokalemia. If K^+ depletion is associated with *severe* metabolic alkalosis, one should suspect accompanying Cl^- depletion, inappropriately high levels of aldosterone or an exogenous source of HCO_3^-. Cl^- depletion is by far the most common cause of moderate or severe metabolic alkalosis.

The generation of K^+ depletion alkalosis is likely due to an intra-cellular shift of H^+. Intracellular acidosis has been noted in many tissues and especially in muscle cells after K^+ depletion (19). K^+ depletion is also associated with enhanced renal production and increased renal excretion of NH_4^+ (34), thus increasing net acid excretion. Renal maintenance of K^+-depletion alkalosis is also associated with enhanced HCO_3^- reabsorption in the proximal tubule, distal convoluted tubule, and in the collecting duct (see Chapter 18).

Combined K^+ and Cl^- depletion can produce metabolic alkalosis, and repletion of both ions is then necessary to achieve correction of alkalosis. Severe K^+ depletion causes impaired renal conservation of Cl^- and negative Cl^- balance (14,16,35–37). Loop and thiazide diuretics can cause negative balances of both K^+ and Cl^- and thus a combined mechanism of maintenance of chronic metabolic alkalosis. Bartter and Gitelman syndromes (38) mimic the effects of the use or abuse of loop and thiazide diuretics, respectively, and also cause normotensive states associated with hyperenine-mic hyperaldosteronism with hypokalemic alkalosis (see Chapter 18). Prolonged vomiting and severe Cl^- depletion can be associated with high cumulative K^+ losses. In these circumstances urine $[K^+]$ falls from its generally high concentration in metabolic alkalosis due to vomiting and this should suggest concomitant severe K^+ depletion.

Metabolic alkalosis is common in primary hyperaldosteronism. Generation of the alkalosis relates to K^+ depletion and likely also to the effects of mineralocorticoid to stimulate H^+ secretion in the collecting ducts (39,40). During continued excess nonphysiological production of aldosterone, there is escape from the Na^+-retaining effects of mineralocorticoid but at the expense of an expanded ECF volume and, eventually, sustained hypertension. There is no escape, however, from the effects of excess aldosterone to continue causing renal K^+ wasting. The differential diagnosis of the syndrome of hypokalemic hypertension with metabolic alkalosis is discussed further in Chapter 18.

CLINICAL FEATURES

The clinical features and adverse consequences of metabolic alkalosis per se are difficult to separate from those of the associated or causative deficits of Cl^-, magnesium, plasma volume and K^+ as well as changes in Ca^{2+} (Table 2).

Neurologic

Apathy, confusion, and neuromuscular irritability (related in part, perhaps, to a low plasma $[Ca^{++}]$) are common when alkalosis is severe. Although neuromuscular irritability may be readily evident, Chvostek and Trousseau signs are seen uncommonly (41).

Cardiovascular

Alkalosis per se has a mild positive inotropic effect on the heart and little or no effect on cardiac rhythm (42). Cardiac arrhythmias occur primarily

Table 2 Major Adverse Consequences of Severe Alkalemia

Cardiovascular
    Arteriolar constriction
    Reduction in coronary blood flow
    Reduction in anginal threshold
    Predisposition to refractory supraventricular and ventricular arrhythmias
Respiratory
    Hypoventilation with attendant hypercapnia and hypoxemia
Metabolic
    Stimulation of anaerobic glycolysis and organic acid production
    Hypokalemia
    Decreased plasma ionized calcium concentration
    Hypomagnesemia and hypophosphatemia
Cerebral
    Reduction in cerebral blood flow

---

because of hypokalemia and encompass a variety of disturbances: atrial and ventricular premature beats, paroxysmal atrial and junctional tachycardias, atrioventricular block and ventricular tachycardia and fibrillation (43); the presence of coronary insufficiency, left ventricular hypertrophy, or digitalis therapy makes these more likely. Alkalosis also intensifies digitalis toxicity (44). ECG changes simulating acute myocardial infarction, which are rarely associated with hyperkalemia, have also been reported during hypokalemia and attributed to a reduction in the intracellular to extracellular ratio for K^+ during replacement (45). Compensatory hypoventilation may contribute to hypoxia or pulmonary infection in very ill or immunocompromised patients.

Metabolic

Increased Organic Acid Production and Organic Anion Excretion

In metabolic alkalosis, production of organic acids such as lactic acid is increased. Lactate production in alkalosis may be enhanced by decreased oxygen delivery due to vasoconstriction (42), decreased oxygen consumption because of impaired mitochondrial (46) and liver (47) metabolism, and impaired tissue oxygen extraction because of increased oxygen–hemoglobin binding, which probably resolves promptly because of an increase in 2,3-DPG (48). Increased production of organic acids has been described teleologically as a response to "compensate" for the alkalemia (49). The increased production likely contributes to the increased anion gap observed in metabolic alkalosis, although the principal cause is the increased negative charge of albumin in alkalemia (50). During treatment of lactic acidosis with $NaHCO_3$, an increase in lactic and keto-acid production occurs (49). Metabolic alkalosis also alters muscle metabolism to increase glycogen utilization (51). Alkalosis increases urinary citrate excretion by inducing changes in mitochondrial tricarboxylate metabolism and may contribute in a quantitatively important way to base excretion, at least in the rat (52). This increase in citrate excretion occurs in the setting of an overall increase in glycolysis during metabolic alkalosis (53).

Effects of K^+ Depletion

When K^+ depletion is severe, muscle weakness may dominate the clinical picture. Polyuria and polydipsia may be present because of a urinary concentrating defect (54). Prolonged hypokalemia and alkalosis, particularly but not exclusively associated with primary aldosteronism is associated with cortical and medullary renal cysts, which can resolve with treatment (55). Whether the renal scarring associated with hypokalemic nephropathy can also resolve is unclear.

Effects on Ionized Calcium

Both respiratory and metabolic alkalosis reduce ionized calcium concentration, and this reduction may contribute to the associated neurological symptoms and cardiac arrhythmias. Metabolic alkalosis also decreases calcium efflux from bone (56).

Renal

ECF volume contraction is a common accompaniment of chronic metabolic alkalosis and has often been believed to be the direct cause of maintenance of metabolic alkalosis; hence the term "contraction alkalosis" (57). Volume contraction may participate in the generation of metabolic alkalosis as in the acute phase of diuretic administration (57,58), but evidence that volume contraction is the single necessary effect to *maintain* alkalosis is lacking (59). Metabolic alkalosis can cause ECF volume contraction by a shift of Na^+ ions from the ECF into cells in the process of buffering via Na^+/H^+ exchange (60,61). Arteriolar constriction may also occur, and these two effects may lead to "alkalotic contraction" of circulating blood volume (62). Thus, metabolic alkalosis and ECF volume contraction can often coexist but the relationship between them is complex. Experimental studies in man, dog, and the rat all suggest that repletion of Cl^- without restoration of ECF or blood volume or of GFR can correct CDA (59) (see Chapter 17).

Just as the clinical features of K^+-depletion alkalosis are in part dependent on the effects of K^+ depletion (e.g., cardiac arrhythmias, nephrogenic diabetes insipidus, and muscle weakness), the effects of Cl^- depletion contribute to the clinical features of Cl^--depletion alkalosis. The limiting factor for absorption of NaCl in the ascending limb of the loop of Henle is Cl^- delivery to that site (63). Thus in Cl^--depletion alkalosis there may be impaired urine concentrating ability (64), impaired response to loop diuretics (65,66) and stimulation of renin via a macula densa mechanism (67,68). Especially in the presence of abundant delivery of $NaHCO_3$ and of high prevailing mineralocorticoid levels, as occur in Cl^--depletion alkalosis, diminished Cl^- delivery to the collecting duct causes enhanced cation exchange, by K^+ and H^+ secretion in response to Na^+ absorption through the electrogenic Na^+ channel (see Chapter 5) (69). As mentioned earlier, prolonged hypokalemia and alkalosis, particularly but not exclusively associated with primary aldosteronism, is associated with cortical and medullary renal cysts, which can resolve with treatment (55). A low luminal $[Cl^-]$ may also increase K^+ secretion in the distal nephron by linked KCl secretion (70).

DIAGNOSIS

The cause of metabolic alkalosis (Table 1) is often evident from the history and physical examination, and determination of serum electrolytes, renal function and arterial blood gases. Figure 1 presents an approach to diagnosing the cause of the many etiologies of metabolic alkalosis. The hierarchy of the proposed tests is not related to the prevalence of the disorders nor are the tests intended to be comprehensive or definitive for the causes that they suggest. The possibility of multiple causes should be kept in mind, e.g., surreptitious diuretic and laxative abuse coupled with bulimia (71), hyperaldosteronism secondary to severe hypertension treated with chloruretic diuretics, hypercalcemia of malignancy with vomiting, etc. The ensuing discussion is aimed particularly at the patient in whom the cause of the metabolic alkalosis is not clear, often because of the deliberate concealment of pertinent historical facts.

Keys to the approach to ferreting out a surreptitious diagnosis include a careful probing history for loss of body fluids, such as vomiting, and an enquiry about appropriate medications, such as diuretics. Diuretic abuse occurs more frequently in women and in those employed in the field of health care delivery with easier access to these drugs. Denial of the use of diuretics is the usual initial response and a persistent and aggressive approach may be needed to establish the diagnosis and any possible underlying psychiatric abnormality.

The emphasis on physical examination should be on the status of ECF volume and the presence or absence of hypertension. Patients with surreptitious vomiting with or without bulimia may have blackened teeth enamel due to repeated exposure to gastric HCl; other clues are scarring of the dorsum of the hand and salivary gland hypertrophy (72). The presence of hypertension is dependent on whether the kidney is Na^+-acquisitive or Na^+-losing. An example of the former is primary aldosteronism, of the latter, Gitelman syndrome or thiazide abuse.

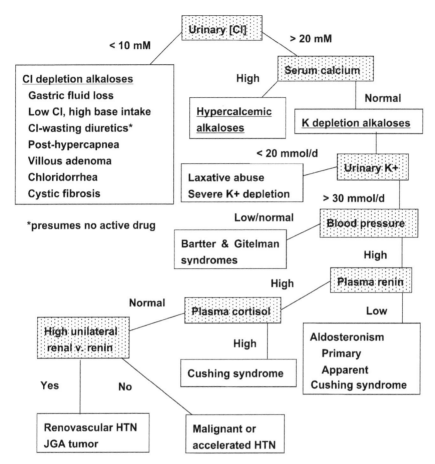

Figure 1 Diagnostic algorithm for metabolic alkalosis. The tests that are recommended (indicated in the stippled boxes) are not definitive, rather they are directive. HTN, hypertension; v, vein.

The diagnosis is usually first noted from the plasma electrolytes and the clinician has to make a decision as to whether to obtain arterial blood gases for the specific acid–base diagnosis. Hypochloremic hyperbicarbonatemia can be due to metabolic alkalosis or *chronic* respiratory acidosis. If one has to guess the acid–base status from the serum electrolytes (a poor substitute for accurate acid–base diagnosis from an arterial blood gas measurement), the presence of hypokalemia and a modest increase in anion gap favors a diagnosis of metabolic alkalosis. Unlike in metabolic acidosis however, the presence of an increased anion gap and its extent is of no value in the differential diagnosis of the cause of metabolic alkalosis. The increase in the gap, which rarely exceeds 8 mEq/L, is due mainly to the increase in the negative charge on albumin induced by the alkaline blood pH (50) and to increased organic anions, mainly lactate, which can be considerable with severe alkalosis (73). Fluctuating severity of alkalosis for obscure reasons should suggest surreptitious causes such as diuretic abuse or concealed vomiting.

Urinary electrolyte determinations prior to therapy, especially [Cl$^-$] and [K$^+$], can be of considerable diagnostic value prior to treatment particularly when the diagnosis is not obvious or the patient is concealing information (bulimia, diuretic abuse, laxative abuse). Urine [Cl$^-$] should be determined precisely; that means distinguished from zero. Very broadly, Cl$^-$ and volume depletion metabolic alkalosis is associated with a random urine [Cl$^-$] <20 mEq/L and often <10 mEq/L. An exception to this finding occurs during the continuing action of an ingested chloruretic diuretic. Urine [K$^+$] is high and often >70 mEq/L (Figure 1). It should be noted that K$^+$ depletion must be severe before efficient renal conservation of K$^+$ develops especially in the presence of factors inducing kaluresis, as with mineralocorticoid excess or Cl$^-$ depletion.

In "saline-unresponsive" metabolic alkalosis, due to mineralocorticoid excess and/or K$^+$ depletion, urine [Cl$^-$] is typically >20 mEq/L, and especially if total body K$^+$ is severely and chronically reduced, urine [K$^+$] may be <30 mEq/L. A urine [K$^+$] <20 mEq/L indicates either extra-renal K$^+$ loss or very severe chronic K$^+$ deprivation. Conversely, a urine K$^+$ excretion >30 mEq/day in the presence of hypokalemia defines urinary K$^+$ wasting and is highly suggestive of excess circulating mineralocorticoid or recent surreptitious diuretic abuse.

The transtubular K$^+$ gradient (TTKG), an index of the appropriateness of the renal response to the serum [K$^+$], is also helpful particularly because a timed collection is unnecessary, thus giving an expeditious determination of the role of the kidney. The TTKG is based on the assumption that no further K$^+$ secretion or reabsorption occurs as water is reabsorbed between the end of the cortical collecting duct and the final urine, which of course is not completely correct. Nonetheless the index is a useful one for the clinical assessment of renal K$^+$ secretion and is calculated as follows: TTKG = Urine [K$^+$]/Serum [K$^+$] × (Serum osmolality/Urine osmolality). In the setting of hypokalemia, a value <3.0 is expected (74). Greater values suggest that the kidney is the cause or route of K$^+$ depletion; however, clinical studies with this index are limited.

With both surreptitious vomiting and diuretic abuse, random urine sampling may reveal widely fluctuating electrolyte concentrations. Commonly used diuretics can be measured in the urine and such measurements are extremely useful when suspicion of the syndrome of surreptitious diuretic abuse is present.

Urine pH varies depending upon the nature and phase of metabolic alkalosis. Alkaline urine can occur intermittently with acute and chronic vomiting and disequilibrium alkalosis. Disequilibrium alkalosis, a phase during or immediately after generation, is characterized by an "alkaline" urine (pH > 6.5) with a urine [Na$^+$] >10 mEq/L, urine [K$^+$] >30 mEq/L, and bicarbonaturia; urine [Cl$^-$] remains low. Bulimia (75) is often associated with episodic disequilibrium alkalosis and a metabolic alkalosis of fluctuating severity. The use of the term "paradoxical aciduria" to describe a normally acidic urinary pH in a setting of a chronic metabolic alkalosis is inappropriate. The urine pH is acidic because renal HCO$_3^-$ reabsorption is complete and the alkalosis is maintained.

Because Bartter and Gitelman syndromes (see Chapter 18) are characterized by normal or low blood pressure, elevated plasma renin activity and secondary hyperaldosteronism, they have been understandably confused with several other forms of metabolic alkalosis such as bulimia and diuretic or laxative abuse. Bartter and Gitelman syndromes are familial; the former mostly diagnosed during childhood, the latter in adulthood. Gitelman syndrome, which mimics thiazide abuse, is more common than Bartter syndrome and causes more symptoms than previously thought (38). Urine Cl$^-$ and K$^+$ excretions are high because of the primary defect. Patients with surreptitious vomiting with or without bulimia have normal renal conservation of Cl$^-$. An intermittently alkaline urine can occur with acute-on-chronic vomiting and disequilibrium alkalosis. Diuretic abuse usually leads to more severe K$^+$ depletion than vomiting; urinary K$^+$ and Cl$^-$ concentrations both will be low unless the diuretic effect is still active; in this setting, random urine sampling may reveal widely fluctuating electrolyte concentrations. With laxative abuse, urine K$^+$ excretion is low unless Na$^+$ depletion is severe in which case secondary hyperaldosteronism may occur and increase kaliuresis (76).

In diarrheal states, stool should be analyzed for electrolyte concentration. The usual tendency is to lose not retain base; thus, in secretory diarrheas such as cholera, metabolic acidosis is the rule. Thus, when metabolic alkalosis is present, the causes are few. Some villous adenomas are associated with metabolic alkalosis due to their secretion of excess Cl$^-$ so that stool [Cl$^-$] is >90 mEq/L. Most are within a few cm of the anus but can be higher in the descending colon. Because of their soft, often sessile nature, they may be difficult to palpate and may be passed over on digital examination.

Congenital chloridorrhea is associated with copious watery diarrhea (1–3 L/day) and a stool [Cl$^-$] > 90 mEq/L, often as high as 145 mEq/L. Stool [Na$^+$] and [K$^+$] are usually normal and their sum is less than Cl$^-$ concentration, unlike normal stool. Urine [Cl$^-$] and [K$^+$] remain low. Laxative abuse is not associated with severe alkalosis despite often profound hypokalemia (77). Urine [K$^+$] and K$^+$ excretion are uniformly low in laxative abuse and plasma [HCO$_3^-$] is rarely above 30–34 mEq/L. The diagnosis may be supported by the findings of phenolphthalein in the feces and urine, or melanosis coli on colonoscopy (78). Proctoscopy and colonoscopy are necessary to distinguish among these possibilities.

Metabolic alkalosis associated with hypertension is most likely associated with an effect of diuretics used for treatment. Unprovoked hypokalemic alkalosis, i.e., without diuretic exposure, coupled with hypertension, which is not malignant or accelerated, is caused by primary hyperaldosteronism about half the time (79). Primary hyperaldosteronism can be screened for by demonstrating an elevated ratio of plasma aldosterone concentration to simultaneously measured plasma renin activity at 8 a.m. (80,81); the actual diagnostic value of this ratio may vary depending on the laboratory employed. The specific diagnosis of this condition and the differentiation between adrenal adenoma and bilateral adrenal hyperplasia as its cause are complex issues and beyond the scope of this chapter.

Unless there is severe renal failure, metabolic alkalosis often accompanies hypokalemia and secondary hyperaldosteronism in accelerated or malignant hypertension especially during diuretic therapy. In contrast to other instances of mineralocorticoid excess, ectopic adrenocorticotropin hormone (ACTH) syndrome may be associated with quite severe metabolic alkalosis even though hypertension is not prominent.

PREVALENCE AND OUTCOME

Data on the prevalence and outcome of metabolic alkalosis are sparse. In a study at one medical center (82), metabolic alkalosis comprised half of all acid–base disorders. Since vomiting, nasogastric suction, and the use of chloruretic diuretics are all common among hospitalized patients, this should not be surprising. The mortality associated with severe metabolic alkalosis is substantial. Wilson et al. (83) determined a mortality rate of 45% in patients with a pH of 7.55 and of 80% when the pH was >7.65; a high mortality (48.5%) for alkalemia >7.60 has been confirmed (84). While this relationship between alkalemia and mortality is not necessarily causal, severe alkalosis should be viewed with concern and should be promptly treated.

REFERENCES

1. Stewart PA. Modern quantitative acid–base chemistry. Can J Physiol Pharmacol 1983; 61:1444–1461.
2. Javaheri S, Kazemi H. Metabolic alkalosis and hypoventilation in humans. Am Rev Respir Dis 1987; 136:1101–1116.
3. Javaheri S, Nardell EA. Severe metabolic alkalosis: a case report. Br Med J 1981; 283:1016–1017.
4. Bear R, Goldstein M, Phillipson E. Effect of metabolic alkalosis on respiratory function in patients with chronic obstructive lung disease. Can Med Assoc J 1977; 117:900–903.

5. Aquino HC, Luke RG. Respiratory compensation to potassium-depletion and chloride-depletion alkalosis. Am J Physiol 1973; 225:1444–1448.

6. Fencl V, Miller TB, Pappenheimer JR. Studies on the respiratory response to disturbances of acid–base balance, with deductions concerning the ionic composition of cerebral interstitial fluid. Am J Physiol 1966; 210:459–472.

7. Penman RW, Luke RG, Jarboe TM. Respiratory effects of hypochloremic alkalosis and potassium depletion in the dog. J Appl Physiol 1972; 33:170–174.

8. Javaheri S, Shore NS, Rose B, Kazemi H. Compensatory hypoventilation in metabolic alkalosis. Chest 1982; 81:296–301.

9. Mithoefer JC, Bossman OG, Thibeault DW, Mead GD. The clinical estimation of alveolar ventilation. Am Rev Respir Dis 1968; 98:868–871.

10. Miller PD, Berns AS. Acute metabolic alkalosis perpetuating hypercarbia: a role for acetazolamide in chronic obstructive pulmonary disease. J Am Med Assoc 1977; 22:2400–2401.

11. Kilburn KH. Shock, seizures, and coma with alkalosis during mechanical ventilation. Ann Intern Med 1966; 65:977–984.

12. Adrogue HJ, Madias NE. Changes in plasma potassium concentration during acute acid–base disturbances. Am J Med 1981; 71:456–467.

13. Kassirer JP, Schwartz WB. Correction of metabolic alkalosis in man without repair of potassium deficiency. Am J Med 1966; 40:19–26.

14. Garella S, Chazan JA, Cohen JJ. Saline-resistant metabolic alkalosis or "chloride-wasting nephropathy". Ann Int Med 1970; 73:31–38.

15. Wall BM, Williams HH, Cooke CR. Chloride-resistant metabolic alkalosis in an adult with congenital chloride diarrhea. Am J Med 1988; 85:570–572.

16. Luke RG, Levitin H. Impaired renal conservation of chloride and the acid–base changes associated with potassium depletion in the rat. Clin Sci 1967; 32:511–552.

17. Seldin DW, Rector FC Jr. The generation and maintenance of metabolic alkalosis. Kidney Int 1972; 1:306–321.

18. Orloff J, Kennedy TJ Jr, Berliner RW. The effect of potassium in nephrectomized rats with hypokalemic alkalosis. J Clin Invest 1953; 32:538–542.

19. Adler S, Fraley DS. Potassium and intracellular pH. Kidney Int 1977; 11:433–442.

20. MacCallum WG, Lintz J, Vermilye HN, Leggett TH, Boas E. The effect of pyloric obstruction in relation to gastric tetany. Bull Johns Hopkins Hosp 1920; 31:1–7.

21. Berger EH, Binger MW. The status of the kidneys in alkalosis. J Am Med Assoc 1935; 104:1383–1387.

22. Haden RL, Orr TG. Chemical changes in the blood of the dog after pyloric obstruction. J Exp Med 1923; 37:377–381.

23. Kirsner JB, Palmer WL. The role of chlorides in alkalosis. J Am Med Assoc 1941; 116:384–390.

24. Cooke RE, Segar WE, Cheek DR, Coville FE, Darrow DC. The extra-renal correction of alkalosis associated with potassium deficiency. J Clin Invest 1952; 31:798–805.

25. Schwartz WB, Cohen JJ. The nature of the renal response to chronic disorders of acid–base equilibrium. Am J Med 1978; 64:417–428.

26. Galla JH, Luke RG. Chloride transport and disorders of acid–base balance. Ann Rev Physiol 1988; 50:141–158.

27. Rosen RA, Julian BA, Dubovsky EV, Galla JH, Luke RG. On the mechanism by which chloride corrects metabolic alkalosis in man. Am J Med 1988; 84: 449–458.

28. Wall BM, Byrum GV, Galla JH, Luke RG. Importance of chloride for the correction of chronic metabolic alkalosis in the rat. Am J Physiol 1987; 87:F1–F9.

29. Emmett M, Seldin DW. Clinical syndromes of metabolic acidosis and metabolic alkalosis. In: Seldin DW, Giebisch G, eds. The Kidney, Physiology and Pathophysiology. New York: Raven Press, 1985:1611–1624.

30. Galla JH, Bonduris DN, Luke RG. Effect of chloride and extracellular fluid volume on bicarbonate reabsorption along the nephron in metabolic alkalosis in the rat: a reassessment of the classical hypothesis of the maintenance of metabolic alkalosis. J Clin Invest 1987; 80:41–50.

31. Durham JH, Brodsky WA. Chloride Reabsorption by the Reptilian (Turtle) Urinary Bladder. Chloride Transport Coupling in Biological Membranes and Epithelia. Amsterdam: Elsevier Science Publishers BV, 1984; 9:249–270.

32. Busk M, Jensen FB, Wang T. Effects of feeding on metabolism, gas transport, and acid–base balance in the bullfrog *Rana catesbeiana*. Am J Physiol 2000; 278:R185–R195.

33. Busk M, Overgaard J, Hicks JW, Bennett AF, Wang T. Effects of feeding on arterial blood gasses in the American alligator Mississippiensis. J Exp Biol 2000; 203:3117–3124.

34. Tannen RL. Relationship of renal ammonia production and potassium homeostasis. Kidney Int 1977; 11:453–465.

35. Gutsche HU, Peterson LN, Levine DZ. In vivo evidence of impaired solute transport by the thick ascending limb in potassium-depleted rats. J Clin Invest 1984; 73:908–916.

36. Luke RG, Wright FS, Fowler N, Kashgarian M, Giebisch GH. Effects of potassium depletion on renal tubular chloride transport in the rat. Kidney Int 1978; 14:414–427.

37. Luke RG, Booker BB, Galla JH. Effect of potassium depletion on chloride transport in loop of Henle in the rat. Am J Physiol 1985; 248:F682–F687.

38. Cruz DN, Shaer AJ, Bia MJ, Lifton RP, Simon DB. Gitelman's syndrome revisited: an evaluation of symptoms and health-related quality of life. Kidney Int 2001; 59:710–717.

39. Garg LC, Narang N. Effects of aldosterone on NEM-sensitive ATPase in rabbit nephron segments. Kidney Int 1988; 34:13–17.

40. Khadouri C, Marsy S, Barlet-Bas C, Doucet A. Short-term effect of aldosterone on NEM-sensitive ATPase in rat collecting tubule. Am J Physiol 1989; 257:F177–F181.

41. Harrington JT, Kassirer JP. Metabolic alkalosis. In: Cohen JJ, Kassirer JP, eds. Acid-Base. Boston: Little, Brown and Co, 1982:242.

42. Mitchell JH, Wildenthal K, Johnson RL Jr. The effects of acid–base disturbances on cardiovascular and pulmonary function. Kidney Int 1972; 1:375–389.

43. Helfant RW. Hypokalemia and arrhythmias. Am J Med 1986; 80(suppl 4A): 13–22.

44. Warren MC, Giannella RE, Cutler RL, Harrison DC. Digitalis toxicity: II. The effect of metabolic alkalosis. Am Heart J 1968; 75:358–363.

45. Madias JE, Madias NE. Hyperkalemia-like ECG changes simulating acute myocardial infarction in a patient with hypokalemia undergoing potassium replacement. J Electrocardiol 1989; 22:93–97.

46. Relman AS. Metabolic consequences of acid–base disorders. Kidney Int 1972; 1:347–359.

47. Goldstein PJ, Simmons DH, Tashkin DP. Effect of acid–base alterations on hepatic lactate utilization. J Physiol (Lond) 1972; 223:261–278.

48. Bellingham AJ, Detter JC, Lenfant C. Regulatory mechanisms of hemoglobin oxygen affinity in acidosis and alkalosis. J Clin Invest 1971; 50:700–706.

49. Hood VL, Tannen RL. Protection of acid–base balance by pH regulation of acid production. N Engl J Med 1998; 339:819–826.

50. Madias NE, Ayus JC, Adrogue HJ. Increased anion gap in metabolic alkalosis; the role of plasma-protein equivalency. N Eng J Med 1979; 300:1421–1423.

51. Hollidge-Horvat MG, Parolin ML, Wong D, Jones NL, Heigenhauser JF. Effect of induced metabolic alkalosis on human skeletal muscle metabolism during exercise. Am J Physiol 2000; 278:E316–E329.

52. Kaufman AM, Kahn T. Complementary role of citrate and bicarbonate excretion in acid–base balance in the rat. Am J Physiol 1988; 255:F182–F187.

53. Lemieux G, Berkofsky J, Lemieux C. Renal tissue metabolism in the rat during chronic metabolic alkalosis: importance of glycolysis. Can J Physiol Pharmacol 1986; 64:1419–1426.

54. Schwartz WB, Relman AS. Effects of electrolyte disorders on renal structure and function. N Engl J Med 1967; 276:383–389.

55. Torres VE, Young WF, Offord KP, Hattery RR. Association of hypokalemia, aldosteronism and renal cysts. N Engl J Med 1990; 322:345–351.

56. Bushinsky DA. Metabolic alkalosis decreases bone calcium efflux by suppressing osteoclasts and stimulating osteoblasts. Am J Physiol 1996; 40:F216–F222.

57. Cannon PJ, Heinemann HO, Albert MS. "Contraction" alkalosis after diuresis of edematous patients with ethacrynic acid. Ann Intern Med 1965; 62:979–990.

58. Wilcox CS, Loon NR, Kanthawatana S, Pham MA, Cannizzaro R. Generation of alkalosis with loop diuretics: roles of contraction and acid excretion. J Nephrol 1990; 2:81–87.

59. Galla JH. Metabolic alkalosis. J Am Soc Nephrol 2000; 11:369–375.

60. Singer RB, Clark JK, Barker ES, Crosley AP Jr, Elkinton JR. The acute effects in man of rapid intravenous infusion of hypertonic sodium bicarbonate solution. I. Changes in acid–base balance and distribution of the excess buffer base. Medicine 1955; 34:51–95.

61. Borkan S, Northrup TE, Cohen JJ, Garella S. Renal responses to metabolic alkalosis induced by isovolemic hemofiltration in the dog. Kidney Int 1987; 32:322–328.

62. Galla JH, Gifford JD, Luke RG, Rome L. Adaptations to chloride-depletion alkalosis. Am J Physiol 1991; 261:R771–R781.

63. Ecelbarger CA, Terris J, Hoyer JR. Localization and regulation of the rat renal Na^+-$K^+$$2Cl^-$ cotransporter, BSC-1. Am J Physiol 1996; 271:F619–F628.

64. Khanh BT, Luke RG. Chloride depletion and hypochloraemia as a cause of renal sodium and water loss in the rat. Clin Sci 1976; 51:353–362.

65. Loon NR, Wilcox CS. Mild metabolic alkalosis impairs the natriuretic response to bumetanide in normal human subjects. Clin Sci 1998; 94:287–292.

66. Fanestil DD, Vaughn DA, Blakely P. Metabolic acid–base influences on renal thiazide receptor density. Am J Physiol 1997; 272:R2004–R2008.

67. Abboud HE, Luke RG, Galla JH, Kotchen TA. Stimulation of renin by acute selective chloride depletion in the rat. Circ Res 1979; 44:815–821.

68. Lorenz JN, Kotchen TA, Ott CE. Effect of Na and Cl infusion on loop function and plasma renin activity in rats. Am J Physiol 1990; 258:F1328–F1335.

69. Harrington JT, Hulter HN, Cohen JJ, Madias NE. Mineralocorticoid-stimulated renal acidification: the critical role of dietary sodium. Kidney Int 1986; 30:43–48.

70. Velazquez H, Ellison DH, Wright FS. Luminal influences on potassium secretion: chloride, sodium, and thiazide diuretics. Am J Physiol 1992; 262: F1076–F1082.

71. Oster JR. The binge–purge syndrome: a common albeit unappreciated cause of acid–base and fluid-electrolyte disturbances. South Med J 1987; 80:58–67.

72. Mitchell JE, Seim HC, Colon E, Pomeroy C. Medical complications and medical management of bulimia. Ann Intern Med 1987; 107:71–77.

73. Bersin RM, Arieff AI. Primary lactic alkalosis. Am J Med 1988; 85:867.

74. Ethier JH, Kamel KS, Magner PO, Lemann J Jr, Halperin ML. The transtubular potassium gradient in patients with hypokalemia and hyperkalemia. Am J Kidney Dis 1990; 15:309–315.

75. Mitchell JE, Seim HC, Colon E, Pomeroy C. Medical complications and medical management of bulimia. Ann Int Med 1987; 107:71–77.

76. Fleischer N, Brown H, Graham DY, Delena S. Chronic laxative-induced hyperaldosteronism and hypokalemia simulating Bartter's syndrome. Ann Int Med 1969; 70:791–798.

77. Cummings JH, Sladen GE, James OGW, Sarner M, Misiewicz JJ. Laxative-induced diarrhea: a continuing clinical problem. Br Med J 1974; 1:537–541.

78. LaRusso NF, McGill DS. Surreptitious laxative ingestion. Delayed recognition of a serious condition: a case report. Mayo Clin Proc 1975; 50:706–708.

79. Kalpan NM. Primary aldosteronism. In: Kaplan NM, ed. Clinical Hypertension. 8th ed. Philadelphia: Lippincott, 2002:455–459.

80. Blumenfeld JD, Sealy JE, Schussel Y, Vaughan ED Jr, Sos TA, Atlas SA, Muller FB, Acevedo R, Ulick S, Laragh JH. Diagnosis and treatment of primary hyperaldosteronism. Ann Int Med 1994; 121:877–885.

81. Gallay BJ, Ahmad S, Xu L, Toivola B, Davidson RC. Screening for primary aldosteronism without discontinuing hypertensive medications: plasma aldosterone–renin ratio. Am J Kidney Dis 2001; 37:699–705.

82. Hodgkin JE, Soeprono FF, Chan DM. Incidence of metabolic alkalemia in hospitalized patients. Crit Care Med 1980; 8:725–728.

83. Wilson RF, Gibson D, Percinel AK, Ali MA, Baker G, LeBlanc LP, Lucas C. Severe alkalosis in critically ill surgical patients. Arch Surg 1972; 105:197–203.

84. Anderson LE, Henrich WL. Alkalemia-associated morbidity and mortality in medical and surgical patients. South Med J 1987; 80:729–733.

Chloride-Depletion Alkalosis

John H. Galla

*Department of Medicine, University of Cincinnati College of Medicine,
Cincinnati, Ohio, U.S.A.*

DEFINITIONS

Chloride-depletion alkalosis (CDA) is the most common form of metabolic alkalosis. It is caused by depletion of body chloride stores and can be corrected solely by a sufficient amount of any chloride-containing compound. The term is synonymous with chloride-responsive alkalosis but serves to emphasize the underlying pathophysiology of all of the etiologies grouped under this rubric. CDA may occur together with other causes of metabolic alkalosis, most commonly K^+ depletion (see Chapter 18). As with other types of metabolic alkalosis, CDA may be divided into three phases: generation, maintenance, and correction (1). During the maintenance phase, low or absent urine Cl^- marks its salient feature (2,3) unless concomitant diuretic administration or severe K^+ depletion has impaired renal tubule function to the extent that Cl^- cannot be appropriately conserved (4).

CLASSIFICATION

Chloride loss, which is fundamental to the pathophysiology of this group of disorders, may occur via several routes: gastric, colonic, renal, or cutaneous (Table 1). Gastric Cl^- loss occurs with vomiting or nasogastric suction or in urine when gastric tissue has been used as an artificial bladder. Urine losses occur primarily because of the use of chloruretic diuretics or in genetically altered Cl^- transport in Henle's loop or the distal convoluted tubule

Table 1 Etiologies of Chloride-Depletion Metabolic Alkalosis

Gastric losses—vomiting, pyloric stenosis, Zollinger–Ellison syndrome, bulimia, mechanical drainage
Gastrocystoplasty
Chloruretic diuretics—bumetanide, ethacrynic acid, chlorothiazide, metolazone, etc.
Diarrheal states—villous adenoma, congenital chloridorrhea
Posthypercapneic state
Dietary chloride deprivation with base loading—chloride-deficient infant formulas
Cystic fibrosis (high sweat chloride)

(DCT); these latter entities are uniformly accompanied by K^+ depletion also (see Chapter 18). Colonic Cl^- loss occurs in patients with villous adenomas that secrete Cl^- or in genetically altered intestinal anion transport. Cutaneous Cl^- losses have been implicated only in cystic fibrosis.

GENERATION

Loss of Gastric Acid

The parietal cell of the gastric epithelium secretes gastric fluid with a $[H^+]$ of 160–170 mEq/L (pH ~1.0), $[Na^+]$ 2–4 mEq/L, $[K^+]$ ~10 mEq/L, and $[Cl^-]$ ~180 mEq/L in a volume of 1.5–2.5 L/day. Gastric acid secretion is not influenced by the state of acid–base balance but is stimulated by histamine, acetylcholine, other cholinergic agents and gastrin, and is inhibited by somatostatin, β-adrenergic agonists and enteroglucagon (5,6). Gastric $[Cl^-]$ is not influenced by serum $[Cl^-]$ (7). Acid secretion increases markedly with food ingestion (8,9). Postprandially serum $[HCO_3^-]$ rises slightly (1–2 mEq/L) and transiently in proportion to the degree of acid secretion (8). Secreted acid enters the duodenum where it stimulates pancreatic HCO_3^- secretion, which buffers the acid and is absorbed distally in the small bowel. Without acid in the duodenum, pancreatic HCO_3^- secretion remains low (10).

HCl secretion by the parietal cell is effected by the gastric isoform of the H^+/K^+ ATPase (HKA) (11) at the luminal membrane; it is inhibited by omeprazole and its congeners and not by digitalis glycosides. At the basolateral membrane, the anion exchanger AE2 transports Cl^- into the cell in a 1:1 exchange for HCO_3^- secretion into the extracellular fluid (ECF) compartment (12,13).

MacCallum et al. first linked Cl^- to alkalosis when they observed hypochloremia and an increase in "alkali reserve" after the loss of gastric fluid due to pyloric obstruction in dogs. When gastric fluid is lost from the body and therefore not absorbed at more distal segments of the gut, alkalosis results (2,14) because the HCO_3^- generated during the production of gastric acid is not subsequently balanced by Cl^- absorption. Although Na^+ and K^+ loss from gastric fluid varies in amount and may rise with protracted vomiting, the deficits of these cations occur predominantly by urine losses, obligated by bicarbonaturia, which is particularly intense during the generation of alkalosis—the disequilibrium phase. Gastric Na^+ losses may be high with achlorhydria.

Vomiting is an accompaniment of a myriad of conditions including obstruction of the gut, inflammatory processes, and central nervous system diseases; it is a well-recognized side effect of many medications including antibiotics, morphine and its congeners, chemotherapeutic agents, nonsteroidal anti-inflammatory agents and alcohol. It may also be self-induced—usually surreptitiously (15). Pyloric stenosis, rare in adults, may be associated with considerable losses of gastric fluid (16). Nasogastric suction is used in a variety of clinical situations to circumvent vomiting secondary to obstruction, ileus, acute pancreatitis, etc., to avoid reflux, or to put the bowel at rest. Regardless of purpose, it results in the loss of total body Cl^- (Fig. 1).

The Zollinger–Ellison syndrome, which is often associated with a severe peptic ulcer diathesis, is caused by the excessive production of gastrin by a non-β islet cell adenoma usually in the pancreas or surrounding organs leading to gastric acid hypersecretion (17). Other extra-pancreatic sites are uncommon (<10%) but 25% are associated with multiple endocrine neoplasia, type 1. Although an elevated serum gastrin concentration is its hallmark, it must be distinguished from gastric atrophy or other states of hypo- or achlorhydria, which themselves lead to high serum gastrin. Diarrhea is a prominent clinical manifestation of this eponymous syndrome.

Gastrocystoplasty

Gastrocystoplasty is used for bladder augmentation in which the acid environment is protective against infection. In the fasted state of patients with gastrocystoplasty, the urinary pH is neutral, there is no titratable acid in the urine, and serum gastrin concentration is normal (18). However after a meal, serum gastrin concentration and urinary acid secretion increase markedly; these can be inhibited by histamine-2 receptor antagonist, a proton pump inhibitor, or an anticholinergic agent. Excessive HCl production may result in urinary losses sufficient to produce alkalosis, which can be severe because of either the extent of secreting gastric epithelium or degree of hypergastrinemia (19,20).

Chloruretic Diuretics

Chloruretic agents all directly produce initial losses of Cl^-, Na^+, K^+, and fluid in the urine. Chlorothiazide and its congeners inhibit the NaCl cotransporter in the luminal membrane of the DCT (21). Furosemide and its congeners and ethacrynic acid inhibit the $Na^+/K^+/2\ Cl^-$ cotransporter in the thick ascending limb (TAL) of Henle's loop; they also increase urinary NH_4^+, titratable acid and net acid excretion (22,23). The weak carbonic

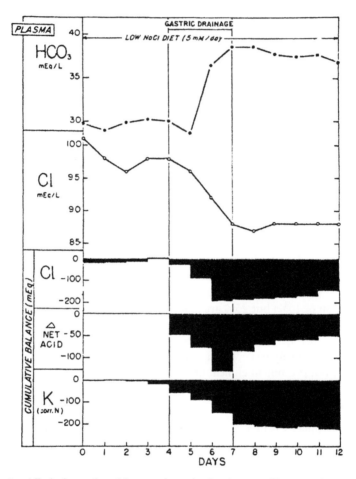

Figure 1 Alkalosis produced by gastric aspiration in man. Plasma anion composition and net Cl, K, and acid balance are shown before, during, and after gastric drainage. Alkalosis was maintained after the generation phase despite dietary K^+ supplementation. *Source*: From Ref. 71.

anhydrase-inhibiting property of furosemide probably accounts for the slight HCO_3^- loss when compared to ethacrynic acid (24). In humans, furosemide given for 2 days induced Cl^- depletion and alkalosis even when K^+ depletion is prevented (25); K^+ balance remained positive until the third day of the maintenance period with stable alkalosis throughout (Fig. 2). Generation was, thus, clearly related to Cl^- depletion. All these chloruretic diuretics commonly cause metabolic alkalosis, more likely when they are used for the treatment of edema than for hypertension (26). Long-term use and higher dosage are more commonly associated with K^+ depletion.

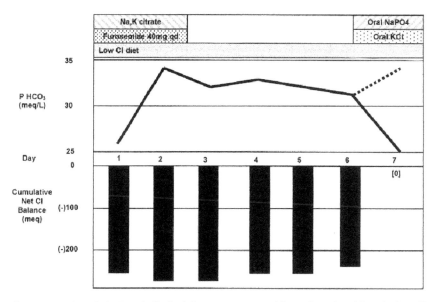

Figure 2 Diuretic-induced alkalosis in man. Furosemide on days 1 and 2 and a low Cl diet induced and maintained chloride depletion and alkalosis; potassium balance was neutral (data not shown). Oral KCl started in the middle of day 6 in six men corrected alkalosis at the end of day 7 with quantitative chloride repletion whereas administration of NaPO₄ in two men (*dashed line*) worsened alkalosis. *Source*: From Ref. 25.

To counteract these diuretic-induced fluid and electrolyte losses, several renal compensatory mechanisms are evoked and may further generate or maintain alkalosis. All diuretics produce some degree of volume depletion but only chloruretic diuretics are associated with alkalosis; K^+-sparing diuretics and carbonic anhydrase inhibitors are associated with metabolic acidosis (27,28). Regardless of mechanism, resultant ECF volume contraction accelerates isotonic fluid reabsorption by the proximal tubule, which returns a fluid rich in HCO_3^- relative to plasma. Volume contraction also stimulates renin and aldosterone secretion. Increased aldosterone can accelerate H^+ secretion and HCO_3^- reabsorption by a Na^+-independent mechanism in the medullary collecting duct (29) and perhaps in other collecting duct segments (30,31).

Chloruretic diuretics accelerate K^+ excretion by several mechanisms and K^+ depletion may contribute to the generation and maintenance of alkalosis. Loop diuretics directly decrease K^+ uptake in the ascending limb of Henle's loop (22). Diuretic-induced increases in Na^+ and fluid delivery to the late distal convolution and collecting duct accelerate K^+ secretion and increased aldosterone further augments K^+ secretion in the collecting duct. Potassium depletion effects a shift of H^+ into cells thereby enhancing alkalosis in the ECF (32). The resultant intracellular acidosis in renal epithelial cells could enhance H^+ secretion with a resultant increase in HCO_3^- reabsorption.

In the proximal tubule, K^+ depletion (33,34), Cl^- depletion and the increase in $PaCO_2$ that occurs as a secondary response to metabolic alkalosis, all may further augment HCO_3^- reabsorption. In the distal tubule, K^+ depletion accelerates HCO_3^- reabsorption independent of load (35). Which of the earlier mechanism(s) primarily engenders renal H^+ loss and generates alkalosis or participates in maintenance has not yet been conclusively established for any of these diuretics.

POSTHYPERCAPNIA

Respiratory acidosis is compensated by sustained increase in renal HCO_3^- reabsorption and a transient increase in net acid and Cl^- excretion, leading to a state of Cl^- depletion with intra- and extracellular acidosis (36,37) (see Chapter 20). Chloruresis begins within a few hours after the onset of respiratory acidosis and is complete usually within 24–48 hr. The responses of individual nephron segments are incompletely understood but HCO_3^- reabsorption in the rat proximal tubule is enhanced (38) and Cl^- reabsorption in the ascending limb of Henle's loop of the rabbit is diminished (39). The collecting duct may also participate: H^+ secreting type A intercalated cells (IC) in the cortical (CCD) and outer medullary collecting ducts (OMCD) are stimulated (40,41), as a result HCO_3^- reabsorption is augmented (42). Messenger RNA for the basolateral anion exchanger of the type A IC is increased (43). When respiratory acidosis is corrected, increased HCO_3^- reabsorption, which is no longer appropriate, persists if insufficient Cl^- intake is available (Fig. 3). The patient with respiratory failure and congestive heart failure managed with NaCl restriction and the successfully treated acute asthmatic infused with only 5% dextrose epitomize this form of metabolic alkalosis.

Villous Adenoma

These tumors are soft, broad-based papillomas, 90% of which are found within the rectosigmoid colon, and have a high degree of malignancy (44). They secrete 1–3 L/day, at times sufficient to produce hypotension or renal failure, contain mucus, and are rich in variable concentrations of Na^+, K^+, and Cl^- (45). Although these adenomas are more commonly associated with metabolic acidosis or a normal serum [HCO_3^-], a minority are associated with metabolic alkalosis (46). The feature(s) of these tumors and mechanism(s) that determine the nature of the acid–base disorder are uncertain. In most instances, the concentrations of Na^+ and Cl^- in the secretions are similar to those in serum. Potassium concentrations in the secretions range broadly from 15 to 120 mEq/L (46). Neither the degree of K^+ depletion nor the magnitude of Cl^- loss appears to be related to the presence of

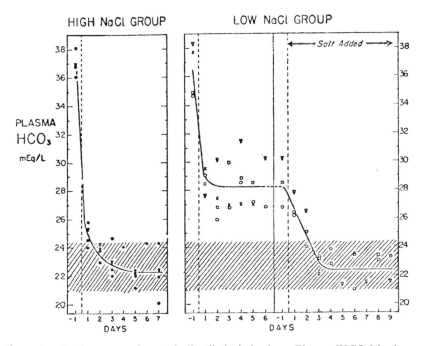

Figure 3 Posthypercapneic metabolic alkalosis in dogs. Plasma [HCO₃] is shown during recovery from chronic respiratory acidosis with a high or a low NaCl diet. When NaCl was restricted during and after respiratory acidosis, a residual metabolic alkalosis persisted after exposure to high CO₂ ceased on day 1. The alkalosis was corrected when NaCl is added to the diet. *Source*: From Ref. 68.

alkalosis or acidosis. Some degree of renal insufficiency is present in many cases as judged by serum urea nitrogen; this is likely due to hypovolemia. Patients with acidosis also appeared to have higher serum urea nitrogen (46). High concentrations of prostaglandins in both the secretions and the tumors may have some role in the pathophysiology (47) but not to the type of acid–base disorder, if present. Conceivably, the relative magnitudes of Cl^-, alkali, and K^+ losses in the secretions—perhaps related to tumor cell type—coupled with the intake of these electrolytes determine the type of associated acid–base disorder.

Chloridorrhea

Defective apical Cl^-/HCO_3^- exchange in the distal ileum and colon is the primary defect that causes congenital diarrhea with alkalosis (48). Gastric and jejunal ion transport are normal. This autosomal recessive disease (49) is caused by a mutation of the down-regulated in adenoma (DRA) gene (50), leading to a loss-of-function defect in the DRA anion exchanger and high fecal [Cl^-] (49). Although fecal [Na^+] and [K^+] are normal, the unremitting copious watery stool results also in Na$^+$, K$^+$, and volume losses. The renal response, mediated by aldosterone, is intense Na$^+$ and water reabsorption at the expense of H$^+$ and K$^+$ secretion thereby further promoting alkalosis. Maternal polyhydramnios and neonatal abdominal distention caused by dilated intestinal loops are important clues to the diagnosis (51).

Dietary Chloride Deficiency

The feeding of infants with formula made from soy protein and deficient in Cl$^-$ can cause metabolic alkalosis (52,53); these are the only reported instances of low dietary intake associated with alkalosis. The extraordinarily low Cl$^-$ content and high alkali content—as potassium citrate—in conjunction with vomiting in some instances resulted in serum [HCO$_3^-$] as high as 50 mEq/L, serum [K$^+$] <3.0 mEq/L, and urine [Cl$^-$] near 0 mEq/L with high urine pH. Infants afflicted by this severe alkalosis appear to have suffered no long-term consequences in either growth and development or renal function after up to 5 years of follow-up (54).

Cystic Fibrosis

This relatively common autosomal recessive disease (55) is associated with hypochloremia (56). Cystic fibrosis is characterized by high [Cl$^-$] in sweat, saliva, and other secretions (57). Skin Cl$^-$ losses due to excessive sweat Cl$^-$ particularly during warm weather can generate metabolic alkalosis; it is unclear whether renal K$^+$ wasting seen during heat stress also participates (58). Alkalosis may even be the presenting feature in adolescence with a few of the several hundred mutations in the cystic fibrosis transmembrane regulator (CFTR) gene (59,60).

MAINTENANCE

General

Before examining the systemic and renal responses to CDA, some intuitively obvious points should be mentioned. First, in any experimental model or clinical example of alkalosis, the manner in which alkalosis is generated must be considered because, if a deficit is not incurred during generation but appears during maintenance, that deficit is a result and not a cause of the alkalosis. In this regard, K$^+$ losses in CDA may be high and with chronic CDA, cumulative K$^+$ depletion may eventually contribute to the maintenance of metabolic alkalosis even though it was not the original cause (61). Likewise, primary K$^+$ depletion, if severe, may lead to renal Cl$^-$ wasting (4,62,63). Thus, cumulative severe deficits of one ion that can cause metabolic alkalosis may cause deficits of another causative ion by separate mechanisms and an alkalosis of dual etiology can develop. Under these circumstances, repletion of both ions, K^+ and Cl^-, is necessary to correct alkalosis completely. Second, retention of excess base during maintenance must be due to factors that, when corrected, result in removal of the excess and recovery to normal. This linkage between maintenance and correction has provided an important axiom for the study of the factors necessary to maintain alkalosis: A specific deficit cannot explain maintenance if alkalosis can be corrected while that deficit persists.

The cessation of events that generate alkalosis, such as the discontinuance of diuretics or nasogastric suction, is not usually accompanied by resolution of the alkalosis, unlike the usual course in metabolic acidosis. To account for the maintenance of metabolic alkalosis in these instances, the kidney must, a priori, retain HCO_3^- by either a decrease in filtered HCO_3^- or an increase in HCO_3^- reabsorption or both (64).

Concurrent deficits of Na^+, K^+ and fluid as well as Cl^- usually occur in CDA; this gives rise to the question as to which of these deficits is responsible for maintenance. In dogs rendered alkalotic by $NaNO_3$ infusion (65), gastric drainage (66), or prior hypercapnia (67–69) and maintained on chloride-deficient diets, the resultant alkalosis has been completely corrected by either NaCl or KCl despite persisting deficits of either Na^+ or K^+; volume contraction also occurred in some models (66). Furthermore, in men given chloruretic diuretics, infused with $NaNO_3$ (70), or selectively depleted of gastric HCl (71), alkalosis occurred despite replacement of Na^+ and K^+ losses and was completely corrected with either NaCl or KCl (71). These studies show that correction of CDA can be effected by the provision of Cl^- without repletion of either K^+ or Na^+; thus deficits of these cations—but not necessarily plasma or ECF volume depletion—cannot be specific causes of maintained alkalosis induced by Cl^- depletion (72). The issue of whether ECF volume depletion plays any role in the maintenance of CDA is discussed as follows.

Volume Hypothesis—Pro

In an effort to separate correction of volume depletion from Cl^- depletion, Cohen (73,74) maintained alkalosis for 5 days in dogs treated with ethacrynic acid by using a NaCl-deficient diet, and then expanded ECF volume with a fluid containing Cl^- and HCO_3^- in concentrations identical to that in the plasma of the alkalemic dogs. This design excluded the possibility that the plasma anion composition would be altered by the infused fluid. These "isometric" infusions completely corrected the alkalosis within 24 hr, without an increase in glomerular filtration rate (GFR) and despite increasing K^+ depletion; Cl^- repletion also occurred (Fig. 4).

Integrating these studies with the contemporarily known characteristics of fluid and electrolyte handling in the various nephron segments, the "volume" hypothesis was proposed in which the intranephronal redistribu-

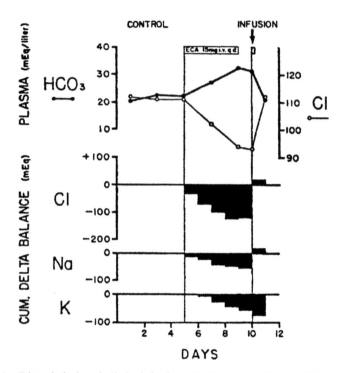

Figure 4 Diuretic-induced alkalosis in dogs. Daily plasma Cl and HCO$_3$ concentrations and cumulative net Na, K, and Cl balances are shown for the generation, maintenance, and correction phases of the study. Isometric volume repletion (infusate
electrolyte composition mirrors that of the ambient plasma composition in the maintenance phase) completely corrected alkalosis produced by ethacrynic acid. Note that
chloride repletion also occurred with this protocol and potassium balance became
more negative with correction. *Source*: From Ref. 73.

tion of fluid reabsorption plays the central role. According to this hypothesis,
ECF volume depletion accompanying alkalosis augments fluid reabsorption
in the proximal tubule where HCO$_3^-$ is preferentially reabsorbed compared
with Cl$^-$. The increased HCO$_3^-$ reabsorption in this segment serves to maintain the alkalosis (75). During correction, volume expansion decreases fluid
reabsorption in the proximal tubule and delivers more HCO$_3^-$ to the distal
nephron (76), where the capacity to reabsorb this anion is limited. As a result,
bicarbonaturia ensues correcting the alkalosis. This hypothesis downplays
any role for the incidental chloride repletion that occurs; volume expansion
is regarded as the impetus to the kidney for correction.

    Volume Hypothesis—Con

The volume hypothesis was advanced before the discovery of HCO$_3^-$ secretion in the collecting duct and identification of neutral Na$^+$-independent

anion exchangers in this segment of the nephron. Notwithstanding this advance, interpretation of the studies of Cohen is confounded in two important ways. First, Cl^- repletion accompanied volume repletion (73), thus vitiating any separation of the pathogenetic role of these two factors. Second, it is uncertain that the effects of volume expansion to increase delivery out of the proximal tubule without an increase in GFR was achieved (74) because aortic clamping before volume expansion is now known not to be associated with decreased proximal tubule fluid reabsorption (77,78). Data differ on whether volume expansion influences Cl^- reabsorption in the proximal tubule differently than it does HCO_3^- (79,80). Moreover, in apparent contradiction to the hypothesis that ECF volume expansion promotes HCO_3^- loss, metabolic acidosis also has been corrected by volume expansion with "isometric" solutions (81).

These concerns led to a reexamination of the volume hypothesis in CDA. Studies were carried out in both acute and chronic CDA produced in humans by diuretics and in rats by peritoneal dialysis that produces selective Cl^- depletion. In rats with CDA given a 70 mEq/L Cl^- solution ad libitum to drink as either a Na^+ or choline salt, acute CDA was completely corrected within 24 hr despite negative Na^+ and K^+ balances, decreased body weight, and, by experimental design, obligatory HCO_3^- loading (82). Chloride infusion did not correct CDA after acute bilateral nephrectomy in this model, showing that correction was dependent on a renal response (83).

To exclude a role for volume in the maintenance or correction in this model in a more rigorous manner, alkalotic rats were infused with 5% dextrose solutions containing either 6% albumin at 2.5 mL/hr/100 g body weight or an 80 mEq/L Cl^- solution as a mixture of Ca^{2+}, Mg^{2+}, Li^+ and K^+ salts at only 0.6 mL/hr/100 g body weight (84). In the rats infused with the albumin-containing solution, alkalosis was maintained despite a 15% plasma volume expansion and a normal GFR, whereas in those infused with the solution containing the Cl^- salts, alkalosis was corrected progressively with increased HCO_3^- excretion despite persisting volume contraction and a decreased GFR (Fig. 5).

In normal men with alkalosis induced by furosemide, maintained by dietary Cl^- restriction for 5 days (25), alkalosis was completely corrected as Cl^- was quantitatively repleted with KCl, similar to the studies of Kassirer et al. (70) (Fig. 2). Plasma volumes estimated serially by ^{131}I-albumin space and plasma albumin concentrations as well as GFR and estimated renal plasma flow decreased after generation and persisted throughout maintenance and correction (25). In five men treated with furosemide without Cl^- restriction, alkalosis did not develop and subsequent oral KCl loading did not produce any change in plasma electrolytes.

In chronic CDA, alkalosis, ECF volume contraction, and decreased GFR were observed in rats maintained for 7–10 days (85). Complete

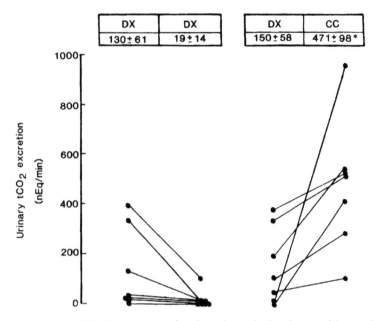

Figure 5 Urinary bicarbonate excretion in volume-depleted rats with or without chloride administration. Rats receiving chloride (CC) increased urinary bicarbonate excretion as alkalosis was corrected (data not shown) whereas those receiving only glucose (DX) had a further decrease while alkalosis was maintained (data not shown). *Source*: From Ref. 84.

correction was achieved over 24 hr with 70 mm choline chloride drinking solution despite negative Na^+ balance, neutral K^+ balance, continued HCO_3^- loading, persistent volume contraction, and a further decrease in GFR. In this chronic model, rats subjected to acute bilateral nephrectomy failed to correct CDA when infused with Cl^- thus excluding an extrarenal mechanism of correction.

Thus, these studies in rats and humans have separated repletion of ECF volume from Cl^- repletion and clearly show that CDA can be corrected by Cl^- administration without repair of ECF volume deficits. Correction occurs by a renal mechanism in both the acute and the chronic CDA model. These results extend the earlier conclusion of Kassirer and Schwartz (71): chloride is necessary and *sufficient* for the correction of CDA.

Other Hypotheses

Others have proposed a "cation-depletion" hypothesis (86,87) and in support of this concept, cite data showing that the low serum $[K^+]$ rises with the correction of alkalosis (25,84). While K^+ metabolism (but not repletion) may have an important role in correction and alkalosis may promote urinary K^+ wasting, the studies cited show persistent or increasing K^+ deficits in the face of the correction of CDA, which is clear evidence against a causative role for K^+ depletion in alkalosis generated in this manner. Early studies suggested that K^+ depletion is a consequence or accompaniment rather than a cause of CDA. Darrow (88) showed that muscle K^+ was replaced with Na^+ in rats rendered alkalotic by peritoneal dialysis with $NaHCO_3$ and Holliday concluded that CDA produced by peritoneal dialysis induced K^+ excretion resulting in intracellular K^+ depletion (89). In humans (25), KCl corrected CDA while equimolar KCl loading in subjects that were Na^+-depleted but not Cl^--depleted and alkalotic produced no change in systemic acid–base balance or in urinary net acid excretion. Furthermore, alkalotic subjects given neutral sodium phosphate experienced an increase in serum $[HCO_3^-]$ while ECF volume was expanded. Much earlier, K^+ depletion had been shown not to be a causative factor in the pathogenesis of CDA (71). Indeed, correction of K^+ depletion after correction of Cl^- depletion actually may induce alkalosis in dogs (90). Chloride with any of several different cations under a variety of conditions has been reported to correct CDA whereas no cation administered without chloride has been shown to do so under any condition.

Volume Distribution

The concept that Cl^- is necessary and sufficient for the correction of CDA should not be construed to indicate that volume and alkalosis are unrelated; they may be associated events. Borkan et al. produced CDA in dogs by isovolemic hemofiltration in which the replacement solution contained HCO_3^- as the only anion (91). Cumulative Na^+ balance was decreased by $23\,mEq/20\,kg$ body weight whereas ECF volume was decreased by $409\,mL/20\,kg$ body weight as estimated by Cl^- space. In similar studies in nephrectomized dogs (38), ECF volume decreased by $360\,mL/20\,kg$ body weight as estimated by ^3H-mannitol space (92). Because urinary losses cannot explain the reduction in ECF volume, the latter must be linked to the movement of solute and fluid from the ECF into the intracellular space in the setting of Cl^- depletion or alkalosis in the ECF.

Although the cellular mechanism(s) by which Cl^- depletion or alkalosis may be associated with fluid shifts between body compartments is unclear, both cell volume and intracellular pH may be regulated by some of the same transport systems (93–95). Furthermore, maintenance of intracellular volume has been associated with transport of both Cl^- and HCO_3^- across the cell membrane. For example, when Cl^- is partially replaced in the medium by an anion with a different reflection coefficient, a different steady state cell volume may be attained (95). The result may be cell shrinkage when the substitute is nonpermeant, such as gluconate, or cell swelling when it is more permeant, such as acetate. While extrapolation from in vitro studies such as these to systemic in vivo events is problematic, it is plausible that alterations in volume detected in both the intracellular and extracellular compartments may occur as a consequence of changes in extracellular anion composition and without an alteration in total body water rather than vice versa. In this context, these shifts may have a role in the corrective response. However, rather than "contraction alkalosis," this association may be more aptly termed "alkalotic contraction."

The foregoing data reinforce the conclusion that Cl^- depletion is necessary and sufficient to maintain CDA by a renal mechanism. Although volume depletion and a fall in GFR are commonly associated phenomenon, CDA is corrected by Cl^- administration by a renal effect even if GFR and ECF volume are declining or, at least, persisting at a level less than normal.

The Role of GFR

The mechanism(s) by which the kidney maintains CDA is not completely understood. A reduction in GFR would serve to maintain alkalosis simply by decreasing filtered HCO_3^-. Although early studies (65,70,71,96) showed no evidence for a decreased GFR in humans and dogs with CDA, more recent studies that focused specifically on GFR have shown a decrease in humans with diuretic-induced alkalosis (25,97). Certainly, the decrease in ECF volume that often accompanies CDA can result in a decrease in GFR. However, with persistent decreases in ECF volume and renal blood flow, GFR does not necessarily return to normal during or immediately after complete correction of CDA by Cl^- administration (25).

In rats with CDA, single nephron GFR decreases linearly as alkalosis and hypochloremia become progressively more severe (98). However, when tubule fluid flow to the macula densa of the juxtaglomerular apparatus is blocked, this effect on single nephron GFR is abolished, supporting the hypothesis that GFR is decreased by regulation through the tubuloglomerular feedback mechanism (99). This mechanism, when activated, decreases GFR and thereby serves to reduce losses of Na^+, K^+, and HCO_3^- during the disequilibrium phase of CDA. The afferent signal for tubuloglomerular feedback to decrease GFR appears to be increased delivery to and reabsorption of Na^+ via luminal membrane Na^+, K^+, $2Cl^-$ and NHE2 transporters (with either Cl^- or HCO_3^-) in the macula densa cells (100,101). Because renin stimulation by the macula densa cells is dependent on Cl^- delivery and uptake, renin and therefore angiotensin levels also remain high in CDA. High angiotensin II levels further increase the tubuloglomerular feedback signal to decrease GFR. Thus, a fall in GFR in CDA appears to be due to a specific intrarenal mechanism and is not necessarily dependent on, or caused by, ECF volume contraction.

In chronic CDA, GFR increases progressively and may exceed normal (102,103) at least in a rat model of diuretic-induced CDA. Because this model is associated with progressive K^+ depletion, a potent stimulus to kidney growth, the role of the chronicity of alkalosis vs. progressive K^+ depletion to effect the return of GFR to normal in prolonged experimental metabolic alkalosis is not settled.

The Renin–Aldosterone Axis

The renin–angiotensin–aldosterone axis is also implicated in the maintenance of CDA (104): Chloride depletion is a potent stimulus to renin release in the rat model of CDA (105) and presumably is associated with high angiotensin II (ANG II) levels, a potent regulator of proximal tubule HCO_3^- reabsorption (106). To examine the importance of the effect of ANG II specifically on CDA, saralasin or enalapril in doses that modestly decrease blood pressure was given to rats with CDA (107). If ANG II were important to maintenance, its blockade should promote correction. However, no correction was noted. In addition, ANG II in subpressor doses (107) was infused into rats in which correction was being effected by the infusion of an $80\,mEq/L$ Cl^- solution. Again, inhibition of the corrective response would be expected but correction was not prevented or blunted. Further, although saralasin infusion may inhibit HCO_3^- reabsorption in the proximal tubule and thereby increase HCO_3^- delivery to the distal convolution and to the urine, alkalosis persists. Thus, ANG II appears to have no notable role in the maintenance or correction of CDA.

Plasma aldosterone levels eventually fall during sustained CDA in humans and administration of excess aldosterone during the maintenance period failed to increase either net acid excretion or the degree of metabolic alkalosis (108). Furthermore, complete correction was effected by NaCl replacement despite continued administration of excess aldosterone (108). In other studies in men with CDA, correction of alkalosis was achieved by KCl despite a marked increase in plasma aldosterone concentrations (25). Thus, high aldosterone levels appear to be unnecessary for maintenance of CDA, and Cl^- administration can correct CDA despite rising concentrations.

The Role of Tubule Reabsorption—The Proximal Tubule

The absence of a clear regulatory role for GFR focuses attention on tubule reabsorptive mechanisms for Cl^- and HCO_3^-. During maintained CDA, the proximal tubule does not adjust Cl^- or HCO_3^- reabsorption to effect a corrective response (84,109–112). Even when GFR and filtered HCO_3^- rise after 3 or 4 weeks of maintained CDA, HCO_3^- reabsorption increases in response to the increase in HCO_3^- delivery (111). Although the proximal tubule reabsorbs most of the filtered load of HCO_3^- and Cl^-, the corrective response and maintenance also appears to be mediated at more distal nephron sites (see below).

Henle's Loop

In the TAL of Henle's loop, HCO_3^- is reabsorbed by an apical Na^+/H^+ exchanger and by a basolateral $Na^+–HCO_3^-$ cotransporter (113) (see Chapter 4 for more detail). In the loop segment in acute CDA (84) and the TAL in chronic CDA (114), HCO_3^- reabsorption decreases in contrast to an increase that occurs during chronic oral $NaHCO_3$ or NaCl loading (114). Nevertheless, fractional HCO_3^- and Cl^- reabsorptions did not differ between normal and alkalotic rats whether alkalosis was being maintained or corrected (84,103,110,112). Thus, HCO_3^- reabsorption in the TAL does not appear to be regulated in CDA.

Distal Convolution

In the DCT, the data on HCO_3^- transport are not consonant. Acute alkalosis does not influence HCO_3^- reabsorption when delivery is controlled (115). However, after 4 weeks of alkalosis, HCO_3^- delivery to and reabsorption in the DCT increased but fractional HCO_3^- reabsorption did not (103). With delivery controlled by in vivo microperfusion, alkali loading induced HCO_3^- secretion in the DCT when fluid and electrolyte deliveries are modified (116). Removal of Cl^- from the perfusion fluid inhibited HCO_3^- secretion and increased HCO_3^- reabsorption while a high Cl^- perfusate caused net HCO_3^- secretion in the usually reabsorbing DCT; this effect occurs in the connecting tubule and early CCD (see later) , segments that are likely included in these in vivo microperfusion studies (115). Thus, while the DCT appears to have the capability to alter HCO_3^- transport under certain conditions, delivery of Cl^- and HCO_3^- to this segment of the nephron in acute CDA does not differ in rats with maintained vs. correcting alkalosis (117). In addition, in acute CDA, delivery of HCO_3^- to the distal nephron determined by micropuncture of the tip of Henle's loop of juxtamedullary nephrons was lower in rats with increased HCO_3^- excretion while correcting the alkalosis (117). Thus, contributions from the DCT are likely to emanate from the connecting tubule or earliest portions of the CCD, which appears to play a dominant role, and both superficial and deep nephrons appear to respond to CDA in a similar manner.

The cortical collecting duct (CCD)—unlike any other nephron segment—can absorb or secrete HCO_3^- depending on the conditions imposed and the species studied (118–121). The CCD contains both type A and type B IC. The type A ICs secrete H^+ into the tubule lumen while reabsorbing HCO_3^- into the blood in exchange for Cl^- across the basolateral membrane; type B ICs secrete HCO_3^- into the tubule lumen in exchange for reabsorbing Cl^- and reabsorb H^+ into the blood across the basolateral

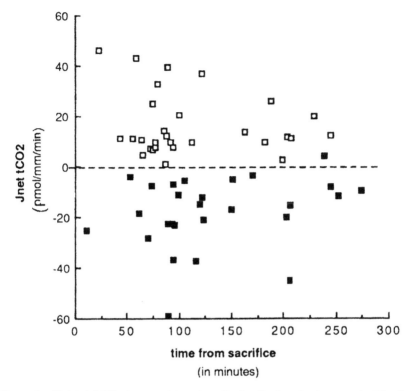

Figure 6 Net total CO_2 transport in rat cortical collecting duct segments. Bicarbonate reabsorption was sustained in tubules from normal rats (□) whereas secretion was sustained in tubules from rats with CDA (■). *Source*: From Ref. 125.

membrane (122–124) (see Chapter 4). The unique capability to alter the magnitude and direction of HCO_3^- transport in the CCD accords a potential paramount importance to this segment for the regulation of renal Cl^- and HCO_3^- excretion.

Certain experimental models may not approximate clinical settings and, therefore, results from them should be interpreted with caution. Oral HCO_3^- or deoxycorticosterone administration may not produce metabolic alkalosis and yet may be associated with alterations in either Na^+ delivery to or transport in the CCD. In contrast, experimental as well as clinical CDA is associated with systemic metabolic alkalosis, and, depending on conditions of the experiment, Na^+ avidity and volume depletion.

CCD obtained from rats with CDA and perfused in vitro show sustained HCO_3^- secretion, a finding that is dependent on luminal $[Cl^-]$, compared to CCD from normal rats, which show sustained HCO_3^- reabsorption, independent of luminal $[Cl^-]$ (Fig. 6) (125). Furthermore, the magnitude and direction of HCO_3^- transport in vitro correlates with in vivo serum $[HCO_3^-]$ and $[Cl^-]$ and Cl^- balance and not with K^+ balance (126). These data suggest that the mechanisms for regulating transport can "sense" the degree of alkalosis or Cl^- balance in vivo. The factors that are responsible for this regulation of HCO_3^- transport in the CCD remain poorly understood. The K_m for $[Cl^-]$ in the CCD luminal anion exchanger in the rabbit has been estimated to be between 20 and 55 mEq/L (127). These concentrations are within the range that would allow changes in Cl^- delivery to the CCD to regulate HCO_3^- secretion.

The OMCD possesses only type A ICs and therefore only reabsorbs HCO_3^- (128). Removal of luminal Cl^- increases HCO_3^- reabsorption in the rabbit OMCD (129); in rats with acute CDA, HCO_3^- uptake is decreased (130). In the inner medullary collecting duct (IMCD) , the initial segment also possesses type A ICs, and HCO_3^- reabsorption decreases in acute and chronic metabolic alkalosis (130,131). In the papillary collecting duct, Cl^- is intensely conserved in animals ingesting a low Cl^- diet (132). In the terminal portion of the IMCD, net HCO_3^- reabsorption occurs even though ICs are not identified in this segment (133). While the role of these medullary segments in the pathophysiology of CDA is unclear, in view of their capacity to transport Cl^- and HCO_3^-, it seems likely that they participate in a coordinated collecting duct response along with the CCD.

The pathways for HCO_3^- reabsorption and secretion in the collecting duct are complex (134) and new ones continue to be identified (135–139). Protons can be secreted by either H^+ ATPase or HKA, both of which appear to be heterogeneous along the collecting duct (see Chapters 4 and 5 for more detail). While H^+ ATPase is present all along the collecting duct, the isoform in the IMCD differs immunohistologically from that in the more proximal segments of the CD (140). At least two isoforms of HKA, gastric (g) and colonic (c) have been identified (134); gHKA is inhibited by Schering 28080 (SCH) but not by ouabain (OUA) and cHKA is inhibited by OUA and not SCH (141,142). A third isoform of HKA is probably present along the CD as well (135,138). Other anion exchangers identified in this segment include pendrin in the CCD, which is likely a luminal HCO_3^-/Cl^- exchanger in the type B IC (136) and AE4, a member of the HCO_3^- transporter superfamily, also in the apical membrane of type B IC (139).

In perfused CCD from rats with acute CDA, SCH completely inhibits HCO_3^- reabsorption, which suggests that some isoform of HKA on the basolateral membrane is primarily responsible for HCO_3^- secretion (125); presently there are no immunohistologic studies to support these functional studies. In the OMCD and IMCD, HCO_3^- reabsorption is decreased in tubules obtained from rats with CDA (143) (In these studies, tubules were perfused and bathed with fluid with containing 100 mm $[Cl^-]$, a much higher concentration than is seen in this segment of the nephron under normal or alkalotic conditions.) Northern hybridization studies show that the cHKA isoform is expressed in the OMCD and the IMCD in tubules from rats with CDA (144) and morphological studies show hypertrophy and increased staining for the H^+ ATPase of the basolateral area in the type B IC of the CCD in CDA rats. Simultaneously, H^+ ATPase is diminished in the luminal membrane of type A ICs but increased in subapical vesicles in both the CCD and OMCD, suggesting removal from the cell membrane. Clearly, the available studies of the role of these transport proteins in the pathophysiology of CDA have only scratched the surface of what is likely to be a complex and highly orchestrated response by the kidney.

In summary, a current overview of the proposed pathophysiology of the maintenance and correction of CDA is as follows. Although the proximal tubule and Henle's loop reabsorb the vast proportion of the filtered Cl^- and HCO_3^-, the primary regulatory adjustments to Cl^- and HCO_3^- transport to maintain or correct CDA appear to occur in the more distal nephron. Prior to the administration of Cl^-, the type B IC is "poised to secrete" HCO_3^- via the luminal anion exchanger with HCO_3^- secretion facilitated by increasing H^+ ATPase activity at the basolateral membrane. When Cl^- is given, this anion corrects CDA without a necessary change in volume or GFR by an effect on the CCD and probably the DCT (103,115,145) to secrete HCO_3^-, and by an effect on the OMCD and IMCD to diminish reabsorption of HCO_3^-. Urine Cl^- excretion in CDA remains low until plasma $[Cl^-]$ approaches normal (98) and, in Cl^- depletion, Cl^- uptake in the collecting duct is greatly accelerated (131,146). In in vivo studies, Cl^- delivery to the CCD increased (84)—albeit not statistically significantly—by an amount consistent in magnitude with the increase in net HCO_3^- secretion seen in CCD harvested from CDA animals (125) and the magnitude of HCO_3^- secretion in vitro, in turn, is comparable to the increase in HCO_3^- excretion (84). While the collecting duct possesses an array of anion and H^+ transporters that respond to acid–base disorders in general and CDA in particular, the integrated response of the several segments to maintain and then correct CDA is not yet understood. A major unresolved question is how the kidney recognizes that Cl^- is being repleted at concentrations at or less than that in ambient plasma (64).

MANAGEMENT

For full correction of Cl^- depletion metabolic alkalosis, the Cl^- deficit must be replaced. Judicious selection of the accompanying cation—Na^+, K^+, H^+ or other—is dependent on assessment of: (i) ECF volume status; (ii) the presence and degree of associated K^+ depletion; and (iii) the degree and reversibility of any depression of GFR (Fig. 7). If the kidney is capable of excreting Na^+ and K^+, HCO_3^- and base equivalents will be excreted with any of those cations and metabolic alkalosis rapidly corrected as Cl^- is

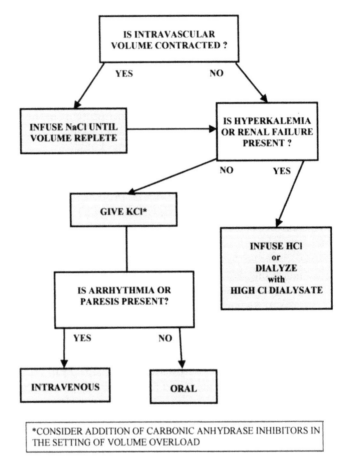

Figure 7 Decision algorithm for the selection of appropriate intervention to correct chloride-depletion alkalosis. See text for details.

made available. When renal function is severely depressed by acute or chronic intrinsic renal disease, or in the presence of intractable congestive cardiac failure, or when hyperkalemia is present, it may be necessary to avoid the administration of Na^+ or K^+.

In the most common clinical setting, Cl^- and ECF volume depletion coexist and administration of isotonic NaCl is the appropriate therapy. It will simultaneously correct both deficits as well as any associated depression in GFR. In patients with overt signs of volume contraction such as hypotension, tachycardia, and diminished skin turgor, the administration of a minimum of 3–5 L of isotonic NaCl is usually necessary to correct both the volume deficit and the metabolic alkalosis. Fluid therapy should be pressed aggressively until signs of hypovolemia are reversed. Replacement of continuing losses of electrolytes (e.g., K^+; see below) must be included in the regimen. As the Cl^- deficit is corrected, a brisk alkaline diuresis should occur with a fall in plasma [HCO_3^-].

If CDA occurs in a setting in which ECF volume is assessed as normal, total body Cl^- deficit can be estimated by the formula: body weight (kg) $\times$ 0.2 $\times$ the desired increment in the plasma [Cl^-] (mEq/L). Although not essential for correction of CDA, correction of K^+ depletion is indicated. Potassium excretion may remain high as plasma volume and GFR are restored to normal. Potassium losses can be replaced conveniently by adding KCl usually in a concentration of 10–20 mEq/L of infused fluid to the regimen; serum [K^+] should be followed carefully. Potassium should not be infused intravenously at rates >20 mEq/hr (147). Recommendations for oral replacement are presented in Chapter 18 (148).

If CDA occurs in the clinical setting of volume overload or congestive heart failure, administration of NaCl is clearly inadvisable. If hypokalemia is present, KCl should be used for Cl^- repletion. If hyperkalemia is present or if the ability to excrete K^+ is of concern due to the presence of renal insufficiency, two therapeutic options are available: (i) infusion of Cl^- as HCl (149) or NH_4Cl, or (ii) provision of Cl^- by peritoneal dialysis, hemodialysis, or hemodiafiltration so that K^+ and Na^+ balance, and plasma volume can be contemporaneously corrected.

Intravenous HCl is indicated if there is an immediate need for correction, such as when arterial pH is >7.55, and when both NaCl and KCl are contraindicated. Some have used HCl infusions to improve oxygenation in respiratory acidosis at lesser degrees of alkalemia (150). The presence of hepatic encephalopathy, cardiac arrhythmia, digitalis cardiotoxicity, or altered mental status all would call for emergency treatment (149). HCl in a 0.1 or 0.2 M solution is appropriate; higher concentrations of HCl have been used (151) but associated with deterioration of some catheter materials and should be avoided (152). The amount of HCl needed to correct alkalosis is calculated by the formula: 0.5 $\times$ body weight (kg) $\times$ desired decrement in plasma [HCO_3^-] (mEq/L); this formula does consider continuing losses. The use of 50% of body weight as the volume of distribution of infused H^+ is based upon the intra- and extracellular buffer response to the added acid (see Chapter 6). Because the goal of HCl administration is to rescue the patient from severe alkalosis, it is prudent to plan initially to restore the plasma [HCO_3^-] halfway toward normal. HCl must be given through a catheter placed in the vena cava or a large vein draining into it. Catheter placement should be confirmed radiographically because leakage of HCl outside the vein can lead to sloughing of perivascular tissue (153); in the mediastinum this would be catastrophic. The infusion rate should not exceed 0.2 mEq/kg body weight/hr (154). The patient is best managed in an intensive care unit with frequent measurement of blood pH, $PaCO_2$ and electrolytes.

An alternative to HCl is NH_4Cl, which may be infused into a peripheral vein; the rate of infusion should not exceed 300 mEq/24 hr. NH_4Cl is contraindicated in the presence of renal or hepatic insufficiency (155). In concurrent renal failure, azotemia is worsened and, in hepatic failure, acute NH_3 intoxication with coma could result. Lysine or arginine HCl should be avoided because these agents can cause dangerous hyperkalemia (156).

If GFR is adequate (serum creatinine concentration <4.0 mg/dL), acetazolamide 250 mg twice or thrice daily orally or 5–10 mg/kg intravenously (157) may be effective in producing a $NaHCO_3$ diuresis, by inhibiting carbonic anhydrase (158,159). Because the distal nephron can avidly reabsorb the excess Na^+ delivery promoted by acetazolamide, which inhibits Na^+ uptake primarily in the proximal tubule, the carbonic anhydrase inhibitors are most effective when used in conjunction with diuretics that have more distal sites of action (160,161). Acetazolamide could also be used intermittently to avoid or lessen CDA in edema-forming states such as congestive heart failure treated with loop diuretics. Plasma electrolyte composition should be followed serially during its administration because acetazolamide is usually associated with high urine K^+ losses.

Acetazolamide is particularly useful, for example, in a patient with chronic obstructive pulmonary disease and cor pulmonale who develops metabolic alkalosis after therapeutic correction of acute CO_2 retention and in the presence of hyperkalemia. Carbonic anhydrase in erythrocytes and along the pulmonary capillary endothelium participates in the dehydration of HCO_3^- to CO_2 and excretion of CO_2 by the lung. In vitro studies of inhibited erythrocytes (162) and lungs inhibited by acetazolamide (163) show significant decreases and delays in CO_2 excretion. While these acute studies have been confirmed in normal humans (164), studies in critically ill patients have shown only minor CO_2 retention (165). Clinicians should be alert to the potential of CO_2 retention with acetazolamide, particularly in patients with impaired respiratory function. In such cases, the goal of treatment is to reduce plasma $[HCO_3^-]$ only to the level appropriate to that patient's chronic hypercapnia and not to normal.

When the kidney is incapable of responding to Cl^- repletion or dialysis is necessary for the control of renal failure, exchange of HCO_3^- for Cl^- by hemodialysis (166) or peritoneal dialysis (167) can correct metabolic alkalosis. The dialysate solutions used for both peritoneal dialysis and hemodialysis contain HCO_3^- or its metabolic precursors, such as lactate, in concentrations ranging from 25 to 40 mEq/L and, thus, have to be modified to lower serum $[HCO_3^-]$ in patients with metabolic alkalosis; the acid concentrate from a two-part HCO_3^- mix has successfully been used to correct alkalosis (168). Hemodiafiltration with a high-flux dialyzer and high volumes of isotonic saline replacement fluid is also effective and seems the most readily available current technique (169). In an emergency, peritoneal dialysis could be performed using sterile 0.15 M NaCl as a bath solution of with appropriate attention to plasma $[K^+]$, $[Ca^{2+}]$ and $[Mg^{2+}]$ by intravenous infusion.

Additional interventions are appropriate in certain specific clinical situations associated with CDA. In the presence of pernicious vomiting or the need for the continual removal of gastric secretions, metabolic alkalosis will continue to be generated and replacement of preexisting deficits will be counteracted by these losses. In such circumstances, administration of an H2-receptor blocker, such as cimetidine (170) or ranitidine, or an H^+/K^+ ATPase inhibitor, such as omeprazole, will blunt acid production by the stomach and thereby decrease gastric HCl losses (171). Omeprazole has been used effectively to treat alkalosis after gastrocystoplasty (172) as well as in the Zollinger–Ellison syndrome. Octreotide has also proven beneficial in controlling hypergastrinemia, thus providing an alternative to surgery (173). Even in the presence of these agents, gastric secretions may contain significant amounts of Na^+, K^+, and Cl^-. An array of antiemetics also are available that may help decrease nausea and vomiting (174). Obviously, medications that promote nausea and vomiting should be omitted whenever possible.

Villous adenomas require surgical removal after correction of the Na^+, Cl^-, K^+, and volume deficits. Chloridorrhea has been responsive to continued repletion of fluid, Cl^- and K^+ losses by dietary supplementation; antidiarrheal agents are ineffective. Omeprazole can decrease stool electrolyte losses in patients with congenital chloridorrhea (175). The proposed mechanism is the reduction in the amount Cl^- delivered to the small intestine.

With diuretic-induced losses, KCl is usually needed when deficits are clinically significant. The role of hypokalemia in the genesis of cardiac arrhythmias (26,176) and the need to supplement K^+ for the amelioration of essential hypertension (177,178) must be balanced against the risks of hyperkalemia; these issues have been the topic of vigorous debate and controversy (26). When chloruretic diuretics are being abused—overtly or surreptitiously—the patient will probably require intensive counseling to effect a behavioral change.

REFERENCES

1. Seldin DW, Rector FC Jr. The generation and maintenance of metabolic alkalosis. Kidney Int 1972; 1:306–321.
2. Gamble JL, Ross SG. The factors in the dehydration following pyloric obstruction. J Clin Invest 1925; 1:403–423.
3. Howe CT, Le Quesne LP. Pyloric stenosis: the metabolic effects. Br J Surg 1964; 51:923–932.
4. Luke RG, Wright FS, Fowler N, Kashgarian M, Giebisch G. Effects of potassium depletion on tubular chloride transport in the rat. Kidney Int 1978; 14:414–427.

5. Gamble JL, McIver MA. The acid–base composition of gastric secretions. J Exp Med 1928; 48:837–847.
6. DelValle J, Lucey MR, Yamada T. Gastric secretion. In: Yamada T, ed. Textbook of Gastroenterology. 2nd ed. Philadelphia: JB Lippincott Co., 1995: 295–326.
7. Ariel IM. The effects of acute hypochloremia on the distribution of body fluid and composition of tissue electrolytes in man. Ann Surg 1954; 140:150–163.
8. Rune SJ. Comparison of the rates of gastric acid secretion in man after ingestion of food and after maximal stimulation with histamine. Gut 1966; 7:344–350.
9. Fordtran JS, Walsh JH. Gastric acid secretion rate and buffer content of the stomach after eating: results in normal subjects and in patients with duodenal ulcer. J Clin Invest 1973; 52:645–657.
10. Preshaw RM, Cooke AR, Grossman MI. Quantitative aspects of response of canine pancreas to duodenal acidification. Am J Physiol 1966; 210:629–634.
11. Wallmark B, Larsson H, Humble L. The relationship between gastric acid secretion and gastric H^+,K^+-ATPase activity. J Biol Chem 1985; 260: 13681–13684.
12. Jons T, Warrings B, Jons A, Drenckhahn D. Basolateral localization of anion exchanger 2 (AE2) and actin in acid-secreting (parietal) cells of the human stomach. Histochemistry 1994; 102:255–263.
13. Stuart-Tilley A, Sardet C, Pouyssegur J, Schwartz MA, Brown D, Alper SL. Immunolocalization of anion exchanger AE2 and cation exchanger NHE-1 in distinct adjacent cells of gastric mucosa. Am J Physiol 1994; 266:C559–C568.
14. MacCallum WG, Lintz J, Vermilye HN, Leggett TH, Boas E. The effect of pyloric obstruction in relation to gastric tetany. Bull Johns Hopkins Hosp 1920; 31:1–7.
15. Oster JR. The binge-purge syndrome: a common albeit unappreciated cause of acid–base and fluid–electrolyte disturbances. South Med J 1987; 80:58–67.
16. Eastwood GL. Stomach: anatomy and structural anomalies. In: Yamada T, ed. Textbook of Gastroenterology. 2nd ed. Philadelphia: JB Lippincott Co., 1995:1312–1313.
17. Weber HC, Orbuch M, Jensen RT. Diagnosis and management of Zollinger–Ellison syndrome. Semin Gastrointest Dis 1995; 6:79–89.
18. Bogaert GA, Mevorach RA, Kim J, Kogan BA. The physiology of gastrocystoplasty: once a stomach, always a stomach. J Urol 1995; 153:1977–1980.
19. Plawker MW, Rabinowitz SS, Etwaru DJ, Glassberg KI. Hypergastrinemia, dysuria–hematuria and metabolic alkalosis: complications associated with gastrocystoplasty. J Urol 1995; 154:546–549.
20. Mingin GC, Stock JA, Hanna MK. Gastrocystoplasty: long-term complications in 22 patients. J Urol 1999; 162:1122–1125.
21. Ellison DH. The physiologic basis of diuretic synergism: its role in treating diuretic resistance. Ann Int Med 1991; 114:886–894.
22. Hropot M, Fowler N, Karlmark B, Giebisch G. Tubular action of diuretics: distal effects on electrolyte transport and acidification. Kidney Int 1985; 28:477–489.
23. Puschett JB, Goldberg M. The acute effects of furosemide on acid and electrolyte excretion in man. J Lab Clin Med 1968; 71:666–677.

24. Stein JH, Wilson CB, Kirkendall WM. Differences in the acute effects of furosemide and ethacrynic acid in man. J Lab Clin Med 1968; 71:654–665.
25. Rosen RA, Julian BA, Dubovsky EA, Galla JH, Luke RG. On the mechanism by which chloride corrects metabolic alkalosis in man. Am J Med 1988; 84:449–458.
26. Kassirer JP, Harrington JT. Diuretics and potassium metabolism: a reassessment of the need, effectiveness and safety of potassium therapy. Kidney Int 1977; 11:505–515.
27. Heller I, Halevy J, Cohen S, Theodor E. Significant metabolic acidosis induced by acetazolamide. Not a rare complication. Arch Int Med 1985; 145:1815–1817.
28. Gabow PA, Moore S, Schrier RW. Spironolactone-induced hyperchloremic acidosis in cirrhosis. Ann Int Med 1979; 90:338–340.
29. Stone DK, Seldin DW, Kokko JP, Jacobson HR. Mineralocorticoid modulation of rabbit medullary collecting duct acidification. J Clin Invest 1983; 72:77–83.
30. Stone DK, Crider BP, Xie X-S. Aldosterone and urinary acidification. Semin Nephrol 1990; 10:375–379.
31. Eiam-Ong S, Kurtzman NA, Sabatini S. Regulation of collecting tubule adenosine triphosphatases by aldosterone and potassium. J Clin Invest 1993; 91:2385–2392.
32. Cooke RE, Segar WE, Cheek DB, Coville FE, Darrow DC. The extrarenal correction of alkalosis associated with potassium deficiency. J Clin Invest 1952; 31:798–805.
33. Chan YL, Biagi B, Giebisch G. Control mechanism of bicarbonate transport across the rat proximal convoluted tubule. Am J Physiol 1982; 242:F532–F543.
34. Soleimani M, Bergman JA, Hosford MA, McKinney TD. Potassium depletion increases luminal Na^+–H^+ exchange and basolateral Na^+:CO_3^-:HCO_3 cotransport in rat renal cortex. J Clin Invest 1990; 86:1076–1083.
35. Capasso G, Jaeger P, Giebisch G, Guckian V, Malnic G. Renal bicarbonate reabsorption in the rat. II. Distal tubule load dependence and effect of hypokalemia. J Clin Invest 1987; 80:409–414.
36. Carter NW, Seldin DW, Teng HC. Tissue and renal response to chronic respiratory acidosis. J Clin Invest 1959; 78:949–960.
37. Levitin H, Branscome W, Epstein FH. The pathogenesis of hypochloremia in respiratory acidosis. J Clin Invest 1958; 37:1667–1675.
38. Cogan MG. Effects of acute alterations in PCO2 on proximal HCO_3^-, Cl^-, and H_2O reabsorption. Am J Physiol 1984; 246:F21–F26.
39. Wingo CS. Effect of acidosis on chloride transport in the cortical thick ascending limb of Henle perfused in vitro. J Clin Invest 1986; 78:1324–1330.
40. Madsen KM, Tisher CC. Cellular response to acute respiratory acidosis in rat medullary collecting duct. Am J Physiol 1983; 245:F670–F679.
41. Verlander JW, Madsen KM, Tisher CC. Effect of acute respiratory acidosis on two populations of intercalated cells in the rat cortical collecting duct. Am J Physiol 1987; 253:F1142–F1156.
42. Laski ME, Kurtzman NA. Collecting tubule adaptation to respiratory acidosis induced in vivo. Am J Physiol 1990; 258:F15–F20.

43. Teixeira da Silva JC, Perrone RD, Johns CA, Madias NE. Rat kidney band 3 mRNA modulation in chronic respiratory acidosis. Am J Physiol 1991; 260:F204–F209.
44. Quan SHQ, Castro EB. Papillary adenomas (villous tumors): a review of 215 cases. Dis Colon Rectum 1971; 14:267–280.
45. Shnitka TK, Freidman MHW, Kidd EG, MacKenzie WC. Villous tumors of the rectum and colon characterized by severe fluid and electrolyte loss. Surg Gynecol Obstet 1961; 112:609–621.
46. Babior BM. Villous adenoma of the colon. Am J Med 1966; 41:615–621.
47. Steven K, Lange P, Bukhave K, Rask-Madsen J. Prostaglandin E2-mediated secretory diarrhea in villous adenoma of rectum: effect of treatment with indomethacin. Gastroenterology 1981; 80:1562–1566.
48. Bieberdorf FA, Gorden P, Fordtran JS. Pathogenesis of congenital alkalosis with diarrhea. Implications for the physiology of normal ileal electrolyte absorption and secretion. J Clin Invest 1972; 51:1958–1968.
49. Holmberg C, Perheentupa J, Launiala K, Hallman N. Congenital chloride diarrhea. Clinical analysis of 21 Finnish patients. Arch Dis Child 1977; 52:255–267.
50. Hoglund P, Haila S, Socha J, Tomaszewski L, Saarialho-Kere U, Karjalainen-Lindsberg ML, Airola K, Holmberg C, de la Chapelle A, Kere J. Mutations of the down-regulated in adenoma (DRA) gene cause congenital chloride diarrhoea. Nat Genet 1996; 14:316–319.
51. Badawi MH, Zaki M, Ismail EA, Majid Molla A. Congenital chloride diarrhea in Kuwait: a clinical reappraisal. J Trop Pediatr 1998; 44:296–299.
52. Roy S III, Arant BS Jr. Alkalosis from chloride-deficient Neo-Mull-Soy. N Engl J Med 1979; 301:615.
53. Wolfsdorf JI, Senior B. Failure to thrive and metabolic alkalosis. Adverse effects of a chloride-deficient formula in two infants. J Am Med Assoc 1980; 243:1068–1070.
54. Malloy MH. The follow-up of infants exposed to chloride-deficient formulas. Adv Pediatr 1993; 40:141–158.
55. National Institutes of Health Consensus Development Conference. Genetic testing for cystic fibrosis. National Institutes of Health Consensus Development Conference Statement on genetic testing for cystic fibrosis. Arch Intern Med 1999; 159:1529–1539.
56. Kessler WR, Anderson DH. Heat prostration in fibrocystic disease of the pancreas and other conditions. Pediatrics 1951; 8:648–655.
57. Koch C, Høiby N. Pathogenesis of cystic fibrosis. Lancet 1993; 339:1065–1069.
58. Bates CM, Quigley R, Baum M. Cystic fibrosis presenting with hypokalemia and metabolic alkalosis in a previously healthy adolescent. J Am Soc Nephrol 1997; 8:352–355.
59. Sojo A, Rodriguez-Soriano J, Vitoria JC, Vazquez C, Ariceta G, Villate A. Chloride deficiency as a presentation or complication of cystic fibrosis. Eur J Pediatr 1994; 153:825–828.
60. Pedroli G, Liechti-Gallati S, Birrer P, Kraemer R, Foletti-Jaggi C, Bianchetti MG. Chronic metabolic alkalosis: not uncommon in young children with severe cystic fibrosis. Am J Nephrol 1995; 15:245–250.

61. Wall BM, Williams HH, Cooke CR. Chloride-resistant metabolic alkalosis in an adult with congenital chloride diarrhea. Am J Med 1988; 85:570–572.
62. Garella S, Chazan JA, Cohen JJ. Saline-resistant metabolic alkalosis or "chloride-wasting nephropathy". Ann Int Med 1970; 73:31–38.
63. Luke RG, Levitin H. Impaired renal conservation of chloride and the acid–base changes associated with potassium depletion in the rat. Clin Sci 1967; 32:511–526.
64. Galla JH, Gifford JD, Luke RG, Rome L. Adaptations to chloride-depletion alkalosis. Am J Physiol 1991; 261:R771–R781.
65. Gulyassy PF, van Ypersele de Strihou C, Schwartz WB. On the mechanism of nitrate-induced alkalosis. The possible role of selective chloride depletion in acid–base regulation. J Clin Invest 1962; 41:1850–1862.
66. Needle MA, Kaloyanides GJ, Schwartz WB. The effects of selective depletion of hydrochloric acid on acid–base and electrolyte equilibrium. J Clin Invest 1964; 43:1836–1846.
67. Polak A, Haynie GD, Hays RM, Schwartz WB. Effects of chronic hypercapnia on electrolyte and acid–base equilibrium. I. Adaptation. J Clin Invest 1961; 40:1223–1237.
68. Schwartz WB, Hays RM, Polak A, Haynie GD. Effects of chronic hypercapnia on electrolyte and acid–base equilibrium. II. Recovery, with special reference to the influence of chloride intake. J Clin Invest 1961; 40:1238–1249.
69. van Ypersele de Strihou C, Gulyassy PF, Schwartz WB. Effects of chronic hypercapnia on electrolyte and acid–base equilibrium. III. Characteristics of the adaptive and recovery process as evaluated by provision of alkali. J Clin Invest 1962; 41:2246–2253.
70. Kassirer JP, Berkman PM, Lawrenz DR, Schwartz WB. The critical role of chloride in the correction of hypokalemic alkalosis in man. Am J Med 1965; 38:172–189.
71. Kassirer JP, Schwartz WB. The response of normal man to selective depletion of hydrochloric acid. Factors in the genesis of persistent gastric alkalosis. Am J Med 1966; 40:10–18.
72. Schwartz WB, van Ypersele de Strihou C, Kassirer JP. Role of anions in metabolic alkalosis and potassium deficiency. N Engl J Med 1968; 279:630–639.
73. Cohen JJ. Correction of metabolic alkalosis by the kidney after isometric expansion of extracellular fluid. J Clin Invest 1968; 47:1181–1192.
74. Cohen JJ. Selective Cl retention in repair of metabolic alkalosis without increasing filtered load. Am J Physiol 1970; 218:165–170.
75. Emmett M, Seldin DW. Clinical syndromes of metabolic acidosis and metabolic alkalosis. In: Seldin DW, Giebisch G, eds. The Kidney, Physiology and Pathophysiology. New York: Raven Press, 1985:1611–1624.
76. Purkerson ML, Lubowitz H, White RW, Bricker NS. On the influence of extracellular volume expansion on bicarbonate reabsorption in the rat. J Clin Invest 1969; 48:1754–1760.
77. Fitzgibbons JP, Gennari FJ, Garfinkel HB, Cortell S. Dependence of saline-induced natriuresis upon exposure of the kidney to the physical effects of extracellular fluid volume expansion. J Clin Invest 1974; 54:1428–1436.

78. Ichikawa I, Brenner BM. Mechanism of inhibition of proximal tubule fluid reabsorption after exposure of the rat kidney to the physical effects of expansion of extracellular fluid volume. J Clin Invest 1979; 64:1466–1474.

79. Cogan MG. Volume expansion predominantly inhibits proximal NaCl rather than NaHCO$_3$. Am J Physiol 1983; 245:F272–F275.

80. Bichara M, Paillard M, Corman B, de Rouffignac C, Level F. Volume expansion modulates NaHCO$_3$ and NaCl transport in the proximal tubule and Henle's loop. Am J Physiol 1984; 247:F140–F150.

81. Hulter HN, Ilnicki LP, Harbottle JA, Sebastian A. Correction of metabolic acidosis by the kidney during isometric expansion of extracellular fluid volume. J Lab Clin Med 1978; 92:602–612.

82. Galla JH, Bonduris DN, Luke RG. Correction of acute chloride-depletion alkalosis in the rat without volume expansion. Am J Physiol 1983; 244: F217–F221.

83. Craig DM, Galla JH, Bonduris DN, Luke RG. Importance of the kidney in the correction of chloride-depletion alkalosis in the rat. Am J Physiol 1986; 250:F54–F57.

84. Galla JH, Bonduris DN, Luke RG. Effects of chloride and extracellular fluid volume on bicarbonate reabsorption along the nephron in metabolic alkalosis in the rat. J Clin Invest 1987; 80:41–50.

85. Wall BM, Byrum GV, Galla JH, Luke RG. Importance of chloride for the correction of chronic chloride depletion metabolic alkalosis in the rat. Am J Physiol 1987; 253:F1031–F1039.

86. Norris SH, Kurtzman NA. Does chloride play an independent role in the pathogenesis of metabolic alkalosis?. Semin Nephrol 1988; 8:101–108.

87. Schwartz WB, Cohen JJ. The nature of the renal response to chronic disorders of acid–base equilibrium. Am J Med 1978; 64:417–428.

88. Darrow DC. Changes in muscle composition in alkalosis. J Clin Invest 1946; 25:324–330.

89. Holliday MA. Acute metabolic alkalosis. Its effect on potassium and acid excretion. J Clin Invest 1955; 34:428–433.

90. Bleich HL, Tannen RL, Schwartz WB. The induction of metabolic alkalosis by correction of potassium deficiency. J Clin Invest 1966; 45:573–579.

91. Borkan S, Northrup TE, Cohen JJ, Garella S. Renal responses to metabolic alkalosis induced by isovolemic hemofiltration in the dog. Kidney Int 1987; 32:322–328.

92. Garella S, Cohen JJ, Northrup TE. Chloride-depletion metabolic alkalosis induces ECF volume contraction via internal fluid shifts in nephrectomized dogs. Eur J Clin Invest 1991; 21:273–279.

93. Chamberlin ME, Strange K. Anisotonic cell volume regulation: a comparative view. Am J Physiol 1989; 257:C159–C173.

94. Hoffman EK, Simonsen LO. Membrane mechanisms in volume and pH regulation. Physiol Rev 1989; 69:315–382.

95. Macknight ADC. Volume maintenance in isoosmotic conditions. In: Kleinzeller A, ed. Current Topics in Membranes and Transport. New York: Academic Press, Inc., 1987; 30:3–34.

96. Atkins EA, Schwartz WB. Factors governing correction of the alkalosis associated with potassium deficiency: the critical role of chloride in the recovery process. J Clin Invest 1961; 41:218–229.

97. Berger BE, Cogan MG, Sebastian A. Reduced glomerular filtration and enhanced bicarbonate reabsorption maintain metabolic alkalosis in humans. Kidney Int 1984; 26:205–208.

98. Galla JH, Bonduris DN, Sanders PW, Luke RG. Volume-independent reductions in glomerular filtration rate in acute chloride-depletion alkalosis in the rat. J Clin Invest 1984; 74:2002–2008.

99. Wright FS, Briggs JP. Feedback regulation of glomerular filtration rate. Am J Physiol 1977; 233:F1–F7.

100. Kovacs G, Peti-Peterdi J, Rosivall L, Bell PD. Angiotensin II directly stimulates macula densa Na-2Cl-K co-transport via apical AT(1) receptors. Am J Physiol Renal Physiol 2002; 282:F301–F306.

101. Peti-Peterdi J, Chambrey R, Bebok Z, Biemesderfer D, St John PL, Abrahamson DR, Warnock DG, Bell PD. Macula densa Na(+)/H(+) exchange activities mediated by apical NHE2 and basolateral NHE4 isoforms. Am J Physiol Renal Physiol 2000; 278:F452–F463.

102. Maddox DA, Gennari FJ. Load dependence of proximal tubular bicarbonate reabsorption in chronic metabolic alkalosis in the rat. J Clin Invest 1986; 77:709–716.

103. Wesson DE. Augmented bicarbonate reabsorption by both the proximal and distal nephron maintains chloride-deplete metabolic alkalosis in rats. J Clin Invest 1989; 84:1460–1469.

104. Luke RG, Galla JH. Chloride-depletion alkalosis with a normal extracellular fluid volume. Am J Physiol 1983; 245:F419–F424.

105. Abboud HE, Luke RG, Galla JH, Kotchen TA. Stimulation of renin by acute selective chloride depletion in the rat. Circ Res 1979; 44:815–821.

106. Liu F-Y, Cogan MG. Role of angiotensin II in glomerulotubular balance. Am J Physiol 1990; 259:F72–F79.

107. Walters EA, Rome L, Luke RG, Galla JH. Absence of a regulatory role of angiotensin II in acute chloride-depletion alkalosis in the rat. Am J Physiol 1991; 261:F741–F745.

108. Kassirer JP, Appleton FM, Chazan JA, Schwartz WB. Aldosterone in metabolic alkalosis. J Clin Invest 1967; 46:1558–1571.

109. Cogan MG, Liu F-Y. Metabolic alkalosis in the rat. Evidence that reduced glomerular filtration rate rather than enhanced tubular bicarbonate reabsorption is responsible for maintaining the alkalotic state. J Clin Invest 1983; 71:1141–1160.

110. Galla JH, Bonduris DN, Dumbauld SL, Luke RG. Segmental chloride and fluid handling during correction of chloride-depletion alkalosis without volume expansion in the rat. J Clin Invest 1984; 73:96–106.

111. Maddox DA, Gennari FJ. Proximal tubular bicarbonate reabsorption and PCO_2 in chronic metabolic alkalosis in the rat. J Clin Invest 1983; 72:1385–1395.

112. Mello Aires M, Malnic G. Micropuncture study of acidification during hypochloremic alkalosis in the rat. Pfleugers Arch 1972; 331:13–24.

113. Krapf R. H/OH/HCO$_3$ transport in the rat cortical thick ascending limb. Evidence for an electrogenic Na/HCO$_3$ cotransporter in parallel with a Na/H Hantiporter.*JClinInvest*1988; 82 : 234–241.

114. Good DW. Bicarbonate absorption by the thick ascending limb of Henle's loop. Semin Nephrol 1990; 10:132–138.

115. Lucci MS, Pucacco LR, Carter NW, DuBose TD Jr. Evaluation of bicarbonate transport in rat distal tubule: effects of acid–base status. Am J Physiol 1982; 243:F335–F341.

116. Levine DZ, Vandorpe D, Iacovitti M. Luminal chloride modulates rat distal tubule bidirectional bicarbonate flux in vivo. J Clin Invest 1990; 85:1793–1798.

117. Galla JH, Bonduris DN, Luke RG. Superficial distal and deep nephrons in the correction of metabolic alkalosis. Am J Physiol 1989; 257:F107–F113.

118. Atkins JL, Burg MB. Bicarbonate transport by isolated perfused rat collecting ducts. Am J Physiol 1985; 249:F485–F489.

119. Garcia-Austt J, Good DW, Burg MB, Knepper MA. Deoxycorticosterone-stimulated bicarbonate secretion in rabbit cortical collecting ducts: effects of luminal chloride removal and in vivo acid loading. Am J Physiol 1985; 249: F205–F212.

120. McKinney TD, Burg MB. Bicarbonate transport by rabbit cortical collecting tubules. J Clin Invest 1977; 77:766–768.

121. Tomita K, Piasona JJ, Burg MB, Knepper MA. Effects of vasopressin and bradykinin on anion transport by the rat cortical collecting duct; evidence for an electroneutral sodium chloride transport pathway. J Clin Invest 1986; 77:136–141.

122. Laski ME, Warnock DG, Rector FC Jr. Effects of chloride gradients on total CO$_2$ flux in the rabbit cortical collecting tubule. Am J Physiol 1983; 244:F112–F121.

123. Schuster VL. Bicarbonate reabsorption and secretion in the cortical and outer medullary collecting tubule. Semin Nephrol 1990; 10:139–147.

124. Star RA, Burg MB, Knepper MA. Bicarbonate secretion and chloride absorption by rabbit cortical collecting ducts. Role of chloride/bicarbonate exchange. J Clin Invest 1985; 76:1123–1130.

125. Gifford JD, Sharkins K, Work J, Luke RG, Galla JH. Total CO$_2$ transport in rat cortical collecting duct in chloride-depletion alkalosis. Am J Physiol 1990; 258:F848–F853.

126. Gifford JD, Ware MW, Luke RG, Galla JH. HCO$_3$ transport in rat CCD: rapid adaptation by in vivo but not in vitro alkalosis. Am J Physiol 1993; 264:F435–F440.

127. Furuya H, Breyer M, Jacobson H. Functional characterization of α and β intercalated cell types in the rabbit cortical collecting duct. Am J Physiol 1991; 261:F377–F385.

128. Madsen KM, Tisher CC. Structural–functional relationships along the distal nephron. Am J Physiol 1986; 250:F1–F15.

129. Stone DK, Seldin DW, Kokko JP, Jacobson HR. Anion dependence of rabbit medullary collecting duct acidification. J Clin Invest 1983; 71:1505–1508.

130. Galla JH, Rome L, Luke RG. Bicarbonate transport in collecting duct segments during chloride-depletion alkalosis. Kidney Int 1995; 48:52–55.

131. Ullrich KJ, Papavassiliou F. Bicarbonate reabsorption in the papillary collecting duct of rats. Pfleugers Arch 1981; 389:271–275.

132. Diezi J, Michoud P, Aceves J, Giebisch G. Micropuncture study of electrolyte transport across papillary collecting duct of the rat. Am J Physiol 1973; 224:623–634.

133. Wall SM, Sands JM, Flessner M, Nonoguchi H, Spring K, Knepper MA. Net acid transport by isolated perfused inner medullary collecting ducts. Am J Physiol 1990; 258:F75–F84.

134. Silver RB, Soleimani M. H^+K^+ATPase: regulation and role in pathophysiological states. Am J Physiol 1999; 276:F799–F811.

135. Nakamura S, Amlal H, Soleimani M, Galla JH. Pathways for HCO_3^- reabsorption in mouse medullary collecting duct segments. J Lab Clin Med 2000; 136:218–223.

136. Soleimani M, Greeley T, Petrovic S, Wang Z, Amlal H, Kopp P, Burnham CE. Pendrin: an apical $Cl^-/OH^-/HCO_3^-$ exchanger in the kidney cortex. Am J Physiol 2001; 280:F356–F364.

137. Wang Z, Conforti L, Petrovic S, Amlal H, Burnham CE, Soleimani M. Mouse Na^+: HCO_3^- cotransporter isoform NBC-3 (kNBC-3): cloning, expression, and renal distribution. Kidney Int 2001; 59:1405–1414.

138. Petrovic S, Spicer Z, Greeley T, Shull GE, Soleimani M. Novel Schering and ouabain-insensitive potassium-dependent proton secretion in the mouse cortical collecting duct. Am J Physiol Renal Physiol 2002; 282:F133–F143.

139. Tsuganezawa H, Kobayashi K, Iyori M, Araki T, Koizumi A, Watanabe S, Kaneko A, Fukao T, Monkawa T, Yoshida T, Kim DK, Kanai Y, Endou H, Hayashi M, Saruta T. A new member of the $HCO_3(-)$ transporter superfamily is an apical anion exchanger of beta-intercalated cells in the kidney. J Biol Chem 2001; 276:8180–8189.

140. Brown D, Hirsch S, Gluck S. Localization of a proton-pumping ATPase in rat kidney. J Clin Invest 1988; 82:2114–2126.

141. Cougnon M, Planelles C, Crowson MS, Shull GE, Rossier BC, Jaisser F. The rat distal colon ATPase α subunit encodes a ouabain-sensitive H–K-ATPase. J Biol Chem 1996; 271:7277–7280.

142. Wallmark B, Briving C, Fryklund K, Munson R, Jackson J, Mendelein J, Rabon E, Sachs G. Inhibition of gastric $H^+–K^+$-ATPase and acid secretion by SCH 28080, a substituted pyridyl (1,2) imidazole. J Biol Chem 1987; 262:2077–2084.

143. Gifford JD, Rome L, Galla JH. $H^+–K^+$-ATPase activity in rat collecting duct segments. Am J Physiol 1992; 262:F692–F695.

144. Nakamura S, Wang Z, Soleimani M, Galla JH. Colonic H–K-ATPase mediates ouabain-sensitive HCO_3^- reabsorption in outer medullary collecting duct in rats with chloride-depletion alkalosis. J Am Soc Nephrol 1998; 9:10a.

145. Wesson DE. Depressed distal tubule acidification corrects chloride-deplete metabolic alkalosis in rats. Am J Physiol 1990; 259:F636–F644.

146. Kirchner KA, Galla JH, Luke RG. Factors influencing chloride reabsorption in the collecting duct segment of the rat. Am J Physiol 1980; 239:F552–F559.

147. Gennari FJ. Hypokalemia. N Engl J Med 1998; 339:451–458.

148. Cohn JN, Kowey PR, Whelton PK, Prisant LM. New guidelines for potassium replacement in clinical practice. Arch Intern Med 2000; 160: 2429–2436.

149. Wagner CW, Nesbit RR, Mansberger AR Jr. The use of intravenous hydrochloric acid in the treatment of thirty-four patients with metabolic alkalosis. Am Surg 1980; 46:140–146.

150. Brimioulle S, Berre J, Dufaye P, Vincent JL, Degaute JP, Kahn RJ. Hydrochloric acid infusion for treatment of metabolic alkalosis associated with respiratory acidosis. Crit Care Med 1989; 17:232–236.

151. Kwun KB, Boucherit T, Wong J, Richards Y, Bryan-Brown CW. Treatment of metabolic alkalosis with intravenous infusion of concentrated hydrochloric acid. Am J Surg 1983; 146:328–330.

152. Kopel RF, Durbin CG Jr. Pulmonary artery catheter deterioration during hydrochloric acid infusion for the treatment of metabolic alkalosis. Crit Care Med 1989; 17:688–689.

153. Jankauskas SJ, Gursel E, Antonenko DR. Chest wall necrosis secondary to hydrochloric acid use in the treatment of metabolic alkalosis. Crit Care Med 1989; 17:963–964.

154. Worthley LI. The rational use of i.v. hydrochloric acid in the treatment of metabolic alkalosis. Br J Anesth 1977; 49:811–817.

155. Martin WJ, Matzke GR. Treating severe metabolic alkalosis. Clin Pharm 1982; 1:42–48.

156. Bushinsky DA, Gennari FJ. Life-threatening hyperkalemia induced by arginine. Ann Int Med 1978; 89:632–634.

157. Marik PE, Kussman BD, Lipman J, Kraus P. Acetazolamide in the treatment of metabolic alkalosis in critically ill patients. Heart Lung 1991; 20:455–459.

158. Fraley DS, Adler S, Bruns F. Life-threatening metabolic alkalosis in a comatose patient. South Med J 1979; 72:1024–1025.

159. Mazur JE, Devlin JW, Peters MJ, Jankowski MA, Iannuzzi MC, Zarowitz BJ. Single versus multiple doses of acetazolamide for metabolic alkalosis in critically ill medical patients: a randomized double-blind trial. Crit Care Med 1999; 27:1257–1261.

160. Kahn MI. Treatment of refractory congestive heart failure and normokalemic hypochloremic alkalosis with acetazolamide and spironolactone. Can Med Assoc J 1980; 123:883–887.

161. Knauf H, Mutschler E. Functional state of the nephron and diuretic dose–response–rationale for low-dose combination therapy. Cardiology 1994; 84(suppl 2):18–26.

162. Crandall ED, Mathew SJ, Fleischer RS, Winter HI, Bidani A. Effects of inhibition of RBC HCO_3/Cl exchange on CO_2 excretion and downstream pH disequilibrium in isolated rat lungs. J Clin Invest 1981; 68:853–862.

163. Schunemann HJ, Klocke RA. Influence of carbon dioxide kinetics on pulmonary carbon dioxide exchange. J Appl Physiol 1993; 74:715–721.

164. Kowalchuk JM, Heigenhauser GJ, Sutton JR, Jones NL. Effect of chronic acetazolamide administration on gas exchange and acid–base control after maximal exercise. J Appl Physiol 1994; 76:1211–1219.

165. Berthelsen P, Gothgen I, Husum B, Jacobsen E. Dissociation of renal and respiratory effects of acetazolamide in the critically ill. Br J Anaesth 1986; 58:512–516.

166. Ayus JC, Olivero JJ, Adrogue HJ. Alkalemia associated with renal failure: correction by hemodialysis with low-bicarbonate dialysate. Arch Int Med 1980; 140:513–515.

167. Vilbar RM, Ing TS, Shin KD, Gandhi VC, Viol GW, Chen WT, Geis WP, Hano JE. Treatment of metabolic alkalosis with peritoneal dialysis in a patient with renal failure. Artif Organs 1978; 2:421–422.

168. Gerhardt RE, Koethe JD, Glickman JD, Ntoso KA, Hugo JP, Wolf CJ. Acid dialysate correction of metabolic alkalosis in renal failure. Am J Kidney Dis 1995; 25:343–345.

169. Kheirbek AO, Ing TS, Viol GW, Vilbar RM, Bansal VK, Gandhi VC, Geis WP, Hano JE. Treatment of metabolic alkalosis with hemofiltration in patients with renal insufficiency. Nephron 1979; 24:91–92.

170. Rowlands BJ, Tindall SF, Elliot DJ. The use of dilute hydrochloric acid and cimetidine to reverse severe metabolic alkalosis. Postgrad Med J 1978; 54:118–123.

171. Barton CH, Vaziri ND, Ness RL, Saiki JK, Mirahmadi KS. Cimetidine in the management of metabolic alkalosis induced by nasogastric suction. Arch Surg 1979; 114:70–74.

172. Kinahan TJ, Khoury AE, McLorie GA, Churchill BM. Omeprazole in post-gastrocystoplasty metabolic alkalosis and aciduria. J Urol 1992; 147:435–437.

173. Tomassetti P, Migliori M, Caletti GC, Fusaroli P, Corinaldesi R, Gullo L. Treatment of type II carcinoid tumors with somatostatin analogues. N Engl J Med 2000; 343:551–554.

174. Ladabaum U, Hasler WL. Novel approaches to the treatment of nausea and vomiting. Dig Dis 1999; 17:125–132.

175. Aichbichler BW, Zerr CH, Santa Ana CA, Porter JL, Fordtran JS. Proton-pump inhibition of gastric chloride secretion in congenital chloridorrhea. N Engl J Med 1997; 336:106–109.

176. Podrid PJ. Potassium and ventricular arrhythmias. Am J Cardiol 1990; 65:33E–44E.

177. Cappuccio FP, MacGregor GA. Does potassium supplementation lower blood pressure? A meta-analysis of published trials. J Hypertens 1991; 9:465–473.

178. Kaplan NM, Carnegie A, Raskin P, Heller JA, Simmons M. Potassium supplementation in hypertensive patients with diuretic-induced hypokalemia. N Engl J Med 1985; 312:746–749.

18

Potassium-Depletion Metabolic Alkalosis

Manoocher Soleimani

Division of Nephrology and Hypertension, University of Cincinnati College of Medicine, Cincinnati, Ohio, U.S.A.

DEFINITION

Potassium-depletion alkalosis is that type of metabolic alkalosis caused by depletion of total body K^+ and corrected solely by the administration of a sufficient amount of K^+. Hypokalemia (defined by a plasma $[K^+]$ of $< 3.5\,mEq/L$)—by contrast—is present in metabolic alkalosis of any type as well as in some types of metabolic acidosis (1). Hypochloremia is also the rule in K^+-depletion alkalosis but administration of Cl^- without K^+, for example, NaCl, exacerbates rather than corrects the K^+ depletion (2,3). The term, "chloride-resistant alkalosis," is often used to describe K^+-depletion alkalosis but that term fails to emphasize the specific underlying pathophysiology of the majority of the disorders grouped under this rubric. Potassium-depletion alkalosis may occur together with other causes of metabolic alkalosis, most commonly Cl^- depletion (see Chapter 17). As with other types of metabolic alkalosis, it may be divided into three phases—generation, maintenance, and correction (4) although the generation and maintenance phases may be difficult to separate. In contrast to Cl^--depletion alkalosis, urinary $[Cl^-]$ is consistently $>20\,mEq/L$ whereas urinary $[K^+]$ vary depending on the cause of the K^+ depletion.

CLASSIFICATION

Potassium depletion, which is hallmark of the pathophysiology of this group of disorders, may occur through either a renal or an intestinal mechanism

(Table 1). Urinary losses occur primarily because of excess mineralocorticoid or with the chronic use of chloruretic diuretics. More uncommonly, they are the result of genetically altered electrolyte transport along the distal nephron that stimulates mineralocorticoid excess; some of these entities may be accompanied by Cl⁻ depletion (see Chapter 17). Intestinal causes are related to the lack of absorption due to severe restriction of K⁺ intake or the binding of K⁺ within the lumen by a variety of substances.

CLINICAL PRESENTATION

Because >97% of total body K⁺ is intracellular, assessment of K⁺ depletion based on serum [K⁺] is difficult. Nevertheless, the magnitude of K⁺ depletion has been roughly related to serum [K⁺] (5) (Table 2). When mild, K⁺ depletion with serum [K⁺] in the range of 3.0–3.5 mEq/L is asymptomatic. With more severe K⁺ depletion (serum [K⁺] of <2.5 mEq/L), generalized weakness, rhabdomyolysis, ascending paralysis, and, rarely, apnea are seen with increasing likelihood as K⁺ depletion becomes more severe (6–8).

Hypokalemia causes characteristic electrocardiographic (EKG) abnormalities include U waves, T-wave depression or inversion and ST segment depression (9). In moderate hypokalemia, changes in EKG are minimal and often limited to the presence of a U wave. Cardiac arrhythmias are common in hypokalemia, particularly in patients with underlying heart disease or on digoxin (10,11).

Hypokalemia and metabolic alkalosis can both cause nephrogenic diabetes insipidus (12–14). Patients with hypokalemia-induced nephrogenic diabetes insipidus present with polyuria and polydipsia. Downregulation of the aquaporin 2 water channel (AQP-2) in the collecting duct may play an

Table 1 Causes of Potassium Depletion/Mineralocorticoid Excess

Primary aldosteronism
Adenoma, idiopathic, hyperplasia, renin-responsive, carcinoma, glucocorticoid-suppressible 17α-hydroxylase deficiency
Secondary aldosteronism
Adrenal corticosteroid excess—primary, secondary, or exogenous
Severe hypertension—malignant, accelerated, renovascular
Hemangiopericytoma, nephroblastoma, renal cell carcinoma
Apparent mineralocorticoid excess
Primary deoxycorticosterone excess — 11β-hydroxylase deficiency
Drugs—licorice (glycyrrhizic acid) as a confection or flavoring, carbenoxolone
Liddle syndrome
Bartter and Gitelman syndromes and their variants
Laxative abuse, clay ingestion, severe dietary K⁺ restriction

Table 2 Estimation of Total Body Potassium Deficit

Serum potassium (mEq/L)[a]	Potassium deficit (mEq)
3.5	100–250
3.0	150–350
2.5	300–600
2.0	500–750

[a]Serum and plasma $[K^+]$ differ by $<10\%$ unless hemolysis or severe thrombocytosis or leukocytosis is present.
Source: Adapted from Ref. 174.

important role in this process (15). It is unclear whether hypokalemia exerts a primary effect on the thirst center (14).

PATHOPHYSIOLOGY

General

The whole body buffering response to metabolic alkalosis of any cause elicits a shift of H^+ from the intracellular to the extracellular compartment, a process linked to K^+ entry into cells (16), thereby promoting hypokalemia. As a result, hypokalemia and mild K^+ depletion occur in nearly all causes of metabolic alkalosis but are not necessarily the proximate cause of the alkalosis (see Chapter 17). External K^+ renal and intestinal losses and the associated hypokalemia, by contrast, promote the entry of H^+ and Na^+ into cells. Because hypokalemia caused by K^+ depletion is associated clinically and experimentally with metabolic alkalosis and metabolic acidosis, the pathophysiological mechanisms by which K^+ depletion is generated and maintained are clearly the critical determinants of the resultant acid–base disorder.

Some notes of caution regarding the interpretation of both experimental and clinical data: The terms, "potassium depletion" and "hypokalemia" are not synonymous and when used to describe the conditions of study may not reflect negative external K^+ balance. For example, hypokalemia can occur without K^+ depletion in a variety of settings in which K^+ shifts into cells (e.g., hyperthyroidism, hypokalemic periodic paralysis). Moreover, an isolated perfused tubule taken from an animal subjected to prior K^+ depletion would not necessarily behave like a tubule from a normal animal studied in a bath with a low $[K^+]$ that approximates in vivo hypokalemia. Furthermore, different species respond differently to K^+ depletion (see following section). Finally, the mechanism by which hypokalemia occurs may result in different acid–base disturbances, for example, diarrhea compared to vomiting.

Generation

Controversy continues to exist over the relative roles of renal and nonrenal causes in the generation of K^+-depletion metabolic alkalosis. Generation of alkalosis by the kidney is attributed primarily to enhanced ammoniagenesis and NH_4^+ excretion, which generates new HCO_3^- and its subsequent absorption in the proximal tubule whereas the nonrenal generation occurs by a shift of H^+ into the intracellular compartment.

Nonrenal: Effect on Proton Shift

In the rat, the generation of metabolic alkalosis by K^+ depletion has been attributed to the intracellular shift of H^+ [17]. Potassium depletion may also cause a shift in the set point for the maintenance of plasma $[HCO_3^-]$ [18]. Intracellular pH in K^+-depleted rats was decreased in kidney cortical cells by nuclear magnetic imaging techniques [19], suggesting that the intracellular H^+ shift in this setting can occur both in the renal and nonrenal cells. While the intracellular H^+ shift in nonrenal cells can increase plasma $[HCO_3^-]$ and thus generate alkalosis, the intracellular acidosis within renal epithelium would enhance HCO_3^- reabsorption and a mechanism for maintaining the alkalosis.

Renal: Effect on Ammoniagenesis

In humans on a low K^+ diet, serum $[HCO_3^-]$ rises modestly suggesting that K^+ depletion per se can generate new HCO_3^- [20]. In this case, metabolic alkalosis is generated because net acid excretion exceeds net acid production (Fig. 1). While new HCO_3^- generation may occur through both renal and nonrenal processes, experiments in rats support an important role for NH_4^+ production and excretion in the generation and maintenance of K^+ depletion-induced metabolic alkalosis.

Renal ammonia production is intimately linked to K^+ homeostasis (21–23) (see Chapter 6). New HCO_3^- can be generated in the kidney by ammoniagenesis, in which the increased excretion of ammonium is accompanied by the transport of new HCO_3^- into the body (24). These studies in both in vivo and in vitro systems indicate that hypokalemia stimulates whereas hyperkalemia suppresses ammonia production (25). Although the specific cellular mechanisms whereby K^+ alters ammoniagenesis remains undefined, the observation that K^+ loading diminishes while K^+ depletion enhances ammonia production supports the supposition that K^+ and NH_3 are linked in a physiologically relevant system.

Potassium depletion causes adaptive increases in several pathways that are involved in ammoniagenesis. Adaptation involves both enhanced glutamine entry into the mitochondria and/or activation of phosphate-dependent glutaminase (25,26). The phosphate-dependent glutaminase pathway in the mitochondria is of primary importance in this regard.

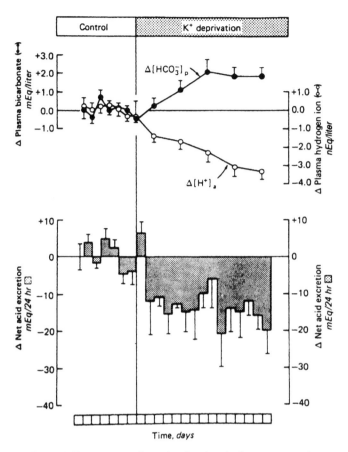

Figure 1 Effect of dietary potassium deprivation in humans on plasma [HCO₃⁻], plasma [H⁺], and net urinary acid excretion. *Source*: From Ref. 20.

Because of this adaptation, the rate of ammoniagenesis in the proximal tubule is increased, which can lead to enhanced acid loss in the form of NH_4^+ (see Chapter 6). As a result, new HCO_3^- is generated in proximal tubule cells and transported to the blood (27). Independent of its effect on ammoniagenesis, K^+ depletion increases the rate of acid secretion and HCO_3^- reabsorption along the nephron.

Effect of Potassium Restriction

Experimental dietary K^+ depletion is associated with modest metabolic alkalosis and increases in intracellular [Na⁺] and [H⁺] in both humans (20,28) and rats (17,18,29). Selective K^+ restriction causes both K^+ depletion and hypokalemia and increases serum [HCO₃⁻] (20,30). The increase in serum [HCO₃⁻] occurs within 2 days of K^+ restriction, is about 2 mEq/L and is associated with increased net acid excretion. Potassium depletion decreases aldosterone secretion as well as plasma aldosterone concentration in man thereby excluding excess mineralocorticoid as a cause for the increase in serum $[HCO_3^-]$ (20,31).

Potassium restriction increased the titratable acid excretion in the distal nephron and decreased urine pH in the isolated perfused rat kidney (32). The decrease in urine pH was not affected by amiloride, an inhibitor of Na channel. These data suggest that enhanced renal acid excretion in hypokalemia is independent of distal nephron Na^+ transport, and is therefore distinct from the mineralocorticoid-stimulated acid secretion (33,34). Taken together, the studies mentioned support the notion that enhanced distal nephron acid secretion that is observed in K^+ depletion is not due to other compounding factors such as excess mineralocorticoids. They provide further evidence that enhanced H^+ secretion in the distal nephron in K^+ depletion is primarily mediated by upregulated proton ATPases as discussed subsequently.

In contrast to rats and humans, K^+ depletion causes metabolic acidosis in dog and rabbit (35,36). In the dog, metabolic acidosis has been attributed to a low plasma aldosterone concentration secondary to K^+ depletion coupled with a putatively more important role for aldosterone in distal HCO_3^- reabsorption (35). In the rat, the generation of alkalosis has been attributed to the intracellular shift of H^+ (29) and to a shift in the "set point" for the maintenance of plasma $[HCO_3^-]$ (37). Whether this new "set point" reflects the upregulation of HCO_3^- reabsorption transporters in the nephron remains to be determined. Net acid excretion does not increase during generation of metabolic alkalosis by K^+ depletion (38). In renal tubular cells, accompanying intracellular acidosis would facilitate HCO_3^- reabsorption and thus maintain alkalosis. An important role of intracellular acidosis is supported by correction of the alkalosis by infusion of K^+ without any suppression of renal net acid excretion (29,38); correction is assumed to occur by intracellular movement of K^+, with movement of H^+ into the ECF where HCO_3^- is titrated. Furthermore, during KDA, the rat excretes an acid load completely while maintaining an elevated plasma $[HCO_3^-]$ (29). Thus, evidence from the rat model of K^+ depletion suggests that the kidney does not generate the alkalosis but does maintain it.

Effects of Mineralocorticoid

Most of the disease states that cause K^+-depletion alkaloses are associated with aldosterone excess (4,5). The increase in aldosterone synthesis and secretion can be primary or secondary via activation of the renin-angiotensin axis. Excess aldosterone increases abnormally the excretion of K^+, leading to K^+ depletion.

Aldosterone also stimulates H^+ secretion in the distal nephron (39). It does so by both Na^+-dependent and Na^+-independent mechanisms, with the Na^+-independent acidification mechanism having a greater capacity (39). In the presence of high Na^+ intake, aldosterone increases acid and K^+ secretion in the distal nephron whereas Na restriction blunts these secretions (33) suggesting that the stimulatory effect of aldosterone on acid secretion depends on the availability of luminal Na^+ in the distal nephron (34). These data are consistent with an electrogenic linkage between H^+ and K^+ secretion and Na^+ reabsorption in the distal nephron.

Mineralocorticoid Excess

The majority of patients with excess aldosterone present with hypokalemia and alkalosis (40,41). Administration of aldosterone causes only a mild alkalosis if hypokalemia is prevented (42). Moreover, the severity of hypokalemia as an index of K^+ depletion in subjects receiving aldosterone directly correlates with the magnitude of alkalosis (42) (Fig. 2). Aldosterone binds to its receptor in the principal cells (PC) of the collecting duct and stimulates the apical Na^+ channel and the basolateral Na^+-K^+ ATPase. The result is enhanced Na^+ reabsorption and increased K^+ and H^+ secretion into the lumen (43,44).

In addition to this indirect stimulation of H^+ secretion through its electrogenic linkage to Na^+ reabsorption, aldosterone directly stimulates H^+

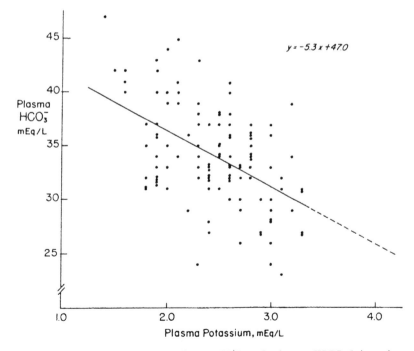

Figure 2 Relationship between plasma $[K^+]$ and plasma $[HCO_3^-]$ in primary aldosteronism. *Source*: From Ref. 5.

secretion by increasing the activity of H^+ ATPase in the collecting duct (45). Increased H^+ secretion enhances HCO_3^- reabsorption in the collecting duct as well as increasing NH_4^+ and titratable acid excretion. The overall effect of aldosterone excess thus is Na^+ retention, hypokalemia and metabolic alkalosis.

Maintenance

An elevated serum $[HCO_3^-]$ can be maintained by either a decrease in filtration rate or an increase in reabsorption or both. The interpretation of studies of renal blood flow and glomerular filtration rate in K^+ depletion are fraught with difficulty and defy comparison for a host of reasons: potassium depletion was induced by the administration of variable dosages of mineralocorticoid in conjunction with low K^+ intake and for different durations; the magnitude of K^+ depletion was not determined by either cumulative K^+ balance or tissue $[K^+]$ or it varied widely among studies; and the well-known effect of K^+ depletion to induce renal growth is not accounted for and thus whole kidney rates were not normalized to kidney size (46,47). Notwithstanding these formidable problems in interpretation, in carefully conducted balance studies of K^+-restricted human subjects on either low or high NaCl intake, glomerular filtration rate was well maintained in the setting of sustained hypokalemia and alkalosis (28). According appropriately considerable weight to this investigation, it seems more likely that the maintenance of metabolic alkalosis in K^+ depletion is due to enhanced HCO_3^- reabsorption along the nephron segment.

EFFECT OF K⁺ DEPLETION AND HYPOKALEMIA ON BICARBONATE REABSORPTION IN NEPHRON SEGMENTS
Proximal Tubule

The proximal tubule is responsible for reabsorption of approximately 85% of the filtered load of HCO_3^- (39) (see Chapters 4 and 6). Segmental analysis of the nephron indicates that K^+ depletion is associated with increased HCO_3^- reabsorption by the proximal tubule (48,49). Molecular and functional studies have demonstrated that HCO_3^- reabsorption in the proximal tubule is predominantly mediated via apical Na^+/H^+ exchanger (NHE-3) and H^+ ATPase and basolateral Na^+:HCO_3^- cotransporter (NBC-1) acting in series (50,51) (see Chapter 5).

Rats on a K^+ free diet for 4 weeks showed metabolic alkalosis (52) with arterial pH 7.51 (7.39 in controls) and serum $[HCO_3^-]$ 33 mEq (24 in controls). In luminal membrane vesicles, amiloride-sensitive Na^+ influx was increased. In basolateral membrane vesicles, HCO_3^--dependent, DIDS-sensitive Na^+ influx increased, suggesting increased basolateral NBC-1 activity. Thus, K^+ depletion appears to upregulate apical and basolateral HCO_3^--absorbing transporters in the proximal tubule.

The molecular mechanisms by which K^+ depletion induces adaptive changes are not certain. The membrane vesicles studies cited above (52) were carried out only after 4 weeks of K^+ deprivation and did not examine the time course of adaptive regulation of luminal NHE-3 and basolateral NBC-1. Thus, whether the upregulation of NHE-3 preceded, followed, or was simultaneous with the enhancement of NBC-1 activity is uncertain. Potassium depletion might increase the elctrochemical driving force for one or both of these transport processes. A primary increase in activity of NHE-3 will increase cell HCO_3^-, thus providing more substrate for the basolateral NBC-1. On the other hand, a primary increase in NBC-1 activity will decrease intracellular pH due to HCO_3^- extrusion across the basolateral membrane, thereby, providing more substrate for the NHE-3 in the luminal membrane. Since proximal tubule cell pH is lower in K^+ depletion (19), it would appear that the luminal NHE-3 is not the primary transporter affected since an alkaline cell pH would be the expected result of a primary increase in activity of this exchanger.

The mechanism(s) responsible for the intracellular acidosis in proximal tubule cells of K^+-depleted rats is not certain. It has been postulated that this may result from H^+ redistribution due to K^+ loss from cells (16,19). However, another plausible explanation is that the intracellular pH falls because of increased HCO_3^- extrusion across the basolateral membrane due to increased activity of the basolateral NBC-1. The NBC-1 with a stoichiometry of $Na^+:3HCO_3^-$ is an electrogenic process and is therefore affected by changes in membrane potential (51) (see Chapter 5). Alpern (53) has shown that increasing peritubular $[K^+]$ from 5 to 50 mEq/L, a maneuver that depolarizes the basolateral membrane, induces cell alkalinization. Studies in basolateral membrane vesicles indicate that the electrical gradient influences the inward flux of HCO_3^- via NBC-1. Thus, the exit of HCO_3^- across the basolateral membrane of proximal tubule cells is sensitive to changes in membrane potential. Given the stoichiometry of NBC-1, membrane depolarization should decrease whereas hyperpolarization should increase the rate of base extrusion. Using a double barrel microelectrode, Cemerikic et al. (54) have shown that K^+ deficiency induces hyperpolarization of the basolateral membrane of proximal tubule cells. Whether changes in membrane potential are responsible for the increased activity of the basolateral NBC-1 cotransporter in K^+ depletion remains speculative.

The increase in NHE activity in apical membrane vesicles isolated from K^+-depleted animals was mostly due to an increase in the transport capacity (V_{max}) of the exchanger (52). Northern hybridization and immunoblot studies have not demonstrated any significant increase in the levels of NHE-3 mRNA or protein, respectively, in K^+ depletion (55). One reasonable conclusion from these studies is that the upregulation of NHE3 in K^+ depletion is a post-translational process. Additional studies however are needed to address this issue.

In addition, the expression of NBC-1 (51,56,57) was examined serially and correlated with its activity in rat proximal tubule in K^+ depletion (58). NBC-1 mRNA levels increased in the superficial cortex by about threefold as early as 72 hr of K^+ deprivation and remained elevated at 21 days of experiment. NBC-1 activity showed ~110% enhancement in proximal tubule suspensions (58). These results indicate that NBC-1 expression is increased early in the course of K deprivation and plays an important role in enhanced HCO_3^- reabsorption. The upregulation of NBC-1 preceded the onset of hypokalemia, indicating that the signal(s) mediating enhanced basolateral NBC-1 is likely intracellular K^+ depletion and not serum $[K^+]$ (58).

In addition to the electroneutral NHE-3, an electrogenic vacuolar H^+-ATPase is expressed on the apical membranes of proximal tubule and participates significantly in H^+ secretion (59,60). It is not clear whether the expression or the activity of H^+-ATPase is altered in K^+ depletion.

Enhanced reabsorption of HCO_3^- in kidney proximal tubule correlates inversely with Cl^- reabsorption, as the sum of Cl^- and HCO_3^- remains unchanged (61,62). In metabolic acidosis, the apical Cl^-/base exchanger is depressed while the apical NHE-3 is stimulated (63). It is plausible that the apical Cl^-/base exchanger is similarly downregulated in K^+ depletion. Indeed, micropuncture studies in rat proximal tubules have demonstrated that Cl^- reabsorption is decreased in K^+ depletion, leading to enhanced excretion of Cl^- in the kidney (64). The downregulation of apical Cl-absorbing transporter(s) in kidney proximal tubule in K^+-depleted animals could contribute to the maintenance of metabolic alkalosis by decreasing Cl^- and increasing HCO_3^- reabsorption. These adaptive changes in apical and basolateral HCO_3^- transporters in kidney proximal tubule cells in response to K^+ depletion are depicted in Fig. 3.

Thick Ascending Limb of Henle

Approximately 5–10% of the filtered HCO_3^- is reabsorbed in the ascending limb of Henle's loop, predominantly via the NHE3 and H^+-ATPase on the luminal membrane (see Chapter 4). The mechanisms of HCO_3^- transport across the basolateral membrane of thick limb seems to be species-specific. Under normal conditions, in the medullary thick ascending limb of Henle's loop (mTAL), a K^+:HCO_3^- cotransporter and Cl^-/HCO_3^- exchanger mediate HCO_3^- exit across the basolateral membrane in rat whereas in mouse, the Na^+:HCO_3^- cotransporter (NBC-1) is responsible for the bulk of HCO_3^- transport (51). However, after 3 days of K^+ deprivation in rat, NBC-1 mRNA was heavily expressed in the inner stripe of outer medulla and remained elevated at 21 days (58). Epithelial cells of mTAL showed induction of NBC-1 mRNA and activity. Thus, K^+ deprivation can induce NBC-1 in the mTAL suggesting enhanced HCO_3^- reabsorption in this nephron segment during K^+ depletion; functional studies have not yet been done.

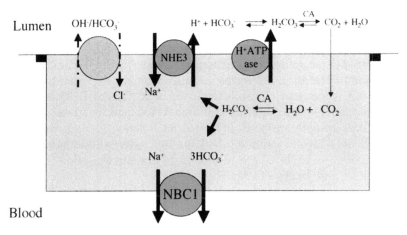

Figure 3 Adaptive regulation of HCO_3^- transporters in kidney proximal tubule cells in K^+ depletion. Bold lines indicate upregulation and dashed lines indicate downregulation of the transporters. Apical Na^+/H^+ exchanger NHE-3 and H^+-ATPase and basolateral $Na^+:3HCO_3^-$ cotransporter (NBC-1) are upregulated and mediate enhanced HCO_3^- reabsorption. The apical Cl^-/base (formate) exchanger is downregulated and therefore allows for HCO_3^- reabsorption to proceed unhindered.

Distal Tubule

The distal tubule reabsorbs 1–3% of the filtered load of HCO_3^-. The mechanism of HCO_3^- reabsorption is likely via an apical H^+-ATPase (65), H^+-K^+-ATPase (66) and an Na^+/H^+ exchanger other than NHE3 (67) (see Chapter 4). During K^+ depletion, net HCO_3^- reabsorption increased significantly in this nephron segment (65,68). Much of this enhanced H^+ secretion was inhibited by Schering 28080, an inhibitor of gastric H^+-K^+-ATPase (66) (see following section). Stimulation of H^+-ATPase may also contribute. In K^+-depleted rats, H^+-ATPase activity is increased in microperfused distal tubule (69,70). Immunocytochemical localization studies showed also that K^+ depletion resulted in an increase in apical staining H^+-ATPase (70).

Cortical Collecting Duct

The cortical collecting duct (CCD) is composed of two different major cell types: the PC and the intercalated cells (IC) (see Chapter 4), which include H^+-secreting (alpha) and HCO_3^--secreting (beta) cells. The alpha IC express both H^+-ATPase and H^+-K^+-ATPase on their apical membranes (66,71) whereas beta IC express only H^+-K^+-ATPase on their apical membrane (66,71). The PC also express H^+-K^+-ATPase on their apical membrane (66,71). Molecular studies indicate the presence of at least two isoforms of H^+-K^+-ATPase in the CCD, the gastric (HKAg) and the colonic (HKAc) (66,72). The H^+-K^+-ATPase that is present in CCD is inhibitable by

Schering 28080 and, therefore, belongs to the HKAg family (66,71). In microperfused CCD, HKAg -like activity is increased with K^+ depletion (66,71,73). While there are no data to indicate that the colonic HKAc plays a role in H^+ secretion or reabsorption under normal conditions, the expression of HKAc in the cortex increases with K^+ depletion (66).

H^+-ATPase activity also is increased in IC cells of CCD in rats with K^+ depletion (74). In addition, immunocytochemical staining with an H^+-ATPase-specific antibody indicated an increase in both the number and intensity of apical staining (74). Thus, in K^+ depletion enhanced HCO_3^- reabsorption in CCD likely results from the upregulation of HKAg, H^+-ATPase and, likely, HKAc.

Medullary Collecting Duct

In the outer medullary collecting duct (OMCD) under normal conditions in rat and rabbit, microperfusion, immunocytochemistry, and Northern hybridization studies show participation of HKAg and H^+-ATPase in HCO_3^- reabsorption and HKAg in K^+ reabsorption (59,66,71,72,75–77).

In K^+ depletion in rat, immunocytochemical studies show that the intensity of H^+-ATPase apical staining is significantly increased in OMCD (59), consistent with enhanced H^+-ATPase activity and HCO_3^- reabsorption. The rate of K^+-dependent pH_i recovery in response to an acute acid load is enhanced in rabbit inner stripe of the OMCD (78). This enhanced rate of K^+-dependent intracellular alkalinization was not completely inhibited with addition of Schering 28080 suggesting that another H^+-K^+-ATPase isoform may be expressed in K^+-depletion (78).

In rats on a K^+-deficient diet for 2 weeks, Northern hybridization and in situ hybridization studies showed that HKAc mRNA was significantly upregulated (55,71,72,79–82). This induction of HKAc was mostly evident in the medulla (55,79–82) but also showed moderate intensity in the cortex (81). In the medulla of K^+-depleted animals, upregulation of HKAc is evident in both outer and inner medulla (39,81,83). This occurs as early as 72 hr after the start of the K^+-deficient diet and precedes the onset of hypokalemia (83), suggesting that the signal may be activated by intracellular K^+-depletion. In contrast, HKAg mRNA and protein abundance remains unchanged in the whole kidney (80), shows mild upregulation in the cortex and downregulation in the inner medulla (66) of K^+-depleted rats. Upregulation of HKAc in K^+-depletion is significantly blocked in hypohysectomized rats, suggesting that pituitary hormones could play an important role on HKAc regulation in K^+-depletion (81).

With an $\sim$30-fold increase in HKAc mRNA expression in the outer medulla in K^+-depletion, HCO_3^- reabsorption ($JtCO_2$) in OMCD was enhanced (81). In normal rats, HCO_3^- reabsorption in OMCD decreased in the presence of 10 µM Schering 28080 and was unchanged in the presence of 1 μM ouabain (81). In contrast, ouabain 1 μM decreased HCO_3^- reabsorption significantly in K^+-depleted rats (81). Although 10 μM Schering 28080 also decreased HCO_3^- reabsorption, the inhibitory effects of Schering 28080 and ouabain were not additive (81). These data suggest that in K^+-depletion, HKAc is induced and mediates increased HCO_3^- reabsorption in OMCD and that in vivo, HKAc is sensitive to both Schering 28080 and ouabain or that a different isoform is also induced (66).

In terminal IMCD, both H^+-ATPase and H^+-K^+-ATPase activities are present on the apical membrane under normal conditions (84–86). Northern hybridization studies, however, provide evidence for the expression of only HKAg and not H^+-ATPase (83). In K^+-depletion in rat, mRNA expression of HKAg is decreased in IMCDt whereas that for HKAc is heavily induced (83).

In K^+-depletion in rat, HCO_3^- reabsorption in the perfused terminal segment was increased due to enhanced SCH-sensitive H^+-K^+-ATPase activity (83). In conjunction with these findings, HCO_3^- reabsorption (JtCO_2 was increased in K^+-depleted rats (27,83). Although in normal rats, ouabain had no effect while 10 μM SCH decreased HCO_3^- reabsorption (27,83), either ouabain or SCH decreased HCO_3^- reabsorption in K^+-depleted rats; these inhibitory effects were not additive suggesting that their effect was on the same transporter (27,81). These results suggest that while HKAg is suppressed in K^+-depletion, HKAc or some other isoform is induced and mediates increased HCO_3^- reabsorption in the terminal IMCD as in the OMCD. The acquisition of SCH sensitivity by HKAc in vivo in K^+-depletion is consonant with the studies of Buffin-Meyer et al. (87). Since this characteristic is at variance with in vitro data (reviewed in 66), further studies will be required to clarify this issue.

The Role of Ammonium

Potassium depletion increases urinary Cl^- (64) and ammonium (NH_4^+) excretion within 2 days of dietary K^+ restriction in rat and before hypokalemia occurs (27,83). Potassium depletion suppresses the apical Na-K-2Cl cotransporter and the apical Na-Cl cotransporter also in this time frame (88), resulting in decreased reabsorption of Na^+ and Cl^- in mTAL and distal convoluted tubule, but only urinary Cl^- and not Na^+ excretion is increased (64), suggesting the possibility of increased NH_4^+ excretion (64). In rats on dietary K^+ restriction for 6 days, NH_4^+ excretion indeed increased (27). In IMCD, which is the [a] major site for NH_4^+ secretion, HKAc was heavily induced whereas the HKAg expression was decreased. Furthermore, ammonium secretion was enhanced and inhibited by ouabain, an inhibitor of HKAc, but not by Schering 28080, an inhibitor of HKAg (27). Induction of HKAc was also closely associated with induction of the secretory K^+ channel, ROMK1 (88). These results are consistent with the possibility that NH_4^+ can replace K^+ on HKAc to mediate the secretion of

NH_4^+ into the lumen facilitated by K^+ recycling by ROMK1. The signal for these changes and their roles in K^+-depletion alkalosis remain speculative and require further studies.

The Integrated Role of Transporters

In K^+-depleted animals, NBC-1 expression is upregulated in the renal papilla (58). Based on the studies in proximal tubule, mTAL and IMCD (58), it has been proposed that NBC-1 likely mediates enhanced HCO_3^- reabsorption in these nephron segments in K^+ deprivation and contributes to the maintenance of metabolic alkalosis in this condition. The roles of HKAc and NBC-1 in HCO_3^- reabsorption and NH_4^+ secretion in terminal IMCD of K^+-depleted rats are proposed in Fig. 4.

Recovery from Metabolic Alkalosis

The recovery from K^+-depletion alkalosis occurs with total body K^+ repletion. Although experimental evidence is lacking, K^+ repletion likely results

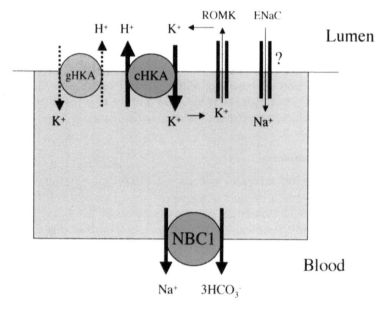

Figure 4 Adaptive regulation of HCO_3^- transporters in kidney inner medullary collecting duct cells in K^+ depletion. Bold lines indicate upregulation and dashed lines indicate downregulation of the transporters. Apical colonic H^+-K^+ ATPase (cHKA) and basolateral Na^+:$3HCO_3^-$ cotransporter (NBC-1) are upregulated and mediate enhanced HCO_3^- reabsorption. ROMK K^+ channel is upregulated and secrets K^+ into the lumen for recycling via HKAc. Apical gastric H^+-K^+ ATPase (gHKA) is downregulated.

in the reversal of the upregulation of NHE-3 and NBC-1 in the proximal tubule, H^+-ATPase in the CCD and HKAc and NBC-1 in the medullary collecting duct. As a result, HCO_3^- reabsorption is decreased along the nephron, leading to excess HCO_3^- excretion and restoration of a normal plasma $[HCO_3^-]$.

SPECIFIC CAUSES

Primary Mineralocorticoid Excess

Among the disease states associated with mineralocorticoid excess are the primary causes of aldosterone excess such as adrenal adenoma, adrenal carcinoma, or bilateral adrenal hyperplasia (40,41,89,90). Increased plasma aldosterone concentration and low plasma renin activity (PRA) characterize this group of diseases. Aldosterone secretion is partially autonomous and cannot be suppressed by volume expansion or increased Na^+ intake (91). Hypertension is a nearly universal clinical feature (92); other clinical features are those associated primarily with K^+ depletion.

In addition to the common causes of primary mineralocorticoid excess, a glucocorticoid-suppressible variety of this group has also been identified (93). This syndrome, now called glucocorticoid-remediable aldosteronism, has been shown to be an autosomal dominant heritable disease that results from the expression of a chimeric gene that comprises the genetic elements that encode two closely related steroidogenic enzymes, 11 beta-hydroxylase and aldosterone synthase (94,95). The regulatory sequences of 11 beta-hydroxylase are responsive to ACTH, and in this genetic chimera, control the expression of the coding sequences of aldosterone synthase. As a result, ACTH stimulates excess aldosterone synthesis.

Classic 17-hydroxylase deficiency, an autosomal recessive disorder originally described in patients with hypertension and sexual infantilism, is due to mutations of the cytochrome P450c17 enzyme; partial and selective forms of P450c17 deficiencies also exist with a variety of mutations (96). These patients demonstrate a range of phenotypes and may present with metabolic alkalosis and hypokalemia. Plasma 11-deoxycorticosterone, corticosterone, and aldosterone are elevated, whereas PRA is suppressed (97).

Secondary Mineralocorticoid Excess

Secondary causes of mineralocorticoid, excess are due to primary increases in PRA, which, in turn, increases aldosterone secretion and plasma aldosterone concentration. Among the causes of secondary hyperaldosteronism are malignant hypertension and renovascular hypertension. In these disorders, mild metabolic alkalosis and hypokalemia are usually mild (98); in this study, only one patient had a serum CO_2 >32 mEq/L in association with serum [K$^+$] of 3.6 mEq/L. Unlike primary aldosteronism, aldosterone secretion can be suppressed by volume expansion (91).

In renovascular hypertension due to either fibromuscular dysplasia or atherosclerotic vascular disease or by a renin-secreting hemangiopericytoma, which is a tumor of the juxtaglomerular apparatus, the increase in PRA may be from only one kidney and may be detected only by bilateral renal vein sampling.

Apparent Mineralocorticoid Excess

Apparent mineralocorticoid excess syndromes are characterized by hypertension, metabolic alkalosis, hypokalemia, low plasma aldosterone concentration and low PRA. These syndromes involve genetic alterations in the enzymatic pathway for adrenosteroid metabolism or in the structure of Na$^+$ channel or drug or tumor effects.

11-Beta-Hydroxysteroid Dehydrogenase (HSD2) Deficiency

Deficiency of the enzyme, HSD2, is a rare autosomal recessive disorder caused by several mutations of the gene, HSD11B2, on chromosome 16 (99). This is the type 2 isoform of the enzyme, 11 beta-hydroxysteroid dehydrogenase, and is present in the principal cell of the CCD as well as other mineralocorticoid target tissue (100,101) HSD2 has high affinity for cortisol and normally shunts cortisol, which can interact with the mineralocorticoid receptor in the principal cell, to the inactive cortisone, which does not interact—the so-called cortisol—cortisone shuttle. Cortisol normally exceeds the concentration of aldosterone by a ratio of ~100:1. The congenital defect of HSD2 prevents inactivation of cortisol and allows it to bind to the promiscuous nuclear mineralocorticoid receptor initiating the signal cascade that leads to Na$^+$ reabsorption and H$^+$ and K$^+$ secretion (102). The result is hypertension, hypokalemia, and metabolic alkalosis. Because cortisol is the "unregulated" mineralocorticoid in this disorder, both aldosterone and renin activity are suppressed.

Licorice Ingestion

Licorice, found in confections (103), chewing tobacco (104), some soft drinks, and herbal preparations, and carbenoxolone (105), a drug used for the treatment of peptic ulcer, contain glycyrrhetinic acid or its derivative, either of which potently inhibit this enzyme leading to a similar clinical presentation (106).

Nasal Spray

Habitual use of large doses of the nasal spray, 9-alpha-fluoroprednisolone, can also result in a similar clinical presentation by the putative direct action on the mineralocorticoid receptor in the principal cell of the CCD. These patients show suppressed plasma aldosterone, cortisol, and ACTH. Cessation of use results in complete resolution of hypokalemia and alkalosis (107).

Liddle Syndrome

Liddle and colleagues in 1963 reported an autosomal dominant form of hypertension characterized by hypokalemia, alkalosis, and suppressed aldosterone excretion rates in a white family (108,109); the disorder has subsequently been described in blacks and Hispanics (110,111) as well as in sporadic cases (112). Mutations in the subunits of Na^+ channel (EnaC) are now known to cause Liddle syndrome and are associated with increased Na^+ channel activity in CCD (113). The reported mutations involve the beta and gamma subunits (114,115) of the epithelial Na^+ channel (116,117). The mutations appear to prevent the binding of a protein, Nedd4, which may normally participate in exocytosis or degradation of the channel (118,119). The consequence is an increased number of functioning channels in the apical membrane leading to increased Na^+ uptake. The low circulating aldosterone concentrations are attributable to plasma volume expansion secondary to the increased Na^+ reabsorption with subsequent suppression of and aldosterone secretion. Enhanced Na^+ reabsorption will at the same time increase H^+ and K^+ secretion into the lumen of CCD, leading to hypokalemia and metabolic alkalosis.

Cushing Syndrome

Cushing syndrome may be caused by pituitary adenomas or adrenal tumors or hyperplasia (120). Although aldosterone production may be increased with adrenocortical adenoma, hypokalemia does not necessarily result (121). The magnitude of metabolic alkalosis in Cushing syndrome parallels the magnitude of hypokalemia (5). Renin substrate is increased but PRA is usually normal (122,123). Aldosterone excretion is typically normal or low (124) whereas the excretion rates of desoxycorticosterone and tetrahydrocorticosterone were several-fold higher than normal in patients with ectopic ACTH syndrome (125,126). Ectopic ACTH production, which leads to Cushing syndrome, is associated with a variety of tumors, most often small cell carcinoma of the lung (127); ACTH is usually not suppressible in this disorder. The more florid manifestations of mineralocorticoid excess in the ectopic ACTH syndrome have been attributed to 11-deoxycorticosterone. In addition, the massive increase in cortisol appears to overwhelm the capacity of the cortisol-cortisone shuttle, thereby allowing cortisol to function in a substantial way as a mineralocorticoid (127–129). Glucocorticoids enhance the expression and activity of NHE3 and NBC1 in the proximal tubule (130); whether this contributes to alkalosis in Cushing syndrome is unknown.

Mineralocorticoid Excess Without Hypertension

Several rare genetic disorders cause abnormalities in electrolyte transport in the kidney that produce hypokalemia and metabolic alkalosis without hypertension but increased serum aldosterone concentration and PRA. These disorders include Bartter (131) and Gitelman syndrome (132). Both disorders are characterized by urinary Na^+ and Cl^- wasting with resultant volume depletion, which, in turn, stimulates the renin–aldosterone axis.

Bartter Syndrome

Bartter syndrome usually presents in young patients, occasionally in the neonatal period. In addition to the aforementioned features, the neonatal variety has been associated with severe hypercalciuria and nephrocalcinosis (133,134). Although long an enigma, its pathophysiology and genetics have now been elucidated by molecular biologic techniques with the identification of at least three transport defects. Both inactivating and regulatory mutations that impair the function of the apical Na-K, 2Cl cotransporter have been identified on chromosome 15 (135–137). The second includes loss-of-function mutations of the apical ROMK channel, which have been identified on chromosome 11 (138,139). The third includes loss-of-function mutations in the basolateral Cl^- channel (CLC2) have been identified on chromosome 1 (140). The clinical presentations of these defects at these three loci are essentially identical because they all impair Na^+ and Cl^- reabsorption in Henle's loop (141). The classical form of Bartter syndrome (as opposed to the neonatal form) the third defect (142,143). Prostaglandin E2 synthesis is secondarily increased in Bartter syndrome but the precise stimulus is unknown. Heterozygotes of the ROMK mutations have been identified; one patient presented with hyperkalemia but a subsequent mild course (144–146).

Gitelman Syndrome

Gitelman syndrome is caused by several loss-of-function mutations in the gene on chromosome 16 encoding the thiazide-sensitive NaCl cotransporter in the distal convoluted tubule (141,147) and to at least one loss-of-function mutation of the chloride channel gene, CLCNKB, on chromosome 1 (148). In contrast with Bartter syndrome, homozygote patients with this disorder presents with hypomagnesemia and hypocalciuria (149,150). These adults typically complain of a panoply of constitutional symptoms likely associated with electrolyte and volume depletion: muscle cramps, weakness, fatigue, dizziness, salt craving, nocturia, polydipsia (151). Heterozygotes have serum electrolytes in the normal range but lower than normal control subjects (141). Potassium depletion can be severe enough to cause acute myoglobinuric renal failure (152).

In both Bartter and Gitelman syndromes, the impaired NaCl reabsorption that occurs before the collecting ducts leads to increased

Na^+ delivery to this nephron site promoting H^+ and K^+ secretion resulting in hypokalemia and metabolic alkalosis. Because not all of the delivered NaCl is reabsorbed, volume depletion ensues. This, in turn, stimulates aldosterone secretion thereby further augmenting Na^+ reabsorption and H^+ and K^+ secretion in the collecting duct.

These presentations can be mimicked by mixed K^+ and Cl^- deficiencies seen in conjunction with chloruretic diuretics or congenital chloridorrhea (153) (see Chapter 17).

Impaired Gut K⁺ Absorption

Laxative abuse has been associated with metabolic alkalosis, which is typically mild, or metabolic acidosis (154–157). The more constant feature is pronounced hypokalemia caused by excess K^+ in stool (see Chapter 8). If the K^+ depletion is chronic and severe, consequent renal failure, nephrogenic diabetes insipidus or renal tubular acidosis may confound or dominate the clinical presentation. Laxative abuse is often surreptitious and may be combined with surreptitious diuretic abuse or vomiting.

Geophagia, particularly in the form of clay ingestion, is uncommon but often associated with clinically significant K^+ depletion due to the K^+ binding capacity of clay (158).

DIAGNOSIS

Potassium depletion is most often heralded by hypokalemia. The most common causes of hypokalemia in clinical practice are due to diuretics and gastrointestinal loss secondary to diarrhea and/or vomiting. Diarrhea, particularly when severe, is usually associated with metabolic acidosis except in villous adenoma, which can present with hypokalemia and metabolic alkalosis (see Chapter 17). These etiologies should therefore be considered first before exhaustive and sophisticated work-up is initiated.

The algorithm in Fig. 5 provides an approach to the differential diagnosis. If the urine $[Cl^-]$ is $>20\,mEq/L$, K^+ depletion is the most likely cause of metabolic alkalosis; miscellaneous causes (see Chapter 19) are much less common. If renal K^+ wasting is the cause of K^+ depletion, urinary K^+ excretion exceeds $30\,mEq/day$ in the presence of hypokalemia. Alternatively, determination of the transtubular K^+ gradient (TTGK) (see Chapter 16) more rapidly can estimate the appropriateness of renal K^+ handling (159). Use of this estimate avoids the necessity of making a 24-hr urine collection and provides a prompt assessment of renal K^+ wasting. The TTGK is calculated by the formula: (urine/plasma $[K^+]$ × plasma/urine osmolality). In the setting of hypokalemia, a TTGK >2.5 (probably >4 in most cases) is consistent with renal K^+ wasting. Low urinary $[K^+]$ ($<15\,mEq/L$) and TTGK (<2.5) suggest gastrointestinal loss.

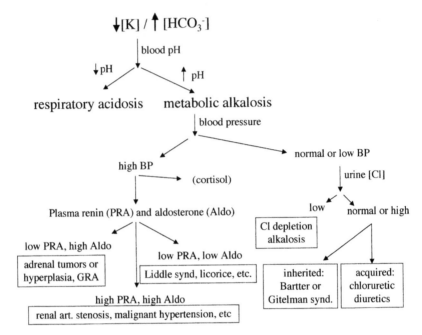

Figure 5 Differential diagnosis of hypokalemia with hyperbicarbonatemia. Chloride-depletion alkalosis and potassium-depletion alkalosis and respiratory acidosis all are shown (see text for discussion).

Determination of blood pressure and of renin, aldosterone and cortisol concentrations under appropriate conditions aid in further differentiating among these etiologies. Hypomagnesemia suggesting magnesium deficiency, which can result in renal K^+ wasting, is seen in Gitelman syndrome as well as in alcoholics who are also nutritionally depleted. Magnesium deficiency can present with metabolic alkalosis (160–162).

Diuretic and/or laxative abuse often mimics Bartter and Gitelman syndromes and should be considered in any adult patient with hypokalemia of unknown etiology and assessed by urinary testing for specific diuretics and stool test for phenolphthalein. The diagnosis of chronic laxative abuse, which is often surreptitious, is particularly difficult. It requires a high index of suspicion in women with chronic diarrhea, abdominal pain, or bizarre illnesses or psychiatric disorders.

MANAGEMENT

Potassium repletion is the primary management goal for K^+-depletion alkalosis. The amount of K^+ needed depends on the severity of the deficit as estimated from the serum $[K^+]$. In general, each $0.3\,mEq/L$ decrement in serum

[K$^+$] below 3.5 mEq/L suggests a decrement of 100 mEq in total body K$^+$. Based on this estimate, a patient with a serum [K$^+$] of 2.6 mEq/L needs at least 300 mEq of K$^+$ for the correction of the deficit. In calculating the total body K$^+$ deficit, one has to consider factors that can independently affect serum [K$^+$] such as pH. A patient with a serum [K$^+$] of 2.6 mEq/L has less total body deficit at blood pH of 7.5 than at pH 7.3. The reason is that alkaline serum pH (i.e., 7.5) can independently lower the serum K$^+$ by intracellular shift.

Potassium can be given orally (in mild to moderate hypokalemia) or intravenously (in severe hypokalemia). With mild to moderate deficits (serum [K$^+$] usually above 2.5), oral replacement will often suffice unless ileus is present. Oral KCl given in the liquid form diluted with fruit juice or in the slow-release form can be given in doses of up to 40–60 mEq four or five times per day. Potassium salts such as citrate, gluconate, or HCO$_3^-$ are not appropriate in K$^+$-depletion alkalosis. Usually, 50–100 mEq of KCl is required per day to maintain serum [K$^+$] within the normal range in patients with increased K$^+$ loss (i.e., in patients receiving diuretic). In addition to KCl, K$^+$ phosphate can be used in patients with combined K$^+$ and phosphate depletion (e.g., alcoholics, patients with liver cirrhosis or diabetic ketoacidosis) (Fig. 5).

If, however, a serious cardiac arrhythmia or generalized paralysis is present, intravenous KCl at rates no higher than 40 mEq/hr can be used. The downregulation of Na, K-ATPase in skeletal muscle with K$^+$ depletion states may slow the entry of the administered K$^+$ into cells (163). Thus, monitoring with electrocardiograms and frequent determinations of serum [K$^+$] are mandatory. Glucose should be omitted from infusions initially because stimulated insulin secretion may cause serum [K$^+$] to decrease even further. However, once repletion is begun, infused glucose will facilitate cellular K$^+$ repletion if insulin release is normal. Because hypokalemic nephropathy may prevent concentration of the urine, plasma [Na$^+$] should also be monitored. If chloruretic diuretics or laxatives are contributing, they should be stopped.

Correction of the K$^+$ deficit reverses the alkalinizing effects of K$^+$ depletion but, when mineralocorticoid excess is responsible, blockade or removal of the source of is essential for definitive correction. If the source of aldosterone excess cannot be removed, K$^+$-sparing diuretics will effectively blunt its effects. Amiloride 5–10 mg daily, triamterene 100 mg twice daily, or spironolactone 25–50 mg in single or divided doses daily all are useful. Spironolactone may produce unacceptable gynecomastia in men. Restriction of Na$^+$ and addition of K$^+$ to the diet will also ameliorate the alkalosis (164) and associated hypertension.

In Bartter and Gitelman syndromes, several therapeutic options should be considered. Correction of K$^+$ depletion is the primary goal so K$^+$ replacement—up to 500 mEq/day may be required—often augmented by K$^+$-sparing diuretics, amiloride, triamterene, or spironolactone (165). Indomethacin to reduce the untoward effects of prostaglandin excess is considered standard therapy (166) but caution is advised since enterocolitis and nephrotoxicity have been reported (167,168). A cylcooxygenase-2 inhibitor may be effective when a nonspecific cylcooxygenase inhibitor is not (169). Converting enzyme inhibitors have been used successfully to ameliorate the symptoms of Bartter syndrome and to correct hypokalemia (170) but blood pressure and glomerular filtration rate should be monitored closely when treatment is initiated.

In most cases of primary aldosteronism due to tumor as opposed to adrenal hyperplasia, surgical ablation is the treatment of choice (91). Correction of hypokalemia in states associated with excess mineralocorticoid significantly reduces the magnitude of alkalosis (42). Indeed, it has been suggested that in patients with primary aldosteronism that are not suitable candidates for surgical removal of the aldosterone-producing adenoma, correction of hypokalemia might be a viable alternative for the treatment of alkalosis (171). With adrenal tumors, adrenalectomy, either unilateral or bilateral as appropriate, may be curative. In the ectopic ACTH syndrome, the ideal treatment of the secreting tumor can rarely be accomplished. In these patients, ketoconazole reduces cortisol and ameliorates hypokalemia and alkalosis (172). Furthermore with ectopic ACTH syndrome and in metastatic adrenal tumors, metyrapone, which inhibits the final step in cortisol synthesis, and aminoglutethimide, which inhibits the initial step in steroid biosynthesis, will blunt the myriad manifestations of hypercortisolism. In those disorders in which curative surgery cannot be carried out, mitotane (p,p-DDD), which produces selective destruction of the zona fasiculata and reticularis and leaves aldosterone production intact, has also been used to control effectively many of the manifestations of the disease. However, to the extent that severe fluid and electrolyte disturbances are due solely to aldosterone production, this drug may not suffice when hypokalemic alkalosis is present; metyrapone or aminoglutethimide would be better choices. Cisplatin has also recently been used in the treatment of adrenal malignancies. With metastatic adrenocortical cancer, radiofrequency ablation is a safe and effective alternative to surgery or mitotane (173).

REFERENCES

1. Seldin DW, Jacobson H. On the generation, maintenance and correction of metabolic alkalosis. Am J Physiol 1983; 245:F425–F432.
2. Relman AS, Schwartz WB. The effect of DOCA on electrolyte balance in normal man and its relation to sodium chloride intake. Yale J Biol Med 1952; 24:540–558.
3. Seldin DW, Welt LG, Cort JH. The role of sodium salts and adrenal steroids in the production of hypokalemic alkalosis. Yale J Biol Med 1956; 29:229–247.

4. Seldin DW, Rector FC Jr. The generation and maintenance of metabolic alkalosis. Kidney Int 1972; 1:306–321.

5. Kassirer JP, London AM, Goldman DM, Schwartz WB. On the pathogenesis of metabolic alkalosis in hyperaldosteronism. Am J Med 1970; 49:306–315.

6. Mohamed SD, Chapman RS, Crooks J. Hypokalaemia, flaccid quadraparesis and myoglobinuria with carbenoxolone (Biogastrone). Brit Med J 1966; 5503:1581–1582.

7. Taylor GJ. Apnoea due to apparent potassium imbalance. Anaesthesia 1963; 18:9–15.

8. Rastegar A, DeFronzo RA. Disorders of potassium and acid–base metabolism in association with renal disease. In: R W Schrier, CW Gottschalk, eds. Diseases of the Kidney 6th ed. Boston: Little, Brown and Co., 1997:2452–2477.

9. Surawicz B, Barum H, Crim WB et al. Quantitative analysis of the electrocardiographic pattern of hypopotassemia. Circulation 1957; 16:750–763.

10. Helfant RH. Hypokalemia and arrhythmias. Am J Med 1986; 80 (suppl 4A):13–22.

11. Packer M, Gottlieb SS, Blum MA. Immediate and long-term pathophysiologic mechanisms underlying the genesis of sudden cardiac death in patients with congestive heart failure. Am J Med 1987; 82 (suppl 3A):4–10.

12. Bank N, Aynedjian HS. A micropuncture study of the renal concentrating defect of potassium depletion. Am J Physiol 1964; 206:1347–1354.

13. Relman AS, Schwartz WB. The kidney in potassium depletion. Am J Med 1958; 24:764–773.

14. Welt LG, Hollander W Jr, Blythe WB. The consequences of potassium depletion. J Chron Dis 1960; 11:213–254.

15. Amlal H, Krane CM, Chen QK, Soleimani M. Early polyuria and urinary concentrating defect in potassium deprivation. Am J Physiol 2000; 279:F655–F663.

16. Adrogue HJ, Madias NE. Changes in plasma potassium concentration during acute acid–base disturbances. Am J Med 1981; 71:456–462.

17. Luke RG, Levitin H. Impaired renal conservation of chloride and the acid–base changes associated with potassium depletion in the rat. Clin Sci 1967; 23:511–526.

18. Struyvenberg A, DeGraeff J, Lameijer, LDF. The role of chloride in hypokalemic alkalosis in the rat. J Clin Invest 1965; 44:326–331.

19. Adams WR, Koretsky AP, Weiner MW. ^{31}P-NMR in vivo measurement of renal intracellular pH: effect of acidosis and K^+ depletion in rats. Am J Physiol 1986; 20:F904–F910.

20. Jones JW, Sebastian A, Hulter HN, Schambelan M, Sutton JM, Biglieri EG. Systemic and renal acid–base effects of chronic potassium restriction in humans. Kidney Int 1982; 21:402–410.

21. Tannen RL, McGill J. Influence of potassium on renal ammonia production. Am J Physiol 1976; 231:F1178–F1184.

22. Sastrasinh S, Tannen RL. Effect of potassium on renal NH_3 production. Am J Physiol 1983; 244:F383–F391.

23. Tannen RL. Relationship of renal ammonia production and potassium homeostasis. Kidney Int 1977; 11:453–465.

24. Hamm LL, Simon EE. Ammonia transport in the proximal tubule in vivo. Am J Kidney Dis 1989; 14:253–257.
25. Tizianello A, Garibotto G, Robaudo C, Saffioti S, Pontremoli R, Bruzzone M, Deferrari G. Renal ammoniagenesis in humans with chronic potassium depletion. Kidney Int 1991; 40:772–778.
26. Sleeper RS, Belanger P, Lemieux G, Preuss HG. Effects of in vitro potassium on ammoniagenesis in rat and canine kidney tissue. Kidney Int 1982; 21:345–353.
27. Nakamura S, Amlal H, Galla JH, Soleimani M. Colonic H^+-K^+ATPase mediates NH_4^+ secretion in inner medullary collecting duct in potassium depletion. Kidney Int 1999; 56:2160–2167.
28. Hernandez RE, Schambelan M, Cogan MG, Colman J, Morris RC Jr, Sebastian A. Dietary NaCl determines severity of potassium depletion-induced metabolic alkalosis. Kidney Int 1987; 31:1356–1367.
29. Kaufman AM, Kahn T. Potassium-depletion alkalosis in the rat. Am J Physiol 1988; 255:F763–F770.
30. Black DAK, Milne MD. Experimental potassium depletion in man. Clin Sci 1952; 11:397–415.
31. Cannon PJ, Ames RP, Laragh JH. Relation between potassium balance and aldosterone secretion in normal subjects and in patients with hypertensive and renal tubular disease. J Clin Invest 1966; 45:865–879.
32. Kornandakieti C, Tannen RL. Hydrogen ion secretion by the distal nephron in the rat: effect of potassium. J Lab Clin Med 1984; 104:293–303.
33. Harrington JT, Hulter HN, Cohen JJ, Madias NE. Mineralocorticoid-stimulated renal acidification: the critical role of dietary sodium. Kidney Int 1986; 30:43–48.
34. Kornandakieti C, Tannen RL. H^+ transport by the aldosterone-deficient rat distal nephron. Kidney Int 1984; 25:629–635.
35. Hulter HN, Sebastian A, Sigala JF, Licht JH, Glynn RD, Schambelan M, Biglieri EG. Pathogenesis of renal hyperchloremic acidosis resulting from dietary potassium restriction in the dog: role of aldosterone. Am J Physiol 1980; 28:F79–F91.
36. McKinney TD, Davidson KK. Effect of potassium depletion and protein intake in vivo on renal bicarbonate transport in vitro. Am J Physiol 1987; 252:F509–F516.
37. Kessaris N, Shotliff K, Nussey SS. Hypokalaemic alkalosis. Postgrad Med J 1998; 74:305–306.
38. Tannen RL. Effect of potassium on renal acidification and acid–base homeostasis. Semin Nephrol 1987; 7:263–273.
39. Hamm LL, Alpern RJ. Cellular mechanisms of renal tubular acidification. In: DW Seldin, G, Giebisch, eds. The Kidney: Physiology and Pathophysiology. 2nd ed. New York: Raven Press, 1992:2581–2717.
40. Conn JW. Presidential address. II. Primary aldosteronism, a new clinical syndrome. J Lab Clin Med 1955; 45:3–17.
41. Conn JW, Cohen EL, Lucas CP, McDonald WJ, Mayor GH, Blough WM, Eveland WC, Bookstein JJ, Lapides J. Primary reninism. Hypertension, hyperreninemia and secondary aldosteronism due to renin-producing juxtaglomerular cell tumors. Arch Intern Med 1972; 130:682–696.

42. Hulter HN, Sigala JF, Sebastian A. K^+ deprivation potentiates the renal alka-losis-producing effect of mineralocorticoid. Am J Physiol 1978; 235:F298–F309.
43. Grunder S, Rossier BC. A reappraisal of aldosterone effects on the kidney: new insights provided by epithelial sodium channel cloning. Curr Opin Nephrol Hypertens 1997; 6:35–39.
44. Cely CM, Contreras G. Approach to the patient with hypertension, unexplained hypokalemia, and metabolic alkalosis. Am J Kidney Dis 2001; 37:E24.
45. Stone DK, Seldin DW, Kokko JP, Jacobson HR. Mineralocorticoid modulation of rabbit medullary collecting duct acidification. J Clin Invest 1983; 72:77–83.
46. Whinnery MA, Kunau RT. Effect of potassium deficiency on papillary plasma flow in the rat. Am J Physiol 1979; 237:F226–F231.
47. Linas SL, Dickmann D. Mechanism of the decreased renal blood flow in the potassium-depleted conscious rat. Kidney Int 1982; 21:757–764.
48. Rector FC Jr, Bloomer HA, Seldin DW. Effect of potassium deficiency on the reabsorption of bicarbonate in the proximal tubule of the rat kidney. J Clin Invest 1964; 43:1976–1982.
49. Kunau RT Jr, Frick A, Rector FC Jr, Seldin DW. Micropuncture study of the proximal tubular factors responsible for the maintenance of alkalosis during potassium deficiency in the rat. Clin Sci (Lond) 1968; 34:223–231.
50. Soleimani M, Singh G. Physiologic and molecular aspects of the Na^+/H^+ exchangers in health and disease processes. J Invest Med 1995; 43:419–430.
51. Soleimani M, Burnham CE. Physiologic and molecular aspects of the $Na:HCO_3^-$ cotransporter in health and disease processes. Kidney Int 2000; 57:371–384.
52. Soleimani M, Bergman JA, Hosford MA, McKinney TD. Potassium depletion increases $Na^+:CO_3^=:HCO_3^-$ cotransport in rat renal cortex. J Clin Invest 1990; 86:1076–1083.
53. Alpern RJ. Mechanism of basolateral membrane $H^+/OH^-/HCO_3^-$ transport in the rat proximal convoluted tubule. A sodium-coupled electrogenic process. J Gen Physiol 1985; 86:613–636.
54. Cemerikic D, Wilcox CS, Giebisch G. Intracellular potential and K^+ activity in rat kidney proximal tubular cells in acidosis and K^+ deprivation. J Membr Biol 1982; 69:159–165.
55. Wang Z, Baird N, Shumaker H, Soleimani M. Potassium depletion and acid–base transporters in rat kidney: differential effect of hypophysectomy. Am J Physiol 1997; 272:F736–F743.
56. Burnham CE, Amlal H, Wang Z, Shull GE, Soleimani M. Cloning and functional expression of a human kidney $Na^+:HCO_3^-$ cotransporter. J Biol Chem 1997; 272:19111–19114.
57. Burnham CE, Flagella M, Wang Z, Amlal H, Shull GE, Soleimani M. Cloning, renal distribution, and regulation of the rat $Na^+-HCO_3^-$ cotranspor-ter. Am J Physiol 1998; 274:F1119–F1126.
58. Amlal H, Habo K, Soleimani M. Potassium depletion upregulates the expression of the renal basolateral $Na^+:HCO_3^-$ cotransporter (NBC-1). Am J Physiol 2000; 279:F532–F543.

59. Bastani B, Haragsim L. Immunocytochemistry of renal H-ATPase. Miner Electrolyte Metab 1996; 22:382–395.
60. Bank N, Aynedjian HS, Mutz BF. Proximal tubule bicarbonate reabsorption independent of Na^+-H^+ exchange: Effect of bicarbonate load. Am J Physiol 1989; 256:F577–F582.
61. Aronson PS. The renal proximal tubule: a model for diversity of anion exchangers and stilbene-sensitive anion transporters. Annu Rev Physiol 1989; 51:419–441.
62. Aronson PS, Giebisch G. Mechanisms of chloride transport in the proximal tubule. Am J Physiol 1997; 273:F179–F192.
63. Wang T, Egbert AL Jr, Aronson PS, Giebisch G. Effect of metabolic acidosis on NaCl transport in the proximal tubule. Am J Physiol 1998; 274: F1015–F1019.
64. Luke RG, Wright FS, Fowler N, Kashgarian M, Giebisch G. Effect of potassium depletion on renal tubular chloride transport in the rat. Kidney Int 1978; 14:414–427.
65. Wang T, Malnic G, Giebisch G, Chan YL. Renal bicarbonate reabsorption in the rat. IV. Bicarbonate transport mechanisms in the early and late distal tubule. J Clin Invest 1993; 91:2776–2784.
66. Silver R, Soleimani M. H^+-K^+-ATPases: regulation and role in pathophysiologic states. Am J Physiol 1999; 276:F799–F811.
67. Biemesderfer D, Pizzonia J, Abu-Alfa A, Markus E, Reilly RF, Igarashi P, Aronson PS. NHE3: a Na^+/H^+ exchanger isoform of renal brush border. Am J Physiol 1993; 265:F736–F742.
68. Capasso G, Jaeger P, Giebisch G, Guckian V, Malnic G. Renal bicarbonate reabsorption in the rat. II. Distal tubule load dependence and effect of hypokalemia. J Clin Invest 1987; 80:409–414.
69. Bailey M, Capasso G, Agulian S, Giebisch G, Unwin R. The relationship between distal tubular proton secretion and dietary potassium depletion: evidence for up-regulation of H^+-ATPase. Nephrol Dial Transplant 1999; 14:1435–1440.
70. Bailey MA, Fletcher RM, Woodrow DF, Unwin RJ, Walter SJ. Upregulation of H^+-ATPase in the distal nephron during potassium depletion: structural and functional evidence. Am J Physiol 1998; 275:F878–F884.
71. Wingo CS, Smolka AJ. Function and structure of H-K-ATPase in the kidney. Am J Physiol 1995; 269:F1–F16.
72. Kone BC. Renal H, K-ATPase: structure, function, and regulation. Miner Elect Metab 1996; 22:349–365.
73. Zhou X, Wingo CS. Mechanisms of rubidium permeation by rabbit cortical collecting duct during potassium restriction. Am J Physiol 1992; 263: F1134–F1141.
74. Silver RB, Breton S, Brown D. Potassium depletion increases proton pump (H^+-ATPase) activity in intercalated cells of cortical collecting duct. Am J Physiol 2000; 279:F195–F202.
75. Wingo CS. Active proton secretion and potassium absorption in the rabbit outer medullary collecting duct. J Clin Invest 1989; 84:361–365.

76. Wingo CS, Armitage F. Rubidium absorption and proton secretion by rabbit outer medullary collecting duct via H^+, K^+-ATPase. Am J Physiol 1993; 263:F849–F857.

77. Gifford JD, Rome L, Galla JH. H^+-K^+-ATPase activity in rat collecting duct segments. Am J Physiol 1992; 262:F692–F695.

78. Kuwahara M, Fu WJ, Marumo F. Functional activity of H-K ATPase in individual cells of OMCD: localization and effect of K^+ depletion. Am J Physiol 1996; 270:F116–F122.

79. DuBose TD, Codina J, Burges A, Pressley TA. Regulation of H^+-K^+-ATPase expression in kidney. Am J Physiol 1995; 269:F500–F507.

80. Kraut JA, Hiura J, Besancon M, Smolka A, Sachs G, Scott D. Effect of hypokalemia on the abundance of HKα1 and HKα2 protein in the rat kidney. Am J Physiol 1997; 272:F744–F750.

81. Nakamura S, Wang Z, Galla JH, Soleimani M. Potassium depletion increases HCO_3^- reabsorption in outer medullary collecting duct by activation of colonic H-K-ATPase. Am J Physiol 1998; 274:F687–F692.

82. Kone BC, Higham SC. A novel N-terminal splice variant of the rat H^+-K^+-ATPase α2 subunit. J Biol Chem 1998; 273:2543–2552.

83. Nakamura S, Amlal H, Galla J, Soleimani M. Colonic H^+-K^+-ATPase is induced and mediates HCO_3^- reabsorption in IMCDt in potassium depletion. Kidney Int 1998; 54:1233–1239.

84. Amlal H, Goel A, Soleimani M. Activation of H^+-ATPase by hypotonicity: a novel regulatory mechanism for H^+ secretion in IMCD cells. Am J Physiol 1998; 275:F487–F501.

85. Alexander EA, Shih T, Schwartz JH. H^+ secretion is inhibited by clostridial toxins in an inner medullary collecting duct cell line. Am J Physiol 1997; 273:F1054–F1057.

86. Alexander EA, Brown D, Shih T, McKee M, Schwartz JH. Effect of acidification on the location of H^+-ATPase in cultured inner medullary collecting duct cells. Am J Physiol 1999; 276:758–763.

87. Buffin-Meyer B, Younes-Ibrahim M, Barlet-Bas C, Chevel L, Marsy S, Doucet A. K depletion modifies properties of SCH-28080-sensitive K-ATPase in rat collecting duct. Am J Physiol 1997; 272:F124–F131.

88. Amlal H, Wang Z, Soleimani M. Potassium depletion downregulates chloride-absorbing transporters in rat kidney. J Clin Invest 1998; 101: 1045–1054.

89. Streeten DH, Tomycz N, Anderson GH Jr. Reliability of screening methods for diagnosis of primary aldosteronism. Am J Med 1979; 67:403–413.

90. Katz FH. Primary aldosteronism with suppressed plasma renin activity due to bilateral nodular adrenocortical hyperplasia. Ann Int Med 1967; 67: 1035–1042.

91. Ganguly A. Primary aldosteronism. N Engl J Med 1998; 339:1828–1834.

92. Kono T, Ikeda F, Oseko F, Imura H, Tanimura H. Normotensive primary hyperaldosteronism: report of a case. J Clin Endocrinol Metab 1981; 52: 1009–1013.

93. Sutherland DJA, Ruse JL, Laidlaw JC. Hypertension, increased aldosterone secretion and low plasma renin activity relieved by dexamethasone. Can Med Assoc J 1966; 95:1109–1119.

94. Lifton RP, Dluhy RG, Powers M, Rich GM, Cook S, Ulick S, Lalouel JM. A chimaeric 11β-hydroxylase/aldosterone synthase gene causes glucocorticoid-remediable aldosteronism and human hypertension. Nature 1992; 355: 262–265.

95. Lifton RP, Dluhy RG, Powers M, Rich GM, Cook S, Ulick S, Lalouel JM. Hereditary hypertension caused by chimaeric gene duplications and ectopic expression of aldosterone synthase. Nat Genet 1992; 2:66–74.

96. Auchus RJ. The genetics, pathophysiology, and management of human deficiencies of P450c17. Endocrinol Metab Clin North Am 2001; 30:101–119.

97. Peter M, Sippell WG, Wernze H. Diagnosis and treatment of 17-hydroxylase deficiency. J Steroid Biochem Mol Biol 1993; 45:107–116.

98. Laragh JH, Ulick S, Januszewicz V, Deming QB, Kelly WG, Lieberman S. Aldosterone secretion and primary and malignant hypertension. J Clin Invest 1960; 39:1091–1106.

99. White PC. 11 β-hydroxysteroid dehydrogenase and its role in the syndrome of apparent mineralocorticoid excess. Am J Med Sci 2001; 322:308–315.

100. Stewart PM, Murry BA, Mason JI. Human kidney 11 β-hydroxysteroid dehydrogenase is a high affinity nicotinamide adenine dinucleotide-dependent enzyme and differs from the cloned type I isoform. J Clin Endocrinol Metab 1994; 79:480–484.

101. Albiston AL, Obeyesekere VR, Smith RE, Krozowski ZS. Cloning and tissue distribution of the human 11 β-hydroxysteroid dehydrogenase type 2 enzyme. Mol Cell Endocrinol 1994; 105:R11–R17.

102. Mantero F, Palermo M, Petrelli MD, Tedde R, Stewart PM, Shackleton CH. Apparent mineralocorticoid excess: type I and type II. Steroids 1996; 61: 193–196.

103. de Klerk GJ, Nieuwenhuis MG, Beutler JJ. Hypokalaemia and hypertension associated with use of liquorice-flavoured chewing gum. BMJ 1997; 314: 731–732.

104. Blachley JD, Knochel JP. Tobacco chewer's hypokalemia: licorice revisited. N Engl J Med 1980; 320:784–785.

105. Davies GJ, Rhodes J, Calcraft BJ. Complications of carbenoxolone therapy. Br Med J 1974; 3:400–402.

106. Farese RV Jr, Biglieri EG, Shackleton CH, Irony I, Gomez-Fontes R. Licorice-induced hypermineralocorticoidism. N Engl J Med 1991; 325: 1223–1227.

107. Mantero F, Armanini D, Opocher G, Fallo F, Sampieri L, Cuspidi B, Ambrosi C, Faglia G. Mineralocorticoid hypertension due to a nasal spray containing 9 alpha-fluoroprednisolone. Am J Med 1981; 71:352–357.

108. Liddle GW, Bledsoe T, Coppage WS Jr. A familial renal disorder stimulating primary aldosteronism but with negligible aldosterone secretion. Trans Assoc Am Physicians 1963; 76:199–213.

109. Botero-Velez M, Curtis JJ, Warnock DG. Brief report: Liddle's syndrome revisited. N Engl J Med 1994; 330:178–181.

110. Gadallah MF, Abreo K, Work J. Liddle's syndrome: an under-recognized entity: a report of four cases including the first report in black individuals. Am J Kidney Dis 1995; 25:924–927.

111. Rodriquez JA, Biglieri EG, Schambelan M. Pseudohypoaldosteronism with renal tubular resistance to mineralocorticoid hormones. Trans Assoc Am Physicians 1981; 94:172–182.

112. Yamashita Y, Koga M, Takeda Y, Enomoto N, Uchida S, Hashimoto K, Yamano S, Dohi K, Marumo F, Sasaki S. Two sporadic cases of Liddle's syndrome caused by de novo ENaC mutations. Am J Kidney Dis 2001; 37: 499–504.

113. Warnock DG. Liddle syndrome: genetics and mechanisms of Na+ channel defects. Am J Med Sci 2001; 322:302–307.

114. Shimkets RA, Warnock DG, Bositis CM, Nelson-Williams C, Hansson JH, Schambelan M, Gill JR, Ulick S, Milora RV, Findling JW. Liddle's syndrome: heritable human hypertension caused by mutations in the β subunit of the epithelial sodium channel. Cell 1994; 79:407–414.

115. Hansson JH, Nelson-Williams C, Suzuki H, Schlid L, Shimkets R, Lu Y, Canessa C, Iwasaki T, Rossier B, Lifton RP. Hypertension caused by a truncated epithelial sodium channel γ subunit: genetic heterogeneity of Liddle syndrome. Nat Genet 1995; 11:76–82.

116. Canessa CM, Horisberger J, Rossier BC. Epithelial sodium channel related to proteins involved in neurodegeneration. Nature 1993; 361:467–470.

117. Canessa CM, Schild L, Buell G, Thorens B, Gautschi I, Horisberger JD, Rossier BC. The amiloride-sensitive epithelial sodium channel is made of three homologous subunits. Nature 1994; 367:463–467.

118. Staub O, Dho S, Henry PC, Correa J, Ishikawa T, McGlade J, Rotin D. WW domains off Nedd4 bind to the proline-rich PY motifs in the epithelial Na$^+$ channel deleted in Liddle's syndrome. EMBO J 1996; 15:2371–2380.

119. Palmer BF, Alpern RJ. Liddle's syndrome. Am J Med 1998; 104:301–309.

120. Orth DN. Cushing's syndrome. N Engl J Med 1995; 332:791–803.

121. Guthrie GP Jr, Kotchen TA. Hypertension and aldosterone overproduction without renin suppression in Cushing's syndrome from an adrenal adenoma. Am J Med 1979; 67:524–528.

122. Krakoff L, Nicolis G, Amsel B. Pathogenesis of hypertension in Cushing's syndrome. Am J Med 1975; 58:216–220.

123. Ritchie CM, Sheridan B, Fraser R, Hadden DR, Kennedy AL, Riddell J, Atkinson AB. Studies on the pathogenesis of hypertension in Cushing's disease and acromegaly. Q J Med 1990; 76:855–867.

124. Mantero F, Armanini D, Boscaro M. Plasma renin activity and urinary aldosterone in Cushing's syndrome. Horm Metab Res 1978; 10:65–71.

125. Biglieri EG, Hane S, Slaton PE, Forsham PH. In vivo and in vitro studies of adrenal secretions in Cushing's syndrome and primary aldosteronism. J Clin Invest 1963; 42:516–524.

126. Rickman T, Garmany R, Doherty T, Benson D, Okusa MD. Hypokalemia, metabolic alkalosis, and hypertension: Cushing's syndrome in a patient with metastatic prostate adenocarcinoma. Am J Kidney Dis 2001; 37: 838–846.

127. Torpy DJ, Mullne N, Ilias I, Nieman LK. Association of hypertension and hypokalemia with Cushing's syndrome caused by ectopic ACTH secretion: a series of 58 cases. Ann NY Acad Sci 2002; 970:134–144.

128. Ulick S, Wang JZ, Blumenfeld JD, Pickering TG. Cortisol inactivation overload: a mechanism of mineralocorticoid hypertension in the ectopic adrenocorticotropin syndrome. J Clin Endocrinol Metab 1992; 74:963–967.

129. Walker BR, Campbell JC, Fraser R, Stewart PM, Edwards CR. Mineralocorticoid excess and inhibition of 11 β-hydroxysteroid dehydrogenase in patients with ectopic ACTH syndrome. Clin Endocrinol 1992; 37:483–492.

130. Ali R, Amlal H, Burnham CE, Soleimani M. Glucocorticoids enhance the expression of the basolateral $Na^+:HCO_3^-$ cotransporter in renal proximal tubules. Kidney Int 2000; 57:1063–1071.

131. Bartter FC, Provone P, Gill JR, MacCardle RC. Hyperplasia of the juxtaglomerular complex with hyperaldosteronism and hypokalemic alkalosis. Am J Med 1962; 33:811–828.

132. Simon DB, Lifton RP. Ion transporter mutations in Gitelman's and Bartter's syndromes. Curr Opin Nephrol Hypertens 1998; 7:43–47.

133. Fanconi A, Schachenmann G, Nussli R, Prader A. Chronic hypokalemia with growth retardation, normotensive hyperrenin-hyperaldosteronism (Bartter's syndrome) and hypercalciuria. Helv Paediatr Acta 1971; 26:144–163.

134. Proesmans W. Bartter syndrome and its neonatal variant. Eur J Pediatr 1997; 156:669–679.

135. Simon DB, Karet FE, Hamdan JM, Di Pietro A, Sanjad SA, Lifton RP. Bartter's syndrome, hypokalemic alkalosis with hypercalciuria, is caused by mutations in the Na-K-2Cl co-transporter NKCC2. Nat Genet 1996; 13: 183–188.

136. Vargas-Poussou R, Feldmann D, Vollmer M, Konrad M, Kelly L, van den Heuvel LPWJ, Tebourbi L, Brandis M, Karolyi L, Hebert SC, Lemmink HH, Deschenes G, Hildebrandt F, Seyberth HW, Guay-Woodford L, Knoers NVAM, Antignac C. Novel molecular variants of the Na-K-2Cl cotransporter gene are responsible for antenatal Bartter syndrome. Am J Hum Genet 1998; 62:1332–1340.

137. Kurtz CL, Karolyi L, Seyberth HW, Koch MC, Vargas R, Feldmann D, Vollmer M, Knoers NVAM, Madrigal G, Guay-Woodford LM. A common NKCC2 mutation in Costa Rican Bartter's syndrome patients: evidence for a founder effect. J Am Soc Nephrol 1997; 8:1706–1711.

138. Simon DB, Karet FE, Rodriguez-Soriano J, Hamdan JH, DiPietro A, Trachtman H, Sanjad SA, Lifton RP. Genetic heterogeneity of Bartter's syndrome revealed by mutations in the K channel, ROMK. Nat Genet 1996; 14:152–156.

139. Vollmer M, Koehrer M, Topaloglu R, Strahm B, Omran H. Two novel mutations of the gene for Kir 1.1 (ROMK) in neonatal Bartter syndrome. Pediatr Nephrol 1998; 12:69–71.

140. Thakker RV. Molecular pathology of renal chloride channels in Dent's disease and Bartter's syndrome. Exp Nephrol 2000; 8:351–360.

141. Shaer AJ. Inherited primary renal tubular hypokalemic alkalosis: a review of Gitelman and Bartter syndromes. Am J Med Sci 2001; 322:316–332.

142. Simon DB, Bindra RS, Mansfield TA, Nelson-Williams C, Mendonca E, Stone R, Schurmann S, Nayir A, Alpay H, Bakkaloglu A, Rodrigeuz-Soriano J, Morales JM, Saniad SA, Taylor CM, Pilz D, Brem A, Trachtman H, Griswold W, Richard GA, John E, Lifton RP. Mutations in the chloride channel gene, CLCNKB, cause Bartter's syndrome type III. Nat Genet 1997; 17:171–178.

143. Konrad M, Vollmer M, Lemmink HH, van den Huevel LPWJ, Jeck N, Vargas-Possou R, Lakings A, Ruf R, Deschenes G, Antignac C, Guay-Woodford L, Knoers NVAM, Seyberth HW, Feldmann D, Hildebrant F. Mutations in the chloride channel gene CLCNKB as a cause of classic Bartter syndrome. J Am Soc Nephrol 2000; 11:1449–1459.

144. Schwalbe RA, Bianchi L, Accili EA, Brown AM. Functional consequences of ROMK mutants linked to antenatal Bartter's syndrome and implications for treatment. Hum Mol Genet 1998; 7:975–980.

145. Lu M, Wang T, Yan Q, Yang X, Dong K, Knepper MA, Wang W, Giebisch G, Shull GE, Hebert SC. Absence of small conductance K^+ channel (SK) activity in apical membranes of thick ascending limb and cortical collecting duct in ROMK (Bartter's) knockout mice. J Biol Chem 2002; 277:37881–37887.

146. Cho JT, Guay-Woodford LM. Heterozygous mutations of the gene for Kir 1.1 (ROMK) in antenatal Bartter syndrome presenting with transient hyperkalemia, evolving to a benign course. J Korean Med Sci 2003; 18:65–68.

147. Simon DB, Nelson-Williams C, Bia MJ, Ellsion D, Karet FE, Molina AM, Vaara I, Iwata F, Cushner HM, Koolen, M, Gainza FJ, Gitelman HJ, Lifton RP. Gitelman's variant of Bartter's syndrome, inherited hypokalemic alkalosis, is caused by mutations in the thiazide-sensitive Na-Cl cotransporter. Nat Genet 1996; 12:24–30.

148. Zelikovic I, Szargel R, Hawash A, Labay V, Hatib I, Cohen N, Nakhoul F. A novel mutation in the chloride channel gene, CLCNKB, as a cause of Gitelman and Bartter syndromes. Kidney Int 2003; 63:24–32.

149. Bettinelli A, Bianchetti MG, Girardin E, Caringella A, Cecconi M, Appiani AC, Pavanello L, Gastaldi R, Isimbaldi C, Lama G, Marchesoni C, Matteucci C, Patriarca P, DiNatale B, Setzu C, Vitucci P. Use of calcium excretion values to distinguish two forms of primary renal tubular hypokalemic alkalosis: Bartter and Gitlelman syndromes. J Pediatr 1992; 20:38–43.

150. Cruz DN, Simon DB, Nelson-Williams C, Farhi A, Finberg K, Burleson L, Gill JR, Lifton RP. Mutations in the Na-Cl cotransporter reduce blood pressure in humans. Hypertension 2001; 37:1458–1464.

151. Cruz DN, Shaer AJ, Bia MJ, Lifton RP, Simon DB. Gitelman's syndrome revisited: an evaluation of symptoms and health-related quality of life. Kidney Int 2001; 59:710–717.

152. Nishihara G, Higashi H, Matsuo S, Yasunaga C. Acute renal failure due to hypokalemic rhabdomyolysis in Gitelman's syndrome. Clin Nephrol 1998; 50:330–332.

153. Wall BM, Williams HH, Cooke CR. Chloride-resistant metabolic alkalosis in an adult with congenital chloride diarrhea. Am J Med 1988; 85:570–572.

154. Schwartz WB, Relman AS. Metabolic and renal studies in chronic potassium depletion resulting from overuse of laxatives. J Clin Invest 1953; 32:258–271.

155. Fleischer N, Brown H, Graham DY, Delena S. Chronic laxative-induced hyperaldosteronism and hypokalemia simulating Bartter's syndrome. Ann Intern Med 1969; 70:791–798.

156. Cummings JH, Sladen GE, James OFW, Sarner M, Misiewicz JJ. Laxative-induced diarrhoea: a continuing clinical problem. Br Med J 1974; 1:537–541.

157. Wright LF, DuVal JW Jr. Renal injury associated with laxative abuse. South Med J 1987; 80:1304–1306.

158. Severance HW, Holt T, Patrone NA, Chapman L. Profound muscle weakness and hypokalemia due to clay ingestion. South Med J 1988; 81:272–274.

159. Ethier JH, Kamel KS, Magner PO, Lemann J Jr, Halperin ML. The transtubular potassium concentration in patients with hypokalemia and hyperkalemia. Am J Kidney Dis 1990; 15:309–315.

160. Solomon R. The relationship between disorders of K^+ and Mg^{++} homeostasis. Semin Nephrol 1987; 7:253–262.

161. Konrad M, Weber S. Recent advances in molecular genetics of hereditary magnesium-losing disorders. J Am Soc Nephrol 2003; 14:249–260.

162. Darr M, Hamburger S, Ellerbeck E. Acid–base and electrolyte abnormalities due to capreomycin. South Med J 1982; 75:627–628.

163. Clausen T, Everts ME. Regulation of the Na, K-pump in skeletal muscle. Kidney Int 1989; 35:1–13.

164. Krishna GG, Kapoor SC. Potassium supplementation ameliorates mineralocorticoid-induced sodium retention. Kidney Int 1993; 43:1097–1103.

165. Guay-Woodford LM. Bartter syndrome: unraveling the pathophysiologic enigma. Am J Med 1998; 105:151–161.

166. Verberckmoes R, Van Damme B, Clement J, Amery A, Michielsen P. Bartter's syndrome with hyperplasia of renomedullary cells. Successful treatment with indomethacin. Kidney Int 1976; 9:302–307.

167. Marlow N, Chiswick ML. Neonatal Bartter's syndrome, indomethacin, and necrotizing enterocolitis. Acta Pediatr Scand 1982; 71:1031–1032.

168. Schachter AD, Arbus GS, Alexander RJ, Balfe JW. Non-steroidal anti-inflammatory drug-associated nephrotoxicity in Bartter syndrome. Pediatr Nephrol 1998; 12:775–777.

169. Mayan H, Gurevitz O, Farfel Z. Successful treatment by cylcooxygenase-2 inhibitor of refractory hypokalemia in a patient with Gitelman's syndrome. Clin Nephrol 2002; 58:73–76.

170. Hene RJ, Koomans HA, Dorhout Mees EJ, vd Stolpe A, Verhoef GE, Boer P. Correction of hypokalemia in Bartter's syndrome by enalapril. Am J Kidney Dis 1987; 9:200–205.

171. Melby JC. Primary aldosteronism. Kidney Int 1984; 26:769–778.

172. Winquist EW, Laskey J, Crump M, Khamsi F, Shepherd FA. Ketoconazole in the management of paraneoplastic Cushing's syndrome secondary to ectopic adrenocorticotropin production. J Clin Oncol 1995; 13:157–164.

173. Abraham J, Fojo T, Wood BJ. Radiofrequency ablation of metastatic lesions in adrenocortical cancer. Ann Intern Med 2000; 133:312–313.

174. Sterns RH, Cox M, Feig PU, Singer IM. Internal potassium balance and the control of plasma potassium concentration. Medicine 1981; 60:339–354.

_____ **19** _____

Metabolic Alkalosis:
Miscellaneous Causes

John H. Galla and Robert G. Luke

*Department of Medicine, University of Cincinnati College of Medicine,
Cincinnati, Ohio, U.S.A.*

INTRODUCTION

Metabolic alkalosis may occur because of a number of factors unrelated to Cl^- or K^+ depletion or to mineralocorticoid excess (Table 1). The pathophysiology, clinical characteristics, and treatment of these disorders are considered in this chapter.

HYPERCALCEMIC DISORDERS

General

Hypercalcemia in humans is associated with both metabolic acidosis and metabolic alkalosis (1–3). Metabolic alkalosis infrequently occurs with disorders of calcium metabolism but may be seen with malignancy, idiopathic or surgical hypoparathyroidism (4), vitamin D intoxication, and sarcoidosis. The milk-alkali syndrome is treated separately.

Pathogenesis—Effects of Parathyroid Hormone

Because both acidosis and alkalosis are seen with hypercalcemia, the elevated serum $[Ca^{2+}]$ per se is not the cause. Rather, the different mechanisms by which hypercalcemia is produced appear to determine the acid–base

585

Table 1 Miscellaneous Causes of Metabolic Alkalosis

Hypercalcemic states
   Hypercalcemia of malignancy
   Acute or chronic milk-alkali syndrome
Other
   Carbenicillin, ampicillin, penicillin
   Bicarbonate ingestion—massive or with renal insufficiency
   THAM
   Recovery from starvation; refeeding
   Hypoalbuminemia
   Exchange resins and antacids
   Recovery from organic acidosis
   Alkaline dialysis

consequences, together with the resultant effects on the kidney and on extracellular buffering. To dissect the factors that produce these acid–base disturbances, hypercalcemia has been induced in human volunteers and other mammalian species by a variety of maneuvers, which are, by and large, peculiar to each particular study. This fact unfortunately confounds analysis of the collective data.

The majority of these studies have been conducted in dogs. In these studies, acute parathyroid hormone (PTH) administration decreased renal HCO_3^- reabsorption and acid excretion (5,6). By contrast, a micropuncture study showed that, after thyroparathyroidectomy (TPTX) and thyroid replacement, intravenous PTH infusion decreased HCO_3^- and fluid reabsorption in the proximal tubule but did not change urine $[HCO_3^-]$ (7). In dogs with isolated hypoparathyroidism, hypocalcemia was sustained despite a high calcium diet and plasma $[HCO_3^-]$ was unchanged (8). PTH administration for 24–48 hr, given either subcutaneously or intravenously, increased plasma $[HCO_3^-]$ and arterial pH modestly (9). With longer periods of PTH administration to TPTX dogs, similar results were noted along with sustained hypophosphatemia, hypercalcemia, and increased net acid excretion (10). Hyperparathyroidism produced by calcium chelation with continuous intravenous EGTA resulted in an even greater degree of alkalosis but without an increase in net acid excretion, suggesting an extrarenal mechanism (10).

In rabbit superficial proximal convoluted and straight tubules perfused in vitro, PTH inhibits both fluid and HCO_3^- uptake, the latter by inhibition of luminal Na^+/H^+ exchange (11–13). Metabolic acidosis would be the expected consequence of this effect.

In rats after TPTX, PTH infusion acutely inhibits fluid and HCO_3^- reabsorption in the proximal tubule with no change in overall renal HCO_3^- reabsorption (14); these data agree substantially with those obtained in dog. Thus, distal nephron segments were apparently able to reabsorb the increased delivery of HCO_3^-; in addition urine net acid excretion increased suggesting stimulation of renal H^+ secretion. In similarly treated anephric rats, PTH was associated with higher blood pH and plasma [HCO_3^-] but not when acetazolamide was given concurrently (15). In addition, administration of EDTA or colchicine, both of which stimulate PTH release, increased plasma [HCO_3^-]. Taken together, these data suggest that PTH enhances extrarenal alkali release by a mechanism that involves the participation of carbonic anhydrase. In chronic hypercalcemia, either multiple grafts of autologous parathyroid gland, which increase PTH, or 1,25(OH)-vitamin D loading, which suppresses PTH, produced mild metabolic alkalosis with increased net acid excretion (16). These observations suggest that hypercalcemia rather than hyperparathyroidism is necessary to generate the alkalosis.

Finally, in humans, PTH infusion produces hypercalcemia with an initial decrease followed by a sustained increase in net acid excretion and a modest increase in serum [HCO_3^-] (17); the respective roles of PTH vs. hypercalcemia were not examined in that study. Collectively, these studies suggest that hypercalcemia produced by several different protocols in different species results in metabolic alkalosis.

The clinical experience is quite different from these experimental data. In treated or untreated hypoparathyroidism, metabolic alkalosis is the rule (1). Although acid–base disorders occur relatively infrequently in the setting of hypercalcemia, metabolic alkalosis is reported in patients with malignancies with or without bone involvement, even with detectable PTH secretion from the neoplasm (18,19). In contrast, hyperchloremic metabolic acidosis is seen in primary hyperparathyroidism (20). Indeed, prior to the widespread availability of PTH measurements, the serum chloride (high) to phosphate (low) ratio was used as a laboratory aid in the diagnosis of primary hyperparathyroidism. Taken together, these clinical observations suggest that hypercalcemia and the presence of suppressed PTH concentrations are the circumstances in which metabolic alkalosis is most likely to occur, e.g., the hypercalcemia of malignancy (21). Whether the presence or concentration of PTH-related protein (PTHrP), which is strongly implicated in the hypercalcemia of malignancy unrelated to bone metastases (22), is related to the presence of alkalosis has not been examined. In the latter circumstances, one might anticipate that endogenous PTH concentrations would be suppressed. Considering the principles of acid–base chemistry (23), the maintained alkalosis may be due, at least in part, to the increase in strong ion difference caused by increased ionized Ca^{2+} per se. A role for enhanced HCO_3^- uptake in the proximal tubule due to suppressed PTH is also possible.

Treatment

Therapy should be directed at the primary cause of the hypercalcemia whenever possible. Mild hypercalcemia usually is not associated with severe alkalosis and treatment need be undertaken only if clinical circumstances dictate (24). With the hypercalcemia of malignancy, volume expansion with saline solutions and the bisphosphonate drugs are the standard treatment (25). In the rare instance of a PTH-secreting renal cell carcinoma, excision of the tumor resulted in resolution of the alkalosis (19).

MILK-ALKALI SYNDROME

General

Renal failure, metabolic alkalosis, and hypercalcemia in the setting of high calcium and alkali intake are the cardinal features of this syndrome (26), which occurs in both an acute and a chronic form. The latter form is often accompanied by low urinary calcium excretion, normal to high serum phosphate, and signs of metastatic calcification (27).

Clinical Presentation

The milk-alkali syndrome originally was linked to alkali treatment for peptic ulcer disease—the so-called Sippy diet (28–31). In the chronic form, the relationship first recognized was renal failure with alkalosis (29); hypercalcemia was not associated until more than 10 years later. Chronicity has been associated with metastatic calcification of the eyes—where it can be seen directly in the cornea as band keratopathy (27), and, to lesser degrees, in kidney, bone, joints, liver, skin, lung, adrenal, vasculature, and brain (32–34). Nephrolithiasis may occur (34). Polydipsia and polyuria are relatively uncommon. Weakness, myalgias, and pruritus are probable accompaniments of muscle and skin involvement. Pancreatitis, which has been reported with a myriad of causes of hypercalcemia, occurs uncommonly in milk-alkali syndrome but may pose a serious complication (35). In the acute form, which can occur after only 7–10 days of calcium and alkali ingestion, alkalosis is often severe. Hypercalcemia may be sufficiently high to produce obtundation or psychosis in addition to the other described features.

With the new emphasis on increasing calcium intake, especially in women, to prevent and treat osteoporosis along with the use of over-the-counter calcium salts, the milk-alkali syndrome is increasing in frequency; in a recent series, it was the third leading cause of hypercalcemia after primary hyperparathyroidism and cancer (36). In this report, the majority of the patients were women (55%) consuming calcium carbonate often supplemented with milk. Of the patients reported in detail, all had adopted these regimens without the knowledge or direction of their physicians. Thus, it is essential to review patients' consumption of over-the-counter medications, many of which may contain calcium carbonate.

In an unusual variation on this theme, betel nut chewing has recently been associated with hypercalcemia, metabolic alkalosis, and acute renal failure (37). Calcium carbonate is apparently combined with betel nut as a paste to blunt its bitter taste. In this report, alkalosis and hypercalcemia resolved with cessation of the agent and the renal function improved significantly. Plasma 1,25-dihydroxycholecalciferol and PTH were low; the latter increased appropriately when plasma [Ca^{2+}] was decreased upon treatment. The factor(s) leading to enhanced calcium absorption are unknown.

With an external source of calcium to produce hypercalcemia, one would anticipate decreased serum PTH concentrations with all cases of milk-alkali syndrome. However, elevated concentrations have been reported (36), leading on occasion to surgical exploration for a parathyroid adenoma (38). It is likely that these elevations were due to determinations of carboxy-terminal PTH concentrations in the setting of renal insufficiency. Advances in the radioimmunoassay of the active moiety of PTH should make this diagnostic misadventure rare.

The timing of the sampling for PTH is critical since elevated concentrations have been reported when treatment of the milk-alkali syndrome resulted in hypocalcemia, producing a so-called rebound increase in PTH (36).

Pathogenesis

The generation of metabolic alkalosis in milk-alkali syndrome is not established but is probably both complex and multifactorial (26). Chloride depletion, hypercalcemia, which may increase HCO_3^- reabsorption or impair urine concentrating ability, a high intake of alkali, and a reduced glomerular filtration rate (GFR), which may be secondary to extracellular fluid (ECF) volume depletion, Cl^- depletion, or nephrocalcinosis, all could play a role.

Gastric aspiration along with the administration of a milk-based diet and nearly continual intake of alkaline powders was a component of the original Sippy diet (28), making Cl^- depletion a likely pathogenic component in early reports. Likewise, vomiting is a common but not universal accompaniment in more recent reports (39,40). As discussed in Chapter 17, Cl^- depletion produces and maintains metabolic alkalosis by several mechanisms, which will not be reiterated here.

There is no evidence for any role for load-independent increases in renal calcium reabsorption to explain the hypercalcemia in milk-alkali syndrome (41). Urine calcium excretion is increased acutely (42), but reduced in the chronic setting (27). Massive alkali intake normally leads to only transient increases in serum [HCO_3^-]. In 20 men ingesting $CaCO_3$, mean serum calcium, phosphorus, and bicarbonate concentrations rose followed by an increase in serum creatinine concentration and a decrease in urinary concentrating ability; one developed milk-alkali syndrome (42). In contrast, chronic oral calcium loading as milk, $CaCl_2$ or $CaCO_3$ had no overall effect on calcium balance. Calcium carbonate ingestion decreased renal acid excretion, whereas milk and $CaCl_2$ ingestion increased acid excretion (43). In normal humans given cimetidine to reduce gastric acid secretion and in one subject with achlorhydria, net calcium absorption was unaffected by the reduction in gastric H^+ secretion (44). However, in another study in patients with achlorhydria, calcium carbonate ingestion was associated with much lower calcium absorption compared to calcium citrate; normal subjects showed no such difference (45). Others have shown that citrate decreases fractional intestinal calcium absorption in normal human subjects (46). In humans given 1 g calcium salts orally, plasma calcium concentration increased slightly (by 6%) but decreased when omeprazole was added; urine calcium excretion also declined with omeprazole (47). Although these data do not permit any clear conclusions, increased calcium ingestion appears to be associated with increased absorption but alkali ingestion or a higher gastric pH may decrease it.

Either hyperparathyroidism or hypervitaminosis D may promote hypercalcemia but neither has been reported in this syndrome although hyperparathyroidism and milk-alkali syndrome can occur simultaneously (48). Serum PTH concentrations are uniformly low and serum 1,25-OH dihydroxyvitamin D (1,25-OH D) are either low or low normal (39). Low PTH concentrations may accelerate HCO_3^- reabsorption in the proximal tubule, potentially promoting alkalosis. While calcium carbonate may not suppress 1,25-OH D in normal humans (49) and its disordered control may play a role in "absorptive" hypercalciuria (50), neither of these conditions are associated with hypercalcemia, alkalosis, or renal failure.

Once hypercalcemia has been established, GFR can be reduced acutely by either vasoconstriction (51) or a reduction in the ultrafiltration coefficient (52). Hypercalcemia also impairs solute transport in the ascending limb of Henle's loop (53,54). Thus, calcium excretion may be further compromised by volume depletion as a consequence of impaired water conservation and vomiting. If the course is prolonged and nephrocalcinosis occurs, scarring may further reduce GFR, often irreversibly.

Treatment

Hypercalcemia in the milk-alkali syndrome typically resolves with a decrease in calcium intake. As with other causes of hypercalcemia, volume expansion with or without the use of loop diuretics is an effective treatment, particularly of the acute form. Correction of accompanying volume depletion is essential. Renal insufficiency usually resolves with the acute syndrome whereas the degree of resolution with chronic variety is dependent on the degree of permanent renal scarring engendered by nephrocalcinosis (39).

OTHER DISORDERS

Antibiotics

Treatment with congeners of penicillin including ampicillin and carbenicillin (the latter no longer available in the United States) have been associated with mild metabolic alkalosis (55). The pathophysiology has not been elucidated but a hypothesis derives from studies of sodium salts of ineffectively reabsorbed anions such as sulfate (56); the observation that sodium sulfate does not sustain an increase in net acid excretion leaves this question open, however. These "nonreabsorbable" anionic antibiotics may simply stimulate K^+ and H^+ excretion through voltage effects in the collecting duct (57).

Hypoalbuminemia

Albumin is the principal protein buffer circulating in the plasma; its buffering capacity is conferred by the numerous histidine groups in its structure (58,59). Thus, hypoproteinemic states by virtue of the decrease in the weak acid concentration also result in a modest degree of metabolic alkalosis (60). This cause of metabolic alkalosis was recognized initially as a decreased anion gap in association with gammopathies (61).

Alkali Intake

Because the normal kidney is so efficient at excreting HCO_3^-, base loading, whether exogenous or endogenous (as in bone dissolution), is rarely a sole cause of significant sustained metabolic alkalosis. Transient acute metabolic alkalosis commonly occurs during and immediately after oral ingestion or intravenous infusion of $NaHCO_3$ or another base equivalent, e.g., citrate in transfused blood or fresh frozen plasma (62,63). Ingestion of $NaHCO_3$ (baking soda) or a metabolic precursor, such as acetate or citrate, does not produce sustained metabolic alkalosis unless intake is massive—in the range of 1000 mEq/day—and prolonged (64,65), GFR is impaired (66), or dietary NaCl is low (67). Typically, the alkalosis resolves spontaneously when alkali intake ceases. Chloride intake may be protective against the development of metabolic alkalosis during base loading (67). A state of transient metabolic alkalosis may also occur after the successful treatment of ketoacidosis or lactic acidosis as these organic anions are metabolized to bicarbonate. Metabolic alkalosis may also occur after refeeding starving subjects with glucose but not with protein or fat (68). The mechanism is not established but may relate to glucose-induced metabolism of ketoacids, previously induced by starvation, to HCO_3^- together with a delay in reducing the enhanced renal acid secretion stimulated by the starvation ketoacidosis. The pathophysiologic responses of the kidney to alkali loading compared to Cl^- depletion have underlined their fundamentally different natures: for example, in the ascending limb of Henle's loop, HCO_3^-

reabsorption decreases with Cl^- depletion but increases with HCO_3^- loading (69) (see Chapter 17).

Citrate infusions are used for regional anticoagulation for both continuous and intermittent hemodialysis primarily when the patient is at increased risk of bleeding or in the setting of heparin-induced thrombocytopenia (70–72). Because the kidney is not participating in dissipating the calcium citrate load in this setting, metabolic alkalosis is more likely to develop (73,74) but it can be prevented by adjusting the buffer content of the dialysate solution (75).

Antacids

Nonabsorbable antacids have also been associated with alkalosis when used together with cation-exchange resins in the setting of renal insufficiency (76); the proposed mechanism is that magnesium or aluminum hydroxides, which normally bind HCl, are bound by the resin in exchange for Na^+. Because the sodium carbonates formed are soluble, HCO_3^- is readily reabsorbed by the intestine (77) and alkalosis ensues because the kidney is unable to excrete the HCO_3^-.

Dialysis

Mild metabolic alkalosis occurs after hemodialysis performed in the conventional prescription of three times per week (see Chapter 24).

REFERENCES

1. Barzel US. Acid–base balance in disorders of calcium metabolism. NY State J Med 1976; 76:234–237.
2. Heinemann HO. Metabolic alkalosis in patients with hypercalcemia. Metabolism 1965; 14:1137–1152.
3. David NJ, Verner JV, Engel FL. The diagnostic spectrum of hypercalcemia. Am J Med 1962; 33:88–110.
4. Barzel US. Systemic alkalosis in hypoparathyroidism. J Clin Endocrinol Metab 1969; 29:917–918.
5. Arruda JAL, Nascimento L, Westenfelder C, Kurtzman N. Effect of parathyroid hormone on urinary acidification. Am J Physiol 1977; 232:F429–F433.
6. Diaz-Buxo JA, Ott CE, Cuche JL, Marchand GR, Wilson DM, Knox FG. Effects of extracellular fluid volume contraction and expansion on the bicarbonaturia of parathyroid hormone. Kidney Int 1975; 8:105–109.
7. Puschett JB, Zurbach P, Sylk D. Acute effects of parathyroid hormone on proximal bicarbonate transport in the dog. Kidney Int 1976; 9:501–510.
8. Hulter HN, Toto RD, Bonner EL Jr, Ilnicki LP, Sebastian A. Renal and systemic acid–base effects of chronic hypoparathyroidism in dogs. Am J Physiol 1981; 241:F495–F501.

9. Licht JH, McVicker K. Parathyroid-hormone-induced metabolic alkalosis in dogs. Miner Electrolyte Metab 1982; 8:78–91.

10. Hulter HN, Toto RD, Ilnicki LP, Halloran B, Sebastian A. Metabolic alkalosis in models of primary and secondary hyperparathyroid states. Am J Physiol 1983; 245:F450–F461.

11. Iino Y, Burg MB. Effect of parathyroid hormone on bicarbonate absorption by proximal tubules in vitro. Am J Physiol 1979; 236:F387–F391.

12. McKinney TD, Myers P. PTH inhibition of bicarbonate transport by proximal convoluted tubules. Am J Physiol 1980; 239:F127–F134.

13. Sasaki S, Marumo F. Mechanisms of inhibition of proximal acidification by PTH. Am J Physiol 1991; 260:F833–F838.

14. Bank N, Aynedjian HS. A micropuncture study of the effect of parathyroid hormone on renal bicarbonate reabsorption. J Clin Invest 1976; 58:336–344.

15. Arruda JA, Alla V, Rubenstein H, Cruz-Soto M, Sabatini S, Batlle DC, Kurtzman NA. Parathyroid hormone and extrarenal acid buffering. Am J Physiol 1980; 239:F533–F538.

16. Mitnick P, Greenberg A, Coffman T, Kelepouris E, Wolf CJ, Goldfarb S. Effects of two models of hypercalcemia on renal acid base metabolism. Kidney Int 1982; 21:613–620.

17. Hulter HN, Peterson JC. Acid–base homeostasis during chronic PTH excess in humans. Kidney Int 1985; 28:187–192.

18. Sanderson PH. Hypercalcemia and renal failure in multiple secondary carcinoma of bone. Br Med J 1959; 2:275–277.

19. O'Grady AS, Morse LJ, Lee JB. Parathyroid hormone-secreting renal carcinoma associated with hypercalcemia and metabolic alkalosis. Ann Int Med 1965; 63:858–868.

20. Mallette LE, Bilezikian JP, Heath DA, Aurbach GD. Primary hyperparathyroidism: clinical and biochemical features. Medicine 1974; 53:127–146.

21. Mundy GR, Yates AJ. Recent advances in pathophysiology and treatment of hypercalcemia of malignancy. Am J Kidney Dis 1989; 14:2–12.

22. Rankin W, Grill V, Martin TJ. Parathyroid hormone-related protein and hypercalcemia. Cancer 1997; 80:1564–1571.

23. Stewart PA. Moderate quantitative acid–base chemistry. Can J Physiol Pharmacol 1983; 61:1444–1461.

24. Bilezikian JP. Clinical review 51: management of hypercalcemia. J Clin Endocrinol Metab 1993; 77:1445–1449.

25. Body JJ. Current and future directions in medical therapy: hypercalcemia. Cancer 2000; 88:3054–3058.

26. Schuman CA, Jones HW III. The "milk-alkali" syndrome: two case reports with discussion of pathogenesis. Q J Med 1985; 55:119–126.

27. Burnett CH, Commons RB, Albright F, Howard JE. Hypercalcemia without hypercalciuria or hypophosphatemia , calcinosis and renal insufficiency. N Engl J Med 1949; 240:788–794.

28. Sippy BW. Gastric and duodenal ulcer: medical cure by an efficient removal of gastric juice corrosion. J Am Med Assoc 1915; 64:1625–1630.

29. Hardy LL, Rivers AB. Toxic manifestations following alkaline treatment of peptic ulcer. Arch Int Med 1923; 31:171–180.

30. McCance RA, Widdowson EM. Alkalosis with disordered kidney functions: observations on case. Lancet 1937; 2:247–249.
31. Kirsner JB, Palmer WL. Alkalosis complicating Sippy treatment of peptic ulcer: analysis of 135 episodes. Arch Int Med 1942; 69:789–807.
32. Kyle LH. Differentiation of hyperparathyroidism and the milk-alkali (Burnett) syndrome. N Engl J Med 1954; 251:1035–1040.
33. Junor BJR, Catto GRD. Renal biopsy in the milk-alkali syndrome. J Clin Pathol 1976; 29:1074–1076.
34. Punsar S, Somer T. The milk-alkali syndrome. A report of three illustrative cases and a review of the literature. Acta Med Scand 1963; 173:435–449.
35. Brandwein SL, Sigman KM. Case report. Milk-alkali syndrome and pancreatitis. Am J Med Sci 1994; 308:173–176.
36. Beall DP, Scofield RH. Milk-alkali syndrome associated with calcium carbonate consumption. Medicine 1995; 74:89–96.
37. Lin S-H, Lin Y-F, Cheema-Dhadli S, Davids MR, Halperin ML. Hypercalcemia and metabolic alkalosis with betel nut chewing: emphasis on its integrative pathophysiology. Nephrol Dial Transplant 2002; 17:708–714.
38. Carroll PR, Clark OH. Milk-alkali syndrome. Does it exist and can it be differentiated from primary hyperparathyroidism?. Ann Surg 1983; 197:427–433.
39. Abreo K, Adlakha A, Kilpatrick S, Flanagan R, Webb R, Shakamuri S. The milk-alkali syndrome. A reversible form of acute renal failure. Arch Int Med 1993; 153:1005–1010.
40. Muldowney WP, Mazbar SA. Rolaids-yogurt syndrome: a 1990s version of milk-alkali syndrome. Am J Kidney Dis 1999; 27:270–272.
41. Schron CM. Vitamins and minerals. In: Yamada T, ed. Textbook of Gastroenterology 2nd ed. Philadelphia: JB Lippincott Co., 1995:477.
42. McMillan DE, Freeman RB. The milk-alkali syndrome: a study of the acute disorder with comments on the development of the chronic condition. Medicine 1965; 44:485–501.
43. Lewis NM, Marcus MS, Behling AR, Greger JL. Calcium supplements and milk: effects on acid–base balance and on retention of calcium, magnesium, and phosphorus. Am J Clin Nutr 1989; 49:527–533.
44. Bo-Linn GW, Davis GR, Buddrus DJ, Morawski SG, Santa Ana C, Fordtran JS. An evaluation of the importance of gastric acid secretion in the absorption of dietary calcium. J Clin Invest 1984; 73:640–647.
45. Recker RR. Calcium absorption and achlorhydria. N Engl J Med 1985; 313:70–73.
46. Rumenapf G, Schwille PO. The influence of oral alkali citrate on intestinal calcium absorption in healthy man. Clin Sci (Lond) 1987; 73:117–121.
47. Graziani G, Como G, Badalamenti S, Finazzi S, Malesci A, Gallieni M, Brancaccio D, Ponticelli C. Effect of gastric acid secretion on intestinal phosphate and calcium absorption in normal subjects. Nephrol Dial Transplant 1995; 10:1376–1380.
48. Wilder WT, Frame B, Haubrich WS. Peptic ulcer in primary hyperparathyroidism: an analysis of fifty-two cases. Ann Int Med 1961; 55:885–893.

49. Adams ND, Gray RW, Lemann J. The effects of oral CaCO₃ loading and dietary calcium deprivation on plasma 1,25-dihydroxyvitamin D concentration in healthy adults. J Clin Endocrinol Metab 1979; 48:1008–1016.
50. Broadus AE, Insogna KL, Lang R, Ellison AF, Dreyer BE. Evidence for disordered control of 1,25-dihydroxyvitamin D production in absorptive hypercalciuria. N Engl J Med 1984; 311:73–80.
51. Zawada ET, TerWee JA, McClung DE. Systemic and renal vascular responses to dietary calcium and vitamin D. Hypertension 1986; 8:975–982.
52. Humes HD, Ichikawa I, Troy JL, Brenner BM. Evidence for a parathyroid hormone-dependent influence of calcium on the glomerular ultrafiltration coefficient. J Clin Invest 1978; 61:32–40.
53. Quamme GA. Effect of hypercalcemia on renal tubular handling of calcium and magnesium. Can J Physiol Pharmacol 1982; 60:1275–1280.
54. Galla JH, Booker BB, Luke RG. Role of the loop segment in the urinary concentrating defect of hypercalcemia. Kidney Int 1986; 29:977–982.
55. Stapleton FB, Nelson B, Vats TS, Linshaw MA. Hypokalemia associated with antibiotic treatment. Am J Dis Child 1976; 130:1104–1108.
56. Lipner HI, Ruzany F, Dasgupta M, Lief PD, Bank N. The behavior of carbenicillin as a nonreabsorbable anion. J Lab Clin Med 1975; 86:183–194.
57. Brunner FP, Frick PG. Hypokalemia, metabolic alkalosis, and hypernatremia due to "massive" sodium penicillin therapy. Br Med J 1968; 4:550–552.
58. Figge J, Rossing TH, Fencl V. The role of serum proteins in acid–base equilibria. J Lab Clin Med 1991; 117:453–467.
59. Figge J, Mydosh T, Fencl V. Serum proteins and acid–base equilibria: a follow-up. J Lab Clin Med 1992; 120:713–719.
60. McAuliffe JJ, Lind LJ, Leith DE, Fencl V. Hypoproteinemic alkalosis. Am J Med 1986; 81:86–90.
61. Frohlich J, Adam W, Golbey MJ, Bernstein M. Decreased anion gap associated with monoclonal and pseudomonoclonal gammopathy. J Can Med Assoc 1976; 114:231–232.
62. Pearl RG, Rosenthal MH. Metabolic alkalosis due to plasmapheresis. Am J Med 1985; 79:391–393.
63. Barcenas CG, Fuller TJ, Knochel JP. Metabolic alkalosis after massive blood transfusion. Correction by hemodialysis. J Am Med Assoc 1976; 236:953–954.
64. Lowder SC, Brown RD. Hypertension corrected by discontinuing chronic sodium bicarbonate ingestion. Subsequent transient hypoaldosteronism. Am J Med 1975; 58:272–279.
65. Goidsenhoven GMT van, Gray OV, Price AV, Sanderson PH. The effect of prolonged administration of large doses of sodium bicarbonate in man. Clin Sci 1954; 13:383–401.
66. Marques MB, Huang ST. Patients with thrombotic thrombocytopenic purpura commonly develop metabolic alkalosis during therapeutic plasma exchange. J Clin Apheresis 2001; 16:120–124.
67. Cogan MG, Carneiro J, Tatsumo J. Normal diet NaCl variation can affect the renal set point for plasma pH- (HCO₃) maintenance. J Am Soc Nephrol 1990; 1:193–199.

68. Veverbrants E, Arky RA. Effects of fasting and refeeding. I. Studies on sodium, potassium and water excretion on a constant electrolyte and fluid intake. J Clin Endocrinol Metab 1969; 29:55–62.

69. Good DW. Bicarbonate absorption by the thick ascending limb of Henle's loop. Semin Nephrol 1990; 10:1850–1862.

70. Pinnick RV, Wiegmann TB, Diederich DA. Regional citrate anticoagulation for hemodialysis in the patient at high risk for bleeding. N Engl J Med 1983; 308:258–261.

71. Mehta RL, McDonald BR, Aguilar MM, Ward DM. Regional citrate anticoagulation for continuous arteriovenous hemodialysis in critically ill patients. Kidney Int 1990; 38:976–981.

72. Evenepoel P, Maes B, Vanwalleghem J, Kuypers D, Messiaen T, Vanrenterghem Y. Regional citrate anticoagulation for hemodialysis using a conventional calcium-containing dialysate. Am J Kidney Dis 2002; 39:315–323.

73. Silverstein FJ, Oster JR, Perez GO, Materson BJ, Lopez RA, Al-Reshaid K. Metabolic alkalosis induced by regional citrate hemodialysis. ASAIO Trans 1989; 35:22–25.

74. Faber LM, de Vries PM, Oe PL, van der Meulen J, Donker AJ. Citrate haemodialysis. Neth J Med 1990; 37:219–224.

75. van der Meulen J, Janssen MJ, Langendijk PN, Bouman AA, Oe PL. Citrate anticoagulation and dialysate with reduced buffer content in chronic hemodialysis. Clin Nephrol 1992; 37:36–41.

76. Madias NE, Levey AS. Metabolic alkalosis due to absorption of "nonabsorbable" antacids. Am J Med 1983; 74:155–158.

77. Schroeder ET. Alkalosis resulting from combined administration of a "nonsystemic" antacid and a cation-exchange resin. Gastroenterol 1969; 56:869–874.

20

Respiratory Acidosis

Horacio J. Adrogué
Baylor College of Medicine, VA Medical Center, Houston, Texas, U.S.A.

Nicolaos E. Madias
*Department of Medicine, Caritas St. Elizabeth's Medical Center,
Tufts University School of Medicine, Boston, Massachusetts, U.S.A.*

INTRODUCTION AND DEFINITIONS

Respiratory acidosis (primary hypercapnia) is initiated by an increase in the CO_2 tension of the body fluids. As a consequence, carbonic acid concentration increases, increasing $[H^+]$. At sea level, a $PaCO_2$ higher than 44 mmHg indicates the presence of respiratory acidosis. In young children (< 3 years old), during pregnancy, in subjects residing at high altitude, or in patients with metabolic acidosis, $PaCO_2$ values < 44 mmHg can be indicative of respiratory acidosis (see Chapters 21 and 22). A special case of respiratory acidosis is the presence of arterial eucapnia, or even arterial hypocapnia, coupled with venous and, therefore, tissue hypercapnia (1). This entity, termed pseudorespiratory alkalosis, can develop in patients with profound depression of cardiac function and pulmonary perfusion who have relative preservation of alveolar ventilation (2). Because body CO_2 stores are increased, respiratory acidosis rather than respiratory alkalosis is present. Complicating acid–base disorders occur frequently in patients with respiratory acidosis (see Chapter 22). In this chapter, we review the pathophysiology, diagnosis, and management of primary hypercapnia.

PATHOPHYSIOLOGY

The ventilatory system is responsible for maintaining $PaCO_2$ within normal limits by adjusting alveolar ventilation ($\dot{V}_A$) to match the rate of CO_2

production ($\dot{V}_{CO_2}$) (see Chapter 3). A reduction in ($\dot{V}_A$) leading to CO_2 retention (i.e., respiratory acidosis) is the dominant mechanism responsible for this acid–base disorder. The determinants of CO_2 retention can be viewed as factors imposing an imbalance between the strength of the respiratory pump and the weight of the respiratory load (Fig. 1). When the respiratory pump is unable to balance the opposing load, respiratory acidosis develops. Decreases in respiratory pump strength, increases in load, or a combination of the two, can result in CO_2 retention (3). Respiratory pump failure can occur because of depressed central drive, abnormal neuromuscular transmission, or respiratory muscle dysfunction. Higher load can be caused by enhanced ventilatory demand, increased dead space ventilation, augmented airway flow resistance, lung stiffness, or pleura/chest wall stiffness.

Respiratory acidosis is categorized into acute and chronic forms, taking into consideration the mode of onset and particularly the duration of the various causes (Tables 1 and 2) (4). Life-threatening acidemia can occur during severe, acute respiratory acidosis, or during respiratory decompensation in patients with chronic hypercapnia. In most clinical settings, the development of hypercapnia is multifactorial, and recognition of each of the underlying mechanisms of CO_2 retention allows for effective patient management (see Tables 1 and 2).

Pseudorespiratory Alkalosis

A marked reduction in pulmonary perfusion in the presence of relative preservation of alveolar ventilation can also result in CO_2 retention leading to the condition referred to as "pseudorespiratory alkalosis." The severely reduced pulmonary blood flow limits the CO_2 delivered to the lungs for excretion, thereby increasing the venous PCO_2. However, the increased ventilation-to-perfusion ratio ($\dot{V}/\dot{Q}$ ratio) causes a larger than normal removal of CO_2 per unit of blood traversing the pulmonary circulation, thereby giving rise to arterial eucapnia or frank hypocapnia. A progressive widening of the arteriovenous difference in pH and PCO_2 develops in such settings of profound cardiac dysfunction, including circulatory failure and cardiac arrest (1,2) (Fig. 2). Severe O_2 deprivation prevails in the tissues in these two disorders, and it can be completely disguised by the reasonably preserved arterial O_2 values. Appropriate monitoring of acid–base composition and oxygenation in patients with advanced cardiac dysfunction requires mixed (or central) venous blood sampling in addition to the sampling of arterial blood.

Enhanced CO_2 Production

Overproduction of CO_2 is seldom the sole cause of CO_2 retention because enhanced $\dot{V}_{CO_2}$ stimulates ventilation, thus increasing CO_2 excretion (3,5) (Chapter 3). Nonetheless, patients with a marked reduction in pulmonary reserve or receiving mechanical ventilation might develop respiratory acidosis

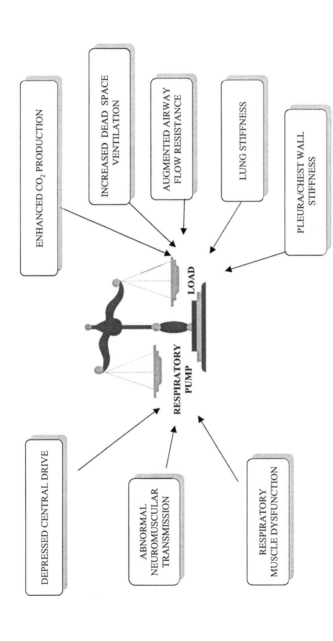

Figure 1 Pathogenesis of respiratory acidosis. When the respiratory pump is unable to balance the opposing load, respiratory acidosis develops. Decreases in respiratory pump strength, increases in load, or a combination of the two can result in carbon dioxide retention. *Source:* Modified from Ref. 175.

Table 1   Causes of Acute Respiratory Acidosis

Increased Load	Depressed Pump
Enchanced ventilatory demand	*Depressed central drive*
High carbohydrate diet	General anesthesia
High carbohydrate dialysate	Sedative overdose
(peritoneal dialysis)	Head trauma
Sorbent-regenerative hemodialysis	Cerebrovascular accident
Increased dead space ventilation	Obesity hypoventilation syndrome
Acute lung injury	Cerebral edema
Multi-lobar pneumonia	Brain tumor
Cardiogenic pulmonary edema	Encephalitis
Pulmonary embolism	Brain-stem lesion
Positive pressure ventilation	Ondine's curse
Supplemental oxygen	*Abnormal neuromuscular transmission*
Augmented airway flow resistance	High spinal cord injury
Upper airway obstruction	Guillain-Barré syndrome
Coma-induced hypopharyngeal	Status epilepticus
obstruction	Botulism; tetanus
Aspiration of foreign body or vomitus	Crisis in myasthenia gravis
Laryngospasm	Familial periodic paralysis
Angioedema	Drugs or toxic agents (e.g., curare,
Inadequate laryngeal intubation	Succinylcholine, aminoglycosides,
Laryngeal obstruction postintubation	Organophosphate poisoning)
Lower airway obstruction	*Muscle dysfunction*
Status asthmaticus	Fatigue
Exacerbation of chronic obstructive	Hyperkalemia
pulmonary disease	Hypokalemia
Lung stiffness	Hypothyroidism
Atelectasis	
Pleura/chest wall stiffness	
Pneumothorax	
Haemothorax	
Flail chest	
Abdominal distension	
Peritoneal dialysis	

because of increased CO_2 production. Clinical settings characterized by increased CO_2 production include carbohydrate loading (6–8), vigorous exercise (9), fever (10), sepsis (11), multi-organ failure (12), burns (13), and hyperthyroidism (14). The effect of hyperthermia can be substantial because CO_2 production increases by approximately 13% for each 1°C increase in body temperature above normal. As a result, a fever to 40°C demands an approximate 40% increase in ventilation to maintain a normal $PaCO_2$.

Table 2 Causes of Chronic Respiratory Acidosis

Increased Load	Depressed Pump
Increased dead space ventilation	*Depressed central drive*
Emphysema	Central sleep apnea
Pulmonary fibrosis	Obesity hypoventilation syndrome
Pulmonary vascular disease	Methadone/heroin addiction
Augmented airway flow resistance	Brain tumor
Upper airway obstruction	Bulbar poliomyelitis
Tonsillar and peritonsillar hypertrophy	Hypothyroidism
Paralysis of vocal cords	*Abnormal neuromuscular transmission*
Tumor of the cords of larynx	High spinal cord injury
Airways stenosis postprolonged intubation	Poliomyelitis
Thymoma, aortic aneursym	Multiple sclerosis
Lower airway obstruction	Muscular dystrophy
Chronic obstructive pulmonary disease	Amyotrophic lateral sclerosis
Lung stiffness	Diaphragmatic paralysis
Severe chronic interstitial lung disease	*Muscle dysfunction*
Pleura/chest wall stiffness	Myopathic disease (e.g., polymyositis)
Kyphoscoliosis	
Thoracic cage disease	
Thoracoplasty	
Obesity	

Additional causes of CO_2 loading include the infusion of bicarbonate-containing solutions, hemodialysis with sorbent regenerative cartridge systems, and insufflation of the peritoneum with CO_2 during endoscopic procedures (15,16).

Increased Dead Space Ventilation

Unless $\dot{V}CO_2$ falls simultaneously, a reduction in $\dot{V}_A$ is always responsible for CO_2 retention (4,5). Alveolar ventilation will fall when total minute ventilation ($\dot{V}_E$) is decreased or when dead space ventilation ($\dot{V}_D$) is increased. An increase in $\dot{V}_D$ can occur in association with decreased, normal, or even increased $\dot{V}_E$. The fraction of inspired gas not reaching the gas exchange surfaces is "wasted" and, therefore, is referred to as dead space volume. The term $\dot{V}_D/\dot{V}_T$ (dead space/tidal volume) refers to the proportion of tidal volume that ventilates dead space; in health this ratio is approximately 0.25–0.35.

Rapid and shallow breathing reduces the fraction of fresh air reaching the alveoli during each respiratory cycle (increased $\dot{V}_D/\dot{V}_T$) but total ventilation is usually increased (17). Conditions associated with a rapid and shal-

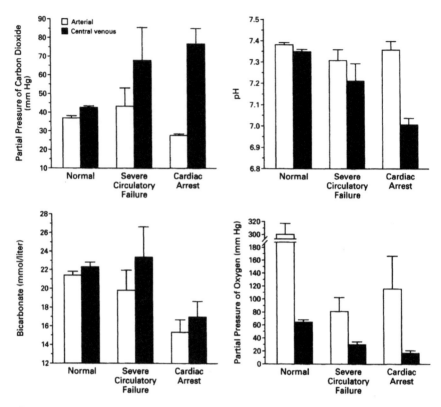

Figure 2 Simultaneous mean (+SE) arterial and central venous values for PCO_2, pH, $[HCO_3^-]$, and PO_2 in 26 patients with normal hemodynamic status, five patients with severe circulatory failure, and five patients with cardiac arrest undergoing cardiopulmonary resuscitation. *Source*: From Ref. 2.

low breathing pattern include many pulmonary diseases, a large fraction of patients with acute respiratory failure, and during failure to wean from mechanical ventilation (17–19). Thus, increased $\dot{V}_D/\dot{V}_T$ in the presence of normal or increased $\dot{V}_E$ is responsible for the CO_2 retention in most patients with respiratory failure (3,5). Advanced chronic obstructive pulmonary disease (COPD) is a typical condition in which increased $\dot{V}_D$ dominates the CO_2 retention observed. The maintenance of eucapnia in patients with less advanced disease results from an increased $\dot{V}_E$, which compensates for the inefficiency of the CO_2 excretion imposed by the $\dot{V}_A/\dot{Q}$ mismatch. The nearly linear shape of the CO_2 dissociation curve over the physiologic range greatly facilitates the excretion of CO_2 in patients with all types of $\dot{V}_A/\dot{Q}$ inequalities, because blood leaving areas with low $\dot{V}_A/\dot{Q}$ ratio (that has a relatively high PCO_2) is counterbalanced when mixed with blood traversing high $\dot{V}_A/\dot{Q}$ units (that has relatively low PCO_2 values) (3). However, if some alveolar units cannot be effectively hyperventilated (high $\dot{V}_A/\dot{Q}$ ratio), respiratory acidosis will develop.

Other Mechanisms of Increased Ventilatory Load

Augmented airway flow resistance, lung stiffness, and pleura or chest wall stiffness, all increase ventilatory load (i.e., work of breathing) and impose an imbalance between the load and the strength of the respiratory pump, thereby predisposing to CO_2 retention. Hyperinflation of the lungs in the course of airway obstruction, whether acute or chronic in nature, increases the respiratory load and impairs the effectiveness of the respiratory muscles. The downward displacement of the diaphragm caused by air trapping causes its flattening; a greater change in pressure must then be generated by the respiratory muscles to achieve a similar change in pulmonary volume and air flow, hastening the onset of respiratory muscle fatigue. With severe pulmonary overinflation, the diaphragm is almost flat at the end of expiration and its contraction causes lung deflation instead of inflation; this phenomenon results in the inward movement of the lower rib cage during inspiration that is known as the "Hoover sign."

Patients with decreased ventilatory drive and respiratory muscle dysfunction in the setting of increased work of breathing develop hypercapnia and hypoxemia ("blue bloater" profile); by contrast, these abnormalities in blood gases are not seen in patients who exhibit a higher ventilatory drive ("pink puffer" profile) (3). In a comparable manner, patients with a history of near fatal asthma demonstrate, during periods of disease quiescence, depressed hypoxic and hypercapnic ventilatory responses as well as reduced perception of dyspnea with added resistive loads (20).

Depressed Central Drive

Morphine derivatives, barbiturates, and benzodiazepines suppress central respiratory drive, and these drugs should be used with caution in patients at risk for CO_2 retention (3,5). When $PaCO_2$ is within normal limits, substantial changes in $\dot{V}_A$ are required to elicit large changes in $PaCO_2$. However, if hypercapnia is already present, small changes in $\dot{V}_A$ result in large deviations in $PaCO_2$ (Chapter 3). Consequently, a major rise in $PaCO_2$ in association with decreases in PaO_2 can be observed in response to sedatives in hypercapnic patients with severe asthma or COPD. By contrast, the suppressive effect of drugs on the central respiratory drive can prove useful in patients with hypocapnia secondary to anxiety, pain, or malignant pleural effusion.

Abnormal Function of Respiratory Muscles

In contrast with respiratory pump depression caused by decreased central drive (i.e., "won't breathe" patients), the global hypoventilation resulting from respiratory muscle weakness is often accompanied by an increased ventilatory drive (i.e., "can't breathe" patients) (21). Primary disorders of the respiratory muscles and of the motor neurons responsible for pulmonary ventilation are classic examples of this pathophysiologic mechanism. However, an even larger and heterogeneous group of patients exists in which fatigue of the respiratory muscles plays a critical role in the development of respiratory acidosis. Such respiratory muscle fatigue is observed with poor nutrition, certain electrolyte disorders (potassium and phosphate depletion), an obligatory high level of ventilation, decreased compliance of the respiratory system, increased resistance to airflow, and alterations in thoracic configuration. Structural and functional changes in the respiratory muscles as well as depletion of their energy stores occur with malnutrition. Respiratory muscle weakness, combined with depression of ventilatory drive, is responsible for the hypoventilation in severe hypothyroidism (22).

Hypercapnia and Hypoxemia

Equation (20.1) presents the simplified form of the alveolar gas equation at sea level and when breathing room air (FiO_2, 21%):

$$P_AO_2 = 150 - 1.25 \, PaCO_2 \qquad\qquad (20.1)$$

In this equation, P_AO_2 is alveolar oxygen tension in mmHg. The P_AO_2 determines the maximum PaO_2, and a decrease in P_AO_2 will always result in a decrease in PaO_2. Equation (20.1) demonstrates that the major threat to life from CO_2 retention in patients breathing room air is the associated obligatory hypoxemia. In the absence of supplemental oxygen, patients suffering respiratory arrest develop critical hypoxemia within a few minutes, long before severe hypercapnia occurs. The alveolar gas equation establishes that patients breathing room air cannot reach $PaCO_2$ levels > 80–90 mmHg because the hypoxemia entailed by higher values ($PaO_2 \leq 40$ mmHg) is incompatible with life (3,5). Thus, extreme hypercapnia occurs only during oxygen therapy, and severe CO_2 retention is often the result of uncontrolled oxygen administration.

The relationship between the severity of the hypoxemia and the level of $PaCO_2$ differs in the two major clinical forms of respiratory insufficiency (3,23,24). Patients with respiratory pump failure exhibit the pattern of "pure alveolar hypoventilation," in which the alveolar–arterial gradient for oxygen ($P_{(A-a)}O_2$) remains normal and the increase in $PaCO_2$ is accompanied by an equivalent decrease in PaO_2. This type of respiratory pump failure is caused by disorders without parenchymal lung disease, in which alveolar gas exchange is normal. In contrast with respiratory pump failure, abnormalities in the lung parenchyma produce the so-called "hypoxemic respiratory failure." In the latter condition, also referred to as "lung failure," the reduction in PaO_2 is a constant finding, whereas $PaCO_2$ is commonly decreased if sufficient ventilatory reserve is present, although hypercapnia can ensue.

SECONDARY PHYSIOLOGIC ADJUSTMENTS

The time course of the changes in acid–base equilibrium associated with respiratory acidosis is depicted in Fig. 3. Hypercapnia increases the carbonic acid concentration of the body fluids and results in a prompt increase in $[H^+]$. Acutely, this acidemia is ameliorated by a secondary adaptive increase in plasma $[HCO_3^-]$ that originates from titration of nonbicarbonate buffers in the body (Fig. 4). During sustained hypercapnia, renal adaptive mechanisms yield a much larger secondary increment in plasma $[HCO_3^-]$ that results in additional amelioration of the acidemia (25) (Fig. 4).

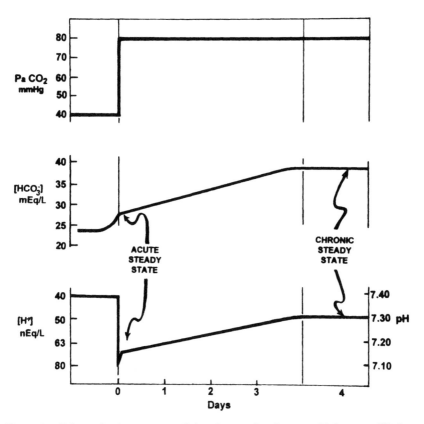

Figure 3   Schematic time course of the changes in plasma acid–base equilibrium during the development of respiratory acidosis. In this scheme, $PaCO_2$ is assumed to rise abruptly from 40 to 80 mmHg and to remain unchanged thereafter. *Source*: Modified from Ref. 74.

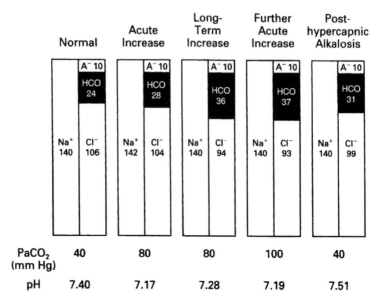

Figure 4   Changes in acid–base and electrolyte composition in patients with respiratory acidosis. From left to right, the panels depict normal acid–base status; adaptation to an acute rise in the partial pressure of arterial carbon dioxide ($PaCO_2$) to 80 mmHg; adaptation to a long-term rise in $PaCO_2$ to 80 mmHg; superimposition of an acute further increment in $PaCO_2$ (to a level of 100 mmHg) in the same patient; and posthypercapnic alkalosis resulting from an abrupt reduction in $PaCO_2$ to the level of 40 mmHg in the same patient. A^- denotes unmeasured plasma anions. The numbers within the bars give ion concentrations in millimoles per liter. *Source*: From Ref. 127.

Acute Respiratory Acidosis

A small increase in plasma $[HCO_3^-]$ is observed within moments following the onset of hypercapnia as H^+ derived from the dissociation of carbonic acid are removed from solution by nonbicarbonate buffers (26). Approximately one-third of the total buffering response to acute respiratory acidosis can be ascribed to red cell and extracellular protein buffering, and the remainder to tissue buffering (27–29). The contribution of hemoglobin is evidenced by Cl^- entry into erythrocytes in exchange for HCO_3^- (the "chloride shift"; see Chapter 1). Tissue buffers abstract H^+ from the extracellular fluid in exchange for Na^+ and K^+. A small fraction of the increment in extracellular $[HCO_3^-]$ can be attributed to net utilization of extracellular lactate, a process that generates HCO_3^-. Barring further changes in $PaCO_2$, this immediate adjustment is completed within 5–10 min and is followed by a stable period of a few hours during which no further changes in acid–base equilibrium are detectable (26–29). Consequently, this period has been designated an "acute steady state" (Fig. 3).

Although the increment in plasma [HCO_3^-] during acute hypercapnia stems almost exclusively from body buffering, renal adaptation begins even during this early phase of the disorder. A fall in urine pH and a small increase in NH_4^+ and titratable acid excretion occurs within minutes after induction of hypercapnia (30,31). Moreover, HCO_3^- reabsorption rate in the proximal convoluted tubules increases in response to acute hypercapnia (32,33).

Figure 5 depicts the 95% confidence limits for plasma [HCO_3^-] and [H^+] in uncomplicated acute respiratory acidosis of graded severity in humans (26). On average, plasma [HCO_3^-] increases by ~0.1 mEq/L for each mmHg increment in $PaCO_2$. Thus, even when $PaCO_2$ is increased to as high as 80–90 mmHg, plasma [HCO_3^-] increases by only a small amount [3–4 mEq/L]. The net effect of this modest increment in plasma [HCO_3^-] elicited by the body's nonbicarbonate buffers is that the plasma [H^+] increases by approximately 0.75 nEq/L for each mmHg increase in $PaCO_2$.

The quantitative aspects of the adaptive response to acute hypercapnia are influenced markedly by the baseline plasma [HCO_3^-] (34,35). Acute hypercapnia induces a larger increment in both plasma [HCO_3^-] and [H^+] in animals with preexisting hypobicarbonatemia (whether due to metabolic acidosis or chronic respiratory alkalosis) than in animals with preexisting hyperbicarbonatemia (whether due to metabolic alkalosis or chronic respiratory acidosis) (Fig. 6). Although these differences might suggest

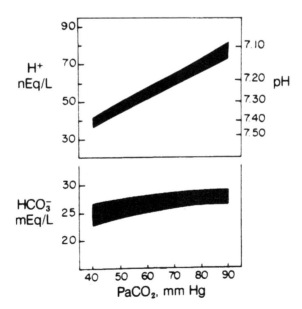

Figure 5 Ninety-five percent confidence limits for plasma [HCO_3^-] (*lower panel*) and plasma [H^+] (*upper panel*) in acute respiratory acidosis. The limits were calculated from data obtained in normal human volunteers. *Source*: From Ref. 26.

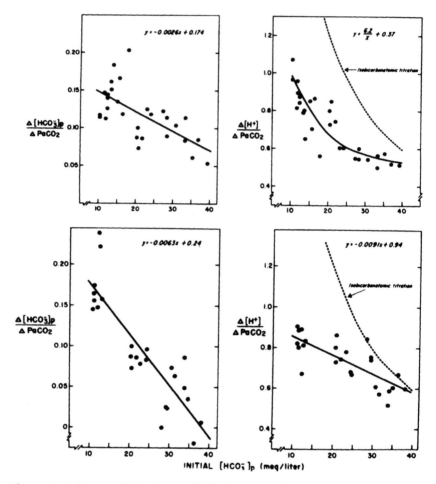

Figure 6 Influence of chronic metabolic (*upper panel*) or respiratory (*lower panel*) acid–base disorders on the acute CO_2 titration curve. Relationship between initial level of $[HCO_3]_p$ and slope of $[HCO_3]_p/PaCO_2$ regression line ($\Delta[HCO_3]_p/\Delta PaCO_2$, left) or slope of $[H^+]/PaCO_2$ regression line ($\Delta[H^+]/\Delta PaCO_2$, right) for all acute CO_2 titration studies is shown. Initial level of $[HCO_3]_p$, rather than of $PaCO_2$, is employed as an index of chronic acid–base status of animals with respiratory disorders (*lower panel*) for reasons of comparison with animals with metabolic acid–base disorders (*upper panel*); initial $[HCO_3]_p$ values of 10 and 40 mEq/L correspond to chronic levels of $PaCO_2$ of about 15 and 100 mmHg, respectively. Equations describing these functions are shown in respective panels. Slope of each relationship is significantly different from 0. Interrupted line (*right*), labeled isobicarbonatemic titration, depicts theoretical values for $\Delta[H^+]/\Delta PaCO_2$ that would be obtained if $[HCO_3]_p$ were to remain constant at its chronic level during acute CO_2 titration. *Source*: From Refs. 34,35.

alterations in the buffering capacity of the body's nonbicarbonate buffers, one can more reasonably ascribe these changes to differences in the fraction of HCO_3^- generated by cellular buffers that is released into the extracellular fluid (34,35). The higher the plasma $[HCO_3^-]$ at the onset of acute hypercapnia, the smaller the increment in plasma $[H^+]$. Thus, hyperbicarbonatemic states are associated both with smaller increments in plasma $[HCO_3^-]$ and with better defense of plasma acidity. The explanation for this paradox resides in the mathematics of the Henderson relationship; despite small increments in $[HCO_3^-]$, high baseline values for plasma $[HCO_3^-]$ limit the change in $[H^+]$ for a given rise in $PaCO_2$. Hypoxemia does not alter the acid–base response to acute respiratory acidosis, but if it is sufficiently severe ($PaO_2 < 40\,mmHg$), it can induce a complicating lactic acidosis (36).

In Vitro vs. In Vivo CO_2 Titration

The modest increase in plasma $[HCO_3^-]$ observed during acute hypercapnia in vivo contrasts sharply with the large increase obtained when PCO_2 is increased to the same degree in isolated whole blood (26,36–38) (Fig. 7). This discrepancy is explained largely by differences in the distribution of the newly generated HCO_3^- in the two circumstances. Bicarbonate generated by hemoglobin and other nonbicarbonate buffers of blood is confined to the plasma phase during in vitro CO_2 titration but diffuses freely into the large, poorly buffered interstitial compartment in vivo. Despite the participation of nonerythrocytic tissue buffers in the living organism, the total quantity of new HCO_3^- generated during acute hypercapnia is insufficient to elevate extracellular $[HCO_3^-]$ in the body to the same extent that plasma $[HCO_3^-]$ is elevated in vitro.

Chronic Respiratory Acidosis

If hypercapnia persists, the plasma $[HCO_3^-]$ increases further as a consequence of significant augmentation of H^+ secretion by the renal tubules (Fig. 4). As a consequence, net acid excretion (largely in the form of NH_4^+) transiently exceeds endogenous acid production, leading to negative H^+ balance and the generation of new HCO_3^- in the body fluids (see Chapters 4 and 6) (39–41). Conservation of the new HCO_3^- is ensured by an augmented rate of renal HCO_3^- reabsorption, a reflection of hypercapnia-induced increment in H^+ secretory rate (41,42). A new steady state emerges for any given level of hypercapnia when the augmented filtered load of HCO_3^- is balanced by the increase in HCO_3^- reabsorption and when net acid excretion returns to the level required to offset daily endogenous acid production. In this new steady state net acid excretion returns to baseline but the mix of acid and HCO_3^- excretion is different that in normal individuals. Ammonium excretion remains persistently increased, but is now coun-

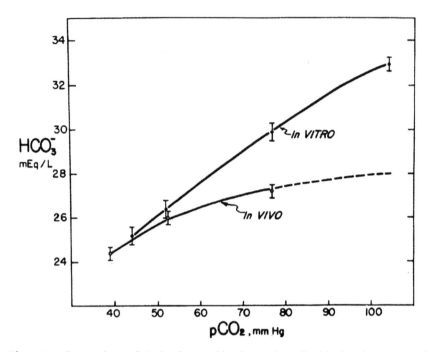

Figure 7   Comparison of the in vitro and in vivo carbon dioxide titration curves of human blood. The dashed portion of the in vivo curve represents a calculated extrapolation. *Source*: From Ref. 26.

terbalanced by an increase in HCO_3^- excretion and suppressed titratable acidity (43).

    As HCO_3^- stores are being augmented by the transient increase in net acid excretion, Cl^- stores are correspondingly depleted by a transient rise in renal Cl^- excretion. Chloruresis appears to outstrip acid excretion during the first 1–2 days of adaptation; the difference is accounted for by an increase in the excretion of Na^+ and K^+. Thus some degree of Na^+ and K^+ depletion typically accompanies adaptation to chronic hypercapnia. The resultant hypochloremia is sustained by persistently depressed renal Cl^- reabsorption (39,40). In dogs, 3–5 days elapse after the onset of a fixed increment in $PaCO_2$ before renal adaptation becomes fully expressed; at that point, plasma $[HCO_3^-]$ ceases to rise and a new steady state of acid–base equilibrium is established. Whether the same temporal pattern applies to the response of humans to a stepwise increase in $PaCO_2$ is unknown.

Mechanism of Renal Adaptation

All segments of the nephron appear to participate in the adaptive response to chronic respiratory acidosis. A substantial increase in H^+ secretion occurs in the proximal tubule during the chronic stage of the disorder (33,42). One study showed parallel increases in the transport rates (V_{max}) of the luminal Na^+/H^+ exchanger and the basolateral $Na^+/3HCO_3^-$ cotransporter in the proximal tubule (44), but stimulation of luminal Na^+/H^+ exchange was not seen in another study (45). Exposure to acute or chronic hypercapnia also induces insertion of H^+-ATPase-containing subapical vesicles into the luminal membrane of both proximal tubule cells and type A intercalated cells of cortical and medullary collecting ducts (46,47). Microdissection studies have shown that after 24 hr of hypercapnia the activity of the H^+-ATPase along the entire nephron and of the H^+–K^+-ATPase in the cortical and medullary collecting tubules is increased (48). Further, chronic hypercapnia increases the steady-state abundance of mRNA coding for the basolateral Cl^-/HCO_3^- exchanger (band 3 protein) of α-intercalated cells in rat renal cortex and medulla (49) (Fig. 8).

The signal that triggers the renal adaptation to persistent hypercapnia remains undefined, but present evidence favors an increase in $PaCO_2$ per se rather than the decrease in systemic pH (25,50,51). Indeed, observations in the dog, summarized in Fig. 9, indicate that a decrement in systemic pH is not a prerequisite for the augmentation of renal HCO_3^- reabsorption required for sustaining the secondary hyperbicarbonatemia characteristic of chronic hypercapnia (51).

Steady-State Relationships in Chronic Hypercapnia

Studies in dogs indicate that a highly predictable relationship exists between the degree of chronic hypercapnia and the levels at which plasma [HCO_3^-] and [H^+] stabilize following full physiologic adaptation (40). Over the entire range of $PaCO_2$ examined (30–120 mmHg), the relationship between plasma [HCO_3^-] and $PaCO_2$ is curvilinear, with successive increments in [HCO_3^-] diminishing in magnitude at higher levels of $PaCO_2$. Over the range of $PaCO_2$ values between 40 and 90 mmHg (which encompass most values encountered clinically) this relationship is closely approximated by a straight line with a slope of 0.3. Hence, over this range, each mmHg chronic increment in $PaCO_2$ is associated, on average, with an approximately 0.3 mEq/L increment in plasma [HCO_3^-]. The corresponding relationship between plasma [H^+] and $PaCO_2$ is strikingly linear, [H^+] rising by 0.32 nEq/L for each mmHg elevation in $PaCO_2$.

Observations in patients with chronic, stable respiratory acidosis appear to confirm the presence of a predictable pattern of response when no complicating acid–base disturbances are present (52–55). In humans, plasma [H^+] rises on average by slightly less than in the dog, 0.12–0.30 nEq/L for each mmHg elevation in $PaCO_2$ (55). Clinical data for levels of $PaCO_2 > 70$ mmHg are scant and somewhat conflicting (56–58). The renal response to chronic hypercapnia is not altered appreciably by the coexistence of such

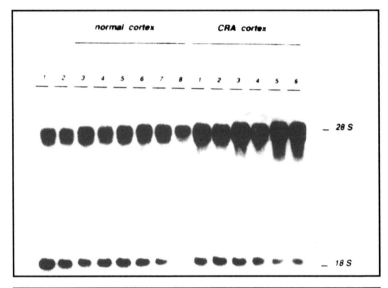

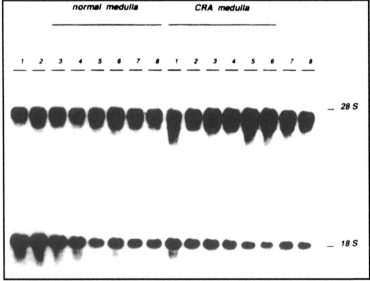

Figure 8 Northern analysis of kidney band 3 (basolateral Cl^-/HCO_3^- exchanger) mRNA in renal cortex (*upper panel*) or renal medulla (*lower panel*) using a $3'$ cDNA probe. Total RNA was obtained from rats exposed to hypercapnia for 5 days and normal controls. Forty micrograms were used in each lane. Densitometric readings disclosed increase of 2.8-fold (renal cortex) or 2.3-fold (renal medulla) in animals with chronic respiratory acidosis after normalization for β-actin signals (18S marker). Band 3 message is at the level of 28S marker. Autoradiograms were exposed as follows: band 3, 48 hr; β-actin, 4 hr. *Source*: From Ref. 49.

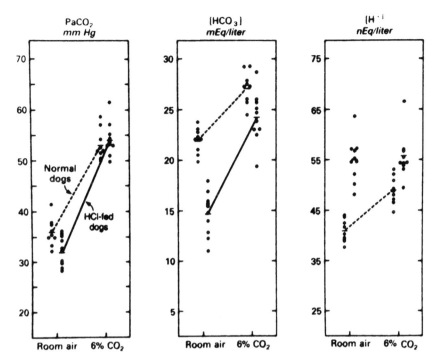

Figure 9 Changes in plasma [HCO₃⁻] and [H⁺] during prolonged exposure to hypercapnia in normal dogs (*dashed lines*) and in dogs with chronic HCl-acidosis (*solid lines*). Note that the large increment in plasma [HCO₃⁻] produced by chronic hypercapnia was associated with a substantial rise in plasma [H⁺] in normal animals but with no detectable change in the level of acidity in HCl-fed animals. *Source*: From Ref. 51.

stresses as hypoxemia (PaO₂ of 45–55 mmHg), dietary Na⁺ or Cl⁻ deprivation, K⁺ depletion, alkali loading, or adrenalectomy (39,41,52,56,59–61).

Return of body HCO₃⁻ stores to normal during recovery from chronic hypercapnia is hampered by Cl⁻ deprivation because the Cl⁻ losses that occurred during the adaptive process cannot be replenished without exogenous intake (62). As a result, a state of "posthypercapnic metabolic alkalosis" is created (Fig. 4, see also Chapter 16). Moderate K⁺ depletion does not interfere with full repair of acid–base equilibrium following the return to eucapnia (61).

Plasma Electrolyte Composition During Respiratory Acidosis

Mild hypernatremia (Δ[Na⁺], 2–4 mEq/L) is typically seen in both acute and chronic hypercapnia (26,40,60). Hypochloremia is a consistent finding in chronic hypercapnia, and it reflects both a shift of chloride into erythrocytes and a loss of chloride in the urine during the adaptive process (40,60) (Fig. 4). Plasma [K^+] increases slightly (by $\sim$0.1 mEq/L for each 0.1 unit fall in pH) during acute hypercapnia, probably because of a shift of this ion out of cells (63); plasma [K^+] does not change appreciably during chronic hypercapnia (39,40,60). Hyperphosphatemia is a characteristic feature of acute hypercapnia and probably reflects a release of phosphate from tissues (26,64); a rise in plasma phosphate is not observed during chronic hypercapnia (39,40,64). No consistent changes in plasma calcium and magnesium have been noted during hypercapnia in limited observations in humans. In animals, calcium concentration increases slightly during acute hypercapnia but returns to baseline in the chronic phase (64,65). Mild increases in plasma magnesium concentration were seen in both acute and chronic hypercapnia (64).

There is little information regarding renal calcium excretion in chronic respiratory acidosis in humans. In animals with chronic hypercapnia, calcium excretion increases independent of changes in parathyroid hormone, and thus appears to be due to a direct depressive effect on renal calcium reabsorption (64,65). In dogs, 1,25 (OH)$_2$ D$_3$ does not change during chronic hypercapnia whereas it falls significantly in the rat (64,65). Plasma lactate and pyruvate concentrations fall during acute hypercapnia, but they are not significantly altered by chronic hypercapnia, even in the presence of moderately severe hypoxemia (27,56,60). No appreciable changes in plasma unmeasured anions occur in either acute or chronic hypercapnia.

Cerebrospinal Fluid Composition During Respiratory Acidosis

Because CO_2 diffuses readily across the blood–brain barrier, increases in $PaCO_2$ are rapidly reflected in the cerebrospinal fluid (CSF), producing a prompt increase in CSF [H^+] (66). During respiratory acidosis, the CSF-arterial PCO_2 difference narrows, most likely due to the associated increase in cerebral blood flow (67). With persistent hypercapnia, CSF [HCO_3^-] increases progressively, so that the rise in CSF [H^+] is ameliorated. In dogs exposed to 12% CO_2 for 5 days, CSF [HCO_3^-] increased during the first day to $\sim$13 mEq/L higher than control and remained unchanged thereafter (68). Plasma [HCO_3^-] rose somewhat more slowly but reached essentially the same level. The fall in steady-state pH was virtually identical in the two compartments. Patients with respiratory acidosis generally have more severe acidification of the CSF than noted in experimental studies (69). This discrepancy may reflect abnormalities in cerebral blood flow and the superimposition of complicating lactic acidosis in clinical studies (70).

Intracellular pH During Respiratory Acidosis

Increases in extracellular PCO_2 exert a prompt acidifying effect on intracellular pH (71). In humans breathing 7% CO_2 in air for 3 hr ($PaCO_2$

55–60 mmHg), "whole-body" intracellular pH fell to a greater extent than did extracellular pH (72). In dog, however, extracellular pH fell to a greater extent (73). In vivo estimates of intracellular pH in various tissues have yielded variable responses to acute hypercapnia. Whereas intracellular pH falls in skeletal muscle and kidney by a magnitude similar to that in the extracellular compartment, smaller changes or no changes in intracellular pH have been noted in cardiac muscle, cerebral cortex, and liver (74). These differences in the apparent buffering capacity of the various tissues have been attributed to the composite effect of differences in physicochemical buffering (inherent buffering characteristics), transmembrane ionic fluxes of H^+ (or OH^-, HCO_3^-), and production of endogenous acids. Renal intracellular pH returns to the normal level during the chronic phase of respiratory acidosis.

CLINICAL MANIFESTATIONS OF RESPIRATORY ACIDOSIS

Because clinical hypercapnia almost always occurs with some degree of hypoxemia, it is often difficult to determine whether a specific manifestation is the consequence of the elevated $PaCO_2$ or the reduced PaO_2. Nevertheless, one should bear in mind several characteristic manifestations of organ dysfunction to diagnose the condition accurately and to treat it effectively.

Neurologic

Most of the clinical manifestations of hypercapnia result from its effects on the central nervous system (CNS). Factors that influence the CNS disturbances in respiratory acidosis are the magnitude of the hypercapnia, the rapidity with which it develops, the severity of the acidemia, and the degree of attendant hypoxemia. Acute respiratory acidosis produces cerebral vasodilation, increasing cerebral blood flow, cerebral blood volume, and intracranial pressure (75). These vascular effects appear to be pH-mediated, as they can be prevented by concomitant HCO_3^- administration (76). As a result of this vasodilation, cerebral blood flow increases in direct relation to the level of $PaCO_2$ up to values of 100 mmHg (77,78). Cerebral blood flow remains increased in chronic hypercapnia, but the increment appears to be less than that occurs with comparable levels of acute hypercapnia (79).

Acute hypercapnia is associated with marked anxiety, severe breathlessness, disorientation, confusion, incoherence, and combativeness (74,80). A transient psychosis can occur, with delusions, hallucinations, episodes of euphoria, delirium, and occasional maniacal behavior. In unusually severe hypercapnia, stupor or coma can result. Hypercapnic coma characteristically occurs in patients with acute exacerbations of chronic respiratory insufficiency, who are treated injudiciously with "high-flow" oxygen (80). In the absence of significant hypoxemia, patients with chronic hypercapnia can manifest levels of $PaCO_2$ as high as 110 mmHg with minimal CNS dysfunction (81). Nevertheless, a narcotic-like effect is not uncommon, and drowsiness, decreased alertness, inattention, forgetfulness, loss of memory, irritability, confusion, and somnolence can occur. Motor disturbances, including tremor, myoclonic jerks, and asterixis, are frequent accompaniments of both acute and chronic hypercapnia. Sustained myoclonus and seizure activity can also develop. Signs and symptoms of increased intracranial pressure (pseudotumor cerebri) are occasionally evident in patients with acute or chronic hypercapnia, related to the vasodilating effects of CO_2 on cerebral blood vessels (82). Headache is a frequent complaint. Blurring of the optic discs and frank papilledema can be found when hypercapnia is severe. Focal neurologic signs (e.g., muscle paresis, abnormal reflexes) have been described. Deep-tendon reflexes can be increased in mild to moderate hypercapnia, but depressed reflexes are usually observed in severe hypercapnia. The plantar response can be extensor. Brain acidosis induced by hypercapnic ventilation attenuates focal ischemic injury, an observation that could have clinical applicability (83).

Cardiovascular

Respiratory acidosis affects cardiovascular function through a variety of mechanisms, including a direct depressing effect on myocardial contractility, systemic vasodilation, increased plasma catecholamine levels, and blunting of receptor responsiveness to catecholamines (84,85). The composite effect of these inputs is such that acute hypercapnia of mild to moderate degree is usually characterized by warm, flushed skin, a bounding pulse, diaphoresis, increased cardiac output, and normal or increased blood pressure (86,87). Severe hypercapnia might be attended by decreases in both cardiac output and blood pressure. The cardiovascular manifestations of acute hypercapnia might well be altered by the effects of concomitant hypoxemia, congestive heart failure, and vasoactive medications, including pharmacologic blockade of β-adrenergic receptors. Chronic respiratory failure is associated with normal cardiac output and blood pressure, unless a complicating disorder such as cor pulmonale supervenes (88,89).

Cardiac arrhythmias occur frequently in patients with acute or chronic respiratory acidosis (90–92), but the specific role of hypercapnia in the generation of these arrhythmias is unclear. Indeed, remarkably little cardiac irritability occurs in extreme hypercapnia in the absence of accompanying hypoxemia and rapid restoration of normal $PaCO_2$ from very high levels is known to trigger cardiac arrhythmias, including those of ventricular origin (93,94). A variety of factors probably contribute to the generation of arrhythmias, including hypoxemia, sympathetic discharge, electrolyte abnormalities, severe acidemia, underlying cardiac disease, and certain medications (such as digitalis, xanthines, and β-adrenergic agonists) (91,92). Myocardial PCO_2 increases to very high levels (e.g., up to 346 mmHg) as does $[H^+]$ (e.g., 440 nEq/L, pH 6.38) after ventricular fibrillation (95), reducing cardiac resuscitability. Because HCO_3^- administration can aggravate PCO_2, leading to further circulatory depression, this agent should be used with caution in the presence of respiratory acidosis (96).

Renal and Metabolic

Mild to moderate hypercapnia results in renal vasodilation, but acute increments in $PaCO_2$ to levels above 70 mmHg induce renal vasoconstriction and hypoperfusion (96–98). Angiotensin II may play a role in the renal vasoconstriction observed during acute respiratory acidosis accompanied by hypoxemia (99).

Acute hypercapnia stimulates renin secretion by augmenting β-adrenergic tone and leads to increased plasma corticosteroid (85) and aldosterone levels (100). Acute hypercapnia also stimulates antidiuretic hormone release and reduces renal Na^+ and water excretion as a result of this stimulation as well as augmented renal adrenergic activity (86,101). Salt and water retention commonly attends sustained hypercapnia, especially in the presence of cor pulmonale. In addition to the effects of heart failure on the kidney, multiple other factors might be at play including the prevailing stimulation of the sympathetic nervous system and the renin–angiotensin–aldosterone axis, increased renal vascular resistance, and elevated levels of antidiuretic hormone and cortisol (101). Respiratory acidosis decreases glucose uptake by tissues by inducing insulin resistance and inhibits anaerobic glycolysis by depressing 6-phosphofructokinase activity (102,103). This effect can have grave consequences during hypoxia, as glycolysis becomes the main source of energy. Uptake of lactate by the liver is curtailed, and the liver can be converted from the premier consumer of lactate to a net producer (104).

Respiratory

Complex shifts in the oxyhemoglobin dissociation curve occur during hypercapnia, because increased $PaCO_2$ shifts the curve to the right (Bohr effect), and acidemia (by decreasing intracellular 2,3-DPG) shifts the curve to the left (105). Further complexity is introduced if chronic hypoxemia is present, because hypoxemia increases intracellular 2,3-DPG level, which again shifts the curve to the right (19,106). The decrease in the 2,3-DPG level that occurs in chronic respiratory acidosis overcomes the initial shift to the right of the dissociation curve resulting in a normal $P50$ level of 26 mmHg in adults at sea level (106). In addition to the effects of hypercapnia on $P50$, erythropoietin production in response to hypoxia is inhibited by respiratory acidosis (107).

Contradictory evidence has been obtained about the effects of acute hypercapnia on pulmonary vascular resistance and pulmonary artery pressure; some studies indicate an increase in these parameters, whereas others have failed to demonstrate any effect (108,109). Respiratory acidosis does not influence hypoxia-induced pulmonary vasoconstriction whereas respiratory alkalosis blunts this response (110). Diaphragm performance decreases during respiratory acidosis in anesthetized dogs but this effect was not observed in other skeletal muscles (111).

Skeletal

Respiratory acidosis causes a smaller net loss of calcium from cultured bone than does metabolic acidosis (112). In these studies, calcium efflux from bone was inversely related to the $[HCO_3^-]$ of the culture medium. Thus, the higher $[HCO_3^-]$ characteristic of respiratory acidosis might explain the differential calcium efflux in the two disorders (113). With respect to the cellular processes involved, respiratory acidosis also differs from metabolic acidosis. Calcium efflux from bone during respiratory acidosis appears to be mediated solely by physicochemical dissolution. By contrast, metabolic acidosis produces calcium efflux through inhibition of osteoblastic bone formation and stimulation of osteoclastic bone resorption (114).

CAUSES OF RESPIRATORY ACIDOSIS

Alveolar hypoventilation can result from disease or malfunction within any element of the regulatory system controlling respiration, including the central and peripheral nervous system, the respiratory muscles, the thoracic cage, the pleural space, the lung parenchyma, and the airways. In Tables 1 and 2, causes are categorized according to the dominant pathophysiologic mechanism at play, although for several disease entities the cause remains a matter of dispute. In most clinical settings, the pathogenesis of hypercapnia involves more than one mechanism.

Acute Respiratory Acidosis

During acute hypercapnia, hypoxemia rather than hypercapnia poses the main threat to life. In the absence of supplemental oxygen, severe hypercapnia ($PaCO_2 > 80$ mmHg) rarely occurs, because patients succumb to the attendant hypoxemia before higher levels of $PaCO_2$ can be achieved. Abrupt cessation of ventilation (e.g., cardiac arrest, airway obstruction) in patients breathing room air leads to death from hypoxia in approximately 4 min. Studies of "apneic oxygenation" (diffusion respiration) in humans have shown that $PaCO_2$ rises at an average rate of 3–5 mmHg/min following ventilatory paralysis (115); consequently, 10–15 min are required before extreme hypercapnia (higher than 90 mmHg) develops.

Increases in respiratory load can occur as a result of an augmented ventilatory demand, a higher airway flow resistance, lung stiffness, and pleura/chest wall stiffness (Table 1). An abnormally high ventilatory demand can be observed in conditions that include the administration of large carbohydrate loads (> 2000 kcal/day) in hyperalimentation solutions to semistarved, critically ill patients (6,7), hemodialysis using sorbent-regenerative cartridge systems (16), and infusion of bicarbonate in the course of treating metabolic acidosis. If any of these conditions occurs in patients whose minute ventilation is fixed by a mechanical ventilator (or those with marked limitation in pulmonary reserve), acute hypercapnia can develop. Multiple causes can lead to acute respiratory acidosis as a result of augmented airway flow resistance. Such causes include sudden obstruction of the airways due to aspiration of a foreign body or gastric contents, laryngospasm, angioedema or generalized bronchospasm (116), and obstructive sleep apnea (117,118). The sudden onset of restrictive defects, such as simple pneumothorax, tension pneumothorax, hemothorax, severe chest injury, or severe pneumonia, can markedly impair alveolar ventilation and lead to CO_2 retention. Respiratory acidosis also can develop with protracted, severe acute respiratory distress syndrome (ARDS), both in infants and adults (3,23,119).

Decreases in pump function can be secondary to depressed central drive, abnormal neuromuscular transmission, and muscle dysfunction (Table 1). The term "Ondine's curse" has been applied to patients with abnormal autonomic control of ventilation, but whose voluntary control remains intact. These patients maintain relatively normal blood gases while awake but they "forget to breath" when they fall asleep (120). Ondine's curse is most frequently caused by a congenital central hypoventilation syndrome but it can also result from surgical incisions in the spinal cord (second cervical segment) to relieve intractable pain (121). Congenital central hypoventilation syndrome is characterized by mild hypercapnia during wakefulness, severe hypercapnia during non-REM sleep (122,123), eucapnia during exercise, and hypocapnia during passive leg cycling (nonchemoreceptive inputs) (124,125).

Acute respiratory acidosis frequently accompanies circulatory catastrophes, notably cardiac arrest; lactic acidosis also occurs frequently in this setting (126). In addition, some patients with severe circulatory failure and pulmonary edema can develop respiratory acidosis; in such patients, coexistent lactic acidosis is frequent (127,128). Acute hypercapnia can result from improperly adjusted mechanical ventilators. When patients dependent on such devices are not closely monitored, $PaCO_2$ can increase markedly. Finally, iatrogenic events, such as malfunction of anesthetic equipment, bronchoscopy-associated obstruction of air flow, and insufflation of the peritoneum with CO_2 during endoscopic procedures, can lead to acute increments in $PaCO_2$ (129,130).

Chronic Respiratory Acidosis

In most patients with chronic respiratory acidosis, carbon dioxide retention is associated with underlying chronic airway obstruction resulting from bronchitis and emphysema (3,131) (Table 2). Hypoxemia is a constant companion of chronic hypercapnia and, in fact, virtually always precedes the development of CO_2 retention in patients with chronic obstructive lung disease. In the earlier stages of the disease, hypercapnia is frequently precipitated by intercurrent infection or congestive heart failure (132); as the disease progresses, however, hypercapnia becomes a constant feature. Chronic respiratory acidosis due to stiffness of the chest wall and/or lungs can result from severe, long-standing restrictive defects, including kyphoscoliosis, interstitial fibrosis, severe chronic pneumonia, and obesity (3,133,134).

Chronic respiratory acidosis can also result from chronic respiratory center depression consequent to chronic sedative overdosage, methadone or heroin addiction (135), primary alveolar hypoventilation (136), the obesity-hypoventilation syndrome (137), tumors, and certain infectious processes (e.g., poliomyelitis, encephalitis, tetanus). Finally, chronic hypercapnia sometimes complicates the course of several neuromuscular disorders, such as poliomyelitis, multiple sclerosis, muscular dystrophy, amyotrophic lateral sclerosis, diaphragmatic paralysis, myxedema, and primary myopathies (21,138).

DIAGNOSIS

One should never rely on clinical examination alone to assess the adequacy of alveolar ventilation. Whenever CO_2 retention is suspected, arterial blood gas determinations should be obtained. Accurate laboratory data are a prerequisite for establishing the diagnosis of respiratory acidosis.

If the patient's acid–base profile reveals hypercapnia in association with acidemia, at least an element of respiratory acidosis must be present. Hypercapnia can be associated with a normal or even an alkaline pH, however, if certain additional acid–base disorders are also present (see Chapter 22). Information from the patient's history, physical examination, and ancillary laboratory data should be used to assess whether part or all of the rise in $PaCO_2$ reflects a secondary response to metabolic alkalosis rather than being primary in origin. For moderate degrees of metabolic alkalosis (plasma $[HCO_3^-] < 40\,mEq/L$), secondary hypoventilation would be expected to raise $PaCO_2$ to levels no higher than about 50 mmHg (see Chapter 27).

Differentiating between acute and chronic hypercapnia can be a difficult task. Neither the level of hypercapnia nor the magnitude of the associated hypoxemia is particularly helpful. If the presence of complicating acid–base disorders can be excluded, the acid–base parameters themselves can be of assistance; acute hypercapnia is associated with a lower plasma $[HCO_3^-]$ and blood pH than is chronic hypercapnia of the same magnitude (see Chapter 28). The utility of this criterion is limited by uncertainty about the coexistence of additional acid–base disturbances, individual variability in the secondary response to hypercapnia, and the fact that insufficient time from the onset of hypercapnia might have elapsed for full expression of the secondary response. In the end, clinical information must be relied on for distinguishing between acute and chronic respiratory acidosis as well as for establishing the underlying etiology.

TREATMENT

Carbon dioxide retention is always associated with hypoxemia in patients breathing room air and hypoxemia, not hypercapnia or acidemia, is the most critical factor that determines morbidity and mortality. Therefore, the greatest emphasis should be placed on ensuring adequate oxygenation. In addition to the maintenance of appropriate oxygenation, the goals of treatment both of acute and chronic respiratory acidosis should include prevention of severe acidemia and amelioration of the hypercapnia (127).

Acute Respiratory Acidosis

Treatment of acute respiratory acidosis must be directed at prompt removal of the underlying cause whenever possible (Fig. 10). Immediate therapeutic efforts should focus on establishing and securing a patent airway, restoring adequate oxygenation by delivering an oxygen-rich inspired mixture, and securing adequate ventilation with the use of mechanical devices if spontaneous breathing is inadequate. At times, prompt removal of the initiating cause might be possible (e.g., foreign body in the airway, maladjusted ventilator, tension pneumothorax), thus enabling swift restoration of oxygenation and ventilation. On other occasions, cause-specific measures might also be available (e.g., cardiogenic pulmonary edema, pleural effusion, atelectasis, paralytic crisis in myasthenia gravis, hypokalemic myopathy, phosphate-depletion myopathy), but in addition to pursuing them aggressively, nonspecific supportive measures should be taken until the underlying disease can be reversed.

Establishing a Patent Airway

In a comatose patient, hypopharyngeal obstruction is common. Restoration of airway patency can often be accomplished by positioning the patient on his or her side, hyperextending the head, displacing the mandible forward, and cleaning the oropharyngeal content manually or by suction. Acute asphyxiation from aspiration of a foreign body should be treated by subdiaphragmatic abdominal thrust (Heimlich maneuver). At times, laryngoscopy or bronchoscopy might be required, particularly if the obstruction is in the lower portion of the upper airway. In an apneic patient, ventilation

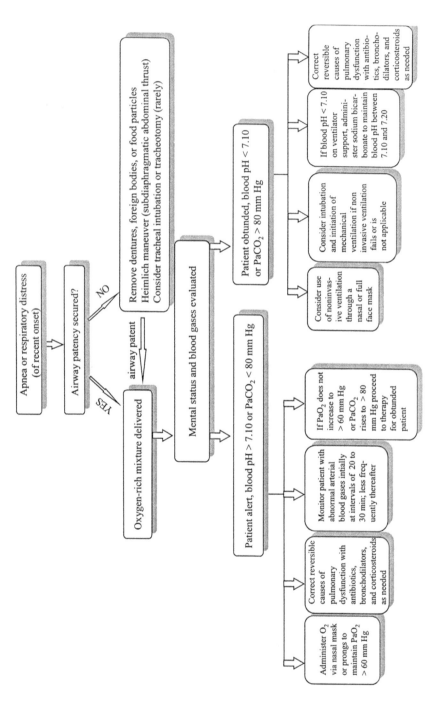

Figure 10 Algorithm for management of acute respiratory acidosis. *Source:* From Ref. 175.

must be immediately restored by either mouth-to-mouth breathing or the use of mechanical devices of pharyngeal intubation. Tracheal intubation should be performed as quickly as possible because it isolates the airway, prevents aspiration, and facilitates oxygenation, ventilation, and removal of secretions. Although tracheotomy is the most reliable way of securing an adequate airway, it has limited indications and should not be attempted by untrained persons. In appropriately selected patients with obstructive sleep apnea, surgical interventions (e.g., tonsillectomy, adenoidectomy, uvulopalatopharyngoplasty) can offer remarkable benefit (118).

Administering Oxygen

If the patient is in coma, severely obtunded, extremely hypercapnic ($PaCO_2 > 80$ mmHg), or severely acidemic (blood pH < 7.10), assisted ventilation should be initiated promptly. If none of these conditions is present, and if the patient has stable cardiovascular status, O_2 can be delivered with a nasal cannula or an air-entrainment mask. Supplemental O_2 is applied to achieve an O_2 saturation of 88–93% or a PaO_2 of 60–70 mmHg (139–142). Further increases in inspired O_2 fraction do not significantly increase the O_2 content of blood but increase the risk of worsening hypercapnia. One should always be mindful of the risk of O_2 toxicity, which increases as a function of the level of inspired fraction of O_2 and the time of exposure. As a rule, the lowest possible inspired fraction of O_2 that achieves the desired hemoglobin saturation should be used, and O_2 support that results in an inspired fraction of $O_2 > 30$–40% should be withdrawn as soon as feasible (143,144). Abrupt removal of supplemental oxygen in patients who develop CO_2 retention with oxygen therapy imposes a serious risk, as the patient's PaO_2 abruptly falls to a level lower than when oxygen therapy was initiated.

High-flow Venturi face masks should be used when possible, as they yield a precise fraction of inspired O_2 and provide a flow that exceeds the full ventilatory requirements (145). The design of the valve ensures that a specific proportion of O_2 and entrained air are mixed and delivered to the patient. Other methods of O_2 delivery can be used, particularly when higher levels of FiO_2 are required. Nasal cannulae, more comfortable devices that permit oral feedings, can provide flow rates of up to 6 L/min and FiO_2 of approximately 44%. Face masks using flow rates of 6–10 L/min provide FiO_2 of up to 55%. Nonrebreather masks can provide FiO_2 of up to 90%. The use of positive end-expiratory pressure (PEEP) or continuous positive airway pressure (CPAP) can enhance the effect of a given level of O_2 administration in patients with pulmonary edema or diffuse pulmonary disease (131,146,147). Development of worsening acidemia (e.g., pH < 7.20) or marked obtundation during oxygen therapy is an indication for mechanical ventilation, although noninvasive positive pressure ventilation (NPPV) might help avoid the need for endotracheal intubation.

Noninvasive Positive Pressure Ventilation

This form of ventilation consists of the mechanical delivery of breaths via a tightly fitting nasal or full facial mask. The salutary effects of NPPV consist of increasing alveolar ventilation, reducing work of breathing and therefore providing rest to the respiratory musculature, and decreasing the rate of intubation (148). The ventilator might deliver only inspiratory pressure (i.e., pressure support mode or PSV) or pressure might be applied during the entire respiratory cycle (i.e., bilevel positive airway pressure) (149). The high success rate of NPPV is well documented in patients with acute respiratory failure caused by decompensated COPD or acute cardiogenic pulmonary edema. It appears that NPPV can also be effectively used in other conditions, including the immunocompromised patient (in whom intubation carries a higher risk of pulmonary infection), in postoperative respiratory failure, after coronary artery bypass grafting or lung resection, as an adjunct to extubation, and to avoid reintubation of previously mechanically intubated patients. Contraindications for the use of NPPV are cardiovascular instability (e.g., hypotension, serious arrhythmias, myocardial ischemia), craniofacial trauma or burns, inability to protect the airway, or the likely need for emergent intubation (149).

Mechanical Ventilation and Permissive Hypercapnia

Acute respiratory failure accounts for about two-thirds of all patients requiring mechanical ventilation. Causes of acute respiratory failure include ARDS, severe heart failure, fulminant pneumonia, sepsis, trauma, and the postoperative state. The remaining one-third of patients require ventilator assistance because of exacerbations of COPD or neuromuscular disorders, or after developing coma.

The objectives of mechanical ventilation are to reverse acute progressive respiratory acidosis or life-threatening hypoxemia unresponsive to conservative management and to decrease the work of breathing (150). The most widely used mode of mechanical ventilation is assist-control ventilation, in which the ventilator delivers a set tidal volume when triggered by the patient's inspiratory effort or independently if such an effort does not occur within a preselected time (147). Another widely used modality is pressure-support ventilation in which 16–30 breaths/min are delivered to augment the patient's spontaneous respiratory effort by a preset level of pressure (rather than volume) (151).

Large tidal volumes with excessively high airway pressures (e.g., plateau levels higher than 25–35 cmH$_2$O) can lead to alveolar overdistension and barotrauma. An alternative approach that uses a protective-ventilation strategy and allows PaCO$_2$ to rise, is "permissive hypercapnia" (or controlled mechanical hypoventilation) (152–155). In this form of treatment, lower tidal volumes and peak inspiratory pressures are used. As expected,

$PaCO_2$ rises but rarely exceeds 80 mmHg, and blood pH can decrease to as low as 7.00–7.10, while blood oxygenation is secured. The increased respiratory drive associated with permissive hypercapnia causes extreme discomfort, making sedation necessary. Because the patient commonly requires neuromuscular blockade as well, accidental disconnection from the ventilator can cause sudden death. Furthermore, after the neuromuscular blocking agent is discontinued, there may be weakness or paralysis for several days or weeks. There are several contraindications to the use of permissive hypercapnia, including cerebrovascular disease, brain edema, increased intracranial pressure, convulsions, depressed cardiac function, cardiac arrhythmias, and severe pulmonary hypertension (127,153). Importantly, most of these entities can develop as adverse effects of permissive hypercapnia itself, especially when hypercapnia is associated with substantial acidemia. In fact, correction of acidemia can attenuate the adverse hemodynamic effects of permissive hypercapnia. It appears prudent, although still controversial, to keep the blood pH at approximately 7.30 by administering intravenous alkali when controlled hypoventilation is prescribed (156).

Strategies of low tidal volume ventilation that often lead to permissive hypercapnia include the "lung-protective ventilation" and "open lung ventilation" (157–159). Lung-protective ventilation consists of the use of a tidal volume of 6 mL/kg, plateau pressure < 30 cmH$_2$O, and high ventilator respiratory rate. Open lung ventilation uses a tidal volume lower than 6 mL/kg, variable PEEP that is adjusted according to the pressure–volume curve, and a respiratory rate lower than 30 breaths/min. These methods of low tidal volume ventilation reduce the rate of barotrauma, mortality, and days of hospitalization in patients with acute respiratory failure of various causes, and facilitate weaning from mechanical ventilation (150).

Improving Pulmonary Function

Swift restoration of $PaCO_2$ to normal levels is advisable in patients with acute hypercapnia. Measures directed against all possible reversible factors responsible for the acute respiratory acidosis should be undertaken. Thus bronchodilator therapy (e.g., xanthines, β-adrenergic agonists, corticosteroids) should be used in patients with bronchospasm (116). Clearing of bronchial secretions might be optimized by proper hydration of the patient, humidification of the inspired air, promotion of cough, and the use of mucolytic agents. Proper care of the airways might necessitate direct removal of bronchial secretions by suction and, under special circumstances, endotracheal intubation, bronchoscopy, or tracheostomy might be required. Pulmonary infections should be treated aggressively; direct examination of bronchial secretions and cultures should guide such therapy. Reversal of the hypercapnia, acidemia, and hypoxemia will usually improve cardiac dysfunction and pulmonary hypertension. With the exception of cor pulmonale in association with low cardiac output, administration of digitalis appears to be of no value in the treatment of the depressed cardiac contractility accompanying severe respiratory acidosis. Close monitoring of the patient's fluid status is crucial, because volume overload increases pulmonary capillary blood pressure and predisposes to the development of pulmonary edema. Diuretics should be used as needed. In appropriate settings, the use of intermittent ultrafiltration/hemodialysis or continuous arteriovenous or venovenous hemofiltration might be required. Administering a larger proportion of nonprotein calories as fat emulsions might aid the weaning process from ventilatory support by decreasing the rate of CO_2 production in comparison with isocaloric amounts of carbohydrate.

Alkali Therapy

Administration of sodium bicarbonate to patients with simple respiratory acidosis breathing spontaneously is not only of questionable efficacy but also involves considerable risk. Concerns include a further, pH-mediated depression of ventilation, enhanced CO_2 production resulting in further aggravation of hypercapnia, and volume expansion causing additional impairment in alveolar gas exchange (127). However, when permissive hypercapnia is utilized in patients maintained on mechanical ventilation and causes blood pH to fall below 7.20, sodium bicarbonate can ameliorate the acidemia and attenuate the adverse hemodynamic effects (156). In addition to the anticipated benefits from the cardiovascular system, moderation of acidemia can improve the responsiveness of bronchi to β-adrenergic agonists. Successful management of intractable asthma in patients with blood pH below 7.00 by administering sufficient sodium bicarbonate to raise blood pH to above 7.20 has been reported (160,161).

Alternative forms of alkali, which do not augment CO_2 generation as much as HCO_3^-, but are effective in ameliorating acidemia include Carbicarb® and *tris*-(hydroxymethyl) aminomethane (THAM). Carbicarb® is an equimolar mixture of sodium carbonate and sodium bicarbonate (162,163). Because carbonate is a stronger base, it is used in preference to bicarbonate for buffering hydrogen ions, generating bicarbonate rather than carbon dioxide in the process ($CO_3^{2-} + H^+ \Rightarrow HCO_3^-$). In addition, the carbonate ion can react with carbonic acid, thereby consuming carbon dioxide ($CO_3^{2-} + H_2CO_3 \Rightarrow 2HCO_3^-$). Yet, the interaction of HCO_3^- with H^+ still generates CO_2. Thus, Carbicarb® limits but does not eliminate the generation of CO_2 (127,164). Clinical experience with Carbicarb® is limited, and this product is not yet commercially available for clinical use.

THAM is a synthetic buffer available as a 0.3 N solution, which at a pH of 7.20–7.40 has a buffer capacity equivalent to that of normal blood (165,166). A distinct property of THAM is its capacity to buffer both metabolic acids (THAM + $H^+ \Rightarrow$ THAM$^+$) and carbonic acid (THAM +

$H_2CO_3 \Rightarrow THAM^+ + HCO_3^-$). Because THAM freely penetrates cells it can be an effective intracellular buffer. Indeed, in vitro and in vivo studies have indicated that both extracellular and intracellular pH rise after THAM administration; in vitro studies have shown that THAM exerts a positive inotropic effect on the ischemic myocardium (165). When used in the experimental treatment of head injury, it reduces brain edema. THAM has been proposed as a substitute for HCO_3^- in treating the acidemia of respiratory acidosis because of its theoretical potential to decrease the $PaCO_2$. However, correction of acidemia with this compound leads to CO_2 retention because of pH-mediated depression of ventilation. In addition, serious adverse effects have been reported with the use of THAM, including hyperkalemia, hypoglycemia, and widespread organ necrosis (165). As a result, THAM is no longer recommended for the treatment of the acidemia of respiratory acidosis, although further studies to examine its potential therapeutic role are warranted.

Chronic Respiratory Acidosis

Patients with chronic respiratory acidosis frequently develop episodes of acute decompensation that can be serious or life-threatening and require immediate care (Fig. 11). The causes of acute decompensation must be aggressively managed.

Improving Pulmonary Function

Pulmonary infections, perhaps the most common cause of respiratory decompensation in patients with COPD, should be treated vigorously with appropriate antibiotics. Bronchodilator therapy aimed primarily at correcting the increased airways resistance might also enhance respiratory drive and improve function of respiratory muscles, often providing substantial benefit. Elimination of retained secretions (by coughing, postural drainage, and chest physiotherapy) can substantially reduce the work of breathing and improve ventilation. Diuretic therapy often reduces the interstitial/ alveolar edema associated with pulmonary vascular congestion and can thus improve gas exchange. Special care must be taken to prevent or repair diuretic-induced metabolic alkalosis (or that induced by any other cause such as gastric losses); even relative alkalemia can dampen ventilatory drive and exacerbate hypercapnia and hypoxemia (167,168). Administration of adequate quantities of chloride (usually as the potassium salt) prevents or corrects this complication. Ventilatory drive can be further optimized by avoiding tranquilizers or sedatives (131,169). Potassium and phosphate depletion should be corrected, because they can contribute to the development or the maintenance of respiratory failure by impairing the function of skeletal muscles. Efforts should be made to return overweight patients toward their ideal weight in order to diminish oxygen consumption and CO_2 production. In addition, this measure might favorably affect a variety

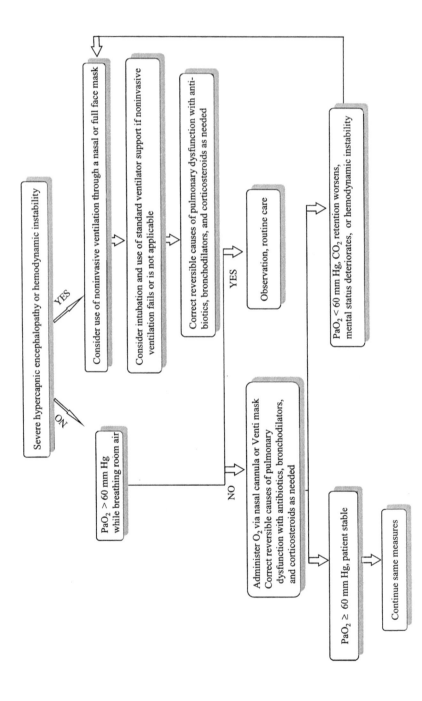

Figure 11 Algorithm for management of chronic respiratory acidosis. *Source:* From Ref. 175.

of other adverse factors, if present, such as central hypoventilation, upper airway obstruction, increased work of respiratory muscles, and $\dot{V}_A/\dot{Q}$ mismatching (131,137,169). The use of pharmacologic stimulants of ventilation has generally been disappointing (170–174).

Administering Oxygen

A substantial reduction in ventilatory drive during O_2 administration can occur in patients with chronic respiratory acidosis, because they gradually acquire insensitivity to the stimulating effects of CO_2 on ventilation and hypoxemia becomes an increasingly important stimulus for ventilation. This risk notwithstanding, careful and controlled O_2 administration can improve oxygenation and symptomatology considerably without substantial aggravation of the hypercapnia (3). The primary goal of O_2 therapy is to maintain an O_2 saturation of 88–93% or a PaO_2 of 60–70 mmHg (139–142).

Assisted Ventilation

The various types of assisted ventilation used in patients with acute respiratory acidosis are also applied to the treatment of chronic hypercapnia (see above). In patients with chronic respiratory acidosis, assisted ventilation should be avoided if adequate oxygenation can be attained by conservative therapy (PaO_2 on the order of 60–70 mmHg and oxygen hemoglobin saturation of 88–93%). As a general rule, if the patient is alert, able to cough, and can cooperate with the treatment program, mechanical ventilation is usually not necessary. Noninvasive positive pressure ventilation is an effective modality for selected patients with acute excerbations of COPD. Contraindications for the use of NPPV include cardiovascular instability (e.g., hypotension, serious arrhythmias, myocardial ischemia), craniofacial trauma or burns, inability to protect the airway, or the likely need for emergent intubation. Progressive obtundation and inability to cough require implementation of endotracheal intubation and mechanical ventilation. If mechanical ventilation is deemed necessary, the goal should be to increase minute ventilation sufficiently to maintain blood pH and $PaCO_2$ at levels that are close to the patient's chronic baseline values.

In the absence of a complicating element of metabolic acidosis and with the possible exception of the severely acidemic patient with intense generalized bronchoconstriction undergoing mechanical ventilation (see previous discussion), there is no role for alkali administration (i.e., $NaHCO_3$, Carbicarb®, THAM) in chronic respiratory acidosis.

REFERENCES

1. Adrogué HJ, Rashad MN, Gorin AB, Yacoub J, Madias NE. Assessing acid–base status in circulatory failure. Differences between arterial and central venous blood. N Engl J Med 1989; 320:1312–1316.

2. Adrogué HJ, Madias NE. Management of life-threatening acid–base disorders. Second of two parts. N Engl J Med 1998; 338:107–111.
3. Adrogué HJ, Tobin MJ. Respiratory Failure. Blackwell's Basics of Medicine. Boston: Blackwell Science, 1997.
4. Madias NE, Adrogué HJ. Respiratory acidosis and alkalosis. In: Seldin DW, Giebisch G, eds. The Kidney: Physiology and Pathophysiology. Philadelphia: Lippincott, Williams & Wilkins, 2000:2131–2166.
5. Epstein SK, Singh N. Respiratory acidosis. Respir Care 2001; 46:366–383.
6. Askanazi J, Rosenbaum SH, Hyman AI, Silverberg PA, Milic-Emili J, Kinney JM. Respiratory changes induced by the large glucose loads of total parenteral nutrition. J Am Med Assoc 1980; 243:1444–1447.
7. Covelli HD, Black JW, Olsen MS, Beekman JF. Respiratory failure precipitated by high carbohydrate loads. Ann Intern Med 1981; 95:579–581.
8. Efthimiou J, Mounsey PJ, Benson DN, Madgwick R, Coles SJ, Benson MK. Effect of carbohydrate rich vs. fat rich loads on gas exchange and walking performance in patients with chronic obstructive lung disease. Thorax 1992; 47:451–456.
9. Wasserman K, Hansen JE, Sue DY, Whipp BJ. Principles of exercise testing and interpretation. Philadelphia: Lea & Febiger, 1987.
10. Manthous CA, Hall JB, Olson D, et al. Effect of cooling on oxygen consumption in febrile critically ill patients. Am J Respir Crit Care Med 1995; 151:10–14.
11. Houtchens BA, Westenskow DR. Oxygen consumption in septic shock: collective review. Circ Shock 1984; 13:361–384.
12. Cerra FB. The hypermetabolism organ failure complex. World J Surg 1987; 11: 173–181.
13. Wilmore DW. Nutrition and metabolism following thermal injury. Clin Plast Surg 1974; 1:603–619.
14. Ben-Dov I, Sietsema KE, Wasserman K. O_2 uptake in hyperthyroidism during constant work rate and incremental exercise. Eur J Appl Physiol Occup Physiol 1991; 62:261–267.
15. Adrogué HJ, Madias NE. Mixed acid–base disorders. In: Jacobson HR, Striker GE, Klahr S, eds. The Principles and Practice of Nephrology. St Louis, MO: Mosby-Year Book, 1995:953–962.
16. Hamm LL, Lawrence G, DuBose TD Jr. Sorbent regenerative hemodialysis as a potential cause of acute hypercapnia. Kidney Int 1982; 21:416–418.
17. Javaheri S, Blum J, Kazemi H. Pattern of breathing and carbon dioxide retention in chronic obstructive lung disease. Am J Med 1981; 71: 228–234.
18. Del Rosario N, Sassoon CS, Chetty KG, Gruer SE, Mahutte CK. Breathing pattern during acute respiratory failure and recovery. Eur Respir J 1997; 10: 2560–2565.
19. Jubran A, Tobin MJ. Pathophysiologic basis of acute respiratory distress in patients who fail a trial of weaning from mechanical ventilation. Am J Respir Crit Care Med 1997; 155:906–915.
20. Kikuchi Y, Okabe S, Tamura G, et al. Chemosensitivity and perception of dyspnea in patients with a history of near-fatal asthma. N Engl J Med 1994; 330:1329–1334.

21. Smith PE, Calverley PM, Edwards RH, Evans GA, Campbell EJ. Practical problems in the respiratory care of patients with muscular dystrophy. N Engl J Med 1987; 316:1197–1205.
22. Zwillich CW, Pierson DJ, Hofeldt FD, Lufkin EG, Weil JV. Ventilatory control in myxedema and hypothyroidism. N Engl J Med 1975; 292: 662–665.
23. Hopewell PC, Murray JF. The adult respiratory distress syndrome. Annu Rev Med 1976; 27:343–356.
24. McFadden ER Jr, Lyons HA. Arterial-blood gas tension in asthma. N Engl J Med 1968; 278:1027–1032.
25. Schwartz WB, Cohen JJ. The nature of the renal response to chronic disorders of acid–base equilibrium. Am J Med 1978; 64:417–428.
26. Brackett NC Jr, Cohen JJ, Schwartz WB. Carbon dioxide titration curve of normal man. Effect of increasing degrees of acute hypercapnia on acid–base equilibrium. N Engl J Med 1965; 272:6–12.
27. Giebisch G, Berger L, Pitts RF. The extrarenal response to acute acid–base disturbances of respiratory origin. J Clin Invest 1955; 34:231–245.
28. Elkinton JR, Singer RB, Barker ES, Clark JK. Effects in man of acute experimental respiratory alkalosis and acidosis on ionic transfers in the total body fluids. J Clin Invest 1955; 34:1671–1690.
29. Cohen JJ, Brackett NC Jr, Schwartz WB. The nature of the carbon dioxide titration curve in the normal dog. J Clin Invest 1964; 43:777–786.
30. Barker ES, Singer RB, Elkinton JR, Clark JK. The renal response in man to acute experimental respiratory alkalosis and acidosis. J Clin Invest 1957; 36: 515–529.
31. Gougoux A, Vinay P, Cardoso M, Duplain M, Lemieux G. Immediate adaptation of the dog kidney to acute hypercapnia. Am J Physiol 1982; 243: F227–F234.
32. Jacobson HR. Effects of CO_2 and acetazolamide on bicarbonate and fluid transport in rabbit proximal tubules. Am J Physiol 1981; 240:F54–F62.
33. Cogan MG. Effects of acute alterations in PCO_2 on proximal HCO_3^-, Cl^-, and H_2O reabsorption. Am J Physiol 1984; 246:F21–F26.
34. Adrogué HJ, Madias NE. Influence of chronic respiratory acid–base disorders on acute CO_2 titration curve. J Appl Physiol 1985; 58:1231–1238.
35. Madias NE, Adrogué HJ. Influence of chronic metabolic acid–base disorders on the acute CO_2 titration curve. J Appl Physiol 1983; 55:1187–1195.
36. Mithoefer JC, Karetzky MS, Porter WF. The in vivo carbon dioxide titration curve in the presence of hypoxia. Respir Physiol 1968; 4:15–23.
37. Shaw LA, Messer AC. The transfer of bicarbonate between the blood and tissues caused by alterations of the carbon dioxide concentration in the lungs. Am J Physiol 1932; 100:122–136.
38. Brown EB Jr, Clancy RL. In vivo and in vitro CO_2 blood buffer curves. J Appl Physiol 1965; 20:885–889.
39. Polak A, Haynie GD, Hays RM, Schwartz WB. Effects of chronic hypercapnia on electrolyte and acid–base equilibrium. I. Adaptation. J Clin Invest 1961; 40:1223–1237.

40. Schwartz WB, Brackett NC Jr, Cohen JJ. The response of extracellular hydrogen ion concentration to graded degrees of chronic hypercapnia: the physiologic limits of the defense of pH. J Clin Invest 1965; 44:291–301.

41. Van Ypersele De Strihou C, Gulyassy PF, Schwartz WB. Effects of chronic hypercapnia on electrolyte and acid–base equilibrium. III. Characteristics of the adaptive and recovery process as evaluated by provision of alkali. J Clin Invest 1962; 41:2246–2253.

42. Cogan MG. Chronic hypercapnia stimulates proximal bicarbonate reabsorption in the rat. J Clin Invest 1984; 74:1942–1947.

43. Adrogué HJ, Madias NE. Renal acidification during chronic hypercapnia in the conscious dog. Pflugers Arch 1986; 406:520–528.

44. Ruiz OS, Talor Z, Arruda JA. Regional localization of renal $Na(+)-H^+$ antiporter: response to respiratory acidosis. Am J Physiol 1990; 259: F512–F518.

45. Northrup TE, Garella S, Perticucci E, Cohen JJ. Acidemia alone does not stimulate rat renal Na^+-H^+ antiporter activity. Am J Physiol 1988; 255: F237–F243.

46. Bastani B. Immunocytochemical localization of the vacuolar $H(+)$-ATPase pump in the kidney. Histol Histopathol 1997; 12:769–779.

47. Schwartz GJ, Al-Awqati Q. Carbon dioxide causes exocytosis of vesicles containing H^+ pumps in isolated perfused proximal and collecting tubules. J Clin Invest 1985; 75:1638–1644.

48. Eiam-ong S, Laski ME, Kurtzman NA, Sabatini S. Effect of respiratory acidosis and respiratory alkalosis on renal transport enzymes. Am J Physiol 1994; 267:F390–F399.

49. Teixera Da Silva JC Jr, Perrone RD, Johns CA, Madias NE. Rat kidney band 3 mRNA modulation in chronic respiratory acidosis. Am J Physiol 1991; 260:F204–F209.

50. Chen LK, Boron WF. Acid extrusion in S3 segment of rabbit proximal tubule. I. Effect of bilateral CO_2/HCO_3. Am J Physiol 1995; 268:F179–F192.

51. Madias NE, Wolf CJ, Cohen JJ. Regulation of acid–base equilibrium in chronic hypercapnia. Kidney Int 1985; 27:538–543.

52. Dulfano MJ, Ishikawa S. Quantitative acid–base relationships in chronic pulmonary patients during the stable state. Am Rev Respir Dis 1966; 93: 251–256.

53. Van Yperselle de S, Brasseur L, De Coninck JD. The "carbon dioxide response curve" for chronic hypercapnia in man. N Engl J Med 1966; 275:117–122.

54. Brackett NC Jr, Wingo CF, Muren O, Solano JT. Acid–base response to chronic hypercapnia in man. N Engl J Med 1969; 280:124–130.

55. Martinu T, Menzies D, Dial S. Re-evaluation of acid–base prediction rules in patients with chronic respiratory acidosis. Can Respir J 2003; 10:311–315.

56. Refsum HE. Acid–base status in patients with chronic hypercapnia and hypoxaemia. Clin Sci 1964; 27:407–415.

57. Eichenholz A, Blumentals AS, Walker FE. The pattern of compensatory response to chronic hypercapnia in patients with chronic obstructive pulmonary disease. J Lab Clin Med 1966; 68:265–278.

58. Engel K, Dell RB, Rahill WJ, Denning CR, Winters RW. Quantitative displacement of acid–base equilibrium in chronic respiratory acidosis. J Appl Physiol 1968; 24:288–295.

59. Luke RG, Levitin H. The renal and electrolyte response to respiratory acidosis in the adrenalectomized rat. Yale J Biol Med 1966; 39:27–37.

60. Sapir DG, Levine DZ, Schwartz WB. The effects of chronic hypoxemia on electrolyte and acid–base equilibrium: an examination of normocapneic hypoxemia and of the influence of hypoxemia on the adaptation to chronic hypercapnia. J Clin Invest 1967; 46:369–377.

61. Makoff D, Rosenbaum BJ. Adaptation to chronic hypercapnia in the potassium-depleted dog. Am J Physiol 1971; 220:1724–1727.

62. Schwartz WB, Hays RM, Polak A, Haynie GD. Effects of chronic hypercapnia on electrolyte and acid–base equilibrium. II. Recovery, with special reference to the influence of chloride intake. J Clin Invest 1961; 40: 1238–1249.

63. Adrogué HJ, Madias NE. Changes in plasma potassium concentration during acute acid–base disturbances. Am J Med 1981; 71:456–467.

64. Canzanello VJ, Bodvarsson M, Kraut JA, Johns CA, Slatopolsky E, Madias NE. Effect of chronic respiratory acidosis on urinary calcium excretion in the dog. Kidney Int 1990; 38:409–416.

65. Canzanello VJ, Kraut JA, Holick MF, Johns C, Liu CC, Madias NE. Effect of chronic respiratory acidosis on calcium metabolism in the rat. J Lab Clin Med 1995; 126:81–87.

66. Nattie EE, Romer L. CSF HCO_3^- regulation in isosmotic conditions: the role of brain PCO_2 and plasma HCO_3. Respir Physiol 1978; 33:177–198.

67. Messeter K, Siesjo BK. Regulation of the CSF pH in acute and sustained respiratory acidosis. Acta Physiol Scand 1971; 83:21–30.

68. Bleich HL, Berkman PM, Schwartz WB. The response of cerebrospinal fluid composition to sustained hypercapnia. J Clin Invest 1964; 43:11–18.

69. Pauli HG, Vorburger C, Reubi F. Chronic derangements of cerebrospinal fluid acid–base components in man. J Appl Physiol 1962; 17:993–998.

70. Siesjo BK. The regulation of cerebrospinal fluid pH. Kidney Int 1972; 1: 360–374.

71. Waddell WJ, Bates RG. Intracellular pH. Physiol Rev 1969; 49:285–329.

72. Manfredi F. Effects of hypocapnia and hypercapnia on intracellular acid–base equilibrium in man. J Lab Clin Med 1967; 69:304–312.

73. Robin ED. Intra- and subcellular aspects of the chemical control of ventilation. In: Cunningham DJC, Lloyd BB, eds. The Regulation of Human Respiration. Oxford: Blackwell, 1963:223–233.

74. Madias NE, Cohen JJ. Respiratory acidosis. In: Cohen JJ, Kassirer JP, eds. Acid–Base. Boston: Little Brown, 1982:307–348.

75. Alberti E, Hoyer S, Hamer J, Stoeckel H, Packschiess P, Weinhardt F. The effect of carbon dioxide on cerebral blood flow and cerebral metabolism in dogs. Br J Anaesth 1975; 47:941–947.

76. Cardenas VJ Jr, Zwischenberger JB, Tao W, et al. Correction of blood pH attenuates changes in hemodynamics and organ blood flow during permissive hypercapnia. Crit Care Med 1996; 24:827–834.

77. Auer LM, Johansson BB. Dilatation of pial arterial vessels in hypercapnia and in acute hypertension. Acta Physiol Scand 1980; 109:249–251.
78. Ellis EF, Wei EP, Cockrell CS, Traweek DL, Saady JJ, Kontos HA. The effect of O_2 and CO_2 on prostaglandin levels in the cat cerebral cortex. Circ Res 1982; 51:652–656.
79. Patterson JL Jr, Heyman A, Duke TW. Cerebral circulation and metabolism in chronic pulmonary emphysema, with observations on the effects of inhalation of oxygen. Am J Med 1952; 12:382–387.
80. Kilburn KH. Neurologic manifestations of respiratory failure. Arch Intern Med 1965; 116:409–415.
81. Neff TA, Petty TL. Tolerance and survival in severe chronic hypercapnia. Arch Intern Med 1972; 129:591–596.
82. Smith RB, Aass AA, Nemoto EM. Intraocular and intracranial pressure during respiratory alkalosis and acidosis. Br J Anaesth 1981; 53:967–972.
83. Simon RP, Niro M, Gwinn R. Brain acidosis induced by hypercarbic ventilation attenuates focal ischemic injury. J Pharmacol Exp Ther 1993; 267:1428–1431.
84. DeGeest H, Levy MN, Zieske H. Reflex effects of cephalic hypoxia, hypercapnia, and ischemia upon ventricular contractility. Circ Res 1965; 17:349–358.
85. Tenney SM. The effect of carbon dioxide on neurohumoral and endocrine mechanisms. Anesthesiology 1960; 21:674–685.
86. Berns AS, Anderson RJ, McDonald KM, Arnold PE. Effect of hypercapnic acidosis on renal water excretion in the dog. Kidney Int 1979; 15:116–125.
87. Price HL. Effects of carbon dioxide on the cardiovascular system. Anesthesiology 1960; 21:652–653.
88. Aber GM, Bayley TJ, Bishop JM. Inter-relationships between renal and cardiac function and respiratory gas exchange in obstructive airways disease. Clin Sci 1963; 25:159–170.
89. Enson Y, Giuntini C, Lewis ML, Morris TQ, Ferrer MI, Harvey RM. The influence of hydrogen ion concentration and hypoxia on the pulmonary circulation. J Clin Invest 1964; 43:1146–1162.
90. Holford FD, Mithoefer JC. Cardiac arrhythmias in hospitalized patients with chronic obstructive pulmonary disease. Am Rev Respir Dis 1973; 108:879–885.
91. Hudson LD, Kurt TL, Petty TL, Genton E. Arrhythmias associated with acute respiratory failure in patients with chronic airway obstruction. Chest 1973; 63:661–665.
92. Sideris DA, Katsadoros DP, Valianos G, Assioura A. Type of cardiac dysrhythmias in respiratory failure. Am Heart J 1975; 89:32–35.
93. Altschule MD, Sulzbach WM. Tolerance of the human heart to acidosis: reversible changes in RS-T interval during severe acidosis caused by administration of carbon dioxide. Am Heart J 1947; 33:458–463.
94. Brown EB Jr, Miller F. Ventricular fibrillation following a rapid fall in alveolar carbon dioxide concentration. Am J Physiol 1952; 169:56–60.
95. Kette F, Weil MH, Gazmuri RJ, Bisera J, Rackow EC. Intramyocardial hypercarbic acidosis during cardiac arrest and resuscitation. Crit Care Med 1993; 21:901–906.

96. Nishikawa T. Acute haemodynamic effect of sodium bicarbonate in canine respiratory or metabolic acidosis. Br J Anaesth 1993; 70:196–200.

97. Simmons DH, Olver RP. Effects of acute acid–base changes on renal hemodynamics in anesthetized dogs. Am J Physiol 1965; 209:1180–1186.

98. Bersentes TJ, Simmons DH. Effects of acute acidosis on renal hemodynamics. Am J Physiol 1967; 212:633–640.

99. Rose CE Jr, Peach MJ, Carey RM. Role of angiotensin II in renal vasoconstriction with acute hypoxemia and hypercapnic acidosis in conscious dogs. Ren Fail 1994; 16:229–242.

100. Anderson WH, Datta J, Samols E. The renin–angiotensin system in patients with acute respiratory insufficiency. Chest 1976; 69:309–311.

101. Rose CE Jr, Godine RL Jr, Rose KY, Anderson RJ, Carey RM. Role of arginine vasopressin and angiotensin II in cardiovascular responses to combined acute hypoxemia and hypercapnic acidosis in conscious dogs. J Clin Invest 1984; 74:321–331.

102. Hood VL, Tannen RL. Maintenance of acid–base homeostasis during ketoacidosis and lactic acidosis: implications for therapy. Diabetes Rev 1994; 2: 177–194.

103. Adrogué HJ, Chap Z, Okuda Y, et al. Acidosis-induced glucose intolerance is not prevented by adrenergic blockade. Am J Physiol 1988; 255:E812–E823.

104. Madias NE. Lactic acidosis. Kidney Int 1986; 29:752–774.

105. Bellingham AJ, Detter JC, Lenfant C. Regulatory mechanisms of hemoglobin oxygen affinity in acidosis and alkalosis. J Clin Invest 1971; 50:700–706.

106. Oski FA, Gottlieb AJ, Delivoria-Papadopoulos M, Miller WW. Red-cell 2,3-diphosphoglycerate levels in subjects with chronic hypoxemia. N Engl J Med 1969; 280:1165–1166.

107. Eckardt KU, Kurtz A, Bauer C. Triggering of erythropoietin production by hypoxia is inhibited by respiratory and metabolic acidosis. Am J Physiol 1990; 258:R678–R683.

108. Kato M, Staub NC. Response of small pulmonary arteries to unilobar hypoxia and hypercapnia. Circ Res 1966; 19:426–440.

109. Horwitz LD, Bishop YS, Stone HL. Effects of hypercapnia on the cardiovascular system of conscious dogs. J Appl Physiol 1968; 25:346–348.

110. Brimioulle S, Lejeune P, Vachiery JL, Leeman M, Melot C, Naeije R. Effects of acidosis and alkalosis on hypoxic pulmonary vasoconstriction in dogs. Am J Physiol 1990; 258:H347–H353.

111. Yanos J, Wood LD, Davis K, Keamy M 3rd. The effect of respiratory and lactic acidosis on diaphragm function. Am Rev Respir Dis 1993; 147:616–619.

112. Bushinsky DA, Sessler NE. Critical role of bicarbonate in calcium release from bone. Am J Physiol 1992; 263:F510–F515.

113. Bushinsky DA, Lam BC, Nespeca R, Sessler NE, Grynpas MD. Decreased bone carbonate content in response to metabolic, but not respiratory, acidosis. Am J Physiol 1993; 265:F530–F536.

114. Bushinsky DA. Stimulated osteoclastic and suppressed osteoblastic activity in metabolic but not respiratory acidosis. Am J Physiol 1995; 268:C80–C88.

115. Frumin MJ, Epstein RM, Cohen G. Apneic oxygenation in man. Anesthesiology 1959; 20:789–798.

116. Braman SS, Kaemmerlen JT. Intensive care of status asthmaticus. A 10-year experience. J Am Med Assoc 1990; 264:366–368.
117. Brouillette RT, Weese-Mayer DE, Hunt CE. Breathing control disorders in infants and children. Hosp Pract (Off Ed) 1990; 25:82–85, 88, 93–96 (passim).
118. Weil JV, Cherniack NS, Dempsey JA, et al. Respiratory disorders of sleep. Pathophysiology, clinical implications, and therapeutic approaches. Am Rev Respir Dis 1987; 136:755–761.
119. Kollef MH, Schuster DP. The acute respiratory distress syndrome. N Engl J Med 1995; 332:27–37.
120. American Thoracic Society. Idiopathic congenital central hypoventilation syndrome: diagnosis and management. Am J Respir Crit Care Med 1999; 160:368–373.
121. Mullan S, Hosobuchi Y. Respiratory hazards of high cervical percutaneous cordotomy. J Neurosurg 1968; 28:291–297.
122. Weese-Mayer DE, Silvestri JM, Huffman AD, et al. Case/control family study of autonomic nervous system dysfunction in idiopathic congenital central hypoventilation syndrome. Am J Med Genet 2001; 100:237–245.
123. Shea SA, Andres LP, Shannon DC, Guz A, Banzett RB. Respiratory sensations in subjects who lack a ventilatory response to CO_2. Respir Physiol 1993; 93:203–219.
124. Shea SA. Life without ventilatory chemosensitivity. Respir Physiol 1997; 110:199–210.
125. Gozal D, Simakajornboon N. Passive motion of the extremities modifies alveolar ventilation during sleep in patients with congenital central hypoventilation syndrome. Am J Respir Crit Care Med 2000; 162:1747–1751.
126. Cohen RD. Lactic acidosis: new perspectives on origins and treatment. Diabetes Rev 1994; 2:86–97.
127. Adrogué HJ, Madias NE. Management of life-threatening acid–base disorders. First of two parts. N Engl J Med 1998; 338:26–34.
128. Aberman A, Fulop M. The metabolic and respiratory acidosis of acute pulmonary edema. Ann Intern Med 1972; 76:173–184.
129. Detmer MD, Chandra P, Cohen PJ. Occurrence of hypercarbia due to an unusual failure of anesthetic equipment. Anesthesiology 1980; 52:278–279.
130. Klein SL, Lilburn JK. An unusual case of hypercarbia during general anesthesia. Anesthesiology 1980; 53:248–250.
131. Elliott GG, Morris AH. Clinical syndromes of respiratory acidosis and alkalosis. In: Seldin DW, Giebisch G, eds. The Regulation of Acid–base Balance. New York: Raven Press, 1989:483–521.
132. Burrows B, Earle RH. Course and prognosis of chronic obstructive lung disease. A prospective study of 200 patients. N Engl J Med 1969; 280:397–404.
133. Gacad G, Hamosh P. The lung in ankylosing spondylitis. Am Rev Respir Dis 1973; 107:286–289.
134. Finlay G, Concannon D, McDonnell TJ. Treatment of respiratory failure due to kyphoscoliosis with nasal intermittent positive pressure ventilation (NIPPV). Ir J Med Sci 1995; 164:28–30.
135. Santiago TV, Pugliese AC, Edelman NH. Control of breathing during methadone addiction. Am J Med 1977; 62:347–354.

136. Farmer WC, Glenn WW, Gee JB. Alveolar hypoventilation syndrome. Studies of ventilatory control in patients selected for diaphragm pacing. Am J Med 1978; 64:39–49.
137. Rapoport DM, Garay SM, Epstein H, Goldring RM. Hypercapnia in the obstructive sleep apnea syndrome. A reevaluation of the "Pickwickian syndrome". Chest 1986; 89:627–635.
138. Rosenow EC 3rd, Engel AG. Acid maltase deficiency in adults presenting as respiratory failure. Am J Med 1978; 64:485–491.
139. Ferguson GT, Cherniack RM. Management of chronic obstructive pulmonary disease. N Engl J Med 1993; 328:1017–1022.
140. Rudolf M, Banks RA, Semple SJ. Hypercapnia during oxygen therapy in acute exacerbations of chronic respiratory failure. Hypothesis revisited. Lancet 1977; 2:483–486.
141. Aubier M, Murciano D, Fournier M, Milic-Emili J, Pariente R, Derenne JP. Central respiratory drive in acute respiratory failure of patients with chronic obstructive pulmonary disease. Am Rev Respir Dis 1980; 122:191–199.
142. Aubier M, Murciano D, Milic-Emili J, et al. Effects of the administration of O_2 on ventilation and blood gases in patients with chronic obstructive pulmonary disease during acute respiratory failure. Am Rev Respir Dis 1980; 122:747–754.
143. American Thoracic Society. Standards for the diagnosis and care of patients with chronic obstructive pulmonary disease. Am J Respir Crit Care Med 1995; 152:S77–S121.
144. Tarpy SP, Celli BR. Long-term oxygen therapy. N Engl J Med 1995; 333: 710–714.
145. Bateman NT, Leach RM. ABC of oxygen. Acute oxygen therapy. Br Med J 1998; 317:798–801.
146. Weinberger SE, Schwartzstein RM, Weiss JW. Hypercapnia. N Engl J Med 1989; 321:1223–1231.
147. Tobin MJ. Mechanical ventilation. N Engl J Med 1994; 330:1056–1061.
148. Mehta S, Hill NS. Noninvasive ventilation. Am J Respir Crit Care Med 2001; 163:540–577.
149. International Consensus Conferences in Intensive Care Medicine. noninvasive positive pressure ventilation in acute respiratory failure. Am J Respir Crit Care Med 2001; 163:283–291.
150. Tobin MJ. Advances in mechanical ventilation. N Engl J Med 2001; 344: 1986–1996.
151. Jubran A, Van de Graaff WB, Tobin MJ. Variability of patient-ventilator interaction with pressure support ventilation in patients with chronic obstructive pulmonary disease. Am J Respir Crit Care Med 1995; 152:129–136.
152. Bidani A, Tzouanakis AE, Cardenas VJ Jr, Zwischenberger JB. Permissive hypercapnia in acute respiratory failure. J Am Med Assoc 1994; 272:957–962.
153. Feihl F, Perret C. Permissive hypercapnia. How permissive should we be? Am J Respir Crit Care Med 1994; 150:1722–1737.
154. Dries DJ. Permissive hypercapnia. J Trauma 1995; 39:984–989.
155. Tuxen DV. Permissive hypercapnic ventilation. Am J Respir Crit Care Med 1994; 150:870–874.

156. Gentilello LM, Anardi D, Mock C, Arreola-Risa C, Maier RV. Permissive hypercapnia in trauma patients. J Trauma 1995; 39:846–852; discussion 852–853.
157. Amato MB, Barbas CS, Medeiros DM, et al. Beneficial effects of the "open lung approach" with low distending pressures in acute respiratory distress syndrome. A prospective randomized study on mechanical ventilation. Am J Respir Crit Care Med 1995; 152:1835–1846.
158. Amato MB, Barbas CS, Medeiros DM, et al. Effect of a protective-ventilation strategy on mortality in the acute respiratory distress syndrome. N Engl J Med 1998; 338:347–354.
159. Hudson LD. Protective ventilation for patients with acute respiratory distress syndrome. N Engl J Med 1998; 338:385–387.
160. Mithoefer JC, Porter WF, Karetzky MS. Indications for the use of sodium bicarbonate in the treatment of intractable asthma. Respiration 1968; 25:201–215.
161. Roncoroni AJ, Adrogué HJ, De Obrutsky CW, Marchisio ML, Herrera MR. Metabolic acidosis in status asthmaticus. Respiration 1976; 33:85–94.
162. Sun JH, Filley GF, Hord K, Kindig NB, Bartle EJ. Carbicarb: an effective substitute for NaHCO₃ for the treatment of acidosis. Surgery 1987; 102:835–839.
163. Leung JM, Landow L, Franks M, et al. Safety and efficacy of intravenous Carbicarb in patients undergoing surgery: comparison with sodium bicarbonate in the treatment of mild metabolic acidosis. SPI Research Group. Study of Perioperative Ischemia. Crit Care Med 1994; 22:1540–1549.
164. Kucera RR, Shapiro JI, Whalen MA, Kindig NB, Filley GF, Chan L. Brain pH effects of NaHCO₃ and Carbicarb in lactic acidosis. Crit Care Med 1989; 17:1320–1323.
165. Tham,tromethamine. Chicago: Abbot Laboratories, 1995.
166. Brasch H, Thies E, Iven H. Pharmacokinetics of TRIS (hydroxymethyl-) aminomethane in healthy subjects and in patients with metabolic acidosis. Eur J Clin Pharmacol 1982; 22:257–264.
167. Bear R, Goldstein M, Phillipson E, et al. Effect of metabolic alkalosis on respiratory function in patients with chronic obstructive lung disease. Can Med Assoc J 1977; 117:900–903.
168. Miller PD, Berns AS. Acute metabolic alkalosis perpetuating hypercarbia. A role for acetazolamide in chronic obstructive pulmonary disease. J Am Med Assoc 1977; 238:2400–2401.
169. Catchlove RF, Kafer ER. The effects of diazepam on respiration in patients with obstructive pulmonary disease. Anesthesiology 1971; 34:14–18.
170. Lyons HA, Huang CT. Therapeutic use of progesterone in alveolar hypoventilation associated with obesity. Am J Med 1968; 44:881–888.
171. Moser KM, Luchsinger PC, Adamson JS, et al. Respiratory stimulation with intravenous doxapram in respiratory failure. A double-blind co-operative study. N Engl J Med 1973; 288:427–431.
172. Sutton FD Jr, Zwillich CW, Creagh CE, Pierson DJ, Weil JV. Progesterone for outpatient treatment of Pickwickian syndrome. Ann Intern Med 1975; 83:476–479.

173. Dull WL, Polu JM, Sadoul P. The pulmonary haemodynamic effects of almitrine infusion in men with chronic hypercapnia. Clin Sci (Lond) 1983; 64: 25–31.

174. Skatrud JB, Dempsey JA, Iber C, Berssenbrugge A. Correction of CO_2 retention during sleep in patients with chronic obstructive pulmonary diseases. Am Rev Respir Dis 1981; 124:260–268.

175. Adrogué HJ, Madias NE. Respiratory acidosis, respiratory alkalosis, and mixed disorders. In: Johnson RJ, Feehally J, eds. Comprehensive Clinical Nephrology. New York: Mosby, 2003:167–182.

21

Respiratory Alkalosis

Reto Krapf

Department of Medicine, Kantonsspital Bruderholz, Basel, Switzerland

Henry N. Hulter

Genentech Inc., South San Francisco, California, U.S.A.

INTRODUCTION AND DEFINITIONS

Respiratory alkalosis is the acid–base disturbance characterized by a primary decrease in the carbon dioxide tension (PCO_2) of the body fluids, i.e., by *primary hypocapnia*. The decrease in PCO_2 has an alkalinizing effect on body fluids, but the magnitude of alkalinization is ameliorated by secondary decrements in plasma $[HCO_3^-]$ that occur by two mechanisms (extra-renal and renal). Acutely (within minutes) hypocapnia elicits a modest decrement in plasma $[HCO_3^-]$ due to extra-renal mechanisms; no further significant changes in plasma acid–base composition occur for several hours, thus establishing an "acute steady state." When hypocapnia persists for a longer period of time, however, renal acid excretion is appreciably decreased, resulting in a further reduction in plasma $[HCO_3^-]$ that further ameliorates the impact of hypocapnia on blood pH. Nevertheless, this adjustment falls short of returning blood $[H^+]$ completely to its preexisting or normal value.

Acute *respiratory alkalosis* is defined by hypocapnia persisting up to several hours, i.e., before signs of renal adaptation are biochemically detectable. The period between several hours from onset up to 48–72 hr is the non-steady-state transition period during which the kidneys retain acid in response to a sustained decrease in arterial carbon dioxide tension ($PaCO_2$).

Chronic *respiratory alkalosis* is judged to be present when the renal adaptation is fully expressed (hypocapnia persisting for >48–72 hr).

PATHOPHYSIOLOGY OF RESPIRATORY ALKALOSIS

Hypocapnia is ordinarily produced by a transient period of negative CO_2 balance, wherein CO_2 excretion exceeds its production rate. Primary increases in CO_2 excretion result mostly from increased alveolar ventilation, but extrapulmonary excretion or removal of CO_2 (dialysis and extracorporeal circulation) may also cause hypocapnia. Primary decreases in CO_2 production (e.g., in hypothyroidism and hypothermia) are ordinarily accompanied by concordant changes in alveolar ventilation (see Chapter 3). Figure 1 illustrates the regulatory roles for ventilatory control of both intrinsic feed-forward factors such as the muscle afferents and CNS centers that drive ventilation as well as feedback regulation by blood gas parameters. This regulatory system is subject to influence by numerous modulators that affect

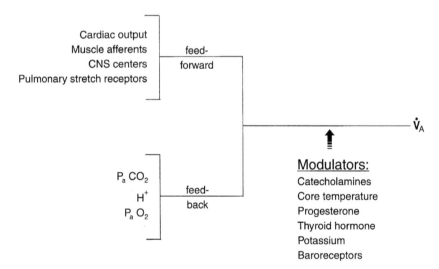

Figure 1 Two classes of respiratory stimuli: feed-forward and feed-backward stimuli (the tightly regulated blood gas parameters) combine to determine ventilation rate. Feed-forward factors are those driving ventilation largely as a tonic physiologic or pathophysiologic stimulus and include the potent muscle afferents and CNS centers. Feed-back factors are those that operate at both CNS and peripheral sites to regulate ventilation largely by feedback inhibition; such control is dominated by $PaCO_2$, $[H^+]$ and PaO_2. Modulating factors are able to affect the magnitude of the ventilatory response to stimuli or provide fine adjustments to the stable resting value of minute ventilation as primarily determined by the feed-forward and feed-back factors. *Source*: Adapted from Ref. 198.

alveolar ventilation rate by virtue of their function as respiratory stimulants (e.g., progesterone, thyroid hormone).

Effect of Hypocapnia on Acid–Base Equilibrium

The acid–base response to a sustained decrease in CO_2 tension can be divided into three phases (Fig. 2). Phases 1 and 2 occur in an overlapping time frame (seconds to several hours) and define acute respiratory alkalosis, while phase 3 initiates the chronic steady-state, termed chronic respiratory alkalosis. The characteristics and temporal occurrence of the three phases are:

1. Acute alkalinization caused by a sudden increase in the ratio of plasma $[HCO_3^-]/PCO_2$ as defined by the Henderson–Hasselbach equation (see following section, seconds to minutes).
2. Rapid secondary buffer response to this acute alkalinization by nonrenal mechanisms, resulting in a reduction in blood pH due to H^+ release from cellular (e.g., hemoglobin) and extracellular

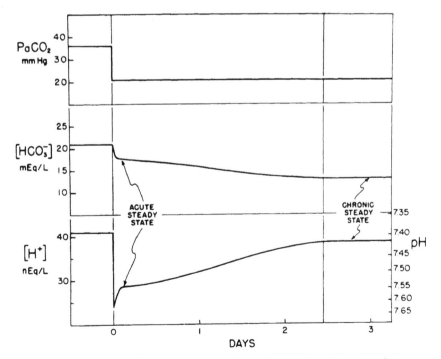

Figure 2 Time course of the response of plasma $[HCO_3^-]$ and blood $[H^+]$ to sustained hypocapnia. See text for description of the different phases of adaptation. *Source:* From Ref. 177.

(e.g., $H_2PO_4^-$) buffers (see following section, 10 min to several hours).

3. Decreased renal acidification (detectable after several hours and manifested as a further decrease in plasma $[HCO_3^-]$) until a chronic steady-state resulting from all three processes is reached after about 48–72 hr.

Acute Respiratory Alkalosis

With the initiation of hypocapnia, $PaCO_2$ is reduced within seconds and extracellular fluid (ECF) is alkalinized immediately as defined by the relationships in the Henderson–Hasselbach equation:

$$pH = 6.1 + \log([HCO_3^-]/PaCO_2 \times 0.03) \qquad (1)$$

The acute adjustments in acid–base equilibrium in reaction to hypocapnia-induced alkalemia are attributed to nonrenal mechanisms and are completed within 5–10 min. This assessment does not indicate that renal mechanisms are not operative during the period of the "acute steady-state," but that their quantitative contribution is too small to be reflected by any change in plasma composition or by whole organism balance studies. An acute "steady-state" response occurs after imposition of hypocapnia-induced alkalemia, characterized by an acidification of ECF that ameliorates the magnitude of initial alkalemia (1).

Several mechanisms contribute to this process:

1. H^+ release from blood, interstitial and tissue buffers consumes ECF HCO_3^- as follows:

   a. $Hbuffer^+ \rightarrow H^+ + Buffer$ (due to $\downarrow [H^+]$)
   b. $HCO_3^- + H^+ + H_2CO_3$ (causing the $\downarrow$ in ECF $[HCO_3]$)
   c. $H_2CO_3 \rightarrow H_2O + CO_2$ (excreted by the lungs)

2. Acute changes in the activities of cellular acid–base transporters
3. Increased organic acid production

Release of H^+ from Blood, Interstitial, and Tissue Buffers

In isolated whole blood, release of H^+ from hemoglobin and plasma proteins in response to acute hypocapnia induces a large decrease in $[HCO_3^-]$. However, in intact organisms, this effect is diminished by a complex interaction with nonerythrocyte cell buffering (e.g., skeletal muscle). The decrease in blood $[HCO_3^-]$ is counterbalanced, in part, by the diffusion of HCO_3^- from the interstitial compartment into blood. This diffusion gradient for HCO_3^- is built up as follows: Due to rapid diffusion of CO_2 across cell membranes, intracellular alkalinization of both erythrocytes and other cells occurs almost instantaneously after the decrease in extracellular CO_2 tension. The much higher intracellular nonbicarbonate buffering capacity of the nonerythrocyte cell mass (in terms of H^+ released per unit pH increase) limits the fall in [HCO_3^-] when compared with the ECF or erythrocytes (2).

Acute Changes in the Activities of Cellular Acid–Base Transporters

Several cellular mechanisms facilitate restoration of cell pH toward normal values. These include inhibition of the rate of turnover of H^+-extruding transporters (i.e., Na^+/H^+ exchange) and activation of base-coupled transporters (i.e., Na^+ and Cl^- - coupled HCO_3^- transporters), which also modulate the extent of an imposed change in cell pH (2). The sudden decrease in ECF PCO_2 can elicit acute cellular effects resulting in delivery of HCO_3^- into the ECF, at least in certain epithelial tissues (2), but this effect is offset by the net supply of H^+ to the ECF from intracellular buffers stimulated by cellular alkalinization. This H^+ efflux, mediated primarily by cell membrane Na^+/H^+ exchange (NHE1) is large; nonerythrocyte intracellular buffering accounts for approximately two-thirds of the net H^+ delivered (total body buffering) to ECF in acute hypocapnia (1,3).

There is considerable uncertainty regarding the magnitude of the increase in cell pH in acute hypocapnia. Human "whole body" intracellular pH estimates using the indirect dimethyl oxazolidinedione (see Chapter 2) method have shown large pH increments similar to those of extracellular pH (4), and similar results are seen with this method in dog and rat muscle (5–7) and in rat brain (8). When intracellular pH is measured by direct in vivo myocardial placement of the sensor coil, using ^{31}P-NMR in dogs, however, hypocapnia-induced increments are very small (9). In fact, acute hyperventilation-induced increases of arterial pH from 7.40 to 7.70 raised myocardial intracellular pH by only approximately 0.10. Such discrepancies are difficult to evaluate at present and await improvements in whole body ^{31}P-NMR technology.

Increased Organic Acid Production

Cell organic acid production increases rapidly in response to hypocapnia-induced alkalemia, providing an additional source of H^+ to accomplish the secondary decrease in ECF [HCO_3^-]. Acute respiratory alkalosis in rats eating a high fat diet results in significant increases in blood ketone body concentrations and large increases in urinary ketone body excretion (10). Although this finding is consistent with early reports of increased blood and urine ketones in humans with respiratory alkalosis (10), systematic studies of ketone metabolism using modern assay methods have not been carried out.

Both passive and voluntary hyperventilation in humans results in small increases in plasma lactate concentration (2–3 mEq/L) (1,4,11,12). During recovery from exercise-induced lactic acid overproduction, blood pH and ^{31}P-NMR-derived intracellular [HCO_3^-] were elevated in alkali-loaded humans compared to controls, in association with accelerated muscle output of lactic acid. Thus, an increase in muscle cell pH or alkali concentration might stimulate lactic acid production and increase plasma lactate levels in alkalemia (13). Although muscle cell pH is known to mediate glycolytic flux, it is unclear whether respiratory alkalosis in vivo modulates pH-sensitive glycolytic enzymes (e.g., phosphofructokinase) and thereby increases lactic acid production (14).

Respiratory alkalosis also activates the sympathetic nervous system in humans, manifested by elevated plasma catecholamines (15). Hepatic sympathetic nerve stimulation in rats, of sufficient magnitude to increase blood catecholamine levels, results in α_1 receptor-mediated increases in lactic acid output. Thus, hypocapnia-induced sympathetic activation might account for the modest elevations of lactic acid production observed with acute hypocapnia (16,17). The effect of experimentally induced respiratory alkalosis on lactic acid production is specific for hypocapnia/alkalemia. Isocapnic (CO_2-supplemented) hyperventilation of the same magnitude (i.e., employing similar muscle work) prevents the increase in lactic acid in humans (18,19). Plasma catecholamine levels also do not increase in isocapnic hyperventilation (15), providing strong evidence that the acid–base disorder, per se, and not augmented respiratory muscle activity/alveolar ventilation rate is the proximate stimulus to both sympathetic activation and increased lactic acid production. The relative contributions of altered cell pH and sympathetic nerve activation in causing the augmented lactic acid output during acute hypocapnia remain to be determined. The time course and the magnitude of systemic acidification attributable to increased organic acid production are poorly defined in both human and animal models of respiratory alkalosis.

Confidence Limits for Changes in [HCO_3^-] and [H^+] in Acute Respiratory Alkalosis

Figure 3 depicts the 95% confidence limits in humans for plasma [HCO_3^-] and [H^+] in uncomplicated acute respiratory alkalosis. These limits represent the range of expected changes in plasma [H^+] and [HCO_3^-] if an acute reduction in $PaCO_2$ were the primary parameter being altered. The data underlying these confidence limits were collected from anesthetized subjects subjected to passive hyperventilation before minor surgical procedures (1). Quantitatively, for each mmHg decrease in $PaCO_2$, plasma [HCO_3^-] falls by 0.2 mEq/L, while blood [H^+] falls by 0.75 nEq/L. Thus, in uncomplicated acute respiratory alkalosis, a reduction in $PaCO_2$ from 40 to 30 mmHg will result in a fall of plasma [HCO_3^-] from 25 to 23 mEq/L, while blood [H^+] will fall from 40 to 32.5 nEq/L (a pH increase from 7.40 to 7.49).

Chronic Respiratory Alkalosis

Figure 4 illustrates the plasma and renal acid–base response to sustained hypocapnia (induced by a hypobaric hypoxic environment, i.e., high altitude

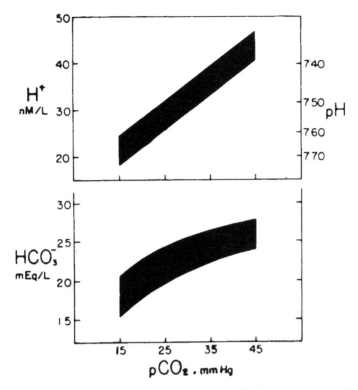

Figure 3 Confidence bands for acute respiratory alkalosis in humans. For any given level of hypocapnia, the bands describe the 95% confidence limits for plasma [H$^+$] (*upper panel*) and [HCO$_3^-$] (*lower panel*) in uncomplicated acute respiratory alkalosis. *Source*: Adapted from Ref. 1.

dwelling) in humans (20). In response to sustained hypocapnia, renal net acid excretion is inhibited transiently to an extent that accounts for the observed additional decrease in plasma [HCO$_3^-$] when compared with acute hypocapnia. This renal response further ameliorates the alkalemia, returning blood pH closer to normal. The decrease in net acid excretion results from an increase in HCO$_3^-$ excretion and a concomitant decrease in titratable acid excretion; NH$_4^+$ excretion is unchanged. In dogs, by contrast, the decrease in net acid excretion was attributable largely to a decrease in NH$_4^+$ excretion (21). Whether suppression of NH$_4^+$ vs. titratable acid is a species difference or due to differences in phosphate intake is unknown. After several days, net acid excretion returns to control levels (the urine is again virtually HCO$_3^-$-free) and plasma [HCO$_3^-$] stabilizes at a lower level. Thus, in chronic respiratory alkalosis in humans, the set point or threshold for renal reabsorption of HCO$_3^-$ is reduced (i.e., the kidney lowers plasma

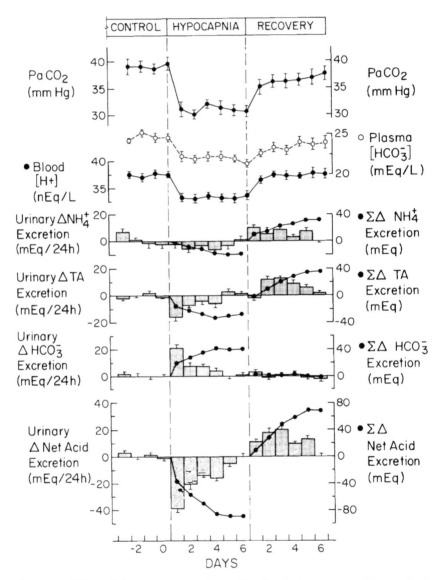

Figure 4 Effect of chronic hypocapnia on blood acid–base composition and urinary ammonium (NH$_4^+$), titratable acid (TA), bicarbonate (HCO$_3^-$) and net acid excretion in normal human volunteers studied under metabolic balance conditions. Urinary Δ values denote the daily deviations from the mean value of the preceding steady-state period, whereas urinary ΣΔ values denote the sum of the daily changes in excretion compared to the preceding steady-state period. Subjects were transported rapidly to a hypoxic, hypobaric environment at an altitude of 3450 m (11,319 feet) above sea level at the research unit on the Jungfraujoch (Switzerland). *Source*: From Ref. 20.

[HCO_3^-]). This new steady-state is characterized by a reduced filtered load of HCO_3^- which is exactly balanced by the decreased rate of renal HCO_3^- reabsorption (i.e., H^+ secretion) again providing the milieu for adjusting net acid excretion to match daily endogenous acid production (12,21–24). The finding in humans that net acid excretion in chronic hypocapnia is essentially identical to corresponding control values suggests that any chronic increase in organic acid production is either of insufficient magnitude for detection or that chronic hypocapnia results in a counterbalancing reduction in other pathways of acid production (e.g., H_2SO_4) (20). Urine SO_4^{2-} values have not been reported in chronic hypocapnia in any species. A single report in dogs has reported dissociation of the acid excretory and hypobicarbonatemic effects of chronic hypocapnia by pretreating the animals with an electrolyte- and phosphate-restricted diet (22). Whether preexisting or ongoing phosphate depletion in that study provided an extrarenal mechanism for full plasma acid–base adaptation in the absence of detectable renal adaptation to hypocapnia remains to be determined.

Changes in Renal H^+ Secretion

Both proximal and distal (collecting duct) H^+ secretion is suppressed during acute hypocapnia (25–30). Bicarbonate reabsorption in the loop of Henle is not affected (31). In chronic hypocapnia, proximal tubule H^+ secretion is decreased in the rat (32); no studies have specifically evaluated distal acidification. The decrease in proximal tubule H^+ secretion (or, equivalently: the decrease in HCO_3^- reabsorption) in acute and chronic hypocapnia is mediated, at least in part, by parallel decreases in the activities of the luminal Na^+/H^+ exchanger (NHE3) and the basolateral Na^+/HCO_3^- cotransporter (2,33,34). The V_{max} of NHE3 (an index of functional transmembrane transporter number) is decreased in hypocapnia (33,34) but total NHE3 protein is unchanged (35). Thus, decreased H^+ efflux is likely due to net retrieval of NHE3 from the apical membrane to a nonfunctional subapical compartment rather than a decrease in transcriptional or translational production of this transport protein.

In addition to the adaptive change in the function of these Na^+-coupled acid–base transporters, H^+-translocating ATPases are also affected by hypocapnia. The disorder induces a K^+- and mineralocortiocoid-independent decrease in H^+-ATPase activities along the entire nephron (35,36) and a decrease in collecting duct H^+/K^+-ATPase activity (36). The mechanism(s) and physiologic relevance of these decreased enzymatic activities in the renal adaptive response to chronic hypocapnia is unclear. In addition to the decrease in total pump number predicted by enzymatic studies (36), it is possible that hypocapnia increases the retrieval rate of H^+-ATPase from the luminal membrane of α-intercalated cells in the collecting duct (36). An increased retrieval rate is induced by low ambient

CO_2, although this effect appears less pronounced than the increased insertion of H^+-ATPase in response to hypercapnia (37). Another intriguing possibility is that hypocapnia reverses the polarity of H^+ and HCO_3^- transporters between the apical and basolateral membranes of intercalated collecting duct cells (38). There is, however, no information about whether hypocapnia increases the number or activity of apical Cl^-/HCO_3^- exchangers in β intercalated cells.

Changes in Renal Na^+ and K^+ Excretion

Renal acid retention in chronic hypocapnia is accompanied by renal Na^+ losses, resulting in a decrease in ECF volume. When dietary Na^+ is restricted, K^+ rather than Na^+ is lost in the urine. Moreover, if both Na^+ and K^+ are restricted, phosphate retention rather than cation wasting is observed in chronic hypocapnia (12,20–22,39). The most likely explanation for these observations is that, in the absence of dietary constraints or phosphate depletion, hypocapnia-induced inhibition of proximal tubule H^+ secretion results in increased HCO_3^- delivery to the distal nephron of sufficient magnitude to overcome the HCO_3^- reabsorptive capacity at that site, resulting in bicarbonaturia and natriuresis.

Nature of the Signal and Potentially Maladaptive Effects of Chronic Hypocapnia

The renal adaptation to hypocapnia is not mediated by a decrease in extra- or intracellular $[H^+]$ but rather by the reduced $PaCO_2$ itself. Irrespective of whether the preexisting plasma $[HCO_3^-]$ and pH are normal, increased or decreased and irrespective of species (dogs and humans), chronic hypocapnia induces a similar reduction in plasma $[HCO_3^-]$, manifested quantitatively by the slope, $\Delta[HCO_3^-]/\Delta PaCO_2$ (12,40,41). Despite the qualitative similarity of the renal response to hypocapnia in dogs and humans, there is an important difference. In dogs, the slope, $\Delta[HCO_3^-]/\Delta PaCO_2$, is -0.54 mEq/L per mmHg fall in $PaCO_2$ over a wide range of plasma $[HCO_3^-]$, dictating that the percent change in $[HCO_3^-]$ becomes greater than the percent change in $PaCO_2$ at initial plasma $[HCO_3^-]$ values below 18 mEq/L. As a result, a sustained reduction in $PaCO_2$ worsens the preexisting acidemia when the initial plasma $[HCO_3^-]$ is < 18 mEq/L, i.e., it is maladaptive (Fig. 5). In humans, however, the slope, $\Delta[HCO_3^-]/\Delta PaCO_2$, is less steep, -0.41 mEq/L per mmHg decrement in $PaCO_2$, over the range of plasma $[HCO_3^-]$ values studied (10–25 mEq/L). As a result, superimposed sustained reductions in $PaCO_2$ do not abolish the adaptive alkalemic effect of this maneuver over this range (Fig. 6). The normal plasma $[HCO_3^-]$ is higher in humans (24–25 mEq/L) than in dogs (21 mEq/L) further accentuating this species difference. If the slope, $\Delta[HCO_3^-]/\Delta PaCO_2$ (-0.41 mEq/L/mmHg), is maintained in humans even at very low initial $[HCO_3^-]$, one can predict that any further sustained decrease in $PaCO_2$ will

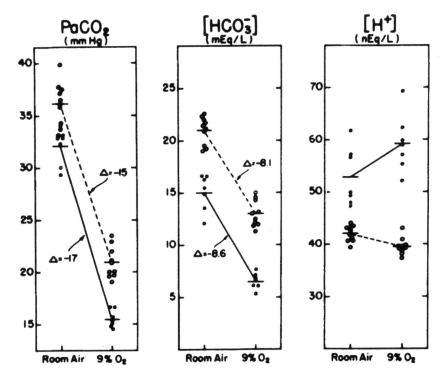

Figure 5 Changes in plasma [HCO₃⁻] and [H⁺] during prolonged exposure to hypocapnia in normal dogs (*dashed lines*) and dogs with chronic HCl-induced metabolic acidosis (*solid lines*). Similar decrements in $PaCO_2$ in the two groups produce nearly equivalent reductions in plasma [HCO₃⁻], despite divergent effects on [H⁺]. *Source*: From Ref. 40.

worsen academia only when the initial plasma [HCO₃⁻] is 6–8 mEq/L (42). Figure 7 illustrates the effects of a sustained decrease of $PaCO_2$ on blood [H⁺] at different baseline [HCO₃⁻] values, and compares the quantitative effect of the different linear slopes between dogs and humans. Based on extrapolation of the available slope data, it is possible that in severe metabolic acidosis (e.g., severe ketoacidosis or cholera) a further sustained decrease in $PaCO_2$ (from the levels that normally occur in response to chronic metabolic acidosis) via mechanical overventilation or additional ventilatory stimulation could be maladaptive and worsen acidemia.

Confidence Limits for Changes in [HCO₃⁻] and [H⁺] in Chronic Respiratory Alkalosis

A new steady-state is achieved within 2–3 days following induction of sustained hypocapnia (Fig. 1). In humans, for each mmHg decrease in $PaCO_2$, plasma [HCO₃⁻] decreases by 0.41 mEq/L, irrespective of the baseline

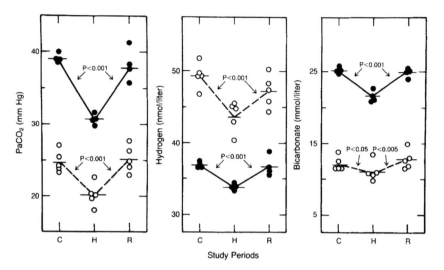

Figure 6 Steady-state changes in plasma [HCO₃⁻] and [H⁺] during chronic hypocapnia in normal humans (*solid lines, filled circles*) and humans with preexisting metabolic acidosis (NH₄Cl feeding) (*dashed, interrupted lines, open circles*). Hypocapnia decreases plasma [HCO₃⁻] in both groups, as observed in dogs but in contrast to dogs (Fig. 5), blood [H⁺] falls irrespective of the prevailing initial plasma [HCO₃⁻]. C, control; H, hypocapnia; R, recovery. *Source*: From Ref. 40.

plasma [HCO₃⁻] (over the range studied). Blood [H⁺] decreases by about 0.4 nEq/L for each mmHg decrease in PaCO₂. Thus, in simple chronic respiratory alkalosis, a decrease of PaCO₂ from 40 to 30 mmHg should result in a reduction in plasma [HCO₃⁻] from 25 to 21 mEq/L and in [H⁺] from 40 to 36 nEq/L.

EFFECTS OF HYPOCAPNIA ON EXTRACELLULAR VOLUME AND ELECTROLYTE BALANCE

Plasma and ECF Volume

In humans, acute respiratory alkalosis induced by voluntary hyperventilation decreases plasma volume due to a shift of protein-free fluid into extravascular compartments, triggered by either increased capillary hydrostatic pressure or enhanced capillary permeability (43,44). Blood volume also decreases in voluntary hyperventilation (45). The reduction in plasma volume is dependent on respiratory alkalosis as isocapnic hyperventilation prevents this change (M. Stäubli, 1998, personal communication).

Chronic respiratory alkalosis induces transient renal Na⁺ wasting, thereby decreasing ECF volume, independent of whether hypoxemia is present as a stimulus for hyperventilation (12,20,21). A chronic decrease in PaCO₂

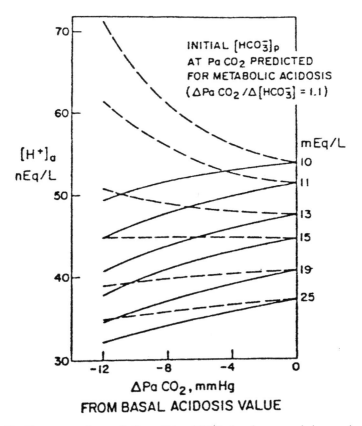

Figure 7 Nomogram for prediction of blood [H$^+$] when hypocapnia is superimposed on chronic metabolic acidosis over a range of initial values for plasma [HCO$_3^-$]. Solid lines represent the [H$^+$] changes for initial plasma [HCO$_3^-$] ranging from 10 to 25 mEq/L and are based on a slope of [HCO$_3^-$]/PaCO$_2$ = 0.41 for humans (56). Dashed lines represent the [H$^+$] changes for initial plasma [HCO$_3^-$] ranging from 10 to 25 mmol/L, and are based on the slope of [HCO$_3^-$]/PaCO$_2$ = 0.54 for dogs. ΔPaCO$_2$ values represent changes in PaCO$_2$ from the initial PaCO$_2$ level. As shown, hypocapnia results in uniform alkalemic response when the human-derived slope is used, whereas a deflection point for acidemic vs. alkalemic response is apparent at initial plasma [HCO$_3^-$] < 18 mEq/L when the canine slope is used. *Source*: From Ref. 42.

from 39 to 31 mmHg in humans induces an Na$^+$ deficit of approximately 150 mEq, without secondary hyperaldosteronism, over a 6-day period (20).

Plasma Electrolytes

Sodium and Chloride

Mild hyponatremia (2–4 mEq/l decrease) occurs in acute (1,3) but not chronic hypocapnia, and has been ascribed to increased cellular uptake of Na$^+$ (46), possibly via an Na^+-coupled H^+ extrusion processes. Hyperchloremia is invariably present in both acute and chronic respiratory alkalosis. In the acute disorder, hyperchloremia is extrarenal and is attributed to a Cl^- shift from erythrocytes (1,3). In chronic hypocapnia, hyperchloremia is the consequence of ECF volume contraction (see preceding section).

Potassium

Studies in humans report conflicting data regarding plasma $[K^+]$ in acute respiratory alkalosis: increases (47,48), no significant changes (12,45,46,49,50) and decreases (52–56) have been reported. When the results in humans are examined without the confounding influences of anesthesia and older analytic methods, acute respiratory alkalosis (induced by voluntary hyperventilation for 20 min) induces a significant and reversible increase in plasma $[K^+]$. Plasma $[K^+]$ increases by ~0.3 mEq/L when $PaCO_2$ is reduced by 16–23 mmHg (15). Hyperkalemia was prevented when HCO_3^- was administered in sufficient amount to block the fall in serum $[HCO_3^-]$ that normally follows acute hypocapnia. Hyperkalemia was prevented by α-adrenergic blockade. Thus, the increase in plasma $[K^+]$ can be attributed to increased α-adrenergic activity induced by hypobicarbonatemia. The magnitude of the increase in plasma $[K^+]$ is partially counterbalanced or attenuated by a concomitant increase in β-adrenergic activity (15).

In chronic respiratory alkalosis in humans, plasma $[K^+]$ falls, regardless of whether the initial plasma $[HCO_3^-]$ is normal or reduced by preexisting metabolic acidosis (20). By contrast, plasma $[K^+]$ is unaffected by chronic respiratory alkalosis in dogs (21). Hypokalemia in humans is maintained by sustained renal K^+ losses without associated changes in urinary aldosterone and cortisol excretion rates (20). The mechanism of this kaliuresis is unknown.

The time course of the plasma $[K^+]$ response to a decrease in $PaCO_2$ is the result of a surprisingly complex sequence of physiologic responses. Acute hypocapnia increases plasma $[K^+]$ due primarily to stimulation of α-adrenergic activity. When hypocapnia persists over several hours, transient kaliuresis and possibly K^+ shifts into cells result in hypokalemia (9,24,57,58). Hypokalemia during the ensuing 72–96 hr is accompanied by a decrease in urinary K^+ excretion, due to the modulation of urinary K^+ excretion by plasma $[K^+]$ (59). Despite persistent hypokalemia, renal K^+ excretion returns to normal (i.e., matching K^+ intake) beyond 72–96 hr of hypocapnia, thus maintaining the hypokalemia by an as yet undefined renal mechanism (21).

Divalent Ions

Hypophosphatemia is a universal finding in acute hypocapnia and results from increased cellular uptake of phosphate. Respiratory alkalosis activates phosphofructokinase, which in turn enhances phosphorylation of glucose as glycolysis is accelerated (60,61). After voluntary hyperventilation (decreases in $PaCO_2$ between 14 and 23 mmHg), a "dose-dependent" decrease in serum [phosphate] of 0.2–0.5 mmol/L occurs (15,49,54). It is unclear whether activation of phosphofructokinase is a consequence of hypocapnia or increases in cell pH. Hypophosphatemia of acute respiratory alkalosis is followed by decreased urinary fractional excretion of phosphate, attributed to increased β-adrenergic activity (62).

Acute voluntary hyperventilation in humans causes no changes in serum total calcium concentration (49,54); however, small but significant decreases in plasma-ionized calcium have been reported in both rats and humans, averaging about 0.4 mmol/L per pH unit. The magnitude of this fall in plasma ionized calcium is similar to that observed in vitro as the net result of counterbalancing pH-induced changes in albumin–Ca^{++} binding and HCO_3^-–Ca^{++} complex formation (63–68). Serum magnesium levels do not change during acute respiratory alkalosis in humans (unpublished observations during performance of studies reported in Ref. 15).

Chronic hypocapnia induces complex changes in divalent ion homeostasis in humans. A reduction in ionized calcium concentration and hyperphosphatemia occur and both are, at least in part, of renal origin, as evidenced by the documented increase in fractional calcium excretion and the decrease in renal phosphate clearance (Fig. 8) (69). The associated decrease in renal cAMP excretion despite unchanged serum PTH levels suggests that chronic hypocapnia induces end-organ insensitivity to PTH. In addition, the failure of PTH to rise in response to hypocalcemia suggests that hypocapnia induces a defect in PTH secretion.

Total plasma magnesium concentration does not change in chronic hypocapnia, but its reabsorption by the kidney increases significantly (hypomagnesuria), a change that could be the result of the acid–base disorder and/or the associated hypocalcemia (Fig. 6) (70). The prolonged reduction in magnesium excretion during hypocapnia (6 days) suggests that fractional intestinal magnesium absorption might also decrease and/or bone magnesium accretion increase (69).

SYSTEMIC AND CLINICAL CONSEQUENCES OF RESPIRATORY ALKALOSIS

Cardiovascular

Acute hypocapnia exerts substantial effects on regional blood flow, which vary with regard to the organ studied and the duration of hypocapnia. For chronic respiratory alkalosis, however, the available hemodynamic data are insufficient for conclusive comments. In acute respiratory alkalosis, myocardial,

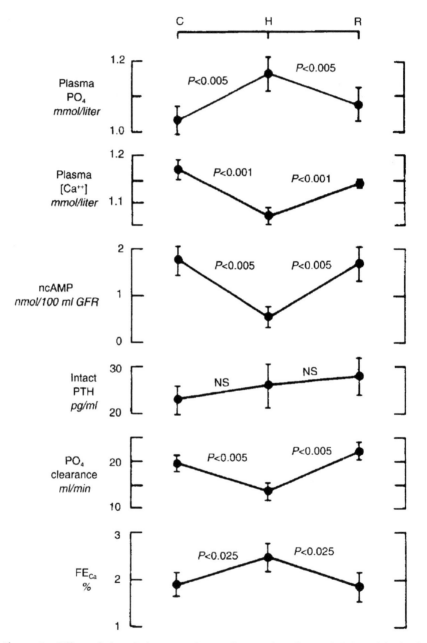

Figure 8 Effect of chronic hypocapnia on plasma phosphorus (PO_4) and ionized calcium (Ca^{++}) concentrations in normal humans. The simultaneous effects on nephrogenous cyclic AMP (ncAMP), intact parathyroid hormone (PTH), PO_4 clearance, and urinary fractional excretion (FE) of calcium are also shown. C, control; H, hypocapnia; R, recovery. *Source*: From Ref. 69.

cerebral, dermal and renal blood flow decrease, and skeletal muscle blood flow increases (71–78). Acute respiratory alkalosis decreases myocardial oxygen supply in both normal subjects and patients with coronary artery disease (79). In addition, chest pain and reversible ST-segment alterations compatible with myocardial ischemia have been described in acutely hyperventilating humans without angiographic evidence for significant coronary artery disease (80–85). The mechanism(s) for these changes is unclear, but might involve hypocapnia-induced vasoconstriction and alkalemia-induced decreases in O_2delivery due to the Bohr effect (see Chapters 1 and 3). Indeed, acute hypocapnia can induce coronary artery spasm and variant angina (86,87). Hyperventilation testing, performed to evaluate chest pain, can be complicated by nitrate-resistant vasopasm (88), ventricular tachycardia (89) and myocardial infarction (90). If coronary spasm occurs, it is typically delayed by several minutes after hyperventilation has ceased (91).

Acute hypocapnia induces a decrease in cardiac output, an increase in peripheral resistance, and a fall in blood pressure in anesthetized humans (92–94), but not in subjects undergoing voluntary hyperventilation, where cardiac output is unchanged or increased (95–98). In isolated perfused heart, a reduction in ambient PCO_2 causes a transient increase in myocardial contractility (99–101), probably due to changes in cell pH and cell calcium concentration (102). In particular, postischemic calcium accumulation in cardiocytes of rat heart is increased by hypocapnia (103).

Central Nervous System

Acute respiratory alkalosis induces a number of well-recognized neurologic symptoms, while the chronic disorder does not cause any clinically detectable changes in neurologic function. The clinical manifestations of acute respiratory alkalosis (hyperventilation) include circumoral and peripheral numbness and paresthesias, muscle cramps, increased deep-tendon reflexes, carpopedal spasms and rarely, generalized seizures. In addition, some patients complain of chest oppression, vertigo, dizziness, or are confused (104). Cerebral vasoconstriction and reduction of cerebral blood flow are well-known consequences of acute hypocapnia (105). Over the range of physiological $PaCO_2$ alterations, a predictable relationship between the severity of hypocapnia and the increase in blood flow velocity (a measure for vasoconstriction) was found in the middle cerebral artery using the transcranial Doppler technique (106). Thus, the neurologic symptoms seem to be caused largely by cerebral hypoperfusion. However, alkalemia-induced decreases in ionized calcium concentration and the alkalemia-induced left shift in the hemoglobin dissociation curve might also contribute. The decrease in cerebral blood flow is likely responsible for the hypocapnia-induced encephalographic changes, which consist of generalized slowing and high-voltage wave forms (107). Probably also as a result of cerebral hypoperfusion, brain and cerebrospinal fluid lactate concentrations are increased to values higher than found in the systemic circulation (108–114). The therapeutic use of hypocapnia-induced vasoconstriction in brain edema has been disappointing: the decrease in intracranial pressure in brain edema is small and transient (115) and clinical outcomes are not demonstrably improved (116,117).

Respiratory

The hypocapnia-induced Bohr effect results in improved capacity for O_2 uptake in the lungs, but impaired capacity for O_2 release in the tissues. Interestingly, O_2 consumption is increased, rather than decreased in passive hyperventilation (paralyzed and anesthetized subjects) (118). Because the hemodynamic and metabolic alterations associated with hypocapnic hyperventilation, such as increased skeletal muscle blood flow, increased adrenergic activity, and increases in cardiac output might obligate an increase in O_2 delivery, ischemia in other organs may ensue.

Hypocapnic hyperventilation in normal subjects has been reported to induce bronchoconstriction, an effect preventable by pretreatment with β-adrenergic agonists (119). Another study did not confirm a significant effect of hypocapnic hyperventilation on airway resistance in normal subjects, but did find a significant bronchoconstrictive effect in asthmatics (120). It is unclear whether the effect is mediated by the biophysical consequences of hyperventilation or by hypocapnia itself. Isocapnic hyperventilation did not affect airway resistance in normal and asthmatic subjects unless dry air was supplied to the latter subjects, suggesting an effect of hypocapnia on airway resistance independent of airway hydration (121,122).

With respect to other alterations in pulmonary function and pathology, it is difficult to differentiate between hypocapnia and hyperventilation-induced changes. Hypocapnia might be an independent risk factor for the development of bronchopulmonary dysplasia in infants with the respiratory distress syndrome (123). Hypocapnia increases microvascular permeability in tracheal mucosa (124), decreases lung compliance (125), and increases production of dysfunctional surfactant (126).

Adrenergic Activity

Hypocapnic hyperventilation increases plasma catecholamine levels, an effect specific for hypocapnia (15,43). Under conditions of isobicarbonatemic hypocapnic hyperventilation, no rise in catecholamines occurs, suggesting that the signal for sympathetic activation is neither hypocapnia nor pH but rather the secondary reduction in plasma $[HCO_3^-]$ (15).

Blood Cell Counts

Acute respiratory alkalosis causes hemoconcentration (due to shift of protein-free plasma fluid out of the vascular compartment) and increases in the concentrations of white blood cells and platelets. The effect depends on hypocapnia, as no significant changes were seen in isocapnic hyperventilation (127).

CAUSES OF ACUTE AND CHRONIC RESPIRATORY ALKALOSIS

Respiratory alkalosis is the most frequently occurring acid–base disorder in humans. In fact, it is so common that the term "disorder" may not be appropriate in many circumstances. Respiratory alkalosis occurs in normal pregnancy, in residents at higher altitudes, during exercise and in normal emotional reactions accompanying common activities. More importantly, respiratory alkalosis, either as a simple or mixed acid–base disorder, is very common in critically ill patients and its detection is of considerable assistance to the clinician in the early diagnosis of an underlying disease which is not yet accompanied by specific signs and symptoms. Important clinical examples are the systemic inflammatory response syndrome (SIRS) or incipient septicemia, salicylate poisoning, pulmonary emboli and psychiatric disease. Table 1 lists the major causes of respiratory alkalosis. The majority result in both acute and chronic respiratory alkalosis depending on the duration of the stimulus, and therefore the following discussion does not separate the acute and chronic conditions.

Pseudorespiratory Alkalosis

In artificially ventilated patients with profoundly decreased cardiac output and pulmonary perfusion (i.e., low output failure, cardiopulmonary resuscitation), substantial misinterpretation of the patient's oxygenation and acid–base status can occur if only arterial blood is analyzed (see Chapter 20). Arterial blood gas analysis in this setting does not adequately assess the corresponding conditions in peripheral tissues but is merely a measure of the efficiency of O_2 uptake and CO_2 elimination across the alveolar-capillary barrier. With marked decreases in pulmonary blood flow during circulatory failure, the amounts of CO_2 eliminated and O_2 taken up decrease sharply, owing to their strict dependence on blood flow. The low blood flow also results in a progressive widening of the arteriovenous difference for pH, PO_2 and PCO_2. Arterial PCO_2 occasionally falls to levels below normal, and the term "pseudorespiratory alkalosis " was created to describe this finding (Fig. 9) (128,129).

Hypoxemia

Decreased O_2 delivery to peripheral chemoreceptors stimulates ventilation (see Chapter 3). As shown in Fig. 10, alveolar ventilation rate increases

Table 1 Causes of Respiratory Alkalosis

Hypoxemia or tissue hypoxia	Drugs and hormones
Decreased inspired O_2 tension	Nikethamide, ethamivan
High altitude	Doxapram
Pneumonia	Xanthines
Aspiration of food, foreign	Salicylates
body, or vomitus	
Laryngospasm	Catecholamines
Near-drowning	Angiotensin II
Cyanotic heart disease	Progesterone
Severe anemia	Dinitrophenol
Left shift deviation of HbO_2 curve	Nicotine
Hypotension	Miscellaneous
Severe circulatory failure	Pregnancy
Pulmonary edema	Septicemia
Pseudorespiratory alkalosis	Hepatic failure
Central nervous system stimulation	Mechanical hyperventilation
Voluntary	Heat exposure
Pain	Recovery from metabolic acidosis
Anxiety-hyperventilation syndrome	Hemodialysis with acetate dialysate
Psychosis	Exercise
Fever/hyperthermia	
CNS diseases (subarachnoid hemorrhage,	
cerebrovascular accident,	
meningoencephalitis, tumor, trauma)	
Pulmonary diseases with stimulation of	
chest receptors	
Pneumonia	
Asthma	
Pneumothorax	
Hemothorax	
Flail chest	
Acute respiratory distress syndrome	
Pulmonary edema	
Pulmonary embolism	
Interstitial lung disease	

Source: Adapted from Ref. 177.

exponentially when PO_2 falls below 60 mmHg (130,131). Examination of the relationship between PaO_2 and $PaCO_2$ shown in this figure is important for clinical assessment of the adequacy of the ventilatory response to hypoxemia. If $PaCO_2$ is lower than expected, additional ventilatory stimuli should be sought; if $PaCO_2$ is higher than predicted, so-called "global respiratory failure" is said to be present (e.g., chronic obstructive lung disease, drug-induced inhibition of ventilatory drive). Hypotension (such as in

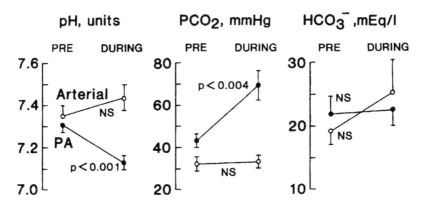

Figure 9 Arterial and mixed venous (pulmonary artery, PA) pH, PCO_2, and HCO_3^- before (pre) and during cardiopulmonary resuscitation in 13 patients. (●) depicts blood gas data from arterial blood, and o the simultaneous blood gas data in mixed venous (PA) blood. *Source*: From Ref. 128.

sepsis, hemorrhage) and severe anemia cause respiratory alkalosis even in the absence of a reduced PaO_2 due to decreased oxygen delivery to the chemoreceptors.

High altitude dwelling is an epidemiologically important cause of respiratory alkalosis. Over 10 million people are estimated to live at an altitude in excess of 10,000 feet and/or ascend to altitudes as high as 20,000 feet on a regular basis (commercial, military, scientific or sports activities). The short-term and long-term ventilatory adaptations to altitude differ. After initial ascent to high altitude, hyperventilation continues to increase and a new steady-state of alveolar ventilation is reached after several days, attributed to hypoxemia and hypobaria. However, after long-term (several years) residence at high altitude, blunting of O_2 sensitivity occurs. As a result, for any given PO_2, minute ventilation is lower and $PaCO_2$ higher in long-term residents than in short-term highlanders (132,133). The blunting of the hypoxic ventilatory response in long-term exposure to high altitude has been attributed to desensitization of the carotid body (134).

Pulmonary Disease

Various upper airway and pulmonary diseases can elicit hyperventilation and thus respiratory alkalosis at least partly independent of hypoxemia (Table 1). Information about ventilatory mechanics, peripheral chemical stimuli and temperature in the entire respiratory tract is transmitted to the brain via afferent fibers running in the olfactory, trigeminal, glossopharyngeal, and vagal nerves. Subepithelial and submucosal receptors in nares, epipharynx, pharynx, larynx, and trachea induce increased inspiration,

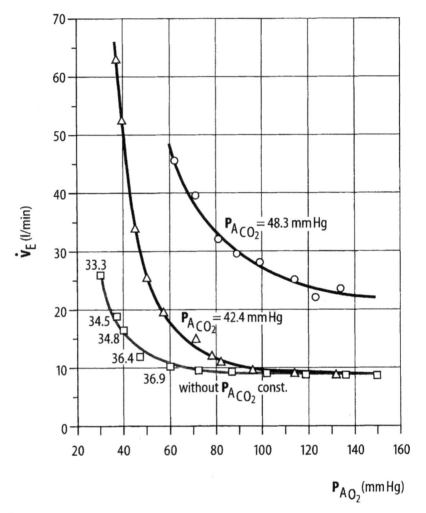

Figure 10   Relationship between alveolar ventilation rate (V_E) and alveolar oxygen tension (P_AO_2): modulation by ambient P_ACO_2. V_E increases exponentially as PaO_2 levels are experimentally reduced to values below 60 mmHg. When P_ACO_2 is fixed experimentally (at either 42.4 or 48.3 mmHg, respectively), the inhibitory effect of progressive hypoxemia-driven hypocapnia on V_E is eliminated, thereby revealing the underlying potency of the hypoxic ventilatory stimulus when unencumbered by coexisting progressive hypocapnia. Figure 1 focuses on the normal ventilatory response to CO_2 when P_AO_2 is fixed, whereas this figure focuses on the normal response to hypoxemia when P_ACO_2 is fixed. Ordinarily, ventilatory responses to either O_2 or CO_2 status are co-modulated by both factors operating in tandem. Both factors are potent within the physiologic range of values and both factors can change substantially as ventilation changes, regardless of the primary perturbation of ventilation. *Source*: From Ref. 199.

expiration or both when stimulated mechanically, chemically (nose and larynx), or by cooling (larynx). In the bronchial system, two types of receptors are present: (i) Subepithelial and intraepithelial "irritant receptors" that sense chemical and mechanical stimuli and induce hyperventilation via vagal afferents. (ii) Bronchial "stretch receptors" located in the lamina propria, which decrease inspiration but stimulate expiration and are responsible for the Hering–Breuer inflation reflex. In the alveoli, a third receptor, termed the J receptor, is located in the juxtacapillary wall. It is stimulated mechanically, chemically and by pulmonary edema, and elicits rapid and shallow breathing mediated by vagal afferents. These receptors stimulate hyperventilation in response to a variety of insults to the lung, including, pneumonia, pulmonary edema, pulmonary embolism, and interstitial lung disease. (see Chapter 3).

Cardiovascular Diseases

Hypotension can induce hyperventilation prior to the onset of hypoxemia and acidosis due to excitation of peripheral chemoreceptors, either directly (135) or via increases in catecholamine and angiotensin II levels. Neurologic symptoms in orthostatic intolerance are prevented by rebreathing of a CO_2-enriched air mixture, suggesting that orthostatic hypotension-induced hypocapnia might be responsible, in part, for cerebral hypoperfusion and associated symptoms (136). Many patients with heart failure are hypocapnic and, not surprisingly, they manifest multiple ventilatory stimuli, including hypoxemia, hypotension, pulmonary congestion, and activation of the sympathoadrenergic axis. Periodic breathing or Cheyne–Stokes respiration during daytime or at night (central sleep apnea) is well recognized to occur in patients with systolic dysfunction. Apnea is triggered by a low $PaCO_2$ but the precise mechanism of periodic breathing is not clear and probably multifactorial. It could involve prolonged circulation time and/or increased ventilatory sensitivity to low $PaCO_2$ values (see below). Periodic breathing intermittently decreases O_2 saturation, increases muscle/nerve activity and heart rate variability, and induces transient hypertension (137). Not surprisingly, Cheyne–Stokes respiration signifies a bad prognosis, but it is unclear whether this is due to the severity of heart failure or whether Cheyne–Stokes respiration itself contributes to progressive deterioration of cardiac function.

The ventilatory response to $PaCO_2$ has recently been studied in more detail in patients with heart failure. Hypocapnic patients manifest enhanced sensitivity to CO_2, i.e., suppression of their ventilatory drive requires subnormal $PaCO_2$ levels. It remains to be shown whether the reported decrease in apnea episodes induced by raising the $PaCO_2$ (via CO_2 inhalation, positive pressure ventilation or possibly by rebreathing) improves outcome in patients with severe heart failure (138).

Central Nervous System Causes of Hypocapnia

Many diseases of the brain can cause hypocapnia. Three types of abnormal breathing patterns are associated with hypocapnia in brain disease. *Central hyperventilation* is characterized by a strikingly regular rhythm, and increased rate and depth of breathing (139,140). Its causes are increased intracranial pressure and/or local lesions in the tegmentum or reticular formation. *Cheyne–Stokes respiration* is characterized by alternating periods of hyperventilation and apnea (see preceding section). After an apnea episode, the depth of respiration increases and decreases in a characteristic crescendo/decrescendo fashion. Cheyne–Stokes respiration is seen in diffuse hemispheric damage or with diencephalic lesions. The periodic breathing pattern is characterized by increased sensitivity to CO_2. Cheyne–Stokes respiration is the paradigm of CO_2-guided ventilation. Ventilation is stimulated at lower prevailing $PaCO_2$ levels, and increases in inspired CO_2 in these patients stimulates alveolar ventilation much more than in normal individuals (141). The third type of abnormal respiration is periodic breathing of the *Biot or cluster type*. This type is rare and characterized by irregular changes from superficial to deep ventilation and apnea episodes; it is observed in lesions involving the dorsolateral medulla oblongata. In contrast to Cheyne–Stokes respiration, hyperpnea consists of four to five deep breaths of the same amplitude with an abrupt beginning and ending.

Anxiety Hyperventilation

Patients with a variety of neurobehavioral disorders (anxiety, panic disorders, stress) can hyperventilate and exhibit the somatic symptoms associated with hypocapnia described earlier. The frequency of psychogenic hyperventilation in anxiety disorders is on the order of 35–83%, and between 5 and 11% among other medical populations (142,143). However, when hyperventilating patients with no obvious cause for hyperventilation were examined in an emergency department, many other, nonpsychogenic causes such as asthma, history of asthma as well as past and present abuse of drugs were found (144). Therefore, anxiety-hyperventilation is essentially a diagnosis of exclusion. Moreover, the hyperventilation test appears to be unreliable for diagnosis of the disorder (145), leaving some doubt about the notion that hyperventilation is the exclusive, causal factor responsible for the symptoms in this disorder. Patients with anxiety hyperventilation complain of shortness of breath despite their overbreathing (and typically increased PaO_2), and hyperventilation is frequently unrecognized by the physician. Acutely, the symptoms can be alleviated rapidly by increasing inspiratory CO_2 (bag rebreathing) and anxiolytic therapy (reassurance, administration of tranquilizers) (146). Chronically, the disorder is more difficult to treat and might respond to psychiatric counseling, "body-oriented" treatment options (autogenic training, hyperventilation provocation training) (147), and drug treatment (i.e., serotonin reuptake inhibitors).

Exercise

During exercise, alveolar ventilation rises in response to a variety of different stimuli (central and peripheral neural afferents, interstitial K^+ content in muscles, plasma $[K^+]$, lactic acidosis and hypoxemia) (148–150). The role of elevated local or systemic $[K^+]$ to stimulate ventilation in exercise is based largely on correlations between plasma $[K^+]$ and ventilatory rates and thus remains controversial. In patients with McArdle's syndrome, (in whom the inability to produce lactic acid due to myophosphorylase deficiency results in an increase in arterial pH with exercise rather than a decrease), however, heavy exercise results in greater increments in ventilation and plasma $[K^+]$ than in normal subjects, suggesting a greater role for K^+ in ventilatory control than for blood acidity (150). In contrast to other species (i.e., equines) which develop frank exercise-induced primary hypocapnia, alveolar ventilation rate in humans is well adjusted to the metabolic demands of mild to moderate exercise. Consequently, most studies have found that PCO_2 rarely decreases by more than 1–3 mmHg from the values at rest (148). The type of exercise appears to determine the acid–base response: while isotonic exercise results in lactic acidemia with secondary hypocapnia, isometric exercise results in primary hypocapnia with no significant increase in lactic acid levels (149).

Endocrine Causes

Progesterone

Progesterone stimulates alveolar ventilation rate and produces hypocapnia. Administration of medroxyprogesterone induces respiratory alkalosis in humans (151,152). During the progesterone-enriched luteal phase of the menstrual cycle, $PaCO_2$ levels actually decrease by 3–8 mmHg due to increased alveolar ventilation (153,154). Similar, but larger changes occur in pregnancy, when increasing plasma progesterone levels lower $PaCO_2$ to 28–30 mmHg in the third trimester (155,156). Hormone replacement therapy using conjugated estrogens and medroxyprogesterone also induces a small ($\sim$5 mmHg) reduction in $PaCO_2$ after 3 months (157). Interestingly, the effects of combined treatment are more pronounced than with equivalent doses during progesterone monotherapy. The potentiating ventilatory effect of estrogens remains to be clarified. Estrogens could act centrally via increased expression of progesterone receptors (158) that are estrogen-dependent (159).

Thyroid Hormone

Thyrotoxic patients have increased O_2 consumption and CO_2 production, which cause a homeostatic increase in alveolar ventilation rate. Most thyrotoxic patients manifest chronic respiratory alkalosis and the ventilatory response to both normoxic hypercapnia as well as to isocapnic hypoxia are increased and independent of the β-adrenergic effects of catecholamines (typically increased in thyrotoxicosis) (160–163). The increased ventilatory drive is associated with a sensation of dyspnea; thyrotoxicosis can worsen dyspnea in preexistent lung disease and/or thyrotoxic myopathy, and it can cause frank respiratory failure in such a setting (164).

Vasoactive Hormones

Type I cells, the most histologically specific cell type in the carotid body, exhibit dense core particles that contain catecholamines (dopamine, norepinephrine, and epinephrine). Catecholamines are probably not essential neurotransmitters, but rather modulators of the chemoreceptor process (Fig. 1). In addition, it is possible that catecholamines act centrally in the medulla (165). Exogenously administered dopamine and epinephrine/norepinephrine depress chemoreceptor discharge but produce complex metabolic changes including increases in O_2 consumption such that alveolar ventilation can either decrease or increase (166–169). Commonly used dopamine infusion doses decrease minute ventilation despite an exacerbation of hypoxemia in patients with heart failure (169). Angiotensin II increases ventilation, probably via a central effect, as the effect is maintained after denervation of carotid chemoreceptors (170). A host of other vasoactive substances (e.g., serotonin, nitric oxide, acetylcholine) can modulate ventilation either as neurotransmitters in the glomus or by central effects, but their in vivo role and clinical relevance remain to be established (166).

Drugs

Salicylate preparations, including salicylic acid, acetylsalicylic acid (aspirin), sodium salicylate and methylsalicylate, stimulate ventilation. As is the case with dinitrophenol, salicylates probably stimulate the respiratory center and increase minute ventilation via uncoupling of oxidative phosphorylation in chemoreceptor cells (171,172). This uncoupling also accelerates O_2 utilization, heat generation and CO_2 production (173). As expected from these effects, salicylate poisoning usually results in a mixed acid–base disturbance, comprising metabolic acidosis and respiratory alkalosis (see Chapter 12).

Aminophylline, a xanthine derivative utilized in the treatment of asthma and chronic obstructive lung disease, stimulates ventilation and can cause respiratory alkalosis. Aminophylline increases the ventilatory response to hypercapnia (174) and attenuates hypoxic central depression of ventilation probably by virtue of its ability to exhibit adenosine receptor antagonism (175,176). Nicotine stimulates ventilation by central and peripheral effects, but generally it does not cause respiratory alkalosis in smokers.

Nikethamide is a respiratory stimulant acting directly on the respiratory center of the brainstem. In addition, it increases the center's sensitivity to CO_2, activates peripheral chemoreceptors and has been used in the treatment of CO_2-retaining disorders. The results obtained with this drug as well as other ventilatory stimulants (e.g., ethamivan, doxapram, almitrine, progesterone, and medroxyprogesterone) have been modest at best (177).

Hepatic Failure/Encephalopathy

Respiratory alkalosis is an almost universal finding in hepatic failure of any cause and the degree of hypocapnia correlates with the severity of hepatic failure (178–180). Hypocapnia might have a homeostatic or even a protective role, because it is reported to restore cerebral blood flow autoregulation in patients with acute liver failure (181). The precise mechanisms causing hyperventilation in liver failure are not clearly delineated, but could involve local brain hypoxia and increased progesterone and ammonia levels. Increases in ammonia levels have been reported to provide the best biochemical predictor of the extent of hypocapnia in hepatic failure, among many candidates examined (179,182).

Septicemia

Septicemia frequently causes respiratory alkalosis due to a multitude of ventilatory stimuli such as fever, hypotension, or hypoxemia. It has been postulated, but not established, that gram-negative sepsis causes respiratory alkalosis independently of these stimuli, with lipopolysaccharides potentially exhibiting independent central stimulating activity (183,184).

Exposure to High or Low Temperatures

Exposure to high ambient temperatures induces acute respiratory alkalosis in humans (185,186). Heat exhaustion and heat stroke can cause respiratory alkalosis of considerable severity ($PaCO_2$ around 20 mmHg). In heat stroke, metabolic acidosis is the most common acid–base disorder, followed by combined metabolic acidosis/respiratory alkalosis and pure respiratory alkalosis in 20% of the cases (187).

Cold exposure has a biphasic effect on ventilation. Acute exposure (i.e., cold water immersion such as in near-drowning) induces hyperventilation for 1–2 min (with increased risk of drowning). Thereafter, ventilation decreases to rates consistent with the metabolic requirements. In severe hypothermia, CO_2 retention leads to the development of respiratory acidosis (188).

Recovery from Chronic Metabolic Acidosis

Hyperventilation can persist for several hours to 1–2 days during recovery from metabolic acidosis. A delay in normalizing cell [H^+] in the medullary respiratory center is presumed to be responsible for hyperventilation despite partial or complete restoration of plasma [HCO_3^-] to normal levels. If plasma [HCO_3^-] is increased too rapidly, postacidosis hyperventilation can result in pronounced alkalemia (189).

Mechanical Overventilation

In the intubated patient on mechanical ventilator support, respiratory alkalosis can be easily produced by inappropriately adjusting the ventilator settings. In such patients who are initiating their own ventilation, abrupt termination of mechanical hyperventilation can result in critical hypoxemia because the prevailing low level of $PaCO_2$ inhibits ventilatory drive (190,191). In a similar fashion, cessation of voluntary hyperventilation can result in hypoxemia due to depressed ventilation or even apnea (192).

DIAGNOSIS

Evaluation of the patient's history, physical examination, and laboratory data are the cornerstones to both the diagnosis of respiratory alkalosis and the rapid identification of its cause(s). Clinical cognizance that hyperventilation can be present without perceptible increases in respiratory effort or rate is important in directing the clinician to an early laboratory assessment of acid–base equilibrium (193).

An arterial or arterialized blood gas measurement is required to confirm the presence of respiratory alkalosis. Both the acute and chronic forms of the disorder are characterized by hypocapnia and hypobicarbonatemia. Because plasma [K^+] changes in a complex manner in respiratory alkalosis (see earlier), abnormalities in [K^+] are not useful in separating respiratory alkalosis from other acid–base disorders. Clinicians should place greatest reliance on the quantitative diagnostic criteria for respiratory alkalosis ($PaCO_2$, [HCO_3^-], [H^+] relationships) using a properly handled blood gas sample (anaerobic, standardized heparin coating, rapid analysis, and use of cooling if processing is delayed beyond 5 min). Such acid–base data taken together with all of the clinical information will almost always provide a precise diagnosis for respiratory alkalosis and its causes.

TREATMENT

Respiratory alkalosis, per se, does not usually produce sufficient symptoms to require treatment. Identification and removal, if possible, of the underlying cause (Table 1) is sufficient treatment in most cases. In severe acute hyperventilation (e.g., in panic disorders) reassurance and/or sedation with a short-acting benzodiazepine and rebreathing into a closed system (paper or plastic bag) will efficiently abrogate the neurologic symptoms induced by hypocapnia and prevent tetanic seizures (194,195).

REFERENCES

1. Arbus GS, Hebert LA, Levesque PR, Etsten BE, Schwartz WB. Characterization and clinical application of the "significance band" for acute respiratory alkalosis. N Engl J Med 1969; 280:117–123.
2. Krapf R, Berry CA, Alpern RJ, Rector FC. Regulation of cell pH by ambient bicarbonate, carbon dioxide tension, and pH in the rabbit proximal convoluted tubule. J Clin Invest 1988; 81:381–389.
3. Giebisch G, Berger L, Pitts RF. The extrarenal response to acute acid–base disturbances of respiratory origin. J Clin Invest 1955; 34:231–245.
4. Manfredi F. Effects of hypocapnia and hypercapnia on intracellular acid–base equilibrium in man. J Lab Clin Med 1967; 69:304–312.
5. Adler S, Roy A, Relman A. Intracellular acid–base regulation. I. Response of muscle cells to changes in CO_2 tension or extracellular bicarbonate concentration. J Clin Invest 1965; 44:8–20.
6. Brown EB Jr., Goott B. Intracellular hydrogen ion changes and potassium movement. Am J Physiol 1963; 204:765–770.
7. Heisler N, Piiper J. Determination of intracellular buffering properties in rat diaphragm muscle. Am J Physiol 1972; 222:747–753.
8. Kjällquist A, Nardini M, Siesjö BK. The regulation of extra- and intracellular acid–base parameters in the rat brain during hyper- and hypocapnia. Acta Physiol Scand 1969; 76:485–494.
9. Katz LA, Swain JA, Portman MA, Balaban RS. Intracellular pH and inorganic phosphate content of heart in vivo: a ^{31}P-NMR study. Am J Physiol 1988; 255:H189–H196.
10. LaGrange BM, Hood VL. Ketoacid production in acute respiratory and metabolic acidosis and alkalosis in rats. Am J Physiol 1989; 256:F437–F445.
11. Eldridge F, Salzer J. Effect of respiratory alkalosis on blood lactate and pyruvate in humans. J Appl Physiol 1967; 22:461–468.
12. Gledhill N, Beirne GJ, Dempsey JA. Renal response to short-term hypocapnia in man. Kidney Int 1975; 8:376–386.
13. Hood VL, Schubert C, Keller U, Muller S. Effect of systemic pH on pH$_i$ and lactic acid generation in exhaustive forearm exercise. Am J Physiol 1988; 255:F479–F485.
14. Hood VL, Tannen RL. Protection of acid–base balance by pH regulation of acid production. New Engl J Med 1998; 339:819–826.
15. Krapf R, Caduff P, Wagdi P, Stäubli M, Hulter HN. Plasma potassium response to acute respiratory alkalosis. Kidney Int 1995; 47:217–224.
16. Ulken V, Puschel GP, Jungermann K. Increase in glucose and lactate output and perfusion resistance by stimulation of hepatic nerves in isolated perfused rat liver: role of α_1, α_2, β_1, and β_2 receptors. Biol Chem Hoppe-Seyler 1991; 372:401–409.
17. Beckh K, Beuers U, Engelhardt R, Jungermann K. Mechanism of action of sympathetic hepatic nerves on carbohydrate metabolism in perfused rat liver. Biol Chem Hoppe-Seyler 1987; 368:379–386.
18. Eichenholz A, Mulhausen RO, Anderson WE, MacDonald FM. Primary hypocapnia: a cause of metabolic acidosis. J Appl Physiol 1962; 17:283–288.

19. Zborowska-Sluis DT, Dossetor JB. Hyperlactatemia of hyperventilation. J Appl Physiol 1967; 22:746–755.

20. Krapf R, Beeler I, Hertner D, Hulter HN. Chronic respiratory alkalosis. The effect of sustained hyperventilation on renal regulation of acid–base equilibrium. N Engl J Med 1991; 324:1394–1401.

21. Gennari FJ, Goldstein MB, Schwartz WB. The nature of the renal adaptation to chronic hypocapnia. J Clin Invest 1972; 51:1722–1730.

22. Gougoux A, Kaehny WD, Cohen JJ. Renal adaptation to chronic hypocapnia: dietary constraints in achieving H^+ retention. Am J Physiol 1975; 229:1330–1337.

23. Stanbury SW, Thomson AE. The renal response to respiratory alkalosis. Clin Sci 1952; 11:357–374.

24. Barker ES, Singer RB, Elkinton JR, Clark JK. The renal response in man to acute experimental respiratory alkalosis and acidosis. J Clin Invest 1957; 36:515–529.

25. Rector FC, Seldin DW, Roberts AD, Smith SS. The role of plasma CO2 tension and carbonic anhydrase activity in the renal reabsorption of bicarbonate. J Clin Invest 1960; 39:1706–1721.

26. Bengele HH, McNamara ER, Schwartz JH, Alexander EA. Acidification adaptation along the inner medullary collecting duct. Am J Physiol 1988; 255:F1155–F1159.

27. Cogan M. Effects of acute alterations in PCO_2 on proximal HCO_3, Cl^-, and H_2O reabsorption. Am J Physiol 1984; 246:F21–F26.

28. Jacobson HR. Effects of CO_2 and acetazolamide on bicarbonate and fluid transport in rabbit proximal tubules. Am J Physiol 1981; 240:F54–F62.

29. Jacobson HR. Medullary collecting duct acidification: Effects of potassium, HCO_3 concentration, and PCO_2. J Clin Invest 1984; 74:2107–2114.

30. Giammarco RA, Goldstein MB, Halperin ML, Stinebaugh BJ. The effect of hyperventilation on distal nephron hydrogen ion secretion. J Clin Invest 1976; 58:77–82.

31. Unwin R, Stidwell R, Taylor S, Capasso G. The effects of respiratory alkalosis and acidosis on net bicarbonate flux along the rat loop of Henle in vivo. Am J Physiol 1997; 273:F698–F705.

32. Santella RN, Maddox DA, Gennari FJ. Delivery dependence of early proximal bicarbonate reabsorption in the rat in respiratory acidosis and alkalosis. J Clin Invest 1991; 87:631–638.

33. Hilden SA, Johns CA, Madias NE. Adaptation of rabbit renal cortical Na^+-H^+ exchange activity in chronic hypocapnia. Am J Physiol 1989; 257:F615–F622.

34. Ruiz OS, Arruda JAL, Talor Z. Na-HCO_3cotransport and Na-H antiporter in chronic respiratory acidosis and alkalosis. Am J Physiol 1989; 256:F414–F420.

35. Soleimani M, Bookstein C, Singh G, Rao MC, Chang EB, Bastani B. Differential regulation of Na/H exchange and H^+ ATPase by pH and $HCO3^-$ in kidney proximal tubules. J Membr Biol 1995; 144:209–216.

36. Eiam-Ong S, Laski ME, Kurtzman NA, Sabatini S. Effect of respiratory acidosis and respiratory alkalosis on renal transport enzymes. Am J Physiol 1994; 267:F390–F399.

37. Schwartz GJ, Al-Awqati Q. Carbon dioxide causes exocytosis of vesicles containing H^+ pumps in isolated perfused proximal and collecting tubules. J Clin Invest 1985; 75:1638–1644.

38. Al-Awqati Q, Vijayakumar S, Hikita C, Chen J, Takito J. Phenotypical plasticity in the intercalated cell: the hensin pathway. Am J Physiol 1998; 275: F183–F190.

39. Gennari FJ, Kaehny WD, Levesque PR, Cohen JJ. Acid–base response to chronic hypocapnia in man. Clin Res 1980; 28:533A.

40. Cohen JJ, Madias NE, Wolf CF, Schwartz WB. Regulation of acid–base equilibrium in chronic hypocapnia. J Clin Invest 1976; 57:1483–1489.

41. Madias NE, Schwartz WB, Cohen JJ. The maladaptive renal response to secondary hypocapnia during chronic HCl acidosis in the dog. J Clin Invest 1977; 60:1393–1401.

42. Krapf R, Hulter HN. Renal response to chronic hypocapnia: qualitative differences between dogs and humans? Clin Chem 1992; 38:443–445.

43. Stäubli M, Rohner F, Kammer P, Ziegler W, Straub PW. Plasma volume and proteins in voluntarily hyperventilation. J Appl Physiol 1986; 60:1549–1553.

44. Steurer J, Schiesser D, Stey C, Vetter W, Elzi MV, Barras JP, Franzeck UK. Hyperventilation enhances transcapillary diffusion of sodium fluorescein. Int J Microcirc Clin Exp 1996; 16:266–270.

45. Straub PW, Bühlmann AA. Reduction of blood volume by voluntary hyperventilation. J Appl Physiol 1970; 29:816–817.

46. Elkinton JR, Singer RB, Barker ES, Clark JK. Effects in man of acute experimental respiratory alkalosis and acidosis on ionic transfers in the total body fluids. J Clin Invest 1955; 34:1671–1690.

47. Yu PN, Yim JB, Stanfield CA. Hyperventilation syndrome. Arch Intern Med 1959; 103:902–913.

48. Hickham JB, Wilson WP, Frayser R. Observations on the early elevation of serum potassium during respiratory alkalosis. J Clin Invest 1956; 35:601–606.

49. Okel BB, Hurst JW. Prolonged hyperventilation in man: associated electrolyte changes and subjective symptoms. Arch Intern Med 1961; 108:157–162.

50. Saltzman HA, Heyman A, Sieker HO. Correlation of clinical and physiological manifestations of sustained hyperventilation. N Engl J Med 1963; 268:1431–1436.

51. Burnell JM, Villamil MF, Uyeno BT, Scribner BH. The effect in humans of extracellular pH change on the relationship between serum potassium concentration and intracellular potassium. J Clin Invest 1956; 35:935–939.

52. Edwards R, Winnie AP, Ramamurthy S. Acute hypocapnic hypokalemia: an iatrogenic anesthetic complication. Anesth Analg 1977; 56:786–792.

53. Finsterer U, Lühr HG, Wirth AE. Effects of acute hypercapnia and hypocapnia on plasma and red cell potassium, blood lactate and base excess during anesthesia. Acta Anaesth Scand 1978; 22:353–366.

54. Mostellar ME, Tuttle EP Jr. The effects of alkalosis on plasma concentration and urinary excretion of inorganic phosphate in man. J Clin Invest 1964; 43:138–149.

55. Sanchez MG, Finlayson DC. Dynamics of serum potassium change during acute respiratory alkalosis. Can Anaesth Soc J 1978; 25:495–498.

56. Stanbury SW, Thomson AE. The renal response to respiratory alkalosis. Clin Sci 1952; 11:357–374.
57. Adrogué HJ, Madias NE. Changes in plasma potassium concentration during acute acid–base disturbances. Am J Med 1981; 71:456–467.
58. Suzuki H, Hishida A, Ohishi K, Kimura M, Honda N. Role of hormonal factors in plasma K alterations in acute respiratory and metabolic alkalosis in dogs. Am J Physiol 1990; 258:F305–F310.
59. Young DB. Quantitative analysis of aldosterone's role in potassium regulation. Am J Physiol 1988; 255:F811–F822.
60. Uyeda K, Racker E. Regulatory mechanisms in carbohydrate metabolism. VII. Hexokinase and phosphofructokinase. J Biol Chem 1965; 240:4682–4688.
61. Brautbar N, Leibovici H, Massry SG. On the mechanism of hypophosphatemia during acute hyperventilation: evidence for increased muscle glycolysis. Miner Electrolyte Metab 1983; 9:45–50.
62. Tucker RR, Berndt TJ, Thotharthri V, Newcome J, Joyner MJ, Knox FG. Propranolol blocks the hypophosphaturia of acute respiratory alkalosis in human subjects. J Lab Clin Med 1996; 128:423–428.
63. Oberleithner H, Greger R, Lang F. The effect of respiratory and metabolic acid–base changes on ionized calcium concentration: in vivo and in vitro experiments in man and rat. Eur J Clin Invest 1982; 12:451–455.
64. Seamonds B, Towfighi J, Arvan DA. Determination of ionized calcium in serum by use of an ion-selective electrode. Clin Chem 1972; 18:155–160.
65. Moore EW. Ionized calcium in normal serum, ultrafiltrates, and whole blood determined by ion exchange electrode. J Clin Invest 1970; 49:318–334.
66. Pedersen KO. The effect of bicarbonate, PCO2, and pH on serum calcium fractions. Scand J Clin Lab Invest 1971; 27:145–150.
67. Schwartz HD, McConville BC, Christopherson EF. Serum-ionized calcium by specific ion electrode. Clin Chim Acta 1971; 31:97–107.
68. Wybenga DR, Ibott FA, Cannon DC. Determination of ionized calcium in serum that has been exposed to air. Clin Chem 1976; 22:1009–1011.
69. Krapf R, Jaeger P, Hulter HN. Chronic respiratory alkalosis induces renal PTH-resistance, hyperphosphatemia and hypocalcemia in humans. Kidney Int 1992; 42:727–734.
70. Coburn JW, Massry SG, Kleeman CR. The effects of calcium infusion on renal handling of magnesium with normal and reduced glomerular filtration rate. Nephron 1970; 7:131–143.
71. Burnum JF, Hickam JB, McIntosh HD. The effect of hypocapnia on arterial blood pressure. Circulation 1954; 9:89–95.
72. Clarke RSJ. The effect of voluntary overbreathing on the blood flow through the human forearm. J Physiol 1954; 118:537–544.
73. Gotoh F, Meyer JS, Takagi Y. Cerebral effects of hyperventilation in man. Arch Neurol 1965; 12:410–423.
74. Kety SS, Schmidt CF. The effects of altered arterial tensions of carbon dioxide and oxygen on cerebral blood flow and cerebral oxygen consumption of normal young men. J Clin Invest 1948; 27:484–491.

75. Richardson DW, Wasserman AJ, Patterson JL. General and regional circulatory response to changes in blood pH and carbon dioxide tension. J Clin Invest 1961; 40:31–43.
76. Rowe GG, Castillo CA, Crumpton CW. Effects of hyperventilation on systemic and coronary hemodynamics. Am Heart J 1961; 63:67–77.
77. Simmons DH, Oliver RP. Effects of acute acid–base changes on renal hemodynamics in anesthetized dogs. Am J Physiol 1965; 209:1180–1186.
78. Wasserman AJ, Patterson JL Jr. The cerebral vascular response to reduction in arterial carbon dioxide tension. J Clin Invest 1961; 40:1297–1303.
79. Bühlmann AA, Angehrn W. Hyperventilation und Sauerstoffversorgung des Myocards. Schweiz Med Wochenschr 1978; 108:708–713.
80. Bass C, Wade C, Gardner WN, Crawley R, Ryan KC, Hutchison DCS. Unexplained breathlessness and psychiatric morbidity in patients with normal and abnormal coronary arteries. Lancet 1983; 1:605–609.
81. Evans DW, Lum LC. Hyperventilation: an important cause of pseudoangina. Lancet 1977; 1:155–157.
82. Jacobs WF, Battle WE, Ronan JA. False-positive ST-T-wave changes secondary to hyperventilation and exercise. Ann Intern Med 1974; 81:479–482.
83. Lary D, Goldschlager N. Electrocardiographic changes during hyperventilation resembling myocardial ischemia in patients with normal coronary arteriograms. Am Heart J 1974; 87:383–390.
84. Magarian GJ. Hyperventilation syndromes: Infrequently recognized common expressions of anxiety and stress. Medicine (Baltimore) 1982; 61:219–236.
85. McHenry PL, Cogan OJ, Elliott WC, Knoebel SB. False-positive ECG response to exercise secondary to hyperventilation: cineangiographic correlation. Am Heart J 1970; 79:683–687.
86. Yasue H, Nagao M, Omote S, Takizawa A, Miwa K, Tanaka S. Coronary arterial spasm and Prinzmetal's variant form of angina induced by hyperventilation and tris-buffer infusion. Circulation 1978; 58:56–62.
87. Ardissino D, De Servi S, Falcone C, Barberis P, Scuri PM, Previtali M, Specchia G, Montemartini C. Role of hypocapnic alkalosis in hyperventilation-induced coronary artery spasm in variant angina. Am J Cardiol 1987; 59:707–709.
88. Ghio S, Angoli L, Bramucci E, de Servi S, Specchia G. Hyperventilation-induced coronary vasospasm refractory to intracoronary nitroglycerin. Am Heart J 1990; 119:957–960.
89. Magarian GJ, Jones S, Calvery T. Hyperventilation testing: induction of spontaneous ventricular tachycardia in association with transmural ischemia without obstructive coronary artery disease. Am Heart J 1990; 120:1447–1449.
90. Fragasso G, Bonetti F, Margonata A, Chierchia S. Non Q-wave myocardialinfarction following hyperventilation test. Eur Heart J 1989; 10:944–946.
91. Goldberg S. Provocative testing for coronary artery spasm: specific methodology. Cardiovasc Clin 1983; 14:99–109.
92. Combes P, Fauvage B. Systemic vasomotor interaction between nicardipine and hypocapnic alkalosis in man. Int Care Med 1992; 18:89–92.

93. Kety SS, Schmidt CF. The effects of active and passive hyoperventilation on cerebral blood flow, cerebral oxygen consumption, cardiac output and blood pressure of normal young men. J Clin Invest 1946; 25:107–119.

94. Prys-Roberts C, Kelman GR, Greenbaum R, Robinson RH. Circulatory influences of artificial ventilation during nitrous oxide anaesthesia in man: II. Results: the relative influence of mean intrathoracic pressure and arterial carbon dioxide tension. Br J Anaesth1967; 39:533–548.

95. Rowe GG, Castillo CA, Crumpton CW. Effects of hyperventilation on systemic and coronary hemodynamics. Am Heart J 1962; 63:67–77.

96. Richardson DW, Wasserman AJ, Patterson JL. General and regional circulatory response to changes in blood pH and carbon dioxide tension. J Clin Invest 1961; 40:31–43.

97. Gotoh F, Meyer JS, Takagi Y. Cerebral effects of hyperventilation in man. Arch Neurol 1965; 12:410–423.

98. Burnum JF, Hickam JB, McIntosh HD. The effect of hypocapnia on arterial blood pressure. Circulation 1954; 9:89–95.

99. McElroy WT Jr, Gerdes AJ, Brown EB Jr. Effects of CO_2, bicarbonate and pH on the performance of isolated perfused guinea pig hearts. Am J Physiol 1958; 195:412–416.

100. Vaughan Williams EM. The individual effects of CO_2, bicarbonate and pH on the electrical and mechanical activity of isolated rabbit auricles. J Physiol 1955; 129:90–110.

101. Wilson RF, Gibson D, Percinel AK, Ali MA, Baker G, LeBlanc LP, Lucas C. Severe alkalosis in critically ill surgical patients. Arch Surg 1972; 105:197–203.

102. Kusuoka H, Backx PH, Camilion de Hurtado M, Azan-Backx M, Marban E, Cingolani HE. Relative roles of intracellular Ca^{++} and pH in shaping myocardial contractile response to acute respiratory alkalosis. Am J Physiol 1993; 265:H1696–H1703.

103. Mosca SM, Gelpi RJ, Borelli R, Cingolani HE. The effects of hypocapnic alkalosis on the myocardial contractility of isovolumic perfused rabbit hearts. Arch Int Physiol Biochem Biophys 1993; 101:179–183.

104. Saltzman HA, Heyman A, Sieker HO. Correlation of clinical and physiological manifestations of sustained hyperventilation. N Engl J Med 1963; 268:1431–1436.

105. Kety SS, Schmidt CF. The effects of altered arterial tensions of carbon dioxide and oxygen on cerebral blood flow and cerebral oxygen consumption of normal young men. J Clin Invest 1948; 27:484–491.

106. Markwalder TM, Grolimund P, Seiler RW, Roth F, Aslid R. Dependency of blood flow velocity in the middle cerebral artery on tidal carbon dioxide partial pressure. J Cereb Blood Flow Metab 1984; 4:368–372.

107. Swanson AG, Stavney LS, Plum F. Effects of blood pH and carbon dioxide on cerebral electrical activity. Neurology 1958; 8:787–792.

108. Van Vaerenbergh PJJ, Demeester G, Leusen I. Lactate in cerebrospinal fluid during hyperventilation. Arch Intern Physiol Biochem1965; 73:738–747.

109. Severinghaus JW, Mitchell RA, Richardson BW, Singer MM. Respiratory control at high altitude suggesting active transport regulation of CSF pH. J Appl Physiol 1963; 18:1155–1166.

110. Plum F, Posner JB, Smith WW. Effect of hyperbaric-hyperoxic hyperventilation on blood, brain and CSF lactate. Am J Physiol 1968; 215:1240–1244.
111. Plum F, Posner JB. Blood and cerebrospinal fluid lactate during hyperventilation. Am J Physiol 1967; 212:864–870.
112. Kazemi H, Valenca LM, Shannon DC. Brain and cerebrospinal fluid lactate concentration in respiratory acidosis and alkalosis. Respir Physiol 1969; 6:178–186.
113. Forster HV, Dempsey JA, Chosy LW. Incomplete compensation of CSF [H$^+$] in man during acclimatization to high altitude (4300 m). J Appl Physiol 1975; 38:1067–1072.
114. Dempsey JA, Forster, HV, DoPico GA. Ventilatory acclimatization to moderate hypoxemia in man. J Clin Invest 1974; 53:1091–1100.
115. Heffner JE, Sahn SA. Controlled hyperventilation in patients with intracranial hypertension: application and management. Arch Intern Med 1983; 143: 765–769.
116. Roberts I, Schierhout G, Alderson P. Absence of evidence for the effectiveness of five interventions routinely used in the intensive care management of severe head injury: a systematic review. J Neurol Neurosurg Psychiatry 1998; 65: 729–733.
117. Dexter F. Research synthesis of controlled studies evaluating the effect of hypocapnia and airway protection on cerebral outcome. J Neurosurg Anesthesiol 1997; 9:217–222.
118. Slater RM, Symreng T, Sum Ping ST, Starr J, Tatman D. The effect of respiratory alkalosis on oxygen consumption in anesthetized patients. J Clin Anesth 1992; 4:462–467.
119. O'Cain CF, Hensley MJ, McFadden ER, Ingram RH. Pattern and mechanism of airway response to hypocapnia in normal subjects. J Appl Physiol 1979; 47:8–12.
120. van den Elshout FJ, Herwaarden CL, Folgering HT. Effects of hypercapnia and hypocapnia on respiratory resistance in normal and asthmatic subjects. Thorax 1991; 46:28–32.
121. Hilberman M, Hogan JS, Peters RM. The effects of carbon dioxide on pulmonary mechanics in hyperventilating, normal volunteers. J Thorac Cardiovasc Surg 1976; 71:268–273.
122. Dejaegher P, Rochette F, Clarysse I, Demedts M. Hypocapnic hyperventilation versus isocapnic hyperventilation with ambient air or with dry air in asthmatics. Eur J Respir Dis 1987; 70:102–109.
123. Garland JS, Buck RK, Allred EN, Leviton A. Hypocarbia before surfactant therapy appears to increase bronchopulmonary dysplasia in infants with respiratory distress syndrome. Arch Ped Adolesc Med 1995; 149: 617–622.
124. Reynolds AM, Zedow SP, Scicchitano R, McEvoy RD. Airway hypocapnia increases microvascular leakage in the guinea pig trachea. Am Rev Resp Dis 1992; 145:80–84.
125. Cutillo A, Omboni E, Perondi R, Tana T. Effects of hypocapnia on pulmonary mechanics in normal subjects and in patients with chronic obstructive lung disease. Am Rev Resp Dis 1974; 110:25–33.

126. Oyarzun MJ, Quijada D. The role of hypocapnia in the alveolar surfactant increases induced by free fatty acid intravenous infusion in the rabbit. Respiration 1986; 49:187–194.
127. Stäubli M, Vogel F, Bärtsch P, Flückiger G, Ziegler WH. Hyperventilation-induced changes in blood cell counts depend on hypocapnia. Eur J Appl Physiol 1994; 69:402–407.
128. Adrogué HJ, Rashad MN, Gorin AB, Yacoub J, Madias NE. Assessing acid–base status in circulatory failure: differences between arterial and central venous blood. N Engl J Med 1989; 320:1312–1316.
129. Adrogué HJ, Rashad MN, Gorin AB, Yacoub J, Madias NE. Arteriovenous acid–base disparity in circulatory failure: studies on mechanism. Am J Physiol 1989; 257:F1087–F1093.
130. Dempsey JA, Forster HV, Birnbaum ML, Reddan WG, Thoden J, Grover RF, Rankin J. Control of exercise hyperpnea under varying durations of exposure to moderate hypoxia. Respir Physiol 1972; 16:213–231.
131. Wade JG, Larson CP, Hickey RF, Ehrenfeld WK, Severinghaus JW. Effect of carotid endarterectomy on carotid chemoreceptor and baroreceptor function in man. N Engl J Med 1970; 282:823–829.
132. Milledge JS, Lahiri S. Respiratory control in lowlanders and Sherpa highlanders at altitude. Respir Physiol 1967; 2:310–317.
133. Severinghaus JW, Bainton CR, Carcelen A. Respiratory insensitivity to hypoxia in chronically hypoxic man. Respir Physiol 1966; 1:308–319.
134. Tatsumi K, Pickett CK, Weil JV. Attenuated carotid body hypoxic sensitivity after prolonged hypoxic exposure. J Appl Physiol 1991; 70:748–755.
135. Heymans C, Bouckaert JJ. Sinus caroticus and respiratory reflexes. J Physiol 1930; 69:254–273.
136. Novak K, Spies JM, Novak P, McPhee BR, Rummmans TA, Low PA. Hypocapnia and cerebral hypoperfusion in orthostatic intolerance. Stroke 1998; 29:1876–1881.
137. van de Borne P, Oren R, Abouassaly C, Anderson E, Somers VK. Effect of Cheyne-Stokes respiration on muscle sympathetic nerve activity in severe congestive heart failure secondary to ischemic or idiopathic cardiomyopathy. Am J Cardiol 1998; 69:254–273.
138. Lorenzi G, Rankin F, Bies I, Douglas Bradley T. Effects of inhaled carbon dioxide and oxygen on Cheyne–Stokes respiration in patients with heart failure. Am J Resp Crit Care Med 1999; 159:1490–1498.
139. Plum F, Swanson AG. Central neurogenic hyperventilation in man. Arch Neurol Psychiatry 1959; 81:535–549.
140. Plum F. Hyperpnea, hyperventilation, and brain dysfunction. Ann Intern Med 1972; 76:328.
141. Brown HW, Plum F. The neurologic basis of Cheyne–Stokes respiration. Am J Med 1961; 30:849–863.
142. Brashear RE. Hyperventilation syndrome. Lung 1983; 161:257–277.
143. Spinhoven P, Onstein EJ, Sterk PJ, Le Haen D. Hyperventilation and panic attacks in general hospital patients. Gen Hosp Psychiatry 1993; 15: 148–154.

144. Saisch SG, Wessely S, Gardner WN. Patients with acute hyperventilation presenting to an inner-city emergency department. Chest 1996; 110:952–957.

145. Hornsveld HK, Garssen B, Fiedeldij D, van Spiegel PI, deHaes JM. Double-blind placebo-controlled study for the hyperventilation provocation test and the validity of the hyperventilation syndrome. Lancet 1996; 348:154–158.

146. Rice RL. Symptom patterns of the hyperventilation syndrome. Am J Med 1950; 8:691–700.

147. Kraft AR, Hoogduin CA. The hyperventilation syndrome. Br J Psychiatry 1984; 145:538–554.

148. Foster HV, Pan LG. Breathing during exercise: demands, regulation, limitations. Adv Exp Med Biol 1988; 227:257–276.

149. Poole DC, Ward SA, Whipp BJ. Control of blood gas and acid–base status during isometric exercise in humans. J Physiol 1988; 396:365–377.

150. Paterson DJ, Friedland JS, Bascom DA, Clement ID, Cunningham DA, Painter R, Robbins PA. Changes in arterial K^+ and ventilation during exercise in normal subjects with McArdle's syndrome. J Physiol 1990; 429:339–348.

151. Skatrud JB, Dempsey JA, Kaiser DG. Ventilatory response to medroxyprogesterone acetate in normal subjects: time course and mechanism. J Appl Physiol 1978; 44:939–944.

152. Lyons HA, Antonio R. The sensitivity of the respiratory center in pregnancy and after the administration of progesterone. Trans Assoc Am Physicians 1959; 72:173–180.

153. Takano N, Sakai A, Iida. Analysis of alveolar PCO2 control during the menstrual cycle. Pfluegers Arch 1981; 390:56–62.

154. Takano N, Kaneda T. Renal contribution to acid–base regulation during the menstrual cycle. Am J Physiol 1983; 244:F320–F324.

155. Fadel HE, Northrop G, Misenheimer HR, Harp RJ. Normal pregnancy: a model of sustained respiratory alkalosis. J Perinat Med 1979; 7:195–201.

156. Lim VS, Katz AI, Lindheimer MD. Acid–base regulation in pregnancy. Am J Physiol 1976; 231:1764–1770.

157. Orr-Walker BJ, Horne AM, Evans MC, Grey AB, Murray MAF, McNeil AR, Reid IR. Hormone replacement therapy causes a respiratory alkalosis in normal postmenopausal women. J Clin Endocrinol Metab 1999; 84: 1997–2001.

158. Shugrue PJ, Lane MV, Merchenthaler I. Regulation of progesterone receptor messenger ribonucleic acid in the rat medial preoptic nucleus by estrogenic and antiestrogenic compounds. Endocrinology 1997; 138:5476–5484.

159. Bayliss DA, Millhorn DE. Central neural mechanisms of progesterone action: application to the respiratory system. J Appl Physiol 1992; 73:393–404.

160. Pino-Garcia JM, Garcia-Rio F, Diez JJ, Gomez-Mendieta MA, Racionero MS, Diaz-Lobato S, Villamor J. Regulation of breathing in hyperthyroidism: relationship to hormonal and metabolic changes. Eur Respir J 1998; 12:400–407.

161. Valtin H, Tenney SM. Respiratory adaptations to hyperthyroidism. J Appl Physiol 1960; 15:1107–1113.

162. Engel LA, Ritchie B. Ventilatory response to inhaled carbon dioxide in hyperthyroidism. J Appl Physiol 1971; 30:173–177.

163. Zwillich CW, Matthay M, Potts DE. Thyrotoxicosis: comparison of effects of thyroid ablation and beta-adrenergic blockade on metabolic rate and ventilatory control. J Clin Endocrinol Metab 1978; 46:491–500.

164. Brussel T, Matthay MA, Chernow B. Pulmonary manifestations of endocrine and metabolic disorders. Clin Chest Med 1989; 10:645–653.

165. Mitchell RA, Loeschcke HH, Severinghaus JW, Richardson BW, Massion WH. Regions of respiratory chemosensitivity on the surface of the medulla. Ann N Y Acad Sci 1963; 109:661–681.

166. Cherniak NS, Widdicombe JG, eds. The respiratory system. Handbook of Physiology. Section 3. Oxford: Oxford University Press1992:Vol. 3.

167. Barcroft H, Basnayake V, Celander O, Cobbold AF, Cunningham DJC, Jukes MGM, Young IM. The effect of carbon dioxide on the respiratory response to noradrenaline in man. Am J Physiol 1957; 137:365–373.

168. Whelan RF, Young IM. The effect of adrenaline and noradrenaline infusions on respiration in man. Br J Pharmacol 1953; 8:98–102.

169. Van de Borne P, Oren R, Somers VK. Dopamine depresses minute ventilation in patients with heart failure. Circulation 1998; 98:126–131.

170. Potter EK, McCloskey DI. Respiratory stimulation by angiotensin II. Respir Physiol 1979; 36:367–373.

171. Tainter ML, Cutting WC. Febrile, respiratory and some other actions of dinitrophenol. J Pharmacol Exp Ther 1933; 48:410–431.

172. Ring T, Anderson PT, Knudsen F, Nielsen FB. Salicylate-induced hyperventilation. Lancet 1985; 1:1450.

173. Millhorn DE, Eldridge FL, Waldorp TG. Effects of salicylate and 2,4 –dinitrophenol on respiration and metabolism. J Appl Physiol 1982; 53:925–929.

174. Stroud MA, Lambertsen CJ, Ewing JH, Kough RH, Gould RA, Schmidt CF. The effects of aminophylline and meperidine alone and in combination on the respiratory response to carbon dioxide inhalation. J Pharmacol Exp Ther 1955; 114:461–474.

175. Georgopoulos D, Holtby SG, Berezanski D, Anthonisen NR. Aminophylline effects on ventilatory response to hypoxia and hyperoxia in normal adults. J Appl Physiol 1989; 67:1150–1156.

176. Yamamoto M, Nishimura M, Kobayashi S, Akiyama Y, Miyamoto K, Kawakami Y. Role of endogenous adenosine in hypoxic ventilatory response in humans: a study with dipyridamole. J Appl Physiol 1994; 76:196–203.

177. Maidas NE, Adrogue HJ. Respiratory alkalosis and acidosis. In: Seldin DW, Giebisch G, eds. The Kidney: Physiology and Pathophysiology. 3rd ed. Philadelphia: Lippincott-Raven Publishers, 2000:2131–2166.

178. Prytz H, Thomsen AC. Acid–base status in liver cirrhosis: disturbances in stable, terminal and porta-caval shunted patients. Scand J Gastroenterol 1976; 11:249–256.

179. Vanamee P, Poppell JW, Glicksman AS, Randall HT, Roberts KE. Respiratory alkalosis in hepatic coma. Arch Intern Med 1956; 97:762–767.

180. Moreau R, Hadengue A, Soupison T, Mamzer MF, Kirstetter P, Saraux JL, Assous M, Roche-Sicot J, Sicot C. Arterial and mixed venous acid–base status in patients with cirrhosis. Liver 1993; 13:20–24.

181. Strauss G, Hansen BA, Knudsen GM, Larsen FS. Hyperventilation restores cerebral blood flow autoregulation in patients with acute liver failure. J Hepatol 1998; 28:199–203.

182. Karetzky MS, Mithoefer JC. The cause of hyperventilation and arterial hypoxia in patients with cirrhosis of the liver. Am J Med Sci 1967; 254: 797–804.

183. Simmons DH, Nicoloff J, Guze LB. Hyperventilation and respiratory alkalosis as signs of gram-negative bacteremia. JAMA 1960; 174:2196–2199.

184. Winslow EJ, Loeb HS, Rahimtoola SH, Kamath S, Gunnar RM. Hemodynamic studies and results of therapy in 50 patients with bacteremic shock. Am J Med 1973; 54:421–432.

185. Gaudio R, Abramson N. Heat-induced hyperventilation. J Appl Physiol 1968; 25:742–746.

186. Boyd AE, Beller GA. Heat exhaustion and respiratory alkalosis. Ann Intern Med 1975; 83:835.

187. Sprung CL, Portocarrero CJ, Fernaine AV, Weinberg PF. The metabolic and respiratory alterations of heat stroke. Arch Intern Med 1980; 140:665–669.

188. Grauberg PO. Human physiology under cold exposure. Arctic Med Res 1991; 50(suppl 6):23–27.

189. Dulfano MJ, Ishikawa S. Quantitative acid–base relationships in chronic pulmonary patients during the steady-state. Am Rev Respir Dis 1966; 93: 25–42.

190. Fink BR, Hanks EC, Holaday DA, Ngai SH. Monitoring of ventilation by integrated diaphragmatic electromyogram: determination of carbon dioxide (CO_2) threshold in anesthetized man. JAMA 1960; 172:1367–1371.

191. Plum F, Brown HW, Snoep E. Neurologic significance of posthyperventilation apnea. JAMA 1962; 181:1050–1055.

192. Raimondi AC, Raimondi GA, Adrogué HJ, Marchissio ML. Hypoxemia after voluntary hyperventilation. Medicina (Buenos Aires) 1973; 33:621 (abstract).

193. Mithoefer JC, Bossman OG, Thibeault DW, Mead GD. The clinical estimation of alveolar ventilation. Am Rev Respir Dis 1968; 98:868–871.

194. Rice RL. Symptom patterns of the hyperventilation syndrome. Am J Med 1950; 8:691–700.

195. Soley MH, Shock NW. The etiology of effort syndrome. Am J Med Sci 1938; 196:840–851.

196. Nielsen M, Smith H. Studies on the regulation of respiration in acute hypoxia. Act Physiol Scand 1952; 24:293–313.

197. Hsia CCW. Respiratory function of hemoglobin. N Engl J Med 1998; 338:239–247.

198. Cunningham DJC, Robbins PA, Wolff CB. Integration of respiratory responses to changes in alveolar partial pressures of CO_2 and O_2 and in arterial pH. In: Handbook of Physiology -The respiratory system II. Oxford University Press, 1992, 475–528.

199. Loeschke HH, Gertz KH. Einfluss des O2 Druckes in der Einatmungsluft auf die Atemtätigkeit des Menschen, geprüft unter Konstanthaltung des alveolären CO2 Druckes. Pflügers Arch 1958; 267:460–477.

22

Mixed Acid–Base Disorders

Asghar Rastegar

*Department of Nephrology, Yale University School of Medicine,
New Haven, Connecticut, U.S.A.*

INTRODUCTION

Mixed acid–base disorders are defined as the simultaneous presence of two or more primary disorders. Identification of these disorders hinges upon a knowledge of the normal secondary responses to single acid–base disturbances, defined by experimental observations in humans and animals (see Chapter 28). Most mixed disturbances are identified by an abnormal secondary response to the primary disturbance. For example a patient with metabolic alkalosis due to vomiting, who also has a primary respiratory acid–base disorder, will have a $PaCO_2$ that is either higher or lower than the expected secondary response to metabolic alkalosis, and the level may even be below normal if a respiratory alkalosis is present. The effect of two or more disorders on arterial blood pH depends on the nature and severity of each disturbance. The resultant pH may be normal or near normal if the two disorders counterbalance each other or highly abnormal if the effect is additive.

Mixed disorders may develop in several ways. The two or more coexisting acid–base disorders may be common features of an underlying illness, as in sepsis-induced respiratory alkalosis and lactic acidosis. Alternatively, a second disorder may develop acutely in a patient who has a stable underlying disorder. For example, a patient with metabolic acidosis due to chronic kidney disease may develop metabolic alkalosis due to vomiting. Another possibility is that two independent acid–base disorders may develop simultaneously, such as metabolic alkalosis due to gastric drainage and respiratory

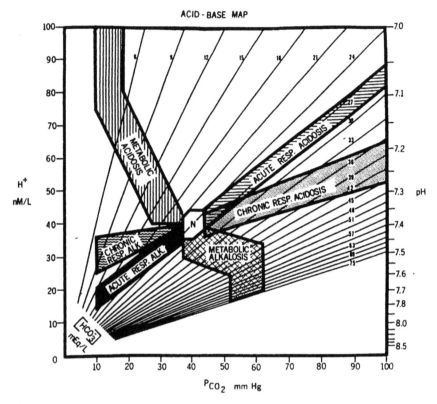

Figure 1   Acid–base "map" showing the confidence bands relating PaCO$_2$, pH (*right-hand ordinate*) and [H$^+$] (*left-hand ordinate*) for the six primary acid–base disturbances. The clear area labeled N in the center represents the range of normal values. *Source*: From Ref. 1.

acidosis due to flail chest in a patient with multiple traumatic injuries. Mixed disorders, even of mild severity, should be recognized promptly to guide therapy as well as to help diagnose underlying diseases. For example, mixed metabolic (lactic) acidosis and alkalosis in a patient with abdominal pain and vomiting should alert one to the diagnosis of bowel ischemia. To assist in diagnosing mixed disorders, one can use an acid–base template (Fig. 1) or rules of thumb (Table 1), but both tools should always be used in conjunction with other clinical data to avoid the pitfalls described below.

APPROACH TO THE PATIENT WITH A MIXED ACID–BASE DISORDER

As outlined in Chapter 28, the approach to the patient suspected of having any acid–base disorder should include a review of all the clinical data and

Table 1 Rules of Thumb for Estimating the Compensatory Response at Bedside

Primary disturbance	Expected compensatory response
Metabolic acidosis	$PaCO_2$ decreases by 1.2 mmHg for each mEq/L decrease in $[HCO_3^-]$
Metabolic alkalosis	$PaCO_2$ increases by 0.7 mmHg for each mEq/L rise in $[HCO_3^-]$
Respiratory acidosis	
Acute	$[HCO_3^-]$ increases by 0.1 mEq/L for each mmHg rise in $PaCO_2$
Chronic	$[HCO_3^-]$ increases by 0.4 mEq/L for each mmHg rise in $PaCO_2$
Respiratory alkalosis	
Acute	$[HCO_3^-]$ decreases by 0.2 mEq/L for each mmHg fall in $PaCO_2$
Chronic	$[HCO_3^-]$ decreases by 0.4 mEq/L for each mmHg fall in $PaCO_2$

not just an evaluation of the acid–base parameters. Diagnostic assessment should include a full evaluation of the history and physical examination, as well as reviewing all the laboratory radiological data, with particular attention to uncovering disorders that impact on acid–base homeostasis. It is important to recognize that acid–base disturbances are dynamic in nature. Therefore whenever possible, evaluation of acid–base and electrolyte data should include several measurements over time. For those interested in acquiring this rewarding diagnostic skill, the best advice is to look at all blood gases as if they represent a mixed disturbance waiting to be discovered. With practice this approach will become second nature ensuring correct diagnosis and management.

TOOLS FOR DIAGNOSING MIXED ACID–BASE DISORDERS

The diagnosis of mixed acid–base disorders hinges on a knowledge of the normal secondary responses to simple acid–base disorders (see Chapter 28). The expected responses to each of the primary acid–base disorders have been combined in a single diagram (Fig. 1) that provides bands, indicating the 95% confidence interval for the expected response (1). These responses can also be assessed with the application of a series of easy to use "rules of thumb" (Table 1). These rules allow for rapid bedside calculation of the expected secondary response for each primary disturbance. One should remember, however, that they define the average rather than the range of expected changes and therefore should be used as a general guide rather than as precise calculations. In many mixed acid–base disorders, the measured $PaCO_2$ or [HCO_3^-] deviates markedly from the normal secondary response, and the diagnosis is readily apparent from consideration of the appropriate rule of thumb. In situations in which the abnormality is questionable, the graph in Fig. 1 can be used to see if the value falls outside the range for the expected secondary response.

Limitations and Cautions

When using either the acid–base diagram (Fig. 1) or the rules of thumb (Table 1), it is important to understand the limitations of these tools. First, the bands reflect steady-state conditions, and therefore data obtained in a patient with a simple disorder during any transition period may be compatible with a mixed disorder (2). Second and more problematic is the normal variation in the response (reflected by the width of the confidence bands in the diagram in Fig. 1). Thus acid–base parameters in patients with mild mixed disturbances will often fall within the normal response band for a single disorder. Patients with more severe mixed disorders affecting acid–base parameters in opposing directions could also have acid–base values that fall within the band for a simple disorder. For example, a patient with acute respiratory acidosis and metabolic alkalosis may present with acid–base values within the compensatory band for chronic respiratory acidosis (see later). In such cases the correct diagnosis can only be made by the use of all clinical and laboratory data, with special attention to dynamic changes in blood pH, $PaCO_2$, and [HCO_3^-]. Although a set of data falling within a compensatory band for a simple disorder may also be compatible with a mixed disturbance, the finding that such a set clearly falls outside these bands indicates a high likelihood that the patient is suffering from more than one disorder.

Anion Gap

The anion gap, an additional tool for identifying the presence of more than one acid–base disturbance, is discussed and defined in Chapters 9 and 28. It is calculated as follows:

$$\text{Anion gap (mEq/L)} = [Na^+] - ([Cl^-] + [HCO_3^-]) \tag{1}$$

The normal value is 8–12 mEq/L, and an increase indicates the presence of a metabolic acidosis in most instances, regardless of the serum [HCO_3^-]. Given the variability in each of the measurements, however, an increase can only be diagnosed with assurance if the value is >17–18 mEq/L (3,4). The use of the anion gap in identifying the presence of a mixed disorder is discussed later under mixed metabolic acid–base disturbances.

Table 2 Classification of Mixed Disorders and Examples

Mixed metabolic and respiratory disorders
Additive
Mixed metabolic and respiratory acidosis
Mixed metabolic and respiratory alkalosis
Counterbalancing
Mixed metabolic acidosis and respiratory alkalosis
Mixed metabolic alkalosis and respiratory acidosis

Mixed metabolic disorders
Counterbalancing
Mixed metabolic acidosis and alkalosis

Mixed respiratory disorders
Additive
Mixed acute and chronic respiratory acidosis
Counterbalancing
Mixed acute respiratory alkalosis and chronic respiratory acidosis

Multiple disorders
Metabolic alkalosis + metabolic alkalosis + respiratory alkalosis or acidosis
Chronic respiratory acidosis + acute respiratory acidosis + metabolic alkalosis

---

CLASSIFICATION OF MIXED ACID–BASE DISORDERS

Given that there are six simple acid–base disturbances (see Chapter 28), the number of possible mixed disturbances is high. Most commonly, mixed disorders reflect the coexistence of two primary disorders, but three and occasionally four disorders may sometimes be present in the same patient. Some combinations, such as mixed acute respiratory acidosis and alkalosis or mixed chronic respiratory acidosis and alkalosis, can be excluded as clinically irrelevant. Others, such as mixed hyperchloremic acidosis and metabolic alkalosis, are difficult to suspect without appropriate history and/or previous laboratory data. In this chapter we will focus primarily on double disorders, which comprise the majority of clinically important mixed disorders.

Mixed acid–base disorders can be classified by the nature of the underlying disturbances (metabolic vs. respiratory disorders) as well as by their impact on serum pH (additive vs. counterbalancing disorders) (Table 2). Additive disorders are those in which the composite changes in $PaCO_2$ and $[HCO_3^-]$ increase the severity of the acidemia or alkalemia, and the counterbalancing disorders are those in which the composite changes decrease the severity of the acidemia or alkalemia.

Mixed Metabolic and Respiratory Disorders

Examples of common clinical settings and laboratory abnormalities in mixed metabolic and respiratory disorders are shown in Figs. 2 and 3. Such

Mixed metabolic and respiratory acid-base disorders:
Clinical settings and typical laboratory values

I. Additive disorders

Metabolic and respiratory acidosis

Exemplary clinical settings:

Cardiopulmonary arrest
Renal and respiratory failure
Cardiogenic shock with pulmonary edema
Chronic respiratory failure and septic shock
Renal tubular acidosis and muscle paralysis

Characteristic acid-base values:	
pH	7.16
PCO$_2$	52 mmHg
[HCO$_3^-$]	18 mEq/L
Anion gap	20 mEq/L

Metabolic and respiratory alkalosis

Exemplary clinical settings:

Hepatic failure with diuretic use and/or vomiting
Severe vomiting in pregnancy
Gastric drainage and sepsis

Characteristic acid-base values:	
pH	7.64
PCO$_2$	22 mmHg
[HCO$_3^-$]	23 mEq/L
Anion gap	16 mEq/L

Figure 2 Examples of mixed metabolic and respiratory acid–base disorders: additive disorders.

Mixed metabolic and respiratory acid-base disorders:
Clinical settings and typical laboratory values

II. Counterbalancing disorders

Metabolic acidosis and respiratory alkalosis

Exemplary clinical settings:

Renal failure and pneumonia
Diabetic ketoacidosis and sepsis
Salicylate toxicity
Septic shock
Severe asthma
Hepatorenal syndrome

Characteristic acid-base values:	
pH	7.45
PCO$_2$	30 mmHg
[HCO$_3^-$]	20 mEq/L
Anion gap	18 mEq/L

Metabolic alkalosis and respiratory acidosis

Exemplary clinical settings:

Chronic respiratory failure treated with diuretics
Chronic respiratory failure on a ventilator
Chronic respiratory failure with vomiting
Acute respiratory failure and nasograstric suction

Characteristic acid-base values:	
pH	7.40
PCO$_2$	58 mmHg
[HCO$_3^-$]	35 mEq/L
Anion gap	14 mEq/L

Figure 3 Examples of mixed metabolic and respiratory acid–base disorders: counterbalancing disorders.

disorders should be suspected if the secondary response is less than or greater than predicted, or in the extreme, moves in the opposite direction. To determine whether a mixed disorder is present, one should first identify the dominant disorder (see Chapters 28 and 29) and then determine whether the response is appropriate. For example, in a patient with an arterial pH and serum [HCO_3^-] lower than normal, metabolic acidosis is the dominant disorder. If the secondary decrease in $PaCO_2$ is less than expected or in the opposite direction, two primary disturbances—metabolic acidosis and respiratory acidosis—exist, one affecting [HCO_3^-] and the other affecting PCO_2, that have an additive effect on the deviation in pH from normal. By contrast, if the reduction in PCO_2 is greater than expected, two disorders—metabolic acidosis and respiratory alkalosis—coexist that minimize the change in pH. In the latter instance, pH may remain at or close to normal range reflecting the countervailing effect of these two disorders. If a clearly dominant disorder is not apparent, one can assume that either disorder is dominant and determine the appropriateness of the secondary response, using the tools in Fig. 1 and Table 1. Examples of additive and countervailing mixed disorders are discussed separately below.

EXAMPLES OF MIXED DISORDERS: DIAGNOSIS AND MANAGEMENT

Additive Metabolic/Respiratory Disorders

Metabolic and Respiratory Acidosis

When metabolic and respiratory acidosis coexist, arterial pH is typically very low, seemingly out of proportion to the change in either $PaCO_2$ or [HCO_3^-]. This mixed disorder is easily recognized when $PaCO_2$ is elevated and serum [HCO_3^-] is reduced, as illustrated by the example in Fig. 2. However, it is important to identify this mixed disorder when one or the other of these parameters appears to be "normal." For example, a patient with a serum [HCO_3^-] of 18 mEq/L and a "normal" $PaCO_2$ of 40 mmHg has a mixed disorder because $PaCO_2$ has not been reduced to the expected range for this degree of metabolic acidosis. Alternatively, serum [HCO_3^-] could be within the normal range and $PaCO_2$ elevated. Such a laboratory result could indicate either the presence of an uncomplicated acute respiratory acidosis, or a mixed disorder with chronic respiratory acidosis combined with metabolic acidosis.

Common Clinical Presentations: The most dramatic presentation of mixed metabolic and respiratory acidosis is in the setting of cardiopulmonary arrest (5). In this setting both runaway lactic acid production and hypercarbia create a vicious combination resulting in severe acidemia. Artificial ventilation and infusion of HCO_3^- may correct arterial pH rapidly but, unless circulatory failure is reversed, tissue hypoperfusion and ongoing production of lactic acid will continue (6–8). Despite the marked acidemia and low serum [HCO$_3^-$], this mixed disorder can be reversed by reestablishing ventilation and cardiac function.

A mixed respiratory and metabolic acidosis can also occur in patients with stable metabolic acidosis (e.g., from chronic renal failure) who subsequently develop ventilatory insufficiency and respiratory acidosis. In pulmonary edema a variety of acid–base problems can occur. Although respiratory alkalosis occurs in a minority of patients with pulmonary edema, the majority develop acute respiratory acidosis or a mixed respiratory and metabolic (lactic) acidosis (9,10). Less common causes of a metabolic acidosis with an increased anion gap combined with respiratory acidosis include diabetic ketoacidosis with exhaustion from prolonged Kussmaul respiration or hypophosphatemia impairing the normal respiratory response. Carbon monoxide and cyanide poisoning can also produce this mixed disorder.

Metabolic acidosis with a normal anion gap combined with respiratory acidosis is a less common event. In patients with type 1 renal tubular acidosis accompanied by severe hypokalemia, respiratory acidosis can develop as a result of muscle weakness and impairment of ventilation (see Case 11 in Chapter 29). Impairment of ventilation can also occur as an independent problem in any patient with renal tubular acidosis, regardless of the type. In this mixed disorder, arterial pH, PaCO$_2$ and [HCO$_3^-$] will fall in the zone between metabolic acidosis and acute respiratory acidosis (Fig. 1).

Treatment: The development of respiratory failure in a patient with metabolic acidosis can rapidly cause profound acidemia and should be dealt with as an emergency. If a rapidly treatable etiology (such as hypokalemia or pulmonary edema) is not quickly identified and reversed, intubation and ventilatory support should be undertaken to reduce PaCO$_2$.

Metabolic and Respiratory Alkalosis

In this mixed disorder, a primary increase in serum [HCO$_3^-$] (metabolic alkalosis) coupled with a simultaneous primary stimulus to hyperventilate (respiratory alkalosis) conspire to cause marked alkalemia. This mixed disorder can easily be missed, as arterial blood gases are often not obtained in patients with mild to moderate elevations in serum [HCO$_3^-$]. With an arterial pH and PCO$_2$ measurement in hand, one proceeds in a systematic way to identify the dominant disorder, if possible, and then determine whether the secondary response is normal. Alternatively, one can start either with the PaCO$_2$ or [HCO$_3^-$], and determine whether the change in the second parameter falls within the expected range. In patients with an elevated serum [HCO$_3^-$], the diagnosis is made if PaCO$_2$ is either reduced, within the "normal" range, or increased to a level less than predicted for the elevation in serum [HCO$_3^-$]. Serum [HCO$_3^-$] may also fall within the "normal" range in this mixed disorder, but may be inappropriate for the prevailing PaCO$_2$. The anion gap is not particularly helpful in sorting out the components of this mixed disorder unless it is markedly elevated (see later under Multiple Acid–Base Disorders). The anion gap may be increased by as much as 4–6 mEq/L in uncomplicated metabolic alkalosis (11) (see Chapter 28).

Common Clinical Presentations: Mixed metabolic and respiratory alkalosis typically develops in a setting in which one of the two disorders has been present for a period of time and the second develops acutely as a result of a new complication (see examples in Fig. 2). For example, a patient with stable respiratory alkalosis due to hepatic cirrhosis may develop metabolic alkalosis due to diuretic therapy and/or vomiting. Because chronic respiratory alkalosis is a normal feature of pregnancy (see Chapter 21), a mixed metabolic and respiratory alkalosis can occur when pregnancy is complicated by nausea and vomiting. An increasingly common scenario is seen in critically ill surgical patients with nasogastric drainage who are artificially ventilated. In one study up to 65% of post-traumatic patients were alkalemic and the majority had mixed metabolic and respiratory alkalosis (12). In another study the severity of alkalemia correlated with mortality rising to 90% when pH increased beyond 7.64 (13). In these critically ill patients, respiratory alkalosis was due to sepsis, primary central nervous system disease or artificially induced hyperventilation while metabolic alkalosis was secondary to nasogastric drainage or massive blood transfusion. Metabolic and respiratory alkalosis can be induced as well in patients with chronic respiratory acidosis or underlying metabolic alkalosis who are overzealously ventilated (14).

Treatment: Recognition of this mixed disorder may uncover and allow prompt treatment of a life-threatening condition. For example, new respiratory alkalosis may be a sign of sepsis or unrecognized pulmonary embolism. Treatment of respiratory alkalosis may be difficult unless secondary to excessive artificial ventilation. Nonetheless, it serves as a key diagnostic clue, drawing attention to its underlying cause, which often can be treated. Metabolic alkalosis can usually be corrected or ameliorated by appropriate therapeutic interventions (e.g., discontinuation of diuretics, K^+ and Cl^- administration, see Chapters 16–19).

Counterbalancing Metabolic/Respiratory Disorders

Metabolic Acidosis and Respiratory Alkalosis

In this dual disorder $PaCO_2$ is lower than expected for the reduction in serum $[HCO_3^-]$, resulting in a pH closer to normal or even within the normal range (Fig. 3). The most challenging diagnostic scenario is when a patient with metabolic acidosis associated with a normal anion gap (e.g., renal tubular acidosis) develops acute respiratory alkalosis. In this setting, the resultant pH, $PaCO_2$ and $[HCO_3^-]$ values are likely to be completely compatible with chronic respiratory alkalosis. The diagnosis often can only be made if previous electrolytes and or arterial pH and $PaCO_2$ measurements are available for comparison. At times presence of underlying renal tubular acidosis can only be established when correction of respiratory alkalosis is not followed by normalization of serum $[HCO_3^-]$ and $[Cl^-]$.

Common Clinical Presentations: Mixed metabolic acidosis/respiratory alkalosis occurs most commonly in patients who have an underlying stable metabolic acidosis, and then develop a superimposed illness that leads to respiratory alkalosis. The superimposed respiratory alkalosis can, if sustained, lower serum $[HCO_3^-]$ even further, minimizing the increase in pH that would otherwise occur (15). Respiratory alkalosis could be secondary to pulmonary emboli, pneumonia, congestive heart failure or sepsis. More rarely, both respiratory alkalosis and metabolic acidosis can develop simultaneously. For example, septic shock could simultaneously result in respiratory alkalosis and metabolic (lactic) acidosis. Metabolic acidosis due to diabetic ketoacidosis could be complicated by respiratory alkalosis due to sepsis or pneumonia. In hepatorenal syndrome, the underlying respiratory alkalosis could be complicated by progressive metabolic acidosis due to acute renal failure. Cirrhosis can be complicated by sepsis and lactic acidosis, resulting in a mixed disturbance.

A mixed metabolic acidosis/respiratory alkalosis is a characteristic feature of salicylate toxicity (see also Chapters 12 and 21). Toxic levels of salicylate stimulate ventilation directly, causing respiratory alkalosis. At the same time salicylate accumulation causes metabolic acidosis by promoting organic acid production. In children, severe metabolic acidosis is usually the predominant component of this mixed disorder, while in adults respiratory alkalosis is often more prominent (16,17).

Treatment: Treatment of metabolic acidosis combined with respiratory alkalosis should always be directed at correcting the underlying cause if possible. Acute treatment with HCO_3^- will often worsen the alkalemia. This dilemma is illustrated by the treatment of salicylate intoxication, for which HCO_3^- administration is recommended to hasten the renal excretion of salicylate (18,19). To the extent that this treatment increases serum $[HCO_3^-]$ in the face of continued hyperventilation, it will also exacerbate the alkalemia. In rare instances, it may be necessary to increase $PaCO_2$ by increasing ventilatory dead space with a rebreathing mask or, in extreme cases, endotracheal intubation and ventilatory control before bicarbonate is infused or dialysis is initiated.

Respiratory Acidosis and Metabolic Alkalosis

The combination of chronic respiratory acidosis and metabolic alkalosis is extremely common, induced in most instances when diuretic therapy is used to treat edema in patients with chronic respiratory acidosis. This mixed disorder can also develop in patients with chronic respiratory acidosis who develop metabolic alkalosis from vomiting or nasogastric drainage, or when $PaCO_2$ is reduced (e.g., by ventilator therapy) in patients ingesting a chloride-restricted diet (see Chapter 17). The diagnosis is easily made when serum $[HCO_3^-]$ is higher than appropriate for the normal compensatory response to chronic respiratory acidosis or, conversely, when $PaCO_2$ is higher than appropriate for the degree of metabolic alkalosis (see Case 3 in Chapter 29).

Treatment: Management of mixed metabolic alkalosis and respiratory acidosis should focus on treatment of underlying disturbances. Steps to improve ventilation and ameliorate the respiratory acidosis should always be coupled with treatment of the metabolic alkalosis, because a reduction in $PaCO_2$ alone will only worsen the alkalemia. Moreover, patients with chronic respiratory acidosis rely in part for their ventilatory drive on an acid pH. Thus concomitant metabolic alkalosis may impair ventilatory drive and impede the ability to improve ventilation.

Mixed Metabolic Acid–Base Disorders

A key tool for identifying the mixture of metabolic alkalosis and acidosis is an analysis of the relationship between the change in serum $[HCO_3^-]$ and the change in anion gap (Δ anion gap) (20–23). The Δ anion gap and its use in diagnosis are discussed in Chapters 28 and 29. It is calculated as follows:

$$\Delta \text{ anion gap (mEq/L)} = ([Na^+] - ([Cl^-] + [HCO_3^-])) - 12 \quad (2)$$

In this calculation 12 is assumed to be the normal value for the anion gap. In settings in which the anion gap is increased and the serum $[HCO_3^-]$ is decreased, the Δ anion gap should correspond roughly with the fall in serum $[HCO_3^-]$ (i.e., $24 - [HCO_3^-]$). If the Δ anion gap is much larger than the reduction in $[HCO_3^-]$, it suggests that serum $[HCO_3^-]$ was $> 24\,\text{mEq/L}$ prior to the induction of metabolic acidosis and the increase in the anion gap, and that a hidden second acid–base disorder, i.e., metabolic alkalosis, is present.

The assumptions underlying this calculation are discussed in Chapter 28, and although not precisely fulfilled in patients with organic acidoses, they are close enough so that large discrepancies between the increase in anion gap and the fall in $[HCO_3^-]$ are diagnostic of a mixed metabolic acid–base disorder. In the case shown in Fig. 4, for example, the Δ anion gap $(30 - 12 = 18\,\text{mEq/L})$ far exceeds the fall in serum $[HCO_3^-]$ $(24 - 20 = 4\,\text{mEq/L})$. To the extent that the assumptions discussed in Chapter 28 hold, one can estimate that the serum $[HCO_3^-]$ would have been $20 + 18$ or $38\,\text{mEq/L}$ prior to the increase in the anion gap. This

Mixed metabolic acidosis and alkalosis: Clinical settings and typical laboratory values

A Counterbalancing disorder

Exemplary clinical settings:	Characteristic acid-base values:	
Alcoholic ketoacidosis and vomiting	pH	7.37
Acute renal failure and nasogastric suction	PCO_2	35 mmHg
Chronic renal failure and diuretic use	$[HCO_3^-]$	20 mEq/L
	Anion gap	30 mEq/L
	Δ Anion gap	18 mEq/L*

*see text

Figure 4   Examples of mixed metabolic acidosis and alkalosis.

constellation of findings often occurs in patients with diabetic ketoacidosis, indicating the presence of a mixed metabolic acidosis and metabolic alkalosis (24–26). Although the mean ratio of change in anion gap to bicarbonate ($\Delta AG/\Delta HCO_3$) in uncomplicated diabetic ketoacidosis is close to 1.0, there is wide variation. As a general rule, a ratio of >1.2 is strongly suggestive of a mixed metabolic acidosis and alkalosis (24,26).

Mixed Metabolic Acidosis and Alkalosis

This mixed disorder can arise from vomiting, aggressive diuresis or use of alkali in patients with underlying metabolic acidosis (27–29). Most commonly, however, this mixture is seen in binge drinkers who first develop metabolic alkalosis from vomiting and then develop an organic acidosis (alcoholic ketoacidosis or lactic acidosis) (30,31).

A mixed metabolic alkalosis and acidosis can also occur without an increase in anion gap. For example a patient with vomiting who then develops severe diarrhea could develop both a metabolic alkalosis (from vomiting) and a metabolic acidosis (from diarrhea). This combination yields a set of electrolytes that provides no clues concerning the presence of two disorders and thus can only be surmised from the history, unless previous laboratory measurements are available demonstrating one or the other disorder.

The acid–base template and rules of thumb discussed earlier are not helpful in diagnosing a mixed metabolic alkalosis and acidosis, as they only describe the expected secondary responses to acid–base disturbances. Nonetheless, one should use these rules in a patient with a mixed metabolic acidosis and alkalosis (diagnosed using the Δ anion gap calculation), to assess whether or not other acid–base disorders are also present (see later under Multiple Acid–Base Disorders).

Treatment: Treatment of mixed metabolic acidosis and alkalosis should address both disorders. Administration of isotonic saline is often effective in reversing both components of this mixed disorder, particularly in the setting of mixed metabolic alkalosis and lactic acidosis. If the metabolic acidosis can also be addressed directly (e.g., diabetic ketoacidosis), then treatment of both disorders should be undertaken simultaneously. In the patient with renal insufficiency or failure, treatment with isotonic saline alone can unmask a significant metabolic acidosis due to impaired acid excretion and/or HCO_3^- reabsorption. Patients with severe renal failure are unable to excrete excess HCO_3^- (or saline) and therefore treatment of the metabolic alkalosis is often very difficult. In this setting, hemodialysis is the most appropriate treatment (32).

Mixed Respiratory Disorders

Acute Respiratory Acidosis Superimposed on Chronic Respiratory Acidosis

Acute CO_2 retention may reflect worsening of underlying pulmonary disease, discontinuation of effective therapy, use of drugs that suppress central nervous system function, or use of an inappropriately high inspiratory O_2 concentration (Fig. 5). Recognition of such a new acute respiratory acidosis in a patient with chronic respiratory acidosis is obviously key for management. Treatment should be directed at improving ventilation and reversing the acute increase in $PaCO_2$.

Acute Respiratory Alkalosis Superimposed on Chronic Respiratory Acidosis Patients with chronic respiratory acidosis can also experience an acute increase in minute ventilation, causing an acute reduction in $PaCO_2$. Such a change may occur spontaneously with improvement in ventilatory function or could represent a new acute disorder, such as sepsis, pulmonary embolus or central nervous system disease (see Chapter 21).

Treatment: Diagnosis of this mixed disorder should trigger a search for the cause of the respiratory alkalosis. If it represents an improvement in pulmonary function, one should ascertain that the serum $[HCO_3^-]$ is falling appropriately. If not, one should take steps to provide adequate chloride and potassium to assure return to more normal values for the new PCO_2 (33,34). If the acute fall represents a new illness, treatment should be directed at the new problem.

Multiple Acid–Base Disorders

A multiple disorder is defined as the coexistence of more than two primary acid–base disturbances in a single individual. When three coexist, the disturbance is termed a triple disorder; when four coexist, it is termed a

Mixed respiratory acid-base disorders: Clinical settings and typical laboratory values

I. Additive disorders

Acute and chronic respiratory acidosis

Exemplary clinical settings:

Chronic respiratory failure with:
    superimposed pneumonia
    superimposed pulmonary edema
        plus high inspired oxygen

Characteristic acid-base values:	
pH	7.27
PCO_2	76 mmHg
$[HCO_3^-]$	34 mEq/L

II. Counterbalancing disorders

Acute respiratory alkalosis and chronic respiratory acidosis

Exemplary clinical settings:

Chronic respiratory failure with:
    sepsis
    excess mechanical ventilation
    spontaneous improvement

Characteristic acid-base values:	
pH	7.50
PCO_2	50 mmHg
$[HCO_3^-]$	38 mEq/L

Figure 5   Examples of mixed respiratory acid–base disorders.

quadruple disorder. Clinically significant multiple acid–base disorders are relatively uncommon and usually occur in patients with many medical problems, often in an intensive care unit setting. The most common multiple disorder is the development of acute respiratory alkalosis or acidosis in a patient who already has a mixed metabolic acidosis and alkalosis. For example, a patient with metabolic acidosis due to renal failure and metabolic alkalosis from vomiting could develop gram-negative sepsis and superimposed respiratory alkalosis, or develop severe pulmonary edema from a cardiac complication resulting in acute respiratory acidosis. Often multiple disorders develop in the setting of cardiac resuscitation. Another setting in which a multiple disturbance can occur is in the patient with chronic respiratory acidosis and metabolic alkalosis (perhaps from diuretics) who develops acute respiratory acidosis as a new complication.

In the patient with a mixed metabolic alkalosis and acidosis with a superimposed respiratory disorder, analysis of the Δ anion gap is a critical step in identifying the two metabolic components of the acid–base disorder. Recognition of the presence of a multiple disorder is important for treatment. Each of the contributing disorders should be taken into consideration in the approach to therapy.

REFERENCES

1. Goldberg M, Green SB, Moss ML, Marbach CB, Garfinkel D. Computerized instruction and diagnosis of acid–base disorders. J Am Med Assoc 1973; 223:269–275.
2. Harrington JT, Cohen JJ, Kassirer JP. Mixed acid–base disturbances. In: Cohen JJ, Kassirer JP, eds. Acid–Base. Boston: Little Brown, 1982:377–390.
3. Goodkin DA, Krishna GG, Narins RG. The role of anion gap in detecting and managing mixed metabolic acid–base disorders. Clin Endocrinol Metab 1984; 13:333–349.
4. Paulson WD, Gadallah MF. Diagnosis of mixed acid–base disorders in diabetic ketoacidosis. Am J Med Sci 1993; 306:295–300.
5. Chazan JA, Stenson R, Kurland GS. The acidosis of cardiac arrest. N Engl J Med 1968; 278:360–364.
6. Weil MH, Rackow EC, Trevino R, Grundler W, Falk JL, Griffel MI. Difference in acid–base state between venous and arterial blood during cardiopulmonary resuscitation. N Engl J Med 1986; 315:153–156.
7. Bishop RL, Weisfeldt ML. Sodium bicarbonate administration during cardiac arrest. Effect on arterial pH, pCO_2 and osmolality. J Am Med Assoc 1976; 235:506–509.
8. Adrogué HJ, Rashad MN, Gorin AB, Yacoub J, Madias NE. Assessing acid–base status in circulatory failure: difference between arterial and central venous blood. N Engl J Med 1989; 320:1312–1316.
9. Avery WG, Samet G, Sachner MA. The acidosis of pulmonary edema. Am J Med 1970; 48:320–324.
10. Aberman A, Fulop M. The metabolic and respiratory acidosis of acute pulmonary edema. Ann Intern Med 1972; 76:173–184.
11. Madias NE, Ayus JC, Adrogué HJ. Increased anion gap in metabolic alkalosis. N Engl J Med 1979; 300:1421–1423.
12. Lyons JH, Moore FD. Posttraumatic alkalosis: incidence and pathophysiology of alkalosis in surgery. Surgery 1966; 60:93–106.
13. Wilson RF, Gibson D, Percinel AK, Ali MA, Baker G, LeBlanc LP, Lucas G. Severe alkalosis in critically ill surgical patients. Arch Surg 1972; 105:197–203.
14. Kilburn KH. Shock, seizure and coma with alkalosis due to mechanical ventilation. Ann Intern Med 1966; 65:977–984.
15. Krapf R, Beeler I, Hertner D, Hulter HN. Chronic respiratory alkalosis. The effect of sustained hyperventilation on renal regulation of acid–base equilibrium. N Engl J Med 1991; 324:1993–1401.
16. Winters RW, White JS, Hughes MC, Ordway NK. Disturbances of acid–base equilibrium in salicylate intoxication. Pediatrics 1959; 23:260–285.
17. Gabow PA, Anderson RJ, Potts DE, Schrier RW. Acid–base disturbances in the salicylate-intoxicated adults. Arch Intern Med 1976; 138:1481–1484.
18. Cummings G, Dukes DC, Widdowson G. Alkaline diuresis in treatment of aspirin poisoning. Br Med J 1964; 2:1033–1036.
19. Prescott LF, Balali-Mood M, Critchley JAJH, Johnstone AF, Proudfoot AT. Diuresis or urinary alkalinization for salicylate poisoning? Br Med J 1982; 285:1383–1386.

20. Adrogué HJ, Brensilver J, Madias NE. Changes in anion gap during chronic metabolic acid–base disturbances. Am J Physiol 1978; 235:F291–F297.
21. Gabow PA, Kaehny WD, Fennesey PV, Goodman SI, Gross PA, Schrier RW. Diagnostic importance of an increased anion gap. N Engl J Med 1980; 303:854–858.
22. DiNubile MJ. The increment in anion gap, overextension of a concept? Lancet 1988; 2:951–953.
23. Salem MM, Mujais SK. Gaps in anion gap. Arch Intern Med 1992; 152:1625–1629.
24. Adrogué HJ, Wilson H, Boyd AE, Suki WN, Eknoyan G. Plasma acid–base pattern in diabetic ketoacidosis. N Engl J Med 1982; 307:1603–1610.
25. Elisaf MS, Tsatoulis AA, Katopodis KP, Siamopoulos KC. Acid–base and electrolyte disturbances in diabetic ketoacidosis. Diabetes Res Clin Pract 1996; 34:23–27.
26. Paulson WD. Anion gap–bicarbonate relation in diabetic ketoacidosis. Am J Med 1986; 81:995–1000.
27. Cronin JW, Kroop SF, Diamond J, Rolla AR. Alkalemia in diabetic ketoacidosis. Am J Med 1984; 77:192–194.
28. Whang R. "Bicarbonate overshoot": an indication for acetazolamide therapy. South Med J 1975; 68:733–734.
29. Walsh CH, Kim KC. Diabetic ketoalkalosis, a readily misdiagnosed entity. Br Med J 1976; 2:19.
30. Halperin ML, Hammeke M, Josse RJG, Jungas RL et al. Metabolic acidosis in alcoholics: a pathophysiological approach. Metabolism 1983; 32:308–315.
31. DeMarchi S, Cechin E, Basile A, Bertotti A, Nardini R, Bartoli E. Renal tubular dysfunction in chronic alcohol abuse—effect of abstinence. N Engl J Med 1993; 329:1927–1934.
32. Ayus JC, Olivero JJ, Adrogué HJ. Alkalemia associated with renal failure. Correction with hemodialysis with low bicarbonate dialysate. Arch Int Med 1980; 140:513–515.
33. Schwartz WB, Hays RH, Polak A, Haynie GD. Effect of chronic hypercapnia on electrolyte and acid–base equilibrium: II. Recovery with special reference to the influence of chloride intake. J Clin Invest 1961; 40:1238–1249.
34. Schwartz WB, van Ypersele de Strihou C, Kassirer JP. Role of anions in metabolic alkalosis and potassium deficiency. N Engl J Med 1968; 279:630–639.

23

Effect of Renal Replacement Therapy on Acid–Base Homeostasis

F. John Gennari

University of Vermont College of Medicine, Burlington, Vermont, U.S.A.

INTRODUCTION

When renal replacement therapy is initiated, regulation of body HCO_3^- stores shifts from a failing biological system (see Chapter 14) to a new process regulated solely by the physical principles of diffusion and convection (1). This switch has major implications for acid–base homeostasis, changing the way one thinks both about both normal and disordered acid balance. In contrast to individuals with functioning kidneys where HCO_3^- stores are continuously replenished by changes in acid excretion to match endogenous production, individuals with end-stage renal disease require exogenous alkali to maintain body stores. Alkali repletion is most often accomplished by adding either HCO_3^- or a HCO_3^- precursor to the dialysis bath solution. With some forms of therapy, HCO_3^- is given intravenously. Regardless of the approach, alkali addition causes a unique new equilibrium to develop in which a biological homeostatic process involving sensors and effectors is replaced by a process determined by factors influencing the movement of HCO_3^- across the dialysis membrane.

NATURE OF THE ACID–BASE EQUILIBRIUM ENGENDERED BY RENAL REPLACEMENT THERAPY

General Principles

Theoretical considerations indicate that once a dialysis prescription is fixed for an individual patient, net alkali addition is linked to endogenous acid production, despite the fact that the dialysis procedure is completely indifferent to body pH (1). This linkage occurs because the net gain or loss of alkali during treatment is directly related to the transmembrane concentration gradient for HCO_3^- (Fig. 1). For any given treatment prescription, the alkali concentration in the bath solution and the membrane permeability for HCO_3^- are fixed, and the delivery rates of blood and dialysate to the membrane are relatively constant. Under these conditions, the initial serum $[HCO_3^-]$ and its rate of change during the procedure are the variables that determine net alkali addition. If the bath contains HCO_3^-, more will be delivered if the patient's initial serum $[HCO_3^-]$ is lower and less will be delivered if it is higher. If the bath has no HCO_3^-, the rate of HCO_3^- loss from the patient to the bath is inversely related to the initial serum $[HCO_3^-]$. The initial serum $[HCO_3^-]$, in turn, is determined by endogenous acid production. This system, although clearly less flexible than functioning kidneys, allows for variations in diet-induced endogenous acid production to be compensated for by variable amounts of alkali delivery during renal replacement therapy, minimizing

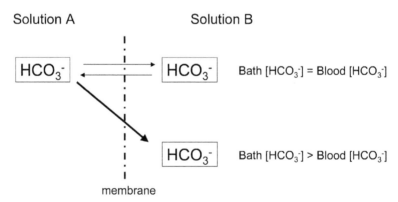

Net HCO_3^- diffusion (A→B) = f(permeability x surface area x Δ concentration)

Figure 1   Schematic representation of the forces controlling HCO_3^- entry from the dialysis bath solution to the patient's blood. If the blood concentration is equal to the bath, no net movement occurs regardless of the permeability of the membrane to HCO_3^-. If the bath concentration is higher than the blood concentration, then HCO_3^- will enter the blood at a rate determined by the permeability of the membrane to HCO_3^-, the surface area of the membrane, and the magnitude of the transmembrane concentration gradient for this anion.

variations in [HCO_3^-]. In addition, the system allows for acid balance to occur despite day-to-day variations in endogenous acid production. These general principles are applied to specific treatment modalities below.

Peritoneal Dialysis

Lactate is used to replenish alkali stores in peritoneal dialysis, with the exception of a rarely used technique that allows for the bath to contain bicarbonate (2,3), described later. Lactate uptake across the peritoneal membrane is directly related to the bath concentration, and the value has been adjusted empirically to 40 mmol/L to optimize serum [HCO_3^-] (4). The lactate in peritoneal dialysis solutions was racemic until recently, containing both D- and L-lactate. The L-lactate is metabolized rapidly, but D-lactate is metabolized more slowly, resulting in minor but measurable levels of this isomer in the blood when the racemic solution is used (5). This delay is of no significance with regard to steady-state [HCO_3^-], but D-lactate is no longer present in peritoneal dialysis solutions.

Figure 2 illustrates the metabolic and physical events relevant to acid–base homeostasis that occur during peritoneal dialysis. Lactate ions diffuse across the peritoneal membrane, enter cells coupled with H^+ and are metabolized to CO_2 and water. These transport and metabolic events generate new HCO_3^- in the extracellular compartment. Because the bath contains no HCO_3^-, a portion of this newly generated HCO_3^- diffuses back across the peritoneal membrane into the bath. Thus, new HCO_3^- is both generated and lost into the bath solution during peritoneal dialysis.

Dynamics of Alkali Transfer

The quantitative aspects of lactate and HCO_3^- movement and metabolism have been carefully studied in peritoneal dialysis using four exchanges a day, each with a 6-hr dwell time (6). During such a dwell, approximately 75% of the lactate delivered is absorbed and metabolized, yielding an equivalent amount of new HCO_3^-. At the same time, HCO_3^- diffuses into the bath so that after 6 hr bath [HCO_3^-] is ~80% of extracellular fluid [HCO_3^-]. Net alkali gain is the sum of these two vectors. From this information, one can easily estimate net alkali gain over a 24-hr period (Fig. 2). In a patient with a serum [HCO_3^-] of 24 mEq/L using four 2-L exchanges and removing 1.5 L of fluid/day, for example, 240 mmol of lactate is added and 182 mEq of HCO_3^- is lost each day, yielding a net alkali gain of 58 mEq.

Because HCO_3^- diffusion from the blood into the bath is directly related to serum [HCO_3^-] (7), one can immediately appreciate the linkage between alkali gain and the prevailing serum level. In a patient with the same dialysis prescription and a serum [HCO_3^-] of 16 mEq/L during the 24 hr of treatment, for example, HCO_3^- loss would fall to 122 mEq with no change in lactate delivery, and net alkali addition would rise to 118

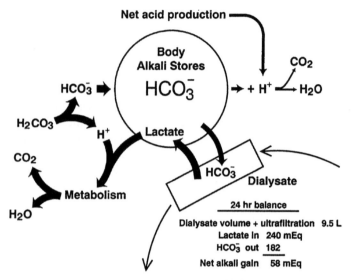

Figure 2   Schematic representation of lactate and HCO_3^- flux during peritoneal dialysis. HCO_3^- is consumed in buffering net acid production and replenished by the addition of lactate from the bath. These lactate anions are metabolized in the body, yielding new HCO_3^-. Because the bath solution contains no HCO_3^-, much of the new HCO_3^- produced diffuses from the patient into the bath solution. The rate of HCO_3^- loss is determined by the transmembrane concentration gradient, resulting in a new steady state at which serum $[HCO_3^-]$ is set — a level at which the difference between lactate added and HCO_3^- lost is equal to daily net acid production. *Source*: From Ref. 9.

mEq/24 hr. If alkali delivery exceeds acid production, serum $[HCO_3^-]$ will rise, limiting net alkali gain. Conversely, if alkali delivery is less than acid production, serum $[HCO_3^-]$ will fall, augmenting net alkali gain. Through iterations of this process at a constant net acid production, serum $[HCO_3^-]$ will settle at a value where alkali addition equals acid production. Note that the patient will then be in a new steady state in which essentially no acid will be retained, i.e., the patient will be in acid balance.

Acid Balance

These theoretical considerations have been tested by measuring acid balance in 19 stable patients receiving peritoneal dialysis (6). The patients had a higher average serum $[HCO_3^-]$ than in the example shown in Fig. 2, and as a result, net alkali addition was only 31 mEq/day. Nonetheless, this small gain equaled net acid production and the patients were in acid balance. A striking finding in these patients is the low rate of sulfate production and the high rate of organic acid production. The latter finding is not surprising, as organic anions (with the exception of lactate) are continuously lost into the bath solution during treatment. As a result, the normal cycle of organic acid production and metabolism is disrupted, and the organic anions lost obviously do not regenerate HCO_3^-. Sulfate generation was less than expected from estimated protein ingestion, a finding that remains unexplained. Organic acid production and loss accounted for approximately 70% of total net acid production in these patients, as compared to <50% in individuals with normal renal function. Sulfate production was entirely counterbalanced by dietary net alkali addition, and dialysis alkali addition matched organic anion loss. Endogenous acid production correlated with net alkali addition, as expected, and with protein catabolic rate, indicating that in the steady state protein catabolic rate, an easily calculated value, is a good index of acid production (see later) (6).

The average steady-state serum [total CO_2] (or [HCO_3^-]) in patients receiving peritoneal dialysis is shown in Table 1. As can be seen, the average values for venous [total CO_2] are generally in the middle of the range of normal. In one study in which arterial measurements were made in patients dialyzed using a lactate-containing bath, however, average serum [HCO_3^-] was only 22 mEq/L, indicating the presence of a mild metabolic acidosis (8).

Overnight Cycling Dialysis

The type of peritoneal dialysis described above has largely been replaced with overnight cycling using an automated exchange device. In this procedure,

Table 1 Steady-State Acid–Base Values in Patients Receiving Peritoneal Dialysis

Type	N	Venous [total CO_2] (mEq/L)	Reference
CAPD[a]	25	27.4 ± 3.3	4
	20	26.3 ± 2.5	48
	8	28.8 ± 3.0	6
	17	24.0 ± 3.1	1
CCPD[b]	13	27.9 ± 2.0	9

Type	N	Arterial [HCO_3^-] (mEq/L)	pH	PCO_2 (mmHg)	Reference
CAPD[a]	69	22.1 ± 3.1			8
CAPD[c]	9	22.0 ± 2.6	7.37 ± 0.04	38 ± 3.3	3
CAPD[d]	9	25.9 ± 2.0	7.42 ± 0.04	39 ± 3.6	3

Values shown are means ± 1 SD.
[a]CAPD, 4 exchanges/day, bath [Lactate] 40 mmol/L.
[b]CCPD, overnight cycling peritoneal dialysis, bath [Lactate] 40 mmol/L.
[c]HCO_3^- bath, [HCO_3^-] = 34 mEq/L.
[d]HCO_3^- bath, [HCO_3^-] = 39 mEq/L.

shorter dwell times are used and a larger volume of fluid is exchanged each day, allowing for better urea clearance. Because the rate of HCO_3^- diffusion across the peritoneal membrane is slightly higher than lactate (see above), shorter dwell times might increase alkali loss relative to lactate addition, and result in a lower serum [HCO_3^-]. Although no formal studies have been carried out, however, this newer form or peritoneal dialysis appears to have no discernible impact on steady-state venous [total CO_2] (Table 1).

HCO_3^--Containing Bath

Bicarbonate is the ideal alkali replacement for all dialysis bath solutions, but has not been used in peritoneal dialysis because of the problem of precipitation with calcium at alkaline pH values. This technical problem has been overcome by using a two-compartment dialysis bath bag (3,8). One compartment contains the HCO_3^- solution and the other, the calcium solution. The two compartments are mixed just as the solution is infused into the peritoneal space, where the prevailing CO_2 tension keeps pH in a range that prevents calcium precipitation. Serum [HCO_3^-] is directly related to bath [HCO_3^-] using a HCO_3^--containing bath, with higher values achieved when the bath concentration is increased from 34 to 39 mEq/L (see Table 1) (3). The increase in serum [HCO_3^-] after the switch to the bath solution with the higher [HCO_3^-] is inversely correlated with endogenous acid production (estimated from protein catabolic rate) (3), demonstrating the dependence of steady-state serum [HCO_3^-] on acid production.

Although venous [total CO_2] is essentially normal in patients using lactate-based peritoneal dialysis solutions (Table 1), it has been argued that [total CO_2] is below the normal range in approximately half the patients, and that the normal average value is due to a small subset of patients with metabolic alkalosis (8). Moreover, average arterial [HCO_3^-] in these patients is lower than normal (8). Despite this argument, the additional expense and inconvenience of the HCO_3^--based solution has not gained wide acceptance. It is very effective in reducing symptoms in patients with infusion pain, perhaps the best argument for its use (2).

Conventional Hemodialysis

Conventional hemodialysis is an intermittent treatment, and therefore, no day-to-day steady-state exists with regard to alkali stores and serum [HCO_3^-].]. Serum [HCO_3^-] increases rapidly as alkali is added during dialysis, and it then falls gradually between treatments as the added alkali is consumed by endogenous acid production (Fig. 3). Given this fluctuation in serum [HCO_3^-], by as much as 7–8 mEq/L from the end of one dialysis to the beginning of the next, it is important to note when acid–base status is assessed (9). By convention, [HCO_3^-] is measured predialysis. Ideally, the nadir predialysis value should be measured (68–70 hr after the last treatment).

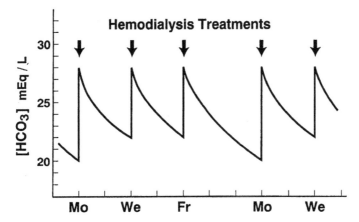

Figure 3 Schematic representation of the changes in serum [HCO$_3^-$] that occur with conventional hemodialysis three times a week. Serum [HCO$_3^-$] is intermittently lower than normal and falls to its nadir once a week at the end of the longest interval between treatments. *Source*: From Ref. 9.

Bath Alkali—Past and Present

When hemodialysis was first developed, HCO$_3^-$ was added to the bath solution in a concentration matching normal serum [HCO$_3^-$] (10). To prevent calcium precipitation, 5% CO$_2$ was continuously bubbled through the bath

Table 2 Predialysis Acid–Base Values in Patients Receiving Conventional Hemodialysis[a]

Year	N	[Total CO$_2$] (mEq/L)	Reference
1990[b]	22	21.4 ± 2.4	48
1993	38	19.0 ± 3.1	26
1996[b]	44	20.4 ± 2.0	1
1999	995	21.6 ± 3.4	28
2000[c]	7123	22.8 ± 3.5	29
2002[b]	80	22.9 ± 3.3	9

Year	N	[HCO$_3^-$]	pH	PCO$_2$ (mmHg)	Reference
1982	10	18.9 ± 2.5	7.37 ± 0.09	33 ± 2.5	20
1983	10	20.2[d]	7.40 ± 0.04	33 ± 1.2	22
1985	16	19.8 ± 1.2	7.37 ± 0.02	36 ± 1.9	13
1987	12	22.1 ± 2.9	7.38 ± 0.04	38 ± 5.1	13

Values shown are means ± 1 SD.
[a]Three times weekly with a bicarbonate bath (final concentration 32–36 mEq/L).
[b]Values obtained after longest interval between treatments.
[c]Mid-week pre-dialysis value.
[d]Calculated from mean pH and PCO$_2$.

solution to keep the pH <7.6. This cumbersome technique required a gas tank for each treatment. Bath [HCO_3^-] was gradually increased from 27 to 35 mEq/L over the ensuing decade to attempt to restore serum [HCO_3^-] to a normal level. In the early 1960s, acetate was shown to be an effective alkali precursor for hemodialysis (11), removing the problem of calcium precipitation. Because it simplified bath preparation, acetate quickly replaced HCO_3^- in the dialysis bath solution.

The dynamics of alkali transfer with a bath solution containing only acetate are impressive. As quickly as the added acetate is metabolized to produce HCO_3^-, the newly produced HCO_3^- is lost back into the bath (12). As a result, the only way to add alkali effectively is to deliver acetate faster than its rate of metabolism. This goal was achieved by setting bath acetate concentration at 37–40 mmol/L. Once dialysis is stopped, the retained acetate is metabolized, increasing serum [HCO_3^-] by 3–4 mEq/L. During an average treatment, approximately 1000 mmol of acetate was added and 800 mEq of HCO_3^- was lost (12).

As dialysis blood flow rates and membrane surface area increased to achieve better urea clearance, the rate of acetate delivery also increased and serum acetate reached toxic levels, causing hypotension and other symptoms (13–15). The increased acetate delivery was matched by increased HCO_3^- loss, so that little was gained in terms of correcting acidosis (16). An additional problem was CO_2 loss into the bath. This new route of CO_2 excretion reduced ventilatory drive, leading to hypoventilation and hypoxemia during dialysis and contributing to symptoms and morbidity (17,18). The problems of acetate toxicity, hypoventilation, and the inherent limitation in the ability to correct metabolic acidosis, led to a return to HCO_3^- in the bath solution in hemodialysis in the 1980s (13,19,20).

Reintroduction of HCO_3^- into the dialysate solution was made possible by a new technology, the use of proportioning pumps that allow continuous production of dialysate from concentrated salt solutions during treatment. Using these concentrates, the problem of calcium precipitation was easily solved by keeping the HCO_3^- solution separate from the calcium-containing solution until just prior to delivery to the patient. In addition, a small amount of acetic acid (3–4 mmol/L) was added to the calcium-containing solution. When the two concentrates are diluted and mixed, the acetic acid immediately reacts with a small fraction of the HCO_3^- producing H_2CO_3 and acetate, the former maintaining pH low during the brief time between mixing and contact with the dialysis membrane, and the latter providing a small additional source of alkali. At a temperature of 37°C, this reaction causes PCO_2 in the solution to rise to 133 mmHg. As soon as the solution comes in contact with blood (across the dialysis membrane), the small amount of CO_2 produced diffuses into the blood and has no detectable impact on systemic PCO_2 (16,21). This new HCO_3^- dialysate system delivered alkali more effectively, increasing predialysis serum [HCO_3^-] by approximately 3 mEq/L (as compared to acetate dialysate), as well as reducing symptoms and ending the problem of CO_2 loss (13,19,22). As a result, HCO_3^- quickly replaced acetate in the hemodialysis bath solution.

The most commonly used hemodialysis bath now is made from two concentrates, one diluting to 39 mEq/L of HCO_3^- and the other to 4 mmol/L of acetic acid. When combined, they create a solution with a $[HCO_3^-]$ of 35 mEq/L and [acetate] of 4 mEq/L. Because acetate enters the blood and is completely metabolized, this combination is equivalent to a total alkali concentration of 39 mEq/L. Bath $[HCO_3^-]$ can now easily be adjusted between 25 and 40 mEq/L, as needed.

Dynamics of Alkali Transfer

Movement of HCO_3^- and acetate across the membrane is dependent on the dialysance of these anions (a function of blood and dialysate flow rates, permeability and surface area) and the transmembrane concentration gradient (ΔC) (Fig. 4). Because the small amount of acetate that enters the blood is rapidly metabolized, ΔC for acetate remains constant and entry is limited only by membrane permeability and delivery rate (dialysance). By contrast, ΔC for $[HCO_3^-]$ changes rapidly during treatment as HCO_3^- is added and increases serum $[HCO_3^-]$. For a given dialysis prescription, HCO_3^- dialysance is fixed by the membrane chosen and by holding blood and dialysate flow rates constant, so that the change in ΔC from moment-to-moment is the main determinant of HCO_3^- entry. The rate of change in ΔC depends on the disposition of the added HCO_3^-. Bicarbonate addition increases systemic pH and, as a result, some of the HCO_3^- is buffered immediately by nonbicarbonate buffers (hemoglobin, plasma proteins, phosphate, and other organic buffers). In addition, the increase in pH stimulates organic acid production, consuming an additional fraction of the added HCO_3^-. The organic anions produced by this reaction are rapidly lost into the dialysis bath solution, thus representing irreversible consumption of alkali (1). The remainder of the added HCO_3^- is added to the body alkali pool and raises serum $[HCO_3^-]$, reducing ΔC (Fig. 4).

The magnitude of the increase in organic acid production and loss during hemodialysis is difficult to measure; values of 30–100 mEq/treatment were estimated to occur in early studies, based on blood and dialysate measurements (23–25). Because only a few organic anions were measured in these studies, total losses were probably higher than reported. In addition, total losses are likely to be higher now due to higher blood flow rates and more efficient dialysis membranes. Using serum lactate levels and the estimated dialysance for this anion, for example, as much as 50 mmol of lactate alone may be lost during a standard treatment with the blood and dialysis flow rates currently used.

The pattern of change in serum $[HCO_3^-]$ during hemodialysis is easier to measure, and reflects the summation of buffer reactions and organic acid

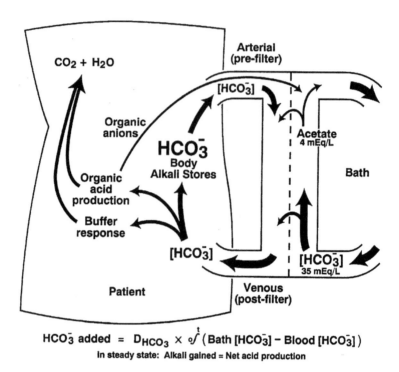

$$\text{HCO}_3^- \text{ added} = D_{\text{HCO}_3} \times \int^t (\text{Bath } [\text{HCO}_3^-] - \text{Blood } [\text{HCO}_3^-])$$

In steady state: Alkali gained = Net acid production

Figure 4 Schematic representation of alkali addition and disposition during conventional hemodialysis. During the treatment, HCO_3^- and acetate are added, each entering down its concentration gradient. The HCO_3^- added, plus that generated by acetate metabolism, is partially consumed by titration with body buffers and by organic acid production. The remainder is added to the body pool and raises the $[\text{HCO}_3^-]$ in the blood re-entering the dialysis circuit, reducing the gradient and decreasing the rate of HCO_3^- entry. The amount of HCO_3^- added during each treatment is a function of its dialysance (D_{HCO_3}) and the integral over time of the transmembrane concentration gradient (bath $[\text{HCO}_3^-]$ – blood $[\text{HCO}_3^-]$). *Source*: From Ref. 9.

production. Strikingly, virtually all the increase occurs during the first 2 hr of treatment in stable dialysis patients (Fig. 5) (9,21). Moreover, end-dialysis serum $[\text{HCO}_3^-]$ uniformly falls far short of bath $[\text{HCO}_3^-]$, despite the high dialysance of this anion and the favorable transmembrane concentration gradient (9,21,26). Three patterns of change in serum $[\text{HCO}_3^-]$ occur in unselected patients (1,9). In the majority of patients, serum $[\text{HCO}_3^-]$ rises rapidly, and then remains essentially stable during the last 2 hr. In a small fraction, serum $[\text{HCO}_3^-]$ continues to rise, although at a slower rate. Finally in some patients, serum $[\text{HCO}_3^-]$ actually falls during the last 2 hr of treatment. When one tries to model the behavior of the system, this variation

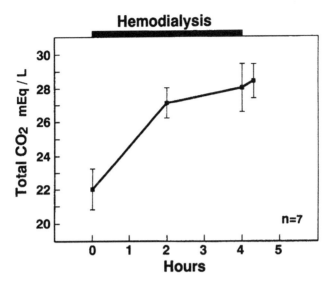

Figure 5   Pattern of change in serum [total CO_2] during 4 hr of hemodialysis in seven stable patients. [Total CO_2] was measured immediately before dialysis, after 2 and 4 hr of dialysis, and 15 min after completing the treatment. The brackets around the data points are equal to ± 1 SE. Note that virtually the entire increase in [total CO_2] occurs during the first 2 hr of treatment. *Source*: From Ref. 9.

can be accounted for differential surges in organic acid production and loss (1), but this postulate remains unproven. Another possibility is that charge constraints (charge balance between cations and anions diffusing across the dialysis membrane) limit HCO_3^- flux during the later part of dialysis. Regardless of the mechanism, serum [HCO_3^-] increases by only 4–8 mEq/L during a typical treatment (9,21,26,27).

Acid Balance

As indicated earlier, alkali addition during hemodialysis is regulated by serum [HCO_3^-] for any fixed dialysis prescription. When predialysis serum [HCO_3^-] is lower, more will be added and when it is higher, less will be added (1). Given this dynamic, it seems likely that a new balance is achieved in the steady state in which alkali addition during dialysis matches alkali consumption in the period between dialysis treatments. If true then continuous acid retention should not occur; that is, patients receiving hemodialysis should be in acid balance (1,12).

    In one study, daily acid production was estimated from the reduction in serum [HCO_3^-] between dialysis treatments (27). In this study, acid production averaged only ~30 mEq/day, a value lower than predicted from protein consumption. The decrease in net acid production is almost certainly due to decreased organic anion excretion. In anephric patients, no organic anions are lost in the urine, and the retained anions inhibit further production. Because acid production was calculated from the fall in serum $[HCO_3^-]$ between treatments and not measured directly in this study, acid balance was present, by definition (i.e., acid production matched alkali delivery during treatment). Although this analysis supports the theoretical concepts presented earlier (1,12), it does not definitively answer the question of whether acid balance occurs. As predicted by this formulation, predialysis serum $[HCO_3^-]$ correlates inversely with protein catabolic rate, a measure of acid production (27–29). Whether acid balance is achieved with intermittent hemodialysis may not be the important issue. The prevailing predialysis serum $[HCO_3^-]$ itself is the important determinant of overall morbidity (30).

The nonsteady-state conditions of hemodialysis raise concerns about bone calcium loss in the period between treatments that may preclude real acid balance from occurring. Titration of bone buffers (calcium carbonate) by retained acid in the period between treatments likely occurs and serves to reduce the magnitude of the fall in serum $[HCO_3^-]$. To the extent that calcium and alkali lost from bone minimizes this fall, less HCO_3^- will be delivered with the subsequent treatment than is needed to restore bone alkali. Although the extent to which titration of bone alkali occurs during the brief period between treatments is unknown, the intermittent acidosis induced by three times a week hemodialysis has been shown to contribute to renal osteodystrophy by promoting bone calcium loss (31,32).

Predialysis Serum $[HCO_3^-]$

Table 2 and Fig. 6 summarize predialysis serum [total CO_2] or $[HCO_3^-]$ values obtained in stable patients receiving three treatments a week. These data indicate that a mild metabolic acidosis is present just prior to treatment in most patients. The ventilatory response to the low serum $[HCO_3^-]$ is normal, minimizing the change in pH that occurs (12,13,25,33). Because it is mild and only intermittent, this metabolic acidosis was not considered to be a problem (12). It is now clear, however, that this mild and intermittent acidosis has adverse effects on bone and muscle metabolism (31,32,34,35). In addition, a low predialysis serum $[HCO_3^-]$ is an adverse factor for patient survival (30).

Factors Influencing Predialysis Serum $[HCO_3^-]$

Predialysis serum $[HCO_3^-]$ is determined primarily by three factors: (i) the specific dialysis prescription, (ii) the daily rate of endogenous acid production, and (iii) the amount of fluid retention between treatments. The specific dialysis prescription determines the amount of alkali delivered and therefore the serum $[HCO_3^-]$ achieved at the end of the dialysis treatment. Endogenous acid production and fluid retention determine the rate

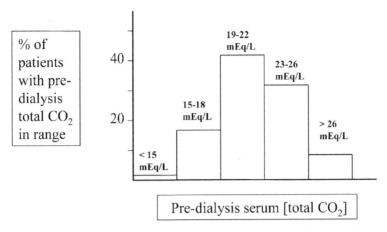

Figure 6 Percentage distribution of predialysis serum [total CO_2] in 995 patients receiving conventional hemodialysis. *Source*: Recalculated from Ref. 28.

of fall from the value achieved at the end of dialysis. Acid production titrates body alkali stores during the period between treatments, and fluid retention without alkali dilutes these stores.

Using some simple assumptions one can estimate the impact of these latter two factors on predialysis serum [HCO_3^-] (Table 3) (1,9). In this model, a patient with an end-dialysis serum [HCO_3^-] of 28 mEq/L, daily endogenous acid production of 40 mEq and an interdialytic fluid gain of 2 L is predicted to have a predialysis [HCO_3^-] of 23.4, whereas predialysis [HCO_3^-] in the same patient will be 6 mEq/L lower (17.3 mEq/L) if his

Table 3 Estimated Effect of Changes in Endogenous Acid Production and Fluid Retention on Predialysis Serum [HCO_3^-] in Patients Receiving Hemodialysis Three Times a Week

Acid production (mEq/day)	Fluid retention[a] (L/interval)	Predialysis [HCO_3^-][b] (mEq/L)
40	2	23.4
80	2	20.4
120	2	17.3
60	0	23.1
60	3	21.3
60	6	19.8

Assumptions: Wt = 70 kg; postdialysis serum [HCO_3^-] = 28 mEq/L; HCO_3^- buffer space = 0.5 × body weight (kg).
[a]Liters retained during longest interval between treatments.
[b]After longest interval between treatments (68 hr).

endogenous acid production rate is 120 mEq/day. This analysis is supported by observations showing an inverse correlation between protein catabolic rate and predialysis serum $[HCO_3^-]$ in hemodialysis patients (27). In addition, predialysis serum $[HCO_3^-]$ can readily be increased by oral alkali administration in the interdialytic period, reducing net acid production (36).

A similar analysis can be made to evaluate the influence of fluid retention (Table 3). For this analysis, endogenous acid production is held constant and fluid retention is varied between 0 and 6 L. This analysis predicts that predialysis serum $[HCO_3^-]$ falls by ~0.5 mEq/L for each liter of fluid retained in the period between treatments. This prediction is also supported by experimental observations showing that retention of as little as 1 L of additional fluid in the interval between treatments reduces predialysis $[HCO_3^-]$ (37).

Influence of Bath $[HCO_3^-]$ on Serum $[HCO_3^-]$

In stable patients, predialysis serum $[HCO_3^-]$ can easily be increased by increasing bath $[HCO_3^-]$ (Table 4). This beneficial change is directly related to the increase in postdialysis serum $[HCO_3^-]$ achieved, which, in the absence of any change in acid production or fluid retention, exerts a parallel effect on the nadir serum $[HCO_3^-]$ prior to the next treatment. Given the wide variation in predialysis serum $[HCO_3^-]$ (Fig. 6), individualizing bath $[HCO_3^-]$ to achieve optimal acid–base values predialysis has been recommended (38). An alternative approach is to increase bath $[HCO_3^-]$ for all patients. Additional long-term studies are needed before these recommendations are accepted.

Daily Hemodialysis

Daily hemodialysis treatments, either in critically ill inpatients or in stable outpatients, readily normalizes serum $[HCO_3^-]$ and pH (39–41). In stable

Table 4 Improving Predialysis Serum $[HCO_3^-]$ in Conventional Hemodialysis: Techniques and Results

N	Duration (months)	$[HCO_3^-]$ (mEq/L)		Technique	Reference
		Baseline	Treatment		
11	18	15.6	24.0	↑ Bath $[HCO_3^-]$ to 40–48 mEq/L	32
38	3	19.0	24.8	↑ Bath $[HCO_3^-]$ to 39 mEq/L	26
8	1	18.6	25.3	↑ Bath $[HCO_3^-]$ to 40 mEq/L	31
6	1	18.5	24.8	↑ Bath $[HCO_3^-]$ to 40 + oral NaHCO$_3$	34
9	1	20.0	25.0	↑ Bath $[HCO_3^-]$ to 40 + oral NaHCO$_3$	49
21	6	20.4	23.3	↑ Bath $[HCO_3^-]$ to 40 mEq/L	35
25	6	22.5	26.7	↑ Bath $[HCO_3^-]$ to 40 mEq/L	35

outpatients receiving daily hemodialysis treatments, the difference between pre- and postdialysis serum [HCO_3^-] is reduced to <1 mEq/L and bath [HCO_3^-] has been reduced to 28–32 mEq/L to avoid metabolic alkalosis (40). These results are not surprising, given the above analysis of the determinants of serum [HCO_3^-].

Continuous Renal Replacement Therapies

Continuous hemofiltration, hemofiltration plus dialysis, and slow low-efficiency hemodialysis are all currently used for the treatment of renal failure in critically ill patients (42,43). With these techniques, the same principles hold with regard to acid–base homeostasis as discussed earlier for conventional hemodialysis. With continuous hemofiltration HCO_3^- loss is related to the serum concentration and the ultrafiltration rate, as well as the ongoing rate of endogenous acid production. Replacement is achieved with a continuous infusion of either a HCO_3^- or lactate-containing solution (43,44), and serum [HCO_3^-] is readily maintained within the range of normal. With continuous slow low-efficiency dialysis, equilibrium between bath and serum [HCO_3^-] occurs and dialysis concentration must be reduced to 24–28 mEq/L, L, *inordertopreventthedevelopmentofmetabolicalkalosis*(42).

Hemofiltration and Hemodiafiltration

Hemofiltration has also been used as an intermittent therapy in stable patients. To achieve adequate clearance, high-volume ultrafiltration occurs during the procedure, requiring rapid infusion of replacement fluids (45). With this procedure, HCO_3^--containing replacement fluids are necessary to maintain a normal predialysis serum [HCO_3^-] (45). Hemodiafiltration combines the convective characteristics of hemofiltration with a bath solution containing acetate or HCO_3^- (46). This procedure has the same complexity as hemofiltration and little advantage over conventional hemodialysis from an acid–base perspective.

Acetate-free biofiltration is a hemodiafiltration technique using a bath solution that contains no HCO_3^- or acetate (47). High-volume ultrafiltration is carried out, and only $NaHCO_3$ needs to be infused into the postfilter blood. Because only HCO_3^- is infused, the concentration can easily be adjusted to increase serum [HCO_3^-] to the level desired in each patient (47). The proposed advantage for acetate-free biofiltration is the absence of acetate in the bath, but there is no evidence that the small amount of acetate currently present in bath solutions has any toxicity.

SUMMARY

In patients without renal function, alkali administration replaces acid excretion as the means to maintain body HCO_3^- stores. Although indifferent to body pH, dialysis therapy varies the rate of alkali delivery in response to variations in serum [HCO_3^-] because net HCO_3^- addition is a function of its transmembrane concentration gradient. Dialysis therapy therefore allows for homeostatic flexibility, with more alkali being added during treatment if serum [HCO_3^-] is low and less if it is high. The change in serum [HCO_3^-] between treatments is dependent on the rate of endogenous acid production and to a lesser extent on fluid retention. Understanding these principles is central for assessment of acid–base homeostasis in patients with end-stage renal disease, and for intervening to change serum [HCO_3^-]. In the following chapter, these principles will be used to detect and treat abnormalities in acid–base homeostasis in this group of patients.

REFERENCES

1. Gennari FJ. Acid–base homeostasis in end-stage renal disease. Semin Dial 1996; 9:404–411.
2. Mactier RA, Sprosen TS, Gokal R, Williams PF, Lindbergh M, Naik RB, Wrege U, Gröntoft KC, Larsson R, Berglund J, Tranaeus AP, Faict D. Bicarbonate and bicarbonate/lactate peritoneal dialysis solutions for the treatment of infusion pain. Kidney Int 1998; 53:1061–1067.
3. Feriani M, Carobi C, La Greca G, Buoncristiani U, Passlick-Deetjen J. Clinical experience with a 39 mmol/L bicarbonate-buffered peritoneal dialysis solution. Perit Dial Int 1997; 17:17–21.
4. Nolph KD, Prowant B, Serkes KD, Morgan L, Baker B, Charytan C, Gham K, Hamburger R, Husserl F, Kleit S, McGuinness J, Moore H, Warren T. Multicenter evaluation of a new peritoneal dialysis solution with a high lactate and a low magnesium concentration. Perit Dial Bull 1983; 3:63–65.
5. Yasuda T, Ozawa S, Shiba C, Maeba T, Kanazawa T, Sugiyama M, Owada S, Ishida M. D-lactate metabolism in patients with chronic renal failure undergoing CAPD. Nephron 1993; 63:416–422.
6. Uribarri J, Buquing J, Oh MS. Acid–base balance in chronic peritoneal dialysis patients. Kidney Int 1995; 47:269–273.
7. Feriani M, Ronco C, La Greca G. Acid–base balance with different CAPD solutions. Perit Dial Int 1996; 16:S126–S129.
8. Feriani M. Use of different buffers in peritoneal dialysis. Semin Dial 2000; 13:256–260.
9. Gennari FJ. Acid–base considerations in end-stage renal disease. In: Henrich WL, ed. Principles and Practice of Dialysis. Baltimore, MD: Williams and Wilkins, 2003:393–407.
10. Murphy WP, Swan RC, Walter CW, Weller JM, Merrill JP. Use of an artificial kidney. III: Current procedures in clinical hemodialysis. J Lab Clin Med 1952; 40:436–444.
11. Mion CM, Hegstrom RM, Boen ST, Scribner BH. Substitution of sodium acetate for sodium bicarbonate in the bath fluid for hemodialysis. Trans Am Soc Artif Intern Organs 1964; 10:110–113.
12. Gennari FJ. Acid–base balance in dialysis patients. Kidney Int 1985; 28:678–688.

13. Hakim RM, Pontzer MA, Tilton D, Lazarus JM, Gottlieb MN. Effects of acetate and bicarbonate dialysate in stable chronic dialysis patients. Kidney Int 1985; 28:535–540.

14. Vinay P, Prud'Homme M, Vinet B, Cournoyer G, Degoulet P, Leville M, Gougoux A, St-Louis G, Lapierre L, Piette Y. Acetate metabolism and bicarbonate generation during hemodialysis: 10 years of observation. Kidney Int 1987; 31:1194–1204.

15. Graefe U, Milutinovich J, Follette WC, Vizzo JE, Babb AL, Scribner BH. Less dialysis-induced morbidity and vascular instability with bicarbonate in dialysate. Ann Intern Med 1978; 88:332–336.

16. Tolchin N, Roberts JL, Hayashi J, Lewis EJ. Metabolic consequences of high mass-transfer hemodialysis. Kidney Int 1977; 11:366–378.

17. Dolan MJ, Whipp BJ, Davidson WD, Weitzman RE, Wasserman K. Hypopnea associated with acetate hemodialysis: carbon dioxide-flow- dependent ventilation. N Engl J Med 1981; 305:72–75.

18. Hunt JM, Chappell TR, Henrich WL, Rubin LJ. Gas exchange during dialysis. Contrasting mechanisms contributing to comparable alterations with acetate and bicarbonate buffers. Am J Med 1984; 77:255–260.

19. Ward RA, Wathen RL, Williams TE. Effects of long-term bicarbonate hemodialysis on acid–base status. Trans Am Soc Artif Intern Organs 1982; 28:295–298.

20. Man NK, Fournier G, Thireau P, Gaillard JL, Funck-Brentano JL. Effect of bicarbonate-containing dialysate on chronic hemodialysis patients: a comparative study. Artif Organs 1982; 6:421–428.

21. Symreng T, Flanigan MJ, Lim VS. Ventilatory and metabolic changes during high efficiency hemodialysis. Kidney Int 1992; 41:1064–1069.

22. Henrich WL, Woodard TD, Meyer BD, Chappell TR, Rubin LJ. High sodium bicarbonate and acetate hemodialysis: double-blind crossover comparison of hemodynamic and ventilatory effects. Kidney Int 1983; 24:240–245.

23. Ward RA, Wathen RL, Williams TE, Harding GB. Hemodialysate composition and intradialytic metabolic, acid–base and potassium changes. Kidney Int 1987; 32:129–135.

24. Gotch FA, Sargent JA, Keen ML. Hydrogen ion balance in dialysis therapy. Artif Organs 1982; 6:388–395.

25. Vreman HJ, Assomull VM, Kaiser BA, Blaschke TF, Weiner MW. Acetate metabolism and acid–base homeostasis during hemodialysis: influence of dialyzer efficiency and rate of acetate metabolism. Kidney Int Suppl 1980; 10: S62–S74.

26. Oettinger CW, Oliver JC. Normalization of uremic acidosis in hemodialysis patients with a high bicarbonate dialysate. J Am Soc Nephrol 1993; 3:1804–1807.

27. Uribarri J, Zia M, Mahmood J, Marcus RA, Oh MS. Acid production in chronic hemodialysis patients. J Am Soc Nephrol 1998; 9:114–120.

28. Uribarri J, Levin NW, Delmez J, Depner TA, Ornt D, Owen W, Yan G. Association of acidosis and nutritional parameters in hemodialysis patients. Am J Kidney Dis 1999; 34:493–499.

29. Chauveau P, Fouque D, Combe C, Laville M, Canaud B, Azar R, Cano N, Aparicio M, Leverve X. Acidosis and nutritional status in hemodialyzed

patients. French Study Group for Nutrition in Dialysis. Semin Dial 2000; 13:241–246.

30. Lowrie EG, Lew NL. Death risk in hemodialysis patients: the predictive value of commonly measured variables and an evaluation of death rate differences between facilities. Am J Kidney Dis 1990; 15:458–482.

31. Graham KA, Hoenich NA, Tarbit M, Ward MK, Goodship TH. Correction of acidosis in hemodialysis patients increases the sensitivity of the parathyroid glands to calcium. J Am Soc Nephrol 1997; 8:627–631.

32. Lefebvre A, de Vernejoul MC, Gueris J, Goldfarb B, Graulet AM, Morieux C. Optimal correction of acidosis changes progression of dialysis osteodystrophy. Kidney Int 1989; 36:1112–1118.

33. Bushinsky DA, Coe FL, Katzenberg C, Szidon JP, Parks JH. Arterial PCO_2 in chronic metabolic acidosis. Kidney Int 1982; 22:311–314.

34. Graham KA, Reaich D, Channon SM, Downie S, Goodship TH. Correction of acidosis in hemodialysis decreases whole-body protein degradation. J Am Soc Nephrol 1997; 8:632–637.

35. Williams AJ, Dittmer ID, McArley A, Clarke J. High bicarbonate dialysate in haemodialysis patients: effects on acidosis and nutritional status. Nephrol Dial Transplant 1997; 12:2633–2637.

36. Kooman JP, Deutz NE, Zijlmans P, van den Wall Bake A, Gerlag PG, van Hooff JP, Leunissen KM. The influence of bicarbonate supplementation on plasma levels of branched-chain amino acids in haemo dialysis patients with metabolic acidosis. Nephrol Dial Transplant 1997; 12:2397–2401.

37. Fabris A, LaGreca G, Chiaramonte S, Feriani M, Brendolan A, Bragantini L, Dell'Aquila R, Pellanda MV, Crepaldi C, Ronco C. The importance of ultra-filtration on acid–base status in a dialysis population. ASAIO Trans 1988; 34:200–201.

38. Thews O. Model-based decision support system for individual prescription of the dialysate bicarbonate concentration in hemodialysis. Int J Artif Organs 1992; 15:447–455.

39. Buoncristiani U. Fifteen years of clinical experience with daily haemodialysis. Nephrol Dial Transplant 1998; 13(suppl 6):148–151.

40. Pierratos A, Ouwendyk M, Francoeur R, Vas S, Raj DS, Ecclestone AM, Langos V, Uldall R. Nocturnal hemodialysis: three-year experience. J Am Soc Nephrol 1998; 9859–868.

41. Zimmerman D, Cotman P, Ting R, Karanicolas S, Tobe SW. Continuous veno-venous haemodialysis with a novel bicarbonate dialysis solution: prospective cross-over comparison with a lactate buffered solution. Nephrol Dial Transplant 1999; 14:2387–2391.

42. Marshall MR, Golper TA, Shaver MJ, Alam MG, Chatoth DK. Sustained low-efficiency dialysis for critically ill patients requiring renal replacement therapy. Kidney Int 2001; 60:777–785.

43. Manns M, Sigler MH, Teehan BP. Continuous renal replacement therapies: an update. Am J Kidney Dis 1998; 32:185–207.

44. McLean AG, Davenport A, Cox D, Sweny P. Effects of lactate-buffered and lactate-free dialysate in CAVHD patients with and without liver dysfunction. Kidney Int 2000; 58:1765–1772.

45. Santoro A, Ferrari G, Bolzani R, Spongano M, Zucchelli P. Regulation of base balance in bicarbonate hemofiltration. Int J Artif Organs 1994; 17:27–36.
46. Biasioli S, Feriani M, Chiaramonte S, Cavallini L, Cesaro A, Fazion S, Petrosino L, Porena P, Zambello A. Different buffers for hemodiafiltration: a controlled study. Int J Artif Organs 1989; 12:25–30.
47. Santoro A, Spongano M, Ferrari G, Bolzani R, Augella F, Borghi M, Briganti M, Cagnoli L, Docci D, Feletti C, Fusaroli M, Gattiani A, Sanna G, Stallone C, Zuchelli P. Analysis of the factors influencing bicarbonate balance during acetate-free biofiltration. Kidney Int Suppl 1993; 41:S184–S187.
48. Gennari FJ. Acid–base disorders in end-stage renal disease: Part I. Semin Dial 1990; 3:81–85.
49. Harris DC, Yuill E, Chesher DW. Correcting acidosis in hemodialysis: effect on phosphate clearance and calcification risk. J Am Soc Nephrol 1995; 6: 1607–1612.

24

Acid–Base Disorders in Dialysis Patients

F. John Gennari

University of Vermont College of Medicine, Burlington, Vermont, U.S.A.

INTRODUCTION

The spectrum of acid–base disorders that can occur in patients receiving renal replacement therapy is narrower and in some ways unique, compared to patients with functioning kidneys (1,2). In the absence of kidney function, one need not consider acid–base disorders induced by changes in renal electrolyte and acid excretion. For the same reason, exogenous alkali administration can induce sustained metabolic alkalosis in these patients. The general approach to identifying acid–base disorders in dialysis patients, nonetheless, is the same as in patients with functioning kidneys (see Chapter 28). The clinician must identify the primary disorder (e.g., metabolic acidosis or alkalosis, respiratory acidosis or alkalosis), determine whether the secondary response is appropriate, assess the anion gap, and determine the cause.

IDENTIFYING AN ACID–BASE DISORDER

The presence of metabolic acidosis or alkalosis is signaled by an abnormal serum [total CO_2] or [HCO_3^-] (Fig. 1). One need not consider respiratory alkalosis or acidosis as causes for the abnormality because serum [HCO_3^-] does not change in these disorders in the absence of renal function. As a result, respiratory disorders must be suspected on clinical grounds and verified by measurements of $PaCO_2$ and pH.

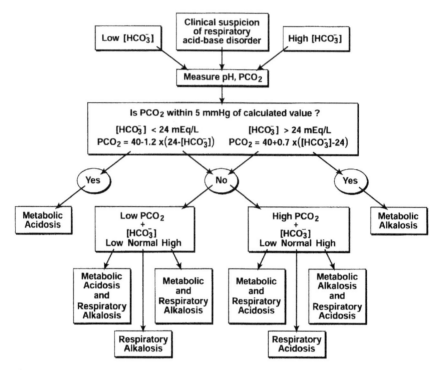

Figure 1 Approach to the recognition and diagnosis of acid–base disorders in patients with end-stage renal disease. The terms "low [HCO₃⁻]" and "high [HCO₃⁻]" refer to serum values that are 3 or more mEq/L lower or higher than the average values found in patients receiving the same dialysis therapy, or a change in [HCO₃⁻] of 3 or more mEq/L when compared with prior values in the same patient. *Source*: From Ref. 6.

In patients with end-stage renal disease, serum [total CO_2] is determined by the form of renal replacement therapy used (see Chapter 23), and thus abnormal values must be defined in the context of the specific treatment. Average "normal" values in patients receiving either conventional hemodialysis (three times weekly) or peritoneal dialysis are shown in Table 1. The average value for hemodialysis is based on predialysis measurements, but recall that serum [HCO₃⁻] rises to as high as 30 mEq/L immediately after dialysis and then falls gradually during the interval between treatments. Thus, the time of measurement in relation to the last treatment is critical for assessment of an abnormality. For patients receiving peritoneal dialysis, serum [HCO₃⁻] is stable from day-to-day and the average values are higher. Because of patient-to-patient variability, the best diagnostic tool for identifying a new metabolic acid–base disorder in any dialysis patient is comparison to a recent prior serum [total CO_2]. If one identifies an abnormally low [total CO_2], one should be certain that the blood sample has been handled in an appropriate manner for analysis before concluding that a new metabolic acidosis is present. Long delays in analysis without appropriate refrigeration or prolonged exposure to air can spuriously reduce serum [total CO_2] by up to 4 mEq/L (3–5).

DIAGNOSIS OF SPECIFIC DISORDERS

Metabolic Acidosis

The vast majority of patients receiving conventional hemodialysis have an intermittent metabolic acidosis. The implications and management of this acidosis are discussed in Chapter 23. The focus of this chapter is to provide tools to diagnose the presence of a new metabolic acidosis, i.e., one that develops independent of the specific dialysis prescription. A new metabolic acidosis is defined empirically as a serum [HCO_3^-] or [total CO_2] that is 3 or more mEq/L below either the average predialysis value in patients receiving hemodialysis or the average steady-state value in patients receiving peritoneal dialysis (one SD for both forms of therapy) (1,6). Comparison with a prior serum [total CO_2] in the same patient provides the most useful information; a new acute metabolic acidosis is manifest by finding an abrupt decrease of 3 or more mEq/L.

Metabolic Alkalosis

Metabolic alkalosis is defined empirically as a serum [HCO_3^-] or [total CO_2] that is 3 or more mEq/L higher than the average predialysis value in patients receiving hemodialysis or the average steady-state value in patients receiving peritoneal dialysis (Table 1) (2,6). The best information, again, is comparison with the patient's own baseline value.

Respiratory Acidosis and Alkalosis

Respiratory acidosis or alkalosis must be suspected on clinical grounds, because $PaCO_2$ is not routinely measured in dialysis patients and serum

Table 1 Average [Total CO_2] Values for Dialysis Patients

	N	mEq/L	Reference
Conventional hemodialysis[a]	995	21.6 ± 3.4	(15)
Peritoneal dialysis[b]	78	26.4 ± 3.0	(16)
Cycling peritoneal dialysis[c]	13	27.9 ± 2.0	(6)

[a]Three to four hours, three times weekly with standard HCO_3^- bath, samples from fistulas and catheters
[b]Four manual exchanges per day, 40 mM lactate bath, venous samples
[c]Nocturnal exchanges using a cycling machine, venous samples

[HCO$_3^-$] does not change notably (2,6). When suspicion is aroused, arterial pH and PaCO$_2$ should be measured and an assessment made as to whether the measured PaCO$_2$ is appropriate for the prevailing serum [HCO$_3^-$]. The ventilatory response to changes in serum [HCO$_3^-$] is normal in patients with renal failure (7). Thus, one can use the formulas shown below and in Fig. 1 to estimate the expected PaCO$_2$ for any given [HCO$_3^-$]. For a serum [HCO$_3^-$] <24 mEq/L:

$$PaCO_2 \, (mmHg) = 40 - 1.2 \times (24 - [HCO_3] \, (mEq/L)) \tag{1}$$

For a serum [HCO$_3^-$] > 24 mEq/L:

$$PaCO_2 \, (mmHg) = 40 + 0.7 \times ([HCO_3] \, (mEq/L) - 24) \tag{2}$$

Because these equations are approximations, one should not consider PaCO$_2$ abnormal unless it is 5 or more mmHg different from the value calculated by the formula. For example, a patient with a predialysis serum [HCO$_3^-$] of 20 mEq/L would be expected to have a PaCO$_2$ of 40 − (1.2 × 4), or 35 mmHg, with a range from 31 to 39 mmHg. Such a patient would have a respiratory alkalosis if the PaCO$_2$ were 30 mmHg or lower, and a respiratory acidosis if the PCO$_2$ were 40 mmHg or higher.

EVALUATION OF THE SECONDARY RESPONSE

In patients with end-stage renal disease, evaluation of the appropriateness of secondary changes induced by acid–base perturbations is simplified because there is no notable change in serum [HCO$_3^-$] in response to respiratory acid–base disorders. The secondary ventilatory response to changes in serum [HCO$_3^-$] is normal, and therefore its appropriateness can be evaluated using Eqs. (1) and (2) above (Fig. 1). One should not consider the PaCO$_2$ abnormal unless it is 5 or more mmHg different from the value calculated by either formula. For example, a dialysis patient with an [HCO$_3^-$] of 15 mEq/L has an expected PaCO$_2$ = 40 − 1.2 × (24 − 15) or 29 mmHg (Formula 1 above). A measured PaCO$_2$ between 25 and 33 mmHg in this patient would be consistent with a simple metabolic acidosis. If PaCO$_2$ is 24 mmHg or lower, a mixed disorder is present, comprising metabolic acidosis and respiratory alkalosis. If PaCO$_2$ is 34 mmHg or higher, a mixed disorder is present, comprising metabolic and respiratory acidosis.

CAUSES AND MANAGEMENT

Metabolic Acidosis

The spectrum of causes of metabolic acidosis in patients with end-stage renal disease is narrower than in patients with functioning kidneys (Table 2). One need not consider any renal causes (e.g., renal tubular acidosis). A new

Table 2 Causes of Metabolic Acidosis in End-Stage Renal Disease

---

Increased anion gap
Diabetic ketoacidosis
Lactic acidosis
Alcoholic ketoacidosis
Toxin ingestions
  Methyl alcohol
  Ethylene glycol
  Salicylates
  Paraldehyde
Other causes
  Catabolic state
  High protein intake
  High fluid retention between treatments
No increase in anion gap
Gastrointestinal alkali loss
  Diarrhea
  Pancreatic drainage
Hemofiltration with NaCl replacement
Ammonium chloride ingestion

---

metabolic acidosis is caused only by the addition and retention of acid or the loss of alkali. The only site for alkali loss is the gastrointestinal tract (e.g., diarrhea, pancreatic drainage). Acid addition in these patients is primarily the result of runaway endogenous acid production such as occurs in uncontrolled diabetes mellitus, lactic acidosis or after exposure to certain toxins.

The causes of metabolic acidosis are subdivided into those with a normal anion gap and those with an increased anion gap (Table 2). In patients with end-stage renal disease receiving hemodialysis, the anion gap is almost always increased (1,6), so this distinction is useful only if one can demonstrate an incremental change. In the absence of prior measurements, an anion gap of >20 mEq/L should be considered abnormally high. In patients receiving peritoneal dialysis, the anion gap is normal or only slightly increased (1). Again the ability to detect a sudden change is the most useful tool in making the diagnosis. As discussed further below, with rare exceptions, the causes of metabolic acidosis in patients with end-stage renal disease are all associated with an increase in anion gap.

Increased Anion Gap

Diabetic Ketoacidosis: Diabetic ketoacidosis is the most common cause of a new metabolic acidosis in patients with end-stage renal disease. Runaway production of β-hydroxybutyric acid in this disorder rapidly titrates

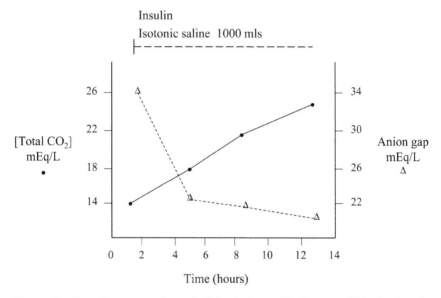

Figure 2 Complete correction of diabetic ketoacidosis over 12 hr by insulin administration in a patient with end-stage renal disease, without the need for dialysis or bicarbonate administration. Note that treatment rapidly reduced the anion gap by 12 mEq/L and that serum [Total CO$_2$] increased by an almost identical amount *Source*: Redrawn from Ref. 1.

body HCO$_3^-$ stores and produces organic anions that increase the anion gap (see Chapter 10). In contrast to patients with functioning kidneys, however, the organic anions produced are all retained unless removed by dialysis. As a result, insulin therapy given between treatments will rapidly restore serum [HCO$_3^-$] to baseline levels by stopping production and promoting metabolism of these organic anions (Fig. 2). In patients receiving peritoneal dialysis or developing ketoacidosis during hemodialysis, however, the disorder may by masked by the rapid loss of β-hydroxybutyrate (and acetoacetate) into the bath solution and its replacement with chloride or HCO$_3^-$. In these patients, the primary manifestation of ketoacidosis will be a very high blood sugar and the systemic symptoms of ketoacidosis (nausea, vomiting, malaise). In all instances, insulin therapy will correct the acidosis without the need for massive fluid volume repletion (unless there are large gastrointestinal losses), because patients with end-stage renal disease do not have the osmotic diuresis that normally accompanies hyperglycemia.

Lactic and Other Organic Acidoses: Sepsis, worsening congestive heart failure or dialysis-induced hypotension can impair tissue oxygen delivery and trigger increased production of lactic acid. In some patients with severe congestive heart failure, this event may occur regularly with during hemodialysis treatments, limiting the normal increase in [HCO$_3^-$] (8). Runaway lactic acid production in patients with end-stage renal disease causes a fall in serum [HCO$_3^-$], and an increase in the anion gap. The lactate anions produced by this disorder are retained unless removed by dialysis, and the acidosis thus is rapidly corrected if the cause can be reversed (e.g., treating sepsis, restoring ECF fluid volume, increasing blood pressure). Hemodialysis treatment can rapidly restore alkali stores, but may stimulate lactic acid production by abruptly increasing systemic pH (9).

In contrast to hemodialysis patients, serum [HCO$_3^-$] remains low in patients receiving peritoneal dialysis with lactic acidosis because their HCO$_3^-$ source is lactate, and generation of [HCO$_3^-$] from lactate is impaired. In a similar fashion, the use of Ringer's lactate as the sole replacement fluid in patients receiving continuous venovenous hemofiltration (with or without dialysis using a lactate containing bath solution) can cause progressive acidosis if the HCO$_3^-$ lost by this procedure is replaced with lactate that cannot be metabolized. Organic acidosis caused by alcohol or other toxins (Table 2) are much rarer events, but can occur in dialysis patients.

Other Causes: Serum [HCO$_3^-$] in patients with end-stage renal disease is inversely related to protein catabolic rate (see Chapter 23). Thus, patients with higher protein intake or increased protein breakdown are more likely to have a lower serum [HCO$_3^-$] and a higher anion gap. Serum [HCO$_3^-$] is also influenced by the amount of fluid retained between treatments. An increase in fluid retention between treatments of as little as 1 L can reduce predialysis [HCO$_3^-$] by 1 mEq/L (10). This form of "dilution acidosis" is unique to end-stage renal disease.

Normal or Unchanged Anion Gap

In patients with end-stage renal disease, metabolic acidosis without a change in anion gap only occurs if there is a loss of HCO$_3^-$ from the body. Gastrointestinal losses of HCO$_3^-$ include severe diarrhea or pancreatic drainage, but the usual alkali addition during dialysis limits the likelihood of such disorders becoming clinically apparent. For such a disorder to develop fully, massive losses would have to occur in the period between hemodialysis treatments, or the losses would have to exceed the ability of alkali replacement with peritoneal dialysis. Severe hyperchloremic metabolic acidosis has been reported in hemodialysis patients after inadvertent replacement of NaHCO$_3$ with NaCl in the bath solution (11). In patients receiving continuous venovenous hemofiltration, replacement solutions containing NaCl without alkali can cause the same problem.

Metabolic Alkalosis

Metabolic alkalosis in patients with end-stage renal disease is produced only by selective loss of HCl from the gastrointestinal tract or addition of excess alkali. Causes induced by changes in renal electrolyte reabsorption and acid excretion such as hyperaldosteronism, pseudohyperaldosteronism, Bartter's and Gitelman's syndromes need not be considered. In contrast to patients with renal function, in whom a change in renal electrolyte handling must occur for excess alkali to be retained, ingested or administered alkali can only be removed by buffer reaction with endogenous acids. Moreover, hemodialysis and peritoneal dialysis are both designed to add HCO_3^- to the body fluids, and will replenish the excess alkali unless serum $[HCO_3^-]$ exceeds 35–40 mEq/L.

Acid Loss

Acid loss occurs with vomiting or nasogastric drainage, and this cause is readily apparent, with the exception of the patient with surreptitious bulimia. In such a patient, pre-dialysis serum $[HCO_3^-]$ may increase by only 3–4 mEq/L, and thus still be in the normal range. The diagnosis of must be suspected and pursued (see Case 15 in Chapter 29).

Addition of Excess Alkali

Potential exogenous sources of alkali include $NaHCO_3$, as well as a wide variety of HCO_3^- precursors such as acetate, lactate and certain anionic amino acids (Table 3). Administration of $NaHCO_3$ is used therapeutically to increase serum $[HCO_3^-]$ in dialysis patients and produces a sustained rise in the pre-dialysis value (see Chapter 23). Citrate, acetate, and cationic amino acids are present in a variety of intravenous supplements, including blood transfusions and pheresis replacement fluids (citrate), and parenteral nutrition (acetate and cationic amino acids). Calcium salts containing carbonate, acetate or citrate are also potential sources of alkali, but only to the extent that these salts are ionized and the anions are absorbed from

Table 3 Causes of Metabolic Alkalosis in End-Stage Renal Disease

Vomiting
Nasogastric drainage
Exogenous alkali/alkali precursor
$NaHCO_3$
$KHCO_3$
$CaCO_3$[a]
Lactate
Acetate
Citrate
Glutamate
Proprionate
Aluminum hydroxide + kayexelate

[a]Calcium salts (carbonate, citrate, or acetate) have little alkalinizing effect.

the gut. In most patients, these agents contribute very little to body alkali stores and their effect on serum [HCO_3^-] is trivial.

With continuous venovenous hemofiltration, serum [HCO_3^-] is controlled by the HCO_3^- content of the replacement solutions and metabolic alkalosis can occur if too much alkali is given. The use of standard hemodialysis bath solutions (which contain 39 mEq/L of total alkali) for daily or slow continuous hemodialysis will cause metabolic alkalosis. This problem is easily resolved by reducing bath [HCO_3^-]. A rare cause of metabolic alkalosis is the combined use of sodium polystyrene sulfonate (kayexelate) and aluminum hydroxide (see Chapter 19).

Clinical Considerations

Metabolic alkalosis is diagnosed when the serum [HCO_3^-] is increased by 3 or more mEq/L in an individual patient or is 3 or more mEq/L higher than the average value for all patients receiving the same form of treatment. In patients receiving conventional hemodialysis, this definition includes values that fall within the normal range for individuals with functioning kidneys. Identification of an increase in serum [HCO_3^-] to 25–30 mEq/L is important, because such values are associated with an increased mortality (12). Hypokalemia, the usual hallmark of metabolic alkalosis, does not occur in patients with end-stage renal disease because this electrolyte abnormality requires renal function. Thus, a low serum [K^+] in dialysis patients requires a separate explanation.

Management

The primary approach to metabolic alkalosis in patients with end-stage renal disease is to search for and remove the cause. Treatment of gastrointestinal losses and/or removal of any sources of exogenous alkali will usually correct the disorder. In the acute care setting, the [HCO_3^-] in hemodialysis bath solutions can easily be reduced, if the elevated serum [HCO_3^-] is a clinical issue. One can also switch to continuous hemofiltration, and add no HCO_3^- to the replacement solution. This technique can safely and rapidly lower serum [HCO_3^-]. In patients receiving peritoneal dialysis, the options are fewer; bath lactate concentration can only be reduced by 5 mmol/L. Fortunately, reducing serum [HCO_3^-] is rarely an emergency; a mild-moderate increase in serum [HCO_3^-] (30–34 mEq/L) has few adverse consequences.

Respiratory Acidosis

In patients with functioning kidneys, the secondary response to respiratory acidosis is an increase in serum [HCO_3^-], initially through titration of non-bicarbonate buffers, and then by renal HCO_3^- generation. In patients with end-stage renal disease, buffer titration occurs but there is no renal response. The prevailing serum [HCO_3^-], moreover, is determined by the dialysis prescription and this process is unaffected by an increase in $PaCO_2$. As a result, none of the laboratory measurements routinely collected will help in the diagnosis of the disorder. The diagnosis can only be made by measuring arterial $PaCO_2$ and determining whether the level is appropriate for the prevailing serum [HCO_3^-] (see earlier). In patients with functioning fistulas or arteriovenous grafts, this determination is simple, as blood taken from these A-V shunts is equivalent to arterial blood (13,14).

Laboratory Findings

A $PaCO_2$ value 5 or more mmHg higher than expected for the prevailing serum [HCO_3^-] indicates the presence of respiratory acidosis (see Fig. 1 and Eqs. 1 and 2). A patient with a serum [HCO_3^-] of 22 mEq/L and a $PaCO_2$ of 45 mmHg, for example, has a respiratory acidosis because the expected $PaCO_2$ for this [HCO_3^-] is only 38 mmHg. In this patient, arterial pH is 7.31, in contrast to someone with functioning kidneys in whom pH will be closer to normal because serum [HCO_3^-] increases adaptively. More severe hypercapnia will result in much lower pH values.

Management

The first step in managing respiratory acidosis is to try to improve alveolar ventilation and reduce $PaCO_2$ if possible. If this cannot be accomplished, then dialysis bath [HCO_3^-] should be increased to the highest level possible, and exogenous alkali given to improve arterial pH. If hypercapnia cannot be ameliorated or reversed, the prognosis for survival on dialysis is grave.

Respiratory Alkalosis

Respiratory alkalosis is caused by a wide variety of pathological processes, including cerebral, cardiac and pulmonary injuries (Table 4), and occurs commonly in hospitalized patients in the intensive care unit. In patients with functioning kidneys, the secondary response is a decrease in serum [HCO_3^-], initially through titration of nonbicarbonate buffers, and then by a reduction in renal H^+ secretion. In patients with end-stage renal disease, buffer titration occurs, but is minimized by increased HCO_3^- delivery during dialysis, and there is no renal response. As a result, none of the laboratory measurements routinely collected help in the diagnosis of the disorder. The diagnosis can only be made by measuring $PaCO_2$ and determining whether the level is appropriate for the prevailing serum [HCO_3^-].

Laboratory Findings

The finding of a $PaCO_2$ value 5 or more mmHg lower than expected for the prevailing serum [HCO_3^-] indicates the presence of respiratory alkalosis (see Fig. 1 and Eqs. 1 and 2). Because no renal adaptation occurs, an

Table 4   Causes of Respiratory Alkalosis

Hypoxemia
Central nervous system disorders
 Anxiety-hyperventilation syndrome
 Stroke
 Infection
 Trauma
 Tumor
Pulmonary disease
 Pneumonia
 Pulmonary edema
 Pulmonary embolus
 Interstitial fibrosis
Other causes
 Gram-negative sepsis
 Hepatic failure
 Pregnancy
Drugs
 Salicylates
 Nicotine

---

increase in alveolar ventilation can produce dangerously high arterial pH values in patients with end-stage renal disease. For example, if $PaCO_2$ falls to 20 mmHg and serum [HCO_3^-] is maintained at 22 mEq/L by dialysis, pH will rise to 7.66. Values as high as 7.90 have been reported (see Case 8 in Chapter 29).

Management

The first approach to managing respiratory alkalosis is to try to reduce ventilation and increase $PaCO_2$. If this cannot be accomplished, an alternative approach is to switch to continuous venovenous hemofiltration and use only saline for replacement. This technique will reduce serum [HCO_3^-] by as much as 8 mEq/L in 12–14 hr, and thereby minimize the alkalemia caused by the hypocapnia. With conventional hemodialysis, bath [HCO_3^-] can be reduced, but not to the levels needed to decrease serum [HCO_3^-] sufficiently. Conventional peritoneal dialysis fluid cannot be adjusted sufficiently to treat respiratory alkalosis.

MIXED ACID–BASE DISORDERS

Mixed acid–base disorders occur when two or more primary disorders are present at the same time (see Fig. 1 and Chapter 22). In patients with end-stage renal disease, the spectrum of possible mixed disorders is narrower

Table 5   Mixed Acid–Base Disorders in End-Stage Renal Disease

---

Mixed metabolic and respiratory disorders
  $\downarrow [HCO_3^-]$
  $PaCO_2 >$ expected^a = metabolic + respiratory acidosis
  $PaCO_2 <$ expected^a = metabolic acidosis + respiratory alkalosis
  $\uparrow [HCO_3^-]$
  $PaCO_2 >$ expected^a = metabolic alkalosis + respiratory acidosis
  $PaCO_2 <$ expected^a = metabolic + respiratory alkalosis
  Metabolic acidosis + alkalosis
  Serum $[HCO_3^-] + \Delta$ anion gap >30 mEq/L (see Chapter 28)
Triple disorders
  Metabolic acidosis + alkalosis + :
  $PaCO_2 >$ expected^a = respiratory acidosis
  $PaCO_2 <$ expected^a = respiratory alkalosis

---

^{a}Using Eqs. 1 and 2 (see text and Fig. 1).

(Table 5) because of the absence of any renal response to respiratory acid–base abnormalities. The most common mixed disorders are combined metabolic and respiratory acid–base disturbances. These are diagnosed by measuring $PaCO_2$ and evaluating whether the value is appropriate for the concomitantly measured serum $[HCO_3^-]$ (see earlier discussion). If the serum $[HCO_3^-]$ is low, and $PaCO_2$ is higher than expected, the patient has both metabolic and respiratory acidosis, and if the $PaCO_2$ is lower than expected, the patient has mixed metabolic acidosis and respiratory alkalosis. More rarely, a mixed metabolic alkalosis and acidosis can occur. The sequence that might cause such a disorder in a dialysis patient would be administration of exogenous alkali, increasing serum $[HCO_3^-]$, followed by the development of a lactic acidosis or diabetic ketoacidosis. Such a sequence might fortuitously result in a serum $[HCO_3^-]$ at or near normal levels, but the disorder is uncovered by finding an increase in the anion gap (see Chapter 22). If the respiratory response to the final serum $[HCO_3^-]$ in such a patient is abnormal, then a triple disorder is diagnosed. Identification of the presence of multiple acid–base disorders coexisting in a patient is important for therapeutic intervention. Most important in this regard is diagnosing the presence of an abnormal respiratory response to a metabolic acid–base disturbance. Such a finding enables one to direct attention to management of the breathing disorder as well as the metabolic acid–base abnormality.

SUMMARY

Recognition and diagnosis of acid–base disorders in patients with end-stage renal disease requires an understanding of the unique new acid base equilibrium that develops when patients receive renal replacement therapy. Because of the lack of kidney function and this new equilibrium, the spectrum of acid–base disorders that can occur is narrower than in individuals with functioning kidneys. No secondary renal response occurs in respiratory acid–base disorders, but the respiratory response to metabolic acid–base disorders is normal. Identification of metabolic acid–base disorders (metabolic acidosis and alkalosis) is simple if one appreciates that baseline serum $[HCO_3^-]$ is often lower than normal in these patients. By contrast, recognition of respiratory disorders requires a clinical suspicion of their presence and measurement of $PaCO_2$ because no telltale changes in $[HCO_3^-]$ occur. With knowledge of the unique aspects of acid–base homeostasis in patients with end-stage renal disease in hand, one can identify the presence of new acid–base disorders, determine whether they are simple or mixed disorders, and intervene appropriately to treat these disorders.

REFERENCES

1. Gennari FJ. Acid–base disorders in end-stage renal disease: Part I. Semin Dial 1990; 3:81–85.
2. Gennari FJ. Acid–base disorders in end-stage renal disease: Part II. Semin Dial 1990; 3:161–165.
3. Bray SH, Tung RL, Jones ER. The magnitude of metabolic acidosis is dependent on differences in bicarbonate assays. Am J Kidney Dis 1996; 28:700–703.
4. Howse ML, Leonard M, Venning M, Soloman L. The effect of different methods of storage on the results of serum total CO2 assays. Clin Sci (Lond) 2001; 100:609–611.
5. Kirschbaum B. Spurious metabolic acidosis in hemodialysis patients. Am J Kidney Dis 2000; 35:1068–1071.
6. Gennari FJ. Acid–base considerations in end-stage renal disease. In: Henrich WL, ed. Principles and Practice of Dialysis. Baltimore: Williams and Wilkins, 2003:393–407.
7. Bushinsky DA, Coe FL, Katzenberg C, Szidon JP, Parks JH. Arterial PCO2 in chronic metabolic acidosis. Kidney Int 1982; 22:311–314.
8. Gennari FJ. Acid–base homeostasis in end-stage renal disease. Semin Dial 1996; 9:404–411.
9. Hood VL, Tannen RL. Protection of acid–base balance by pH regulation of acid production. N Engl J Med 1998; 339:819–826.
10. Fabris A, LaGreca G, Chiaramonte S, Feriani M, Brendolan A, Bragantini L, Dell'Aquila R, Pellanda MV, Crepaldi C, Ronco C. The importance of ultrafiltration on acid–base status in a dialysis population. ASAIO Trans 1988; 34:200–201.
11. Brueggemeyer CD, Ramirez G. Dialysate concentrate: a potential source for lethal complications. Nephron 1987; 46:397–398.
12. Lowrie EG, Lew NL. Death risk in hemodialysis patients: the predictive value of commonly measured variables and an evaluation of death rate differences between facilities. Am J Kidney Dis 1990; 15:458–482.

13. Gennari FJ. Acid–base balance in dialysis patients. Kidney Int 1985; 28: 678–688.
14. Santiago-Delpin EA, Buselmeier TJ, Simmons RL, Najarian JS, Kjellstrand CM. Blood gases and pH in patients with artificial arteriovenous fistulas. Kidney Int 1972; 1:131–133.
15. Uribarri J, Levin NW, Delmez J, Depner TA, Ornt D, Owen W, Yan G. Association of acidosis and nutritional parameters in hemodialysis patients. Am J Kidney Dis 1999; 34:493–499.
16. Gennari FJ, Feriani M. Acid–base problems in hemodialysis and peritoneal dialysis. In: Lameire N, Mehta RL, eds. Complications of Dialysis. New York: Marcel Dekker, 2000:361–376.

Acid–Base Considerations in Infants and Children

George J. Schwartz

Departments of Pediatrics and Medicine, University of Rochester School of Medicine, Rochester, New York, U.S.A.

INTRODUCTION

This chapter presents a review of maturational acid–base physiology and a variety of specific problems of acid–base balance that are unique to infants and children. Much of the material underscores the different physiology of the infant compared to the adult. The kidney of the premature infant is unable to compensate for the frequent respiratory and metabolic disturbances encountered in the nursery. Thus, acid–base balance is very precarious for the sick low-birth-weight infant. The process of growth is also unique to infants and children and requires special understanding and management. Growth induces an additional acid load that must be handled by a maturing kidney, thus placing the newborn at continual risk for metabolic acidosis. Metabolic acidosis and alkalosis impair growth and cause failure to thrive, so that correction of these disorders is urgent and critical in pediatrics. Acid–base disorders specific to the pediatric population also include inherited metabolic and tubular transport problems. Such patients have not often been seen by internists, in part because they failed to live to adulthood. Now more and more affected children are living longer and enjoying a better quality of life. As adults, they will require medical care by internists and other physicians not familiar with pediatric diseases. Therefore, this review should provide information that will improve the care of young adults with inherited tubulopathies, errors of metabolism, and other acid–base disturbances.

MATURATION OF ACID–BASE HOMEOSTASIS

Infants maintain lower values of blood pH and [HCO_3^-] than do older children and adults (Fig. 1) (1,2). In addition, the infant is prone to the development of acidosis during periods of sickness and poor dietary intake. Although the neonatal kidney can maintain acid–base homeostasis, it is limited in its response to exogenous acid loads (3). The lower levels of buffer base concentration in the blood of infants can be explained in part by the inability to completely excrete the byproducts of growth and metabolism (3,4).

At birth, the acid–base state of the neonate reflects that of the fetus, which is controlled by the placenta (5,6). Fetal blood pH is lower than maternal pH by 0.1–0.2 units and $PaCO_2$ is 10–15 mmHg higher, whereas no differences are apparent in [HCO_3^-] (5,7,8). Shortly after birth, the term neonate is in a state of mild metabolic acidosis with an average blood pH of 7.30 (1,2,9). By 24 hr of age, the term infant has a blood pH that is comparable to that of the adult (~7.39), but lower $PaCO_2$ (~34 mmHg) and [HCO_3^-] (~20 mEq/L) prevail due in large part to a centrally driven hyperventilation (1). Premature infants take longer to attain normal childhood blood pH and [HCO_3^-] (Fig. 2) (10,11). By adult standards, the newborn

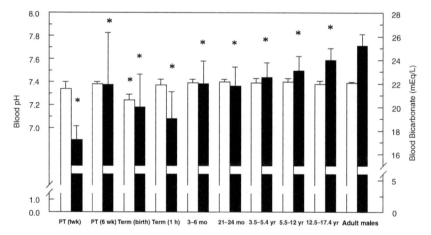

Figure 1   Blood acid–base measurements as a function of age (open bars, pH; filled bars, [HCO_3^-]). *Significantly different from adult males. Data given as mean ± SD. *Source*: Data taken from Sulyok E, et al. (Biol Neonate 1971; 19:200); Graham BD, et al. (Pediatrics 1951; 8:68); Smith CA (In: The Physiology of the Newborn Infant, Springfield: Thomas CC, ed., 1959); Cassels DE, et al. (J Clin Invest 1953; 32:824); and Madias NE et al. (Kidney Int 1979; 16:612).

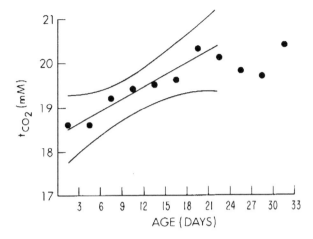

Figure 2 Regression and confidence limits of plasma total CO_2 concentration as a function of age in low-birth-weight infants. *Source*: From Schwartz GJ, et al. (J Pediatrics 1979; 95:102).

has a mixed acid–base disturbance of metabolic acidosis and respiratory alkalosis; as the kidney matures, the respiratory drive diminishes (3).

OVERVIEW OF ACID–BASE HANDLING BY THE NEONATAL KIDNEY

Bicarbonate Reabsorption

Plasma [HCO_3^-] is determined predominantly by the renal threshold for HCO_3^-, a set point of the proximal tubule (12). Infants have a lower HCO_3^- threshold despite having maximal rates of HCO_3^- reabsorption during acute alkali loading that are in the range reported for adults ($\sim$2.5 mEq/dL glomerular filtrate) (13–16) (Fig. 3). During the first year of life, the plasma [HCO_3^-] is $\sim$22 mEq/L compared with $\sim$26 mEq/L in adults (1,14). The plasma [HCO_3^-] is even lower in preterm infants, ranging from 16 to 19 mEq/L during the first three weeks of life (15–18) (Fig. 4). Thus the intrinsic capacity of the proximal tubule to reabsorb HCO_3^- during the first year of life, as measured by the acute loading experiments shown in Fig. 3, exceeds the rate of HCO_3^- reabsorption observed at threshold, and relative to the prevailing glomerular filtration rate, appears to be more than adequate to handle the filtered load of HCO_3^- (19).

Net Acid Excretion

In response to a comparable acid load, infants exhibit a larger fall in blood pH and [HCO_3^-], a smaller and less rapid fall in urinary pH, and much

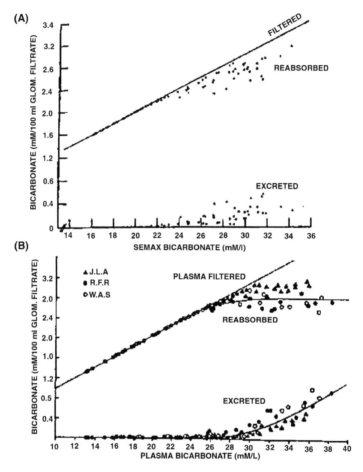

Figure 3   Reabsorption and excretion of filtered HCO_3^- in (**A**) infants and (**B**) adults undergoing a HCO_3^- titration. Infants have a lower threshold for HCO_3^- reabsorption, despite comparable rates of maximal HCO_3^- reabsorption per mL GFR. *Source*: From Edelmann CM Jr, et al. (J Clin Invest 1967; 46:1309), and Pitts RF, et al. (J Clin Invest 1949; 28:35).

smaller increases in urinary titratable acid and ammonium (NH_4^+) excretion per m^2 body surface area than do older children (Fig. 5) (10,20–22). Similar results have been noted in animal studies (5,23).

The renal response to acid loading increases with both gestational and postnatal ages. Titratable acid and NH_4^+ excretion both increase by ~50% during the first three weeks of life (10,11,24). Premature infants born at 31–35 weeks of gestational age (1.3–2.3 kg birth weight) show excretion rates for titratable acid, NH_4^+, and net acid that are about half those of term babies at 1–3 weeks postnatal age (24). In addition, the urine pH of premature

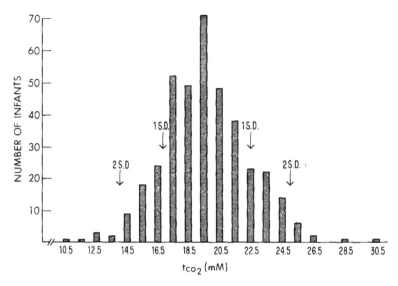

Figure 4 Frequency distribution of serum HCO_3^- values in 114 preterm infants. *Source*: From Schwartz GJ, et al. (J Pediatrics 1979; 95:102).

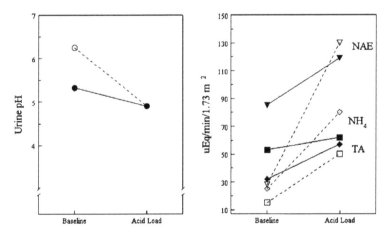

Figure 5 Comparison of urinary responses to acute acid load in infants (*solid lines and closed symbols*) vs. children (*dotted lines and open symbols*). Left panel shows urine pH at baseline and then after acid loading. Right panel shows baseline and acid loading values for titratable acid (*squares*), ammonium (*diamonds*) and net acid excretion (*triangles*). Data given as mean ± SD for baseline and after acid loading. *Source*: Data taken from Edelmann, CM, Jr et al. (J Clin Invest 1967; 46:1309).

infants seldom falls below 5.9 until the second postnatal month of life, whereas in 1- to 3-week-old term infants, urine pH falls below 5.0 after acid loading (11,15,17,18,25). Ammonium excretion is limited to a greater extent than titratable acid excretion in premature infants (Fig. 5).

Effect of Growth on Acid–Base Homeostasis

Compared to adults, infants have a higher rate of endogenous H^+ released during the metabolism of protein and deposition of Ca^{2+} into the growing skeleton (26,27), which can be exacerbated by loss of alkali from the intestine (21,27,28). Incorporation of Ca^{2+} into the skeleton causes the release of $0.5–1.0\,mEq/kg/day$ of H^+ that must be excreted by the kidney or be neutralized by gastrointestinal absorption of base (27,29). This H^+ load is added to the H^+ load generated by endogenous acid production and urinary organic anion excretion, which amounts to $\sim 2\,mEq/kg/day$ (27,29). As a result, endogenous acid production per kilogram body weight in infants and growing children is 50–100% higher than in adults.

Despite growth and the attendant release of H^+ into the extracellular fluid (ECF) (27,29) as well as the limited ability to increase renal net acid excretion (14,24,30) most infants are still able to maintain external acid–base balance because of the dietary input of base (27,28). Thus, in the neonate gastrointestinal absorption of dietary base helps to neutralize H^+ released during deposition of Ca^{2+} into the skeleton (28). A reduction in milk intake, a major source of net base, or in the absorption of base by the gut (such as occurs with diarrhea) can readily result in metabolic acidosis reflecting the limited H^+ excreting capacity of the immature kidney. Thus, infants operate at close to the maximum rate of net acid excretion (Fig. 5) due in part to the acid-generating process of growth. The renal response to acid loading increases with both gestational and postnatal ages (10,11,24).

SITES OF ACID–BASE TRANSPORT ALONG THE DEVELOPING NEPHRON

Proximal Tubule

One- to four-week-old puppies have acid–base values similar to those of newborn human infants: blood pH 7.24 ± 0.02, $[HCO_3^-]$ $18.2 \pm 0.6\,mEq/L$, and $PaCO_2$ $44 \pm 1\,mmHg$ (31). The mean HCO_3^- threshold is $18\,mEq/L$ compared with $23–26\,mEq/L$ in adult dogs. Gastric aspiration increases plasma $[HCO_3^-]$ and increase the HCO_3^- threshold to $25.2 \pm 1.1\,mEq/L$. The reduced threshold in puppies is not due to a limitation in intrinsic capacity for HCO_3^- reabsorption, but may reflect greater nephron heterogeneity or low fractional reabsorption of HCO_3^- in the immature kidney. The larger proportion of total body water in the infant coupled with a slightly lower serum albumin could contribute to decreased fractional HCO_3^- reabsorption (32).

In maturing rats, the tubular fluid:plasma ultrafiltrate concentration ratio for Cl^- (TF:UF Cl^-) at the end of the proximal tubule was 0.98 ± 0.03 at 13–15 days of age and increased to 1.20 ± 0.03 at 30–39 days of age (33). This result indicates that the immature superficial proximal tubule cannot generate or maintain a concentration gradient for Cl^-, indirectly implying a lower rate of HCO_3^- reabsorption in immature proximal tubules.

Comparison of proximal tubule HCO_3^- reabsorption between neonates and adults is complicated by the heterogeneity of nephron development. The kidney displays a centrifugal pattern of nephron growth and differentiation, wherein the juxtamedullary nephrons develop first and are relatively mature at birth (34). In rats, mice, rabbits and other animal species, as well as in humans born before 36 weeks of gestation, nephrogenesis is still occurring in the outer cortex at birth. The excessive splay in HCO_3^- titration studies performed in infants might well reflect this heterogeneity of nephron development, i.e., populations of maturing nephrons with varying capacities for HCO_3^- reabsorption (14). In isolated rabbit juxtamedullary proximal convoluted tubules obtained during the first three weeks of life and perfused, the rate of HCO_3^- absorption is one-third of that observed in the adult. Reabsorption rate then rises abruptly, so that near-mature levels are reached during the sixth week of life (Fig. 6) (35). The 160%

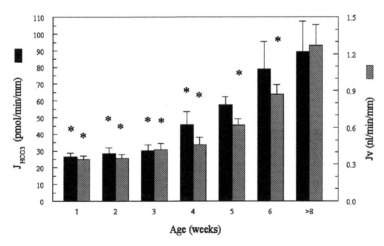

Figure 6   Rates of net HCO_3^- [J_{HCO3}, in pmol/min/mm (*filled bars*)] and fluid absorption [Jv, in pmol/min/mm (*slashed bars*)], as a function of age of animal, in isolated perfused juxtamedullary proximal convoluted tubules. * = Significant difference from > 8 week tubules (right column). *Source*: Drawn from data of Schwartz GJ, Evan AP (Am J Physiol 1983; 245:F382).

increase in HCO_3^- absorption observed between the third and sixth weeks of life was paralleled by a similar increase in fluid absorption. The Na^+,K^+-ATPase inhibitor, ouabain, impaired both fluid and HCO_3^- transport at all ages, indicating that both processes are primarily Na^+ dependent.

Bicarbonate permeability in rabbit juxtamedullary proximal convoluted tubules was several-fold lower in neonatal tubules than in mature segments (36). Thus, the lower rate of HCO_3^- reabsorption and the smaller HCO_3^- gradient observed in the neonatal juxtamedullary proximal convoluted tubule cannot be explained by increased HCO_3^- backleak, but rather by decreased HCO_3^- uptake (due to decreased rates of H^+ secretion, see below).

H^+ Secretion

The activity of the apical membrane Na^+/H^+ exchanger in the proximal tubule epithelium increases with maturation (37–39). In isolated perfused juxtamedullary proximal convoluted tubules, the rate of Na^+/H^+ exchange activity in tubules from 1- to 2-week-old rabbits was one-third of the adult level, and it doubled during the third week of life (38). Mature levels were reached at 6 weeks. The maturation of apical Na^+/H^+ exchange activity parallels that of net HCO_3^- absorptive flux (35). When brush border membrane vesicles from late gestation fetal and adult rabbit kidney cortex were compared, a 2.4- to fourfold maturational increase in Na^+/H^+ exchange activity occurs without any change in affinity (39). The molecular identity of the principal apical Na^+/H^+ exchanger in the proximal tubule is NHE3 (see Chapter 5) (40). Renal cortex obtained from neonatal rabbits (1-week-old) had approximately one-quarter of the NHE3 mRNA and protein abundance of adult rabbits (41). By contrast, there was no significant maturation of the basolateral housekeeping Na^+/H^+ exchanger (NHE1) mRNA or protein.

Maturational studies of the H^+-ATPase in the proximal tubule have not been as extensively characterized. Approximately 50% of the recovery of cell pH after an acid load in mature juxtamedullary proximal convoluted tubules is Na^+-independent, whereas in neonates most is Na^+-dependent and due to the apical Na^+/H^+ exchanger (37). These studies suggest a maturational increase in a Na^+-independent H^+ secretory mechanism, presumably the H^+-ATPase.

The rate of basolateral Na^+–$3HCO_3^-$ cotransport in the rabbit juxtamedullary proximal convoluted tubule was $\sim$60% of the adult level during the first month of life (38). Adult levels were achieved by 6 weeks of age. Thus, the basolateral Na^+–$3HCO_3^-$ cotransport activity in the newborn was more comparable to the mature rate than was the apical Na^+/H^+ exchanger activity, suggesting that the basolateral cotransporter is not rate limiting for HCO_3^- reabsorption early in life.

Na$^+$,K$^+$-ATPase

Renal cortical Na$^+$,K$^+$-ATPase activity also increases with maturation (39,42). The activity of Na$^+$,K$^+$-ATPase in rabbit juxtamedullary early proximal convoluted tubules during the first week of life was one-third of the adult level and rose by 70% during the next five weeks before a final surge in week 7 to nearly the adult level (43). Maturation of Na$^+$,K$^+$-ATPase activity lagged behind that of fluid (Na$^+$) and HCO$_3^-$ reabsorption (Fig. 7), suggesting that the increase in transport might drive the maturation of Na$^+$,K$^+$-ATPase activity. The rate of ATP production does not appear to be limiting, as there are only small differences between neonatal and adult animals in the rate of oxygen consumption (44,45). Moreover, in proximal tubule cells in culture, an increase in Na$^+$/H$^+$ exchange activity results in increased cell Na$^+$ concentration and a resulting stimulation of Na$^+$,K$^+$-ATPase activity (46). Similarly, chronic increases in Na$^+$/H$^+$ anti-porter activity in proximal tubules isolated from weanling rats (but not

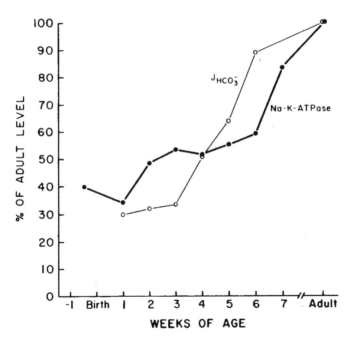

Figure 7 Development of Na$^+$/K$^+$-ATPase activity (*closed circles*) and net HCO$_3^-$ absorption [J_{HCO_3} (*open circles*)] in isolated rabbit renal juxtamedullary proximal convoluted tubules. Each weekly mean is expressed as a percent of the average value observed in tubules taken from adult rabbits. *Source*: From Schwartz GJ, Evan AP (Am J Physiol 1984; 246:F845).

from adult rats) stimulate Na^+,K^+-ATPase activity, also by increasing cell Na^+ activity (47).

Carbonic Anhydrase

The HCO_3^- transport rate in the neonatal juxtamedullary proximal convoluted tubule (35) is expected to accommodate the estimated filtered load of HCO_3^- during maturation (19). Thus, it is possible that the low threshold for HCO_3^- is due to an imbalance between HCO_3^- filtration and reabsorption in newly developing superficial nephrons, leading to a greater degree of splay (14,19). This imbalance might be manifested by heterogeneous expression of key transporter proteins or enzymes, which would limit tubular HCO_3^- reabsorption. Such a key enzyme is carbonic anhydrase (CA).

Most renal CA is cytosolic (isoform II) and this isoform is present in proximal tubule cells (48,49). Deficiency of CA II results in proximal renal tubular acidosis (RTA) (50) and inhibition of CA II markedly diminishes proximal tubular HCO_3^- reabsorption (51–53). An additional isoform, CA IV, comprises approximately 5% of renal CA and has been found on both the apical and basolateral membranes of proximal tubule cells (54,55). The limitation in neonatal HCO_3^- reabsorption could be due to low activity of CA II or CA IV, or another membrane-bound CA, in neonatal proximal tubules.

Carbonic anhydrase activity is present at low levels in the early human fetal kidney (56,57). The newborn kidneys of several animal species (58) harbor distinctly less CA activity than do mature kidneys and there is a substantial maturation in the early postnatal period (59). Total cortical CA II activity in rabbit kidney doubles during maturation,(58) with about one-half the increase occurring by 3 weeks of age (55). Carbonic anhydrase II protein abundance in the rat proximal tubule at 1 week of age is 11% of the level at 12 weeks (60); of this ninefold maturational increment, a major increase occurs between weeks 2 and 3 to 41% of mature levels, with a more gradual increase occurring between 3 and 7 weeks to 93% of mature levels. The concentration of CA II at 7 weeks of age is higher in S1 than in S2 and S3 segments of proximal tubules (60).

Carbonic anhydrase IV activity in the maturing kidney cortex increases by 230% during maturation with half the increase occurring by 3 weeks of age (55). Carbonic anhydrase IV protein abundance in the neonatal rabbit kidney cortex is 15–30% of adult levels during the first two weeks of life before increasing to adult levels by 5 weeks of age (55). Most of the increase occurs before 4 weeks of age. By immunohistochemistry, there is a large increase in CA IV labeling of apical and basolateral membranes with maturation (55,61). These major increases in both CA II and CA IV activities likely contribute to the threefold maturation of HCO_3^- reabsorption in the maturing proximal tubule.

Distal Nephron

Thick Ascending Limb of Henle's Loop

There are no published data concerning the maturation of HCO_3^- transport in the loop of Henle in any species.

Cortical Collecting Duct

The mature cortical collecting duct (CCD) can secrete H^+ or HCO_3^- depending on the acid–base status of the animal (see Chapters 4–6) (62,63). Proton and HCO_3^- secretion are mediated primarily by α- and β-intercalated cells, respectively. Intercalated cells comprise 20–35% of total cells in the CCD, with the remainder being principal cells. The number of intercalated cells per mm tubular length doubles during maturation, most of this increase occurring after the first four weeks of life (64,65). The increase in total intercalated cells is associated with a doubling of β-intercalated cells (65). Indeed, neonatal CCDs show no intercalated cells in the outer cortex (66), consistent with the pattern of centrifugal nephron development (64,66–68).

Immunostaining of 18-day fetal rat kidneys showed simultaneous appearance of CA II and the vacuolar H^+-ATPase in a subpopulation of cells in the connecting segment of the distal tubule and in the medullary collecting duct (66). These data suggest that intercalated cells differentiate from two separate foci, one in the connecting segment and another in the collecting duct. Both α and β intercalated cells were seen at each focal site, indicating they differentiate simultaneously during development. Whereas band 3 labeling (a marker for the Cl^-/HCO_3^- exchange protein in intercalated cells) was weak in the fetal kidney, staining was increased at 3 days of age, indicating an activation of H^+-secreting intercalated cells soon after birth.

An ultrastructural study showed α-intercalated cells in the inner medulla and renal pelvis in 19-day rat fetuses and neonates (69). Two weeks after birth, the α-intercalated cells disappeared from these regions and populated outer medullary collecting ducts (OMCDs) and to a lesser extent CCDs. β-intercalated cells began to appear 3 weeks after birth in the CCD (69). Imposed maternal alkalosis resulted in an earlier appearance and an increase in the number of β-intercalated cells in newborn and 2-week-old rats (70).

Not only do intercalated cells increase in number with development, but they also manifest maturational changes in morphology and function. The pH of intercalated cells of CCDs from the midcortex of newborn rabbits is about 0.15 pH units less alkaline than that of mature CCDs (64). Compared to the mature segment, the neonatal CCD exhibits less labeling for H^+-ATPase and the basolateral Cl^-/HCO_3^- exchanger, as well as for CA and β-intercalated cell surface markers (65–67,71). Carbonic anhydrase

II expression in rat CCDs increased ninefold during maturation, with nearly half the increase occurring during the first three weeks of life (60). Ultrastructurally, intercalated cells from newborn rabbit CCDs show smaller apical perimeters and markedly reduced vesicular profiles and mitochondrial volume (68). Differentiation proceeds such that a nearly mature ultrastructural appearance is achieved by 24 days of age; however, at this age the number of intercalated cells per mid- or outer-cortical zone is still only about one-half of what is observed at maturity (68).

Functional studies of β-intercalated cells reveal a lower cell pH during the first month of life (65) and a markedly reduced activity of the apical Cl^-/HCO_3^- exchanger (65). When intercalated cells are alkali loaded, the initial rate of Cl^--dependent luminal alkali extrusion is three times higher in mature CCDs compared with CCDs from newborn rabbits (65). Accordingly, CCDs during the first month of life fail to show spontaneous HCO_3^- secretion despite a mild metabolic alkalosis of the neonatal rabbit, whereas CCDs from 6-week and adult rabbits show net HCO_3^- secretion (Fig. 8) (72). Removal of bath Cl^-, which stimulates HCO_3^- secretion in mature CCDs, failed to do so in CCDs from newborn and 4-week-old rabbits (72).

Outer Medullary Collecting Duct

The mature OMCD is comprised of principal cells and α-intercalated cells. The latter represent 10–20% of total cells in the outer stripe and one-third to one-half in the inner stripe of the outer medulla (64,68,73,74). This segment regularly secretes H^+ at high rates (75,76). OMCDs from newborn rats and

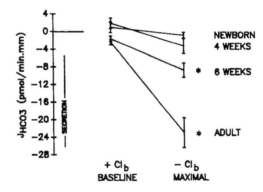

Figure 8 Effect of bath Cl^- removal ($-Cl_b$) on net HCO_3^- transport (J_{HCO_3}) in maturing rabbit CCDs. Data are mean ± SE. Baseline transport was net HCO_3^- secretion only at age 6 weeks and adult, and these segments were the only ones to consistently show significant stimulation of HCO_3^- secretion by removal of bath Cl^- (*). Maximal HCO_3^- secretion in adult CCDs significantly exceeded that observed in segments from each age group of younger animals. *Source*: From Mehrgut FM, et al. (Am J Physiol 1990; 259:F801).

rabbits show fainter and less apical polarization of H^+-ATPase and less basolateral polarization of the Cl^-/HCO_3^- exchanger as compared to 3-week-old and adult rabbits (66,67). Carbonic anhydrase II expression in rat OMCD increases sevenfold during maturation, with nearly half the increase occurring during the first three weeks of life (60). Carbonic anhydrase II activity in outer medullary homogenates doubles during maturation, with most of the increase occurring after 4 weeks of age (58). Carbonic anhydrase IV protein, expressed primarily by medullary collecting ducts, increases 4–10-fold, with more than one-half of the increase occurring before 4 weeks of age (55).

Immunostaining of 18-day fetal rat kidneys showed CA II and H^+-ATPase in cells throughout the medullary collecting duct and papillary surface (66). After birth, the immunostaining disappears from the terminal inner medullary collecting duct and papillary surface. Intercalated cells with apical H^+-ATPase or CA IV labeling (α-intercalated cells) are extruded from the epithelium into the lumens (55,77). Cells with basolateral H^+-ATPase labeling (β-intercalated cells) gradually disappear from the OMCD and initial inner medullary collecting duct. These intercalated cells are deleted by apoptosis and subsequent phagocytosis by neighboring principal cells or inner medullary collecting duct cells (77).

The expression of differentiated proteins by the immature OMCD appears to be more advanced than in the CCD (66–68). This is confirmed by cell pH studies, which show that neonatal medullary intercalated cells have a pH ($\sim$7.27) similar to that of mature cells (64). Ultrastructural studies of intercalated cells in the outer stripe confirm their presence in mature numbers, but the cells contain slightly smaller vesicular and mitochondrial volumes and much smaller apical perimeters as compared to mature segments (68). Microperfusion studies indicate that the neonatal OMCD secretes H^+ at 70% of the mature rate (72). Each of these studies indicates the relative maturity of α-intercalated cells (both in number and function) in the neonatal OMCD.

Inner Medullary Collecting Duct

There are no published maturational acid–base studies in the inner medullary collecting duct. However, there is a clear maturation of CA IV expression in this segment (55).

Summary of Segmental Acid–Base Transport in the Neonatal Kidney

The neonatal kidney is faced with a large endogenous acid load due to the process of growth superimposed on daily metabolic needs. There is good evidence for immaturity of several transport systems in the proximal tubule, but because of the low glomerular filtration rate prevailing at this stage of development, the fractional reabsorption of HCO_3^- attains adult levels. The distal nephron is limited in its ability to acidify the urine, in part due to low rates of NH_4^+ synthesis in the proximal tubule, as well as limited excretion of phosphate. Some compensation occurs in the intestine, where absorption of organic anions partially offsets the accumulation of endogenous acid. The result is that the newborn operates at a near-maximum rate of renal net acid excretion, and is dependent on intestinal absorption of organic anions to assist in base regeneration. It is not difficult to perceive how systemic metabolic acidosis can easily develop if the endogenous acid load is increased or if base is lost via the intestine (or kidney).

SPECIFIC ACID–BASE PROBLEMS OF INFANTS AND CHILDREN

Metabolic Acidosis

Severe metabolic acidosis in the newborn is generally suspected from the clinical presentation and history of predisposing conditions, such as perinatal asphyxia (hypoxic–ischemic encephalopathy), respiratory distress, blood loss, sepsis, or congenital heart disease associated with poor systemic perfusion or cyanosis (78,79). However, in infants and children, other pathological processes should be investigated thoroughly. As in adults, the causes of metabolic acidosis are separated into two groups, based on calculation of the anion gap: normochloremic (high anion gap) organic acidosis and hyperchloremic (normal anion gap) acidosis caused by excessive HCO_3^- loss or inadequate renal acid excretion (Table 1). The anion gap is normally $< 15\,mEq/L$ in infants and children and consists primarily of the negative charges on plasma proteins. This value should be adjusted downward in a setting of hypoalbuminemia, such as in a sick malnourished child. On the other hand, premature infants might normally exhibit an anion gap as high as $22\,mEq/L$ (80).

Causes: General Overview

Metabolic acidosis is produced by selective HCO_3^- loss, by excess acid production or by impaired acid excretion either alone or in combination. Examples of these three pathogenetic processes are discussed below.

Loss of HCO_3^-: Sodium is usually lost with HCO_3^- leading to a state of hyperchloremia with a normal anion gap. Causes of this type of metabolic acidosis in infants include diarrhea, proximal RTA, and congenital adrenal hyperplasia (salt-losing form). Urinary losses of HCO_3^- can also occur in conditions such as the use of CA inhibitors and ureteroenterostomy. Regarding the latter entity, ileum and colon are the bowel segments generally used; they secrete Na^+ and HCO_3^-, and reabsorb ammonia, protons, and Cl^- when exposed to urine (81). Drainage of alkaline pancreatic or biliary secretions can also lead to a hyperchloremic metabolic acidosis. Substantial decrements

Table 1 Causes of Metabolic Acidosis Categorized on the Basis of the Anion Gap Level

---

Normal anion gap
Bicarbonate loss
  Diarrhea
  Drainage from small bowel, biliary or pancreatic tube/fistula
  Ureteroenterostomy
  Proximal renal tubular acidosis
  Carbonic anhydrase inhibitors
Distal renal tubular acidosis
Acid load (NH_4Cl, arginine hydrochloride, HCl, $CaCl_2$, $MgCl_2$)
Dilution of extracellular fluid compartment
High protein formulas
Hyperalimentation
Aldosterone deficiency
  Type IV renal tubular acidosis
  21-Hydroxylase deficiency
Posthypocapnia
High anion gap
Lactic acidosis (major ion: lactate)
  Hypoxemia, shock, sepsis
  Inborn errors of carbohydrate or pyruvate metabolism
    Primary lactic acidosis
    Pyruvate dehydrogenase deficiency
    Pyruvate carboxylase deficiency
    Mitochondrial respiratory chain defects
    Leigh's encephalopathy
    Glycogen storage disease (type I)
Uremic acidosis (major ions: sulfate, phosphate, urate, hippurate)
Ketoacidosis (major ion: β-hydroxybutyrate)
  Inborn errors of amino acid or organic acid metabolism
    Propionic acidemia
    Methylmalonic acidemia
    Isovaleric acidemia
    Branched chain aminoacidemia
    Multiple carboxylase deficiency
Ingestions
  Salicylate (major ions: ketoacids, salicylate, lactate)
  Methanol (major ion: formate)
  Ethylene glycol (major ion: glycolate, oxalate)
  Ethanol
  Paraldehyde (organic anions)
Massive rhabdomyolysis

Source: Adapted from Rose BD, Post TW (Clinical Physiology of Acid–Base and Electrolyte Disorders. 5th ed. New York: McGraw-Hill, 2001:584), and Kappy MS, Morrow G (A diagnostic approach to metabolic acidosis in children. Pediatrics 1980; 65:353).

in plasma [HCO_3^-] and reductions in blood pH can occur in infants with infusions of large amounts of saline (dilutional acidosis).

Excess Production or Ingestion of Acid: In the neonatal period, inborn enzymatic abnormalities lead to defective metabolism of amino and organic acids and a metabolic acidosis with an increased anion gap ($\geq 16\,\text{mEq/L}$) (82). Many of these inborn errors of metabolism are associated with the accumulation of acidic metabolites in the plasma, which are readily detectable in the urine (Fig. 9). Some of these inborn errors are also associated with hypoglycemia due to inhibition of gluconeogenesis, which results in further mobilization of fat and protein as energy sources and consequent ketoacidosis. Specific entities include methylmalonic acidemia, propionic acidemia, and isovaleric acidemia. Defects in pyruvate metabolism or in the respiratory chain might cause a primary lactic acidosis in infancy, which presents as a severe metabolic acidosis, but in this case the urine contains normal amounts of organic acids with the exception of high concentrations of lactate.

In infancy, ingestion of excessive protein or potential nonvolatile acid in commercial formulas or cow's milk might also cause metabolic acidosis. Premature babies are particularly susceptible, developing what is termed the "late metabolic acidosis of prematurity." Another cause of excessive acid

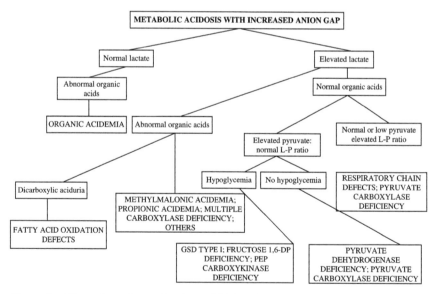

Figure 9   Flow chart for evaluation of high-anion-gap metabolic acidosis in the young infant. In this flow chart, lactic acid is not considered to be an organic acid. Fructose-1,6-DP, fructose-1,6-diphosphatase; L/P, lactate/pyruvate. *Source:* From Burton BK (Pediatrics 1998; 102:e69).

production in childhood is the ingestion of toxins that are acid precursors (e.g., methanol, acetylsalicylic acid) (83). Also, many of the errors in glyco-genolysis and gluconeogenesis that lead to fasting hypoglycemia, as well as diabetic ketoacidosis, can result in high-anion-gap metabolic acidosis due to the excessive production of acetoacetate and β-hydroxybutyrate. Increased lactate production in the absence of hypoglycemia, hyperammonemia, or ketosis can also result from substantial tissue necrosis, such as ischemic bowel (84). A normal-anion-gap acidosis can result from the ingestion of acidifying agents such as NH_4Cl and arginine hydrochloride, or the provision of cationic amino acids in parenteral hyperalimentation.

Inadequate Renal Acid Excretion: Impaired acid excretion can result from damage or hypoperfusion of the kidneys, as with shock, hypoxic renal damage, or congenital heart diseases (79,83). These conditions are generally associated with an elevated blood urea nitrogen (BUN) level. Severe malnu-trition or anorexia may result in hypophosphatemia and can interfere with renal titratable acid excretion by reducing the urinary excretion of phos-phates. Prolonged renal failure is usually associated with the accumulation of sulfate, phosphate, and other anions, resulting in a metabolic acidemia with an increased anion gap. Renal tubulopathy (distal RTA) causes a hyperchloremic metabolic acidosis (see Chapter 13).

Causes: Specific Entities

Specific causes of metabolic acidosis in infants and children deserving special emphasis are discussed below.

Neonatal Metabolic Acidosis: Preterm and term infants have a reduced ability to increase acid excretion in response to an acid load. Com-plex disorders of acid–base metabolism are found more frequently in the early neonatal period than in any other pediatric age group. Metabolic acidosis in newborn infants is usually normochloremic, with an increased serum anion gap. Most common is lactic acidosis, generally due to asphyxia, ischemia, hypoxemia, local tissue damage, or congenital heart disease (79) (Table 2) (80). Other causes include congenital metabolic disorders and acute renal failure. Hyperchloremic conditions are less common but usually are caused by losses of HCO_3^- from the gastrointestinal or urinary tract; insufficient renal proton secretion also causes hyperchloremic acidosis. Underexcretion of acid might be due to acute renal failure or insufficient dis-tal Na^+ delivery, the latter associated with volume contraction accompany-ing the gastrointestinal losses of base in diarrhea. Buffering of a chronic acidosis by bone might lead to loss of growth potential and to an increased incidence of orthopedic problems in growing children (85).

Diagnosis requires a detailed perinatal and obstetric history, serial physical examinations, and extensive laboratory studies. Laboratory studies include arterial/arterialized blood gases, serum electrolytes, osmolality, urea

Table 2   Clinical Conditions Most Commonly Associated with Acidosis in Newborn Infants

Term infants
  Perinatal asphyxia/hypoxia
  Poor peripheral circulation
  Hemorrhage (infant/maternal)
  Septicemia
Preterm infants
  Perinatal asphyxia/hypoxia
  Poor peripheral circulation
  Hemorrhage (infant/maternal, includes intraventricular hemorrhage)
  Septicemia
  Acute renal failure
  Transient/permanent renal tubular dysfunction
  Hyperalimentation issues (excessive protein, insufficient cation, etc.)
  Necrotizing enterocolitis
  Patent ductus arteriosus
  Late metabolic acidosis
  Gastroenteritis (usually later presentation)

Sources: Data from Moore ES, Evans MS (The newborn kidney and acid–base homeostasis. In: Pediatric Nephrology. Brodehl J, Ehrich JHH, eds. Berlin: Springer-Verlag, 1984:72–75) and unpublished observations from the University of Rochester Golisano Children's Hospital at Strong Neonatal Intensive Care Unit.

nitrogen and creatinine, urinalysis, urine electrolytes and pH, and urine culture; no single test will suffice for evaluation of acid–base disorders in infants (80). Because most acid–base disorders are extrarenal in origin and some renal causes are transient (reflecting delayed maturation), clinically stressful studies such as ammonium chloride loading or HCO_3^- titration studies are not generally performed in newborn infants (80). Inability to acidify the urine in the setting of acidosis might be due to renal tubular immaturity in the very low-birth-weight infants, lack of available urine buffers in term infants during the first week of life, or the presence of a urinary tract infection in infants of any age.

Perinatal Asphyxia (Hypoxic–Ischemic Encephalopathy):   Perinatal asphyxia usually results in a normochloremic metabolic acidosis with a rapid fall in blood pH and rise in $PaCO_2$ along with tissue oxygen debt (79,86). The prevalence of metabolic acidosis (base deficit $> 12\,mEq/L$) at birth is 20 per 1000 births and for severe metabolic acidosis (base deficit $> 16\,mEq/L$) is 5 per 1000 births (87). Indeed, term infants born with an umbilical artery base deficit exceeding $12\,mEq/L$ (umbilical artery pH < 7.0) are much more likely to develop moderate and severe newborn encephalopathy (lethargy progressing to coma, abnormal tone, and seizures) and respiratory complications requiring mechanical ventilation (87). Infants with more severe acidosis develop cardiovascular complications and kidney problems, including oligo/anuria, acute renal failure, acute tubular necrosis, and hyperkalemia. The base deficit rises initially in parallel with blood lactate concentrations but subsequently outstrips the rise in lactate, such that lactate only accounts for a third of the base deficit (86). It is clear that correction of the underlying disorder (restoration of adequate ventilation and tissue perfusion) is the mainstay of treatment.

A study that followed 102 premature infants during the first week of postnatal life revealed that most healthy infants have an acid–base status that is comparable to that of normal term infants (88). The typical disturbance of the remaining premature infants tends to be a mixed metabolic and respiratory acidosis, a disturbance resulting in severely reduced blood pH values. In general, the higher the blood $PaCO_2$, the more severe is the metabolic acidosis and clinical course. Asphyxiated newborn infants almost always show a mixed acidosis, which is usually associated with cyanosis and hypoventilation. Asphyxia usually leads to a metabolic acidosis, which is reversible upon proper oxygenation of the tissues. In some infants with respiratory distress, the acid–base disturbance is predominately a metabolic acidosis, which likely results from the hypoxia. In these cases, hypoxia is not associated with significant CO_2 retention (88). The early metabolic acidosis is likely secondary to the accumulation of organic acids during hypoxia. While respiratory acidosis is occasionally observed during the first 24 hr of life, in nearly all cases of protracted hypoxia metabolic acidosis supervenes.

Sodium bicarbonate therapy should not be given if ventilation is inadequate because its administration results in an increase in $PaCO_2$ with no improvement in blood pH. Nevertheless, most neonatologists will give $NaHCO_3$ slowly in diluted form when there is documented metabolic acidosis with adequate ventilation, and will try to correct the disorder to a blood pH of 7.3 (79).

Patent Ductus Arteriosus: Metabolic acidosis occurring early in the newborn period can be due to patent ductus arteriosus. The ductus normally closes after 32 weeks gestation as normal pulmonary circulation is established. In premature infants of < 30 weeks gestation, the ductus is open, so that a large left-to-right shunt develops across it, causing increased pulmonary blood flow, pulmonary edema, apnea, and congestive heart failure. Examination shows bounding pulses, systolic murmur, widened pulse pressure, active precordium and cardiomegaly; renal insufficiency often develops. Babies with the most symptomatic form of the condition might develop a severe metabolic acidosis (89). Presumably, the acidosis reflects compromised tissue perfusion due to hypoxia and ineffective cardiac output leading to anaerobic metabolism.

Respiratory Distress and Respiratory Distress Syndrome: Within the first hour after delivery the healthy infant attains normal acid–base status (Fig. 1). Many babies who do not make a normal cardiorespiratory adjustment following birth are tachypneic and cyanotic, with expiratory grunting and retractions on inspiration. Initially, these infants have a respiratory acidosis due to impaired ventilation. When this condition progresses to respiratory failure it is referred to as respiratory distress syndrome and comprises a mixed respiratory and metabolic acidosis (90). Respiratory distress syndrome, an affliction of very premature babies (23–27 weeks gestation), is associated with both impaired ventilation and perinatal asphyxia. In this condition, surfactant deficiency results in pulmonary atelectasis, increased pulmonary vascular resistance, poor lung compliance, and decreased lymphatic drainage (79). The primary finding is hypoxia with hypercapnia due to decreased alveolar ventilation with mismatching of ventilation and perfusion in some alveoli. As the $PaCO_2$ rises, so does the plasma $[HCO_3^-]$; however, renal compensation is limited by tubular immaturity (90) and the relatively large ECF volume of the premature infant.

The acidosis of respiratory distress syndrome is typically a mixed metabolic and respiratory acidosis. The metabolic component generally indicates insufficient cardiac output. Efforts to improve myocardial contractility and systemic blood flow, and to reduce afterload should be started immediately. Treatment of the acidosis involves a slow infusion of glucose water with 50–100 mm $NaHCO_3$ (79). Rapid correction of the acidosis using hypertonic $NaHCO_3$ over 3 hr is associated with increased mortality due to brain hemorrhage (90).

Diarrheal Dehydration: Diarrhea with dehydration remains an important and common problem in pediatrics. The pathophysiology of acidosis in diarrhea in infancy is multifactorial (91). First, stool water losses contain more base than the ECF, so a selective loss of HCO_3^- occurs. Second, the accompanying starvation ketosis leads to the accumulation of β-hydroxybutyric acid and acetoacetic acid in the body fluids. Third, enteric organisms produce metabolic acid, which is absorbed. Fourth, reduced tissue perfusion due to volume depletion leads to lactic acid production. Fifth, renal excretion of nonvolatile acid is impaired due to the decreased vascular volume and renal blood flow. Sixth, infantile acid excretion is already near-maximal. And seventh, intestinal absorption of organic anions is reduced. Thus, diarrhea and dehydration in infants is frequently associated with metabolic acidosis, and an elevated anion gap can sometimes be present.

Treatment is to restore volume by giving Na^+, with 20–35% of the anion being HCO_3^- depending on the severity of acidosis (91). Only in rare cases of severe acidosis should specific base replacement be calculated. When necessary, this calculation should assume 30% of the body weight as a distribution space for quick changes in plasma [HCO_3^-] and 50% of body weight for more chronic (>4 hr) changes (91).

Hyperalimentation: Some problems occurring in the neonate are consequences of management. The unstable premature infant is frequently unable to tolerate oral feedings and is required to receive hyperalimentation therapy. Whereas the need for calories and amino acids is very large, the premature infant is also undergoing an obligate loss of retained ECF during the first postnatal days of life (32,91). Although "physiological," this loss of ECF is associated with negative Na^+ balance; with poor intake, signs of dehydration will occur. Volume depletion will delay the postnatal rise in glomerular filtration and subsequent renal tubular maturation, including renal acidification mechanisms.

Acidosis might result from the administration of excessive amounts of cationic amino acids, such as arginine and lysine. These are metabolized to urea, CO_2, and H^+. This acid load is in addition to that stemming from the sulfur-containing amino acids in the solution (92). Further, to allow the "physiologic" loss of ECF in the newborn and maintain adequate ventilation, some clinicians do not provide much Na^+ in the hyperalimentation fluid, and therefore not as much anion, such as acetate, which is metabolized to HCO_3^-. Clearly, the optimal management is to limit cationic amino acids and liberalize Na^+ intake.

Late Metabolic Acidosis of the Neonate: Feeding large amounts of protein can lead to metabolic acidosis in otherwise healthy premature infants (93). Such "feeding acidosis" might be due to the inadequate ability of the immature kidney to excrete the acid released by the catabolism of excessive amounts of protein. The reduction of protein to 3–4 g/kg body weight per day has essentially eliminated this condition.

A subtler type of metabolic acidosis can occur in premature infants receiving only a modest amount of milk protein. Such infants are otherwise entirely healthy and are considered to have "late metabolic acidosis" (94). This term was coined to describe a condition in a population of apparently healthy preterm infants receiving cow's milk formula, who, when investigated at 1–3 weeks of age, were found to have low values for whole blood base excess and a tendency for a low $PaCO_2$, findings consistent with a metabolic acidosis. In addition to generally receiving cow's milk formulas (3–4 g protein/kg body weight per day), many such infants showed a delayed start of postnatal weight gain with increased renal net acid excretion (78). Late metabolic acidosis is usually associated with impaired weight gain (78,95). Estimates of the prevalence of late metabolic acidosis range from 8% to 40% of preterm infants, and this variation depends in part on diagnostic criteria, feeding practices, and native characteristics of the population studied (78).

Modification of formulas with reduced protein and minerals, particularly phosphate, has markedly diminished the numbers of infants with late metabolic acidosis. The decrease in dietary acid load reflects the recent "humanization" of cow's milk formulas so that the acid load approaches that of human milk (0.8 mmol/kg body weight per day) (95). Moreover, many infants previously diagnosed as having late metabolic acidosis do not lose weight and have plasma [HCO_3^-] levels that are within 2 standard deviations of the mean normal value (17). Nowadays, most babies developing late metabolic acidosis either have impaired renal acidification, other renal tubular disorders, or sequelae of postnatal asphyxia or septicemia. The process is self-healing with the maturation of renal transport mechanisms. Very low-birth-weight infants after intensive care therapy can be assumed to be at risk for at least a transient reduction of renal acid excretion capability, which could lead to acid retention and impaired growth, or late metabolic acidosis. Demonstration of persistently low blood and urine pH, lethargy, and evidence for failure to grow, inadequate weight gain, or frank weight loss would warrant the empiric treatment with $NaHCO_3$ at 2 mEq/kg body weight per day (96) for approximately a week or a further reduction in the acid load of the formula (95).

Goat's milk acidosis has also been described in a term infant, who presented with tachypnea, growth failure, hyperkalemia, hyperchloremia, and a plasma [HCO_3^-] of 4 mEq/L (97). This acidosis is not due to excessive protein contained in the goat's milk, but rather the high KCl content.

Renal Tubular Acidosis: All types of RTA are encountered in infants and children, and are discussed below (see also Chapter 13).

Proximal RTA. Proximal RTA (type II) is caused by decreased HCO_3^- reabsorption in the proximal tubule. It should be suspected in infancy or childhood when the plasma [HCO_3^-] is found to be low for age and the urinary pH is insufficiently low in the setting of a mild to moderate metabolic acidosis. Proximal RTA can occur as an isolated defect or be accompanied by other tubular dysfunction, resulting in the Fanconi syndrome (98). The diagnosis is established by documenting a reduced renal threshold for HCO_3^- in a HCO_3^- titration study. Defects in luminal proton pumps, basolateral anion transporters, or CA could be responsible for the impairment in HCO_3^- reabsorption in this disorder. Cases of proximal RTA have been described with CA II deficiency (50,99,100) and recently with a defect in the kidney sodium–bicarbonate transporter, kNBC1 (101,102). Mice with the sodium-proton antiporter gene (NHE3) knocked out show reduced HCO_3^- reabsorption in the proximal tubule and proximal RTA (103). Bicarbonate wasting results in metabolic acidosis once the HCO_3^- rejected by the proximal tubule overwhelms the reabsorptive capacity of the distal nephron. A neonatal form of proximal RTA occurs that is characterized by polyuria with episodes of dehydration, failure to thrive, vomiting, serum biochemical abnormalities, and a history of polyhydramnios.

Table 3   Inherited Causes of Fanconi Syndrome in Infancy

Idiopathic
Cystinosis (AR)
Deal syndrome (AR)
Disorders of energy metabolism
  Pearson's marrow-pancreas syndrome (maternal inheritance)
  Fatal infantile mitochondrial myopathy
  Mitochondrial cytopathy
  Cytochrome *c* oxidase deficiency
  Pyruvate carboxylase deficiency
  Carnitine palmitoyl transferase I deficiency
  Phosphoenolpyruvate carboxykinase deficiency
Galactosemia (AR)
Glycogneosis (AR)
Hereditary fructose intolerance (AR)
Oculocerebrorenal syndrome of Lowe (X-linked)
Tyrosinemia type I (AR)
Vitamin D-dependent rickets
Wilson disease

AR, autosomal recessive.
Source: Data modified from Brion LP, Satlin LM, Edelmann CM Jr (Renal disease. In: Textbook of Neonatology. Avery G, ed. Philadelphia: JP Lippincott, 1999:887–974).

Fanconi syndrome is a generalized proximal tubular dysfunction, characterized by proximal RTA, and in addition impaired reabsorption of Na^+, glucose, phosphate, uric acid, amino acids, and small molecular weight proteins. Fanconi syndrome occurs most often sporadically, but also in association with a variety of congenital disorders the most common of which is cystinosis (Table 3). The clinical presentation of Fanconi syndrome in infants and children includes polyuria, polydipsia, dehydration, and failure to thrive. Signs are acidosis, hypophosphatemia, rickets, generalized aminoaciduria, and glucosuria in the absence of hyperglycemia.

Carnitine depletion occurs in Fanconi syndrome because the proximal tubule fails to reabsorb free carnitine (104). Carnitine mediates the transport of coenzyme A-conjugated organic acids, including fatty acids, into the mitochondrial matrix for further metabolism. Tissues with high energy demands, such as the brain, muscle, liver, and kidney, are particularly sensitive to carnitine deficiency.

Distal RTA.   In distal RTA (type I) the tubular secretion of H^+ in the distal nephron is impaired, resulting in reduced net acid excretion and inability to lower urinary pH below 5.5 (105,106). The primary form of distal RTA is uncommon, and is due to specific gene defects (see also Chapter 13). Autosomal recessive forms generally present early in life, usually as severe growth retardation, and are often associated with parental consanguinity (107).

Other features might include deafness, rickets, mental retardation, hypokalemia, nephrocalcinosis, and renal calculi (105,106). One of the most endearing characters in English literature, Tiny Tim, the son of Ebenezer Scrooge's clerk Bob Cratchit in Charles Dicken's *"A Christmas Carol,"* may represent an example of this disorder. His short stature, crippling, and progressive weakness strongly suggest that Tiny Tim had distal RTA, complicated by osteomalacia, rickets, pathologic fractures, short stature, hypokalemic muscle weakness, and progression to renal failure (108). Interestingly, with the available tonics and solutions of that day (plus some prescient financial support from Scrooge to provide sufficient calories and fresh air), Tiny Tim might have been prescribed enough doses of "alkalies" and citrates to restore his growth, strength, skeletal mass, and kidney function.

Autosomal dominant forms sometimes present in childhood, but are generally less severe and do not cause as much growth retardation. Unlike adults, many infants and children with distal RTA show HCO_3^- wasting, such that the fractional excretion of HCO_3^- at normal plasma $[HCO_3^-]$ ranges from 5% to 15% of the filtered load (109,110). The magnitude of this HCO_3^- wasting presumably reflects proximal tubular immaturity as well as a distal inability to reabsorb HCO_3^- (109), and is the major determinant of the amount of alkali required to correct the acidosis. This combination of distal RTA and HCO_3^- wasting used to be called type III RTA (see below under mixed RTA); however, it is now recognized to be a characteristic feature of infantile distal RTA. In general, this HCO_3^- wasting diminishes by age 4–6 years (111,112).

The genetic basis for distal RTA can be considered in the context of the major transporters of the acid-secreting α-intercalated cell of the collecting duct. Mutations in the basolateral anion exchanger AE1 generally cause the autosomal dominant form of distal RTA (113,114); however, some autosomal recessive cases of distal RTA have also been observed (115,116). Autosomal recessive forms are consistently encountered with mutations in the genes coding for cytosolic CA II and vacuolar proton pumps. The CA II deficiency syndrome results from at least 12 different mutations in CA II on chromosome 8 (107) and is characterized by RTA, osteopetrosis and cerebral calcification (99,100). The majority of reported cases come from the Middle East (107,117). The CA II-deficient phenotypes may be distal, proximal, or hybrid types of RTA (118,119).

Distal RTA is also seen with mutations in the apical H^+-ATPase in the distal nephron, and most cases present in the first two years of life (120). At least 15 mutations have been found in the *ATP6B1* gene that encodes the B1 (ATPase) subunit of the vacuolar H^+-ATPase in α-intercalated cells. Bilateral sensorineural deafness is present in most patients with distal RTA due to these mutations (120). Other patients have distal RTA with normal hearing due to a mutation in a gene coding for a different subunit of H^+-ATPase (121,122).

The role of the H^+,K^+-ATPase in acid–base homeostasis has been controversial. However, we recently described an infant who presented with failure to thrive in association with severe hypokalemia, distal RTA, and normal gastric acidification (123). He most likely has a defect in a nongastric form of H^+,K^+-ATPase in the medullary collecting duct. Indeed, vanadate, an inhibitor of the H^+,K^+-ATPase, causes a similar condition in rats (124).

While hyperammonemia is frequently found with organic acidemias, it can also occur in distal RTA (125). Presumably, in response to acidosis, the proximal tubules increase ammonia synthesis, but much of this newly synthesized ammonia is not excreted, because the urine cannot be acidified in the collecting ducts. With correction of the acidosis, blood ammonia levels fall to normal (125).

Hyperkalemic distal RTA. Primary hyperkalemic RTA (type IV) has been described in some infants and children, who present with failure to thrive and frequent vomiting but without nephrocalcinosis (106). These patients have distal RTA with hyperkalemia, but with no impairment in ability to lower urine pH; acquired obstructive uropathy and tubulointerstitial disease are commonly present. The acidosis might be due to a combined rate-limited secretory defect caused by a lack of direct stimulation of H^+-ATPase by aldosterone, a voltage defect from decreased Na^+ reabsorption, and impaired ammonium production. Type IV RTA can be the only indication of the presence of obstructive uropathy (126). It has also been observed in long-term survivors of inborn errors of metabolism. Children with methylmalonic academia can develop chronic interstitial nephritis and a syndrome of hyporeninemic hypoaldosteronism, possibly due to accumulation of metabolites that are toxic to the kidney tubules (127).

Type IV RTA is associated with hypoaldosterone states, such as primary hypoaldosteronism with congenital adrenal hyperplasia (primarily 21-hydroxylase deficiency in children) or primary adrenal insufficiency, and pseudohypoaldosteronism (types I and II). Type I pseudohypoaldosteronism is associated with failure to thrive, dehydration, hyponatremia, hyperkalemia, metabolic acidosis, and high plasma aldosterone and renin levels (128). It is unresponsive to mineralocorticoids because of mutations in the subunits of the amiloride-sensitive epithelial Na^+ channel of the distal nephron (128).

The most common form of congenital adrenal hyperplasia is 21-hydroxylase deficiency, an autosomal recessive disorder occurring in one of every 14,000 births (129). There is decreased mineralocorticoid and cortisol synthesis, and the latter leads to increased ACTH release with enhanced adrenal androgen synthesis and virilization through the accumulation of 17-hydroxyprogesterone (129). Infants with the classic syndrome present with salt wasting, hyperkalemia, and metabolic acidosis.

In addition, a hyperkalemic variant of type II distal RTA occurs, which is due to a voltage defect and not associated with hypoaldosteronism or aldosterone resistance. Unlike the latter form of type IV RTA, the urinary pH in the variant with a voltage defect does not decrease below 5.5.

Mixed RTA. In some cases of infantile RTA, both proximal and distal components are present; this hybrid form used to be known as mixed RTA or type III. Typically, the HCO_3^- wasting disappears after 6 years of age. Very low-birth-weight infants during the first weeks of life might have a mixed RTA with lower normal values of plasma $[HCO_3^-]$ and higher urinary pH despite the acidosis. This picture might reflect delayed maturational physiology. Patients with CA II deficiency may also have mixed RTA (117–119), but in these patients the HCO_3^- wasting persists (117).

Diagnosis of RTA: The diagnosis of RTA should be considered in any infant or child with growth failure and persistent hyperchloremic metabolic acidosis with a normal anion gap (see also Chapter 13, "Renal Tubular Acidosis"). Before making the diagnosis, it is critical to assure that the patient is well-hydrated, well-nourished, and without other sources of HCO_3^- loss, such as chronic diarrhea. Because the full renal adaptation to acidosis takes several days, follow-up studies are always required. First, one confirms the presence of metabolic acidosis by an arterial blood gas (Fig. 10). A venous blood gas (VBG) can be adequate for follow-up, if it is unlikely that a primary respiratory alkalosis is present. The calculated plasma $[HCO_3^-]$ of the VBG should agree to within 10% of the measured $[HCO_3^-]$ on the electrolyte panel (98). If not, one should suspect an apparent decrease in plasma $[HCO_3^-]$ associated with poor blood drawing or sample handling technique (Table 4). In addition, the presence of a normal serum anion gap needs to be confirmed. Any condition associated with substantial abnormalities in an unmeasured cation or an anion can give a normal-appearing anion gap (and falsely rule out a high-anion-gap acidosis, Table 4).

Next, the renal response to acidosis is evaluated. Measurement of urinary pH is a necessary first step, but it is not sufficient for evaluation of RTA. Alkaline urine is characteristic of distal RTA, whereas both proximal RTA and type IV RTA can present with acidic urine. Other conditions causing high urine pH during metabolic acidosis include: (i) urinary infections with urea-splitting organisms; (ii) severe K^+ depletion stimulating ammoniagenesis and generating excessive ammonia to buffer free luminal protons; and (iii) gastrointestinal losses producing avid salt retention with decreased distal Na^+ delivery, leading to an abnormal distal luminal electrochemical gradient and subsequent increased urinary pH (98).

The gold standard for assessing the renal response to metabolic acidosis is measurement of titratable acid and NH_4^+ excretion. Because most laboratories do not routinely measure these parameters, alternatives have been suggested. The urine anion gap (UAG, actually cation gap), defined as UAG = Urine $[Na^+] + [K^+] - [Cl^-]$, provides a good estimation of urine $[NH_4^+]$ in the setting of metabolic acidosis (105,130,131). A negative UAG

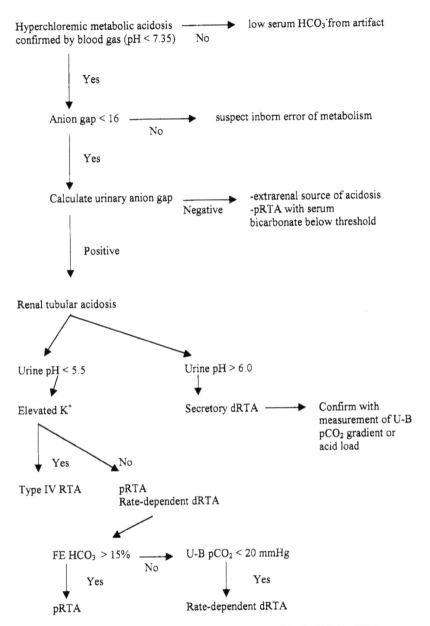

Figure 10 Algorithm for diagnosing renal tubular acidosis (RTA). VBG, venous blood gas; pRTA, proximal RTA; dRTA, distal RTA. *Source*: From Gregory MJ, Schwartz GJ (Sem Neph 1998; 18:317).

Table 4   Factors Interfering with the Diagnosis of RTA

Factors responsible for artificially decreasing serum [HCO_3^-]
   Prolonged tourniquet use
   Use of heel stick with poor blood flow to obtain blood
   Underfilling of blood vial
   Delay between time blood obtained and time blood processed
   Blood gas specimen with large amount of heparin in syringe
Factors responsible for artificially reducing serum anion gap to normal
   Decreased concentration of unmeasured anion, principally albumin
   Retained nonsodium cations (calcium, magnesium)
   Lithium intoxication
   Severe hypernatremia (>170 mEq/L)

---

is the appropriate response, indicating that sufficient NH_4^+ is present; a positive gap suggests an inappropriate absence of NH_4^+ and a defect in urinary acidification. The UAG cannot be used in high-anion-gap acidosis (because of excessive urinary organic anions) or in severe volume depletion with avid Na^+ retention (because of decreased distal delivery). Caution should be used when interpreting the UAG in neonates (132). If excessive unmeasured urine anions are suspected, urine [NH_4^+] can be estimated from the difference between measured and calculated urine osmolalities (133), as follows (131):

$$\text{Urine}[NH]_4^+ = 0.5 \times \{\text{Osmolality} - (2 \times ([Na^+]$$
$$+ K^+]) + [\text{urea}] + [\text{glucose}])\},$$

where osmolality is the measured value in mOsm/kg H_2O, and the concentration of each urine solute is in mmol/L.

Once the diagnosis is established, further evaluation is needed to determine the tubular defect responsible. Low urinary pH (< 5.5) indicates appropriate distal urinary acidification and suggests one of the following defects: abnormal proximal reabsorption of HCO_3^-, an abnormal renin–aldosterone axis, or a rate-limited secretory distal defect. A urine pH of > 5.5 points to a defect in distal acidification (classic distal RTA). Tests that can further define the tubular defect are measurement of the urine-blood PCO_2 (U-B PCO_2) under conditions of alkali loading (see Chapter 13) (134) and measurement of titratable acid and NH_4^+ (or pH and UAG) after an acute acid (NH_4Cl) load (105,131). The presence of RTA and hyperkalemia suggests type IV RTA. These children need careful evaluation for the presence of underlying renal disease or renal structural anomalies. If no abnormality is found, then an evaluation of the renin–aldosterone axis should be done.

Therapy of RTA: All children with RTA require alkali replacement. In classic distal RTA, the accompanying hypokalemia makes potassium (rather than sodium) citrate or bicarbonate the preferred supplement. Also, the use of potassium salts reduces the hypercalciuria of distal RTA by preventing volume expansion with sodium. A good starting dose of alkali for distal RTA is 3 mEq/kg/day given in divided doses, followed by titration upward until acidosis is corrected. As growth velocity increases in response to alkali therapy, increasing doses are often needed (98,109,135). Infants require larger doses of alkali per kg body weight than older children because of the associated HCO_3^- wasting and the more rapid rate of skeletal growth, which generates more H^+ (see earlier) (111,135).

For proximal RTA, alkali treatment usually starts at 5 mEq/kg/day given in divided doses and can increase to as high as 20 mEq/kg/day (135,136). Combinations of sodium and potassium citrate or bicarbonate are generally used for treatment. Correction of acidosis usually results in catch-up growth (80,136). If the dose of alkali required for correction of the acidosis is prohibitively large, a thiazide (hydrochlorothiazide 1–2 mg/kg or chlorothiazide 10–20 mg/kg/day) can be added to permit correction of the acidosis with lower dose of administered alkali. Additional treatment of the Fanconi syndrome includes supplements of sodium, water, potassium, phosphate, and carnitine (104).

Treatment of type IV RTA depends on its etiology. With underlying renal pathology, one corrects acidosis with alkali supplements (1–2 mEq/kg/day) and restricts dietary K^+. A loop diuretic is often added to facilitate urinary K^+ loss. Aldosterone deficiency is treated with synthetic mineralocorticoid (fludrocortisone, 0.05–0.2 mg/day), whereas patients with pseudohypoaldosteronism can often be treated with sodium supplements and potassium-binding resins.

Metabolic Alkalosis

Metabolic alkalosis results from either a gain of HCO_3^- by the ECF or a loss of acid from that fluid (Table 5). Usually, the latter occurs because the renal ability to alkalinize the urine is impaired by concomitant Na^+, K^+ and/or Cl^- deficiency. The most common cause is loss of acid in the course of vomiting, and this is observed in infants with hypertrophic pyloric stenosis. Other presentations that are unique to pediatric practice include metabolic alkalosis due to dietary Cl^- deficiency, Bartter's syndrome, and congenital chloride-losing diarrhea. Long-term complications of metabolic alkalosis include the risk for sensorineural hearing loss in low-birth-weight infants (137) and failure to thrive (see below).

As in adults, the urine $[Cl^-]$ is useful in differentiating among the various causes of metabolic alkalosis. Children with metabolic alkalosis due to pyloric stenosis, vomiting, low Cl^- intake, congenital chloride-losing diarrhea, cystic fibrosis, or late after diuretic therapy should have maximum urinary Cl^- conservation (urine $[Cl^-] < 25$ mEq/L), due to the normal renal

Table 5 Causes of Metabolic Alkalosis in Infants and Children

---

Loss of protons
Gastrointestinal loss
  Gastric secretions (pyloric stenosis, nasogastric suction, vomiting)[a]
  Stool secretions (congenital chloridorrhea, Cl^--losing diarrhea)
Renal loss
  Diuretics (loop or thiazide-type)[a]
Mineralocorticoid excess (primary hyperaldosteronism or hyperreninemia)[a]
Chloride deficiency (dietary chloride deficiency syndrome, congenital chloridorrhea, Bartter-type syndromes)
Postchronic hypercapnia
High-dose nonreabsorbable anion delivery (carbenicillin, penicillin-derivatives)
Cellular shifts
Hypokalemia
Retention of bicarbonate
HCO_3^- (intravenous $NaHCO_3$ therapy)
Citrate (extensive blood transfusion, plasma protein fractions)
Carbonate (antacids, milk-alkali syndrome)
Acetate (hyperalimentation, peritoneal dialysate)
Lactate (intravenous fluids)
Contraction alkalosis
Loop or thiazide-type diuretics[a]
Sweat losses in cystic fibrosis

---

[a]Most common causes.
Source: Some data from Rose BD, Post TW (Clinical Physiology of Acid–Base and Electrolyte Disorders. 5th ed. New York: McGraw-Hill, 2001:552).

response to Cl^- and/or ECF volume depletion. Children with metabolic alkalosis due to mineralocorticoid excess, alkali or organic anion loading, severe hypokalemia, or shortly after diuretic therapy should have urine $[Cl^-] > 40$ mEq/L and signs of volume expansion. Urine $[Cl^-]$ is also high in Bartter's syndrome and Bartter-like syndromes, even though signs of hypervolemia might be absent. Note that urine $[Cl^-]$ might not be as useful in low-birth-weight infants who cannot conserve Cl^- early in life (132).

Causes

Dietary Chloride Deficiency: A severe hypochloremic hypokalemic metabolic alkalosis with failure to thrive was identified in infants fed chloride-deficient soybean formulas manufactured in the United States in 1978–79 (Neo-Mull-Soy; Syntex Laboratories) and in Spain in 1981 (Aptamil-1, Milupa S.A.) (138–141). None of the affected babies had hypertension despite having high plasma renin and aldosterone levels (138,140). The Cl^- content of many batches of formula was below 1.0 mEq/L (139,141) compared to breast milk, which ranges from 8 to 12 mEq/L. Indeed, Cl^- was absent from the urine of these babies (139,140) indicating that they were able to conserve it, and establishing that a deficiency of dietary Cl^- was responsible for the metabolic alkalosis.

Pyloric Stenosis: Nearly all infants with hypertrophic pyloric stenosis are alkalemic (142), whereas blood pH might be alkaline, normal, or acidic in those who are vomiting from other causes. The reason is that when infants vomit with an open pylorus, the vomitus is comprised of alkaline intestinal juices in addition to acidic gastric fluid, and the resulting acid–base state depends on the balance of these losses (bile staining indicates intestinal juices). The vomiting of pyloric stenosis is clearly acidic, without addition of intestinal juices, causing large losses of H^+ and Cl^-. As HCO_3^- rises in the blood, it is excreted in the urine in the company of K^+, so that hypokalemia accompanies the volume contraction and metabolic alkalosis. Hypokalemia causes a transcellular shift of K^+ out of cells and H^+ into cells, resulting in an intracellular acidosis, which in turn stimulates both proximal and distal tubule H^+ secretion. The initial response of the kidney is to produce an alkaline urine; that is, to excrete HCO_3^- in conjunction with Na^+ and K^+. As the body stores of Na^+, K^+ and Cl^- fall (because of ongoing losses and with vomiting precluding their replenishment from the diet), the kidney then avidly reabsorbs Na^+, largely in exchange for H^+ rather than the deficient K^+. At this point urine pH again falls to acid levels (the so-called "paradoxical acidura"), contributing to maintenance of the alkalosis (see Chapter 17).

Treatment includes cessation of oral intake, restoration of ECF with intravenous NaCl (often 10–15 mEq/kg body weight), and replacement of K^+ losses with KCl (3–5 mEQ/kg body weight per day) (142). Correction of the metabolic alkalosis over a few days is necessary to prepare such infants for surgery, because an unstable acid–base status heightens the risk of complications during anesthesia.

Bartter Syndrome: Bartter syndrome is characterized by hypochloremic alkalosis with severe hypokalemia and intravascular volume depletion, hyperreninemia, secondary hyperaldosteronism and normal blood pressure (143). Pathologically, the kidneys demonstrate hypertrophy and hyperplasia of the juxtaglomerular apparatus. It is a hereditary autosomal recessive disease associated with mutations in transport systems located in the thick ascending limb of Henle's loop and collecting duct. Clinical disease is attributable to defective NaCl reabsorption in the thick ascending limb, where approximately 30% of the filtered salt is reabsorbed (98,144–146). Transport of Na^+, K^+, and Cl^- ions across the apical membrane of the thick ascending limb is mediated by the Na–K–2Cl cotransporter. Recycling of K^+ from the cell back into the lumen is via the K channel ROMK. Chloride and Na^+ traverse the basolateral membrane into the bloodstream via a Cl^- channel and the Na^+,K^+-ATPase, respectively (146). Mutations in the activity of any of these processes could be expected to reduce the reabsorption of NaCl in the thick ascending limb and lead to the clinical presentation of Bartter syndrome.

Three distinct phenotypes have been identified, each associated with a hypokalemic metabolic alkalosis. The neonatal variant (formerly termed hyperprostaglandin E syndrome) presents in the newborn period with dehydration, failure to thrive, dysmorphic facies, and a history of polyhydramnios and premature delivery (145,147). Infants with this disorder usually have significant Na^+ wasting, polyuria, and hypercalciuria, elevated urinary prostaglandin E levels, and normal serum magnesium levels. Nephrocalcinosis is usually present at birth. This syndrome is caused by mutations in the gene encoding the $Na^+/K^+/2Cl$ cotransporter (NKCC2 or BSC1, Bartter type I) (146,148) or in the gene encoding the ATP-regulated K^+ channel (ROMK, Bartter type II) (147,149), both of which are expressed in the thick ascending limb of Henle's loop.

The second phenotype is classic Bartter's syndrome which presents in infants and children (< 5 years) often as failure to thrive with signs of severe intravascular volume depletion. Loss-of-function of the renal Cl^- channel (ClCNKB, Bartter type III) (146) causes most of the cases of the classic phenotype (144,150). Compared to the neonatal form, urine calcium is less elevated and nephocalcinosis is absent (146).

Gitelman syndrome. The third phenotype of hypokalemic metabolic alkalosis is now known as Gitelman syndrome and is due to mutations in the thiazide-sensitive NaCl cotransporter (NCCT or TSC) in the distal convoluted tubule (151). This form presents in childhood or later; it is not usually associated with growth retardation, salt craving, or bouts of dehydration, and might be asymptomatic. This subgroup comprises the Bartter-type patients having hypomagnesemia and hypocalciuria. Although serum calcium values are normal, the combination of hypomagnesemia and alkalosis tend to cause recurrent episodes of muscle spasm and tetany.

Treatment of the Bartter/Gitelman syndromes is focused on correcting the electrolyte abnormalities and preventing dehydration. Potassium chloride therapy is required to fully address the K^+ imbalance and NaCl helps manage the defect in Cl^- reabsorption. Spironolactone, a K^+ sparing diuretic, is often helpful. Indomethacin inhibits prostaglandin production and decreases renin and aldosterone production. Despite these treatments, neonatal Bartter patients often have persistent hypokalemia. Patients with Gitelman syndrome require magnesium salts ($MgCl_2$ also compensates for the Cl^- losses). In these patients, the hypokalemia is treated with KCl and/or spironolactone or amiloride (98,150). Volume resuscitation and prostaglandin synthase inhibition are not required.

Other patients with chronic hypokalemic metabolic alkalosis do not have Bartter-like syndromes but rather a state of Cl^- depletion due to either extrarenal causes (administration of a Cl^--deficient formula, bulimia with cyclic vomiting, congenital chloridorrhea, laxative abuse, cystic fibrosis) or surreptitious use of diuretics (150). Such patients are grouped under the heading "pseudo-Bartter syndrome." Diagnosis can be readily made if one demonstrates a low urinary [Cl⁻] or the presence of diuretics in the urine (150).

Congenital Enteric Chloride Wasting

Infants have been described with congenital Cl⁻ losses in the stool. Because enteric fluids distal to the stomach are alkaline, this type of diarrhea leads to metabolic acidosis. However, the rare defect, congenital chloridorrhea, is associated with a specific intestinal defect in Cl⁻ absorption and HCO_3^- secretion, resulting in a high fecal [Cl⁻], substantial fecal K^+ content, and low fecal pH (152,153). The defective protein is closely related to the sulfate transporter family and is a membrane glycoprotein located in the apical brush border of colonic mucosal epithelial cells that functions as a Cl^-/HCO_3^- or a Cl^-/OH^- antiporter (154,155). Infants are usually born prematurely with polyhydramnios and develop severe dehydration and electrolyte disorders soon after birth. Loss of Cl⁻-rich fluid leads to increased serum [HCO_3^-] and a metabolic alkalosis with hypokalemia, not unlike Bartter's syndrome, but urinary [Cl⁻] is very low. The same electrolyte defect might also occur in cystic fibrosis of the pancreas (156). Management requires supplemental KCl at 3–5 mEq/kg/day (91).

Mixed Acid–Base Disturbances

Mixed acid–base disorders are defined as the coexistence of two or more primary acid–base disorders (see Chapter 22 for a full discussion of mixed disorders). Several mixed disorders occur in infants and children. A frequently encountered mixed disorder is chronic metabolic alkalosis and respiratory acidosis, which occurs in low-birth-weight infants with bronchopulmonary dysplasia on long-term diuretic treatment. Other examples include salicylate poisoning and metabolic diseases of the urea cycle in children in whom the organic acidosis coexists with the centrally driven respiratory alkalosis. These entities are discussed below.

Bronchopulmonary Dysplasia

This condition is frequently associated with low gestational age and birth weight (extreme prematurity), severe hyaline membrane disease of the newborn with oxygen toxicity, patent ductus arteriosus, barotrauma from mechanical ventilation, and insufficient nutrition. These infants retain excess interstitial lung fluid due to the nonspecific inflammatory process that continues in their lungs. Fluid boluses and positive Na^+ and fluid balance promote lung fluid accumulation and ductal patency, and are associated with an increased incidence and severity of bronchopulmonary dysplasia. These infants initially have a chronic respiratory acidosis, but with prolonged and aggressive diuretic treatment, they develop a mixed disturbance of respiratory acidosis and metabolic alkalosis; the net effect on blood pH depends on the dominant component. Occasionally, a normal blood pH results. Thus, in hypercapnic newborns undergoing diuretic therapy, a normal or elevated blood pH indicates the coexistence of a metabolic alkalosis with depletion of K^+ and Cl^-. At times, a diuretic-induced metabolic alkalosis may go unrecognized as the premature infant retains more CO_2.

Diuretic-induced hypochloremic metabolic alkalosis is also associated with growth failure and may contribute to the poor outcome of infants with bronchopulmonary dysplasia (157). Growth failure is caused primarily by the decrease in cell proliferation and diminished DNA and protein synthesis in association with intracellular alkalosis (158). Chronic hyponatremia with a negative Na^+ balance might further inhibit normal growth in premature infants (80).

Bronchopulmonary dysplasia treated with diuretics is usually accompanied by hyponatremia, as Na^+ shifts into the intracellular space to replace K^+. In this situation, KCl, rather than NaCl, at 3–7 mEq/kg/day corrects the abnormalities (79). Moreover, administration of Na^+ can aggravate respiratory failure. Because Cl^- deficiency is the predominant cause of the increased blood pH, ammonium chloride or arginine chloride can be used to correct the alkalosis.

Salicylate Intoxication: Accidental ingestion of aspirin is generally seen in the toddler age group, in a child who is mobile and previously well. The usual findings in severe salicylism include hyperventilation, vomiting, dehydration, and polyuria followed by oliguria (159). There is a clear age-dependent difference in the response to salicylate intoxication (see also Chapter 12). Children 0–4 years of age tend to have a blood pH below 7.35, whereas older children tend to show a pH above 7.4 and only rarely have acidemia (159). The stimulating effect of salicylates on oxidative metabolism drives oxygen consumption and CO_2 production, while the direct effect of salicylates to stimulate the respiratory center causes hyperventilation and decreased $PaCO_2$; the latter effect dominates in older children, resulting in a respiratory alkalosis. In the younger child, there is a third effect of salicylates to increase production of organic acids (ketone bodies and others) resulting in a mixed acid–base disturbance: respiratory alkalosis and metabolic acidosis (159). The metabolic acidosis is a high anion gap disturbance, the decrease in plasma $[HCO_3^-]$ being largely due to an increase in ketoacids (β-hydroxybutyric and acetoacetic acids) with a small contribution from the ingested acetylsalicylic acid. The relative intensities of the metabolic and respiratory perturbations determine the final blood pH. In severely poisoned toddlers, the increased production of organic acids outweighs the respiratory stimulation, resulting in an acidemia along with profuse ketonuria. In some patients, these processes are balanced resulting in a normal blood pH in the presence of reduced levels of plasma [HCO_3^-] and $PaCO_2$. Treatment includes induction of emesis, rehydration, alkalinization of the urine, and in severe cases, removal of salicylate by dialysis.

Metabolic Disorders: Another problem unique to pediatrics is the case of a child with a urea cycle disorder and evolving hyperammonemic coma (82). Such patients exhibit central hyperventilation, which leads to an initial respiratory alkalosis; metabolic acidosis is not a typical feature of urea cycle defects. Then, as the child becomes sicker, dehydration and starvation ensue, resulting in a metabolic acidosis. Clearly, for some of these mixed disturbances, the time of blood pH sampling is most critical in making the diagnosis. Sampling too early might miss the metabolic component that ultimately offsets the central hyperventilation seen in salicylism and some inborn errors of metabolism.

ACKNOWLEDGMENTS

Work from my laboratory has been supported by grants from the NIH (DK-50603) and from the American Heart Association. I am grateful to Dr R. Guillet and Dr C.-T. Fong for thought-provoking discussions and critical reviews of the manuscript.

REFERENCES

1. Smith CA. The Physiology of the Newborn Infant. Springfield: Thomas,C.C., 1959.
2. Weisbrot IM, James LS, Prince CE, Holaday DA, Apgar V. Acid–base homeostasis of the newborn infant during the first 24 hours of life. J Pediatr 1958; 53:395–403.
3. Schwartz GJ. Acid–base homeostasis. In: Edelmann CM Jr, ed. Pediatric Kidney Disease. Boston: Little, Brown and Company, 1992:201–230.
4. Edelmann CM Jr, Spitzer A. The maturing kidney: a modern view of well-balanced infants with imbalanced nephrons. J Pediatr 1969; 75:509–519.
5. Vaughn D, Kirschbaum TH, Bersentes T, Dilts PV Jr, Assali NS. Fetal neonatal response to acid loading in the sheep. J Appl Physiol 1968; 24:135–141.
6. Smith FG, Schwartz A. Response of the intact lamb fetus to acidosis. Am J Obstet Gynecol 1970; 106:52–58.
7. Yamada N. Respiratory environment and acid–base balance in the developing fetus. Biol Neonate 1970; 16:222–242.
8. Kesby GJ, Lumbers ER. Factors affecting renal handling of sodium, hydrogen ions, and bicarbonate by the fetus. Am J Physiol 1986; 251:F226–F231.
9. Graham BD, Wilson JL, Tsao MU, Baumann ML, Brown S. Development of neonatal electrolyte homeostasis. Pediatrics 1951; 8:68–78.

10. Kerpel-Fronius E, Heim T, Sulyok E. The development of the renal acidifying processes and their relation to acidosis in low-birth-weight infants. Biol Neonate 1970; 15:156–168.

11. Sulyok E, Heim T. Assessment of maximal urinary acidification in premature infants. Biol Neonate 1971; 19:200–210.

12. Alpern RJ, Stone DK, Rector FC Jr. Renal acidification mechanisms. In: Brenner BM, Rector FC Jr, eds. The Kidney. Philadelphia: WB Saunders, 1996:408–471.

13. Pitts RF, Ayer JL, Schiess WA. The renal regulation of acid–base balance in man. III. The reabsorption and excretion of bicarbonate. J Clin Invest 1949; 28:35–44.

14. Edelmann CM Jr, Rodriguez-Soriano J, Boichis H, Gruskin AB, Acosta M. Renal bicarbonate reabsorption and hydrogen ion excretion in infants. J Clin Invest 1967; 46:1309–1317.

15. Svenningsen NW. Renal acid–base titration studies in infants with and without metabolic acidosis in the postneonatal period. Pediatr Res 1974; 8: 659–672.

16. Tudvad F, McNamara H, Barnett HL. Renal response of premature infants to administration of bicarbonate and potassium. Pediatrics 1954; 13:4–16.

17. Schwartz GJ, Haycock GB, Edelmann CM Jr, Spitzer A. Late metabolic acidosis: a reassessment of the definition. J Pediatr 1979; 95:102–107.

18. Sulyok E. The relationship between electrolyte and acid–base balance in the premature infant during early postnatal life. Biol Neonate 1971; 17:227–237.

19. Spitzer A, Schwartz GJ. The kidney during development. In: Windhager EE, ed. Handbook of Physiology. Section 8: Renal Physiology. New York: Oxford University Press, 1992:475–544.

20. Hatemi N, McCance RA. Renal aspects of acid–base control in the newly born. III. Response to acidifying drugs. Acta Paediatr Scand 1961; 50:603–616.

21. McCance RA, Hatemi N. Control of acid–base stability in the newly born. Lancet 1961; 1:293–297.

22. Fomon SJ, Harris DM, Jensen RL. Acidification of the urine by infants fed human milk and whole cow's milk. Pediatrics 1959; 23:113–120.

23. Cort JH, McCance RA. The renal response of puppies to an acidosis. J Physiol 1954; 124:358–369.

24. Svenningsen NW, Lindquist B. Postnatal development of renal hydrogen ion excretion capacity in relation to age and protein intake. Acta Paediatr Scand 1974; 63:721–731.

25. Sulyok E, Heim T, Soltesz G, Jaszai V. The influence of maturity on renal control of acidosis in newborn infants. Biol Neonate 1972; 21:418–435.

26. Svenningsen NW, Lindquist B. Incidence of metabolic acidosis in term, preterm and small-for-gestational age infants in relation to dietary protein intake. Acta Paediatr Scand 1973; 62:1–10.

27. Kildeberg P, Engel K, Winters RW. Balance of net acid in growing infants: endogenous and transintestinal aspects. Acta Paediatr Scand 1969; 58: 321–329.

28. Wamberg S, Kildeberg P, Engel K. Balance of net base in the rat. II. Reference values in relation to growth rate. Biol Neonate 1976; 28:171–190.
29. Kildeberg P, Winters RW. Balance of net acid: concept, measurement, and applications. Adv Pediatr 1978; 25:349–381.
30. Kleinman LI. The kidney. In: Stave U, ed. Perinatal Physiology. New York: Plenum, 1978:589–616.
31. Moore ES, Fine BP, Satrasook SS, Vergel ZM, Edelmann CM Jr. Renal reabsorption of bicarbonate in puppies: effect of extracellular volume concentration on the renal threshold for bicarbonate. Pediatr Res 1972; 6:859–867.
32. Friis-Hansen B. Body water compartments in children: changes during growth and related changes in body composition. Pediatrics 1961; 28:169–181.
33. Lelievre-Pegorier M, Merlet-Benichou C, Roinel N, De Rouffignac C. Developmental pattern of water and electrolyte transport in rat superficial nephrons. Am J Physiol 1983; 245:F15–F21.
34. Evan AP, Gattone VHI, Schwartz GJ. Development of solute transport in rabbit proximal tubule. II. Morphological segmentation. Am J Physiol 1983; 245:F391–F407.
35. Schwartz GJ, Evan AP. Development of solute transport in rabbit proximal tubule. I. HCO_3^- and glucose absorption. Am J Physiol 1983; 245:F382–F390.
36. Quigley R, Baum M. Developmental changes in rabbit juxtamedullary proximal convoluted tubule bicarbonate permeability. Pediatr Res 1990; 28:663–666.
37. Baum M. Developmental changes in rabbit juxtamedullary proximal convoluted tubule acidification. Pediatr Res 1992; 31:411–414.
38. Baum M. Neonatal rabbit juxtamedullary proximal convoluted tubule acidification. J Clin Invest 1990; 85:499–506.
39. Beck JC, Lipkowitz MS, Abramson RG. Ontogeny of Na/H antiporter activity in rabbit renal brush border membrane vesicles. J Clin Invest 1991; 87:2067–2076.
40. Biemesderfer D, Rutherford PA, Nagy T, Pizzonia JH, Abu-Alfa AK, Aronson PS. Monoclonal antibodies for high-resolution localization of NHE3 in adult and neonatal rat kidney. Am J Physiol 1997; 273:F289–F299.
41. Baum M, Biemesderfer D, Gentry D, Aronson PS. Ontogeny of rabbit renal cortical NHE3 and NHE1: effect of glucocorticoids. Am J Physiol 1995; 268:F815–F820.
42. Aperia A, Larsson L, Zetterstrom R. Hormonal induction of Na–K-ATPase in developing proximal tubular cells. Am J Physiol 1981; 241:F356–F360.
43. Schwartz GJ, Evan P. Development of solute transport in rabbit proximal tubule. III. Na–K-ATPase activity. Am J Physiol 1984; 246:F845–F852.
44. Caldwell T, Solomon S. Changes in oxygen consumption of kidney during maturation. Biol Neonate 1975; 25:1–9.
45. Dicker SE, Shirley DG. Rates of oxygen consumption and of anaerobic glycolysis in renal cortex and medulla of adult and newborn rats and guinea-pigs. J Physiol 1971; 212:235–243.
46. Harris RC, Seifter JL, Lechene C. Coupling of Na–H exchange and Na–K pump activity in cultured rat proximal tubule cells. Am J Physiol 1986; 251:C815–C824.

47. Fukuda Y, Aperia A. Differentiation of Na^+-K^+ pump in rat proximal tubule is modulated by Na^+-H^+ exchanger. Am J Physiol 1988; 255:F552–F557.

48. Brion LP, Zavilowitz BJ, Suarez C, Schwartz GJ. Metabolic acidosis stimulates carbonic anhydrase activity in rabbit proximal tubule and medullary collecting duct. Am J Physiol 1994; 266:F185–F195.

49. Dobyan DC, Bulger RE. Renal carbonic anhydrase. Am J Physiol 1982; 243:F311–F324.

50. Sly WS. The carbonic anhydrase II deficiency syndrome: osteopetrosis with renal tubular acidosis and cerebral calcification. In: Scriver CR, Beaudet AL, Sly WS, Valle D, eds. The Metabolic Basis of Inherited Disease. New York: McGraw-Hill, 1989:2857–2866.

51. Burg M, Green N. Bicarbonate transport by isolated perfused rabbit proximal tubules. Am J Physiol 1977; 233:F307–F314.

52. DuBose TD Jr, Lucci MS. Effect of carbonic anhydrase inhibition on superficial and deep nephron bicarbonate reabsorption in the rat. J Clin Invest 1983; 71:55–65.

53. Cogan MG, Maddox DA, Warnock DG, Lin ET, Rector FC Jr. Effect of acetazolamide on bicarbonate reabsorption in the proximal tubule of the rat. Am J Physiol 1979; 237:F447–F454.

54. Brown D, Zhu XL, Sly WS. Localization of membrane-associated carbonic anhydrase type IV in kidney epithelial cells. Proc Natl Acad Sci USA 1990; 87:7457–7461.

55. Schwartz GJ, Olson J, Kittelberger AM, Matsumoto T, Waheed A, Sly WS. Postnatal development of carbonic anhydrase IV expression in rabbit kidney. Am J Physiol 1999; 276:F510–F520.

56. Day R, Franklin J. Renal carbonic anhydrase in premature and mature infants. Pediatrics 1951; 7:182–185.

57. Lonnerholm G, Wistrand PJ. Carbonic anhydrase in the human fetal kidney. Pediatr Res 1983; 17:390–397.

58. Brion LP, Zavilowitz BJ, Rosen O, Schwartz GJ. Changes in soluble carbonic anhydrase activity in response to maturation and NH_4Cl loading in the rabbit. Am J Physiol 1991; 261:R1204–R1213.

59. Maren TH. Carbonic anhydrase: chemistry, physiology and inhibition. Physiol Rev 1967; 47:595–781.

60. Karashima S, Hattori S, Ushijima T, Furuse A, Nakazato H, Matsuda I. Developmental changes in carbonic anhydrase II in the rat kidney. Pediatr Nephrol 1998; 12:263–268.

61. Winkler CA, Kittelberger AM, Watkins RH, Maniscalco WM, Schwartz GJ. Maturation of carbonic anhydrase IV expression in rabbit kidney. Am J Physiol 2001; 280:F895–F903.

62. Schwartz GJ, Barasch J, Al-Awqati Q. Plasticity of functional epithelial polarity. Nature 1985; 318:368–371.

63. McKinney TD, Burg MB. Bicarbonate transport by rabbit cortical collecting tubules. J Clin Invest 1977; 60:766–768.

64. Satlin LM, Schwartz GJ. Postnatal maturation of the rabbit renal collecting duct: intercalated cell function. Am J Physiol 1987; 253:F622–F635.

65. Satlin LM, Matsumoto T, Schwartz GJ. Postnatal maturation of rabbit renal collecting duct. III. Peanut lectin-binding intercalated cells. Am J Physiol 1992; 262:F199–F208.
66. Kim J, Tisher CC, Madsen KM. Differentiation of intercalated cells in developing rat kidney: an immunohistochemical study. Am J Physiol 1994; 266: F977–F990.
67. Matsumoto T, Fejes-Toth G, Schwartz GJ. Postnatal differentiation of rabbit collecting duct intercalated cells. Pediatr Res 1996; 39:1–12.
68. Evan AP, Satlin LM, Gattone VH II, Connors B, Schwartz GJ. Postnatal maturation of rabbit renal collecting duct. II. Morphological observations. Am J Physiol 1991; 261:F91–F107.
69. Narbaitz R, Vandorpe D, Levine DZ. Differentiation of renal intercalated cells in fetal and postnatal rats. Anat Embryol 1991; 183:353–361.
70. Narbaitz R, Kapal VK, Levine DZ. Induction of intercalated cell changes in rat pups from acid- and alkali-loaded mothers. Am J Physiol 1993; 264: F415–F420.
71. Holthofer H. Ontogeny of cell type-specific enzyme reactivities in kidney collecting ducts. Pediatr Res 1987; 22:504–508.
72. Mehrgut FM, Satlin LM, Schwartz GJ. Maturation of HCO_3^- transport in rabbit collecting duct. Am J Physiol 1990; 259:F801–F808.
73. Schuster VL, Fejes-Toth G, Naray-Fejes-Toth A, Gluck S. Colocalization of H^+ ATPase and band 3 anion exchanger in rabbit collecting duct intercalated cells. Am J Physiol 1991; 260:F506–F517.
74. Kaissling B, Kriz W. Structural analysis of the rabbit kidney. Adv Anat Embryol Cell Biol 1979; 56:1–123.
75. Stone DK, Seldin DW, Kokko JP, Jacobson HR. Anion dependence of rabbit medullary collecting duct acidification. J Clin Invest 1983; 71:1505–1508.
76. Tsuruoka S, Schwartz GJ. Metabolic acidosis stimulates H^+ secretion in the rabbit outer medullary collecting duct (inner stripe) of the kidney. J Clin Invest 1997; 99:1420–1431.
77. Kim J, Cha J-H, Tisher CC, Madsen KM. Role of apoptotic and nonapoptotic cell death in removal of intercalated cells from developing rat kidney. Am J Physiol 1996; 270:F575–F592.
78. Kildeberg P. Late metabolic acidosis of premature infants. Winters RW, ed. The Body Fluids in Pediatrics. Medical, Surgical, and Neonatal Disorders of Acid–Base Status, Hydration, and Oxygenation. Boston: Little, Brown and Company, 1973:338–348.
79. Seri I, Evans J. Acid–base, fluid, and electrolyte management. In: Taeusch HW, Ballard RA, eds. Avery's Diseases of the Newborn. Philadelphia: W.B. Saunders Company, 1998:372–393.
80. Brion L, Satlin LM. Renal disease. In: Avery G, ed. Textbook of Neonatology. Philadelphia: J.B. Lippincott, 1999:887–974.
81. McDougal WS. Metabolic complications of urinary intestinal diversion. J Urol 1992; 147:1199–1208.
82. Burton BK. Inborn errors of metabolism in infancy: a guide to diagnosis. Pediatrics 1998; 102(e69):1–9.

83. Kappy MS, Morrow G III. Pediatrics for the clinician. A diagnostic approach to metabolic acidosis in children. Pediatrics 1980; 65:351–356.
84. Ein SH, Superina R, Bagwell C, Wiseman N. Ischemic bowel after primary closure for gastroschisis. J Pediatr Surg 1988; 23:728–730.
85. Mundy AR. Metabolic complications of urinary diversion. Lancet 1999; 353:1813–1814.
86. James LS. Pathophysiology of birth asphyxia and resuscitation. In: Winters RW, ed. The Body Fluids in Pediatrics. Boston: Little, Brown and Company, 1973:215–233.
87. Low JA, Lindsay BG, Derrick EJ. Threshold of metabolic acidosis associated with newborn complications. Am J Obstet Gynecol 1997; 177:1391–1394.
88. Kildeberg P. Disturbances of hydrogen ion balance occurring in premature infants. I. Early types of acidosis. Acta Paediatr 1964; 53:505–516.
89. Nair UR, King H, Walker DR. Surgical ligation of the patent ductus arteriosus in low birth weight pre-term infants. J Cardiovasc Surg 1985; 26:577–580.
90. Sinclair JC. Pathophysiology of hyaline membrane disease. In: Winters RW, ed. The Body Fluids in Pediatrics. Medical, Surgical, and Neonatal Disorders of Acid–Base Status, Hydration, and Oxygenation. Boston: Little, Brown and Company, 1973:279–302.
91. Finberg L. Fluid, electrolyte, and acid–base abnormalities in pediatrics. In: Maxwell MH, Kleeman CR, eds. Clinical Disorders of Fluid and Electrolyte Metabolism. New York: McGraw-Hill, 1980:1563–1580.
92. Heird WC, Dell RB, Driscoll JM Jr, Grebin B, Winters RW. Metabolic acidosis resulting from intravenous alimentation mixtures containing synthetic amino acids. N Engl J Med 1972; 287:943–948.
93. Darrow DC, DaSilva MM, Stevenson SS. Production of acidosis in premature infants by protein milk. J Pediatr 1945; 27:43–58.
94. Kildeberg P. Disturbances of hydrogen ion balance occurring in premature infants. II. Late metabolic acidosis. Acta Paediatr 1964; 53:517–526.
95. Manz F, Kalhoff H, Remer T. Renal acid excretion in early infancy. Pediatr Nephrol 1997; 11:231–243.
96. Kalhoff H, Manz F, Diekmann L, Kunz C, Stock GJ, Weisser F. Decreased growth rate of low-birth-weight infants with prolonged maximum renal acid stimulation. Acta Paediatr 1993; 82:522–527.
97. Harrison HL, Linshaw MA, Sierk Bergen J, McGeeney T. Goat milk acidosis. J Pediatr 1979; 94:927–929.
98. Gregory MJ, Schwartz GJ. Diagnosis and treatment of renal tubular disorders. Semin Nephrol 1998; 18:317–329.
99. Sly WS, Whyte MP, Sundaram V, Tashian RE, Hewett-Emmett D, Guibaud P, Vainsel M, Baluarte HJ, Gruskin A, Al-Mosawi M, Sakati N, Ohlsson A. Carbonic anhydrase II deficiency in 12 families with the autosomal recessive syndrome of osteopetrosis with renal tubular acidosis and cerebral calcification. N Engl J Med 1985; 313:139–145..
100. Sly WS, Hewett-Emmett D, Whyte MP, Yu Y-SL, Tashian RE. Carbonic anhydrase II deficiency identified as the primary defect in the autosomal recessive syndrome of osteopetrosis with renal tubular acidosis and cerebral calcification. Proc Natl Acad Sci USA 1983; 80:2752–2756.

101. Igarashi T, Inatomi J, Sekine T, Seki G, Shimadzu M, Tozawa F, Takeshima Y, Takumi T, Takahashi T, Yoshikawa N, Nakamura H, Endou H. Novel nonsense mutation in the Na^+/HCO_3^- cotransporter gene (SLC4A4) in a patient with permanent isolated proximal renal tubular acidosis and bilateral glaucoma. J Am Soc Nephrol 2001; 12:713–718..

102. Shiohara M, Igarashi T, Mori T, Komiyama A. Genetic and long-term data on a patient with permanent isolated proximal renal tubular acidosis. Eur J Pediatr 2000; 159:892–894.

103. Schultheis PJ, Clark LL, Meneton P, Miller ML, Soleimani M, Gawenis LR, Riddle TM, Duffy JJ, Dolmetsch RE, Wang T, Giebisch G, Aronson PS, Lorenz JN, Shull GE. Renal and intestinal absorptive defects in mice lacking the NHE3 Na^+/H^+ exchanger. Nat Genet 1998; 19:282–285..

104. Gahl WA, Bernardini IM, Dalakas MC, Markello TC, Krasnewich DM, Charnas LR. Muscle carnitine repletion by long-term carnitine supplementation in nephropathic cystinosis. Pediatr Res 1993; 34:115–119.

105. Rodriguez-Soriano J, Vallo A. Renal tubular acidosis. Pediatr Nephrol 1990; 4:268–275.

106. McSherry E. Renal tubular acidosis in childhood. Kidney Int 1981; 20: 799–809.

107. Batlle D, Ghanekar H, Jain S, Mitra A. Hereditary distal renal tubular acidosis: new understandings. Annu Rev Med 2001; 52:471–484.

108. Lewis DW. What was wrong with Tiny Tim?. Am J Dis Child 1992; 146:1403–1407.

109. McSherry E, Sebastian A, Morris RC Jr. Renal tubular acidosis in infants: the several kinds, including bicarbonate-wasting, classic renal tubular acidosis. J Clin Invest 1972; 51:499–514.

110. Rodriguez-Soriano J, Vallo A, Garcia-Fuentes M. Distal renal tubular acidosis in infancy: a bicarbonate wasting state. J Pediatr 1975; 86: 524–532.

111. Rodriguez-Soriano J, Vallo A, Castillo G, Oliveros R. Natural history of primary distal renal tubular acidosis treated since infancy. J Pediatr 1982; 101:669–676.

112. Caldas A, Broyer M, Dechaux M, Kleinknecht C. Primary distal tubular acidosis in childhood: clinical study and long-term follow-up of 28 patients. J Pediatr 1992; 121:233–241.

113. Bruce LJ, Cope DL, Jones GK, Schofield AE, Burley M, Povey S, Unwin RJ, Wrong O, Tanner MJ. Familial distal renal tubular acidosis is associated with mutations in the red cell anion exchanger (Band 3, AE1) gene. J Clin Invest 1997; 100:1693–1707.

114. Karet FE, Gainza FJ, Gyory AZ, Unwin RJ, Wrong O, Tanner MJ et al. Mutations in the chloride–bicarbonate exchanger gene AE1 cause autosomal dominant but not autosomal recessive distal renal tubular acidosis. Proc Natl Acad Sci USA 1998; 95:6337–6342.

115. Tanphaichitr VS, Sumboonnanonda A, Ideguchi H, Shayakul C, Brugnara C, Takao M et al. Novel AE1 mutations in recessive distal renal tubular acidosis. Loss-of-function is rescued by glycophorin A. J Clin Invest 1998; 102:2173–2179.

116. Vasuvattakul S, Yenchitsomanus PT, Vachuanichsanong P, Thuwajit P, Kaitwatcharachai C, Laosombat V et al. Autosomal recessive distal renal tubular acidosis associated with Southeast Asian ovalocytosis. Kidney Int 1999; 56:1674–1682.

117. Whyte MP. Carbonic anhydrase II deficiency. Clin Orthop 1993; 294: 52–63.

118. Ohlsson A, Cumming WA, Paul A, Sly WS. Carbonic anhydrase II deficiency syndrome: recessive osteopetrosis with renal tubular acidosis and cerebral calcification. Pediatrics 1986; 77:371–381.

119. Aramaki S, Yoshida I, Yoshino M, Kondo M, Sato Y, Noda K, Jo R, Okue A, Sai N, Yamashita F. Carbonic anhydrase II deficiency in three unrelated Japanese patients. J Inher Metab Dis 1993; 16:982–990.

120. Karet FE, Finberg KE, Nelson RD, Nayir A, Mocan H, Sanjad SA, Rodriguez-Soriano J, Santos F, Cremers CWRJ, Di Pietro A, Hoffbrand BI, Winiarski J, Bakkaloglu A, Ozen S, Dusunsel R, Goodyer P, Hulton SA, Wu DK, Skvorak AB, Morton CC, Cunningham MJ, Jha V, Lifton RP. Mutations in the gene encoding B1 subunit of H^+-ATPase cause renal tubular acidosis with sensorineural deafness. Nat Genet 1999; 21:84–90.

121. Karet FE, Finberg KE, Nayir A, Bakkaloglu A, Ozen S, Hulton SA, Sanjad SA, Al-Sabban EA, Medina JF, Lifton RP. Localization of a gene for autosomal recessive distal renal tubular acidosis with normal hearing (rdRTA2) to 7q33–34. Am J Hum Genet 1999; 65:1656–1665.

122. Smith AN, Skaug J, Choate KA, Nayir A, Bakkaloglu A, Ozen S, Hulton SA, Sanjad SA, Al-Sabban EA, Lifton RP, Scherer SW, Karet FE. Mutations in ATP6N1B, encoding a new kidney vacuolar proton pump 116-kD subunit, cause recessive distal renal tubular acidosis with preserved hearing. Nat Genet 2000; 26:71–75.

123. Simpson AM, Schwartz GJ. Distal renal tubular acidosis with severe hypokalaemia, probably caused by colonic H^+–K^+-ATPase deficiency. Arch Dis Child 2001; 84:504–507.

124. Dafnis E, Spohn M, Lonis B, Kurtzman NA, Sabatini S. Vanadate causes hypokalemic distal renal tubular acidosis. Am J Physiol 1992; 262:F449–F453.

125. Miller SG, Schwartz GJ. Hyperammonaemia with distal renal tubular acidosis. Arch Dis Child 1997; 77:441–444.

126. Rodriguez-Soriano J, Vallo A, Oliveros R, Castillo G. Transient pseudohypoaldosteronism secondary to obstructive uropathy in infancy. J Pediatr 1983; 103:375–380.

127. Rodriguez-Soriano J, Vallo A, Sanjurjo P, Castillo G, Oliveros R. Hyporeninemic hypoaldosteronism in children with chronic renal failure. J Pediatr 1986; 109:476–482.

128. Chang SS, Grunder S, Hanukoglu A, Rösler A, Mathew PM, Hanukoglu I, Schild L, Lu Y, Shimkets RA, Nelson-Williams C, Rossier BC, Lifton RP. Mutations in subunits of the epithelial sodium channel cause salt wasting with hyperkalaemic acidosis, pseudohypoaldosteronism type 1. Nat Genet 1996; 12:248–253.

129. White PC, New MI, Dupont B. Congenital adrenal hyperplasia. N Engl J Med 1987; 316:1519–1524.

130. Batlle DC, Hizon M, Cohen E, Gutterman C, Gupta R. The use of the urinary anion gap in the diagnosis of hyperchloremic metabolic acidosis. N Engl J Med 1988; 318:594–599.

131. Carlisle EJF, Donnelly SM, Halperin ML. Renal tubular acidosis (RTA): recognize the ammonium defect and pH or get the urine pH. Pediatr Nephrol 1991; 5:242–248.

132. Sulyok E, Guignard J-P. Relationship of urinary anion gap to urinary ammonium excretion in the neonate. Biol Neonate 1990; 57:98–106.

133. Dyck RF, Asthana S, Kalra J, West ML, Massey KL. A modification of the urine osmolal gap: an improved method for estimating urine ammonium. Am J Nephrol 1990; 10:359–362.

134. Donckerwolcke RA, Valk C, van Wijngaarden-Penterman MJG, van Stekelenburg GJ. The diagnostic value of the urine to blood carbon dioxide tension gradient for the assessment of distal tubular hydrogen secretion in pediatric patients with renal tubular disorders. Clin Nephrol 1983; 19:254–258.

135. McSherry E, Morris RC Jr. Attainment and maintenance of normal stature with alkali therapy in infants and children with classic renal tubular acidosis. J Clin Invest 1978; 61:509–527.

136. McSherry E. Acidosis and growth in nonuremic renal disease. Kidney Int 1978; 14:349–354.

137. Leslie GI, Kalaw MB, Bowen JR, Arnold JD. Risk factors for sensorineural hearing loss in extremely premature infants. J Paediatr Child Health 1995; 31:312–316.

138. Garin EH, Geary D, Richard GA. Soybean formula (Neo-Mull-Soy) metabolic alkalosis in infancy. J Pediatr 1979; 95:985–987.

139. Grossman H, Duggan E, McCamman S, Welchert E, Hellerstein S. The dietary chloride deficiency syndrome. Pediatrics 1980; 66:366–374.

140. Reznik VM, Griswold WR, Mendoza SA. Neo-Mull-Soy metabolic alkalosis: a model of Bartter's syndrome? Pediatrics 1980; 66:784–786.

141. Rodriguez-Soriano J, Vallo A, Castillo G, Oliveros R, Cea JM, Balzategui MJ. Biochemical features of dietary chloride deficiency syndrome: a comparative study of 30 cases. J Pediatr 1983; 103:209–214.

142. Winters RW. Metabolic alkalosis of pyloric stenosis. Winters RW, ed. The Body Fluids in Pediatrics. Medical, Surgical, and Neonatal Disorders of Acid–Base Status, Hydration, and Oxygenation. Boston: Little Brown and Company, 1973:402–414.

143. Bartter FC, Pronove P, Gill JR Jr, MacCardle RC, Diller E. Hyperplasia of the juxtaglomerular complex with hyperaldosteronism and hypokalemic alkalosis. A new syndrome. Am J Med 1962; 33:811–828.

144. Dell KM, Guay-Woodford LM. Inherited tubular transport disorders. Semin Nephrol 1999; 19:364–373.

145. Proesmans W. Bartter syndrome and its neonatal variant. Eur J Pediatr 1997; 156:669–679.

146. Simon DB, Bindra RS, Mansfield TA, Nelson-Williams C, Mendonca E, Stone R, Schurman S, Nayir A, Alpay H, Bakkaloglu A, Rodriguez-Soriano J, Morales JM, Sanjad SA, Taylor CM, Pilz D, Brem A, Trachtman H, Griswold W, Richard GA, John E, Lifton RP. Mutations in the chloride channel

gene, *CLCNKB*, cause Bartter's syndrome type III. Nat Genet 1997; 17: 171–178.

147. Karolyi L, Konrad M, Kockerling A, Ziegler A, Zimmermann DK, Roth B, Wieg C, Grzeschik K-H, Koch MC, Seyberth HW, Vargas R, Forestier L, Jean G, Deschaux M, Rizzoni GF, Niaudet P, Antignac C, Feldmann D, Lorridon F, Cougoureux E, Laroze F, Alessandri J-L, David L, Saunier P, Deschenes G, Hildebrandt F, Vollmer M, Proesmans W, Brandis M, van den Heuvel LPWJ, Lemmink HH, Nillesen W, Monnens LAH, Knoers NVAM, Guay-Woodford LM, Wright CJ, Madrigal G, Hebert SC. Mutations in the gene encoding the inwardly-rectifying renal potassium channel, ROMK, cause the antenatal variant of Bartter syndrome: evidence for genetic heterogeneity. Hum Mol Genet 1997; 6:17–26.

148. Simon DB, Karet FE, Hamdan JM, Di Pietro A, Sanjad SA, Lifton RP. Bartter's syndrome, hypokalaemic alkalosis with hypercalciuria, is caused by mutations in the Na–K–2Cl cotransporter *NKCC2*. Nat Genet 1996; 13: 183–188.

149. Simon DB, Karet FE, Rodriguez-Soriano J, Hamdan JH, DiPietro A, Trachtman H, Sanjad SA. Genetic heterogeneity of Bartter's syndrome revealed by mutations in the K^+ channel, ROMK. Nat Genet 1996; 14:152–156.

150. Rodriguez-Soriano J. Bartter and related syndromes: the puzzle is almost solved. Pediatr Nephrol 1998; 12:315–327.

151. Simon DB, Nelson-Williams C, Bia MJ, Ellison D, Karet FE, Molina AM, Vaara I, Iwata F, Cushner HM, Koolen M, Gainza FJ, Gitelman HJ, Lifton RP. Gitelman's variant of Bartter's syndrome, inherited hypokalaemic alkalosis, is caused by mutations in the thiazide-sensitive Na–Cl cotransporter. Nat Genet 1996; 12:24–30.

152. Darrow DC. Congenital alkalosis with diarrhea. J Pediatr 1945; 26:519–532.

153. Gamble JL, Fahey KR, Appleton J, McLachlan E. Congenital alkalosis with diarrhea. J Pediatr 1945; 26:509–518.

154. Moseley RH, Hoglund P, Wu GD, Silberg DG, Haila S, de la Chapelle A, Holmberg C, Kere J. Downregulated in adenoma gene encodes a chloride transporter defective in congenital chloride diarrhea. Am J Physiol 1999; 276:G185–G192.

155. Byeon MK, Westerman MA, Maroulakou IG, Henderson KW, Suster S, Zhang XK, Papas TS, Vesely J, Willingham MC, Green JE, Schweinfest CW. The down-regulated in adenoma (DRA) gene encodes an intestine-specific membrane glycoprotein. Oncogene 1996; 12:387–396.

156. Beckerman RC, Taussig LM. Hypoelectrolytemia and metabolic alkalosis in infants with cystic fibrosis. Pediatrics 1979; 63:580–583.

157. Perlman JM, Moore V, Siegel MJ, Dawson J. Is chloride depletion an important contributing cause of death in infants with bronchopulmonary dysplasia?. Pediatrics 1986; 77:212–216.

158. Heinly MM, Wassner SJ. The effect of isolated chloride depletion on growth and protein turnover in young rats. Pediatr Nephrol 1994; 8:555–560.

159. Winters RW. Salicylate intoxication. In: Winters RW, ed. The Body Fluids in Pediatrics. Medical, Surgical, and Neonatal Disorders of Acid–Base Status, Hydration, and Oxygenation. Boston: Little Brown and Company, 1973:483–498.

26

Measurement of Acid–Base Status

Horacio J. Adrogué

Baylor College of Medicine, VA Medical Center, Houston, Texas, U.S.A.

Nicolaos E. Madias

Department of Medicine, Caritas St. Elizabeth's Medical Center, Tufts University School of Medicine, Boston, Massachusetts, U.S.A.

INTRODUCTION

Assessment of acid–base status requires reliable data on both the measured parameters as well as the values derived from these measurements (1). The measurements include blood pH and PCO_2, and total CO_2 concentration (2). Plasma bicarbonate concentration ($[HCO_3^-]$) and other measures of the "metabolic" component of acid–base status are usually calculated from pH and PCO_2, but they can also be calculated from the measured pH and [total CO_2]. The analytical methods, the errors and limitations of these methods, and the definition, utility, and limitations of derived acid–base parameters are examined in this chapter. In addition, blood sampling and specimen handling are described.

BLOOD GAS ANALYZERS

The pH Electrode

The basis for pH measurement is the electrical potential that develops when a membrane selectively permeable to H^+ separates two solutions of differing concentrations of this ion. The relationship between voltage (electrical potential) and pH is described by the modified Nernst equation, which indi-

775

cates that for one pH unit difference between the two solutions (a 10-fold difference in the activity of H^+) an electrical potential of 61.5 mV develops at 37°C (3). The pH electrode compares the voltage generated on exposure to a solution of unknown acidity with the voltage obtained with a solution of known acidity. The pH displayed on the pH meter is derived from conversion of this electrical potential difference to pH units (see Chapter 1).

Figure 1 depicts the basic principle of the glass pH electrode (4). A standard buffered reference solution fills the interior of the electrode (represented on the left side of the electrode in the figure), and the sample to be tested bathes its exterior (represented on the right side of the electrode). Two additional electrodes, an Ag/AgCl electrode and an Hg/HgCl electrode, are used for measuring the voltage generated by the solutions of known (reference) and unknown acidity, respectively. The pH-sensitive glass electrode

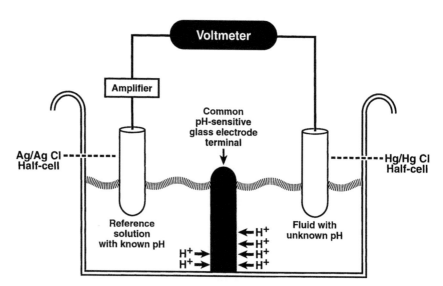

Figure 1   Diagram illustrating the basic principle of the glass pH electrode. A reference solution of known pH fills the interior of the pH-sensitive glass electrode (represented on the left side of the electrode) and provides a reference voltage to compare with the voltage generated by the test solution of unknown pH that bathes the exterior of the pH electrode (represented on the right side of the electrode). An Ag/AgCl electrode and an Hg/HgCl electrode are used for measuring the voltage generated by the reference solution and the solution of unknown acidity, respectively. The relationship between voltage and ΔpH is described by the modified Nernst equation; for each pH unit difference between the two solutions, a difference of 61.5 mV develops. The voltmeter converts electrical voltage to pH units based on the Nernst equation and displays the measured pH of the sample. A high impedance amplifier placed between the voltmeter and the reference solution prevents actual electron flow between the two sides, thereby allowing measurement of small differences in voltage.

functions as a common electrode terminal for both solutions. Hydrogen ions migrate from the solutions toward the glass surface and occupy cationic sites (i.e., the glass membrane acts as a cation exchanger). Because the two glass surfaces are in contact with solutions of differing acidity, an electrical potential difference is established, which is measured by the voltmeter. A high impedance amplifier ($>10^9$ ohm) is placed between the voltmeter and the reference solution, which prevents actual electron flow (current) between the two sides, thereby allowing measurement of small differences in voltage. Standard solutions of known pH are used to calibrate the system.

The pH electrode has two major components (4). One component, often referred to as the "working or measuring electrode," has a thin glass membrane (i.e., glass pH electrode) at the tip and an $Ag/AgCl$ half-cell inside it. The second component, called the "reference electrode," has an electrode terminal made of $Hg/HgCl$ (calomel). The terms "measuring electrode" and "reference electrode" of the pH meter are misnomers since the former is in contact with the reference solution (with known pH) (Fig. 1, left side), and the latter is immersed in fluid with unknown pH (Fig. 1, right side). This electrode terminal interfaces with a platinum wire that transmits the change in voltage to the voltmeter. The nature of the glass (e.g., Corning 015) ensures that the electrode responds almost selectively to H^+. Materials other than glass are currently used in pH electrodes and operate on the same principle. Such pH sensors are polyvinyl chloride-based ion-selective electrodes that are selectively permeable to H^+. They are comparable to those used for measurement of other electrolytes, such as Na^+, K^+, and Ca^{++}. Instruments are currently available that measure pH, PCO_2, PO_2, and electrolytes from a single blood sample.

The temperature of all solutions (calibrating and rinsing) used for the operation of the pH meter must be maintained at the normal body temperature of $37.0 \pm 0.1°C$. The pH electrode is typically calibrated by the two-point method using a low pH buffer (pH 6.84) and a high pH buffer (pH 7.384) (5). The accuracy of these high and low standards is ± 0.005 pH units. Care must be taken to avoid contamination of the standards with saline or cross-contamination, since such practices can introduce errors. The pH measurement is the most accurate and reliable measurement among the blood gas determinations, its accuracy being approximately ± 0.01 units.

Commonly observed problems include protein buildup on the pH glass electrode, incorrect concentration of KCl in salt bridge, insufficient KCl solution, dehydrated or defective glass membrane, air bubble trapped in salt bridge, and electrode temperature deviating from 37°C (4).

The PCO₂ Electrode

The PCO_2 electrode is a modified version of the pH electrode, which is now positioned behind a membrane permeable to CO_2 molecules but not to

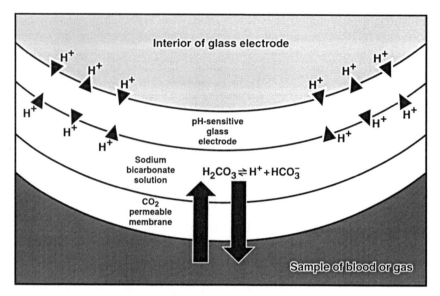

Figure 2   Diagram illustrating the basic principle of the PCO_2 electrode. The PCO_2 of the test sample equilibrates with the sodium bicarbonate solution in the thin layer immediately adjacent to the pH-sensitive glass electrode. The change in pH of this layer produces an electrical potential difference; the relationship between pH and voltage is linear but that between PCO_2 and pH or PCO_2 and voltage is logarithmic. The blood-gas analyzer contains an antilogarithmic amplifying unit that produces a linear relationship between PCO_2 of the sample and the values of voltage/pH obtained on the analyzer display gauge.

water or electrolytes. Between this membrane and the pH electrode is a very thin layer of sodium bicarbonate solution (usually 5 mmol/L) (3) (Fig. 2). The bicarbonate solution is also in contact with an Ag/AgCl electrode terminal. Consequently, the PCO_2 electrode has two Ag/AgCl electrode terminals but no salt bridge because blood is not in direct contact with the electrode terminals. The rationale behind the PCO_2 electrode is that exposure of a bicarbonate-containing solution to various PCO_2 levels results in highly predictable changes in pH. In fact, a straight line is obtained when the $\log PCO_2$ is charted against the measured pH values. The coordinate system of $\log PCO_2$ (abscissa) and pH (ordinate) that graphically expresses the Henderson–Hasselbach equation, depicted in Fig. 3, is characterized by the presence of isobicarbonate straight lines with a slope of -1.0 (i.e., 45° angle) (6). A 10-fold increase in the PCO_2 of the sample being tested will increase the acidity of the HCO_3^- layer adjacent to the pH-sensitive membrane by one pH unit, whereas $[HCO_3^-]$ will remain essentially unchanged.

The PCO_2 electrode is calibrated by the two-point method using 5% and 10% CO_2 gases. Concentration of the CO_2 cylinders should be certified

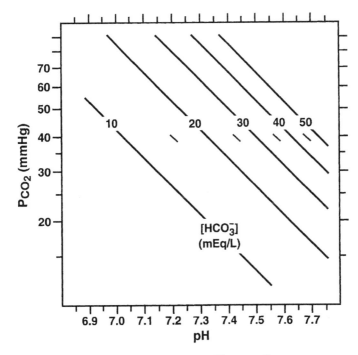

Figure 3 pH/log PCO_2 coordinate system. The coordinate system graphically expresses the Henderson–Hasselbalch equation. The isobicarbonate lines are straight lines with a slope of -1 (i.e., 45° angle). *Source*: From Ref. 6.

to within $\pm 0.03\%$. The approximate accuracy of the PCO_2 electrode is ± 3 mmHg (7,8). This electrode is slightly more stable than the blood pH electrode because the pH-sensitive element is not exposed directly to blood (3). Inaccurate measurements of PCO_2 can result from incorrect calibration, improperly certified gas tanks, cooling of electrode due to high gas flow rate, inadequately flushed gas lines, or diffusion of room air into gas tubing lines.

Derived Parameters

Because only pH and PCO_2 can be measured directly with blood gas analyzers, determination of the nonrespiratory (metabolic) component of acid–base status is based on derived parameters (9). The most relevant among these parameters are plasma bicarbonate concentration ($[HCO_3^-]$), standard bicarbonate concentration (SBC), whole blood buffer base (BB), and base excess (BE). Other measures, including alkali reserve, CO_2-combining power, and nonrespiratory pH, are not described in this chapter, since they are not currently in use (10).

Bicarbonate Concentration

The plasma [HCO_3^-], also known as actual bicarbonate concentration, is the most widely used metabolic parameter of acid–base status (9). It is considered the most reliable because its value depends exclusively on the physicochemical constraints of the relationship between pH and PCO_2, the two directly measured variables. Thus, plasma [HCO_3^-] can be calculated reliably from measured pH and PCO_2 using the Henderson–Hasselbalch equation (see Chapter 1). For this calculation, a pK'_a of 6.10 is used for the carbonic acid–bicarbonate buffer system (6,11). Although temperature, pH, and ionic strength of blood can each modify the pK'_a, their composite effects are very minor in the ranges compatible with life, and therefore such corrections are unnecessary in the clinical setting (12–14).

Just as with other "metabolic parameters" (see following text), the actual [HCO_3^-] is altered by the in vivo response to changes in the respiratory component of acid–base status (15). Hypercapnia increases, whereas hypocapnia decreases, the plasma [HCO_3^-] due to titration of nonbicarbonate buffers (see Chapters 20 and 21). In addition to CO_2 titration-mediated changes in the plasma [HCO_3^-], changes in renal acidification modulate this parameter in response to deviations in the respiratory component (16–18) (see Chapters 4 and 23).

Standard Bicarbonate

Standard bicarbonate concentration (SBC) is defined as the concentration of HCO_3^- in the plasma of fully oxygenated whole blood after equilibration in vitro with a partial pressure of CO_2 equal to 40 mmHg at 37°C. Therefore, standard bicarbonate is simply a measure of the plasma [HCO_3^-] under standard conditions of PCO_2, PO_2, and temperature (6,9). This value can be determined by interpolation after tonometric equilibration of the blood sample at two levels of CO_2 tension (see below, the CO_2 equilibration method), using the log PCO_2/pH diagram with HCO_3^- isopleths (6) (Fig. 4). Because the level of oxygenation of hemoglobin alters its buffer value (see Chapter 1), measurement of standard bicarbonate requires standardization of the oxygen level of the sample. The average normal value of standard bicarbonate is 24 mEql/L, which is identical to the mean normal value of actual plasma [HCO_3^-] in a patient with an average normal level of $PaCO_2$. Standard bicarbonate can also be obtained with the use of nomograms and equations that require knowledge of the patient's buffer base or base excess and hemoglobin concentration (see following text).

Standard bicarbonate was conceived in the search for an estimate of the metabolic component of acid–base status that is truly independent of the respiratory component (19). Unfortunately, standard bicarbonate, an in vitro determination, is not independent of the respiratory component in vivo. In fact, changes in standard bicarbonate occur in vivo with respiratory

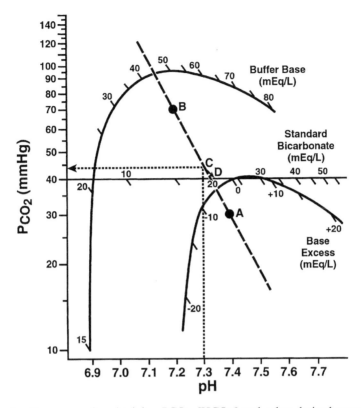

Figure 4 Nomogram for obtaining PCO_2, $[HCO_3^-]$ and other derived parameters from pH using the CO_2 equilibration method. In the example shown, the pH of a blood sample is 7.39 after equilibration at a PCO_2 of 30 mmHg (pointA) and 7.19 after equilibration at a PCO_2 of 70 mmHg (pointB). The slope of the straight line joining points (**A**) and (**B**) is dependent on the buffer value of the blood sample (15). Prior to equilibration, the pH of the sample was 7.30. The location of this pH value on line (**A**)(**B**) at point (**C**) defines the PCO_2 of the sample (44 mmHg). The $[HCO_3^-]$ of the sample is obtained by extending a line from point (**C**) to the standard bicarbonate line (point**D**) on a 45° angle from the pH isobar. The nomogram also indicates the standard bicarbonate, buffer base excess, and buffer base values of the sample. *Source*: From Ref. 6.

disturbances (i.e., primary hypercapnia or hypocapnia) because of redistribution of the newly generated or consumed HCO_3^- between blood and the rest of the extracellular fluid volume. Consequently, standard bicarbonate does not offer advantages when compared with actual bicarbonate (19).

Whole Blood Buffer Base

Whole blood buffer base (BB) represents the sum of "reaction-dependent" anions of blood within the pH range of 6.8–7.8 (6,10). Considering all the blood anions, only HCO_3^-, plasma proteins, hemoglobin, and phosphate behave as "reaction-dependent" anions (i.e., H^+ acceptors or donors) within this pH range. Precise measurement of the anionic equivalency of the BB demands a detailed analysis of the blood electrolyte composition, a task that cannot be performed routinely in a clinical laboratory (6,10,20). However, determination of the BB for clinical purposes can be done by means of the CO_2 equilibration method and plotting the data on the log PCO_2/pH nomogram (Fig. 4). Alternatively, BB can be obtained from measurement of blood pH, the total CO_2 concentration of plasma, and hemoglobin concentration; with this information, a graphic determination of the BB is obtained using the Singer–Hastings or other nomograms (6).

Normal whole blood buffer base (NBB) is the buffer base of blood when the PCO_2 is 40 mmHg and the pH is 7.4; its value can be obtained as follows:

$$NBB \ (mmol/L) = 41.7 + 0.42 \times [Hb]$$

where 41.7 is the contribution of buffers other than hemoglobin (mostly HCO_3^- and plasma proteins) and hemoglobin is expressed in g/dL of blood. If the hemoglobin concentration is expressed in mmol/L, the multiplication factor is 0.67 instead of 0.42. Because BB is independent of the oxygen saturation, its value is identical in arterial and venous blood.

Base Excess

The blood base excess (BE) represents the amount of acid or alkali that must be added to 1 L of whole blood exposed in vitro to a PCO_2 of 40 mmHg at normal temperature (37°C) to achieve a normal pH of 7.40 (6,9). When the initial blood pH is higher (more alkaline) than normal, acid must be added to titrate the blood to normal pH; thus, the blood sample under evaluation has a positive base excess or simply, base excess. On the other hand, if the initial blood pH is lower (more acidic) than normal, alkali must be added to titrate the blood to normal pH; thus, the blood sample under evaluation has a negative base excess or simply, a base deficit. The blood BE is expressed in mmol/L and has either a positive or negative sign preceding its value that indicates "base excess" or "base deficit," respectively. Under normal circumstances, BE is zero, as no deviation in the metabolic component from normal is observed in the presence of normal values for blood pH and respiratory component.

Determination of BE can be performed by means of the CO_2 equilibration method and plotting the data on the log PCO_2/pH nomogram (6) (Fig. 4). Alternatively, nomograms and computer programs (that sometimes are incorporated in the blood-gas analyzer itself) can provide the BE based on the pH and PCO_2 of the blood sample. The alignment nomogram of Siggaard-Anderson (21) is very useful when both PCO_2 and pH have been measured directly with specific electrodes.

The blood BE is equal to the difference between the observed buffer base (BB) and the normal buffer base (NBB):

$$BE = \Delta BB = BB - NBB$$

Although BB and NBB vary with hemoglobin concentration, BE (or ΔBB) is independent of this variable. As a result BB itself is not commonly used in clinical practice, yet base excess (BE) is widely used.

Base excess can vary in disease states within the limits of approximately -30 to $+30$ mmol/L (6). Venous blood has a higher BE than arterial blood (on the order of 2–2.5 mmol/L) because of the lower oxygen saturation of hemoglobin. However, if venous blood is oxygenated in vitro it acquires the same BE as arterial blood.

The relationship between BE and changes in SBC is not entirely linear and varies with the hemoglobin concentration. For a normal hemoglobin concentration, the relationship can be expressed as follows:

$$BE = 1.3 \times \Delta SBC$$

Base excess, like standard bicarbonate, was conceived as an estimate of the metabolic component of acid–base status that is truly independent of the respiratory component. In fact, both base excess and standard bicarbonate are truly independent of PCO_2 *only* within the closed in vitro system in which they are estimated (19,22). This is the case because in vitro any CO_2-induced increase in $[HCO_3^-]$ is stoichiometrically equivalent to the decrease in the anionic equivalency of nonbicarbonate buffers that results from binding the H^+ released from carbonic acid; the opposite reactions occur during in vitro decreases in PCO_2 such that the "metabolic component" again remains constant. In vivo, however, neither BE nor SBC is independent of the respiratory component.

During in vivo acute hypercapnia plasma $[HCO_3^-]$ rises because of CO_2-induced titration of nonbicarbonate buffers (largely hemoglobin), a process similar to that occurring in vitro in which HCO_3^- generation is stoichiometrically equivalent to the consumption of buffer base from the non-bicarbonate blood buffers. However, in vivo, a fraction of the newly generated HCO_3^- will exit the plasma toward the interstitial compartment in response to a concentration gradient. This loss of HCO_3^- from plasma leads to a decrease in base excess and standard bicarbonate in acute hypercapnia, a process known as "pseudometabolic acidosis." The higher the hemoglobin concentration and the larger the interstitial compartment, the greater the degree of "pseudometabolic acidosis," for a given level of acute hypercapnia.

The above-mentioned considerations led Schwartz and Relman to publish an influential critique of the use of standard bicarbonate and base excess in the analysis of clinical acid–base disturbances (19). This critique clearly established that these parameters offer no advantages in the evaluation of the metabolic component of acid–base status when compared with the actual plasma [HCO_3^-]. In fact, it is unnecessary to include both BE (or standard bicarbonate) and plasma [HCO_3^-] in a given blood gas report. This practice has its origin from "The Great Trans-Atlantic Acid–Base Debate" between the Boston and Copenhagen schools about 40 years ago (22). The Boston school advocated the use of plasma [HCO_3^-] as the most appropriate metabolic parameter, whereas the Copenhagen school advocated the use of BE. Mindful of the decrease in BE during in vivo acute hypercapnia (pseudometabolic acidosis), the Copenhagen school proposed the use of yet another index, the in vivo BE or "standard base excess" (SBE) that considers the hemoglobin level and the size of the interstitial fluid compartment (22). However, the latter metabolic parameter has failed to gain substantial acceptance.

Considering that patients can be managed properly by using different metabolic parameters, clinicians should have a complete understanding of the advantages and limitations of the metabolic index that they select for the diagnosis and management of acid–base disorders. In this book we make use of plasma [HCO_3^-], as we consider it the most direct and straightforward metabolic index of acid–base status.

Autoanalyzer and Other Estimates of Plasma [HCO_3^-]

Because plasma [HCO_3^-] cannot be readily quantified, measurement of total CO_2 concentration ([Total CO_2]) is used as a substitute. Plasma [Total CO_2] refers to the aggregate of free and bound CO_2, including dissolved CO_2, carbonic acid, carbamates, and HCO_3^-, with HCO_3^- representing approximately 95% of the total value. Consequently, [Total CO_2] provides a good estimate of plasma [HCO_3^-] and is routinely measured when serum electrolytes are determined in a venous blood sample (23).

The autoanalyzer technique currently used in most clinical laboratories measures [Total CO_2] in plasma using a colorimetric process to detect the CO_2 released from the sample after the addition of a strong acid; its major attribute is great efficiency. Plasma [Total CO_2] can also be measured with enzymatic assays (e.g., phosphoenolpyruvate carboxylase) or electrometric methods (e.g., CO_2 diffusion through a membrane that is monitored by a pH electrode) (24).

Loss of CO_2 from a sample exposed to air is largely caused by the breakdown of HCO_3^- due to release of lactic acid from red cells when delays in centrifugation of the blood sample occur and in the initiation of analysis (25). Such a loss of CO_2 can be largely prevented if the sample is promptly spun and stored at 4°C (26).

The CO_2 Equilibration Method

The acid–base status of the blood can also be determined with great precision by means of the CO_2 equilibration method (6). This technique takes advantage of the nearly linear relationship between pH and log PCO_2 in biologic fluids. Thus, if the pH of a blood sample is measured after the sample is equilibrated sequentially at two or more CO_2 tensions, a straight line can be drawn that relates pH and log PCO_2 values. Using the same straight line, the PCO_2 of the original sample is given by the value corresponding to the pH of the sample measured prior to CO_2 equilibration. In addition, the $[HCO_3^-]$ of the sample is read on a 45° angle over the standard bicarbonate line (Figs. 3 and 4). The nomogram also indicates the standard bicarbonate, buffer base, and base excess of the sample. The points of intersection of the pH/log PCO_2 straight line with the nomogram lines for standard bicarbonate, buffer base, and base excess define the respective values of these parameters for the blood sample (Fig. 4).

The Astrup apparatus, developed for the practical application of the CO_2 equilibration method, consists of a pH electrode system coupled with a tonometer thereby facilitating pH measurements before and after equilibration with known CO_2 concentrations. The sample to be analyzed is equilibrated with two gas mixtures, one with a CO_2 tension below and one with a CO_2 tension above the expected PCO_2 of the sample. When proper technique is followed, the error of the CO_2 equilibration method is ± 3% over the range encountered in clinical practice. The greater simplicity of operation of blood gas analyzers and autoanalyzers compared with the CO_2 equilibration method is largely responsible for the overwhelming dominance of the first two methods in assessing the acid–base status of patients worldwide.

Blood Sampling and Specimen Handling

Arterial Blood

An arterial blood sample is routinely used for determination of acid–base status. Arterial sampling is considered to provide a reliable index of acid–base status in the tissues and, in addition, allows evaluation of pulmonary gas exchange. Nonetheless, firm evidence that an arterial sample provides a reliable index of acid–base status in the tissues exists only in the normal state (27–29). No systematic data exist about the relationship between the arterial and mixed venous blood acid–base profile in various abnormal states, with the exception of circulatory failure. In this setting, assessment of the acid–base status of the tissues can be misleading if only arterial blood is examined. The degree of misrepresentation worsens with the severity of circulatory compromise, and it becomes extreme during cardiac arrest (28,29). Therefore, information on venous as well as arterial blood gases is required for reliable monitoring of the critically ill patient (see Chapter 20). It has been shown that acid–base data derived from central and mixed venous blood sampling are practically interchangeable. Because mixed venous blood is obtained through a more risky, technically demanding, and expensive procedure, we recommend sampling of central venous blood in this clinical setting.

In the adult, the radial, brachial, and femoral arteries are most commonly punctured. The carotid artery should be avoided because of the risk for cerebral air embolism or damage to other vital structures. In the newborn, the umbilical arteries are easily accessible, whereas in the infant, the radial and temporal vessels are recommended. Complications of arterial puncture include vasovagal responses, external bleeding, hematoma, thrombosis, peripheral nerve damage, and infection.

There are several additional concerns about blood sampling for monitoring acid–base status. Obtaining arterial blood requires an invasive procedure consisting of either an arterial puncture or insertion of an indwelling catheter. Because blood sampling is intermittent, transient alterations in acid–base composition can remain undetected. There is often a considerable lag time between ordering the test and obtaining the result, which can impede prompt diagnosis and treatment of a serious condition. Further, deterioration of the arterial blood gas profile can occur relatively late in the patient's downhill course, thereby limiting its utility as a monitoring tool.

Capillary and Venous Blood

Acid–base parameters in capillary blood and venous blood samples vary as a function of blood flow and local tissue metabolism (30). However, capillary blood from the earlobe, finger, or heel can be substituted for arterial blood, particularly in infants and small children, if the capillary bed is dilated by heating the area for 10–15 min before sampling. The results of pH and PCO_2 determinations from such samples are virtually identical to those in arterial blood except in clinical situations characterized by low capillary blood flow. Thus, this sampling technique should be avoided in patients with marked peripheral vasoconstriction or overt circulatory collapse.

Standard venipuncture techniques using a peripheral vein provide the least reliable sample for the assessment of acid–base status. However, if an occluding tourniquet is not being used; the muscles of the arm from which the blood is drawn are relaxed; and blood flow is adequate, venous pH is generally 0.02–0.04 unit lower and venous PCO_2 6–8 mmHg higher than simultaneous values in arterial blood. Alternatively, venous blood sampled from the dorsum of the hand just after heating the hand for 10–15 min (so-called arterialized venous blood) can be used, a method that provides acid–base data virtually identical to those of arterial blood (see Chapter 27).

Specimen Handling

Blood samples for acid–base measurement should be collected with anticoagulant, under anaerobic conditions, and be promptly processed or cooled to 4°C if delays are expected. When liquid heparin is used, a small amount should be drawn into the syringe, securing that it coats the inner walls of the syringe but expelling any excess. Excessive amounts of sodium heparin solution can have a dilutional effect leading to spurious hypocapnia and hypobicarbonatemia (31). Some blood gas syringes are prepackaged with dry lyophilized heparin thereby eliminating the need of adding liquid heparin.

Careful handling of the blood sample is important for optimal results. Any sample obtained with more than minor air bubbles should be discarded because contamination of the blood with air can alter blood gas values. After expelling any excess air, the sample must be quickly sealed by removing the needle and capping the syringe in an airtight fashion. The sample should be mixed with the anticoagulant by rolling the syringe between the hands and by inverting the sample repeatedly, and then placed on ice immediately, a procedure that maintains blood gas values fairly stable for 1–2 hr. Uncooled blood samples are best analyzed within 20 min.

REFERENCES

1. Kraut JA, Madias NE. Approach to patients with acid–base disorders. Respir Care 2001; 46:392–403.
2. Shapiro BA, Harrison RA, Cane RD, Kozlowski-Templin R. Clinical Application of Blood Gases. 4th ed. Chicago: Year Book Medical Publishers, 1989.
3. Adams AP, Hahn CEW. Principles and Practice of Blood-Gas Analysis. Edinburgh: Churchill Livingstone, 1982.
4. Malley WJ. Clinical Blood Gases. Application and Non-invasive Alternatives. Philadelphia: WB Saunders, 1990.
5. Durst RA. Blood pH, gases, and electrolytes. Proceedings on the Workshop on pH and Blood Gases held at the National Bureau of Standards, Gaithersburg, MD, July 7–8, 1975. US Department of Commerce. Issued June 1977.
6. Siggaard-Andersen O. The Acid–Base Status of the Blood. 4th ed. Baltimore: Williams & Wilkins, 1974.
7. Flenley DC, Millar JS, Rees HA. Accuracy of oxygen and carbon dioxide electrodes. Br Med J 1967; 2:349–352.
8. Bartschi F, Haab P, Held DR. Reliability of blood PCO_2 measurements by the CO_2-electrode, the whole-blood C_{CO2}/pH method and the Astrup method. Respir Physiol 1970; 10:121–131.
9. Adrogué HJ, Wesson DE. Acid–Base. Blackwell's Basics of Medicine. Boston: Blackwell Science, 1994.
10. Singer RB, Hastings AB. An improved clinical method for the estimation of disturbances of the acid–base balance of human blood. Medicine (Baltimore) 1948; 27:223–242.
11. Siggaard-Andersen O. The first dissociation exponent of carbonic acid as a function of pH. Scand J Clin Lab Invest 1962; 14:587–597.
12. Hastings AB, Sendroy J. The effect of variation in ionic strength on the apparent first and second dissociation constants of carbonic acid. J Biol Chem 1925; 65:445–455.

13. Severinghaus JW, Stupfel M, Bradley AF. Variations of serum carbonic acid pK' with pH and temperature. J Appl Physiol 1956; 9:197–200.

14. Rispens P, Dellebarre CW, Eleveld D, Helder W, Zijlstra WG. The apparent first dissociation constant for carbonic acid in plasma between 16 and 42.5°. Clin Chim Acta 1968; 22:627–637.

15. Adrogué HE, Adrogué HJ. Acid–base physiology. Respir Care 2001; 46:328–341.

16. Bracket NC Jr, Cohen JJ, Schwartz WB. Carbon dioxide titration curve of normal man: effect of increasing degrees of acute hypercapnia on acid–base equilibrium. N Engl J Med 1965; 272:6–12.

17. Madias NE, Adrogué HJ. Influence of chronic metabolic acid–base disorders on the acute CO_2 titration curve. J Appl Physiol 1983; 55:1187–1195.

18. Adrogué HJ, Madias NE. Influence of chronic respiratory acid–base disorders on acute CO_2 titration curve. J Appl Physiol 1985; 58:1231–1238.

19. Schwartz WB, Relman AS. A critique of the parameters used in the evaluation of acid–based disorders. "Whole-Blood Buffer Base" and "Standard Bicarbonate" compared with blood pH and plasma bicarbonate concentration. N Engl J Med 1963; 268:1382–1388.

20. Dill DB, Edwards HT, Consolazio WV. Blood as a physicochemical system. XI, Man at rest. J Biol Chem 1937; 118:635–648.

21. Siggaard-Anderson O. Blood acid–base alignment nomogram. Scales for pH, PCO_2, base excess of whole blood of different hemoglobin concentrations, plasma bicarbonate, and plasma total-CO_2. Scand J Clin Lab Invest 1963; 15:211–217.

22. Astrup P, Severinghaus JW. The History of Blood Gases, Acids and Bases. Copenhagen: Munksgaard, 1986.

23. O'Leary TD, Langton SR. Calculated bicarbonate or total carbon dioxide? Clin Chem 1989; 35:1697–1700.

24. Miller AL. Plasma bicarbonate assays – time for a new look?. Ann Clin Biochem 1993; 30:233–237.

25. Kirschbaum B. Spurious metabolic acidosis in hemodialysis patients. Am J Kidney Dis 2000; 35:1068–1071.

26. Howse MLP, Leonard M, Venning M, Soloman L. The effect of different methods of storage on the results of serum total CO_2 assays. Clin Science 2001; 100:609–611.

27. Adrogué HJ, Madias NE. Management of life-threatening acid–base disorders. Second of two parts. N Engl J Med 1998; 338:107–111.

28. Adrogué HJ, Rashad MN, Gorin AB, Yacoub J, Madias NE. Arteriovenous acid–base disparity in circulatory failure: studies on mechanism. Am J Physiol 1989; 257:F1087–F1093.

29. Adrogué HJ, Rashad MN, Gorin AB, Yacoub J, Madias NE. Assessing acid–base status in circulatory failure: differences between arterial and central venous blood. N Engl J Med 1989; 320:1312–1316.

30. Gambino SR. Comparisons of pH in human arterial, venous, and capillary blood. Am J Clin Pathol 1959; 32:298–300.

31. Bloom SA, Canzanello VJ, Strom JA, Madias NE. Spurious assessment of acid–base status due to dilutional effect of heparin. Am J Med 1985; 79: 528–530.

$$27$$

Normal Acid–Base Values

Horacio J. Adrogué

Baylor College of Medicine, VA Medical Center, Houston, Texas, U.S.A.

Nicolaos E. Madias

*Department of Medicine, Caritas St. Elizabeth's Medical Center,
Tufts University School of Medicine, Boston, Massachusetts, U.S.A.*

INTRODUCTION

This chapter reviews the normal values for acid–base parameters in humans. As will be discussed, the pH of the body fluids is maintained at a relatively alkaline level, with vanishingly low levels of free H^+, controlled by the interplay between the CO_2 tension and the bicarbonate concentration (see Chapters 6 and 8). Despite the tight control of pH, significant interindividual variations exist among normal humans, and some of the causes for such variability are discussed in this chapter. First we address the terminology for defining the amount of free H^+ in the body fluids.

SCALES OF ACIDITY: pH vs. HYDROGEN ION CONCENTRATION

Blood acidity can be expressed either in pH units or in terms of hydrogen ion concentration ($[H^+]$). As discussed in Chapter 1, neither is a completely precise description of the activity of this elusive cation, but by convention, the activity of H^+, estimated by a H^+-specific electrode is expressed either in pH units or as $[H^+]$ in nEq/L or nmol/L. The major difference between these ways of defining acidity is that the latter is in an arithmetic scale, and the former is in a logarithmic scale. More precisely, pH is the negative

Table 1   Relationship Between pH and [H$^+$]

pH	[H$^+$] (nEq/L)
7.80	16
7.75	18
7.70	20
7.65	22
7.60	25
7.55	28
7.50	32
7.45	35
7.40	40
7.35	45
7.30	50
7.25	56
7.20	63
7.15	71
7.10	79
7.05	89
7.00	100
6.95	112
6.90	126
6.85	141
6.80	159

[H$^+$] (nEq/L) = antilog (9 − pH).

decimal logarithm of the estimated H$^+$ activity measured by the pH electrode—where H$^+$ activity is expressed in mol/L or Eq/L. The reason for introducing the calculated [H$^+$] in nEq/L is that when acidity is expressed in pH units, conceptualization of quantitative changes in acidity is difficult. For example, a change in blood pH from 7.40 to 7.10 might appear modest, but it actually represents a doubling of [H$^+$] from 40 to 80 nEq/L. Considering that log of 2 equals 0.3, [H$^+$] doubles for every 0.3 decrease in blood pH. Table 1 presents the conversion of pH to [H$^+$] (in nEq/L) over the range of blood acidity encountered in human beings.

Because the conversion table might not be immediately available at the patient's bedside, the physician can use anyone of three different methods to achieve the same goal (1). The first and most precise method can be accomplished with a simple hand-held calculator and uses the following equation:

$$[\text{H}^+](\text{nEq/L}) = \text{antilog}(9 - \text{pH})]$$

Using this equation, the calculated [H$^+$] for a pH of 7.15, for example, is the antilog of 9 − 7.15, or 1.85, [10$^{1.85}$], which equals 71. Thus a pH of 7.15

Table 2 Comparison of Methods of Interconversion of pH and [H$^+$]

| | Hydrogen ion concentration (nEq/L) | | |
| | | Derived values | |
pH	Actual values	0.01 Rule	% Method
7.80	16		16
7.75	18		18
7.70	20		20
7.65	22		23
7.60	25		26
7.55	28	25	29
7.50	32	30	32
7.45	35	35	36
7.40	40	40	40
7.35	45	45	45
7.30	50	50	50
7.25	56	55	56
7.20	63		63
7.15	71		71
7.10	79		80
7.05	89		90
7.00	100		100
6.95	112		113
6.90	126		125
6.85	141		140
6.80	159		156

is equivalent to a [H$^+$] of 71 nEq/L. This method was used to construct Tables 1 and 2 (column 2). The rationale for subtracting the pH of interest from 9 when expressing acidity in nEq/L is that pH 9 represents the start of the scale, as it corresponds to 1 nEq/L [10^{-9} Eq/L]. To convert [H$^+$] (nEq/L) to pH units, one solves the same equation for pH:

$$pH = 9 - \log[H^+]$$

For example, the pH for a [H$^+$] of 95 nEq/L is derived by calculating log(95), which is 1.98; 9 − 1.89 equals 7.02; thus a [H$^+$] of 95 nEq/L is equivalent to a pH of 7.02. The availability of pocket computers with a software program for automatic conversion of H$^+$ from pH further facilitates this calculation.

A second method is to apply the rule whereby for each 0.01 pH unit below or above its average normal value of 7.40, 1 nEq/L is added to or subtracted from the corresponding [H$^+$] value of 40 nEq/L, respectively

(Table 2, column 3). Therefore, pH values of 7.35 and 7.45 correspond to $[H^+]$ of 45 and 35 nEq/L, respectively. This conversion rule is only relatively accurate for a limited range of pH of about 0.15 units below and above the average normal value (i.e., 7.25–7.55). Utilization of this rule for larger deviations of pH yields considerable inaccuracies and should be avoided.

A third method of converting pH values to $[H^+]$ in nEq/L is the so-called percent method; it is applicable to any blood pH value and does not require a calculator with a logarithmic capability. Hydrogen ion concentration is derived from pH by sequentially multiplying the preceding $[H^+]$ by 0.8 for each increment in pH of 0.1 unit, or by 1.25 for each decrement in pH of 0.1 (Table 2, column 4). This method, of course, requires remembering the $[H^+]$ in nEq/L for a single pH value, that is, for example, a pH of 7.40 corresponds to a $[H^+]$ of 40 nEq/L. Thus, the $[H^+]$ for a pH of 7.60 is 26 nEq/L ($40 \times 0.8 = 32$; $32 \times 0.8 \simeq 26$) and that of a pH of 7.20 is 63 nEq/L ($40 \times 1.25 = 50$; $50 \times 1.25 \simeq 63$). Memorizing additional interconversions, for example, that pH values of 8 and 7 correspond to $[H^+]$ of 10 and 100 nEq/L, respectively, adds expediency to the method. Thus, the $[H^+]$ for a pH of 7.80 is 16 nEq/L [$10 \times 1.25 = 12.5$; $12.5 \times 1.25 \simeq 16$, where the starting value of 10 nEq/L corresponds to pH of 8 and that for a pH of 7.10 is 80 nEq/L ($100 \times 0.8 = 80$, where the starting value of 100 nEq/L corresponds to pH of 7.00). The $[H^+]$ for pH values that are intermediate between those calculated by this method must be estimated by interpolation. The percent method is generally accurate and has practical value. The different methods of translating pH into $[H^+]$ (nEq/L) are compared in Table 2.

THE RANGE OF NORMAL VALUES

The $[H^+]$ of extracellular fluid is maintained at exceptionally low levels—actually, in the alkaline range—by physiologic mechanisms that result on average in a 20:1 ratio of $[HCO_3^-]$ to $[H_2CO_3]$, when the values are expressed in mmol/L (see Chapters 1–8) (2–5). The normal blood acid–base composition in adult humans at sea level is shown in Table 3. As shown in the table, a relatively wide range of normal values for each of the acid–base parameters is observed—7.36–7.44 for arterial pH (36–44 nEq/L for $[H^+]$); 36–44 mm Hg for the partial pressures of CO_2 in arterial blood ($PaCO_2$); and 21–27 mEq/L for arterial $[HCO_3^-]$. Despite this apparent variability, acid–base composition is remarkably stable in a given individual. Daily variations in resting values for $PaCO_2$ and $[HCO_3^-]$ rarely exceed 2–3 mmHg and 1–2 mEq/L, respectively.

Interrelationships Between PCO_2, $[H^+]$ and $[HCO_3^-]$

According to conventional methodology, acid–base equilibrium is judged to be normal when the values for PCO_2, plasma $[HCO_3^-]$, and $[H^+]$ (or pH),

Table 3 Normal Acid–Base Composition at Sea Level

	pH	[H$^+$] (nEq/L)	PCO$_2$ (mmHg)	[HCO$_3^-$] (mEq/L)	Base excess[a] (mEq/L)
Arterial blood	7.40 (7.36–7.44)	40 (36–44)	40 (36–44)	24.0 (21.0–27.0)	0 (−2.4 to +2.2)
Capillary blood	7.40 (7.36–7.44)	40 (36–44)	40 (36–44)	24.0 (21.0–27.0)	0 (−2.4 to +2.2)
Arterialized venous blood	7.39 (7.35–7.43)	41 (37–45)	41 (37–45)	25.2 (22.2–28.2)	0 (−2.4 to +2.2)
Peripheral venous blood	7.38 (7.34–7.42)	42 (38–46)	46 (42–50)	26.0 (23.0–29.0)	0 (−2.4 to +2.2)

[a]All base excess values correspond to fully oxygenated blood in vitro; otherwise, its value in venous blood is approximately 1.1 mEq/L higher than in arterial blood.

Values given are mean (range). (*Source:* Data compiled from Ravel R (Clinical Laboratory Medicine. 6th ed. St Louis, Mo: Mosby, 1995); Cohen JJ, Kassirer JP Acid-Base. Boston: Little, Brown, 1982, Siggaard-Anderson O (The Acid-Base Status of the Blood. 4th ed. Baltimore: Williams & Wilkins, 1974).

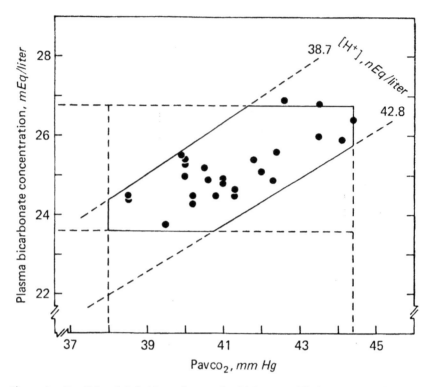

Figure 1   Traditional definition of normal acid–base equilibrium. The broken lines emanating from the ordinate and abscissa encompass the normal steady-state ranges (mean ± 2 SD) for plasma bicarbonate concentration and carbon dioxide tension in arterialized venous blood ($PavCO_2$). The diagonal lines encompass the normal steady-state range for plasma hydrogen ion concentration. The area of overlap is defined by the solid hexagonal zone in the center and corresponds to the traditional definition of the normal domain. The solid circles indicate data obtained in 25 healthy male subjects. *Source*: From Ref. 7.

each examined independently, fall within their respective normal ranges (Fig. 1). This approach to the definition of the normal domain is methodologically erroneous for two reasons (6,7): first, on a priori grounds, the equilibrium kinetics that govern this system permit only two of these "variables" to change independently; the third necessarily acquires the value predicted by the Henderson relationship. Second, the actual in vivo variables in this system—CO_2 tension and $[HCO_3^-]$—are themselves interrelated (1–3). As a result, the set point at which blood acidity is controlled in normal subjects results from the influence of both respiratory and metabolic determinants.

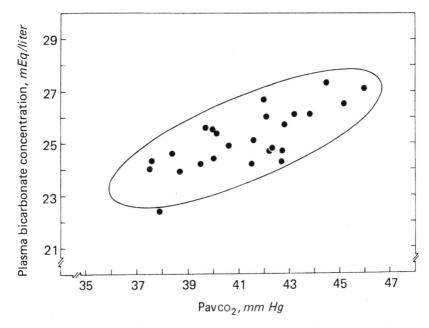

Figure 2 Dependence of bicarbonate concentration on partial pressure of carbon dioxide in arterialized venous blood ($PavCO_2$) in the normal state. The 90% joint confidence region for assessing new values for $PavCO_2$ and plasma bicarbonate concentration obtained from a single sample is shown. The points depict values obtained in 25 healthy male subjects. A single set of acid–base data obtained from a normal man can, with 90% probability, be expected to fall within this elliptical region. *Source*: From Ref. 7.

Having recognized this interrelationship, we proposed that the interindividual differences in plasma [HCO_3^-] in normal subjects are accounted for in part by differences in the level at which PCO_2 is regulated by the respiratory system (7). Studies summarized in Fig. 2 and Table 4 provide support for the primacy of PCO_2 in regulating [H^+]. As shown, values for plasma [HCO_3^-] *within the normal range* are highly dependent on the prevailing PCO_2. In these studies, 50% of the variability in plasma [HCO_3^-] in arterialized venous blood was attributable simply to variations in PCO_2. Thus, in normal humans, a variation of 1 mmHg in PCO_2 of arterialized venous blood is associated with 0.36 mEq/L change in the same direction in plasma [HCO_3^-]. Limits of the 90% joint confidence region for plasma acid–base values at different levels of arterialized venous PCO_2 show that in normal individuals with PCO_2 of 44 mmHg, the expected [HCO_3^-] and blood pH are 25.4–27.0 mEq/L and 7.37–7.39, respectively, whereas in subjects with PCO_2 of 38 mmHg, the expected [HCO_3^-] and blood pH are in the range of 23.5–24.7 mEq/L and 7.40–7.42, respectively.

Table 4   Normal Plasma Acid–Base Values in Arterialized Venous Blood at
Different Carbon Dioxide Tension Levels[a]

PavCO$_2$	[HCO$_3^-$] (mEq/L)	[H$^+$] (nEq/L)	pH
Mean steady-state values			
38	23.5–24.7	40.1–38.2	7.40–7.42
39	23.4–25.4	41.4–38.1	7.38–7.42
40	23.6–25.9	42.1–38.3	7.38–7.42
41	23.9–26.4	42.6–38.5	7.37–7.41
42	24.3–26.7	42.9–39.0	7.37–7.41
43	24.8–26.9	43.0–39.7	7.37–7.40
44	25.4–27.0	43.0–40.4	7.37–7.39
Values from a single blood sample			
36	22.9–23.6	39.0–37.8	7.41–7.42
37	22.6–24.7	40.6–37.2	7.39–7.43
38	22.6–25.4	41.7–37.1	7.38–7.43
39	22.8–25.9	42.4–37.4	7.37–7.43
40	23.0–26.4	43.1–37.6	7.37–7.42
41	23.4–26.8	43.5–38.0	7.36–7.42
42	23.7–27.1	44.0–38.5	7.36–7.42
43	24.2–27.4	44.1–38.9	7.36–7.41
44	24.7–27.6	44.2–39.6	7.35–7.40
45	25.2–27.8	44.3–40.2	7.35–7.40
46	26.0–27.7	43.9–41.2	7.36–7.39

[a]Limits of the 90% joint confidence region for plasma acid–base values at different levels of PavCO$_2$ in normal humans. *Source*: From Ref. 7.

Effects of Diet and Age on Normal Values

In addition to variations in PCO$_2$, metabolic factors appear to play a role in determining the interindividual differences in plasma [HCO$_3^-$], and thus plasma acidity, in normal subjects (3,8). Diet influences the acid–base status, at least in part, through changes in endogenous acid production. Consequently, a small but detectable decrease in [HCO$_3^-$] is observed when consuming a meat diet as compared with a vegetable diet (8,9). It has been proposed that ingestion of a diet abundant in cereal grains (that supply H$^+$ precursors in excess of HCO$_3^-$ precursors) and meager in plant foods (that are rich in HCO$_3^-$ precursors) promotes the occurrence of a low plasma [HCO$_3^-$] in otherwise healthy adult humans. A detailed evaluation of the impact of the diet on acid–base status is presented in Chapter 8.

Acid–base composition is also influenced by age (9–12) (see also Chapters 8 and 25). Infants and young children (up to age 3) have PaCO$_2$ values of 33–37 mmHg. In older children PaCO$_2$ gradually increases; by age 15, the

Table 5 Normal Acid–Base Values in Pregnancy and Childhood

		pH	$[H^+]$ (nEq/L)	PCO_2 (mmHg)	$[HCO_3^-]$ (mEq/L)
Pregnancy (arterial blood)	8–19 weeks	7.47 ± 0.02	34 ± 2	34 ± 2	23.8 ± 1.2
	20–29 weeks	7.48 ± 0.01	33 ± 1	32 ± 2	23.0 ± 1.7
	30 weeks	7.47 ± 0.03	34 ± 2	29 ± 3	20.4 ± 3.2
Childhood (capillary blood)	6 hr	7.38 ± 0.04	42 ± 4	37 ± 4	21.4 ± 1.9
	24 hr	7.41 ± 0.04	39 ± 4	37 ± 4	21.7 ± 1.9
	72 hr	7.42 ± 0.04	38 ± 4	36 ± 5	22.2 ± 3.1
	3 months–2 years	7.40 ± 0.03	40 ± 3	34 ± 4	20.1 ± 1.9
	1–3 years	7.38 ± 0.03	42 ± 3	34 ± 4	19.5 ± 1.4
	3–15 years	7.41 ± 0.03	39 ± 3	37 ± 3	22.7 ± 1.4

All values are mean $\pm$ SD.
Source: Data compiled from Refs. 3,9,12–14.

range rises to 35–40 mmHg, and the average and range are identical to adults at age 17. Table 5 presents the normal acid–base values in childhood (11–13). In adults, plasma $[HCO_3^-]$ falls and $[H^+]$ increases with age; the change is quite small but highly significant for both variables. In a careful study carried out in 64 normal subjects ranging in age from 17 to 74 years, mean $[HCO_3^-]$ fell from 25.2 mEq/L at age 20 to 23.5 mEq/L at age 65, and $[H^+]$ increased from 38 to 40 nEq/L (9). The direction of these subtle age-related changes indicates that they reflect a metabolic effect, as opposed to one driven by variations in $PaCO_2$.

Physiologic Effects on Normal Values

Several physiologic factors can influence acid–base status. Compared with the recumbent position, sitting or standing lowers $PaCO_2$ by about 2 and 4 mmHg, respectively. Women have $PaCO_2$ values about 2–4 mmHg lower, plasma $[HCO_3^-]$ is about 1 mEq/L lower, and pH about 0.01–0.02 higher than men (2,3). During the luteal phase of the menstrual cycle this hypocapnia is more evident, reflecting the direct effect of progesterone to stimulate ventilation, with decreases in $PaCO_2$ of 3–8 mmHg [14, see also Chapter 21]. Even larger decreases are observed during pregnancy (15), most notably in the last trimester, with $PaCO_2$ values of 29 ± 3 mmHg, with the expected secondary decreases in $[HCO_3^-]$ and increases in pH [20.4 ± 3.2 mEq/L and 7.47 ± 0.03 pH units, respectively] (Table 5). Both in the luteal phase of the normal menstrual cycle and in pregnancy, the reduction in $PaCO_2$ is caused by progesterone secretion, and lead to the expected changes in plasma

[HCO₃⁻] and blood pH. Estrogens appear to enhance the ventilatory effects of progesterone (see Chapter 21). High-altitude residents or individuals ascending to high altitudes also increase ventilation, secondary to hypoxemia, and the acid–base values reflect primary hypocapnia (see Chapter 21).

Arterial vs. Venous Blood

The difference in acid–base composition between arterial and venous blood from a resting extremity is small under normal conditions; venous blood pH is 0.01–0.03 lower, PCO_2 about 6 mmHg higher, and [HCO₃⁻] about 2 mEq/L higher than the respective values of arterial blood (Table 3). The higher PCO_2 and [HCO₃⁻] in venous blood than in arterial blood reflect the interposition of body tissues, which add CO_2 to venous blood. As discussed in Chapters 20 and 26, however, the difference in acid–base composition between venous and arterial blood can vary depending on venous blood flow rate and the rate of CO_2 addition to the venous blood. As a result venous blood samples are not a reliable way to assess systemic acid–base status. To minimize the difference between venous and arterial blood, venous blood can be "arterialized" in vivo by warming up the hand at 45°C for 10 min, an intervention that markedly increases venous blood flow rate. This procedure renders arteriovenous acid–base differences negligible.

REFERENCES

1. Adrogué HJ, Wesson DE. Introductory concepts. In: Adrogué HJ, Wesson DE, eds. acid–base. Blackwell's Basics of Medicine. Boston: Blackwell Science, 1994:1–47.
2. Siggaard-Andersen O. The acid–base Status of the Blood. 4th ed. Baltimore: Williams & Wilkins, 1974.
3. Gennari FJ, Cohen JJ, Kassirer JP. Normal acid–base values. Cohen JJ, Kassirer JP, eds. Acid–Base. Boston: Little, Brown, 1982:107–110.
4. Moller B. The hydrogen ion concentration in arterial blood. Acta Med Scand 1959; 348(suppl):1.
5. Valtin H, Gennari FJ. Acid–Base balance in health. In: Valtin H, Gennari FJ, eds. Acid–Base Disorders. Boston: Little, Brown, 1987:1–36.
6. Madias NE, Adrogué HJ, Cohen JJ, Schwartz WB. Effect of natural variations in PaCO₂ on plasma [HCO₃⁻] in dogs: a redefinition of normal. Am J Physiol 1979; 236:F30–F35.
7. Madias NE, Adrogué HJ, Horowitz GL, Cohen JJ, Schwartz WB. A redefinition of normal Acid–Base equilibrium in man: carbon dioxide tension as a key determinant of normal plasma bicarbonate concentration. Kidney Int 1979; 16: 612–618.
8. Kurtz I, Maher T, Hulter HN, Schambelan M, Sebastian A. Effect of diet on plasma acid–base composition in normal humans. Kidney Int 1983; 24: 670–680.

9. Frassetto L, Morris RC, Sebastian A. Effect of age on blood acid–base composition in adult humans: role of age-related renal functional decline. Am J Physiol 1996; 271:1114–1122.

10. Frassetto L, Sebastian A. Age and systemic acid–base equilibrium: analysis of published data. J Gerontol 1996; 51A:B91–B99.

11. Cassels DE, Morse M. Arterial blood gases and acid–base balance in normal children. J Clin Invest 1953; 32:824.

12. Malan AF, Evans A, Heese HD. Serial acid–base determinations in normal, premature and full-term infants during the first 72 hours of life. Arch Dis Child 1965; 40:645.

13. Albert MS, Winters RW. Acid–base equilibrium of blood in normal infants. Pediatrics 1966; 37:728.

14. Takano N, Kaneda J. Renal contribution to acid–base regulation during the menstrual cycle. Am J Physiol 1983; 244:F320–F324.

15. Lucius H, Gahlenbeck H, Kleine Ho, Fabel H, Bartels H. Respiratory functions, buffer system and electrolyte concentrations of blood during human pregnancy. Respir Physiol 1970; 9:311.

28

Tools for Clinical Assessment

Horacio J. Adrogué

Baylor College of Medicine, VA Medical Center, Houston, Texas, U.S.A.

Nicolaos E. Madias

*Department of Medicine, Caritas St. Elizabeth's Medical Center,
Tufts University School of Medicine, Boston, Massachusetts, U.S.A.*

INTRODUCTION

Acid–base status is assessed, as a first step, by direct evaluation of blood acidity. The level of blood acidity is determined by the prevailing "respiratory component" (i.e., carbonic acid concentration, $[H_2CO_3]$, a function of carbon dioxide tension, PCO_2) and "metabolic component" (i.e., actual bicarbonate concentration, $[HCO_3^-]$), as stipulated by the Henderson–Hasselbalch equation (Chapter 26). Although only blood pH and the "respiratory component" ($PaCO_2$) are usually directly measured, the physicochemical constraints of the Henderson–Hasselbalch equation obligate a unique level of $[HCO_3^-]$. Thus, $[HCO_3^-]$ stands alone among the various estimates of the "metabolic component" (i.e., standard bicarbonate and base excess, see below) as the only one whose level derives from direct measurements of the patient's blood sample. Further, plasma $[HCO_3^-]$ can almost be equated to the directly measured level of total CO_2 content in plasma (Chapter 26).

DEFINITION OF TERMS

Deviations from normal blood acidity are termed "acidemia" (increased $[H^+]$ or decreased pH) and "alkalemia" (decreased $[H^+]$ or increased pH). On the other hand, "acidosis" refers to a pathophysiologic process tending to acidify body fluids, whereas "alkalosis" refers to a process tending to alkalinize body fluids. Importantly, patients can have acidosis or alkalosis without being acidemic or alkalemic, because of the simultaneous presence of both processes (1–3).

Deviations of the "respiratory component" are termed "hypocapnia" (decreased PCO_2) and "hypercapnia" (increased PCO_2). Deviations of actual $[HCO_3^-]$ (i.e., the "metabolic component") are termed "hypobicarbonatemia" (reduced $[HCO_3^-]$) and "hyperbicarbonatemia" (elevated $[HCO_3^-]$). The terms "correction" and "repair" describe the restoration to normal levels of the initiating, primary abnormality responsible for the acid–base disturbance.

SIMPLE ACID–BASE DISORDERS (TABLE 1)

A "simple acid–base disorder" is characterized by a primary or initiating abnormality in either the "respiratory component" ($PaCO_2$) or the "metabolic component" (plasma $[HCO_3^-]$) accompanied by an appropriate secondary change in the other component. The four cardinal simple acid–base disorders are metabolic acidosis, respiratory acidosis, metabolic alkalosis, and respiratory alkalosis (Fig. 1).

Disturbances of acidity initiated by changes in the "respiratory component" are termed "respiratory acidosis" (i.e., primary hypercapnia) and "respiratory alkalosis" (i.e., primary hypocapnia)[a] Disturbances of acidity initiated by changes in the "metabolic component" are termed "metabolic acidosis" (primary reduction of plasma $[HCO_3^-]$, standard bicarbonate, or base excess) and "metabolic alkalosis" (primary elevation of plasma $[HCO_3^-]$, standard bicarbonate, or base excess) (3,6–8).

Changes in the "respiratory component" occurring in response to primary changes in the "metabolic component" (i.e., the ventilatory responses to metabolic acid–base disorders) are termed "secondary hypercapnia" (or secondary hypoventilation) in the case of metabolic alkalosis, and "secondary hypocapnia" (or secondary hyperventilation) in the case of metabolic acidosis. Changes in the "metabolic component" occurring in response to primary changes in the "respiratory component" (i.e., the changes in $[HCO_3^-]$ in response to respiratory acid–base disorders) are termed "secondary hyperbicarbonatemia" (or secondary increase in $[HCO_3^-]$) in the case of respiratory acidosis, and "secondary hypobicarbonatemia" (or secondary decrease in $[HCO_3^-]$) in the case of respiratory alkalosis.

---

[a]Pseudorespiratory alkalosis is an idiotypic form of respiratory acidosis in which hypercapnia is not detected in arterial blood but is present only in central or mixed venous blood; arterial blood features eucapnia or frank hypocapnia. This entity occurs in patients with profound depression of cardiac function and pulmonary perfusion but with relative preservation of alveolar ventilation (4,5) (see Chapter 20).

Table 1 The Four Simple Acid–Base Disturbances

Disturbance	Primary change	Secondary response	Mechanism of secondary response
Metabolic acidosis	Decrease in plasma [HCO_3^-]	Decrease in $PaCO_2$	Hyperventilation
Metabolic alkalosis	Increase in plasma [HCO_3^-]	Increase in $PaCO_2$	Hypoventilation
Respiratory acidosis	Increase in $PaCO_2$	Increase in plasma [HCO_3^-]	Acid titration of tissue buffers; transient rise in acid excretion and sustained increase in HCO_3^- reabsorption by the kidneys
Respiratory alkalosis	Decrease in $PaCO_2$	Decrease in plasma [HCO_3^-]	Alkaline titration of tissue buffers; transient reduction in acid excretion and sustained decrease in HCO_3^- reabsorption by the kidneys

SECONDARY RESPONSES

The term "uncomplicated" is used to refer to an abnormal state of acid–base equilibrium produced by a single acid–base disturbance (e.g., uncomplicated metabolic acidosis), including the secondary physiologic response to the primary change (1). Tables 1 and 2 catalogue the primary change and secondary response of each of the four simple acid–base disturbances. Although the term "compensatory" has been widely used as a substitute for "secondary", we consider the latter term more appropriate because the secondary response can be non-compensatory or even "maladaptive" when sustained (9,10). Furthermore, terms "compensated" and "uncompensated" imply success and failure in returning the level of acidity to normal, and secondary physiologic responses evoke amelioration but never complete restoration of systemic acidity to control levels.

MIXED ACID–BASE DISORDERS

A "mixed acid–base disorder" denotes the simultaneous presence of two or more simple acid–base disturbances. Combinations might include two or more simple acid–base disorders (e.g., metabolic acidosis and respiratory alkalosis), two or more forms of a simple disturbance having different time

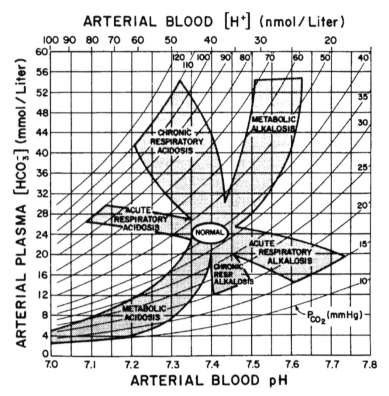

Figure 1   Acid–base template. This nomogram depicts the 95% confidence limits for graded degrees of severity of each of the four simple acid–base disorders. The ellipse near the center of the figure indicates the normal range for the acid–base parameters. If one assumes the presence of a steady-state, values falling within the areas depicted are consistent with, but not diagnostic of, the corresponding simple acid–base disorders. Acid–base values falling outside these areas denote the presence of a mixed acid–base disturbance *Source*: Modified from Fig. 13.3, Brenner BM, Rector FC. (The Kidney. Vol. 1 3rd ed. Philadelphia: W.B. Saunders Company, 1986).

course or pathogenesis (e.g., acute and chronic respiratory acidosis, or high anion gap and hyperchloremic metabolic acidosis), or a mixture of the previous two forms.

SYSTEMATIC APPROACH TO ACID–BASE DIAGNOSIS

Proper diagnosis of acid–base status requires the systematic approach outlined in Table 3 (11,12). The importance of adherence to these principles cannot be overemphasized. Even experienced physicians risk misdiagnosing the patient's acid–base status by bypassing the steps outlined below and in Table 3.

Table 2 Secondary Responses to Alterations in Acid–Base Status

Disturbance	Initiating mechanism	Expected response	Maximal level of response
Respiratory acidosis	$\uparrow PaCO_2$		
Acute		$\uparrow[HCO_3^-] \approx 0.1\ \Delta PaCO_2$	30 mEq/L
Chronic		$\uparrow[HCO_3^-] \approx 0.3\ \Delta PaCO_2$	45 mEq/L
Respiratory alkalosis	$\downarrow PaCO_2$		
Acute		$\downarrow[HCO_3^-] \approx 0.2\ \Delta PaCO_2$	16–18 mEq/L
Chronic		$\downarrow[HCO_3^-] \approx 0.4\ \Delta PaCO_2$	12–15 mEq/L
Metabolic acidosis	$\downarrow[HCO_3^-]_p$	$\downarrow PaCO_2 \approx 1.2\ \Delta[HCO_3^-]$	10 mm Hg
Metabolic alkalosis	$\uparrow[HCO_3^-]_p$	$\uparrow PaCO_2 \approx 0.7\ \Delta[HCO_3^-]$	No maximum[a]

[a]PCO_2 values as high as 85–90 mm Hg have been reported in severe metabolic alkalosis ($[HCO_3^-] > 80$ mEq/L).

Table 3 Systematic Approach to the Analysis of Acid–Base Disorders

1. Assess the internal consistency of the acid–base data and the reliability of blood sampling.
2. Obtain clinical information, including history and physical examination, for clues to a particular acid–base disorder.
3. Assess the expected secondary response to determine whether a simple or mixed acid–base disorder is present.
4. Establish the cause of the acid–base disorder by evaluating other laboratory parameters, as appropriate, including:
   A. Calculation of the serum anion gap: $[Na^+] - ([Cl^-] + [HCO_3^-])$ and measurement of serum $[K^+]$.
   B. Measurement of other laboratory parameters as appropriate (e.g., ketones, lactate, methanol).
   C. Calculation of serum osmolal gap if toxic exposure is suspected.
   D. Measurement of urine electrolytes, pH, and calculation of urine anion gap if an element of normal anion gap metabolic acidosis is present.
   E. Measurement of urine $[Cl^-]$ and urine pH if metabolic alkalosis is suspected.
   F. Calculation of urine osmolal gap if toxic exposure is suspected.

ASSESSMENT OF THE ACCURACY OF THE ACID–BASE MEASUREMENTS AND THE RELIABILITY OF BLOOD SAMPLING

The first step is verification of the accuracy of the acid–base data by ensuring that the values for pH, $PaCO_2$, and plasma $[HCO_3^-]$ satisfy the mathematical constraints of the Henderson equation,

$$[H^+] = 24 \times PaCO_2/[HCO_3^-] \tag{1}$$

where [H$^+$] is in nEq/L, PaCO$_2$ is in mmHg, and [HCO$_3^-$] is in mEq/L, or its logarithmic derivative, the Henderson–Hasselbalch equation,

$$pH = 6.1 + \log([HCO_3^-]/0.03 \times PaCO_2) \qquad (2)$$

To make certain that the individual acid–base parameters adhere to the expected mathematical relationship, either equation can be used. If independently measured values for blood pH, PaCO$_2$, and plasma [HCO$_3^-$] (or [total CO$_2$]) are available and do not fit reasonably well into these equations, an error in one or more of the values must be present and repeat determinations should be performed. Recall that [total CO$_2$] is 2–3 mmol/L higher in venous blood than in arterial blood. Not rarely, acid–base values that appear to pose major diagnostic challenges and lead interpreters to propose the most complex mixed acid–base disorders are merely sets of parameters that lack internal consistency (11,12).

An assessment of the acid–base status of the tissues in patients with circulatory failure may be misleading if only arterial blood is sampled (see Chapter 26) (4,5). The degree of misrepresentation worsens with the severity of circulatory compromise, and becomes extreme during cardiac arrest. Therefore, acid–base measurements on central or mixed venous blood as well as arterial blood are required for reliable assessment of the acid–base status in patients with circulatory failure.

ROLE OF CLINICAL INFORMATION TO IDENTIFY THE ACID–BASE DISORDER (TABLE 3)

After internal consistency of the acid–base values has been verified, the next step is to obtain relevant clinical information, including history and physical examination, for clues to a particular acid–base disorder. The importance of these tasks becomes apparent by considering that normal acid–base parameters are not in themselves sufficient to exclude the presence of acid–base disorders; indeed, normal values might be the fortuitous result of two simultaneous and counteracting acid–base disorders (e.g., high-anion-gap acidosis treated with alkali infusion or diarrhea-induced metabolic acidosis in conjunction with vomiting-induced metabolic alkalosis). More broadly speaking, a given set of acid–base values is never diagnostic of a particular acid–base disorder, whether simple or mixed in nature, but rather it is consistent with a range of acid–base abnormalities (13–17).

Clinical History

Information from the patient's history often provides the key information necessary to diagnose the prevailing acid–base status (Table 4). This principle

Table 4 Diagnosing Acid–Base Disorders: Examples on the Role of History and Physical Examination

Clues	Potential acid–base disorder
Volume depletion, circulatory failure, shock	Lactic acidosis
Diarrhea	Hyperchloremic metabolic acidosis
Vomiting, nasogastric suction	Metabolic alkalosis
Loop or thiazide diuretics	Metabolic alkalosis
Acetazolamide	Hyperchloremic metabolic acidosis
Chronic obstructive pulmonary disease	Respiratory acidosis; posthypercapnic alkalosis
Eating disorder	Metabolic alkalosis
Laxative abuse	Metabolic acidosis; metabolic alkalosis
Chronic renal failure	Metabolic acidosis
Type 1 diabetes mellitus	Diabetic ketoacidosis
Hepatic coma, sepsis	Respiratory alkalosis
Pregnancy, ascent to high altitude, anxiety attack	Respiratory alkalosis
$CaCO_3$ abuse	Milk-alkali syndrome
Alcoholism	Alcoholic ketoacidosis; metabolic alkalosis; respiratory alkalosis; methanol/ethylene glycol intoxication
Hearing loss, tinnitus	Salicylate intoxication
Optic papillitis	Methanol intoxication
Urine calcium oxalate monohydrate crystals	Ethylene glycol intoxication
Metformin	Lactic acidosis
Short bowel syndrome	D (-) lactic acidosis

is especially important in the diagnosis of mixed acid–base disturbances, because clinical experience indicates that these disorders most commonly occur in a limited number of settings (11) (Chapter 22).

Physical Examination

Table 4 provides examples on the role of history and physical examination in the diagnosis of acid–base disorders. Essentially, a clinical setting-focused approach enables the clinician to formulate diagnostic hypotheses and then to proceed with their confirmation or refutation by utilizing acid–base and other ancillary laboratory data (11,12). We believe this approach not only allows for a more accurate and prompt diagnosis of simple and mixed acid–base disorders but also fosters the anticipation of their development and thus the potential for prevention.

IDENTIFICATION OF THE PRIMARY OR DOMINANT ACID–BASE DISORDER (TABLE 3)

Use of Serum [HCO_3^-]

To identify the primary or dominant acid–base disorder, one can first evaluate the serum [HCO_3^-] (or [total CO_2]). A high value represents either metabolic alkalosis or the secondary response to respiratory acidosis. If blood pH is elevated, metabolic alkalosis is the primary disorder. If blood pH is reduced, respiratory acidosis is the primary disorder. If serum [HCO_3^-] exceeds 45 mEq/L, at least a component of metabolic alkalosis can be diagnosed with certainty even in the absence of measurement of blood pH, because the secondary response to even the most severe respiratory acidosis never exceeds this level.

A low serum [HCO_3^-], conversely, signifies metabolic acidosis or the secondary response to respiratory alkalosis. If hypobicarbonatemia is accompanied by a reduced blood pH, metabolic acidosis is the primary disorder. If the blood pH is high, respiratory alkalosis is the primary disorder. If serum [HCO_3^-] is <10 mEq/L, an unequivocal diagnosis of at least a component of metabolic acidosis can be made irrespective of blood pH, because hypobicarbonatemia of such severity never occurs in response to the most marked respiratory alkalosis.

Use of Base Excess/Deficit

If the clinician uses base excess instead of plasma [HCO_3^-] to assess the metabolic component of acid–base status (Chapter 26), two major caveats must be remembered. First, acute respiratory disturbances can alter base excess as a result of redistribution between the vascular and the interstitial compartment of titration-induced changes in plasma [HCO_3^-]. Second, base deficit is not pathognomonic of metabolic acidosis and base excess is not pathognomonic of metabolic alkalosis (see Chapter 26). Base deficit only indicates the existence of a bicarbonate-depleting state, which occurs both in metabolic acidosis and chronic respiratory alkalosis. In a comparable manner, base excess only indicates the presence of a bicarbonate-rich state, which occurs both in metabolic alkalosis and chronic respiratory acidosis.

ASSESS THE EXPECTED SECONDARY RESPONSE TO DETERMINE WHETHER A SIMPLE OR MIXED ACID–BASE DISORDER IS PRESENT

Table 2 presents the equations describing the mean, steady-state, whole-body secondary responses to the four cardinal acid–base disturbances. As a general rule, deviation of $PaCO_2$ values by >5 mmHg, or [HCO_3^-] by >3 mEq/L, from those predicted by the equations indicate that a mixed disorder is present. The relationships embodied in these equations have been used to construct acid–base templates (with the empirical range of variability depicted as "confidence bands") that present schematically the limits of the secondary response to each of the simple acid–base disturbances. These templates can be used as aids to the diagnostic process (Fig. 1), but their use requires a clear understanding of the following caveats:

1. A certain time interval is required for each secondary adaptive response to reach completion or to be eradicated once the initiating primary disturbance has vanished. Thus, a mixed acid–base disturbance might be diagnosed incorrectly because insufficient time has elapsed for the secondary response to a simple disturbance to develop or to resolve.

2. Assuming that a steady-state is present, an accurate set of acid–base data that falls outside the expected limits for each simple acid–base disorder denotes the presence of a mixed acid–base disturbance. By contrast, acid–base data falling within the limits of the expected secondary response to a simple disorder are consistent with, but not diagnostic of the particular disorder. Thus, reaching a diagnosis with reasonable certainty will require careful examination of the acid–base values in light of all relevant clinical information (including the patient's history, physical examination, and ancillary laboratory data).

3. Mild acid–base disorders pose particular diagnostic difficulty because of the considerable overlap of values for the simple disturbances near the range of normal. In such circumstances, any one of several simple disorders or a variety of mixed disturbances might fully account for the acid–base data under evaluation. Again, careful correlation of all available clinical information should guide the diagnostic process.

ESTABLISH THE CAUSE OF THE ACID–BASE DISORDER BY EVALUATING OTHER LABORATORY PARAMETERS

Calculation of the Serum Anion Gap

The serum concentration of unmeasured anions, or anion gap, is calculated from the measured serum electrolytes, as $[Na^+] - ([Cl^-] + [HCO_3^-])$, all in mEq/L (18–20). This derived parameter provides important insights into the nature of the prevailing changes in plasma $[HCO_3^-]$. Once calculated, the value should be compared with the normal level at the local laboratory. Although the average normal value has historically been set at 10–12 mEq/L, new methodologies for measuring serum electrolytes, used by some clinical laboratories, yield lower values. Furthermore, the range of normal for the calculated anion gap is substantial (on the order of 8 mEq/L) as a

consequence of biological and measurement variability of serum electrolytes. Because of these considerations, the best approach is to compare the
anion gap with previous values in the same patient obtained at a time when
neither acid–base nor electrolyte disturbances were present, if such values are
available.

Effect of Serum Albumin and pH on Anion Gap

Serum proteins are polyanions and account for the largest fraction of the
serum unmeasured anions. Accordingly, substantial abnormalities in serum
albumin concentration are associated with appreciable parallel changes in
the serum anion gap. The adjustment ("normalization") of the anion gap
for this effect is approximated by subtracting or adding 2.5 mEq/L for each
1 g/dL of serum albumin below or above the normal value of 4 g/dL (21).
Thus, the average "normal" serum anion gap is 7 mEq/L when serum albumin is 2 g/dL (e.g., nephrotic syndrome, cirrhosis of the liver), but it extends
to 17 mEq/L when serum albumin is 6 g/dL (e.g., severe volume depletion).
In these examples, normal serum anion gap is assumed to be 12 mEq/L for
an albumin level of 4 g/dL.

In addition, the prevailing pH affects the serum anion gap because of
pH-dependent changes both in protein charge and the serum levels of
organic acids (18,19). Acidemia reduces the anionic charge of proteins
and the acid products of glycolysis, and alkalemia has the opposite effect.
The effects of alkalemia on pyruvate and lactate metabolism are more pronounced than those of acidemia. The composite effect of these two influences is a decrease in anion gap of 1–3 mEq/L in acidemic states and an
increase of 3–5 mEq/L in alkalemic states, depending on the severity of
the deviation in blood acidity (3). As an example, the expected "normal"
value for the serum anion gap in a patient with moderately severe metabolic
alkalosis (blood pH, 7.50, serum albumin concentration, 5 g/dL) would be
17 mEq/L, if one assumes a normal anion gap of 12 mEq/L in a patient with
blood pH of 7.40 and serum albumin of 4 g/dL.

Excess Anion Gap (Table 5)

The difference between the observed serum anion gap and the adjusted
normal value generates a new parameter termed the excess anion gap or
delta (Δ) anion gap. If the Δ anion gap is positive (i.e., the observed anion
gap is greater than the adjusted normal value), the presence of an element of
high-anion-gap metabolic acidosis is diagnosed. This diagnosis is based on
the assumption that the anions of the acids that have replaced HCO_3^- in
the body fluids have a similar space of distribution. Because of this assumption and potential errors in analysis, the degree of confidence in the diagnostic value of this finding is greatly increased when the excess anion gap
exceeds 5 mEq/L.

Table 5 Utility of the Relationship Between Δ Anion Gap and Δ[HCO$_3^-$] in the Evaluation of Metabolic Acidosis and Mixed Acid–Base Disorders

Blood composition	Normal	Normal anion-gap acidosis	High anion-gap acidosis	High anion-gap and normal anion-gap acidosis	High anion-gap acidosis and metabolic alkalosis	High anion-gap acidosis and chronic respiratory acidosis
pH	7.40	7.26	7.29	7.28	7.38	7.12
PaCO$_2$	40	23	30	26	35	70
[HCO$_3^-$]	24	10	14	12	20	22
Anion gap	12	12	22	18	28	23
Δ[HCO$_3^-$]	0	−14	−10	−12	−4	−2
Δ Anion gap	0	0	+10	+6	+16	+11
[HCO$_3^-$] after correction of Δ AG	24	10	24	18	36	33

PaCO$_2$, mm Hg; [HCO$_3^-$] and anion gap, mEq/L; AG, anion gap.

The quantitative relationship between the decrement in plasma [HCO$_3^-$] and the excess anion gap also permits an assessment of whether the retention of fixed acids is fully or only partially responsible for the observed metabolic acidosis. For example, if the prevailing Δ anion gap corresponds to only 50% of the decrement in plasma [HCO$_3^-$], then only 50% of the decrement is attributable to high-anion-gap metabolic acidosis. The remaining 50% is accounted for by a hyperchloremic hypobicarbonatemic process (normal-anion-gap metabolic acidosis or respiratory alkalosis). Adding the Δ anion gap to the prevailing serum [HCO$_3^-$] allows estimation of the [HCO$_3^-$] value that existed prior to the development of the high-anion-gap metabolic acidosis. For example, if the Δ anion gap is 16 mEq/L in a patient with a serum [HCO$_3^-$] of 20 mEq/L, one can estimate that serum [HCO$_3^-$] was approximately 36 mEq/L (20 + 16 mEq/L) prior to the development of the high-anion-gap metabolic acidosis. Such calculations are of practical importance because they allow anticipation of the plasma [HCO$_3^-$] that would result following eradication of the complicating high-anion-gap metabolic acidosis (21,22). Table 4 depicts the utility of comparing the change in anion gap with the change in plasma [HCO$_3^-$] from their respective normal values in evaluating metabolic acidosis and some forms of mixed acid–base disorders.

Measurement of Serum Potassium Concentration ([K$^+$]) (Table 3)

The serum [K$^+$] can be very helpful in the differential diagnosis of normal anion gap (hyperchloremic) metabolic acidosis (see also Chapter 13). In patients with a high-anion-gap metabolic acidosis, serum [K$^+$] can be high, normal, or low, and therefore it is of no particular help in the differential diagnosis of the cause of this disorder. Hypokalemia accompanies all forms of metabolic alkalosis and, while the presence of this abnormality should alert one to the possibility that metabolic alkalosis may be present, it is not pathognomonic nor is it helpful in the differential diagnosis of the cause. Respiratory acid–base disturbances can also alter serum [K$^+$] but the abnormalities induced are generally mild; therefore, marked deviations in serum [K$^+$] usually suggest the presence of a metabolic acid–base disturbance.

Measurement of Other Laboratory Parameters as Appropriate (Table 3)

In patients with high-anion-gap metabolic acidosis, determination of serum glucose, lactate, ketones and creatinine concentration will usually identify lactic acidosis, ketoacidosis, or renal failure as causes of the acidosis. Precise quantification of the cause of the increase in the serum anion gap, however, is often not possible. In investigating for evidence of ketosis, as an example, the nitroprusside reaction detects only acetoacetate and not β-hydroxybutyrate, the predominant ketoanion. In alcoholic ketoacidosis, in particular, there is a shift away from the formation of acetoacetate and toward β-hydroxybutyrate, and therefore the nitroprusside reaction can be negative or only mildly positive (see Chapter 10).

Serum Osmolal Gap

A laboratory screen of blood or urine for certain toxins is very useful in detecting salicylate, methanol, or ethylene glycol in patients with a high anion gap metabolic acidosis. If such an analysis is not readily available on a timely basis, measurement of serum osmolality and comparison of this value to the value calculated from the measured concentrations of the substances in serum that normally contribute to serum osmolality can be of great value in the initial assessment of intoxications caused by various alcohols or glycols. The quantitatively dominant moieties contributing to serum osmolality are Na^+ (and its counterbalancing anions, Cl^- and HCO_3^-), glucose, and urea. Thus, serum osmolality can be estimated as follows:

$$S_{osm} = 2 \times [Na^+] + [glucose]/18 + [BUN]/2.8 \qquad (3)$$

where $[Na^+]$ is in mEq/L and [glucose] and blood urea nitrogen ($[BUN]$) are expressed in mg/dL. An osmolal gap (defined as the difference between the measured and estimated serum osmolality) of $>10\,mOsm/kg\ H_2O$ signifies the presence in serum of additional osmotically active particles and suggests a diagnosis of intoxication with a low-molecular-weight solute, such as methanol, ethylene glycol, or ethanol (causing alcoholic ketoacidosis, see Chapter 10).

MEASUREMENT OF URINE ELECTROLYTES, pH, AND CALCULATION OF URINE ANION GAP (TABLE 3)

Urine Electrolytes

Measurement of urine electrolytes can be helpful in distinguishing the causes of various acid–base disorders (13,14,23), but this evaluation is seriously hampered by previous or concomitant administration of loop or thiazide diuretics. Thus, before embarking on this assessment, one should determine whether diuretics have been administered. In patients with metabolic alkalosis, measurement of urine $[Cl^-]$ and $[Na^+]$ can be a valuable tool in the evaluation of the cause. On the basis of urine $[Cl^-]$, metabolic alkaloses are classified into chloride-responsive (low urine $[Cl^-]$, $<20\,mEq/L$) and chloride-resistant (high urine $[Cl^-]$, $>20\,mEq/L$) forms (see Chapter 16) (2,3,6). In normal anion-gap metabolic acidosis, the urine anion gap, calculated from urine electrolyte measurements, can assist in distinguishing the cause as well (see below).

Urine pH

A pH meter should be utilized always for the measurement of urine pH since dipsticks can be inaccurate and misleading. In individuals with normal anion gap metabolic acidosis, urine pH along with an estimation of urinary ammonium excretion can aid in the detection and/or further characterization of metabolic acidosis resulting from defects in renal acidification. Urine collection under mineral oil (to prevent loss of CO_2) is not necessary if urine pH is measured promptly on freshly voided "first morning" urine. The presence of a urinary tract infection with a urea-splitting organism (i.e., urea $\rightarrow NH_3 + CO_2$) increases urine pH in the absence of an acidification defect.

Urine Anion Gap

Urine $[NH_4^+]$ is not measured in most clinical laboratories, but the value can be estimated from the concentrations of Na^+, K^+ and Cl^- by calculating the urine anion gap (defined as $[Na^+] + [K^+] - [Cl^-]$) (see Chapter 13). This calculation is only useful in a setting in which NH_4^+ excretion should normally be stimulated, i.e., the presence of metabolic acidosis (serum $[HCO_3^-] < 18\,mEq/L$. Additional requirements for using this calculation are that the urine does not contain unusual anions (e.g., ketone bodies, carbenicillin) and that HCO_3^- excretion is low (urine pH < 6.5). Ammonium is an unmeasured cation, so an increase in its excretion as NH_4Cl will cause an increase in the urine Cl^- excretion and yield a negative value for the urine anion gap, i.e., $[Cl^-]$ exceeds the sum of $[Na^+]$ and $[K^+]$. A negative urine anion gap indicates that the urine contains substantial quantities of NH_4^+ and provides evidence against impaired NH_4^+ excretion as the major factor in the pathogenesis of the acidosis. By contrast, a positive value in the range of $20\text{–}30\,mEq/L$ indicates that NH_4^+ excretion is low and implicates this reduction as an important factor in the production of metabolic acidosis.

Despite adequate quantities of NH_4^+ being present in a urine of low pH, a positive urine anion gap can be seen when there is increased excretion of unusual unmeasured anions, such as β-hydroxybutyrate and acetoacetate with ketoacidosis, or hippurate with toluene intoxication. These anions obligate the excretion of Na^+ (and K^+), thereby producing the positive urine anion gap. Under these circumstances, urine NH_4^+ excretion can be estimated from calculation of the urine osmolal gap, as described below.

Urine Osmolal Gap

The urine osmolal gap is defined as follows:

$$\text{Urine osmolal gap} = \text{measured osmolality} - \text{calculated osmolality}$$

$$(4)$$

And the calculated osmolality in urine is:

$$\text{Calculated osmolality} = 2 \times ([Na^+] + [K^+])$$
$$+ [\text{urea nitrogen}]/2.8 + [\text{glucose}]/18 \quad (5)$$

where $[Na^+]$ and $[K^+]$ are in mEq/L and [urea nitrogen] and [glucose] are measured in mg/dL. The gap between the measured and calculated urine osmolality should primarily reflect excretion of ammonium salts (23). An appropriate urine osmolal gap in an acidotic patient is >150–200 mOsm/kg H_2O, whereas in patients with low NH_4^+ excretion, the urine osmolal gap is usually < 50–100 mOsm/kg H_2O. Approximately one half of the calculated osmolal gap is accounted for by NH_4^+, and the remainder is accounted for by its accompanying anions.

REFERENCES

1. Cohen JJ. Towards a physiologic nomenclature for in vivo disturbances of acid–base balance. National Bureau of Standards Special Publication 450. Proceedings of a workshop on pH and blood gases held at NBS, Gaithersburg, MD, July 7–8, 1975. Issued June 1977, 127–129.
2. Valtin H, Gennari FJ. Acid–Base Disorders. Basic Concepts and Clinical Management. Boston: Little, Brown, 1987.
3. Adrogué HJ, Wesson DE. Acid–Base. Blackwell's Basics of Medicine. Boston: Blackwell Science, 1994.
4. Adrogué HJ, Rashad MN, Gorin AB, Yacoub J, Madias NE. Assessing acid–base status in circulatory failure: differences between arterial and central venous blood. N Engl J Med 1989; 320:1312–1316.
5. Adrogué HJ, Rashad MN, Gorin AB, Yacoub J, Madias NE. Arteriovenous acid–base disparity in circulatory failure: studies on mechanism. Am J Physiol 1989; 257:F1087–F1093.
6. Laski ME, Kurtzman NA. Acid–base disorders in medicine. Dis Month 1996; 42:51–125.
7. Siggaard-Andersen O. The acid–base status of the blood. 4th ed. Baltimore: Williams & Wilkins, 1974.
8. Howorth PJN. Base excess. Why reopen the acid–base debate? National Bureau of Standards Special Publication 450. Proceedings of a workshop on pH and blood gases held at NBS, Gaithersburg, MD, July 7–8, 1975. Issued June 1977, 127–129.
9. Madias NE, Schwartz WB, Cohen JJ. The maladaptive renal response to secondary hypocapnia during chronic HCl acidosis in the dog. J Clin Invest 1977; 60:1393–1401.
10. Madias NE, Adrogue HJ, Cohen, JJ. Maladaptive renal response to secondary hypercapnia in chronic metabolic alkalosis. Am J Physiol 1980; 238:F283–F289.
11. Adrogué HJ, Madias NE. Mixed acid–base disorders. In: Jacobson HR, Striker GE, Klahr S, eds. The Principles and Practice of Nephrology. 2nd ed. Philadelphia: BC Decker, 1995:953–962.

12. Kraut JA, Madias NE. Approach to the diagnosis of acid–base disorders. In: Massry SG, Glassock RJ, eds. Textbook of Nephrology. Philadelphia: Lippincott, Williams & Wilkins, 2001:436–443.
13. Gennari FJ, Rimmer JM. Acid–base disorders in end-stage renal disease. Semin Dial 1990; 3:81–85 (Pt. 1), 161–165 (Pt. 2).
14. Madias NE, Perrone RD. Acid–base disorders in association with renal disease. In: Schrier RW, Gottschalk CW, eds. Diseases of the Kidney. 5th ed. Boston: Little, Brown, 1993:2669–2699.
15. Cohen JJ. Minimal acceptance criteria for acid–base nomograms. National Bureau of Standards Special Publication 450. Proceedings of a Workshop on pH and Blood Gases held at NBS, Gaithersburg, MD, July 7–8, 1975. Issued June 1977, 131–132.
16. Howorth PJN. Use of in vivo CO_2 titration curves in the physiological assessment of acid–base balance. National Bureau of Standards Special Publication 450. Proceedings of a Workshop on pH and Blood Gases held at NBS, Gaithersburg, MD, July 7–8, 1975. Issued June 1977, 57–66.
17. Harrington JT, Cohen JJ, Kassirer JP. Mixed acid–base disturbances. In: Cohen JJ, Kassirer JP, eds. Acid/Base. Boston: Little, Brown, 1987:377–390.
18. Adrogué HJ, Brensilver J, Madias NE. Changes in the plasma anion gap during chronic metabolic acid–base disturbances. Am J Physiol 1978; 235:F291–F297.
19. Madias NE, Ayus JC, Adrogué HJ. Increased anion gap in metabolic alkalosis: the role of plasma protein equivalency. N Engl J Med 1979; 300:1421–1423.
20. Adrogué HJ, Wilson H, Boyd AE, Suki WN, Eknoyan G. Plasma acid–base patterns in diabetic ketoacidosis. N Engl J Med 1982; 307:1603–1610.
21. Gabow PA. Disorders associated with an altered anion gap. Kidney Int 1985; 27:472–487.
22. Emmett M, Narins RG. Mixed acid–base disorders. In: Maxwell MH, Kleeman CR, Narins RG, eds. Clinical Disorders of Fluid and Electrolyte Metabolism. New York: McGraw-Hill, 1994:991–1007.
23. Kamel KS, Ethier JH, Richardson RM. Urine electrolytes and osmolality: when and how to use them. Am J Nephrol 1990; 10:89–102.

29

Illustrative Cases

F. John Gennari
University of Vermont College of Medicine, Burlington, Vermont, U.S.A.

John H. Galla
Department of Medicine, University of Cincinnati College of Medicine, Cincinnati, Ohio, U.S.A.

Horacio J. Adrogué
Baylor College of Medicine, VA Medical Center, Houston, Texas, U.S.A.

Nicolaos E. Madias
Department of Medicine, Caritas St. Elizabeth's Medical Center, Tufts University School of Medicine, Boston, Massachusetts, U.S.A.

INTRODUCTION

This chapter is devoted to a series of clinical vignettes, followed by questions, chosen to illustrate the approach to diagnosing and managing acid–base disorders. The cases were selected by the editors as examples of disorders we have seen in our practices, in the hope that they will provide concrete clinical instances to reinforce the principles elucidated in the preceding chapters.

CASE 1

A previously healthy 30-year-old nurse developed profound weakness after an aerobics class. In the emergency room, she is unable to rise from a chair or lift her arms over her head. Laboratory measurements are in Table 1.

Table 1   Laboratory Measurements (Case 1)

Venous serum	
Creatinine	0.8 mg/dL
Urea nitrogen	15 mg/dL
Sodium	136 mEq/L
Potassium	1.8 mEq/L
Chloride	82 mEq/L
Total CO_2	39 mEq/L
Urine	
Sodium	12 mEq/L
Potassium	17 mEq/L
Chloride	21 mEq/L
Arterial blood	
pH	7.52
$[H^+]$	30 nEq/L
$PaCO_2$	50 mmHg
PaO_2	100 mmHg

Questions for Case 1

1. Are the acid–base data internally consistent?
2. Considering the history and acid–base findings, what is the dominant acid–base disorder?
3. Is it a simple or mixed disorder?
4. What is the likely cause for this acid–base disorder?

Answers for Case 1

1. For the acid–base data to be consistent, serum $[HCO_3^-]$ calculated from the measured arterial PCO_2 ($PaCO_2$) and pH should be within 3 mEq/L of the measured venous [total CO_2], with few exceptions (see Chapter 28). Rearranging the Henderson equation and converting pH to $[H^+]$ to make this calculation:

$$[HCO_3^-] = 24 \times PaCO_2/[H^+] = 24 \times 50/30 = 40\,mEq/L \qquad (1)$$

   The calculated and measured values differ by only 1 mEq/L, and therefore the data are internally consistent.
2. The history gives few clues as to the nature of this disorder, but the acid–base measurements showing an abnormally high pH, $[HCO_3^-]$ and $PaCO_2$ indicate that metabolic alkalosis is the dominant acid–base disorder.
3. To determine whether metabolic alkalosis is the only acid–base disturbance present (simple disorder), one must evaluate whether the secondary ventilatory response is appropriate. To assist in

Table 2 Laboratory Measurements (Case 2)

Venous serum	
Creatinine	1.2 mg/dL
Urea nitrogen	35 mg/dL
Sodium	133 mEq/L
Potassium	3.5 mEq/L
Chloride	78 mEq/L
Total CO_2	37 mEq/L
Anion gap	18 mEq/L
Urine	
Sodium	35 mEq/L
Potassium	44 mEq/L
Chloride	4 mEq/L
Arterial blood	
pH	7.66
$[H^+]$	22 nEq/L
$PaCO_2$	32 mmHg
PaO_2	100 mmHg

making this judgment, rules of thumb have been developed from steady-state observations in humans and animals, defining the expected response (see Chapter 28, Table 2). In the case of metabolic alkalosis, the expectation is that $PaCO_2$ increases by 0.7 mmHg for each mEq/L rise in $[HCO_3^-]$. Assuming the baseline $PaCO_2$ is 40 mmHg and the baseline serum $[HCO_3^-]$ is 24 mEq/L, the expected $PaCO_2 = 40 + 0.7 \times ([HCO_3^-] - 24)$. In this case $PaCO_2 = 40 + 0.7 \times (39 - 24) = 51$ mmHg. Because of variability in the secondary ventilatory response, a calculated value within 5 mmHg of the measured value is considered consistent with expectation. In this instance the calculated and measured values are virtually identical. Thus the data suggest that no independent respiratory acid–base disorder is present. It should be emphasized that one cannot exclude a complex respiratory problem on the basis of this simple analysis (see Chapters 20 and 28), but taken together with the history and physical examination, one can reasonably exclude an underlying pulmonary problem. The final step to exclude a mixed disorder is to evaluate the anion gap (see answers to Case 2). In this case, the patient has an uncomplicated metabolic alkalosis.

4. The classification that helps one sort out the causes of metabolic alkalosis is based on whether Cl^- depletion is responsible (see Chapter 16). If Cl^- depletion is responsible, the urine should be virtually Cl^--free. In this case, urine $[Cl^-]$ is 21 mEq/L, somewhat

higher than expected in a Cl⁻-depletion alkalosis. This patient has severe hypokalemia, caused by urinary losses because the urine [K⁺] is higher than expected if hypokalemia of this severity were due to extrarenal losses. With severe K^+ depletion, renal Cl^- wasting can occur, regardless of the cause of the metabolic alkalosis (see Chapter 17). Pure K^+ losses, mineralocorticoid excess or the use of a chloruretic diuretic could produce these findings. The clinical presentation (i.e., severe muscle weakness) is consistent with profound K^+ depletion. This patient used both diuretics and laxatives surreptitiously.

CASE 2

A 72-year-old man with a history of coronary artery disease and hypertension is intubated and on ventilatory support following a partial colectomy for colon cancer. He is on continuous gastric drainage via a nasogastric tube, and is receiving Ringer's lactate with added KCl (15 mEq/L) at 50 mL/hr intravenously. Laboratory measurements on the second postoperative day are in Table 2.

Questions for Case 2

1. Are the acid–base data internally consistent?
2. Considering the patient's history and acid–base data, what is the dominant acid–base disorder?
3. Is this a simple or mixed disorder?
4. Does the increased anion gap indicate the presence of a metabolic acidosis?
5. What is the cause of the acid–base disorder?
6. What treatment interventions should be undertaken based on your diagnosis?

Answers for Case 2

1. The data are consistent. Serum [HCO₃⁻] calculated from arterial pH and PaCO₂ is: $[HCO_3^-] = 24 \times 32/22 = 35$ mEq/L. This value, 35 mEq/L, is essentially the same as the measured [total CO₂], 37 mEq/L.
2. The history of nasogastric suction, as well as the alkaline pH and elevated [HCO₃⁻] all point to metabolic alkalosis as the dominant acid–base disorder, but one should note immediately that PaCO₂ is low, a finding inconsistent with the usual secondary ventilatory response to metabolic alkalosis.
3. This is a mixed disorder. The expected ventilatory response to this increase in serum [HCO₃⁻] (∼10 mEq/L) should increase PaCO₂

by $\sim 7\,mmHg$. In this case, the $PaCO_2$ is not increased at all, but is decreased by $8\,mmHg$. Therefore two separate and independent disorders, metabolic alkalosis and respiratory alkalosis, are present.

4. Assessment of the anion gap is primarily of use in the differential diagnosis of metabolic acidosis, but a high value can indicate the presence of a "hidden" metabolic acidosis in patients with a normal or high serum $[HCO_3^-]$. In this case, the anion gap is somewhat high ($18\,mEq/L$), but it is unlikely that a concurrent metabolic acidosis is present. The anion "gap" is due to unmeasured anions in serum, of which approximately 50% are accounted for the net negative charge on albumin (see Chapter 28). The value for this charge is pH-dependent, increasing as pH rises. The very alkaline pH in this patient could account for a large part of the high anion gap. In addition, alkalemia stimulates organic acid production, increasing the concentration of organic anions in plasma. The combination of these two pH-dependent events could easily account for the anion gap of $18\,mEq/L$. The gap is also affected by the serum albumin concentration, varying by $\sim 2.5\,mEq/L$ for each g/dL deviation from $4\,g/dL$ (see Chapter 28). In patients with severe Cl^--depletion metabolic alkalosis, the associated ECF volume depletion and hemoconcentration can increase albumin concentration, contributing to an increase in the anion gap. In this postoperative patient with underlying cancer, however, it is more likely that the serum albumin concentration is low.

5. Nasogastric suction leads to loss of HCl, which in turn induces metabolic alkalosis (see Chapter 17). In this instance, however, the expected secondary hypoventilation has been blocked by machine-controlled ventilation, which is set inappropriately high. Thus the complicating respiratory alkalosis is iatrogenic.

6. Resetting the ventilator (or increasing dead space) to increase $PaCO_2$ will correct the respiratory component in this mixed disorder. Intravenous NaCl will repair the Cl^- depletion and correct the metabolic component. If continued nasogastric suction is required, loss of HCl can be minimized by administering an H^+/K^+ ATPase inhibitor such as omeprazole.

CASE 3

A 64-year-old woman with a history of chronic asthma and hypertension has been vomiting for the past 5 days. Several members of her household have also been afflicted with the same symptoms. The patient uses inhalers for her respiratory problems, but the medications in the inhalers are unknown. In the emergency room, laboratory measurements were obtained (Table 3).

Table 3 Laboratory Measurements (Case 3)

Venous serum	
Creatinine	1.1 mg/dL
Urea nitrogen	22 mg/dL
Sodium	130 mEq/L
Potassium	3.2 mEq/L
Chloride	80 mEq/L
Total CO_2	35 mEq/L
Anion gap	15 mEq/L
Urine	
Sodium	15 mEq/L
Potassium	35 mEq/L
Chloride	6 mEq/L
Arterial blood	
pH	7.42
$[H^+]$	38 nEq/L
$PaCO_2$	55 mmHg
PaO_2	60 mmHg

Questions for Case 3

1. Are the acid–base data internally consistent?
2. Considering the patient's history and the acid–base data, what is the likely dominant acid–base disorder?
3. Is this a simple or mixed disorder?
4. What is the likely cause for this acid–base disorder, and how should it be treated?

Answers for Case 3

1. The acid–base data are consistent: $[HCO_3^-] = 24 \times 55/38 = 35$ mEq/L. The calculated $[HCO_3^-] =$ the measured [total CO_2].
2. Based on the history in this patient, the dominant disorder could either be metabolic alkalosis due to the vomiting or respiratory acidosis resulting from exacerbation of bronchial asthma. The laboratory data are also compatible with the dominant disorder being either metabolic alkalosis or respiratory acidosis; the $PaCO_2$ and the serum $[HCO_3^-]$ are both high, but blood pH is normal.
3. This is a mixed disorder. One can begin this analysis either from the perspective of metabolic alkalosis or respiratory acidosis. Starting with metabolic alkalosis, the expected ventilatory response to an increase in serum $[HCO_3^-]$ of 11 mEq/L (from a baseline of 24–35 mEq/L) is to increase $PaCO_2$ by $11 \times 0.7 = 8$ mmHg. Assuming a baseline $PaCO_2$ of 40 mmHg, the expected

$PaCO_2 = 40 + 8 = 48$ mmHg. This patient's $PaCO_2$ is 55 mmHg, more than 5 mmHg greater than expected, indicating that a respiratory acid–base disorder has caused an additional increment in $PaCO_2$. One obtains the same result if one begins the analysis with respiratory acidosis. In this case, one assesses whether the serum $[HCO_3^-]$ is increased as expected by body buffers for acute hypercapnia or by the kidney for chronic hypercapnia (see Chapter 20). One can immediately exclude uncomplicated acute respiratory acidosis in this case as the expected buffer response should increase serum $[HCO_3^-]$ by only 1 mEq/L above the normal value of 24 mEq/L. The rule for uncomplicated chronic respiratory acidosis is that serum $[HCO_3^-]$ should increase by 3 mEq/L for each 10 mmHg increment in $PaCO_2$ (see Table 2, Chapter 28). Using this rule, serum $[HCO_3^-]$ should rise by only $\sim$5 mEq/L in this patient, much less that the 11 mEq/L increment observed. Thus one reaches the same conclusion; a mixed metabolic alkalosis and respiratory acidosis is present.

4. Vomiting has caused a Cl^--depletion metabolic alkalosis (see Chapter 17), manifested by the very low urine $[Cl^-]$. The metabolic alkalosis is complicated in this patient, who either has chronic respiratory acidosis, or who has developed acute CO_2 retention due an exacerbation of her asthma. Because of the superimposed metabolic alkalosis, we cannot determine with certainty whether the respiratory acidosis is acute or chronic. Chloride repletion with KCl is recommended in this patient to avoid fluid overload, and the asthma should obviously also be treated with appropriate inhaler therapy.

CASE 4

A 28-year-old man, previously healthy, comes in with a 1–2 week history of polyuria and polydipsia that has progressed to lethargy and weakness in the last 1–2 days. On arrival in the ER, the patient is poorly responsive with obvious Kussmaul ventilation. His blood pressure is 90/50 mmHg. Initial laboratory measurements are shown in Table 4.

Questions for Case 4

1. Is this a simple or mixed disorder?
2. Is the change in anion gap (Δ anion gap) accounted for by the fall in serum $[HCO_3^-]$?
3. What is the likely cause for this acid–base disorder, and how should it be treated?
4. What has led to the lethargy and weakness?

Table 4 Laboratory Measurements (Case 4)

	Initial measurements	8 hr later
Venous serum		
Creatinine	4.5 mg/dL	1.3 mg/dL
Urea nitrogen	120 mg/dL	40 mg/dL
Sodium	127 mEq/L	138 mEq/L
Potassium	4 mEq/L	3.7 mEq/L
Chloride	88 mEq/L	118 mEq/L
Total CO_2	<5 mEq/L	10 mEq/L
Anion gap	>34 mEq/L	10 mEq/L
Glucose	1400 mg/dL	
Acetone	Positive 1:4 dilution	
Arterial blood		
pH	6.91	
$[H^+]$	123 nEq/L	
$PaCO_2$	8 mmHg	
PaO_2	130 mmHg	
$[HCO_3^-]$	1.6 mEq/L	

Answers for Case 4

1. The history and physical examination in this case, coupled with the very low arterial pH, serum $[HCO_3^-]$ and $PaCO_2$, indicate that the dominant acid–base disorder is metabolic acidosis. Assessment of the expected ventilatory response is complicated by the fact that with severe metabolic acidosis one cannot use the usual rule of thumb with confidence (Chapter 28, Table 2), as this rule is based on observations in patients with serum $[HCO_3^-]$ values >6 mEq/L. This patient's $PaCO_2$ is 8 mmHg, a near-maximal ventilatory response. Thus, his respiratory response can be deemed appropriate, and one can reasonably exclude any complicating respiratory acid–base disorder. Next, one must assess whether a preexisting metabolic alkalosis has complicated the acid–base picture. To evaluate for this possibility, the Δ anion gap is evaluated, as discussed below.

2. The anion gap ($[Na^+] - [Cl^-] + [HCO_3^-]$) calculated in this patient is 37 mEq/L. To assess whether this high value is completely accounted for by the fall in serum $[HCO_3^-]$, one estimates the rise in the anion gap that occurred during the development of acidosis (Δ anion gap, see Chapter 28). Assuming a baseline gap of 12 mEq/L, the value has risen by 37–12 or 25 mEq/L. If we assume that each mEq/L rise in the gap is due to the consumption of 1 mEq/L of HCO_3^-, then addition of the Δ anion gap to the

prevailing serum [HCO_3^-] should yield an estimate of serum [HCO_3^-] prior to the development of metabolic acidosis. In this case, $25 + 1.6 = 26.6\,mEq/L$, essentially a normal value. Even if one assumes a baseline anion gap of $10\,mEq/L$, due to the low pH, one still only gets a value for [HCO_3^-] of 28.6. As discussed in Chapter 28, the Δ anion gap calculation is based on several assumptions and must always be viewed as a loose estimate. As a general rule, one should not conclude that the preexisting serum [HCO_3^-] is high unless the calculated value is $>32\,mEq/L$. In this case, the Δ anion gap appears to fully account for the fall in [HCO_3^-] from a normal value, making it unlikely that a metabolic alkalosis preceded the metabolic acidosis.

3. This patient has severe, but uncomplicated metabolic acidosis due to diabetic ketoacidosis. Treatment should include ECF volume and K^+ repletion with intravenous saline and K^+, along with insulin to block further organic acid production. Despite severe acidosis, intravenous HCO_3^- is not necessary (although it was given in this case), as the patient has high concentrations of keto-anions in his blood, which will rapidly generate new HCO_3^- once adequate insulin is supplied (see Chapter 10).

4. The change in mental status is probably not caused by metabolic acidosis. The patient has severe hyperglycemia, leading to an increase in serum osmolality, which in turn causes an encephalo-pathy characterized by lethargy and weakness.

Follow-up Observations in Case 4

The patient was treated aggressively with intravenous isotonic saline, K^+, insulin, and was given $200\,mEq$ of $NaHCO_3$ as well. The results of repeat venous blood work 8 hr after initiating treatment are in Table 4.

Additional Questions for Case 4

1. What acid–base disorder is now present?
2. What accounts for the change in the anion gap in this patient?
3. What is the expected change in serum [HCO_3^-] for the amount of $NaHCO_3$ given?

Answers to Additional Questions for Case 4

1. Although we do not have complete information (arterial pH and $PaCO_2$ are missing), the patient now almost certainly has a meta-bolic acidosis with a normal anion gap. The acid–base data reflect a typical transition seen in the treatment of diabetic ketoacidosis (see Chapter 10).

2. Repletion of ECF volume with isotonic saline has led to the excretion of ketoanions before they can be metabolized to generate new HCO_3^- in the body fluids. These ketoanions have been replaced by Cl^- in the ECF, restoring the anion gap to normal. Loss of ketoanions in the urine limits the ability to increase serum $[HCO_3^-]$ through metabolism, resulting in a prolongation of the metabolic acidosis. Nonetheless this transition is essential for survival, as repletion of ECF volume with NaCl is a first priority, more important than rapid correction of metabolic acidosis.

3. To answer this question we need to know the patient's weight and the apparent space of distribution of administered HCO_3^-. Although the clinical rule of thumb dictates that this "space" is $\sim$50% of body weight, this fraction only applies when the serum $[HCO_3^-]$ is at or near-normal levels prior to HCO_3^- administration. As discussed in Chapters 6 and 28, the space of distribution (as a fraction of body weight) increases as serum $[HCO_3^-]$ falls, and is essentially equal to 100% of body weight when serum $[HCO_3^-]$ is very low. Assuming he weighs 70 kg, administration of 200 mEq should therefore have only increased serum $[HCO_3^-]$ by 200/70, or $\sim$3 mEq/L. This patient's serum $[HCO_3^-]$ however increased by a much larger amount, 8 mEq/L, indicating endogenous generation of new HCO_3^- from retained and metabolized ketoanions. In fact the rate of correction of the metabolic acidosis caused by uncontrolled diabetes is unaffected by HCO_3^- administration (see Chapter 10).

CASE 5

A 69-year-old man with a 3-day history of an upper respiratory infection and headache is found unresponsive in bed, with evidence that he had a seizure. He is brought to the ER and intubated on arrival. On examination he has no edema, his BP is 140/80 mmHg, and he is responsive only to painful stimuli. Laboratory measurements obtained after intubation are in Table 5.

Questions for Case 5

1. Is this a simple or mixed disorder?
2. Is the change in anion gap (Δ anion gap) accounted for by the fall in serum $[HCO_3^-]$?
3. What are the possible causes for this acid–base disorder?
4. What treatment is indicated for this disorder?

Table 5 Laboratory Measurements (Case 5)

Venous serum	
Creatinine	1.3 mg/dL
Sodium	143 mEq/L
Potassium	4.5 mEq/L
Chloride	94 mEq/L
Total CO_2	6 mEq/L
Anion gap	43 mEq/L
Arterial blood	
pH	6.90
$[H^+]$	126 nEq/L
$PaCO_2$	22 mmHg
PaO_2	450 mmHg on 100% FiO_2
$[HCO_3^-]$	4.2 mEq/L

Answers for Case 5

1. It is most likely a mixed disorder. The history here, including a seizure, and the acid–base data (low pH, $PaCO_2$, and $[HCO_3^-]$) indicate that metabolic acidosis is the dominant disorder. The expected ventilatory response to a reduction in serum $[HCO_3^-]$ from a baseline value of 24 mEq/L to 4 mEq/L is estimated using the rule of thumb for metabolic acidosis ($\Delta PaCO_2/\Delta[HCO_3^-]=1.2$, Chapter 28, Table 2). Using this rule: $PaCO_2 = 40 - 1.2 \times (24 - 4) = 16$ mmHg. As noted earlier, this rule is derived from observations in humans with lesser reductions in serum $[HCO_3^-]$ than in this case, but clinical observations suggest that the expected response to a metabolic acidosis of this severity would be to decrease $PaCO_2$ to at least 16 mmHg. This patient's $PaCO_2$ of 22 mmHg is therefore higher than expected, indicating an inadequate ventilatory response. The only caveat to this analysis is whether adequate time has elapsed since the patient's seizure to allow a steady-state ventilatory response.

2. No, the Δ anion gap is much larger than the estimated fall in $[HCO_3^-]$, suggesting the presence of a hidden metabolic alkalosis. In this case, the anion gap is 43 mEq/L, 31 mEq/L greater than the assumed baseline, 12 mEq/L (Δ anion gap = 31). Assuming that a 1 mEq/L increase in anion gap is equal to a 1 mEq/L fall in serum $[HCO_3^-]$ (see Chapter 28), the estimated serum $[HCO_3^-]$ prior to development of metabolic acidosis is obtained by adding the Δ anion gap to the prevailing serum $[HCO_3^-]$. In this case the calculation yields $31 + 4 = 35$ mEq/L. See Answer 2 to Case 4 and Chapter 28 for the limitations of this analysis. Thus, a mixed metabolic disorder—metabolic acidosis and metabolic

alkalosis—coexist along with respiratory acidosis making this a triple disorder. When the patient became more responsive, he was able to give a history of vomiting, supporting the diagnosis of metabolic alkalosis made by our anion gap calculation.

3. We cannot know for certain, but a likely scenario is that the patient developed nausea and persistent vomiting, causing a severe chloride-depletion metabolic alkalosis. This disorder then could have precipitated the seizure that caused both a lactic acidosis and obtundation, impairing the usual ventilatory response. He did not have diabetes mellitus.

4. The treatment for this individual should include intubation, because of the impaired ventilatory response (which was done appropriately on arrival to the ER), and intravenous isotonic saline to replete ECF volume and body chloride stores. Bicarbonate administration is not necessary in this patient, because he has large amounts of potential HCO_3^- precursors in the form of organic anions in his body. These anions will be rapidly metabolized, yielding new HCO_3^- once the underlying organic acidosis is treated. He had a presumed lactic acidosis (lactic acid levels were not measured), as he responded rapidly to saline administration.

CASE 6

A 36-year-old man is admitted to the hospital with a 2-week history of continuous nausea and vomiting. These symptoms followed a several week binge of heavy alcohol intake. He was brought to the hospital by friends, lethargic and poorly responsive. On examination he responds to vocal stimuli, BP is 160/80 mmHg, and he is afebrile; respiratory rate is 5/min. He is not jaundiced and has no liver enlargement, ascites or peripheral edema. Asterixis is present. Laboratory measurements are shown in Table 6.

Questions for Case 6

1. Considering the patient's history and laboratory data, what is the dominant acid–base disorder?
2. Is this a simple or mixed disorder?
3. What is the likely cause for this acid–base disorder, and how should it be treated?

Answers for Case 6

1. The history of vomiting and the acid–base data showing an elevated arterial pH, $PaCO_2$ and $[HCO_3^-]$ all point to metabolic alkalosis as the dominant disorder.

Table 6 Laboratory Measurements (Case 6)

Venous serum	
Creatinine	1.5 mg/dL
Urea nitrogen	34 mg/dL
Sodium	134 mEq/L
Potassium	2.2 mEq/L
Chloride	58 mEq/L
Total CO_2	55 mEq/L
Anion gap	21 mEq/L
Arterial blood	
pH	7.54
$[H^+]$	29 nEq/L
$PaCO_2$	70 mmHg
PaO_2	63 mmHg on 1.5 L/min nasal O_2
$[HCO_3^-]$	58 mEq/L

2. To assess whether this is a mixed disorder, the first step is to determine whether the ventilatory response is appropriate. Unfortunately, for this severe a metabolic alkalosis (serum $[HCO_3^-]$ = 58 mEq/L), the rule of thumb for estimating the expected $PaCO_2$ is based only on isolated clinical observations. Nonetheless, the relationship $\Delta PaCO_2/\Delta[HCO_3^-] = 0.7$ appears to hold. Using this ratio in this case, the expected $PaCO_2 = 40 + 0.7 \times (58 - 24) = 64$ mmHg. The patient's $PaCO_2$ is 6 mmHg higher than that, 70 mmHg, suggesting a superimposed respiratory acidosis. Certainly, his obtundation or the severe hypokalemia could have contributed to an impaired respiratory response. In this case, treatment of the metabolic alkalosis alone led to a return of the patient's $PaCO_2$ to normal, without the need for ventilatory assistance. The next step is to evaluate the anion gap, in this case, 21 mEq/L. Given this value, one cannot exclude with certainty the simultaneous presence of an organic acidosis, but recall that the anion gap is increased in severe metabolic alkalosis due to an increase in serum albumin concentration coupled with pH effects on its net anionic charge. In this case, the patient most likely has a simple (but severe) metabolic alkalosis.

3. When the serum $[HCO_3^-]$ is >50 mEq/L, essentially the only cause is vomiting or nasogastric suction, causing Cl^- depletion metabolic alkalosis. The treatment is isotonic saline administration coupled with vigorous K^+ repletion, both of which this patient received.

CASE 7

A 54-year-old woman with known cirrhosis is admitted to the hospital with confusion, ascites and jaundice. On examination she is alert but only oriented to person, BP = 90/50 mmHg. She is afebrile with obvious jaundice and ascites, but no peripheral edema. She has asterixis. Laboratory results are in Table 7.

Questions for Case 7

1. Considering the history and laboratory data, what is the likely dominant acid–base disorder?
2. Is this a simple or mixed disorder?
3. What is the likely cause for this acid–base disorder, and how should it be treated?

Answers for Case 7

1. The patient has hepatic cirrhosis, a disorder associated both with respiratory alkalosis and metabolic acidosis. Her confused state makes it likely that respiratory alkalosis is dominant here, and the acid–base data showing a low $PaCO_2$ and serum $[HCO_3^-]$ with an arterial pH > 7.40 support this conclusion.
2. To answer this question, one must decide whether the serum $[HCO_3^-]$ is in the expected range for the degree of hypocapnia present. This question has two components because respiratory alkalosis has an acute form, characterized by a fall in serum $[HCO_3^-]$ due to titration by nonbicarbonate buffers, and a chronic

Table 7   Laboratory Measurements (Case 7)

Venous serum	
Creatinine	0.7 mg/dL
Urea nitrogen	15 mg/dL
Albumin	3 g/dL
Sodium	124 mEq/L
Potassium	3.2 mEq/L
Chloride	92 mEq/L
Total CO_2	16 mEq/L
Anion gap	16 mEq/L
Arterial blood	
pH	7.44
$[H^+]$	36 nEq/L
$PaCO_2$	24 mmHg
PaO_2	75 mmHg
$[HCO_3^-]$	16 mEq/L

form, characterized by a change in renal HCO_3^- handling (see Chapter 21). With acute respiratory alkalosis, the expected buffer response should reduce serum $[HCO_3^-]$ by 2 mEq/L for every 10 mmHg fall in $PaCO_2$. With chronic respiratory alkalosis, the renal response reduces serum $[HCO_3^-]$ by 4 mEq/L for the same reduction in $PaCO_2$. In this patient, $PaCO_2$ has fallen by 16 mmHg (assuming a baseline value of 40 mmHg). The expected serum $[HCO_3^-]$ in uncomplicated acute respiratory alkalosis of this degree $= 24 - (16 \times 0.2) = 21$ mEq/L, a much higher value than in our patient. For chronic respiratory alkalosis, the expected serum $[HCO_3^-]$ $= 24 - (16 \times 0.4) = 18$ mEq/L, much closer to the observed value of 16 mEq/L. Recall that by "chronic", we mean persisting for >72 hr. Thus the data are most consistent with an uncomplicated chronic respiratory alkalosis. One cannot exclude, however, a complicating metabolic acidosis (e.g., due to alcoholic ketoacidosis). The anion gap is not helpful in this regard, as it increases by ~3 mEq/L in chronic respiratory alkalosis.

3. Hepatic encephalopathy causes hyperventilation, although the mechanism is not fully understood. No specific treatment is required for the respiratory alkalosis. Treatment of the hepatic encephalopathy should reduce ventilatory rate and correct the respiratory alkalosis, and it did in this patient.

CASE 8

A 45-year-old man with end-stage renal disease and type 1 diabetes mellitus, receiving regular hemodialysis, is admitted to the hospital with confusion and lethargy. He enters the hospital on the morning after his last hemodialysis. Admission laboratory results are in Table 8. A diagnostic evaluation for mental status changes was undertaken and yielded negative blood cultures, negative CT of the head and abdomen (without contrast), and normal liver function tests save for a serum albumin of 2.8 g/dL. On the following day, the patient received his usual hemodialysis treatment. Immediately after dialysis, he became more lethargic and was noted to have a respiratory rate of 30/min. Laboratory measurements 2 hr after completing dialysis are in Table 8.

Questions for Case 8

1. Are the acid–base data internally consistent?
2. What is the reason for the increase in serum [total CO_2] between the two blood samples?

Table 8 Laboratory Measurements (Case 8)

	Admission results	2 hr after hemodialysis
Venous serum		
Creatinine	7.2 mg/dL	4.3 mg/dL
Urea nitrogen	55 mg/dL	22 mg/dL
Sodium	142 mEq/L	140 mEq/L
Potassium	4.5 mEq/L	3.5 mEq/L
Chloride	102 mEq/L	98 mEq/L
Total CO_2	24 mEq/L	30 mEq/L
Anion gap	16 mEq/L	12 mEq/L
Arterial blood		
pH		7.90
$[H^+]$		13 mEq/L
$PaCO_2$		15 mmHg
PaO_2		105 mmHg
$[HCO_3^-]$		28 mEq/L

4. Considering the history and acid–base data, what is the dominant acid–base disorder?
5. Is this a simple or mixed disorder?
6. What management problem does this acid–base disorder entail?

Answers for Case 8

1. This amazing set of arterial acid–base values is indeed consistent with the venous values, and occurred in one of our dialysis patients. The serum $[HCO_3^-]$ calculated from arterial pH and $PaCO_2$, 28 mEq/L, is almost identical to the venous [total CO_2], 30 mEq/L.

2. Between the two blood samples, the patient received hemodialysis, a therapy designed to deliver HCO_3^- to the patient (see Chapter 23). As a result serum [total CO_2] increased from 24 to 30 mEq/L, as expected. This dialysis-induced increment is dependent only on the predialysis serum $[HCO_3^-]$ and the alkali content of the dialysate. It is affected little if at all by respiratory acid–base perturbations.

3. The history here, save for confusion, provides little help in guessing at the acid base disorder, but the blood gases obtained after hemodialysis demonstrate extreme alkalemia in association with hypocapnia, indicating that respiratory alkalosis is the dominant disorder. Respiratory alkalosis was probably present before the dialysis treatment, and likely accounted for the patient's confused state on admission. The unusual finding in this case, however, is

the high serum [HCO$_3^-$]. In dialysis patients, there are rarely any hints from blood chemistries that a respiratory alkalosis is present. There is no renal adaptation (see Chapters 23 and 24). In the face of severe hypocapnia, the dialysis-determined serum [HCO$_3^-$] has caused severe alkalemia.

4. Using the normal rules for assessing acid–base disorders, this is a mixed metabolic and respiratory alkalosis, with the metabolic alkalosis caused by the hemodialysis treatment. However, one could regard this as a simple respiratory alkalosis in a patient with serum [HCO$_3^-$] set by his dialysis therapy. From an operational point of view, one faces the task of trying to increase his PaCO$_2$ and/or decreasing serum [HCO$_3^-$] (see next answer).

5. This is a difficult management problem because the patient needs dialysis but also needs his serum [HCO$_3^-$] decreased if the hyperventilation cannot be stopped. The standard dialysis bath [HCO$_3^-$] is high because it is designed to deliver HCO$_3^-$ to the patient. In order to lower serum [HCO$_3^-$], therefore, one must reduce the [HCO$_3^-$] in the dialysis bath solution. With current dialysis technology, this intervention is relatively simple but is rarely undertaken because the respiratory alkalosis is usually not recognized. In this case, urgent attention was directed at trying to uncover the cause of the hyperventilation and to correct it. No cause was found, and the patient expired within 2 days.

CASE 9

A 60-year-old man is admitted to the hospital with somnolence and confusion following a flu-like syndrome and production of purulent sputum. He is known to have severe chronic obstructive lung disease, with a baseline PaCO$_2$ of ~60 mmHg and serum [HCO$_3^-$] of ~30 mEq/L. On examination, the patient has myoclonic jerking and asterixis. He is afebrile, BP 170/95 mmHg, and he has clubbing, peripheral cyanosis and edema. Laboratory data obtained after oxygen administration are in Table 9.

Questions for Case 9

1. Considering the history and laboratory data, what acid–base disorder is present?
2. Is it a simple or mixed disturbance?
3. What is the nature of the adaptive response in this acid–base disorder?
4. What treatment is indicated?

Table 9   Laboratory Measurements (Case 9)

Arterial blood	
pH	7.22
$[H^+]$	60 nEq/L
$PaCO_2$	80 mmHg
PaO_2	75 mmHg
$[HCO_3^-]$	32 mEq/L
Venous serum	
Sodium	141 mEq/L
Potassium	4.3 mEq/L
Chloride	97 mEq/L
Total CO_2	35 mEq/L
Anion gap	9 mEq/L

Answers for Case 9

1. The patient is known to have chronic respiratory acidosis, and now has a high $PaCO_2$ and serum $[HCO_3^-]$ with a low blood pH, all indicating that respiratory acidosis is present.

2. A mixed disorder, acute respiratory acidosis superimposed on chronic respiratory acidosis. This diagnosis is based on history as well as the acid–base data. We know that the patient has a chronically elevated $PaCO_2$ with a serum $[HCO_3^-]$ around 30 mEq/L, numbers consistent with an uncomplicated chronic respiratory acidosis (see Chapters 20 and 28). On admission, however, $PaCO_2$ is markedly higher, 80 mmHg, while serum $[HCO_3^-]$ is only very slightly increased at 32 mEq/L. The small increase in $[HCO_3^-]$ is consistent with the acute response to an increase in $PaCO_2$, as this response is confined to titration of nonbicarbonate body buffers, a process that generates little new HCO_3^-. Given the history and these findings, the above mixed disorder is most likely. One should note, however, that other possibilities cannot be excluded. For example, the patient may have developed a chronic increase in $PaCO_2$ (>72 hr in duration) to 80 mmHg. Testing for this possibility using the rule of thumb (see Table 2 in Chapter 28), serum $[HCO_3^-]$ should increase to 36–38 mEq/L, a value not that different from venous [total CO_2], 35 mEq/L. A likely possibility is that the patient is in a transition between the acute and chronic response to this elevation in $PaCO_2$. A complicating metabolic acidosis (acting to reducing serum $[HCO_3^-]$) is unlikely given the normal anion gap.

3. As indicated above, the adaptive response to an acute increase in $PaCO_2$ is generation of new HCO_3^- by titration of non-HCO_3^-

buffers. The major buffer available for this response is hemo-globin, which binds H^+ in a pH-dependent manner. Other buffers contribute as well, but the net effect of all these buffer events is to increase serum $[HCO_3^-]$ by only 1 mEq/L for each 10 mmHg increase in $PaCO_2$. By contrast, the response to a sustained increase in $PaCO_2$ involves a transient increase in renal acid excretion, generating new HCO_3^-, and a sustained increase in renal HCO_3^- reabsorption, maintaining the resultant increase in serum $[HCO_3^-]$ (see Chapter 20).

4. Treatment should obviously be directed at improving the patient's ventilation. Such treatment might reasonably include ventilatory assistance, but in this case, the patient was managed without this intervention, using inhalers and antibiotics. With treatment, the patient's $PaCO_2$ returned to its baseline value of 60 mmHg.

CASE 10

A 45-year-old man is admitted to the hospital after returning from a visit to Central America, where he developed severe diarrhea . He attempted to control the symptoms but did not seek medical care. His stools continued at a rate of 20–30/day. After several days, he returned home and headed to the nearest emergency room. On examination he appeared obviously volume depleted with a BP of 90/60 mmHg supine, unobtainable on standing. He was afebrile, pulse rate, 120/min, respiratory rate, 24/min. Laboratory data are in Table 10.

Questions for Case 10

1. Considering the history and laboratory data, what acid–base disorder is present?
2. Is it a simple or mixed disorder?
3. What treatment is indicated?

Answers for Case 10

1. Given the history of severe diarrhea and the acid–base findings (low arterial pH, $PaCO_2$ and $[HCO_3^-]$), metabolic acidosis is the dominant disorder.
2. This is an uncomplicated metabolic acidosis. The expected $PaCO_2$ for a serum $[HCO_3^-]$ of 11 mEq/L is 24 mmHg, virtually identical to the observed value. The anion gap is normal, and therefore there are no Δ anion gap issues.
3. This is a hyperchloremic metabolic acidosis, presumably due to selective HCO_3^- losses from diarrhea (see Chapters 9 and 15).

Table 10   Laboratory Measurements (Case 10)

	Initial measurements	After treatment
Venous serum		
Creatinine	2.5 mg/dL	1.3 mg/dL
Urea nitrogen	50 mg/dL	15 mg/dL
Sodium	133 mEq/L	140 mEq/L
Potassium	3.2 mEq/L	3.3 mEq/L
Chloride	110 mEq/L	112 mEq/L
Total CO_2	13 mEq/L	20 mEq/L
Anion gap	10 mEq/L	8 mEq/L
Arterial blood		
pH	7.26	7.35
$[H^+]$	55 nEq/L	45 nEq/L
$PaCO_2$	25 mmHg	34 mmHg
PaO_2	95 mmHg	98 mmHg
$[HCO_3^-]$	11 mEq/L	18 mEq/L

The anion gap is normal in this case, indicating that there are no significant HCO_3^- precursors in the circulation. In this setting, exogenous alkali is necessary to assist in correction of the acidosis. Because NaCl is lost as well as alkali, replacement fluid should include both NaCl and $NaHCO_3$.

Follow-up Observations in Case 10

The patient was treated with intravenous isotonic saline and K^+ replacement, and was also given 200 mEq of $NaHCO_3$ intravenously. He weighs 60 kg. Laboratory measurements obtained after treatment are shown in Table 10.

Additional Questions for Case 10

1. Is the change in serum $[HCO_3^-]$ in the range expected after HCO_3^- administration in this patient?
2. What acid–base disorder is present?

Answers to Additional Questions for Case 10

1. To answer this question, one must assess the "space of distribution" of the administered HCO_3^-, i.e., the extent to which it remained in the extracellular fluid and the extent which it was consumed in buffering endogenous acids. The patient weighs 60 kg and received 200 mEq of HCO_3^- intravenously. After treatment,

serum [HCO_3^-] increased by 7 meq/L, from 11 to 18 meq/L. From this information, we can calculate the space of distribution by dividing the total amount of HCO_3^- given by the Δ serum [HCO_3^-] (see Chapter 6). Dividing 200 meq by 7 meq/L = 29 L, a value equal to 48% of his body weight. This estimate is close to the expected space (50–60% when one starts from a serum [HCO_3^-] of 11 meq/L), indicating that the increase in serum [HCO_3^-] can be accounted for by the treatment. Moreover, it suggests that no additional HCO_3^- was either lost in the stool or urine, and that none was generated by endogenous alkali precursors.

2. The patient still has a mild metabolic acidosis, with $PaCO_2$ in the expected range for the serum [HCO_3^-]. In some patients with severe metabolic acidosis, rapid correction can be associated with persistent hypocapnia, presumed to be due to a transient disequilibrium between extracellular pH and the pH in the cerebrospinal fluid bathing the cells regulating ventilation. In this patient such a complication was prevented by only partially correcting the low serum [HCO_3^-]. Over time the patient gradually returned to normal acid–base balance.

CASE 11

A 35-year-old woman is brought to the emergency room in a comatose state. According to her sister, she had been complaining of progressive weakness for 2 months. On examination, the patient was responsive only to painful stimuli, blood pressure was 110/70 and respiratory rate was 10 and shallow; she had no peripheral edema. The deep tendon reflexes were absent; muscle strength was not testable. Initial laboratory measurements are shown in Table 11.

Questions for Case 11

1. Considering the history and laboratory data, what acid–base disturbance is present?
2. What is the most likely underlying diagnosis?
3. Why is the respiratory response lacking?

Answers for Case 11

1. This is a mixed metabolic and respiratory acidosis. The history is not revealing, but the absence of Kussmaul ventilation on exam is striking. Given the low pH and serum [HCO_3^-], metabolic acidosis is certainly the dominant disorder. However, one is struck

Table 11 Laboratory Measurements (Case 11)

Venous serum	
Creatinine	0.9 mg/dL
Sodium	135 mEq/L
Potassium	1.5 mEq/L
Chloride	118 mEq/L
Total CO$_2$	7 mEq/L
Anion gap	10 mEq/L
Urine	
Specific gravity	1.010
pH	6.5
Protein	1+
Sodium	50 mEq/L
Potassium	10 mEq/L
Chloride	52 mEq/L
Arterial blood	
pH	6.88
[H$^+$]	132 nEq/L
PaCO$_2$	40 mmHg
PaO$_2$	95 mmHg
[HCO$_3^-$]	7 mEq/L

mmediately by the PaCO$_2$ of 40 mmHg, a value distinctly abnormal for this severe acidosis. In response to this degree of metabolic acidosis, the expected PaCO$_2$ should be: $40 - 1.2 \times (24 - 7)$, or 23 mmHg. Thus two acid–base disorders are present, respiratory and metabolic acidosis, both of which require immediate attention.

2. The acid–base and electrolyte abnormalities in this patient suggest the presence of type 1 renal tubular acidosis (RTA). This diagnosis is suggested by the following constellation of findings: (i) metabolic acidosis with a normal anion gap, (ii) a urine pH of 6.5 in the face of severe acidosis, and (iii) associated severe hypokalemia. The diagnosis is further supported by calculation of the urinary anion gap (see Chapters 13 and 28). In response to metabolic acidosis, the kidney normally increases NH$_4^+$ excretion, adding increased amounts of this unmeasured cation to the urine. Thus, if metabolic acidosis were due, for example, to diarrhea, the sum ([Na$^+$] + [K$^+$] − [Cl$^-$]) should yield a negative value, reflecting the presence of large amounts the unmeasured cation, NH$_4^+$, counterbalancing [Cl$^-$] in the urine. In this case, however, [Na$^+$] + [K$^+$] is greater than [Cl$^-$], yielding a urine anion gap of +8, indicating an abnormal renal response. This result is typically found in patients with type 1 RTA (see Chapter 13).

3. The severe hypokalemia in this otherwise healthy young woman has caused respiratory muscle weakness, leading to an impaired respiratory response to metabolic acidosis. In this case, the diagnosis was known, and K^+ was rapidly administered intravenously (in addition to HCO_3^-). Almost immediately after receiving K^+ the patient developed characteristic Kussmaul ventilation with marked improvement in her blood pH and increased responsiveness. Intubation was not necessary.

CASE 12

A 40-year-old man is seen in a clinic with a history of renal failure as a teenager from glomerulonephritis . He received a kidney transplant from his father 22 years ago. The graft worked well for 17 years, but over the last 5 years he has developed progressive renal insufficiency due to chronic transplant nephropathy. His only medications are prednisone and azathiaprine. He is asymptomatic and working full time. His BP is130/70 and has no peripheral edema. Laboratory data are in Table 12.

Questions for Case 12

1. Considering the history and laboratory data, what is the most likely acid–base disturbance in this patient?
2. What additional information is needed to confirm the diagnosis?
3. How would you manage this acid–base disorder?

Answers for Case 12

1. Metabolic acidosis. The finding of a low venous [total CO_2] in a patient with chronic renal insufficiency, who is otherwise well,

Table 12 Laboratory Measurements (Case 12)

Venous serum	
Creatinine	3.2 mg/dL
Sodium	143 mEq/L
Potassium	5.2 mEq/L
Chloride	115 mEq/L
Total CO_2	16 mEq/L
Anion gap	12 mEq/L
Urine	
Specific gravity	1.010
pH	5.0
Protein	1+

most commonly indicates the presence of metabolic acidosis due to impaired acid excretion (see Chapter 14).

2. To confirm this diagnosis and assure there are no other superimposed acid–base disorders requires arterial blood measurements of pH and $PaCO_2$. Such testing is not routinely done in asymptomatic stable patients with chronic renal insufficiency, however, and it was not done in this patient. The findings of a normal anion gap and hyperkalemia, coupled with the low [total CO_2] and elevated serum creatinine concentration make the diagnosis of type 4 RTA very likely, and this is supported by the acid urine (pH = 5.0).

3. Patients with type 4 RTA have impaired ability to excrete the endogenous acids produced each day, and as a result can develop bone disease and have increased muscle catabolism. These effects can be reversed by adding a daily oral HCO_3^- supplement in sufficient amount to increase serum $[HCO_3^-]$ to normal levels. Supplemental HCO_3^- (or a HCO_3^- precursor such as acetate or citrate) should be given at 30–60 mEq/day in divided doses. Although beneficial, the therapy is often poorly tolerated and in some patients is ineffective because of renal HCO_3^- wasting.

CASE 13

A 54-year-old man with a known history of alcohol abuse is brought to the emergency room by friends, confused and disoriented. According to his friends, he was drinking heavily until about 1 week ago when he developed nausea and vomiting. He has been unable to keep anything down for the last several days. On examination, the patient is oriented only to person. His BP is 90/50 mmHg. He is afebrile with a respiratory rate of 22/min, has asterixis and no ascites or edema. Laboratory measurements are in Table 13.

Questions for Case 13

1. Considering the history and laboratory data, what is the most likely dominant acid–base disturbance in this patient?
2. Are there coexistent acid–base disorders?
3. What treatment is indicated?

Answers for Case 13

1. Although the history and physical exam are suggestive of a Cl^--depletion metabolic alkalosis from vomiting, the high arterial pH and low $PaCO_2$ and serum $[HCO_3^-]$ indicate that respiratory alkalosis the dominant disorder at this time.

Table 13 Laboratory Measurements (Case 13)

Venous serum	
Creatinine	0.9 mg/dL
Sodium	129 mEq/L
Potassium	2.9 mEq/L
Chloride	78 mEq/L
Total CO_2	19 mEq/L
Anion gap	32 mEq/L
Arterial blood	
pH	7.50
$[H^+]$	32 nEq/L
$PaCO_2$	24 mmHg
PaO_2	95 mmHg
$[HCO_3^-]$	18 mEq/L

2. The first step in this determination is to evaluate whether the expected secondary renal response to respiratory alkalosis has occurred. For a sustained reduction in $PaCO_2$ to 24 mmHg, serum $[HCO_3^-]$ in the chronic steady-state should be: $24 - (16 \times 0.4) = 18$ mEq/L (see Chapter 28, Table 2), identical to the observed value in arterial blood. Thus this analysis is seemingly consistent with an uncomplicated chronic respiratory alkalosis. However, this conclusion does not fit with the historical data, nor with the very high anion gap, 32 mEq/L. The high anion gap indicates that an organic acidosis is present and, when one calculates and adds the Δ anion gap to the prevailing serum $[HCO_3^-]$, one gets $18 + (32 - 12) = 38$ mEq/L (see above, Case 2, Answer 4, and Chapter 28). This computation indicates that the initial disorder was indeed metabolic alkalosis (serum $[HCO_3^-] \sim 38$ mEq/L), presumably from vomiting, which was then complicated by an organic acidosis. If this analysis is correct, the urine $[Cl^-]$ should be low (< 20 mEq/L), reflecting the pathogenesis of metabolic alkalosis due to vomiting-induced loss of hydrochloric acid. The respiratory alkalosis most likely developed as the final complication. The serum $[HCO_3^-]$ at the time the patient was seen thus is the fortuitous result of this acid–base history, and has nothing to do with the response to respiratory alkalosis. In this setting, we cannot even deduce whether the respiratory disorder is acute or sustained. Only the history can help us in that regard. This is a triple disturbance, metabolic alkalosis and acidosis, and respiratory alkalosis.

3. Treatment with isotonic NaCl, in addition to repletion of body K^+ stores, should correct both metabolic acid–base disorders,

assuming the organic acidosis was a lactic acidosis. The organic acidosis could also be due alcoholic ketoacidosis, which would be manifested by positive serum ketone levels. If so, intravenous glucose is indicated as well to reverse the acidosis. If the respiratory alkalosis was caused by the underlying disease, this acid–base disorder should correct with this treatment as well. One should be alert to other more life-threatening causes, however, such as sepsis or a pulmonary embolism (see Chapter 21). In this patient saline administration, with added K^+, was all that was needed to correct all the acid–base disturbances.

CASE 14

You are asked to see a 39-year-old man with hypertension and hypokalemia. He has a strong family history of hypertension. The patient is asymptomatic, specifically denying diarrhea, vomiting, or recent diuretic use. On examination, the only abnormality is a BP of 155/95. Laboratory measurements are in Table 14 .

Questions for Case 14

1. Considering the history and laboratory data, what is the most likely acid–base disturbance in this patient?
2. What is the likely cause for this disorder?
3. What is the recommended treatment?

Answers for Case 14

1. The history is unhelpful in this case, but the most likely acid–base disorder is metabolic alkalosis. An elevated serum [total CO_2] coupled with a low serum [K^+] is most commonly indicative of metabolic alkalosis (see Chapter 16). Measurement of arterial pH and $PaCO_2$ is necessary to confirm the diagnosis, but in this asymptomatic patient is not indicated.
2. The absence of a history of vomiting, nasogastric suction or diuretic use, coupled with the presence of hypertension and the finding of more than adequate amounts of Cl^- in the urine, raise the possibility of primary hyperaldosteronism in this patient, the most common cause of Cl^--resistant metabolic alkalosis. This diagnosis was pursued appropriately, but surprisingly both the renin and aldosterone levels are very low. The strong family history of early-onset hypertension then led to a search for a genetic cause for these findings. The patient was found to have Liddle syndrome (see Chapter 18).

Table 14 Laboratory Measurements (Case 14)

Venous serum	
Creatinine	0.9 mg/dL
Sodium	143 mEq/L
Potassium	2.9 mEq/L
Chloride	100 mEq/L
Total CO_2	33 mEq/L
Anion gap	10 mEq/L
Renin activity	0.05 ng/mL/min
Aldosterone	1 ng/mL
Urine	
Specific gravity	1.010
pH	5.0
Protein	Negative
Sodium	45 mEq/L
Potassium	25 mEq/L
Chloride	80 mEq/L

3. Liddle syndrome is caused by a genetic defect that prevents down-regulation of the epithelial Na^+ channel, ENaC, in the collecting duct, mimicking hyperaldosteronism. Because of the sustained high activity of ENaC in this disorder, Na^+ reabsorption in the collecting duct is increased, promoting excess K^+ and H^+ secretion, and resulting in ECF volume expansion and hypertension, as well as hypokalemia and metabolic alkalosis. As a result of the volume expansion, both renin and aldosterone levels are suppressed to very low levels. The syndrome responds to amiloride, a drug which, in low dosage, specifically inhibits ENaC. This drug blocks the channel and thereby prevents the excess Na^+ reabsorption that causes the hypertension, hypokalemia and metabolic alkalosis.

CASE 15

A 38-year-old woman with end-stage renal disease due to glomerulonephritis is receiving hemodialysis therapy. She has a distant history of bulimia, but denies any recent vomiting. The results of routine monthly labs obtained just before dialysis (through an arteriovenous fistula) 2 months ago are shown in Table 15. Her predialysis weight was 47 kg then. Today you notice that her weight has dropped to 42 kg. She is asymptomatic and has no complaints. In fact she appears quite healthy and her serum albumin has increased from 3.9 to 4.8 g/dL. Blood pressure predialysis is 120/80,

Table 15 Laboratory Measurements (Case 15)

Predialysis values	2 months ago	Now
Urea nitrogen	85 mg/dL	60 mg/dL
Sodium	135 mEq/L	130 mEq/L
Potassium	4.5 mEq/L	4.2 mEq/L
Chloride	98 mEq/L	78 mEq/L
Total CO$_2$	18 mEq/L	27 mEq/L
Anion gap	19 mEq/L	25 mEq/L

unchanged from 2 months ago. Her current predialysis laboratory measurements are also in Table 15.

Questions for Case 15

1. What acid–base disorder was present 2 months ago?
2. Considering the history and laboratory data, what, if any, acid–base disorder is present now?
3. What is the likely cause for the increase in serum [total CO$_2$] in the second set of data? What accounts for the increase in anion gap?

Answers for Case 15

1. The initial acid–base data are consistent with a metabolic acidosis with an increased anion gap. Such findings are common in patients receiving hemodialysis three times weekly (see Chapter 23), and relate to the intermittent nature of the therapy, the rate of endogenous acid production and the bath [HCO$_3^-$]. The [total CO$_2$] of 18 mEq/L is lower than the expected value of 20–21 mEq/L, and probably reflects a high rate of endogenous acid production in this active young woman. Efforts should be made to find the specific cause and to increase serum [total CO$_2$] by appropriate intervention (see Chapters 23 and 24).
2. At first glance, the patient appears to have completely corrected the metabolic acidosis, with her serum [total CO$_2$] now increased to a "normal" value, 27 mEq/L. However, this 9 mEq/L increase occurred without any therapeutic intervention and is accompanied by an increase in anion gap from 19 to 25 mEq/L and a 5-kg weight loss. Given these data, one can be confident that a metabolic alkalosis is present.
3. The metabolic alkalosis is likely due to renewed bulimia. Note that in patients with end-stage renal disease, one does not need to determine whether this disorder is Cl$^-$-responsive or not. In

the absence of kidney function, metabolic alkalosis, once generated, will be sustained by the dialysis treatment, which exposes the patient to a bath $[HCO_3^-]$ of 35 mEq/L on a regular basis. The increase in anion gap is likely due to the increase in serum albumin concentration and the accompanying change in pH (not measured). The patient eventually admitted to renewed vomiting, and received counseling which resolved the problem. She now has a functioning kidney transplant with normal electrolytes.

CASE 16

You are asked to see a 40-year-old woman with a 1–2 year history of weakness and associated hypokalemia. The weakness has recently been severe enough to keep her home from work on many occasions. She denies diarrhea, vomiting, or diuretic usage. She has been treated with oral K^+ supplements, without notable improvement in her symptoms. On physical exam, her BP is 110/75 falling to 100/65 on standing, without symptoms. She has difficulty rising from the seated position. The remainder of the examination is unremarkable. Laboratory results are in Table 16.

Questions for Case 16

1. Considering the history and laboratory data, what is the most likely acid–base disturbance in this patient?
2. What are the possible causes of this acid–base disorder?
3. What further tests should be obtained?
4. What treatment would you recommend?

Answers for Case 16

1. Metabolic alkalosis. The history is not helpful in this case. As indicated earlier (see Case 14), an elevated serum [total CO_2] coupled with a low serum $[K^+]$ is most commonly the result of metabolic alkalosis (see Chapter 16). Measurement of arterial pH and $PaCO_2$ is necessary to confirm the diagnosis, but is not indicated in this patient.
2. The finding of a high urine $[Cl^-]$ (Table 16) suggests the presence of a Cl^--resistant metabolic alkalosis, with the caveat that surreptitious diuretic use can produce a high urine $[Cl^-]$ even in the face of Cl^- depletion. The normal blood pressure is an important finding that distinguishes this patient from Case 14, and also from the more common causes of Cl^--resistant metabolic alkalosis. In this normotensive patient the possible causes include laxative abuse,

Table 16   Laboratory Measurements (Case 16)

Venous serum	
Creatinine	0.7 mg/dL
Sodium	139 mEq/L
Potassium	2.1 mEq/L
Chloride	100 mEq/L
Total CO_2	33 mEq/L
Anion gap	10 mEq/L
Urine	
Specific gravity	1.010
pH	5.0
Protein	Negative
Sodium	45 mEq/L
Potassium	25 mEq/L
Chloride	80 mEq/L

surreptitious vomiting, diuretic abuse, and Bartter and Gitelman syndromes. Laxative abuse is possible but unlikely as a serum $[HCO_3^-]$ this high is relatively uncommon. Surreptitious vomiting is also unlikely given the lack of significant postural hypotension and the high urine $[Cl^-]$. Bartter syndrome is a hereditary disorder caused by several genetic mutations that impair the function of the $Na^+/K^+/2Cl^-$ cotransporter in the ascending limb of Henle's loop (see Chapters 18 and 25). However, this disorder is almost always diagnosed at a very young age and is usually associated with severe volume depletion. Thus, a realistic differential diagnosis is limited to diuretic abuse or Gitelman syndrome. Gitelman syndrome is also a hereditary genetic disorder caused by one of several mutations that inactivate the thiazide-sensitive Na^+/Cl^- cotransporter in the early distal tubule (see Chapters 18 and 25). Thus, this hereditary disease mimics the effect of chronic thiazide diuretic use, promoting K^+ secretion in the collecting duct and producing metabolic alkalosis.

3. The only way to differentiate these two diagnoses is to obtain a urine screen for diuretics. In this case, the screen was negative. A characteristic feature of Gitelman syndrome that separates it from Bartter syndrome is hypocalciuria. In this case, the 24-hr urine calcium excretion was low (39 mg), supporting the diagnosis of Gitelman syndrome. Her age at presentation is also characteristic, but no family history could be elucidated.

4. There is no ideal treatment for this disorder. Along with K^+ supplementation, amiloride or triamterene can help blunt the renal K^+ losses causing both the metabolic alkalosis and her symptoms.

CASE 17

A 29-year-old man is brought to the emergency room by his family because of unresponsiveness. According to the family, the patient has a history of alcohol abuse and of suicide attempts. On examination, the patient is responsive only to painful stimuli. His BP is 110/80, he is afebrile and his respiratory rate is 24/min and labored. The remainder of the exam is unremarkable. Laboratory measurements are in Table 17.

Questions for Case 17

1. Considering the history and laboratory data, what is the dominant acid–base disorder?
2. Is this a simple or mixed disorder?
3. What is the likely cause of this disorder?
4. How should this disorder be treated?

Answers for Case 17

1. Metabolic acidosis. The history, the labored breathing on physical examination and the low arterial pH, $PaCO_2$, and serum $[HCO_3^-]$ all suggest this disorder.
2. The acid–base data are consistent with an uncomplicated metabolic acidosis. The expected ventilatory response to a primary reduction in serum $[HCO_3^-]$ from a baseline value of $24\,mEq/L$ to $8\,mEq/L$ is: $PaCO_2 = 40 - 1.2 \times 16 = 21\,mmHg$. Although lower than the observed $PaCO_2$, $25\,mmHg$, the difference is

Table 17 Laboratory Measurements (Case 17)

Venous serum	
Creatinine	$1.2\,mg/dL$
Urea nitrogen	$30\,mg/dL$
Sodium	$148\,mEq/L$
Potassium	$4.7\,mEq/L$
Chloride	$108\,mEq/L$
Total CO_2	$10\,mEq/L$
Anion gap	$30\,mEq/L$
Glucose	$110\,mg/dL$
Ketones	Negative
Osmolality	$380\,mOsmol/kg\ H_2O$
Arterial blood	
pH	7.13
$[H^+]$	$74\,nEq/L$
$PaCO_2$	$25\,mmHg$
PaO_2	$125\,mmHg$
$[HCO_3^-]$	$8\,mEq/L$

within the range of variability. Calculation of the Δ anion gap in this case, 18 mEq/L, results in a presumed preacidosis serum [$HCO_3=$] of 26 mEq/L, indicating no evidence of a hidden metabolic alkalosis (see Answer 2, Case 4).

3. The patient has a high anion gap (30 mEq/L) metabolic acidosis. The differential diagnosis for this acid–base disorder in someone with normal renal function includes diabetic and alcoholic ketoacidosis, lactic acidosis, and ingestions of certain toxins. This man did not have diabetes, ketonemia or any apparent reason to have lactic acidosis. Given the history of alcohol abuse and suicide attempts, one should immediately consider ingestions of low-molecular-weight toxins, such as methyl alcohol and ethylene glycol, as candidates for causing the metabolic acidosis. This possibility is strengthened by the large discrepancy between the measured osmolality (380 mOsmol/kg H_2O) and the value calculated from the serum [Na^+], urea and glucose concentrations (see Chapter 28): 2×148 + urea/2.8 + glucose/18 = 312 mOsmol/kg H_2O. The difference, termed the osmolal gap, is 68 mOsmol/kg H_2O. While this large a gap is usually seen with a low molecular weight toxin such as methyl alcohol, in this instance the toxin was ethylene glycol. The patient had an extremely high ethylene glycol level in his blood (60 mmol/L), essentially accounting for the entire osmolal gap.

4. Treatment should be directed at preventing metabolism of ethylene glycol to its toxic metabolites, using the metabolic inhibitor fomepizole, administering saline to maintain renal perfusion and to promote renal excretion of the toxin and its metabolites and, in this case, initiating hemodialysis as soon as possible to assist in removing the potentially lethal amount of ethylene glycol ingested. These treatments were undertaken rapidly, and the patient survived with no renal injury.

Index

T - #0287 - 071024 - C2 - 229/152/39 - PB - 9780367392345 - Gloss Lamination